Medication Safety in Pregnancy and Breastfeeding

NOTICE

Medicine is an ever-changing science. As new research and clinical experience broaden our knowledge, changes in treatment and drug therapy are required. The authors and the publisher of this work have checked with sources believed to be reliable in their efforts to provide information that is complete and generally in accord with the standards accepted at the time of publication. However, in view of the possibility of human error or changes in medical sciences, neither the authors nor the publisher nor any other party who has been involved in the preparation or publication of this work warrants that the information contained herein is in every respect accurate or complete, and they are not responsible for any errors or omissions or for the results obtained from use of such information. Readers are encouraged to confirm the information contained herein with other sources. For example and in particular, readers are advised to check the product information sheet included in the package of each drug they plan to administer to be certain that the information contained in this book is accurate and that changes have not been made in the recommended dose or in the contraindications for administration. This recommendation is of particular importance in connection with new or infrequently used drugs.

MEDICATION SAFETY IN PREGNANCY AND BREASTFEEDING

Gideon Koren, MD, FRCPC, FACMT

Professor and Director, The Motherisk Program
The Hospital for Sick Children and University of Toronto,
Holder, The Ivey Chair in Molecular Toxicology
The University of Western Ontario
Toronto, Ontario, Canada

McGraw-Hill
HEALTH PROFESSIONS DIVISION

New York St. Louis San Francisco Auckland Bogotá Caracs Lisbon London Madrid
Mexico City Milan Montreal New Delhi San Juan Singapore Sydney Tokyo Toronto

The McGraw·Hill Companies

MEDICATION SAFETY IN PREGNANCY AND BREASTFEEDING

1 2 3 4 5 6 7 8 9 0 CCW/CCW 0 9 8 7

ISBN 0-0714-4828-4

This book was set in Times by International Typesetting and Composition.
The editors were James Shanahan, Kim J. Davis, and Regina Y. Brown.
The production supervisor was Sherri Souffrance.
The cover designer was Elizabeth Pisacreta.
The index was prepared by Robert Swanson.
Kendallville was printer and binder.

This book is printed on acid-free paper.

Library of Congress Cataloging-in-Publication Data

The book is dedicated to my
family and to members of the Motherisk team at
The Hospital for Sick Children in Toronto

CONTENTS

Section 2: Maternal Morbidities

Section 3: Alcohol, Caffeine, Cocaine and Environmental Exposure

Section 4: Use of Vitamins, Contraceptives and Therapeutic Drugs

CONTRIBUTORS

Antonio Addis
Ufficio Informazione sui Farmaci
Agenzia Italiana del Farmaco (AIFA)
Rome, Italy

Alaa Ali, MD, MSc, PhD
Lecturer, National Research Center
Ain Shams University Hospitals
Cairo, Egypt
Clinical Fellow
Mount Sinai Hospital
Department of Pediatrics, NICU
Toronto, Ontario, Canada

Yedidia Bentur, MD
Director, Israel Poison Information Center
Rambam Health Care Campus
The Bruce Rapapport Faculty of Medicine
Technion – Israel Institute of Technology
Haifa, Israel

Enkelejda Bollano, MD
PGY1 Resident, Family Practice
University of Toronto
Toronto, Ontario, Canada

Heather Boon, BScPhm, PhD
Associate Professor
Leslie Dan Faculty of Pharmacy
University of Toronto
Toronto, Ontario, Canada

Gerald F. Chernoff, PhD
California Environmental Protection Agency
Human and Ecological Risk Division
Sacramento, California

David Chitayat, MD, FABMG, FACMG, FCCMG, FRCPC
Professor, Departments of Pediatrics, Molecular and Medical Genetics, Obstetrics and Gynecology, Laboratory Medicine and Pathobiology,
Medical Director, The MSc Program in Genetic Counseling
University of Toronto
Head, The Prenatal Diagnosis and Medical Genetics Program
Department of Obstetrics and Gynecology, Mount Sinai Hospital
Staff, Division of Clinical Genetics and Metabolism, The Hospital for Sick Children
Toronto, Ontario, Canada

Orna Diav-Citrin, MD
The Israeli Teratology Information Service
Israel Ministry of Health
Jerusalem, Israel

Adrienne Einarson, RN
Assistant Editor
Assistant Director, The Motherisk Program
The Hospital for Sick Children
University of Toronto
Toronto, Ontario, Canada

Noah Farber
Student, Honors Specialization in Biology
University of Western Ontario
London, Ontario, Canada

Yaron Finkelstein, MD
PregTox Network, Division of Clinical Pharmacology and Toxicology
Department of Pediatrics
The Hospital for Sick Children
University of Toronto School of Medicine
Toronto, Ontario, Canada

Michael Gallo, BSc
The Motherisk Program
Division of Pharmacology and Toxicology
The Hospital for Sick Children
Toronto, Ontario, Canada

Shital Gandhi, MD, MPH, FRCP(C)
Staff Physician, Mount Sinai Hospital
Assistant Professor, Department of Medicine
University of Toronto
Toronto, Ontario, Canada

Joey N. Gareri, HBSc, MSc
Motherisk Laboratory
Division of Clinical Pharmacology and Toxicology
The Hospital for Sick Children
Toronto, Ontario, Canada

Christelle Gedeon, HBSc
University of Toronto
The Hospital for Sick Children
Toronto, Ontario, Canada

Ruth R. Geist, MD
Department of Obstetrics and Gynecology
Shaare Zedek Medical Center
Jerusalem, Israel
Ben Gurion University of the Negev
Beer-Sheva, Israel

Y. Ingrid Goh, HBSc
Graduate Student
Department of Pharmaceutical Sciences and Toxicology
University of Toronto
Toronto, Ontario, Canada

Yana Izmaylov
Research Student
The Motherisk Program
Division of Pharmacology and Toxicology
The Hospital for Sick Children
Toronto, Ontario, Canada

Sanjog Kalra, MSc
Graduate Student
The Motherisk Program
Division of Pharmacology and Toxicology
The Hospital for Sick Children
Toronto, Ontario, Canada

Julia Klein, MSc
The Motherisk Program
Division of Pharmacology and Toxicology
The Hospital for Sick Children
Toronto, Ontario, Canada

Dafna Knittel-Keren, MA
Motherisk Program
The Hospital for Sick Children
Toronto, Ontario, Canada

David C. Knoppert, MScPHm, FCCP, MSc
Liaison Pharmacist – Neonatology
St. Joseph's Hospital
Scientist, Children's Health Research Institute
Adjunct Professor, Departments of Paediatrics and Medicine
University of Western Ontario, London, Ontario, Canada

Gideon Koren, MD, FRCPC, FACMT
Professor and Director, The Motherisk Program
The Hospital for Sick Children and University of Toronto,
Holder, The Ivey Chair in Molecular Toxicology
The University of Western Ontario
Toronto, Ontario, Canada

Doreen Matsui, MD, FRCPC
FRAME Program, Children's Hospital of Western Ontario
Associate Professor, Department of Pediatrics
University of Western Ontario
London, Ontario, Canada

Myla E. Moretti, MSc
Assistant Director
The Motherisk Program
Project Director, Research Institute
The Hospital for Sick Children
Toronto, Ontario, Canada

Alejandro A. Nava-Ocampo, MD
Assistant Editor
The Motherisk Program
Division of Pharmacology and Toxicology
The Hospital for Sick Children
Toronto, Ontario, Canada

Irena Nulman, MD
Associate Professor in Pediatrics
Division of Pharmacology and Toxicology
The Hospital for Sick Children
Toronto, Ontario, Canada

Lori E. Ross, PhD
Research Scientist
Women's Mental Health and Addiction Research Section
Centre for Addiction and Mental Health
Academic Leader, Reproductive Life Stages Program
Women's College Hospital
Assistant Professor, Department of Psychiatry
University of Toronto
Toronto, Ontario, Canada

Lavínia Schüler-Faccini
Teratogen Information Service - Porto Alegre
Genetics Department, Universidade Federal do Rio Grande do Sul
Brazil

Alon Shrim, MD
The Motherisk Program
Division of Clinical Pharmacology and Toxicology
The Hospital for Sick Children
The University of Toronto
Toronto, Ontario, Canada

Anna G. Sivojelezova, MSc
Counselor
The Motherisk Program
The Hospital for Sick Children
Toronto, Ontario, Canada

Arthur Staroselsky, MD
Clinical Fellow
Division of Clinical Pharmacology and Toxicology
University of Toronto
Toronto, Ontario, Canada

Meir Steiner, MD, PhD, FRCPC
Professor of Psychiatry and Behavioural Neurosciences and Obstetrics and Gynecology
McMaster University
Professor, Department of Psychiatry and Institute of Medical Sciences
University of Toronto
Adjunct Scientist, The Hospital for Sick Children, Toronto
Foundation Director, Women's Health Concerns Clinic
St. Joseph's Healthcare
Hamilton, Ontario, Canada

Reuven Sussman, BSc
Clinical Research Coordinator
Division of Pharmacology and Toxicology
The Hospital for Sick Children
Toronto, Ontario, Canada

Nobuko Taguchi, MD
The Hospital for Sick Children
Toronto, Ontario, Canada

Haleh Talaie, MD, MPH
The Motherisk Program
Division of Clinical Pharmacology & Toxicology
The Hospital for Sick Children
Toronto, Ontario, Canada;
Shahid Beheshti University of Medical Sciences
Poison Center of Loghman General Hospital
Tehran, Iran

PREFACE

Approximately one fetus is aborted for every two or three children born in Western countries. Since the thalidomide diaster over four decades ago, medicine has been practiced as if every drug were a potential human teratogen. Women exposed to nonteratogens commonly believe they have a high teratogenic risk. Their physicians often encourage them to terminate their pregnancies, yet only about 30 drugs and chemicals have been proven to be teratogenic.

Every year scores of new drugs and hundreds of new chemicals are introduced into the market. In neither case are human reproductive effects known. Furthermore, according to different studies, between 40% and 90% of pregnant women consume one or more medications during gestation. Finally, despite hundreds of scientific studies published yearly on reproductive effects of xenobiotics, little has been done in the past to crystallize a clinical approach to deal with these issues.

No single medical specialty is equipped to deal with the complex issues of reproductive toxicology. While geneticists commonly deal with congenital malformations, it is unlikely that they have the experience of pharmacologists in tailoring alternative therapy. Neither group is trained to evaluate such factors as occupational exposures. A multidisciplinary team of pharmacologists, toxicologists, geneticists, obstetricians, neonatologists, occupational and addiction specialists, drug information specialists, psychologists, sonographers, and epidemiologists is needed.

In September 1985, we counseled the first patient in the Motherisk clinic in Toronto. This program was designed to inform, counsel, and follow up pregnant women exposed to drugs, chemicals, or radiation in pregnancy. In order to perform these tasks, new approaches and clinical tools had to be developed by our multidisciplinary team; these are presented in this volume.

Much of the confusion surrounding the counseling process sterns from the well-understood "do not use in pregnancy" statements commonly found in the *Physicians' Desk Reference, Compendium of Phannaceuticals and Specialties* or their equivalents. Since many women are inadvertently exposed to medications *before* finding out they have conceived, the "do not use in pregnancy" statements are easily translated into "harmful" or "teratogenic." While the exact rate of pregnancy termination due to fears of adverse fetal effects of xenobiotics is not known, there is indirect evidence that this is not uncommon. Similarly disturbing are the many cases where women are exposed to drugs and chemicals known to adversely affect the fetus without being appropriately informed.

The goal of this book is to assist the large number of health professionals who are asked by women and their families to provide answers on potential reproductive effects of xenobiotics and radiation. These include general physicians, obstetricians, poison control specialists, geneticists, occupational specialists, pediatricians, pharmacologists, toxicologists, pharmacists, nurses, and others. With increasing public awareness of environmental toxins, it is likely that concerns surrounding reproductive toxicology will increase over the next few decades. We hope that an appropriate clinical approach will help put the issue in its correct perspective, by avoiding both understatements and ambiguity.

In the 6 years that have elapsed since publication of the third edition of *Maternal-Fetal Toxicology: A Clinician's Guide,* the field of teratology information has seen an exponential growth, both in terms of quantity and quality of knowledge. The Motherisk Program in Toronto, in collaboration with several American services, has initiated and brought to completion large-scale, prospective studies on the safety of drugs in pregnancy, some of which are presented in this volume. In this text, we have assembled for the first time all systematic reviews and meta analyses published by us in the peer review literature. We hope that this will evolve to become a living document such as the Cochrane Reviews and other similar efforts.

Finally, I wish to thank the members of the Motherisk team, my students, fellows, and colleagues for being active in generating new knowledge in the field of maternal-fetal toxicology, and making any edition obsolete within a few years. Special thanks to the two Assistant Editors of this volume: Ms. Adrienne Einarson and Dr. Alejandro Nava-Ocampo.

Gideon Koren

PART I

MATERNAL FETAL TOXICOLOGY

CHAPTER 1

DRUGS IN PREGNANCY: ACKNOWLEDGING CHALLENGES-FINDING SOLUTIONS

Gideon Koren

Due to obvious ethical issues of experimenting drugs during fetal development, women and their unborn babies are commonly excluded from drug trials. As a result, these two groups of patients are commonly orphaned from the revolution in drug therapy witnessed in the last generation.

The removal of Bendectin from the American market despite being safe in pregnancy sent a chilling signal to drug companies, essentially discouraging them from studying pregnant patients. Even in areas, which are exclusively typical of pregnancy (e.g., morning sickness or tocolysis) no new drug trials are performed. Consequently, the advance in therapeutics in pregnancy lags substantially behind the same conditions or drugs in nonpregnant women, or men.

However, this approach is highly unwarranted, as uncontrolled maternal conditions may affect adversely both the mother and her fetus. Hence, a rational approach must also incorporate estimation of the risks of the untreated maternal condition. This has been highlighted painfully in recent years, where anxiety of yet unproven fetal risks of selective serotonin reuptake inhibitors (SSRIs) have received much attention, leading many women to discontinue these drugs, but with very little attention to the tremendous risk of untreated maternal depression.

Because embryogenesis is completed by the end of the first trimester of pregnancy, if a drug is not affecting brain development (which continues throughout gestation), there is no apparent reason not to study it during the second and third trimesters of pregnancy.

Several recent developments may mark important milestones in changing the approach to drug trials in pregnancy.

CHANGES IN DRUG DISPOSITION IN LATE PREGNANCY

During the last few years, a large body of evidence has suggested that in late pregnancy there is substantial increase in the clearance rate of various drugs, due to increase function of different cytochrome P-450 enzymes, including nicotine (2A6), fluoxetine and citalopram (2D6), and protease inhibitors (3A4).[1,2] This means that women may need larger doses to achieve therapeutic steady-state concentrations. For example, using nicotine replacement therapy has failed to prevent smoking in late pregnancy when compared to placebo, probably because the dose regimen used in late pregnancy was insufficient.

Similarly, many women with depression are not controlled clinically in late pregnancy, possibly at least in part because doses that were adequate before pregnancy are grossly inappropriate in late pregnancy.[3]

Late pregnancy is also characterized by major changes in glomerular filtration rate (GFR), hepatic blood flow, protein binding and altered drug compliance. These changes lead, in most instances, to lower systemic exposure to medications, both hepatically and renally eliminated.

LEARNING FROM THE GLYBURIDE MILESTONE

Gestational diabetes (GD) affects up to 5% of late pregnancies. Left untreated, it may adversely affect pregnancy outcome. The hallmark of therapy is dietary control and insulin, as this naturally occurring hormone does not cross the placenta appreciably. However, insulin therapy is expensive, unavailable in many areas, and is associated with low compliance rates.

The use of oral hypoglycemic drugs has been largely contraindicated, because these drugs cross the placenta causing fetal hyperinsulinism and increasing the risk of neonatal hypoglycemia.[4]

In 1994, using the *ex-vivo* placental perfusion studies, Elliot and colleagues documented that unlike other "older" sulfonylurea glyburide did not cross the placental barrier from the mother to the fetus.[5]

In 2000, the same group published the results of a randomized controlled trial comparing pregnancy outcome comparing insulin to glyburide. The offspring were not different in any outcome characteristics, including birth weight, rates of hypoglycemia, or mortality. Critically, while maternal glyburide levels were in the therapeutic ranges (50–150 ng/mL), the drug was undetected in any of the umbilical blood samples.[6]

The mechanisms preventing a relatively small nonpolar molecule from crossing the placenta has not been elucidated yet. It has been hypothesized that this may be a combination of relatively short half-life with extremely high protein binding. We have recently shown that glyburide is effluxed from the fetal to the maternal circulation by several placental ATP binding cassette (ABC) transporters, including breast cancer resistance protein (BCRP) and multidrug resistant protein 3 (MRP3).[7]

A Proposed Framework for Drug Trials in Pregnancy

The objective of this section is to synthesize known principles and concepts of maternal-fetal clinical pharmacology, and to propose a framework for trials of medicines in pregnancy.

Principles

1. Studies should be conducted first in the second–third trimester of pregnancy, when embryopathy is not an issue. This may not be relevant to drugs affecting brain development, as fetal brain continues to develop until birth.
2. High priority should be given to studies of agents, which can be expected to address an unmet maternal/fetal risk or improve maternal or fetal outcomes compared to existing therapy. Some examples include glyburide and metformin for GD or labetalol for hypertension.
3. High priority should be given to agents not likely to affect central nervous system (CNS) development, which continues throughout gestation.

4. A pharmacokinetic study should precede an efficacy-effectiveness study, as in late pregnancy women may need larger dose due to a faster clearance rate.
5. Before a study is initiated during the first trimester of pregnancy, human safety data should be available. Such data should be prospective observational data with an unexposed comparison group. Because half of all pregnancies are unplanned, and due to the fact that programs collecting such studies exist, there is no excuse not to collect and analyze such data.
6. Participants in studies should consent after being made aware of the available safety data and their limitations, including the risk of the untreated condition, as well as the known risks-benefits of available data on alternative therapeutics.

The recent breakthrough in pediatric drug trials in the United States, secondary to enacting financial benefits through extension of exclusivity to products studied in children, should logically lead to a similar move for drug trials in pregnancy. However, the legal-ethical equation in pregnancy is much more complex than in childhood, and it seems less likely that the pharmaceutical industry will agree to participate in the very litigious climate of today.

REFERENCES

1. Dempsey D, Jacob P, Benowitz NZ. Accelerated metabolism of nicotine and cotinine in pregnant smokers. *J Pharmacol Exp Ther.* 2002; 301:594–598.
2. Heikkinen T, Ekblad U, Palo P, et al. Pharmacokinetics of fluoxetine and norfluoxetine in pregnancy and lactation. *Clin Pharmacol Ther.* 2003;73:330–337.
3. Bonari L, Bennett H, Einarson A, et al. Risks of untreated depression during pregnancy. *Can Fam Physician.* 2004;50:37–39.
4. Koren G. *Maternal-Fetal Toxicology: A Clinician's Guide.* 3rd ed. New York, NY: Marcel Dekker; 2001.
5. Elliott BD, Schenker S, Langer O, et al. Comparative placental transport of oral hypoglycemic agents in humans. *Am J Obstet Gynecol.* 1994;171:653–660.
6. Langer O, Conway DL, Berkus MD, et al. A comparison of glyburide and insulin in women with gestational diabetes mellitus. *N Engl J Med.* 2000;343:1134–1138.
7. Garcia-Bournissen F, Feig DS, Koren G. Maternal-fetal transport of hypoglycemic drugs. *Clin Pharmacokinet.* 2003;42:303–313.

CHAPTER 2

GESTATIONAL CHANGES IN DRUG DISPOSITION IN THE MATERNAL-FETAL UNIT

Christelle Gedeon and Gideon Koren

A large number of pregnant women suffer from medical conditions that require ongoing or episodic drug treatment such as asthma, epilepsy, or hypertension. Moreover, pregnancy can induce conditions such as nausea and vomiting, which may need to be treated. Pharmacologically, while the woman's well-being is at the heart of any medical treatment, placental transfer of drugs leading to potential toxicity to the fetus is a major concern in the pharmacological management of the pregnant patient. Hence, when managing a pregnant patient with medication, the treatment of two individual patients, mother and fetus, should be considered independently and the decision must be based on the risk/benefit assessment of both. While the use of prescription drugs has sometimes increased fetal risk of teratogenicity, some medical conditions such as gestational diabetes, hyperthyroidism, or hypertension may require drug therapy in order to ensure optimal health of the mother and fetus.

Of the thousands of available drugs, relatively few have been shown to adversely affect the fetus. For example, the use of most traditional anticonvulsants, while necessary for the treatment of mother, may cause structural defects as well as impaired neurocognitive development.[27,28] Thus, a potential maternal-fetal conflict brings to light the need to identify drugs that can effectively treat the mother without adversely affecting the fetus.

Placental passage of a drug is a function of multiple factors such as protein-binding, lipid solubility, and ionization constant (pKa), but fetal exposure to drugs also depends on maternal pharmacokinetics including the volume of distribution, the rate of metabolism and excretion by the placenta, the pH difference between maternal and fetal fluids, and the effect of hemodynamic changes in the mother during pregnancy (Table 2-1). Ideally, one may wish to identify drugs that will not cross the placental barrier. However, with the exception of drugs with large molecular weights, such as heparin or insulin, most drugs appear to cross the placenta and are associated with varying degrees of fetal exposure.

Recently we have been witnessing a pharmacological breakthrough—glibenclamide (Glyburide),[10,12,13] a drug used to treat gestational diabetes, does not appear to demonstrate significant maternal-fetal transfer. In vitro, studies by Elliott et al. have demonstrated negligible levels of glibenclamide in the fetal compartment even when maternal concentrations were eight times greater than therapeutic concentrations.[13] Glibenclamide's poor maternal-fetal transfer may be due to its high protein binding (99.8%), its short elimination half-life (6 hours)[1,11,18] and more importantly the role of specific placental transporters such as *P*-glycoprotein (*P*-gP), multidrug resistance protein 1 (MRP1), multidrug resistance protein 2 (MRP2), or multidrug resistance protein 3 (MRP3).[24,25] Indeed, in a recent placental perfusion study, we have documented that glibenclamide is transferred from the fetal to the maternal circulation against its concentration gradient. This may be the first generation of drugs on the journey toward an ideal drug specifically designed for pregnancy. The objective of this conceptual paper is to identify the characteristics that render drugs capable of staying in maternal circulation while obviating fetal exposure and risk, making them optimal for use in pregnancy.

TRANSPLACENTAL TRANSPORT MECHANISMS

Typically discoid, the human placenta consists of the chorionic villi having attendant blood vessels and connective tissues. Viewed from the basal surface, the placenta displays slightly raised areas denoted as maternal lobes or cotyledons. Each maternal cotyledon is associated with several fetal cotyledons allowing for maternal circulation to be nearly superimposed on to fetal circulation. Considering the movement of materials from the mother to the fetus, molecules are carried by the maternal bloodstream in one of three ways: in free form dissolved in plasma, bound to carrier proteins, or bound to red blood cells. As a molecule crosses from the maternal-fetal bloodstream, the solutes must cross the syncytiotrophoblast either by passing through the cytoplasm of the trophoblast or via a network of transporters (Fig. 2-1). Thus, transport across the placenta involves the movement of molecules between three compartments: the maternal blood, the cytoplasm of the syncytiotrophoblast, and the fetal blood. Solute levels in each of these compartments will play a key role in controlling the rate by which substances cross the placenta and are largely dependent on the initial absorption of the drug into the maternal bloodstream.

PHYSIOLOGICAL CHANGES IN PREGNANCY

During pregnancy, the maternal gastrointestinal absorption of drugs may be altered because of changes in gastric secretion and motility. Changes in gastric pH influence the degree of ionization and solubility of many drugs, where their absorption rate is modified thereby altering drug bioavailability. Once absorbed, maternal drug metabolism may be altered due to elevation of endogenous hormones such as progesterone. This can stimulate the hepatic microsomal oxidase system where elevated rates of hepatic metabolism may result in increased transformation of drugs such as phenytoin.[27,28] Conversely, theophylline and caffeine experience reduced hepatic elimination as a consequence of elevated estradiol, which may inhibit microsomal drug metabolizing enzymes. Therapeutic concentrations of the active drug may also be affected by hemodynamic changes that take place throughout pregnancy. Cardiac output and blood volume increase by 40% primarily due to an increase in plasma volume.[17] Total body water also increases by 5–8%, due to the expansion of the extracellular fluid space and the growth of new tissue.[27,28] Body water also accumulates in the fetus, placenta, and amniotic fluid, which collectively contributes to an increase in volume of distribution and may lower the concentration of drugs and increase their elimination half-life (Table 2-2).

Table 2-1
Physiological Changes in Pregnancy

FUNCTION	CHANGE
Cardiac output	Increased
Tidal volume	Increased
Pulmonary blood flow	Increased
Gastric ph	Increased
Glomerular filtration rate	Increased
Renal drug elimination	Increased
Hepatic drug elimination	Increase, decrease, or unchanged
Clearance	Increased
Total body water	Increased
Volume of distribution	Increased
Steady-state plasma concentration	Decreased
Peak serum concentration	Decreased
Intestinal motility	Decreased
Protein-binding capacity	Decreased

SOURCE: [21] and [28].

PROTEIN BINDING IN PREGNANCY

Protein-binding alterations may also occur in pregnancy as a result of changes in the concentration of specific proteins as well as changes in protein-binding affinity. Decreases in maternal serum albumin may lead to corresponding increases in the free fraction of drug.[4,7] Increased levels of free fatty acids and total lipids together with the hormonal changes in pregnancy can also decrease the binding capacity of drugs to the protein. This may have important implications to maternal-fetal drug transfer, since binding changes may influence the maternal plasma concentration of free drug available to partition across the placental barrier. Furthermore, there is a lower concentration of specific binding proteins and altered binding affinity of drugs in the fetus; albumin concentration in the cord blood of neonates is markedly lower than the maternal levels.[22] In addition, there is a threefold lower level of α_1-acid glycoprotein in the fetus compared to the mother.[4] Should free drug cross the placenta, the fetus will experience larger concentrations of the free drug, due to its diminished protein-binding capacity.

GESTATIONAL pH CHANGES

Lipid solubility, the pH of the maternal and fetal fluids, the ionization constant of the drug (pKa), and the molecular weight also influence the passage of the drug across the placenta. In general, uncharged, unionized molecules with high lipid solubility and lower molecular weight penetrate the cell membranes more readily than hydrophilic ionized drug molecules.[21]

The transfer of weak acids and bases is influenced by the pH gradient between the maternal and fetal circulations and by the pKa of the drug. Since fetal plasma is slightly more acidic, 0.1 lower than maternal plasma pH, for weak bases, the unionized free drug crossing the placenta becomes ionized and is "trapped" in the more acidic fetal circulation.[22,27] The pH of the amniotic fluid is also

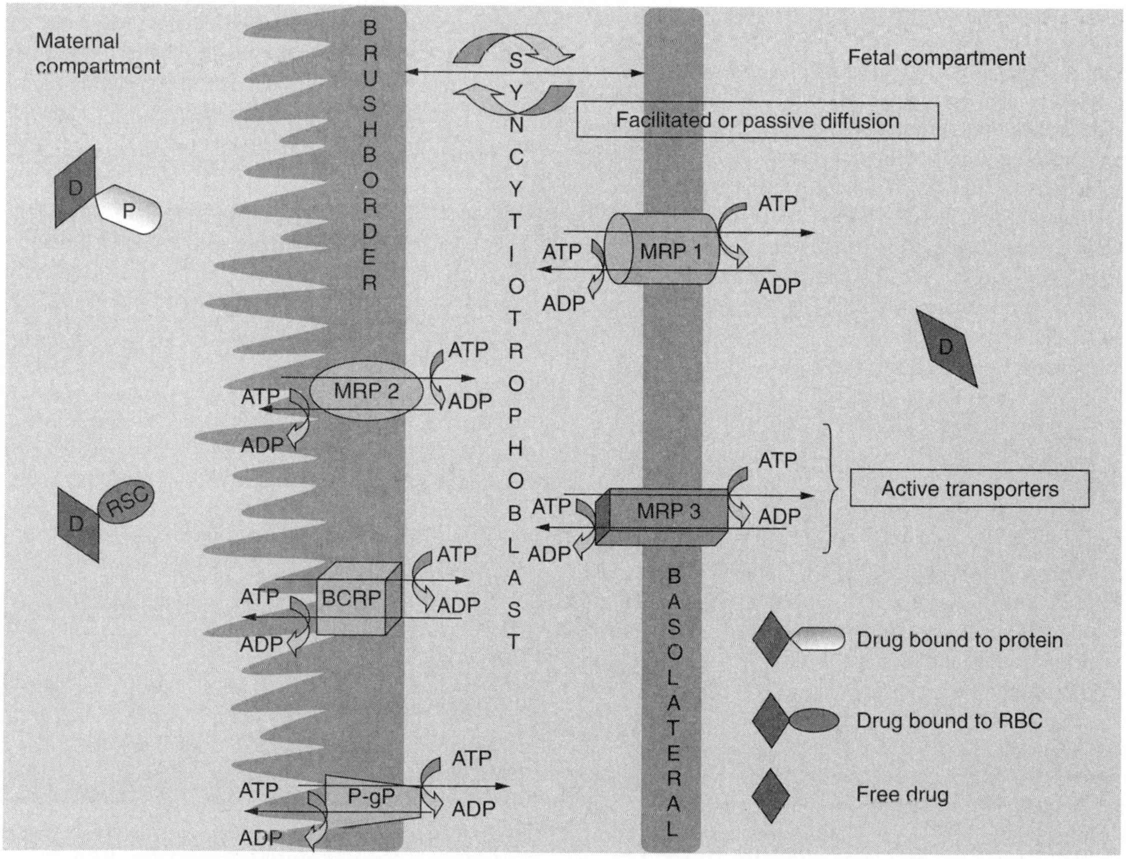

Figure 2-1. Transport across the placental barrier.

Table 2-2
Pregnancy-Induced Pharmacokinetic Changes for Selected Drugs

	$T^{1/2}$		Vd (l)		CL (mL/min)	
DRUGS	PREGNANT	NONPREGNANT (min)	PREGNANT	NONPREGNANT (min)	PREGNANT	NONPREGNANT
Ampicillin	54.2 ± 3.9	69.6 ± 6.1	32.8 ± 2.5	34.5 ± 2.7	450 ± 31	370 ± 30
Cefuroxime	44 ± 5	58 ± 8	17.8 ± 1.9	16.3 ± 2.1	282 ± 34	198 ± 27
Imipenem	36 ± 8	41 ± 16	47.1 ± 14.8	18.9 ± 5.8	973 ± 47	338 ± 85
Piperacillin	46.5 ± 10	53.7 ± 4.6	67.6 ± 11.8	41.9 ± 6.2	1538 ± 362	540 ± 75
Azlocillin	65.4	72	15.4	24.7	126.1	195.7
Nifedipine	81 ± 18	360			266 ± 105	27 ± 15
Labetalol	102 ± 16	160			1704 ± 531	1430
Sotalol	396 ± 36	558 ± 42	106.4 ± 8.1	87.3 ± 7.2	196 ± 24	109 ± 7
Phenytoin	900 ± 314					

SOURCE: [32], [34], [35], [36] and [37].

lower than that of maternal plasma. Therefore, the more acidic environment of both fetal blood and amniotic fluid favor ionization and accumulation of basic drug due to "ion trapping" often resulting in fetal drug concentrations that may exceed maternal plasma concentrations and lead to toxicity.

Finally, at the placental cytoplasmic barrier, free drug can cross either by simple or facilitated diffusion or by active transport. Diffusion, simple or facilitated, depends upon the transmembrane concentration gradient, where it moves from a higher concentration compartment to an area of lower concentration. Active transport depends not only on solute concentration but also on a steady supply of adenosine triphosphate (ATP). In addition, the placenta itself contributes to maternal-fetal drug transfer since it possesses metabolizing enzymes capable of oxidation, reduction, hydrolysis, and conjugation, which can potentially convert an inactive drug into an active metabolite and vice versa.

Clearly, the transfer of drugs across the placental membrane will vary, depending on the apparent volume of distribution, the degree of protein binding, acid-base equilibrium, metabolic and excretory mechanisms in the placenta and fetus as well as hemodynamic alterations.

Placental ATP Binding Cassette Transporters and Pregnancy

The trophoblast is the interface of exchange between the maternal and fetal circulations. As a barrier, the trophoblast has abundant expression of ATP binding cassette (ABC) transporters such as *P*-gP and MRP1, MRP2, and MRP3, respectively. Powered by ATP, these transporters actively extrude substrates from the placenta (Table 2-3).[23] Particularly, *P*-gP and MRP2 have been shown to be expressed on the brush border (maternal side) of the human placental trophoblast,[42] while MRP1 and MRP3 are on the basal membrane (fetal side).[19,34] Multidrug resistance transporters may result in a lower cellular concentration of drug via an efflux mechanism, thus creating pharmacological sanctuaries. For example, MRP1 and MRP3 preferentially transport organic anions, promote the excretion of glutathione/glucuronide metabolites, and thus prevent their entry into fetal blood.

P-gP is also an active drug transporter of the ABC transporter family with a wide range of substrates.[19] Abundant in the apical membrane of the placental trophoblast, *P*-gP transports its substrates in an outward (extracellular) direction. Since it can be detected in placental trophoblast from the first trimester of pregnancy,[14,42] it is likely that it protects the fetus from amphipathic xenotoxins.[10] Thus, fetal tolerance to maternal concentrations of drugs, which are considered to be good *P*-gP substrates, will be higher than that for drugs considered to be poor *P*-gP substrates. Thus, it may be preferable to treat pregnant women with drugs that are good *P*-gP substrates such as during antineoplastic chemotherapy where drugs, such as Paclitaxel, may be preferred over other antineoplastic agents that cross the placenta more easily.

Antiretrovirals in Pregnancy

In contrast, there are clinical situations where it is desirable to increase the penetration of drugs in order to treat the unborn child. An important example is antiretroviral treatment of human immunodeficiency virus (HIV)-infected pregnant women. Data suggest that nucleoside reverse transcriptase inhibitors rapidly cross the placenta (Table 2-4). Cord blood concentrations of Zidovudine and Lamivudine tend to equal maternal concentrations at the time of delivery, whereas cord blood concentrations of didanosine and zalcitabine are approximately 50% that of maternal concentrations.[38,39] Non-nucleotide reverse transcriptase inhibitors, such as nevirapine, have also been shown to cross the placenta.[31,38] Several factors may account for their passage including the drug's lower protein binding (60%), low molecular weights, favorable degree of lipophilicity (log octanol/water coefficient 1.81).[43] As well, the majority are not *P*-gP substrates. Hence, these drugs passively diffuse across the placenta and are administered in sufficient doses to cross the placenta and prevent maternal-fetal transmission of HIV during labor.

Conversely, protease inhibitors (PI) do not cross the placenta to a clinically appreciable extent.[30] Nelfinavir, ritonavir, saquinavir, and lopinavir undergo incomplete transplacental transfer.[33] Low PI placental transfer can be attributed to high protein binding (98%) and that these drugs are substrates for placental *P*-gP transporter.[23] For example, Saquinavir is a *P*-gP substrate with a high molecular weight (767 g/mol), high protein binding (98%), and partition coefficient (octanol/water 4.1 $\log_{10}$), which may contribute to the small amount that crosses the placenta.[16] Other PI, which follow similar placental kinetics, include indinavir, ritonavir, lopinavir, and nelfinavir. *P*-gP's relative affinity to different PI drugs varies three- to fourfold.[24] Nelfinavir has become a commonly used protease inhibitor during pregnancy because of its tolerability and

Table 2-3
Drug Efflux Transporters and Substrates

SUBSTRATES		TRANSPORTER
Actinomycin D	Etoposide	*P*-glycoprotein (MDR1)
Doxorubicin	Daunorubicin	
Irinotecan	Mitomycin C	
Mitoxantrone	Paclitaxel	
Teniposide	Topotecan	
Vinblastine	Vincristine	
Morphine	Loperamide	
Dexamethasone	Ketoconazole	
β-Acetyldigoxin	Alpha methyldigoxin	
Digitoxin	Quinidine	
Amprenavir	Indinavir	
Nelfinavir	Saquinavir	
Ritonavir	Cyclosporine A	
Tacrolimus	Erythromycin	
Levofloxacin	Sparfloxacin	
Atorvastatin	Lovastatin	
Cerivastatin	Simvastatin	
Diltiazem	Mibefradil	
Verapamil	D617, D620	
Aldosterone	Bisantrene	
Calcein-M	Citalopram	
Colchicine	Corticosterone	
FK 560	Loperamide	
Ondansetron	Paclitaxel	
Phenytoin	Prednisolone	
Quinidine	Rifampin	
Terfenadine	(99 m)-Tc-tetrofosmin	
PSC833		
Adriamycin	Etoposide	MRP1
Glutathione	Mitoxantrone	
Methotrexate	Organic anions	
Aflatoxin B1	Cisplatinum	
Paclitaxel	Topotecan	
Vincristine	Colchicine	
Dehydroepiandrosterone		
Etoposide	Fluorescein	
17-β-glucuronyl estradiol		
S-Glutathionyl Prostaglandin A2		
Methotrexate		
Methotrexate	Cisplatin	MRP2
Vinblastine	Vincristine	
Ceftriaxone	Grepafloxacin	
Rifampicin	Saquinavir	
Ritonavir	Indinavir	
Estradiol	Octreotide	
Temocaprilate	Furosemide	
Pravastatin	Flavonoids	
Heavy metals	Arsenite	
Food carcinogens		
Doxorubicin	Sulphinpyrazone	
Epirubicin	Etoposide	
Phenytoin		

Table 2-3
Drug Efflux Transporters and Substrates (*Continued*)

SUBSTRATES		TRANSPORTER
Acetaminophen	Glucuronide	MRP3
Etoposide	Leukotriene C4	
Methotrexate	Teniposide	
Topotecan	9-Aminocamptotecin	BCRP
Doxorubicin	Irinotecan	
Daunorubicin	Epirubicin	
Zidovudine	Idrubicinol	
Lamivudine	Flavopiridol	
Mitoxantrone	Prazosin	
Methotrexate	Indolocarbazol	
MTX-glu	Pheophorbide	
Adriamycin	Etoposide	

MDR1—multidrug resistant protein 1; MDR2—multidrug resistant protein 2; MDR3—multidrug resistant protein 3; BCRP—breast cancer resistance protein.

Table 2-4
Pharmacokinetic Changes in Human Immunodeficiency Virus Drugs during Pregnancy

DRUG CLASS	DRUG	HALF-LIFE	CLEARANCE	PROTEIN BINDING (%)	BIOAVAILABILITY	PLACENTAL TRANSFER
Nucleoside reverse transcriptase inhibitors	Zidovudine	No change (1.1 hours)	Increases	<25	63%	Cross by diffusion
	Lamivudine	No change (6 hours)	No change	10–50	55%	Cross by diffusion
	Didanosine	No change (1.5 hours)	Increases		45%	Cross by diffusion
	Stavudine	No change			86%	Cross by diffusion
Non-nucleoside reverse transcriptase inhibitors	Nevirapine	Unchanged	Prone to induction	60	90%	Cross by diffusion
	Efavirenz **Delavirdire**	Neural tube defect: not used in pregnancy				
Protease inhibitors	Nelfinavir	Unchanged (3–5 hours)		98		Not detectable in cord blood
	Ritonavir					5.3% maternal detected in cord blood
	Lopinavir	Unchanged (5–6 hours)		99		
	Amprenavir	Unchanged (6 hours)		98		6–8% of maternal in cord blood
	Saquinavir			98		Not detectable in cord blood
	Hydroxicarbamide: not recommended in pregnancy					

SOURCE: [29], [31], [33], [39], [40], [41], [42] and [42].

potency; however, it has also been demonstrated to exhibit a more rapid development of viral resistance and less durable suppression of viral replication leading to a greater likelihood of HIV transmission to the fetus. Saquinavir monotherapy is not adequate and often requires "boosting with low-dose ritonavir." Ritonavir is rarely used in pregnancy owing to its frequent and severe gastrointestinal adverse effects.[30] Only 5.3% of maternal plasma concentrations of ritonavir are detected in fetal cord blood. Ritonavir's well-documented interaction and perhaps inhibition of *P*-gP and MRP1 may account for its exclusion from the placenta.[1] However, ritonavir's inhibition of these transporters is disadvantageous since it gives rise to drug exclusions, altered bioavailability, and changes in drug distribution resulting in a decreased efficacy of treatment with time. This requires the initiation of combination therapies to achieve clinically beneficial and sustained viral suppression. Consequently, polytherapy is usually accompanied by decreased adherence. However, if certain PI are effluxed by the placenta, and not reaching the fetus, future use of the appropriate ABC inhibitor may allow for greater concentrations in the fetal compartment and the prevention of maternal-fetal HIV transmission.

As the use of combination antiretroviral regimens becomes increasingly common among HIV-infected pregnant women and the rate of transmission decreases, the safety, toxicity, and teratogenicity of these agents become paramount. For example, a common toxicity with zidovudine is bone marrow suppression, and decreases in hemoglobin in infants exposed to zidovudine at 3 weeks of age.[19] As a class, nucleoside reverse transcriptase inhibitors have been suggested to cause fetal hepatic microsomal damage in infants exposed perinatally.[5] Additionally, combination therapy has been suggested to trigger glucose intolerance. In particular, zidovudine in combination with lamivudine and nelfinavir fosters a reduction in neonatal insulin similar to that observed in type I diabetes.[9] These data may indicate an early damaging effect on fetal pancreas such as inhibition of proinsulin conversion to insulin due to the activity of these PI. Cumulative damaging effects on pancreatic β-cells may culminate in the death of these cells and consequent insulinopenia followed by clinical diabetes.

Glibenclamide's Interaction with the ABC Transporter Family

Recently, we have shown using the placental perfusion model that glibenclamide is actively transferred from the fetal to the maternal circulations against a concentration gradient. Overall, there was a net decrease (63%) of glibenclamide in fetal to maternal concentration ratios despite equal initial concentrations (200 ng/mL) in both maternal and fetal circulation.[15,26] Undoubtedly, placental active transporters such as the ABC transporter family should be considered in the movement of glibenclamide from fetal to maternal circulation.

From an in vitro perspective, glibenclamide is well known to interact with *P*-gP. However, the emerging thought is that glibenclamide may represent a general inhibitor for ABC transporters, both *P*-gP and MRPs alike and other placental homologue, in that it may bind to some conserved motif.[19] Yet, the belief that glibenclamide is simply an inhibitor of these transporters is contradictory to in vivo findings. Elliott et al's[13,25–27] dually perfused human placental model showed virtually no appearance of glibenclamide in the fetal circulation. Even when maternal concentrations were eightfold greater than therapeutic peak levels (1000 ng/mL), a relatively large concentration gradient facilitating the possibility for diffusion, only minimal concentrations of glibenclamide were seen in fetal blood.

Diffusion, simple or facilitated, cannot explain the negligible presence of glibenclamide in the fetal compartment. As a substrate of certain members of the ABC transporter family, glibenclamide may be actively pumped back to maternal circulation, and can both maintain maternal steady state concentrations and normoglycemia while decreasing fetal exposure and risk of hypoglycemia. Perhaps the possibility should be considered that glibenclamide is not an inhibitor of the ABC transporters but rather a substrate.

LIMITATION AND CHALLENGES

In summary, for pregnancy, future drugs should be sought, which can effectively treat the maternal condition, all the while minimizing fetal exposure. Ideally, the drug should possess a high protein binding, a short elimination half-life, and a small volume of distribution. Identification of drugs, which interact with placental efflux transporters, will allow the possibility of minimizing fetal exposure (e.g., glibenclamide) in the treatment of maternal conditions. Conversely, these transporters also allow the possibility for treating fetal conditions (e.g., PI) through their inhibition and modulation. As for future research, the endeavor of understanding the exact protein motif to which drugs such as glibenclamide interact with placental transporters should include techniques such as vector construction and site-directed mutagenesis. Replicating the binding sites and incorporating them into already existing drugs used in pregnancy allows for the possibility of altering transporter binding affinity. Ultimately, this may allow for drugs specifically designed for pregnancy to come into being.

REFERENCES

1. Agarwal M, Punnose J. Recent advances in the treatment of gestational diabetes. *Expert Opin Investig Drugs.* September 2004;13(9):1103–1111.
2. Elliot B, Langer O, Schenker S, et al. Insignificant transfer of glyburide occurs across the human placenta. *Am J Obstet Gynecol.* October 1991;165(4 Pt 1):807–812.
3. Bawdon RE. The ex vivo human placental transfer of the anti-HIV antinucleoside inhibitor abacabir and the protease inhibitor amprenavir. *Infect Dis Obstet Gynecol.* 1998;6(6):244–246.
4. Beck F. Comparative placental morphology and function. *Dev Toxicol.* 1981;2:35–54.
5. Blanche S, Tardieu M, Rustin P, et al. Persistent mitochondrial dysfunction and perinatal exposure to antiretroviral nucleoside analogues. *Lancet.* 1999;354:1084–1099.
6. Holcberg G, Tsadkin Tamir M, Sapir O, et al. New aspects in placental drug transfer. *Placental Drug Transfer.* 2003;5:873–876.
7. Boyd J, Hamilton W. *The Human Placenta.* 1st ed. Heffer, Cambridge; 1970.
8. Smit JW, Huisman MT, Cantellingen O, et al. Absence or pharmacological blocking of placental P-glycoprotein profoundly increases fetal drug exposure. *J Clin Invest.* 1999;104:1441–1447.

9. Connor E, Sperling R, Gelber R. Reduction of maternal-infant transmission of human immunodeficiency virus type 1 with zidovudine treatment. *N Engl J Med.* 1994;331:1173–1180.
10. Conway D, Gonzales O, Skiver D. Use of glibenclamide for the treatment of gestational diabetes: San Antonio experience. *J Matern Fetal Neonatal Med.* 2004;15:51–55.
11. De Lange E. Potential role of ABC transporter as a detoxification system at the blood–CSF barrier. *Adv Drug Deliv Rev.* 2004;56:1793–1809.
12. Elliott B, Schenker S, Langer O. et al. Comparative placental transport of oral hypoglycemic agents in humans: a model of human placental drug transfer. *Am J Obstet Gynecol.* 1994;171:653–660.
13. Elliott B, Langer O, Schenker S, et al. Insignificant transfer of glyburide occurs across the human placenta. *Am J Obstet Gynecol.* October 1991;165(4):807–812.
14. Faber J, Thornburg K. *Placental Physiology.* 1st ed. Raven Press, New York; 1983.
15. Feig D, Kraemer J, Klein J, et al. Transfer of glyburide into breast milk. [abstract] *Clin Pharmacol Ther.* 2004;75:28.
16. Forestier F, De Renty P, Peytavin G, et al. Maternal–fetal transfer of saquinavir studied in the ex vivo placental perfusion model. *Am J Obstet Gynecol.* 2001;185(1):178–181.
17. Bournissen G, Feig D, Koren G. Maternal–fetal transport of hypoglycemic drugs, *Clin Pharmacokinet.* 2003;42(4):303–313.
18. Gluek C, Goldenberg N, Streicher P, et al. The contentious nature of gestational diabetes: diet, insulin, glyburide and metformin. *Expert Opin Pharmacother.* November 2002;3(11):1557–1568.
19. Gottesman MM, Pastan I, Ambudkar S. P-glycoprotein and multidrug resistance. *Curr Opin Genet Dev.* 1996;6:610–617.
21. Heikkila A, Renkonen OV, Erkkola R. Pharmacokinetics and placental passage of imipenem during pregnancy. *Antimicrob Agents Chemother.* 1992;36:2652–2655.
22. Holcberg G, Tsadkin Tamir M, Sapir O, et al. New aspects in placental drug transfer. *Placental Drug Transfer.* 2003;5:873–876.
23. Huisman M, Smit J, Schinkel A. Significance of P-glycoprotein for the pharmacology and clinical use of protease inhibitors. *AIDS.* 2000;14:237–242.
24. Jones K, Hoggard PG, Sales SK, et al. Differences in the intracellular accumulation of HIV protease inhibitors in vitro and the effect of active transport. *AIDS.* 2001;15:675–681.
25. Koren G. Glyburide and fetal safety; trans-placental pharmacokinetic considerations. *Reprod Toxicol.* 2001;15:227–229.
26. Kramer J, Feig D, Klein J, et al. The transport of glyburide in the human placenta: implication for treatment of gestational diabetes [submitted for publication. August, 2005.
27. Langer O, Conway D, Berkus M, et al. A comparison of glyburide in insulin in women with gestational diabetes mellitus. *N Engl J Med.* October 2000;343:1134–1138.
28. Lobstein R, Lalkin A, Koren G. Pharmacokinetic changes during pregnancy and their clinical relevance. *Maternal fetal toxicology a clinician guide.* 3rd ed. (2001), Marcel Dekker Inc. pp. 1–21.
29. Marsolini C, Rudin C, Decosterd LA, et al. Swiss mother + child HIV cohort study. Transplacental passage of protease inhibitors at delivery. *AIDS.* 2002;16(6):889–893.
30. Maarten T, Huisman J, Smit J, et al. P-glycoprotein limits oral available brain and fetal penetration of saquinavir even with high doses of ritonavir. *Mol Pharmacol.* 2001;59(4):806–813.
31. Mirochnick M. Antiretroviral pharmacology in pregnant women and their newborns. *Ann N Y Acad Sci.* 2000;918:287–297.
32. O'Hara MF, Leahey W, Murraghan GA. Pharmacokinetics of sotalol during pregnancy. *Eur J Clin Pharmacol.* 1983;24(4):521–524.
33. Owen A, Chandler B, Back DJ. The implication of P-glycoprotein in HIV: friend or foe? *Fundam Clin Pharmacol.* 2005:283–296.
34. Pacifi GM, Nottoli R. Placental transfer of drugs administrated to the mother. *Clin Pharmacokinet.* 1995;28:235–269.
35. Page K. The physiology of the human placenta. (1993), UCL Press Limited, University College London.
36. Perucca E, Richens A, Ruprah M. Serum protein binding of phenytoin in pregnant women. *Proc Br Pharmacol Soc.* 1981;11:409–410.
37. Philipson A, Stiernstede G. Pharmacokinetics of cefuroxime in pregnancy. *Am J Obstet Gynecol.* 1982;142:823–828.
38. Rogers RC, Sibai BM, Whybrew WD. Labetolo pharmacokinetics in pregnancy induced hypertension. *Am J Obstet Gynecol.* 1990; 162(2):362–366.
39. Sanberg JA, Slikker W. Developmental pharmacology and toxicology of anti-HIV therapeutic agents: dideozynuclosides. *FASEB J.* 1995;9: 1157–1163.
40. Shelley H. Transfer of carbohydrate, *Placental transfer.* (1979), Pitman Medical, Tunbridge Wells. pp. 118–141.
41. Sibley C, Boyd R. Control of transfer across the mature placenta, *Oxford reviews of reproductive biology*, (1988), Oxford University Press, Oxford. pp. 382–435.
42. Smit JW, Huisman MT, Cantellingen O, et al. Absence or pharmacological blocking of placental P-glycoprotein profoundly increases fetal drug exposure. *J Clin Invest.* 1999;104:1441–1447.
43. Voit R, Schroder S, Peiker G. Pharmacokinetics studies of azlocillin and piperacillin during late pregnancy. *Chemotherapy.* 1985;31:417–424.

CHAPTER 3

DEVELOPMENTAL RISK ASSESSMENTS

Gerald F. Chernoff

Originally presented as a workshop at the 5th International Conference of Teratogen Information Services, March 1992.

The material presented in this chapter represents the views of the author and does not necessarily reflect the policy of the Office of Environmental Health Hazard Assessment (OEHHA).

INTRODUCTION

For those on the front line communicating risk information to pregnant women, one of the more frustrating questions that can be asked regards the risk of exposures to occupational chemicals and environmental hazards. Whereas, information about pharmaceuticals is available from central sources such as the *Catalog of Teratogenic Agents.*[1] information on occupational and environmental exposures is often available only from government agencies such as the U.S. Environmental Protection Agency.[2] The information provided by these agencies can be quite limited, consisting of only permissible emission levels (PELs), maximum concentration limits (MCLs), acceptable daily intakes (ADIs), or some other regulatory number derived from a formal risk assessment. What is a risk assessment? What do the regulatory numbers mean? How can they be used in the risk communications process?

In this chapter, we investigate some of these questions. The intent is not to provide a formula for instant expertise on risk assessments but rather to broaden the reader's appreciation for how these assessments can be used and misused in counseling concerned individuals. To accomplish this task, we review briefly the basic principles of each of the four steps in the risk assessment process: hazard identification, reference dose determination or dose-response assessment, exposure assessment, and risk characterization.[3] After each step has been reviewed, a database of fictional studies on the imaginary chemical A VOID is presented. This database will help illustrate the types of study available for risk assessments and will provide an opportunity to apply the principles of risk assessment to representative data. Finally, questions germane to the evaluation of the A VOID data are listed and the issues that generate the most controversy are discussed briefly.

HAZARD IDENTIFICATION

Principles

1. The purposes of hazard identification are to identify the types of adverse health effect that may be associated with exposure to an agent and to characterize the quality and strength of evidence supporting this identification. For the purpose of this exercise only developmental (teratogenic) adverse effects induced by A VOID are considered.
2. Human studies are generally considered to be the best source of information, since ultimately it is the human population that we are attempting to protect. Unfortunately, for most chemicals of concern, good human studies are lacking; even when data do exist, establishing a causal link between the exposure and developmental endpoint is seldom possible. Human developmental studies can generally be divided into two categories, descriptive and analytical.[4]
   - **a.** Descriptive studies, which are useful for generating hypotheses, include case reports, surveillance systems, and ecological and cluster studies.
   - **b.** Analytical studies, which test a hypothesis to examine cause-effect relationships, include case control, cohort, and human experimental studies.
3. Studies with experimental animals are often the best source of information for hazard identification. These studies can be either regulatory or experimental.
   - **a.** Regulatory studies are those that are prescribed or recommended by agencies such as the U.S. Environmental Protection Agency and the Food and Drug Administration; they include single- and multigeneration reproductive studies, continuous breeding studies, and developmental studies with exposure in the embryonic and fetal periods or in the perinatal period.[5–10] These studies have the advantage of consistent protocols, with full reporting of all the collected data. Unfortunately, they apply to only a limited spectrum of agents, and they are generally not reported in the open scientific literature.
   - **b.** Experimental studies are those conducted to investigate a hypothesis of interest to the investigator; as such, they do not conform to any one protocol. The results of these studies are reported in the open literature and often are your only source of information for hazard identification.
4. In evaluating the individual human and animal studies, several important factors should be taken into consideration:
   - **a.** Exposure parameters such as the route, time, and duration of exposure, and the actual or estimated dose of exposure should be well defined; for animal studies, these doses should be within the realm of expected human exposures.
   - **b.** The endpoints evaluated should be described, and the methodology used in the evaluation should be appropriate.
   - **c.** The presence of maternal toxicity should be evaluated.[11]
   - **d.** Appropriate statistical procedures should be used to demonstrate the significance of the adverse effect.[12] For human studies, the strength of the association and study power should be discussed.[13–15]
   - **e.** The results should be evaluated for the presence of a dose-response relationship.
   - **f.** The quality of each paper should be assessed using the foregoing considerations.
5. The evaluation of each individual study should lead to one of three conclusions:
   - **a.** The study provides data indicative of an adverse effect.

   b. The study provides data indicative of no adverse effect. For a chemical to be placed in this category, it is essential that the study design be adequate to detect an adverse effect if one is present.
   c. The study provides inconclusive data. The reasons for placing a study in this category are many but usually involve inadequate or inappropriate study designs or incomplete reporting of the data.
6. After the individual studies have been evaluated, it is necessary to assess the total body of evidence. This is usually accomplished by evaluating the animal data separately from the human data. The following factors should be taken into consideration:
   a. Consistent adverse findings in two or more studies that use different study designs and populations are generally regarded as evidence of a causal relationship.
   b. The evidence that an agent is a developmental toxicant may be strengthened by demonstrating biological plausibility of a causal relationship. This is an especially important consideration in evaluating a group of epidemiological studies.
   c. Pharmacokinetic and pharmacogenetic differences that may account for differences between studies should be evaluated.
   d. Structural relationships and other evidence for chemical similarity may in some cases be useful in drawing inferences of potential developmental toxicity.
7. The final step in hazard identification is a weight of evidence determination. Different agencies use different schemes, which range from the very simple to the very complex.[16,17] Most of these schemes can be reduced to three basic categories:
   a. *Sufficient human evidence:* Data from human studies provide sufficient evidence for the scientific community to judge that a causal relationship is or is not supported. Supporting animal data mayor may not be available.
   b. *Sufficient experimental animal evidence/limited human data:* Data from experimental animal studies and/or limited human data that provide sufficient evidence for the scientific community to judge that the potential for developmental toxicity does or does not exist.
   c. *Insufficient evidence:* Data are not available or the data that are available are based on human or experimental animal studies that are flawed in design.

Database

Eight studies on A VOID, three in humans and five in animal, make up the database available for the hazard identification step. Each study is briefly summarized below.

Study 1. There have been a series of anecdotal reports from the union health and safety committee at the formulation and packaging facility, as well as from rural health clinics, suggesting that pregnant workers exposed to A VOID experience a high incidence of spontaneous abortion. These reports have not been published or reviewed in any scientific forum.

Study 2. A paper on accidental and purposeful poisoning with A VOID was recently published in a reputable peer-reviewed medical journal. Forty cases were described, and six involved women who were estimated to be in their first trimester of pregnancy at the time of the poisoning. The poisoning was attributed to unsuccessful suicide attempt by A VOID ingestion in five of the cases and to attempted homicide with A VOID-poisoned food in one case. The clinical symptoms recorded at the time of admission to the emergency room for the poisoning and the pediatrician's evaluation of each newborn in the perinatal period are shown in Table 3-1.

Table 3-1
Clinical Symptoms and Newborn Evaluations Reported in Study 2

CASE	CLINICAL SYMPTOMS	NEWBORN EVALUATION
1	Sweating, tremors	Normal physical and growth
2	Sweating, tremors	Normal physical and growth
3	Sweating, tremors	Spina bifida with myeloschisis
4	Sweating, tremors, convulsions	Normal physical; pre- and postnatal growth retardation
5	Sweating, tremors, convulsions	Fetal alcohol syndrome
6	Sweating, tremors, coma	Normal physical and growth

Study 3. An epidemiological study was conducted in a plant where A VOID was formulated and packaged. The study, which was conducted for the plant owners by investigators from Cosmic University, has never been published. The study population consisted of women who had worked in the packaging section of the plant for at least 6 months between 1981 and 1985. Over this 4-year period, the mean combined dose of A VOID from respiration and dermal absorption was estimated to be less than 0.07 mg/kg/day in the packaging department. The highest combined dose during this same period was estimated at 0.26 mg/kg/day. The control group consisted of female clerical staff who worked in plant offices, where it was assumed that there was no exposure to A VOID. After identifying the study and control populations, the investigators sent each woman a questionnaire regarding any pregnancies she may have had while working at the plant. Included were questions on each respondent's length of time working in the plant, her work location, and the outcome of pregnancy. Response rates to the questionnaire were 37% for the study group and 42% for the controls. Table 3-2 gives the major results as reported by the investigative team.

Study 4. In an unpublished study conducted for the manufacture of A VOID, groups of 20 C57 mated mice were administered A VOID in their diets at doses of 0, 25, or 75 mg/kg/day from days 6–18 of gestation. At the high dose tested, there was a significant decrease in maternal food consumption between days 6 and 12, and several of the females exhibited convulsions. Fetal resorptions and exencephaly were significantly increased. At the mid-dose, there was a nonsignificant increase in cleft palate. Major study results are summarized in Table 3-3.

Study 5. A meeting abstract reported that groups of five C3H mice administered A VOID by intraperitoneal injection at 5 mg/kg/day on

Table 3-2
Summary of Major Results Reported in Study 3

GROUP	STUDY	CONTROL
Respondents	56	48
Pregnancies	110	86
Abortions		
Therapeutic	10 (9%)	1 (1%)
Spontaneous	10 (9%)	9 (10%)
Stillbirths	1(1%)	0
Live births	89 (81%)	76 (88%)
Normal	85 (96%)	74 (97%)
Abnormal	4 (4%)	2 (3%)
Anencephaly	1	0
Extra finger	1	0
Heart defect	1	1
Holoprosencephaly	1	0
Trisomy 21	0	1

days 10, 11, and 12 of gestation exhibited a significant increase in cleft palate (86%) compared to controls. No mention was made of maternal toxicity or the presence of any other malformations in the treated group.

Study 6. In an unpublished teratology study conducted for the manufacturer of A VOID, groups of 20 pregnant SD rats were administered A VOID in their diets at doses sufficient to provide 0, 0.2, 2, or 20 mg/kg/day from days 6–20 of gestation. At the high dose, several females died between days 10 and 18 of gestation; between days 7 and 15, maternal food consumption and weight gain were significantly depressed, and a statistically significant increase in fetal resorptions and exencephaly was noted. At 2 mg/kg/day, there was a significant increase in microphthalmia and wavy ribs. Wavy ribs were also noted at 0.2 mg/kg/day, but the incidence did not reach statistical significance. The key results of this study are summarized in Table 3-4.

Study 7. In an unpublished study conducted for the manufacturer, groups of 20 pregnant CR rats were exposed to A VOID by inhalation at doses of 0, 0.16, 0.3, or 0.64 mg/m^3 for 6 hours/day from days 6 to 20 of gestation. At the high dose there was a slight decrease in maternal food consumption between days 6 and 7 of gestation and a significant increase in microphthalmia. No significant findings were reported at the other doses tested. The key results of this study are summarized in Table 3-5.

Table 3-3
Summary of Major Results Reported in Study 4

	NUMBER OF CASES PER DOSE (mg/kg/day) GROUP		
	0	25	75
Mated	20	20	20
Pregnant	15	13	20
Resorbed litters	0	0	10[a]
Live litters	15	13	10
Live fetuses	125	99	52[a]
Resorbed fetuses	7	6	37[a]
Abnormal fetuses	4	9	42[a]
Delayed ossification	4	3	7
Cleft palate	1	7	0
Exencephaly	0	0	38
Anophthalrnia	0	0	2

[a] Significantly different from control ($p < 0.05$).

Table 3-4
Summary of Major Results Reported in Study 6

	NUMBER OF CASES PER DOSE (mg/kg/day) GROUP			
	0	0.2	2.0	20
Mated	20	20	20	20
Pregnant	19	20	18	20
Resorbed litters	1	0	0	6[a]
Live litters	18	20	18	6[a]
Live fetuses	175	182	179	32[a]
Resorbed fetuses	10	5	7	38[a]
Abnormal fetuses	6	13	27[a]	32[a]
Delayed ossification	4	5	3	32[a]
Wavy ribs	4	7	15[a]	5
Exencephaly	1	0	0	29[a]
Microphthalmia	1	0	12[a]	2

[a] Significantly different from controls ($p < 0.05$).

Study 8. The final animal study was an unpublished report using groups of 20 NZW rabbits administered A VOID by oral gavage at doses of 0, 0.2, 20, or 200 mg/kg/day from days 7 to 19 of gestation. Maternal toxicity was observed at the high dose, with a significant decrease in body weight and increase in liver weight. At this dose there was also a statistically significant increase in resorptions and exencephaly. No significant findings were reported at any of the other dose levels tested.

Questions to Ask When Evaluating Hazard Identification Data

1. How do these data conform (or not conform) to the principles used in hazard identification?
2. What is the most sensitive endpoint of potential teratogenicity in the animal and human studies?

Table 3-5
Summary of Major Results Reported in Study 7

	NUMBER OF CASES PER DOSE (mg/m^3) GROUP			
	0	0.16	0.3	0.64
Mated	20	20	20	20
Pregnant	20	17	17	20
Resorbed litters	1	0	2	0
Live litters	19	17	16	20
Live fetuses	193	180	169	198
Resorbed fetuses	7	9	4	5
Abnormal fetuses	7	10	3	25[a]
Delayed ossification	3	2	3	4
Wavy ribs	7	5	0	3
Microphthalmia	1	4	0	21[a]

[a] Significantly different from controls ($p < 0.05$).

3. Should the wavy ribs in rodents be considered relevant to low exposure risks to humans?
4. Should the data obtained by IP injection treatment be considered relevant to human exposure?
5. Should the evidence for maternal toxicity at high doses in the animal studies negate considering the adverse effects seen in the fetuses as true developmental effects?
6. From the data given, is there any way to determine whether responses in humans are likely to be similar to those in the experimental animals?
7. Do the data provide sufficient evidence to convince you that A VOID should be considered to be a teratogen?

There are no simple or straightforward answers to these questions, and the underlying issues continue to be debated. One area of lively controversy is the role of maternal toxicity in interpreting study results.[11,18–20] Can a 20% decrease in maternal weight gain in the early part of organogenesis negate the finding of a high incidence of cleft palate or decreased fetal weight? These issues remain unresolved. Similarly, the importance of skeletal variations, such as wavy ribs or partially ossified sternebra remains controversial and as yet unresolved.[21–23]

At the conclusion of the hazard identification step in the risk assessment process, a choice must be made. It must be decided which of the following conclusions the data support: (1) A VOID is teratogenic in humans, (2) it is highly likely that A VOID is a teratogen in humans, (3) A VOID is a potential human teratogen, or (4) A VOID is not classifiable as to human teratogenicity.

REFERENCE DOSE DETERMINATION

Principles

1. The reference dose (RfD) is defined as an estimate (with uncertainty spanning perhaps an order of magnitude) of a daily exposure to the human population (including sensitive subgroups) that is assumed to be without appreciable risk of deleterious developmental effects.[24]
2. The Rill is usually derived from the "no observed adverse effect level" (NOAEL) or the "lowest observed adverse effect level" (LOAEL).
3. The most appropriate NOAEL is determined from the body of evidence examined in the hazard identification stage.
4. Dose-response data from human studies are generally preferred over animal data provided that the human data are sufficiently quantitative.
5. Data on the most sensitive relevant endpoint should be used.
6. To calculate the Rill, the NOAEL is divided by an overall uncertainty factor (UF) ranging from 10 to 10,000.[25] The total UP is calculated by multiplying together appropriate individual UPs of 10.
7. UF for intraspecies variability = 10.
8. UF for interspecies variability = 10.
9. UP for different exposure scenarios = 10.
10. UF when using the LOAEL rather than NOAEL = 10.
11. The Rill may be further reduced by applying a modifying factor greater than zero but less or equal to 10, which may be used to reflect qualitative professional judgments about scientific uncertainties such as the completeness of the overall database and the number of species and animals tested.

Database

The data to be used in this section consist of the same eight studies used in the hazard-identification step.

Questions to Ask When Evaluating Reference Dose Data

1. What study is the most appropriate for deriving a NOAEL for A VOID?
2. What do you consider to be the appropriate NOAEL?
3. Is the observed NOAEL from the studies a true "no-effect" level? Could it simply reflect the fact that in experiments with relatively small numbers, the failure to observe a statistically significant increase in adverse developmental effects is an artifact of the experimental design, not a true absence of biological effect?
4. What uncertainty factors should be applied to the NOAEL for A VOID?
5. What is the appropriate RfD for A VOID?
6. Does the RfD adequately account for the uncertainties associated with the NOAEL?
7. Is it appropriate to use an RfD derived from a study using one route of exposure for all routes of exposure?
8. Is the RfD a reliable indicator of human risk? Are there any other conditions that should be applied to this number?

Again, there are no simple or straightforward answers to these questions. Of greatest controversy is the use of NOAELs and safety factors.[26] It is now generally recognized that the determination of a NOAEL is highly dependent on the sample size and dose levels used. Methods using various mathematical models that are less sensitive to sample size and utilize the full dose-response curve have been proposed as alternatives to the NOAEL/UF approach.[27–31] No one method has yet gained favor and the majority of risk assessments still utilize the NOAEL-derived RfD.

After completing the RfD-determination step in the risk-assessment process, you may conclude that the RfD you calculated, and the NOAEL from which it was derived, are sufficient to determine the developmental risks associated with exposure to A VOID. Alternatively, you may wish to conclude that RfDs are of little value and in fact create a false sense of precision in an area involving tremendous uncertainty. A third possible conclusion is that while risks from developmental toxicants cannot be quantified, they should be described in qualitative terms.

EXPOSURE ASSESSMENT

Principles

1. An exposure assessment serves to identify the magnitude of human exposure to an agent, the frequency and duration of that exposure, and the routes by which humans are exposed.[32] It may be useful to identify the number of exposed people along with other characteristics of the exposed population, such as age, genetic history, and exposure to (other) known teratogens.
2. Exposure may be based on quantitative or qualitative measurements in various media such as air, water, or food.
    a. Daily intake of individual and combined media exposures should be determined.
    b. When individuals may be exposed by contact with several media, it is important to consider total intake from all media.

   c. Daily intake under different conditions of activities in different locations should be determined.
3. Sampling and monitoring of individual exposures is usually conducted by contractors for either the responsible parties or regulatory bodies.
4. Usually only a limited amount of monitoring and only a limited number of samples of various media can be taken for measurement.
   a. The representativeness of measured values is usually uncertain.
   b. The degree to which data for a given medium are representative of that medium should be estimated.
5. When data are incomplete or lacking, mathematical models may be used to estimate air and water concentrations. The validity of the model should be checked in context of the exposure scenario.
6. Standard average values and ranges for human intake of various media are available and are generally used unless data on specific agents indicate that such values are inappropriate.[33]
   a. Adults drink approximately 2 L water/day.
   b. The average adult inhales 23 m^2/day of air.

Database

Four monitoring studies have been conducted on A VOID: two were conducted in workplace settings, one on air and one on water. A brief description is provided below.

Study 1. In conjunction with the epidemiology study reported earlier, a 3-day study was conducted in the plant during which time workers packaging A VOID were monitored for exposure via the inhalation and dermal routes. The data collected were used to estimate the mean combined dose, which was calculated to be 0.07 mg/kg/day. The highest dose received by a single worker on any one day was 0.26 mg/kg.

Study 2. A study was conducted by a state regulatory agency that used passive dosimetry to monitor field worker exposure to A VOID. From the data collected, the absorbed dosage was calculated. The relative contributions of the inhalation and dermal routes of exposure were back-calculated from the total absorbed dosage, assuming that a certain proportion of A VOID exposure was through inhalation. This proportion was based on measured concentrations of A VOID in the air, standard respiratory rate and retention, and 100% absorption. The calculated absorbed exposure dosage for a person weighing 70 kg expressed μg/kg/day is shown in Table 3-6.

Table 3-6
Exposure Levels Reported in Study 2

	ROUTE OF EXPOSURE	
WORKERS	DERMAL	INHALATION
Pilots	0.50	1.13
Aerial mix/load	0.02	0.53
Flagger	0.53	1.73
Ground mix/load	0.05	0.85
Ground applications	0.02	0.37
Combined mix/load/ applications	0.10	1.77
Gofer	0.03	0.70

Table 3-7
Sampling Results Reported in Study 3

	LOCATION			
	1	2	3	4
Mean	62	132	152	630
Range	2–142	<1.4–280	76–415	145–1720

Study 3. An air-monitoring study was conducted in four rural communities near fields where A VOID was being used. Twenty-four-hour collections were conducted over three 4-day periods in 1987. The mean concentrations (ng/m^3) of airborne A VOID over the 12 sampling days, along with the range of values, were published in a reputable peer-reviewed journal and are shown in Table 3-7.

Study 4. A water-monitoring study was conducted using samples collected from the major river that runs through the agricultural area and past several metropolitan areas downstream. Samples were collected near each of the metropolitan areas, one per month from May through September 1989. The results of the study, which appear in a government report, indicate that only trace amounts of A VOID were detected. The validity of this study has been challenged by several environmental advocacy groups.

Questions to Ask When Evaluating Exposure Data

1. Do the monitoring data adequately describe exposures to A VOID in all possible media? If not, what additional media need to be considered, and why?
2. Should the different types of exposure data be treated the same for purposes of characterizing human risk?
3. Is the mean concentration in the various media the appropriate summary statistic to use to characterize human exposure? Should the upper range or statistical upper confidence limit be used as an alternative?
4. Are the various assumptions about human intake and average exposure to various media valid?
5. Should exposure and risk to workers at the production facility be considered in the same context as exposure and risk to field-workers or residents in exposed communities?

It should come as no surprise that there are no simple or straightforward answers to these questions. Debate continues on the use of various models for estimating exposures, but generally the issue of greatest concern is the method of extrapolating from one route of exposure to another.[34,35] This is typified by the debate over the various routes of exposure following an animal whole-body versus nose-only exposure. With whole-body exposure, it must be decided how much of the agent enters via the respiratory route, how much via the dermal route, and how much via ingestion from grooming behavior and contaminated food. The rates of absorption for these various routes may differ rather dramatically. With nose-only exposures, the majority of the exposure is considered to be respiratory, but dermal adsorption from the nose area and ingestion by swallowing cannot be ruled out.

After the exposure-assessment step in the risk-assessment process has been completed, you may conclude that although different exposure estimates are based on different data and assumptions, they are all adequate and sufficient for assessing risks. Alternatively, you may wish to conclude that none of the exposure data are adequate for use in risk assessment and that no quantitative risk assessment should be developed until better information is available.

RISK CHARACTERIZATION

Principles

1. The purpose of risk characterization, the final step of the risk assessment, is to integrate the information collected and analyzed in the first three steps to characterize the excess risk to humans.
2. An explicit numerical RfD should be included in the characterization.
3. Compare the exposures experienced or expected for different groups of individuals.
4. Estimate the margin of exposure (MOE) for each group by dividing the NOAEL from the critical study used to estimate the RfD by the exposure for each group.
5. Describe risks qualitatively for each population group.
6. Describe the statistical and biological uncertainties in estimating the extent of adverse health effects.

Database

The data used in the risk-characterization step are those accumulated in the preceding steps of the risk-assessment process.

The risk characterization can be thought of as the conclusion of the risk assessment, summarizing the information from the preceding steps (hazard identification, RfD determination, and exposure assessment). As such, the issues of controversy discussed earlier also apply to this final step.

CONCLUSION

Having gained some appreciation of risk assessments, we can now consider how they can be used in the risk-communication process. Paul Peters (personal communications) has observed that there are two types of risk information: "ready-made" and "tailor-made."

The RfDs developed in the risk assessment process are applicable to all individuals in the population, and as such, represent "ready-made" information. They serve as a powerful public health tool in defining the exposure level below which it can be assumed that no adverse developmental effects will occur. In contrast, individual risk counseling requires tailor-made information. Typically, this information is based on interpreting the results of human and animal studies in the context of a pregnant woman's age, parity, genetic background, and exposure to other chemicals of concern.

The ready-made information from the risk assessment can have value beyond the public health perspective. While using an RfD as the sole basis for individual risk counseling is never appropriate, the studies that served as the basis for obtaining the NOAEL on which the RfD is based can serve as the starting material for crafting the tailor-made information needed to communicate risk information to individual pregnant women.

ACKNOWLEDGMENTS

I am indebted to the U.S. Environmental Protection Agency's workshop on risk and decision making, which served as a model for the workshop on which this chapter is based. I am also grateful to Linda Chernoff and Dr. Paul Peters for their help and insight in planning this project, and to Dr. Gideon Koren for his encouragement to complete the project.

REFERENCES

1. Shepard TH. *Catalog of Teratogenic Agents,* 6th ed. Baltimore: Johns Hopkins University Press, 1989.
2. U.S. Environmental Protection Agency. Integrated Risk Information Service (IRIS). Online. Washington, DC: Office of Health and Environmental Assessment, 1991.
3. National Research Council. Risk Assessment in the Federal Government: Managing the Process. Committee on the Institutional Means for the Assessment of Risks to Public Health. Commission on Life Sciences, National Research Council. Washington, DC: National Academy Press, 1983, pp 17–83.
4. Erickson ill. Epidemiology and developmental toxicology. In: Kimmel CA, Buelke-Sam J, eds. Developmental Toxicology. New York: Raven Press, 1981, pp 289–301.
5. U.S. Environmental Protection Agency. Pesticide assessment guidelines, subdivision F. Hazard evaluation: Human and domestic animals, EPA-540/9-82-025. Washington, DC: Office of Pesticides and Toxic Substances, 1982. Available from NTIS, Springfield, VA.
6. U.S. Environmental Protection Agency. Toxic Substances Control Act test guidelines; final rules. *Fed Reg.* 1985;50:39426–39428 and 39433–39434.
7. U.S. Environmental Protection Agency. Pesticide Assessment guidelines, subdivision F. Hazard evaluation: Human and domestic animals, EPA 540/09-91 123. Addendum 10: Neurotoxicity, series 81 83. Washington, DC: Office of Pesticides and Toxic Substances. 1991. Available from NTIS, Springfield, VA.
8. Organization for Economic Cooperation and Development. Guidelines for Testing of Chemicals' Teratogenicity, OECD, 1981.
9. U.S. Food and Drug Administration. Guidelines for reproduction and studies for human use. Rockville, MD: Bureau of Drugs, 1966.
10. U.S. Food and Drug Administration. Advisory Committee on Protocols for Safety Evaluation. Panel on reproduction-Studies in the safety evaluation of additives and pesticide residues. *Toxicol Appl Pharmacol.* 1970;16:264–296.
11. Kimmel GL, Kimmel CA, Francis EZ, eds. Evaluation of maternal and developmental toxicity. *Teratogenesis Carcinog Mutagen.* 1987; 7:203–338.
12. Kimmel CA, Kimmel GL, Frankos V, eds. Interagency Regulatory Liaison Group Workshop on Reproductive Toxicity Risk Assessment. *Environ Health Perspect.* 1986;86:193–221.
13. Bloom AD. Guidelines for reproductive studies in exposed human populations. Report of Panel II. In: Bloom AD, ed. Guidelines for Studies of Human Populations Exposed to Mutagenic and Reproductive Hazards. White Plains, NY: March of Dimes Birth Defects Foundation, 1981, pp 37–110.
14. Stein Z, Kline J, Shrout P. Power in surveillance. In: Hemminki K, Sorsa M, Vaninio H, eds. Occupational Hazards and Reproduction. Washington, DC: Hemisphere, 1985, pp 203–208.
15. Greenland S. Quantitative methods in the review of epidemiologic literature. *Epidemiol Rev.* 1987;9:1–30.

16. U.S. Environmental Protection Agency. Guidelines for developmental toxicity risk assessment. *Fed Reg.* 1991;56:63798–63826.
17. California Department of Health Services. Draft guidelines for hazard identification and dose-response assessment of agents causing developmental and/or reproductive toxicity, Sacramento, CA: Office of Environmental Health Hazard Assessment, 1991.
18. Schardein JL. Approaches to defining the relationship of maternal and developmental toxicity. *Teratogenesis Carcinog Mutagen.* 1987;7: 255–271.
19. Johnson E, Christian M. When is a teratology study not an evaluation of teratogenicity? *J Am Coll Toxicol.* 1984;3:431–434.
20. Black DL, Marks TA. Role of maternal toxicity in assessing developmental toxicity in animals: a discussion. *Regul Toxicol Pharmacol.* l992;16:189–201.
21. Kimmel CA, Wilson JG. Skeletal deviations in rats: malformations or variations? *Teratology.* 1973;8:309–316.
22. Chernoff N, Rogers JM, Thrner CI, et al. Significance of supernumerary ribs in rodent developmental toxicity studies: postnatal persistence in rats and mice. *Fundam Appl Toxicol.* 1991;17:448–453.
23. Palmer AK. Incidence of sporadic malformations, anomalies and variations in random-bred laboratory animals. In Neubert D, Merker HJ, Kwasigroch TE, eds. Methods in Prenatal Toxicology. Stuttgart: Thieme, 1977, pp 52–71.
24. Barnes DG, Dourson M. Reference dose (Rill): Description and use in health risk assessments. *Regul Toxicol Pharnlacol.* 1988;8:471–486.
25. Dourson M, Stara I. Regulatory history and experimental support of uncertainty (safety) factors. *Regul Toxicol Pharnlacol.* 1983;3:224–238.
26. Gaylor DW. Incidence of developmental defects at the no observed adverse effect level (NOAEL). *Regul Toxicol Pharnlacol.* 1992;15: 151–160.
27. Crump KS. A new method for determining allowable daily intakes. *Fundarn Appl Toxicol.* 1984;4:854–871.
28. Gaylor DW. Quantitative risk analysis for quantal reproductive and developmental effects. *Environ Health Perspect.* 1989;79:243–246.
29. Kimmel C, Gaylor D. Issues in qualitative and quantitative risk analysis for developmental toxicology. *Risk Anal.* 1988;8:15–20.
30. Kodell RL, Howe RB, Chen II, et al. Mathematical modeling of reproductive and developmental toxic effects for quantitative risk assessment. *Risk Anal.* 1991;11:583–590.
31. Ryan L. The use of generalized estimating equations for risk assessment in developmental toxicity. *Risk Anal.* 1992;12:439–447.
32. U.S. Environmental Protection Agency. Guidelines for exposure assessment. *Fed Reg.* 1986;51:34042–34054.
33. U.S. Environmental Protection Agency. Exposure Factors Handbook, EPA-600/8-89-043. Washington, DC: Office of Health and Environmental Assessment, 1989. Available from NTIS, Springfield, VA.
34. Sachsse K, Zbinden K, Ullman L. *Significance of mode of exposure in aerosol inhalation toxicity studies: Head-only versus whole-body exposure.* Arch Toxicol Suppl 1980;4:305–311.
35. Iwasaki M, Yoshida M, Ikeda T, et al. Comparison of whole-body versus snout- only exposure in inhalation toxicity of fenthion. *Jpn J Vet Sci.* 1988;50:23–30.

CHAPTER 4

TERATOGENIC DRUGS AND CHEMICALS IN HUMANS

Irena Nulman, Yana Izmaylov, Arthur Staroselsky, and Gideon Koren

INTRODUCTION

Since the thalidomide disaster, drugs and chemicals have been scrutinized carefully for their potential human teratogenicity. However, despite valiant efforts in this direction, several objective limitations hinder our ability to detect human teratogens.

1. Most birth defects occur rarely; therefore, even an increased risk posed by a teratogen may not be easily identified. While thalidomide caused more than 20% of major malformations following first-trimester exposure, most suspected teratogens increase the baseline risk of major malformations very slightly (1–3%), even when significantly increasing the risk of a specific pattern. For example, valproic acid increases 200-fold the risk for neural tube defects (NTDs), yet its impact on the overall risk for major malformations is less than 0.5%.[1] Consequently, a woman exposed to valproic acid may still have better than a 95% chance of having a healthy baby.

   As a result it may be necessary to study a large number of infants exposed in utero to a certain drug to prove or disprove its teratogenic potential. Most studies are limited in their statistical power because their numbers are not large enough.
2. For obvious reasons, pharmaceutical manufacturers warn the public not to use drugs in pregnancy owing to a lack of information about their safety. Consequently, the accumulation of data on a specific drug is often sketchy and uncontrolled. While most manufacturers try to record and follow up voluntary reports of exposures in pregnancy, it has to be recognized that such data are incomplete and may be biased. For example, it is conceivable that disproportionately high numbers of families having malformed children will report their drug exposure to the manufacturer or to the regulatory agencies, whereas families with healthy babies are less likely to do so. This tendency was recently documented in a large study on the teratogenicity of retinoic acid. In the prospective section of that cohort, 38% of the infants were malformed, whereas 80% of those reporting retrospectively cited major malformations. This means that a large number of families having normal children after first-trimester exposure to retinoic acid did not report voluntarily to either the manufacturer or the Centers for Disease Control (CDC).[2,3]
3. As part of the regulatory process, the teratogenic potential of drugs has to be tested in animals. The failure of animal models to detect the teratogenicity of thalidomide before the human disaster occurred has resulted in a growing feeling that we cannot extrapolate from animal studies to humans. Differences in pharmacokinetics, metabolism, embryology, target organ sensitivity, and other factors may account for such discrepancies. Yet almost all known human teratogens have been shown to cause similar effects in animals, warfarin (Coumadin) being the exception.[4] Moreover, in the case of retinoic acid (Accutane), the most potent human teratogen currently available, animal data clearly prevented a postmarketing disaster similar to that of thalidomide.[5]

CASE REPORTS

Cases associating in utero exposure to a certain drug or chemical with an adverse outcome may be either most helpful or useless, depending on the following statistical considerations.

In a case of a drug that is rarely used in pregnancy, a small number of cases showing the same pattern of malformations may be most indicative, since these cases may already exceed manyfold the baseline risk for the occurrence of such malformations. For example, if a new drug has been reported to cause 10 cases of cleft palate out of the total 100 known cases of first-trimester exposure, then it has a 10% risk of causing cleft palate. This calculated risk exceeds by 100-fold the known risk of cleft palate, which is 0.1%. Based on this approach, several human teratogens, including warfarin and retinoic acid, were incriminated long before prospective studies confirmed these associations.

At the other extreme, it will be impossible to prove teratogenicity based on case reports when the drug is commonly used (e.g., salicylates) and the malformation is not rare. Salicylates are consumed by thousands of pregnant women every year; therefore, based on statistical chance only, one would expect to find within this group offspring with any described malformation.

Bendectin (the combination of pyridoxine and doxylamine) was for decades one of the most widely used antiemetic drugs to cope with pregnancy-associated morning sickness. The drug was wrongly incriminated as causing congenital malformations based on case reports: hundreds of thousands of pregnant women were exposed to this drug; 1–3% of their offspring would have had major malformations, just because of their baseline risk. Subsequently, controlled studies (both case control and prospective) failed to confirm an association between Bendectin and human teratogenicity; however, the American manufacturer withdrew the drug from the market owing to excessive insurance costs. In Canada, this antiemetic is available under the trade name Diclectin, and recently the Canadian Health Protection Branch has specifically labeled it as an antiemetic appropriate for use in pregnancy.

EPIDEMIOLOGICAL STUDIES

Several approaches are commonly employed in studying the potential reproductive effects of drugs and chemicals.

The retrospective study tries to identify women exposed in pregnancy to the drug in question and to evaluate the outcome of the exposed offspring. A variety of methodological problems may complicate the interpretation of such data.

It may not be possible to identify and assess all cases, and it is conceivable that cases with an adverse outcome will be overrepresented. For example, the Danish lithium registry is a voluntary reporting system of exposure to the drug in pregnancy. Of its 300 cases reported by 1993, about 10% represented cardiac malformation; however, it is probable that parents of healthy babies born after such exposures had less motivation to report to the registry than those with an adverse outcome.[6]

Another major disadvantage of such cohorts, owing to the rare occurrence of most congenital anomalies, is the need for very large numbers of individuals exposed to the drug. To overcome this shortcoming, the case control study focuses on offspring with a specific malformation and tries to assess maternal exposure to the drug in question. The percentage of maternal use is then compared to a group of mothers of infants not having the tested malformation. A major problem with all retrospective studies, both cohorts and case control, is the need to rely on maternal recall of drug exposure (i.e., time and dose). In a recent study, mothers we had interviewed first at the time of their exposure in pregnancy tended not to remember significant parts of this information when questioned again after giving birth.[7] Mitchell has significantly improved the reliability of case control studies by developing questionnaires that reduce the effect of maternal recall characteristic of the previously used open-ended questionnaire.[8]

In prospective studies, the information about exposure and other possible pregnancy risk factors is collected at the time of exposure or soon after it. Although this is likely to be the most accurate approach to assess potential teratogenicity, such studies are lengthy and costly because very large numbers of test subjects are needed to overcome the rareness of most congenital malformations.

Whereas, full discussion of methodological problems associated with each approach is beyond the scope of this chapter, it is clear that proving the teratogenicity of a specific drug in humans may be a complex process, demanding a high degree of scrutiny. In many cases, evidence is accumulated through several different approaches (e.g., case reports, case control, and prospective studies).

The combination of increased awareness to human teratogenicity with the above-mentioned difficulties in differentiating normal background from slightly increased rates of malformations has led to unjustified incrimination of useful medications, which were later found out to be nonteratogenic. These include oral contraceptive hormones, diazepam, Bendectin, and spermicides. Typically, a devastating potential, as reflected above in the case of Bendectin, may result from wrong incrimination of a nonteratogen, as many women may terminate an otherwise wanted pregnancy. Presently it is felt that a number of criteria must be met before an agent is incriminated as human teratogen.[9] (1) Exposure to the drug at the critical time or times; (2) Consistent findings by epidemiologic studies; (3) Case reports, especially of a specific defect or syndrome; (4) A rare exposure associated with a rare defect; (5) Evidence that the frequency of the specific outcomes is associated with the introduction or withdrawal of the agent; (6) Teratogenicity in animals at doses equivalent to those in humans; and (7) Biologic plausibility. A drug does not have to meet all of the criteria to establish it as a human teratogen. Sheppard[9], thought that at least three of the criteria (1, 2, and 3 or 1, 3, and 4) were essential for proof of human teratogenicity, as well as abrupt increase in the frequency of a particular defect or association of defects (syndrome), coincidence of this increase with a known environmental change, such as widespread use of a new drug or sudden exposure to a chemical, known exposure to the environmental change early in pregnancy yielding characteristically defective infants, absence of other factors common to all pregnancies yielding infants with the characteristic defect(s).

COUNSELING WOMEN ABOUT KNOWN TERATOGENS

Table 4-1 presents details of drugs and chemicals known to be teratogenic in humans, with a major reference for each.

When a clinician confronts an exposure of a pregnant patient to a known teratogen, it is important to convey the available information to the family in a way that will prevent both understatements and ambiguity. An accurate estimate of the risk for an adverse outcome should be provided because pregnant women tend to have an unrealistically high perception of teratogenic risk even when exposed to nonteratogens (see Chap. 23).

In the Motherisk Program, we find that the same estimated risk may be unacceptably high for some families and reasonable for others. For example, epileptic women who are well controlled with phenytoin and have failed to have their epilepsy controlled with other anticonvulsants are often reluctant to change their medication in pregnancy. Conversely, we recently consulted the mother of three healthy children who was treated briefly with phenytoin following a single seizure. When it became apparent that she was pregnant again, an electroencephalogram was taken. The results were normal, and it was planned to discontinue the drug. For this patient, the teratogenic risk of phenytoin was perceived as unacceptable.

Not included in Table 4-1 are scores of drugs that cause direct fetal toxicity consistent with their pharmacological effects. These are detailed in Chap. 8.

Proven human teratogens are by no means a homogeneous group of compounds; however, they can be divided by several criteria into subgroups.

Obsolete Drugs

Diethylstilbestrol and trimethadione are currently unlikely to create a problem in pregnancy because they are not used clinically. Thalidomide, which was banned after the disaster three decades ago, is an important drug for some forms of leprosy. It is presently used in South America for leprosy in women who receive injectable forms of contraceptive hormone. However, recently there have been reports of a new wave of malformed children due to inappropriate use. Retinoic acid, which bears a rate of teratogenicity similar to that of thalidomide, is widely used, mostly for treatment of cystic acne in adolescents and young adults, who are the most likely group to fail contraceptives. In fact, the U.S. Food and Drug Administration (FDA) is reevaluating conflicting reports on the number of pregnancies and birth defects associated with retinoic acid in order to decide the future of this drug in the American market.

Existence of Alternative Therapy

Several teratogenic drugs may have value as alternative therapies in pregnancy; however, each case is characterized by unique problems.

Although there are alternatives to lithium carbonate (e.g., tricyclics or valproic acid) for manic-depressive disorders. Some patients may not respond favorably to the replacement drug (tricyclic) or the replacement drug is a more potent teratogen (valproic acid). Moreover, recent evidence suggests lithium to be safe during

Table 4-1
Drugs and Chemicals Proven to Be Teratogenic in Humans

DRUG/CHEMICAL	FETAL ADVERSE EFFECTS	RELATIVE RISK FOR TERATOGENICITY	CLINICAL INTERVENTION	REF.
Alcohol	Consumption of alcohol during pregnancy leads to a spectrum of structural growth, neurocognitive and behavioral impairments currently termed *Fetal Alcohol Spectrum Disorder (FASD)*. The spectrum ranges from complete phenotype, *Fetal Alcohol Syndrome (FAS)*, to the partial FAS, the alcohol-related birth defects (ARBD), and the alcohol-related neurodevelopmental disorder (ARND). FAS includes facial anomalies, presence of pre- and/or postnatal growth deficiency and neurodevelopmental anomalies. ARND is characterized by a complex pattern of neurodevelopmental abnormalities such as behavioral, temperament and cognitive deficits.	In alcohol-dependent women consuming above 2 g/kg/day ethanol over first trimester: two- to three-fold higher risk for congenital malformations (about 10%).	Documentation of alcohol consumption at any point during gestation is essential for the diagnostic categories of the spectrum. Screen for alcohol use with validated screening tools (TACE, TWEAK). Meconium fatty acid ethyl esters levels may be used as biological markers of chronic prenatal exposure to alcohol. *Prospective:* to discontinue exposure, if a woman is addicted to alcohol, refer to addiction center. *During pregnancy:* to alleviate fears in mild or occasional drinkers who may terminate pregnancy based on unrealistic perception of risk. Level 2 ultrasound to rule out visible malformation.	10, 11, 12, 13, 14, 15, 16
Alkylating agents (busulfan, chloram bucil, cyclophosphamide, mechlorethamine)	Growth retardation, cleft palate, microphthalmia hypoplastic ovaries, cloudy corneas, agenesis of kidney, malformations of digits, cardiac defects, multiple other anomalies.	Based on case reports, between 10 and 50% of cases were malformed following different alkylating agents. It is possible that adverse outcome was over represented.	Level 2 ultrasound to rule out visible malformations.	4
Antimetabolic agents (aminopterin azauridine, cytarabine, 5-FU, 6-MP, methotrexate)	Hydrocephalus, meningocephalocele, anencephaly, malformed skull, cerebral hypoplasia, growth retardation, eye and ear malformations, malformed nose and cleft palate. malformed extremities and fingers *Aminopterin syndrome:* Cranial dysostosis, hydrocephalus, hypertelorism, anomalies of external ear, micrognathia, posterior cleft palate.	Based on case reports 7–75% of cases were malformed. It is possible that adverse outcome was overrepresented.	Level 2 ultrasound to rule out visible malformations and supplement folic acid to women receiving antifolates (e.g., methotrexate).	4
Benzodiazepines	Increased risk for oral cleft alone.	Meta-analysis of case control studies showed an association between major malformation and/or oral cleft alone (odds ratios 3.01; 95% CI, 1.32–6.84).	Level 2 ultrasound to rule out visible malformations. Avoid withdrawal by tapering the drug.	17, 18

(*Continued*)

Table 4-1
Drugs and Chemicals Proven to Be Teratogenic in Humans (*Continued*)

DRUG/CHEMICAL	FETAL ADVERSE EFFECTS	RELATIVE RISK FOR TERATOGENICITY	CLINICAL INTERVENTION	REF.
Carbamazepine	Increased risk for neural tube defects (0.5–1%) and major congenital malformations estimated at 2.3%. May cause kinked ribs, cleft palate and anophthalmos as well as lower body weight, length and head circumference. Normal intelligence.	An NTD estimates at 1% with carbamazepine doses greater than 1200 mg/day.	Periconceptional folate; maternal and/or amniotic α-feto-protein; ultrasound to rule out NTD.	19, 20, 21, 22, 23
Carbon monoxide	Cerebral atrophy, mental retardation, microcephaly, convulsions, spastic disorders, intrauterine or postnatal death.	Based on case reports, when mother is severely poisoned, high risk for neurological sequelae; no risk in mild accidental exposures.	Measure maternal carboxyhemoglobin levels. Treat with 100% oxygen for 5 hours after maternal carboxyhemoglobin returns to normal because fetal equilibration takes longer. If hyperbaric chamber available, should be used, as elimination $T_{1/2}$ of CO is more rapid. Fetal monitoring by an obstetrician; sonographic follow-up.	24, 25
Cocaine	Gestational period is, on average, 2 weeks shorter. Decreased uterine blood flow and induced uterine contractions. Growth retardation and small head circumference, low birth rate, intracranial bleeding, fetal distress, and congenital anomalies involving the heart, limbs, genitourinary tract and face. May also lead to neurobehavioral impairment in the neonatal period, sudden infant death syndrome.	A dose-response relationship was found between cocaine use and perinatal outcome. Often used with other substances.	Level 2 ultrasound for measurement of fetal head size and to rule out visible malformations or intraventricular haemorrage.	21, 26, 27, 28
Corticosteroids	Cleft palate, cataracts, polycystic kidney disease, reduction in birth weight and head circumference, spontaneous abortions. Higher risk for first trimester use.	Dose response relationship. Odds Ratio (OR) 2.5 (CI 1.5–4.4) meta-analysis. Antenatal Exposure at 24 weeks or later causes up to a 9% reduction ($p < 0.014$) in birth weight and up to 4% reduction ($p < 0.0024$) in head circumference.	Level 2 ultrasound to rule out visible malformations.	29, 30, 31

Diethylstilbestrol (DES)	*Female offspring:* clear cell adenocarcinoma in young female adults exposed in utero (before 18th week): irregular menses (oligomenorrhea), reduced pregnancy rates, increased rate of preterm deliveries, increased perinatal mortality and spontaneous abortion. *Male offspring:* cysts of epididymis, cryptorchidism, hypogonadism, diminished and/impair spermatogenesis, varicocele.	Exposure before 18 weeks of gestation: = 1.4\1000 of exposed female with carcinoma. Congenital morphological changes in vaginal epithelium in 39% of exposures.	*Diagnosis:* direct observation of mucosa and Shiller's test. *Treatment:* mechanical excitement or destruction in relatively confined area. Surgery and radiotherapy for diffused tumor.	32
Lead	Impaired child long-term neurodevelopment.	Higher risk when maternal lead is above 10 μg/dL.	*Maternal lead levels* > 10 μg/dL: investigate for possible source of contamination. *Levels* > 25 μg/dL: consider chelation.	33
Lithium Carbonate	Cardiovascular defects and possibly higher risk for Ebstein's anomaly; no detectable higher risk for other malformations		Women who need lithium should continue therapy, with sonographic follow-up (level 2 ultrasound and fetal cardioechography at 18–20 week). Patients may need higher doses because of increased clearance rate. The level of the drug should be monitored closely.	6, 21
Methyl mercury, mercuric sulfide	Microcephaly, eye malformations, cerebral palsy, mental retardation, malocclusion of teeth.	Women of affected babies consumed 9–27 ppm mercury; greater risk when ingested at 6–8 gestational months. Relative risk was not elucidated but 13\220 babies born in Minamata, Japan, at time of contamination had severe disease.	Good correlation between mercury concentrations in maternal hair follicles and neurological outcome of the fetus. Hair mercury content above 50 ppm was used successfully as a cut point for termination. In acute poisoning, the fetus is 4–10 times more sensitive than the adult to methylmercury toxicity.	34, 35
Misoprostol	Spontaneous abortions, fetal death. Möbius syndrome (paralysis of sixth and seventh cranial nerves). Vascular disruption, hemorrhages, and cell death.	RR 3.15; CI 1.20–8.27 OR 25.7; CI 8.30–89.4	Increase awareness of teratogenicity of the drug.	36, 37, 21
Organic solvents	Increased risk for major malformations without a single pattern, increased risk for miscarriage.	13% (1.8–99.5) OR 1.64 (CI 1.16–2.30) for major malformations OR 1.25 (0.99–1.58) for spontaneous abortions.	Minimize exposure, avoid toxicity by protection and ventilation.	38, 29

(*Continued*)

Table 4-1
Drugs and Chemicals Proven to Be Teratogenic in Humans (*Continued*)

DRUG/CHEMICAL	FETAL ADVERSE EFFECTS	RELATIVE RISK FOR TERATOGENICITY	CLINICAL INTERVENTION	REF.
PCBs	*Stillbirth Signs at birth:* white eye discharge, 30% (32/108); teeth present, 8.7% (11/127); irritated/swollen gums, 11% (11/99); hyperpigmentation ("cola" staining), 42.5% (54/127); deformed/small nails, 24.6% (30/122); acne, 12.8% (16/125). *Subsequent history:* bronchitis or pneumonia, 27.2% (30/124); chipped or broken teeth, 35.5% (38/107); hair loss, 12.2% (14/115); acne scars, 9.6% (11/115); generalized itching, 27.8% (32/1150). *Developmental:* Impaired child long-term neurodevelopment.	4% (6 of 159)–20% (8 of 39)	These figures, which are from cases poisoned by high consumption of PCB-contaminated rice oil, cannot be extrapolated to cases in which maternal poisoning has not been verified. Women working near PCBs (e.g., hydroelectric facilities) should use effective protection	40
Penicillamine	Skin hyperelastosis, cleft lip and palate.	Few case reports; risk unknown.		41
Phenobarbital	Microcephaly, sexual dysfunction, cardiac defects. Long-term child neurocognitive delay.	Risk is two to three times greater than base line.	The drug should be used at the lowest therapeutical level. The newborn should be carefully monitored for sedation.	21, 42, 43, 44
Phenytoin	*Fetal Hydantoin Syndrome:* low nasal bridge, inner epicanthal folds, ptosis, strabismus, hypertelorism, low set or abnormal ears, wide mouth, large fontanels, anomalies and hypoplasia of distal phalanges and nails, skeletal abnormalities, microcephaly, growth deficiency, neuroblastoma, lymphangioma, cardiac defects, cleft palate/lip. Lower language, locomotor and full scale child IQ.	5–10% of typical syndrome; about 30% of partial picture. Relative risk of 7 for IQ less than 84 in exposed children.	Neurologist should consider changing to other medications. Keep phenytoin concentrations at lower effective levels. Close monitoring of the drug level as well as level of folic acid is strongly advised. Level 2 ultrasound to rule out visible malformations. Vitamin K to mother during last 4 weeks of pregnancy and to the neonate right after delivery.	50
Systemic retinoids (Isotretinoin, Etretinate)	Spontaneous abortions; deformities of cranium, ears, face, heart, limbs, liver; hydrocephalus, microcephalus, heart defects. Cognitive defects even without dysmorphology	For Isotretinoin: 38% risk: 80% of malformations are CNS.	Treated women should have an effective method of contraception. Pregnancy termination. If diagnosed too late, sonographic follow-up to rule out confirmed malformations.	2
Thalidomide	Limb phocomelia, amelia, hypoplasia, congenital heart defects, renal malformations, cryptorchidism, abducens paralysis, deafness, microtia, anotia.	About 26% risk when exposure to drug occurs in days 34–50 of gestation.	Thalidomide is an effective drug for some forms of leprosy. Treated women should have an effective mode of contraception 1 month prior to therapy initiation.	45, 21

Tetracycline	Yellow, gray-brown, or brown staining of deciduous teeth, with exposure during 5–6 months of gestation, destruction of enamel.	From 4 months of gestation and on, occurs in 50% of fetuses exposed to tetracycline: 12.5% to oxytetracycline.	If there is exposure between 14 and 16 weeks of gestation, no known risk.	46
Valproic acid/Sodium Valproate	Up to 2,9% risk for NTD (lumbosacral spina bifida, meningomyelocele). CNS defects (microcephaly); cardiac, urogenital, skeletal and skin-muscle defects. Neurodevelopmental delay in children. Intrauterine growth retardation.	Fetal exposure to doses greater than 1000 mg/day is associated with child long-term neurocognitive impairment. Doses greater than 1500 mg/day are associated with increased risk for neural tube defects.	Level 2 ultrasound and maternal α-fetoproteins or amniocentesis to rule out neural tube defects. Diagnosed NTD deliver by cesarean section.	1, 47, 20, 21, 23, 48
Warfarin	*Fetal Warfarin Syndrome:* nasal hypoplasia, chondrodysplasia punctata, brachydactyly, skull defects, abnormal ears, malformed eyes, CNS malformations, microcephaly, hydrocephalus, skeletal deformities, mental retardation, optic atrophy, spasticity, Dandy Walker malformations.	6% of exposed fetuses have malformations; another 3% hemorrhages; 8% stillbirths.	*Prospective:* switch to heparin for the first trimester. Women should be followed up in a high-risk perinatal unit.	49

pregnancy.[6] The same argument is valid for phenytoin and valproic acid, and in each case the physician caring for the woman planning pregnancy should evaluate other alternatives. Heparin, which does not cross the placenta, may substitute warfarin during the first trimester; the former must be injected, however, and compliance may become a major problem.

Form a pharmacological standpoint, in very few instances is there no alternative drug for human teratogens; retinoic acid, however, appears to be very efficacious in complicated types of acne, and no other compound shares the same mechanisms of action. This is a strong argument in favor of not removing the drug from the market despite its known teratogenic risk. Thousands of patients would thus be deprived of an irreplaceable therapy. Clearly, this drug is completely contraindicated in pregnancy.

Alkylating agents and antimetabolites (azathioprine, chlorambucil, etc.) represent a specific therapy that may need to be continued uninterrupted. The main teratogenic effects of these drugs are associated with first-trimester exposure; current analysis done by us in Toronto reveals that in most cases, when cancer is diagnosed early in pregnancy, the women choose to terminate the pregnancy. However, to date there is increasing use of some of these agents in collagen diseases and nephritis as well as after organ transplants; it is likely that the number of women seeking prospective advice on these drugs will increase.

Magnitude of the Public Health Issue

Alcohol is undoubtedly the most common human teratogen. Because 10 million Americans are alcoholics, large numbers of fetuses are exposed to the amount of alcohol associated with fetal alcohol syndrome (FAS). It has been estimated that 1 baby in every 2500 live births has FAS, which means 1600 new cases in the United States per year.[10] The combined rate of FAS and alcohol-related neurodevelopmental disorder is estimated to be at least 9.1 per 1000, nearly 1 in every 100 live births.[50] Clearly the number of consumers of this teratogen is several orders of magnitude larger than for any other teratogenic compound. With increasing public awareness of the adverse fetal outcome associated with alcohol, many women and families fear the potential adverse effects of alcohol consumed before conception was realized, even when much smaller amounts than that associated with FAS are involved. Although there is some preliminary evidence of a dose-response relationship of alcohol teratogenicity in humans,[11] even up to two drinks a day during embryogenesis has not been associated with increased morphological or developmental risks.[12] The problem of verifying the degree of drinking is major. Recently, for example, we documented that women who have had an adverse outcome of their pregnancy tend to decrease the amount of alcohol reported postnatally compared to their initial report during pregnancy.[7]

The commonly used anticonvulsants are established human teratogens. Congenital heart defects, cleft lip and/or palate, genitourinary defects, and cognitive impairments were associated with use of anticonvulsant medication.[20] Interaction of valproic acid and carbamazepine with folic acid may lead to NTDs (2.9% and 1% respectively).[22,51] Valproic acid was also found to be associated with cognitive and behavioral impairment in school-age children.[47,52–55] Phenytoin is undoubtedly another drug that, through its common use, creates a public health issue. It has been estimated by Hanson et al.[40] that between 5 and 10% of fetuses exposed in utero to the drug will exhibit the full picture of fetal hydantoin syndrome (FHS). Since 0.5% of pregnant women are epileptic, and about half of them are treated with phenytoin, the rate of FHS should be somewhere between 0.019% and 0.025% of births.[41] This means that with an annual birthrate of 4 million in the United States, between 500 and 100 newborns every year suffer from this serious syndrome. The risk for major malformations is increasing with the number of anticonvulsive medications used. Lindhout et al. reported a 5% risk of birth defects in children of women with epilepsy who took two drugs concomitantly, 10% in those who took three drugs, and more than 20% when four drugs were used.[56] However, proper seizure control is the primary goal in treating women with epilepsy. Patients should understand the risks associated with uncontrolled seizures as well as the potential for teratogenicity of the anticonvulsive medication.

Retinoic acid, evolving as a commonly used drug for acne in young adults, has the potential of becoming a similar public health issue, if not a worse one. However, no peer-reviewed data have been published on the number of pregnancies occurring while women are being treated with Accutane. Unlike phenytoin, which may be essential in pregnancy, the use of retinoic acid is absolutely contraindicated in pregnancy, and treatment of acne can be postponed without risk to the mother.

Benzodiazepines are commonly used for anxiety, insomnia, drug withdrawal, and epilepsy. Bergman et al. found that 2% of pregnant women in the United States receive benzodiazepines during pregnancy.[57] Antepartum exposure to benzodiazepines has been found to be associated with an increased risk for fetal cleft lip and/or cleft palate in some studies but not in others. These contradictory results have led to a meta-analysis that found a small but significantly increased risk for major malformation or oral cleft alone according to data from the case-controlled studies.[45] Until more research is reported, level 2 ultrasonography should be used to rule out visible forms of cleft lip.

Many women of child bearing age are occupationally exposed to organic solvents. The most common female-dominated occupations are the health care professions and the clothing and textile industries. In the occupational setting, exposure to a multitude of solvents usually occurs. Because exposure usually involves more than one agent and different circumstances, adequate human epidemiological studies are difficult to interpret. The counseling of women who have been exposed to organic solvents is problematic because it is difficult to estimate the airborne or blood levels, the predominant chemicals and/or their by-products, the odor threshold, and the circumstances of exposure. Smelling organic solvents is not indicative of a significant exposure, as the olfactory nerve can detect levels as low as several parts per million, which is not necessarily associated with toxicity. Many organic solvents are teratogenic and embryotoxic in laboratory animals. The various malformations described include hydrocephaly, anencephaly, skeletal defects, cardiovascular defects, cardiovascular abnormalities, blood changes, and neurodevelopmental deficits. In some of these studies, exposure levels were high enough to cause maternal toxicity, which biologically may be a source of fetal toxicity as well.

Because many human studies are subject to top recall and response bias, not always controlled for confounders, and not powerful, they are not confirmative enough. A meta-analysis concluded that maternal occupational exposure to organic solvents is associated with a tendency toward an increased risk for spontaneous abortions (n = 2899 patients; OR 1.25, CI 0.99–1.58) and major malformations (n = 7036 patients; OR 1.64, CI 1.16–2.30).[28] Another prospective controlled study found that occupational exposure to organic solvents during pregnancy is associated with an increased risk for major malformations (RR 13; CI 1.8–99.5) in women who experienced symptoms of toxicity during exposure. Symptomatic exposure appears to predict higher fetal risk for malformations. More of these exposed women had previous miscarriages while working with organic solvents than did the comparison women who were not exposed (46.2% vs. 19.2%).[58]

Corticosteroids are used widely as agents for a variety of conditions. They are known to cross the placenta (both animal and human) and to exert teratogenic effects, including cleft palate in animals. Prospective follow-up studies failed to show an association between first trimester exposure to corticosteroids and major birth defects. However, a meta-analysis of epidemiological studies pulled out clustering of cleft palate cases in the exposed group compared to controls. Those findings suggest a lower, but yet significant, teratogenic potential of corticosteroids.[29] Moreover, French et al. in a prospective study followed up 477 infants who were exposed to corticosteroids at 24 weeks' gestation or later (due to high risk or premature birth). This study showed that repeated corticosteroid courses were associated with reductions in birth weight and head circumference. At the age of 3 years though, growth and severe disability outcomes did not appear to be related to increasing number of corticosteroid courses.[30] Taking into consideration that there is evidence based increased risk for cleft palate and birth weight, corticosteroids should not be the drugs of first choice in pregnancy. Since the risk is not as great as that associated with other known human teratogens, those pregnant women who have an inadvertent exposure to corticosteroids should be reassured.

Misoprostol, a prostaglandin E1 analog, has been indicated for use in preventing gastrointestinal lesions induced by nonsteroidal anti-inflammatory drugs and in treating duodenal and gastric ulcers. However, misoprostol has been abused because of its known side effect of inducing abortion. In Brazil, where elective abortions are illegal and misoprostol is available over the counter, it has been estimated that 10% of all pregnant women use it as abortifacient. Although a prospective observational cohort study on this population did not find an association with an increased risk for major malformations, it did find that the rate of miscarriages and fetal death were significantly higher among fetuses exposed to misoprostol in utero.[36] In addition, an analytical case-control study suggested that gestational misoprostol use is associated with an increased risk for Möbius sequence.[37] Since the drug has been used on purpose to abort an unplanned or unwanted pregnancy, there is little to be done to protect the unborn.

Cocaine use has increased rapidly over the last two decades for recreational purposes. It is now estimated that more than 10 million Americans currently use cocaine. As a rapid increase in use has occurred in women of childbearing age, much concern has been expressed about the potential effects of the drug during pregnancy. Animal studies show that cocaine affects fetal growth and brain development. The human studies confirmed that that fetuses exposed to cocaine in utero have increased rate of stillbirth, smaller head circumference, lower birth weight, and increased rates of intracranial bleeding. Significant depression of interactive behavior and a less effective organizational response to environmental stimuli—suggestive of effects on neurologic integrity—were found in children of preschool age.[26] Although prenatal cocaine exposure was not found to be associated with lower full-scale, verbal or performance IQ scores, an association with an increase risk for specific cognitive impairments (visual-spatial skills, general knowledge, and arithmetic skills) and lower likelihood of IQ above the normative mean at 4 years was reported.[59] The exposures' effects on fetal development should be clearly outlined in counseling women of reproductive age on cocaine.

Environmental Contamination

The common denominator of methyl mercury, carbon monoxide, and polychlorinated biphenyls (PCBs) is that their human teratogenic effect has been shown only following maternal exposure to excessive amounts. Extrapolation from these exposures to the background amounts of carbon monoxide or PCBs in the environment is not justified. Yet, because the lower part of the dose-response curves has not been described, it is possible that moderate exposure may have clinical implications: heavy smokers, for example, have a carboxyhemoglobin level of 10% and even more; such levels have been shown to be associated with lower birth weights, and according to preliminary reports, with a less favorable developmental outcome.[58]

Environmental lead may differ from the compounds above; recent studies suggest adverse developmental effects even with levels within the subtoxic range (above 10 μg/dL but below 25 μg/dL).[33]

REFERENCES

1. Fabro S, Brown NA, Scialli AR. Valproic acid and birth defects. *Reprod Toxicol.* 1983;2:9–11.
2. Lammer EJ, Chen DT, Hoar RM, et al. Retinoic acid embryopathy. *N Engl J Med.* 1985;313:837–841.
3. Koren G. Retinoic acid embryopathy. *N Engl J Med.* 1986;315:262.
4. Schardein J. Chemically induced birth defects. Marcel Dekker, New York, 1985.
5. Rosa FW, Wilk AL, Kelsey FO. Vitamin A congeners. In Teratogen Update (Sever JL, Brent RL, eds), Liss, New York, 1986, pp 61–70.
6. Jacobson SJ, Jones K, Johnson K, et al. A prospective multicenter study of pregnancy outcome following lithium exposure during the first-trimester of pregnancy. *Lancet.* 1992;339:530–533.
7. Feldman Y, Koren G, Mattice D, Shear H, Pellegrini E, MacLeod SM. Determinants of recall and recall bias in studying drug effects in pregnancy. *Teratology.* 1989;40:37–46.
8. Mitchell AE, Cottler LB, Shapiro S. Effect of questionnaire design on recall of drug exposure in pregnancy. *Am J Epidemiol.* 1986; 123:670–676.
9. Shepard TH. Catalog of Teratogenic Agents. 10th ed. Baltimore: Johns Hopkins University Press; 2001.
10. Rosett HZ, Weiner L. Alcohol and the Fetus. Oxford University Press, New York, 1984.
11. Graham JM. Hanson JW, Darby BL, Barr HM, Streissguth AP. Independent dysmorphology evaluation at birth and 4 years of age for children exposed to varying amounts of alcohol in utero. *Pediatrics.* 1988;81:772–778.
12. Mills JL, Graubard BI. Is moderate drinking during pregnancy associated with an increased risk of malformations? *Pediatric.* 1987;80:309–314.
13. Sampson PD, Streissguth AP, Bookstein FL, et al. Incidence of fetal alcohol syndrome and prevalence of alcohol-related neurodevelopmental disorder. *Teratology.* 1997;56:317–326.

14. Albert E Chadley, Julianne Conry, Jocelynn L, et al. Fetal alcohol spectrum disorder: Canadian guidelines for diagnosis. *CMAJ.* 2005; 172(5 suppl).
15. Chan D, Bar-Oz B, Pellerin B, et al. Population baseline of meconium fatty acid ethyl esters among infants of non-drinking women in Jerusalem and Toronto. *He Drug Monit.* 2003;25(3):271–278.
16. Stratton K, Howe C, Battaglia FC. Fetal alcohol syndrome: diagnosis, epidemiology, prevention, and treatment. Washington: Institute of Medicine (IOM) and National Academy Press; 1996.
17. Bergman U, Rosa FW, Baum C, et al. Effects of exposure to benzodiazepine during fetal life. *Lancet.* 1992;340:694–696.
18. Dolovich LR, Addis A, Vaillancourt JMR, et al. Benzodiazepine use in pregnancy and major malformations or oral cleft: meta-analysis of cohort and case control studies. *BMJ.* 1998;34:288–292.
19. Rosa FW. Spina bifida in infants of women treated with carbamazepine during pregnancy. *N Engl J Med.* 1991;324:674–676.
20. Delago-Escueta AV, Janz D. Consensus guidelines: preconception counseling, management, and care of the pregnant woman with epilepsy. *Neurology.* 1992;42(4 suppl 5):149–160.
21. Briggs GG, Freeman RK, Yaffe SJ. Drugs in Pregnancy and Lactation. 7th ed 2005;217–225.
22. Rosa FW. Spina bifida in infants of mothers taking carbamazepine. *N Engl J Med.* 1991;325:664–665.
23. Epilepsy Registry, (UK- GSK, European Pregnancy Registry (EURAP). Medscape 2004.
24. Longo LD. The biological effects of carbon monoxide on the pregnant woman, fetus and newborn infant. *Am J Obstet Gynecol.* 1977; 129:69–103.
25. Koren G, Sharav T, et al. A multicenter prospective study of reproductive outcome following carbon monoxide poisoning in pregnancy. *Reprod Toxicol.* 1991;5:397–403.
26. Koren G, Nulman I, Rovet J, et al. Long-term neurodevelopmental risks in children exposed in utero to cocaine. *Ann NY Acad Sci.* 1998; 846:306–313.
27. Chasnoff IJ, Chisum GM, Kaplan WE. Maternal cocaine use and genitourinary tract malformations. *Teratology.* 1988;37:201–204.
28. Doberczak TM, Shanzer S, Kandall SR. Neonatal effects of cocaine abuse in pregnancy (abstract). *Pediatr Res.* 1987;21:359A.
29. Diav-Citrin O, Park L, Pastuszak A, et al. Pregnancy outcome following maternal exposure to corticosteroids: a prospective controlled cohort study and a meta-analysis of epidemiological studies. *Teratology.* 1998;57:188.
30. French NP, Hagan R, Evans SE, et al. Repeated antenatal corticosteroids: size at birth and subsequent development. *Am J Obstet Gynecol.* 1999;180(1):114–121.
31. Gur C, Diav-Citrin O, Shechtman, et al. Pregnancy outcome after first trimester exposure to corticosteroids: a prospective controlled study. *Reprod Toxicol.* 2004;18:93–101.
32. Herbst AL, Uffelder H, Posbanzer DC. Adenocarcinoma of the vagina: association of maternal stilbestrol therapy with tumor appearance in young girls. *N Engl J Med.* 1971;284:878–881.
33. Bellinger D, et al. Longitudinal analysis of prenatal and postnatal lead exposure and early cognitive development. *N Engl J Med.* 1987; 316:1037–1043.
34. Amin-Zakil, Majeed MA, Greenwood MR, et al. Methylmercury poisoning in the Iraqi suckling infant: a longitudinal study over 5 years. *J Appl Toxicol.* 1981;1:210–214.
35. Harada M. Congenital Minamata disease: intrauterine methyl mercury poisoning. *Teratology* 1978;18:285–288.
36. Schller L, Pastuszak AL, Sanseverino MT, et al. Pregnancy outcome after abortion attempt with misoprostol. *Teratology.* 1997;55:36.
37. Pastuszak AL, Schller L, Coelho KA, et al. Misoprostol use during pregnancy is associated with an increased risk for Moebius sequence. *Teratology.* 1997;55:36.
38. McMartin KI, Chu M, Kopecky E, et al. Pregnancy outcome following maternal organic solvent exposure: meta-analysis of epidemiologic studies. *Am J Industr Med.* 1998;34:288–292.
39. Khattak S, Moghtader G, McMartin K, et al. Pregnancy outcome following gestational exposure to organic solvents: a prospective controlled study. *JAMA.* 1999;281:1106–1109.
40. Rogan WJ, Gladen BC, Kun-Long H, et al. Congenital poisoning by polychlorinated biphenyls and their contaminants Taiwan. *Science.* 1988;241:334–336.
41. Rosa FW. Teratogen update: penicillamine. *Teratology.* 1986;22: 127–131.
42. Rovet J, Cole S, Nulman I, et al. Effects of maternal epilepsy on children's neurodevelopment. *Child Neuropsychol.* 1995;1(2):150–157.
43. Shapiro S, Hartz SC, Siskind V, Mitchell AA, Slone D, Rosenberg L, et al. Anticonvulsants and parental epilepsy in the development of birth defects. *Lancet.* 1976;1(7954):272–275.
44. Wide K, Henning E, Tomson T, et al. Psychomotor development in preschool children exposed to antiepileptic drugs in utero. *Acta Paediatr.* 2002;91(4):409–414.
45. Newman CGH. Clinical aspects of thalidomide embryopathy—a continuing preoccupation. *Teratology.* 1985;32:133–144.
46. Cohlan SQ. Tetracycline staining of the teeth. *Teratology.* 1977; 15:127–130.
47. Koch S, Jager-Roman E, Losche G, et al. Antiepileptic drug treatment in pregnancy: drug side effects in the neonate and neurological outcome. *Acta Paediatr.* 1996;85(6):739–746.
48. Mawer G, Clayton-Smith J, Coyle H, et al. Outcome of pregnancy in women attending an outpatient epilepsy clinic: adverse features associated with higher doses of sodium valproate. *Seizure.* 2002 Dec;11(8):512–518.
49. Iturbe-Alessio J, Fonesca MDC, Mutchiniko Santos MA, et al. Risks of anticoagulant therapy in pregnant women with artificial heart valve. *N Engl J Med.* 1986;315:1390–1393.
50. Hansen JW. Fetal hydantoin syndrome. *Teratology.* 1976;13:185–188.
51. Wyszynski D, Nambisan M, Surve T, et al. For the Antiepileptic Drug Pregnancy Registry. Increased risk of major malformations in offspring exposed to valproate during pregnancy. *Neurology.* 2005;961–965.
52. Adab N, Kini U, Vinten J, et al. The longer term outcome of children born to mothers with epilepsy. *J Neurol Neurosurg Psychiatry.* 2004; 75:1575–1583.
53. Shorvon SD. Longer term outcome of children born to mothers with epilepsy. *J Neurol Neurosurg Psychiatry.* 2004;75:1517–1518.
54. Dean JCS, Hailey H, Moore SJ, et al. Long term health and neurodevelopment in children exposed to antiepileptic drugs before birth. *J Med Genet* 2002;39:251–259.
55. Mawer G, Clayton-Smith J, Coyle H, et al. Outcome of pregnancy in women attending an outpatient epilepsy clinic: adverse features associated with higher doses of sodium valproate. *Seizure.* 2002;11:512–518.
56. Lindhout D, Hoppener RJ, Meinardi H. Teratogenicity of antiepileptic drug combinations with special emphasis on epoxidation (of carbamazepine). *Epilepsia.* 1984;25(1):77–83.
57. Goldman AS, Zachai EH, Yaffe SJ. Fetal trimethadione syndrome. *Teratology.* 1978;17:103–106.
58. Sexton MJ, Fox NL, Hebel JR. the effects of neonatal exposure to tobacco on behavioral outcomes in three-year-old children. *Teratology.* 1988;37:491.
59. Singer LT, Minnes S, Short E, et al. Cognitive outcomes of preschool children with prenatal cocaine exposure. *JAMA.* 2004;291: 2448–2456.

CHAPTER 5

EPILEPSY AND PREGNANCY

Irena Nulman and Gideon Koren

INTRODUCTION

Pregnant women with epilepsy represent 0.5% of all pregnancies. Proper seizure control is the primary goal in treating these women. The commonly used antiepileptic drugs (AEDs) are established human teratogens. Factors such as epilepsy, AED-induced teratogenicity, the patient's genetic predisposition, and the severity of her convulsive disorder may contribute to the adverse outcome of an epileptic woman's pregnancy. The interaction of an AED with folic acid and vitamin K metabolism may lead to an increased risk for neural tube defect (NTD) and early neonatal bleeding. Psychological, hormonal, and pharmacokinetic changes in pregnancy may escalate seizure activity. Preconceptional counseling should include patient education as to the risks of uncontrolled seizures and the possible teratogenicity of AEDs. Genetic counseling should be performed if both parents have epilepsy or the disease is inherited. Seizure control should be achieved at least 6 months prior to conception and, if clinically possible, by the lowest effective dose of a single AED according to the type of epilepsy. The new AEDs require further research to prove their safety to humans. In addition, 4.0–5.0 mg/day of folic acid should be administered 3 months preconceptionally and during the first trimester to prevent malformations induced by inadequate levels of folic acid. The benefits of pharmacotherapy should not be underestimated, the risk of abrupt drug discontinuation should be stressed, and the AED compliance should be monitored. The AED-treatment should be changed during pregnancy only if clinically indicated for seizure control. Antenatal management should include an assessment of the patient for AED-associated birth defects through detailed ultrasound examination and levels of maternal serum a-fetoproteins. Therapeutic drug monitoring should be performed monthly or as clinically indicated. If enzyme inducing AEDs are administered, maternal vitamin K supplementation should begin 4 weeks before the expected date of delivery. In order to prevent convulsions during 1abor, proper seizure control should be achieved during the third trimester. A benzodiazepine or phenytoin is found to be effective for seizure cessation during labor and delivery. Vitamin K should be administered to the newborn immediately after birth. The neonate should be examined carefully for AED-associated dysmorphology. Advising the mother on postpartum management regarding AED-dose adjustment, contraception, and breast-feeding will help maximize the best possible postnatal outcome for the newborn and the mother. With proper preconceptional, antenatal, and postpartum management, up to 95% of these pregnancies have been reported to show favorable results. Epilepsy, although not common among pregnant women, is the most common neurological disorder during gestation. Increased public awareness of the progress in diagnosis and management of epilepsy have enabled many epileptic women to bear children and manage careers.[1,2] Pregnant women with epilepsy constitute 0.5% of all pregnancies, and medical professionals should be aware that—with appropriate selection of treatment and prudent preconceptional, antenatal, and postpartum management—up to 95% of these pregnancies have been reported to have favorable results.[3] The evaluation of the risk and safety of pregnancy in such women is complicated by a variety of factors. Women with epilepsy are at risk for menstrual abnormalities, reproductive endocrine disorders, and reduced fertility.[4] Polycystic ovaries as well as hypo- or hypergonadotrophic hypogonadism are more common in women with epilepsy than in general population. The investigators relate those abnormalities to the effect of seizures on the hypothalamic–pituitary-gonadal axis[5] and to the possible side effect of AEDs.[6,7] Even when not exposed in utero to medications, infants of mothers with epilepsy have higher rates of major and minor malformations[8,9] when compared to the general population. On the other hand, a resent meta-analysis of 10 studies and 400 women with untreated epilepsy showed that risk for major malformations in children with untreated maternal epilepsy was not significantly higher than among control children. This report also showed a probable publication bias associated with 5 previous reports including 101 children from untreated epileptic mothers.[10] These results should be interpreted with caution because the severity of maternal epilepsy and the type and frequency of seizures during pregnancy are incomparable with those in women taking AEDs. To add to the complexity, commonly used AEDs are established human teratogens. Table 5-1 presents congenital malformations in humans caused by AEDs for which there is consensus among scientists. Research indicates that the incidence of malformations is influenced by the number of anticonvulsant medications, the dose of the drug, timing of use during gestation, pharmacogenetics, and differences in metabolism.[8,11] Some investigators hypothesize that anticonvulsant-induced teratogenicity occurs in genetically predisposed individuals.[12] Other researchers have reported that epilepsy per se, the type, and severity of the seizure disorder also contributes to the dysmorphology.[13] The mechanism of neurocognitive impairment of children of mothers with epilepsy exposed to AEDs is not clear yet, but seizure severity, type of epilepsy, toxicity of AEDs and genetic predisposition has been proposed. Considering the complex interaction between genetic and environmental factors, it is difficult to attribute congenital abnormalities in children of epileptic mothers to any single factor[14] especially in view of the lack of large enough studies with sufficient power to control for such determinants.

PREGNANCY-INDUCED PHARMACOKINETIC CHANGES OF ANTIEPILEPTIC DRUGS

The plasma concentration of anticonvulsant drugs tend to fall during pregnancy as a result of a 50% expansion in plasma volume, decrease in protein binding[15], increased clearance rate, and a tendency to decrease in patient compliance due to fears of teratogenicity.

As most anticonvulsant drugs are acidic or neutral, they are highly bound to serum albumin. During late pregnancy, albumin levels fall, with a corresponding decrease in the fraction of bound drug, which leads to total (unbound and protein bound) plasma concentration to fall. The decrease in plasma protein binding makes

TABLE 5-1
Congenital Malformations in Humans Caused by Antiepileptic Drugs

MALFORMATIONS	PHENYTOIN	VALPROIC ACID	CARBAMAZEPINE	PHENOBARBITAL
Congenital heart defects	+	+	+	+
Cleft lip and/or palate	+	+	−	+
NTD[1]	−	+	+	−
Genitourinary defects	+	+	+	+
Cognitive impairment	+	+	±	±
Dysmorphic syndrome	+	+	+	+

[1] NDT, neural tube defect, ±, inconclusive evidence.

more free drug available for biotransformation and clearance. Although the AED free levels fall much less than the total levels, they often do decline significantly during pregnancy.[16,17]

Monitoring the total plasma concentrations of these drugs can, therefore, be misleading. In complex clinical cases therapeutic drug monitoring that can measure both protein-bound and unbound drug concentrations can be helpful. The measurement of free drug concentrations of highly bound drugs should be considered in cases where seizure control is not achieved. It should be remembered that the constant, or even higher free drug concentration, may provide appropriate antiepileptic control, as it is the free drug that reaches the brain. The increase in GFR[18] and renal plasma flow[19] may theoretically enhance the clearance rate of renally excreted drugs, such as gabapentin and vigabatrin. However, presently there are no studies available regarding the pharmacokinetics of these agents during human pregnancy.

Carbamazepine

Carbamazepine has a relatively slow absorption, with 70 to 80% protein binding to albumin. Hepatic metabolism is the main route of elimination, and there may be a decrease in serum concentrations during the first months of therapy as a consequence of auto-induction of metabolism. Dosage intervals and sample time are critical in interpreting serum concentrations and large peak-trough fluctuations can be minimized by using a control-led-release formulation.[20] As drug levels tend to be lower in pregnancy, and bioavailability may be lower than with conventional carbamazepine, higher dosages may be required when a control-led-release medication is used.[21] The concentration of the active metabolite (carbamazepine-10, 11-epoxide) was reported to increase during pregnancy, possibly as a result of the increased carbamazepine metabolism and impaired conversion of carbamazepine-10, 11-epoxide to carbamazepine-10, 11 *trans*-diol. This increase is of potential importance as the metabolite (10, 11-epoxide) is believed to have comparable pharmacological activity to the parent drug.[22]

Oxcarbazepine

Oxcarbazepine does not produce the active 10, 11-epoxide metabolites which may play a role in pharmacokinetics and drug interaction, and teratogenicity.

Phenytoin

Phenytoin follows nonlinear pharmacokinetics and has a narrow therapeutic window.[23] It is highly bound to protein (90 to 93%)[24,25] and cleared mainly by saturable hepatic metabolism. A substantial increase in 8-hydroxylation during pregnancy may be responsible, at least partially, for its increased clearance rate and consequently decreased serum concentrations.[26] Generally, a fall in total serum phenytoin concentrations may cause lack of seizure control and may require increases in dose. However, as indicated above, the total concentration by itself may not indicate a fall in free drug concentrations. The decrease in the protein binding of phenytoin may be an important mechanism for decreasing total drug concentrations in pregnancy as it is the free drug that is available for the enhanced metabolism.

Valproic Acid

Valproic acid is rapidly absorbed and highly protein bound to plasma albumin (88 to 92%).[27] The interpretation of its pharmacokinetics is limited by large fluctuations in the concentration-time profile, wide therapeutic index and concentration-dependent protein binding.[28,29] Analysis of unbound valproic acid is not routine and similarly there is no established therapeutic range. Dose adjustments during pregnancy are best made by clinical observation in combination with therapeutic drug monitoring. Divided doses are preferred to avoid high peaks of valproic acid serum concentrations.[16]

Phenobarbital

Phenobarbital has been less frequently prescribed during the last years because of its tendency to produce sedation and impaired cognitive function. It has a high oral bioavailability (90%) and is only 50% protein-bound. Similar to phenytoin and carbamazepine, it induces hepatic microsomal oxidative enzymes and may interact with therapeutic efficacy of other drugs.

Neonates exposed prenatally to phenobarbital should be monitored for withdrawal symptoms for 2–6 weeks starting at day 7 of life due to its long elimination half life (100 hours).

TERATOGENICITY, MECHANISMS AND CLINICAL IMPLICATIONS

Fetal risk for major malformations (MM) with older-generation of AEDs is higher than in general population (1.25–11.5% vs 1–2.5%) as was shown in most studies and registries.[3,30–42] The most common MMs are similar to those reported in general population such as heart defects, hypospadias, club foot, and orofacial clefts.[14] The highest rates are in treated versus nontreated epilepsy and in polytherapy.[32–35,41–43] The rates of MM in polytherapy was reported to be from 8 to 25%.[44]

No specific pattern of malformations are associated with AEDs, with the exception of neural tube defect (NTD) which is more common in offspring exposed to valproic acid (1–5%) and carbamazepine (0.5–1%).[45–50] Because the vast majority of NTDs can be ruled out by maternal or amniotic fluid α-fetoproteins combined with ultrasound, these examinations should be routinely performed in women taking carbamazepine or valproic acid.

Pregnancy registries, although employed different methodologies, explore the risk associated with individual AEDs.[32–35,41–43] Although previous studies reported lower rates, analysis of 77 cases exposed to phenobarbital revealed a malformation rate of 6.5% compared to 2.9% in pregnancies exposed to other AEDs (North American Registry).[36] Reduction in 7[51] and 11[52] points in Global IQ and language impairments, even after controlling for socioeconomic status (SES), matching, and the drug-dose, have been shown in school-age children and adult men exposed in utero to Phenobarbital.

Exposure to phenytoin was associated with malformation rates ranged between 2.4 to 9.1%[37,38]; however, Holmes et al. in a prospective cohort study found lower then 2.4% MM rates,[39] and in the UK Registry the rates to be 3.7% in monotherapy.[32] A prospective, controlled Motherisk study showed a 10, 6 points decrease in Global IQ in 34 exposed in utero to phenytoin preschool children matched for age and gender, and controlled for maternal intelligence and SES.[53] This study supported previous finding of Hanson et al. on Fetal Hydantoin Syndrome.[54] A study of 21 phenytoin-exposed children did not find differences between matched healthy controls.[52]

Malformation rates of 8% following in utero carbamazepine exposure have been reported in a recent meta-analysis.[40] The Australian Registry of Antiepileptic Drugs in Pregnancy reported rates of 4.5%,[43] and rates of 2.2% have been found in UK Registry.[32] Wide and colleagues (Swedish Registry) found the risks to be significantly lower.[41] In regards of cognitive development of children exposed prenataly to carbamazepine, although the previous studies have found differences between the exposed and not exposed children,[55,56] recent prospective studies[53,57] better powered[57,58] and better methodologically performed[53,57] have not found differences among carbamazepine exposed children, those who were not exposed to medications, and healthy controls.

Valproic acid teratogenicity has been assessed in a number of studies and data concerning dose-dependent brain toxicity have remarkable consistency. The highest MM rates have been consistently associated with valproic acid. In most recent studies in monotherapy the ORs ranged from 2.59 to 4.24[48,33,41,42] and 6.2%.[32] In polytherapy the rates were found to be 13% in Australian Registry of Antiepileptic Drugs in Pregnancy[43] and with Lamotregine the rates were found to be 12.5%.[33] Several studies have shown a dose response effect with exposure to valproic acid. With doses above 800–1000 mg/day the increase in malformation rates was repeatedly most evident.[30,32,42,43] This dose-effect relationship was supported by higher maternal serum concentrations of valproic acid in children born with a defect than in those without malformation.[33] Valproic acid behavioral teratogenicity has been assessed in a number of studies and data concerning dose-dependent brain toxicity have remarkable consistency. Koch et al.[59] showed that valproic acid-exposed children had higher rates of neurological dysfunction. Serum concentrations of valproic acid at birth correlated with the degree of neonatal hyper excitability and the degree of dysfunction when the children were reexamined at the age of 6. The following studies, although underpowered, showed developmental delay, learning difficulties, additional educational needs and low Verbal IQ in exposed children.[60–63,49]

New Antiepileptic Drugs

The new AEDs, which are low- (topiramate, felbamate, oxcarbazepine) or nonprotein bounded (gabapentin, vigabatrin), are eliminated from the body through renal clearance (vigabatrin, gabapentin), have no effect on the cytochrome P-450 enzyme system (gabapentine, lamotrigine, vigabatrin), no antifolate effects, no arene oxide metabolites, and if given in monotherapy may be considered for use for women with epilepsy, but there is little information regarding their pharmacokinetics and safety during pregnancy.

Animal studies have been extremely beneficial in understanding of mechanisms of adverse effects and teratogenicity of new AEDs. They are very informative in testing hypotheses, assessing nutrition and environmental factors which may interfere with or modify normal embryonic or fetal development. Although animal studies help to clarify pharmacokinetic changes in pregnancy and to define the risk factors associated with birth defects,[64] they may be imperfect predictors of human teratogenicity. Animals may be more sensitive because of higher than in humans dose ranges (tiagabine)[65] or species—specific effect (topiramate, zonosamide)—but today reports regarding animal reproductive toxicology of new AEDs appear to be promising (gabapentine, levetiracetam).[66] Although results of animal studies regarding teratogenic effects of the new AEDs are encouraging, it is too early to conclude whether such data will apply to humans.

The International Lamotrigine Pregnancy Registry contains a description of all prenatal exposure to lamotrigine voluntarily and prospectively reported to the registry. MM rates of 2.95% in monotherapy have been found in 414 pregnancies outcomes.[33] Slightly higher rates of 3.2% have been reported by the UK Registry in 647 women. Significantly higher rates of 12.55 were reported in polytherapy with valproic[32] and 5.4% with a total daily dose of more the 200 mg.[32]

Novarties safety database and other pregnancy registries reported outcome of 248 oxcarbazepine pregnancies with MM rates of 2.4% in monotherapy and 6.6% in 61 women exposed to polytherapy.[67] No MM were found in a retrospective cohort of 101 women on monotherapy in Finland.

The UK Registry reported 7.1% MM in 28 offspring exposed to topiramate monotherapy and Yerby found 5 cases of hypospadias in 89 pregnancies.[68]

The UK Registry reported 1 malformation in 31 pregnancies with gabapentin.[32] No malformations were found in 19 pregnancies in Gabapentin Registry,[69] and in 11 cases reported by Wilton et al.[70]

Numbers reported for the rest of newer AEDs were very small. No MM were found in 22 levetiracetam-exposed pregnancies.[32]

The behavioral teratogenicity of AEDs, the long-term neurocognitive development of exposed children, is insufficiently addressed in research and is one of the most difficult areas to study and about which to counsel women.

Mechanisms of Teratogenicity

Several mechanisms have been proposed for AED-induced teratology. Some anticonvulsant medications (e.g., phenytoin) form intermediate oxide metabolites that are known to be embryotoxic. Free active oxide radicals have been shown to bind to proteins and nucleic and may interfere with DNA and RNA synthesis. Critical amounts of free radicals may increase the risk of perinatal death, intrauterine growth retardation, and malformations.[71]

Scavenging enzymes capable of conjugating these free radicals to inactive substances may prevent fetal damage, and variabilities in such enzymes may explain variable fetal outcome. Unstable intermediates can also be metabolized to nonreactive hydrodiones by epoxide hydrolase. It has been proposed that fetuses with low levels of free radical scavenging enzymes and low activity of epoxide hydrolase are at increased risk to develop malformations associated with phenytoin. Polytherapy may lead to excessive amounts of unstable epoxides, such as arene oxides, and inhibit epoxide metabolism, especially in fetuses with a genetic defect in fetal epoxide hydrolase activity.[72]

Evidence for increased risk for major malformations with an increased number of AEDs comes from several epidemiological studies. Lindhout et al.[73] reported a 5% risk for birth defects in children of epileptic women who took two drugs concomitantly, 10% in those who took three drugs, and more than 20% when four drugs were used. The authors reported a malformation risk of only 3% (versus 2–2.5% as in untreated epileptic women or in general population) when the seizures were controlled with only one AED.

The occurrence of specific malformations depends on the timing of exposure during embryogenesis.[11,74] Neural tube defects (NTDs) occur before closure of the neural tube, between days 21 and 28 after the first day of the last menstrual period (LMP). Cleft lip occurs with exposure before day 35 and cleft palate before day 70, whereas congenital heart defects occur with exposure before day 42 post-LMP.[16] Exposure after the first trimester should not affect rates of dysmorphology except for the toxic effects on the brain, which develops throughout pregnancy.[75]

Minor anomalies that were described as a part of the fetal hydantoin syndrome[54] were later hypothesized to be associated with maternal epilepsy and not necessarily with the AEDs.[9,76,77] Different patterns of minor anomalies have been found to be caused by phenytoin. carbamazepine, and untreated epilepsy.[9]

Another mechanism that has been implicated in AED-mediated teratogenicity is folate deficiency.[11] Up to a 90% reduction in serum folate levels was reported in patients treated with phenytoin, carbamazepine, and barbiturates. Conversely, valproic acid did not reduce levels of folate directly but interfered with its metabolism.[78,79] Folate supplementation was found to be effective in preventing several malformations, in particular NTDs. The Medical Research Council study[80] reported a 70% reduction of NTD recurrence among pregnant women who were supplemented with 4 mg of folic acid before conception and during gestation. The current recommendations call for 5 mg of folic acid per day in women being treated with valproic acid or carbamazepine.[2,81] Although there are no data at present to document the efficacy of this regimen in women with epilepsy, the potential benefit of such approach outweighs the theoretical risk of high levels of folate.[82] Vitamin B 12 levels should be assessed before folic acid supplementation is begun so as to avoid neurological symptoms of vitamin B 12 deficiency.[83]

The genetic influence of the maternal epileptic syndrome and seizure effects on fetal development in regards of congenital malformation are not well defined. A control group with a large enough sample size of unmedicated women with epilepsy was not assessed by any research group. If collected, healthy women and women with epilepsy should be comparable, and women with epilepsy might represent less severe forms of epilepsy with low frequency of seizures.

The effect of seizure activity during pregnancy on fetal wellbeing has been investigated by several groups.[84] Isolated, short seizures are generally not believed to have an adverse effect on the fetus. Spontaneous abortions, injury to the mother and fetus, fetal hypoxia, bradycardia, and antenatal death were reported[3,85,86] with repeated tonic-clonic seizures, complex partial seizures, and status epilepticus. There is ample evidence that physiological changes during pregnancy may affect the duration and frequency of seizures. Seizure rates have been reported to increase in 17–37% of women with epilepsy.[2,85] When seizures recur in a well-controlled woman during pregnancy, they most often appear during the first and second trimesters.[82] Holmes et al. reported increase in MM rates in women with uncontrolles epilepsy.[39]

Poor patient compliance, sleep disturbances, nausea, vomiting, and decreased levels of free (unbound) drugs are the main risk factors believed to decrease seizure control.[16,87] Increases in estrogen levels during pregnancy may reduce seizure threshold levels.[88] Progesterone reduces intestinal motility, thus interfering with the secretion of mucus as well as gastric pH, and it may affect drug absorption.[87] Changes in seizure frequency during pregnancy may also stem from fluid and sodium retention, hyperventilation, and emotional and psychological problems.[89] A potential problem in the management of seizures may also arise from altered pharmacokinetics of AEDs associated with pregnancy.

Effect of AEDs on Vitamin K

The association between maternal anticonvulsant therapy and neonatal hemorrhage was reported 40 years ago[90] and supported by a number of subsequent studies and reports.[91] These hemorrhages, which typically occur during the first 24 hours after birth (in contrast to the classic neonatal bleeding which occurs on day 2 or 3 after delivery,[92] may be severe, involving the skin as well as the brain, pleural, and peritoneal cavities.

The mechanism and origin of these hemorrhages is not fully understood, but vitamin K deficiency was observed in neonates exposed in utero to enzyme-inducing AEDs such as carbamazepine, phenytoin, phenobarbital, and primidone. These medications readily cross the placenta and induce liver enzymatic pathways, resulting in increased degradation of vitamin K, and they produce proteins that are induced by vitamin K absence (PIVKA). These proteins are present when vitamin K is absent in neonates exposed in utero to AEDs. The decarboxylated form of prothrombin, PIVKA II, is the most sensitive marker for vitamin K deficiency[93] and was proven informative in studies of neonatal vitamin K levels. Although vitamin K does not easily cross the placenta from the maternal to the fetal circulation, prenatal supplementation of vitamin K results in valuable effects in preventing neonatal bleeding.[94]

The consensus guidelines[11] regarding women receiving enzyme-inducing AEDs called for antenatal maternal vitamin K supplementation at 20 mg orally throughout the last 4 weeks of gestation and 1 mg of vitamin K parenterally to the neonate immediately after delivery. If PIVKA are found in cord blood specimens, fresh frozen plasma should be given at a dose of 20 mL/kg over a period of 1–2 hours.[11] Some experts debate the value of maternal antenatal supplementation during the last month of pregnancy. Kaaja et al.[95] found no increase in rates of bleeding in 662 neonatal of mothers taking enzyme inducing AEDs when compared with 1324 controls. Based on this study the NICE recommendations[96] were against the need for prenatal vitamin K supplementation, although the Kaaj's numbers may be insufficient to show effect.[97]

Preconceptional Counseling

Women should be counseled about the potential risk of increased seizure activity during pregnancy so as to make sure that they do not avoid taking their medication. Poor compliance, resulting in increased seizure activity, has tangible risks. Preconceptional counseling should optimally begin at least 3 month before conception to allow for adequate supplementation of folic acid. Adequate patient education regarding the increased incidence of major malformations[98] and possible adverse effects of AEDs to the fetal central nervous system[53,99] should be achieved. Genetic counseling should be offered if both partners have epilepsy or the epileptic disorder is inherited. Gradual drug discontinuation (over at least 3 months) should be considered if the patient has been seizure-free for 2 or more years. An epileptic woman who is planning a pregnancy should be encouraged to quit smoking, maintain good nutrition, and get enough sleep.[16]

If treatment with anticonvulsant medications cannot be avoided, proper seizure control should be achieved by the lowest effective dose of the single AED that best controls seizures in the given patient or, alternatively, pregnancy should be delayed until seizure control is reached. It should be remembered that poly therapy and/or higher daily doses of AEDs are associated with higher rates of congenital malformation.

Valproid acid should be avoided to be given to women planning a pregnancy. If valproic acid is indicated, divided doses are preferred to avoid high levels of valproic acid in plasma[16,30] and levels below 1000 mg/day are preferable. The combination of valproic acid, carbamazepine, and phenobarbital has been reported to be more teratogenic than other combinations, as well valproic acid and lamotrigine.[82,33]

Lamotrigine should be kept on daily doses below 200 mg, if clinically possible.

The risk for MM associated with carbamazepine appears to be similar to lamotrigine.

Folate supplementation at 5 mg/day should start 3 months before conception and continue until the end of the first trimester. If possible, serum folate levels should be monitored to confirm sufficient supplementation.

ANTENATAL MANAGEMENT

More than 50% of all pregnancies are unplanned[100]; if the pregnancy is diagnosed while the woman is seizure-free, there is no proven benefit to changing the patient's drug because any morphological teratogenic effects will be irreversible by 10 weeks of gestation.[16] The patient should be advised regarding appropriate prenatal diagnosis for AED-associated abnormalities. For example, targeted fetal ultrasound examination at 18 weeks can diagnose up to 95% of fetuses with open NTD[101,102] as well as other anomalies.[103]

Early transvaginal ultrasonography at 11–13 weeks to assess for NTD is presently possible.[82] Detailed sonographic imaging of the fetal heart at 18–20 weeks, followed by fetal echocardiography, which can identify up to 85% of cardiac defects. Imaging of the fetal face for cleft lip at 18–20 weeks may be performed, but the sensitivity of this assessment has yet to be established.[82]

Amniocentesis with amniotic fluid a-fetoprotein and acetylcholinesterase may support blood serum findings caused by structural malformations.

Epoxide hydrolase activity in amniocytes has been suggested to predict those fetuses at risk for phenytoin-mediated anomalies; however, this test has not yet been confirmed for routine clinical use. Vitamin K supplementation of the mother is recommended, as detailed above.

Optimally, therapeutic drug monitoring should be performed every 1–2 months or more frequently if seizure control is not achieved.

LABOR, DELIVERY, AND BIRTH

Tonic-clonic seizures occur during labor or after delivery in 1–2% of women with epilepsy.[16] Monitoring plasma AED levels during the third trimester and regular administration of medication(s) are essential to prevent seizures due to inappropriately low serum concentrations.[3]

Convulsive seizures at the time of labor and delivery are commonly treated with intravenous administration of benzodiazepines or phenytoin. Intravenous administration of phenytoin should be given under cardiac monitoring to detect possible dysrhythmias.[101]

Emergency cesarean section is often performed in the case of status epilepticus or when there are repeated tonic-clonic, psychomotor, or absence seizures.[86] Obstetric intervention in the form of induction of labor, mechanical rupture of membranes, forceps delivery, or cesarean section is more common among women with epilepsy, as are such obstetric complications as vaginal bleeding, anemia, and preeclampsia.[3]

MANAGEMENT DURING THE PUERPERIUM

Vitamin K should be administered to the newborn immediately after birth. The neonate should be examined carefully for AEDs and epilepsy-associated dysmorphology. If the neonate was exposed to phenobarbital or primidone, observation for withdrawal symptoms should be performed during the first 7 months of life.

Maternal anticonvulsant drug levels should be carefully maintained with appropriate changes in dosage, bearing in mind that the lower volium of distribution and the decreased clearance rate postnatally may be associated with toxicity.

The patient should be counseled regarding postpartum contraception. There are no contraindications to use no hormonal methods of contraception. All contraception agents are suitable for women treated with nonenzyme-inducing anticonvulsant (valproic acid, gabapentine, vigabatrine, tiagabine, leviteracetam). The use of oral contraceptives with higher hormonal doses are recommended for women on enzyme-inducing AEDs. The progesterone only pill is unlikely to be effective, the medroxyprogesteron may be beneficial.

The issues of breast-feeding should also be discussed with the mother, as most women with epilepsy can breast-feed. Phenytoin and valproic acid are highly protein-bound; therefore, only low levels of these drugs are present in breast milk. Carbamazepine and phenobarbital are present in higher concentrations. Because of the sedative effect of phenobarbital, breast-feeding by women taking this drug is not recommended. When the mother is taking phenobarbital and breast-feeding, the infant must be monitored for the risk of lethargy and poor suck.

CONCLUSIONS

Proper seizure control is the primary goal in treating women with epilepsy. Patients should understand the risks associated with uncontrolled seizures as well as the teratogenicity of the anticonvulsive medication in question. If AEDs cannot be avoided, a first-line drug for the seizure type should be used at the lowest effective dose and in monotherapy if clinically possible. Judicious preconceptional, antenatal, and postpartum management leads to favorable maternal and neonatal outcome in the vast majority of patients.

REFERENCES

1. Dansky LV, Andennann E, Andennann F. Marriage and fertility in epileptic patients. *Epilepsia.* 1980;21(3):261–271.
2. Byme B. Epilepsy and pregnancy. *Ir Med J.* 1997;90:173–174.
3. Yerby MS. Pregnancy and epilepsy. *Epilepsia.* 1991;32(suppl 6): S51–S59.
4. Medeiros YS, Calixto JB. Inhibitory effect of diphenylhydantoin on myometrium from pregnant women in vitro: A comparative study with nicardipine and trifluoperazine. *Pharmacol Res.* 1990;22(5): 597–603.
5. Nappi C, Meo R, Di Carlo C, et al. Reduced fertility and neuroendocrine dysfunction in women with epilepsy. *Gynecol Endocrinol.* 1994;8:133–145.
6. Isojarvi N, Laatikainen TJ, Pakarinen AJ, et al. Menstrual disorders in women with epilepsy receiving carbamazepine. *Epilepsia.* 1995; 36:676–681.
7. Isojarvi N, Laatikainen TJ, Pakarinen AJ, et al. Polycystic ovaries and hyperandrogenism in women taking valproate for epilepsy. *N Engl J Med.* 1993;329:1383–1388.
8. Kaneko S. Antiepileptic drug therapy and reproductive consequences: functional and morphological effects. *Reprod Toxicol.* 1991;5(3):179–198.
9. Nulman I, Scolnik D. Chitayat D, et al. Findings in children exposed in utero to phenytoin and carbamazepine monotherapy: independent effects of epilepsy and medications. *Am J Med Genet.* 1997;68(1): 18–24.
10. Fried S, Kozer E, Nulman I, et al. Malformation rates in children of women with untreated epilepsy: a meta-analysis. *Drug Saf.* 2004; 27:197–202.
11. Kaneko S, Otani K, Fukushima Y, et al. Teratogenicity of antiepileptic drugs: analysis of possible risk factors. *Epilepsia.* 1988;29: 459–467.
12. Janz D. On major malformations and minor anomalies in the offspring of parents with epilepsy: review of the literature. In: Janz D, Dam M, Richeus A, et al., eds. Epilepsy, Pregnancy, the Child. New York: Raven Press, 1982:211–222.
13. Majewski F, Steger M, Richter B, et al. The teratogenicity of hydantoins and barbiturates in humans, with considerations on the etiology of malformations and cerebral disturbances in the children of epileptic parents. *Int J Bio Res Pregnancy.* 1981;2(1):37–45.
14. Dansky LV, Finnell RH. Parental epilepsy, anticonvulsant drugs, and reproductive outcome: epidemiologic and experimental findings spanning three decades. 2: Human studies. *Reprod Toxicol.* 1991; 5(4):301–335.
15. Fried S, Kozer E, Nulman I, et al. Plasma volume in normal first pregnancy. *J Obstet Gynaecol Br Comrnonw.* 1973;80(10):884–887.
16. Delgado-Escueta AV, Janz D. Consensus guidelines: preconception counseling, management, and care of the pregnant woman with epilepsy. *Neurology.* 1992;42(4 suppl 5):149–160.
17. Yerby MS, Freil PN, McConnick K. Antiepileptic drug disposition during pregnancy. *Neurology.* 1992;42(suppl 5):12–16.
18. Davison JM, Hytten FE. Glomerular filtration during and after pregnancy. *J Obstet Gynaecol Br Commonw.* 1974;81(8):588–595.
19. Dunihoo DR. Maternal Physiology. In: Dunihoo DR, ed. Fundamentals of Gynecology and Obstetrics. Philadelphia: Lippincott, 1992, pp 280–284.
20. Yerby MS, Friel PN, Miller DQ. Carbamazepine protein binding and disposition in pregnancy. *Ther Drug Monit.* 1985;7(3):269–273.
21. Tomson T, Almkvist 0, Nilsson BY, et al. Carbamazepine-lO, ll-epoxide in epilepsy: a pilo study. *Arch Neurol.* 1990;47(8):888–992.
22. Bourgeois BFD, Wad N. Individual and combined antiepileptic and neurotoxic activity of carbamazepine and carbamazepine-I 0, ll-epoxidejn mice. *J Pharmacol Exp Ther.* 1984;231;411–415.
23. Annijo JA, Cavada E. Graphic estimation of phenytoin dose in adults and children. *Ther Drug Monit.* 1991;13(6):507–510.
24. Brodie MJ. Management of epilepsy during pregnancy and lactation. *Lancet.* 1990;336(8712):426–427.
25. Perucca E, Richens A, Ruprah M. Serum protein binding of phenytoin in pregnant women. *Proc Br Phannacol Soc.* 1981;1I:409P–4IOP.
26. Bologa M, Tang B, Klein J, et al. Pregnancy-induced changes in drug metabolism in epileptic women. *J Phannacol Exp Ther.* 1991; 257(2):735–740.
27. Thomson AH, Brodie MJ. Phannacokinetics optimisation of anticonvulsant therapy. *Clin Pharmacokinet.* 1992;23(3):216–230.
28. Henriksen 0, Johannessen SI. Clinical and phannacokinetic observations on sodium valproate: a 5-year follow-up study of 100 children with epilepsy. *Acta Neurol Scand.* 1982;65(5):504–523.
29. Pugh CB, Garnett WR. Current issues in the treatment of epilepsy. *Clin Phannacol.* 1991;10(5):335–358.
30. Samren EB, van Duijn CM, Koch S, et al. Maternal use of antiepileptic drugs and the risk of major congenital malformations: a joint European prospective study of human teratogenesis associated with maternal epilepsy. *Epilepsia.* 1997;38:981–990.
31. Tomson T, Perucca E, Battino D. Navigating toward fetal and maternal health: the challenge of treating epilepsy in pregnancy. *Epilepsia.* 2004;45:1171–1175.
32. Morrow JI, Russell A, Gutherie E, et al. Malformation risks of antiepileptic drugs in pregnancy: A prospective study from the UK Epilepsy and Pregnancy Register. J *Neurol Neurosurg Psychiatry.* 2005. (published online Sep doi.10.1136/jnnp.2005.074203)
33. Cunnington M, Tennis P. Lamotrigine and the risk of malformations in pregnancy. *Neurology.* 2005;64:955–960.
34. Tomson T, Battino D, Bonizzoni E, et al. EURAP: an international registry of antiepileptic drugs and pregnancy. *Epilepsia.* 2004;45: 1463–1464.
35. Holmes LB, Wyszynski DF. North American antiepileptic drug pregnancy registry. *Epilepsia.* 2004;45:1465.
36. Holmes LB, Wyszynski DF, Lieberman E. The AED (antiepileptic drug) pregnancy registry: a 6-year experience. *Arch Neurol.* 2004;61:673–678.
37. Kaaja E, Kaaja R, Hiilesmaa V. Major malformations in offspring of women with epilepsy. *Neurology.* 2003;60:575–579.
38. Kaneko S, Battino D, Andermann E, et al. Congenital malformations due to antiepileptic drugs. *Epilepsy Res.* 1999;33(2–3):145–158.
39. Holmes LB, Harvey EA, Coull BA, et al. The teratogenicity of anticonvulsant drugs. *N Engl J Med.* 2001; 344(15):1132–1138.
40. Matalon S, Schechtman S, Goldzweig G, et al. The teratogenic effect of carbamazepine: a meta-analysis of 1255 exposures. *Reproductive Toxicology.* 2002;16(1):9–17.
41. Wide K, Winbladh B, Kallen B. Major malformations in infants exposed to antiepileptic drugs in utero, with emphasis on carbamazepine and valproic acid: a nation-wide, population-based register study. *Acta Paediatr.* 2004;93:174–176.
42. Artama M, Auvinen A, Raudaskoski T, et al. Antiepileptic drug use of women with epilepsy and congenital malformations in offspring. *Neurology.* 2005;64:1874–1878.
43. Vajda FJ, O'Brien TJ, Hitchcock A, et al. Critical relationship between sodium valproate dose and human teratogenicity: results of the Australian register of anti-epileptic drugs in pregnancy. *J Clin Neurosci.* 2004;11:854–858.
44. Pennell PB. The importance of monotherapy in pregnancy. *Neurology.* 2003;60:S31–S38.
45. Rosa FW. Spina bifida in infants of women treated with carbamazepine during pregnancy. *N Engl J Med.* 1991;324(10):674–677.
46. Omtzigt JG, Los FJ, Grobbee DE, et al. The risk of spina bifida aperta after first-trimester exposure to valproate in a prenatal cohort. *Neurology.* 1992; 42(4 suppl 5):119–125.
47. Lindhout D, Omtzigt JG. Teratogenic effects of antiepileptic drugs: implication for the management of epilepsy in women of childbearing age. *Epilepsia.* 1994;35(suppl 4):S19–S28.

48. Wyszynski DF, Nambisan M, Surve T, et al. Increased rate of major malformations in offspring exposed to valproate during pregnancy. *Neurology.* 2005;64:961–965.
49. Mawer G, Clayton-Smith J, Coyle H, et al. Outcome of pregnancy in women attending an outpatient epilepsy clinic: adverse features associated with higher doses of sodium valproate. *Seizure.* 2002;11: 512–518.
50. Omtzigt JG, Los FJ, Grobbee DE, et al. The risk of spina bifida aperta after first-trimester exposure to valproate in a prenatal cohort. *Neurology.* 1992;42(4 Suppl 5):119–125.
51. Reinisch JM, Sanders SA, Rubin DB. In utero exposure to Phenobarbital and intelligence deficits in adult men. *JAMA.* 1995; 724:1518–1525.
52. Adams J, Harvey EA, Holmes LB. Cognitive deficits following gestational monotherapy with Phenobarbital and carbamazepine. *Neurotoxicol Teratol.* 2000;22:466.
53. Scolnik D, Nulman I, Rovet J, et al. Neurodevelopment of children exposed in utero to phenytoin and carbamazepine monotherapy. *JAMA.* 1993;271(10):767–770.
54. Hanson JW, Myrianthopoulos NC, Harvey MA, et al. Risks to the offspring of women treatec with hydantoin anticonvulsants, with emphasis on the fetal hydantoin syndrome. *J Pediatr.* 1976:89(4):662–668.
55. Ornoy A, Cohen E. Outcome of children born to epileptic mothers treated with carbamazepinl during pregnancy. *Arch Dis Child.* 1996; 75(6):517–520.
56. Jones KL, Lacro RV, Johnson KA, et al. Pattern of malformations in the children of women treated with carbamazepine during pregnancy. *N Engl J Med.* 1989;320(25):1661–1666.
57. Gaily E, Kantola-Sorsa E, Hiilesmaa V, et al. Normal intelligence in children with prenatal exposure to carbamazepine. *Neurology.* 2004; 62:28–32.
58. Loring DW, Meador KJ, Thompson WO. Neurodevelopment effects of phenytoin and carbamazepine. *JAMA.* 1994;271:767–770.
59. Koch S, Jager-Roman E, Losche G, et al. Antiepileptic drug treatment in pregnancy: side effects in the neonate and neurological oncome. *Acta Paediatr.* 1996;85(6):739–746.
60. Adab N, Jacoby A, Smith D, et al. Additional educational needs in children born to mothers with epilepsy. *J Neurol Neurolsurg Psychiatry.* 2001;70:15–21.
61. Adab N, Kini U, Vinten J, et al. The longer term outcome of children born to mothers with epilepsy. *J Neurol Neurosurg Psychiatry.* 2004; 75:1575–1583.
62. Shorvon SD. Longer term outcome of children born to mothers with epilepsy. *J Neurol Neurosurg Psychiatry.* 2004;75:1517–1518.
63. Dean JCS, Hailey H, Moore SJ, et al. Long term health and neurodevelopment in children exposed to antiepileptic drugs before birth. *J Med Genet.* 2002;39:251–259.
64. Wilson JG. Current status of teratology-general principles and mechanisms derived from animal studies. In: Wilson JG, Fraser FC, eds. Handbook of Teratology, vol. 1. New York: Plenum Press, 1977, pp 47–74.
65. Gabitril package insert, Abbott Laboratories. September 2, 1998.
66. Morrow JI, Craig JJ. Anti-epileptic drugs in pregnancy: current safety and other issues. *Expert Opin Pharmacother.* 2003;4:445–456.
67. Montouris G. Safety of the newer antiepileptic drug oxcarbazepine during pregnancy. *Curr Med Res Opin.* 2005;21:693–701.
68. Yerby MS. Clinical care of pregnant women with epilepsy: neural tube defects and folic acid supplementation. *Epilepsia.* 2003;44 Suppl 3:33–40.
69. Montouris G. Gabapentin exposure in human pregnancy: results from the Gabapentin Pregnancy Registry. *Epilepsy Behav.* 2003;4:310–317.
70. Wilton LV and Shakir S. A postmarketing surveillance study of gabapentin as add-on therapy for 3,100 patients in England. [comment]. *Epilepsia.* 2002;43(9):983–992.
71. Finnel RM, Buehler BA, Kerr BM, et al. Clinical and experimental studies linking oxidative metabolism to phenytoin-induced teratogenesis. *Neurology.* 1992;42(4 suppl 5):25–31.
72. Buehler BA, Delimout D, Van Waes M, et al. Prenatal prediction of risk of the fetal hydantoin syndrome. *N Engl J Med.* 1990;322(22): 1567–1572.
73. Lindhout D, Hoppener RJ, Meinardi H. Teratogenicity of antiepileptic drug combinations with special emphasis on epoxidation (of carbamazepine). *Epilepsia.* 1984;25(1):77–83.
74. Sulik KK, Johnston MC, Daft PA, et al. Fetal alcohol syndrome and DiGeorge anomaly: critical ethanol exposure periods for craniofacial malformations as illustrated in an animal model. *Am J Med Genet.* 1986;(suppl 2):97–112.
75. Spreen 0, Tupper D, Risser A, et al. Chronology of neural development. In: Human Developmental Neuropsychology. New York: Oxford University Press, 1984, pp 26–28.
76. Gaily E, Granstrom ML. Minor anomalies in children of mothers with epilepsy. *Neurology.* 1992;42(4 suppl 5):128–131.
77. Gaily E, Granstrom ML, Hiilesmaa V, et al. Minor anomalies in the offspring of epileptic mothers. *J Pediatr.* 1988;112:520–529.
78. Ogawa Y, Kaneko S, Otani K, et al. Serum folic acid levels in epileptic mothers and their relationship to congenital malformations. *Epilepsy Res.* 1991;8(1):75–78.
79. Dansky LV, Rosenblatt DS, Andermann E. Mechanisms of teratogenesis: folic acid and antiepileptic therapy. *Neurology.* 1992;42 (4 suppl 5):32–42.
80. MRC Vitamin Study Research Group. Prevention of neural tube defects: results of the Medical Research Council Vitamin Study. *Lancet.* 1991;338(8760):131–137.
81. Brodie MJ, Dichter MA. Antiepileptic drugs. *N Engl J Med.* 1996; 334(3):168–175.
82. Malone FD, D'Alton ME. Drugs in pregnancy: anticonvulsants. *Semin Perinatol.* 1997;21(114–123).
83. Shuster EA. Epilepsy in women (Symposium on Epilepsy-Part VII). *Mayo Clin Proc.* 1971;(10):991–999.
84. Yerby M, Koepsell T, Daling J. Pregnancy complications and outcomes in a cohort of won with epilepsy. *Epilepsia.* 1985;26: 631–635.
85. Lopes-Cendes I, Andennann E, Candes F, et al. Risk factors for changes in seizure frequently during pregnancy of epileptic women: A cohort study (abstr). *Epilepsia.* 1992;33(suppl 57).
86. Hiilesmaa VK. Pregnancy and birth in women with epilepsy. *Neurology.* 1992;42(4 suppl):8–11.
87. Loebstein R, Lalkin A, Koren G. Phannacokinetic changes during pregnancy and their clinical relevance. *Clin Phannacokinet.* 1997; 33(5):328–343.
88. Morrell MJ. Honnones, reproductive health and epilepsy. In: Wyllie E, ed. The Treatment Epilepsy: Principles and Practice, 2nd ed. Baltimore: Williams & Wilkins, 1997.
89. Koren G. Changes in drug disposition in pregnancy and their clinical implications. In: Koren G, ed. Maternal-Fetal Toxicology: A Clinician's Guide, 2nd ed. New York: Marcel Dekker 1994, pp 3–13.
90. Van Creveld S. Nouveau aspects de la maladie heimorragique du nouveau-vie. *Arch Fr Pediatr.* 1958;6:721–735.
91. Moslet U, Hansen ES. A review of vitamin K, epilepsy and pregnancy. *Acta Neurol Scand.* 1992;85(1):39–43.
92. Sutor AH. Vitamin K deficiency bleeding in infants and children. *Semin Thromb Hemostas.* 1995;21(3):317–329.
93. Anai T, Hirota Y, Oga M, et al. PIVKA-I! (protein induced by vitamin K absence-I!) status in newborns exposed to anticonvulsant drugs in utero. *Nippon Sanka Fujinka Gakkai Zasshi.* 1991;43(3):347–350.
94. Cornelissen M, Steegers-Theunissen R, Kollee L, et al. Supplementation for vitamin K in pregnant women receiving anticonvulsant therapy prevents neonatal vitamin K deficiency. *Am J Obstet Gynecol.* 1993; 168(3 part 1):884–888.
95. Kaaja E, Kaaja R, Matila R, et al. Enzyme inducing antiepileptic drugs in pregnancy and the risk of bleeding in the neonate. Neurology 2002;58:549–553.
96. Stokes T, Shaw EJ, Juarez-Garcia A, et al. Clinical Guidelines and Evidence Review for the Epilepsies: diagnosis and management in adults and children in primary and secondary care. *NICE Clinical Guideline no CG20.* 2004. Royal College of General Practitioners.

97. O'Brien MD, Gilmar-White SK. Management of epilepsy in women. *Postgrad Med J.* 2005;81:278–285.
98. Nakane Y, Okuma T, Takahashi R, et al. Multi-institutional study on the teratogenicity and fetal toxicity of antiepileptic drugs: a report of a collaborative study group in Japan. *Epilepsia.* 1980;21(6):663–680.
99. Fujioka K, Kaneko S, Hirano T, et al. A study of the psychomotor development of the offspring of epileptic mothers. In: Sato T, Shinagawa S, eds. Antiepileptic Drugs and Pregnancy. *Amsterdam: Excerpta Medica.* 1984, pp 196–206.
100. Sophocles AM, Brozovich EM. Birth control failure among patients with unwanted pregnancies: 1982–1984. *J Fam Pract.* 1986; 22(1):45–48.
101. American Collage of Obstetricians and Gynecologists. Seizure Disorders in Pregnancy. ACOG educational bulletin No. 231, December 1996. Committee on Educational Bulletins of the International Journal of Gynaecology and Obstetrics. *Int J Obstet Gynaecol.* 1997;56(3): 279–286.
102. Mattson RH, Cramer JA, Darney PD, et al. Use of oral contraceptives by women with epilepsy. *JAMA.* 1986;256(2):238–240.
103. Koren G, Nulman I. Fetal malformations associated with drugs and chemicals: visualization by sonography. In Koren G, ed. Maternal-Fetal Toxicology: A Clinician's Guide. 2nd ed. New York: Marcel Dekker, 1994, pp 627–639.

CHAPTER 6

FETAL MALFORMATIONS ASSOCIATED WITH DRUGS AND CHEMICALS: VISUALIZATION BY SONOGRAPHY/FETAL MRI

Irena Nulman, Reuven Sussman, Noah Farber, David Chitayat, and Gideon Koren

INTRODUCTION

The ability to detect fetal malformations antenatally is important both in order to allow women to terminate affected pregnancies if they so wish and to plan for optimal fetal/neonatal management if pregnancy continues.

Since the thalidomide disaster in the 1950s, an increasing number of drugs and chemicals have been incriminated as causing teratogenicity or fetal toxicity. As the majority of pregnant women are exposed to at least one medication during pregnancy, either before or after realizing that they are pregnant[1], the need to determine the relative risk for fetal malformations associated with pregnancy exposure is of the utmost importance.

Data on chemically induced teratogenic risk are derived from animal studies, human case reports, and epidemiological studies. While such information is essential for assigning a relative risk for a potential teratogen, it may be of little help for drug therapy in a specific case. Sonography has emerged as a powerful tool for antenatal detection of structural fetal anomalies. It is conceivable therefore that more and more pregnant women exposed to drugs and chemicals will be referred for fetal ultrasound to rule out or diagnose fetal abnormalities associated with exposure to these agents. In the last few years fetal MRI have been used in addition to ultrasound in cases with poor visibility due to maternal habitus and cases with oligohydramnios, when the fetal ultrasound does not provide a clear picture of the fetal abnormalities. Furthermore, fetal MRI can provide us with important information regarding the intrauterine growth and development of the fetal brain, including conditions such as cerebral ventriculomegaly, posterior fossa lesions, and callosal anomalies. It also helps in the diagnosis of lesions such as diaphragmatic hernias and genitourinary abnormalities. This additional information can be of utmost importance in prenatal decision making.

Currently, pregnant women who attend the Motherisk clinic for antenatal counseling of drug-chemical exposure are scheduled for a detailed fetal ultrasound at 18–19 weeks of pregnancy if there is an increased risk for malformations. If indicated by the ultrasound findings, fetal MRI may be considered.

This guide aims at providing the radiologist/sonographer with a practical list of malformations that have been reported in association with specific drugs or chemicals. It is an updated version of our original publication several years ago.[1]

METHODOLOGICAL CONSIDERATION

Two groups of agents are included.[1] Common drugs and chemicals that have been associated with malformations are listed. In many cases the incriminating data are controversial; hence the inclusion of a certain malformation in this guide by no means suggests that we are convinced that the agent is a teratogen. This guide does not claim to prove teratogenicity of all of the drugs listed. It is to be used only to raise the awareness of the ultrasonographer. Because of the controversy of the data, the source of information is mentioned (for instance, case reports, retrospective or prospective studies). Drugs and chemicals that have been proven beyond doubt as teratogens are marked (see Table 6-1).

Table 6-1 includes only malformations that can be visualized by current ultrasonographic techniques and cannot be used as a complete list of drug-induced teratogenicity. The data in this guide have been extracted from currently available literature.

Certain points with respect to the ultrasound examination itself should be stressed. The ultrasound is possibly best carried out by a physician ultrasonographer who has had significant experience in looking at fetuses. A very meticulous technique and high resolution, real-time equipment should be used. The examination is best recorded on videotape so that it can be reviewed as needed. A great deal of patience is required in this type of study, especially when one is examining the brain, spinal cord, face, limbs, and heart. When a cardiac abnormality is suspected an attempt should be made to refer the mother for an echocardiography, if possible done by a specialist in fetal cardiology. At the outset of the examination it should be explained to the patient that the assessment may take some time to complete, may be done by more than one person and that more than one sitting may be required.

Table 6-1
Common Drugs

▶	#	MEDICATION NAME	CENTRAL NERVOUS SYSTEM	CARDIOVASCULAR	SKELETON	EXTREMITIES	GASTROINTESTINAL	GENITOURINARY	CRANIOFACIAL	MISCELLANEOUS	DESIGN	REF#
▶ - **Proven teratogen**												
	1	5-ASA				Aphakia					PS, pop PS	2, 3
	2	Acebutolol (see Atenolol)										
	3	Acetaminophen	NTD	Pulmonic stenosis, VSD	congenital hip dislocation	Limb Reductions, syndactyly, band constriction, clubfoot, polydactyly	Gastroschisis, small intestinal atresia, hydronephrosis		Craniofacial anomalies		CCS, CCS, CCS, PS, CPP CR, SS	4–11, 12–15
	4	Acetazolamide			Sacrococcygeal teratoma						CR	4–11
	5	Acetylsalicylic Acid		VSD							RS	16
	6	Acyclovir	NTD, diastematomyelia, hydrocephalus, calcified foci in the CNS	Ascites, cardiomegaly, VSD	Hip dysplasia, micrognathia, absence of right fibula	Lower limb deformities, hypoplasia congenita ossis, adactyly	Pyloric stenosis, diaphragmatic hernia	Undescended testis, bladder-based diverticulum, hydronephrosis, hypospadias	Cleft palate	Hemangiomas, IUGR	PS/RS, CR, SS	4–11, 17–18
	7	Albuterol	NTD	Tachycardia		Polydactyly					CR, CS, SS	4–11
▶	8	Alcohol	Microcephaly	VSD, cardiac defects		Upper limb reduction, adactyly		Renal agenesis	Craniofacial anomalies	IUGR	PS, CR, CR, PS	19–22
	9	Alpha Carotene (lack of)					Gastroschisis				RS	23
	10	Alprazolam		VSD		Clubfoot			Oral clefts		PS, CR, MA	4–11, 24
	11	Amantadine		Cardiac defects		Limb-reduction defects					CR, SS	4–11
	12	Amiloride						Hypospadias		IUGR	CR, SS	4–11
▶	13	Aminopterin	Brachycephaly, hydrocephaly, NTD		Cranial anomalies, incomplete skull ossification	Hypoplasia of thumb and fibula, short forearms, sydactyly, talipes		Hypospadias	Low-set ears	IUGR	CR, SS, CR	4–11
	14	Amiodarone		Bradycardia, cardiac defects	hypertelorism					Goiter, IUGR	CR, CS	4–11

15	Amitriptyline	Hydrocephaly, microcephaly	Cardiac defects	Anomalous mandible	Foot deformaties, limb-reduction defects, polydactyly		Ambiguous genitalia, hypospadias	Oral clefts	Anopthalmia	CR, SS	4–11
16	Amlodipine	Hydrocephalus with widely open sutures, small posterior fossa, agenesis of the corpus callosum			Adactyly, phalanges were absent, camptodactly of all digits			Low-set ears, rotated and crumpled ears, ear lacking opening		CR	25
17	Amobarbital	NTD	Cardiac defects		Clubfoot, polydactyly, limb deformities		Genitourinary malformations, hypospadias	Accessory auricle, oral clefts	Nuchal edema	CPP, SS	4–11
18	Amoxicillin		VSD	Congenital dislocation of hip	Clubfoot			Oral clefts	Tracheo-oesophageal fistula	PS, PS, SS	4–11, 15, 26
19	Amphetamine	Brain abnormalities, intracranial hemorrhage, microcephaly, NTD, porencephaly	VSD, cardiac defects, tachycardia		Clinodactyly, limb deformity	Hydronephrosis	Ambiguous genitalia, genitourinary malformations	Eye abnormalities, oral clefts	IUGR	PS, CR, PS, RS	4–11, 22
20	Ampicillin		Cardiac defects	Pectus excavatum	Polydactyly		Hypospadias	Oral clefts	Esophageal atresia	pop CCS, PS, CCS, RS, SS	4–11, 27–29
21	Aspirin	Intracranial hemorrhage	Cardiac defects			Small intestinal atresia, gastroschisis	Hypospadias		IUGR	CCS, RS, SS	4–11, 12
22	Atenolol		Bradycardia, cardiac defects		Limb-reduction defects		Hypospadias	Oral clefts	IUGR	PS, RS, RS, PS, RS, PS, SS	4–11, 30–34
23	Atorvastatin	NTD			Limb reduction defects			Cleft palate	esophageal atresia, tracheo-esophageal fistula	CS	35
24	Atropine	NTD			Limb-reduction defects, polydactyly					CR, SS	4–11
25	Azatadine				Limb-reduction defects				Oral clefts	SS	4–11
▶ 26	Azathioprine	Plagiocephaly	Pulmonary stenosis, cardiac defects		Aphakia, rudimentary thumb, clubfeet, pes equinovarus, polydactyly	Agenesia of bile conducts	Hypospadias, urinary tract abnormalities		Lung dysplasia, IUGR, single umbilical artery, umbilical hernia	pop PS, PS, CS, RS, RS/ PS,CR, SR	4–11, 3, 36 39

(*Continued*)

Table 6-1
Common Drugs (*Continued*)

▶ #	MEDICATION NAME	CENTRAL NERVOUS SYSTEM	CARDIOVASCULAR	SKELETON	EXTREMITIES	GASTROINTESTINAL	GENITOURINARY	CRANIOFACIAL	MISCELLANEOUS	DESIGN	REF#
27	Azithromycin					Pyloric stenosis				RS	40
28	Baclofen		VSD							RS	16
29	Beclomethasone (see also Corticosteroids)	Intraventricular hemorrhage			Rocker bottom feet		Hypospadias, large abnormal kidney	Hypoplastic bones of skull vault, widened cranial sutures, defective ossification of roof of calvarium, oral clefts	IIUGR	CR, RCT, CCS, MA	4–11, 41–43
30	Belladonna						Hypospadias	Eye and ear anomalies		CPP	4–11
31	Benazepril (see Captopril)										
32	Benzodiazepine						Renal dysplasia			PS	24
33	Benzthiazide (See Chlorothiazide, Hydrochloro-thiazide)										
34	Benztropine		Cardiac defects			Gastrointestinal anomalies				CR, SS	4–11
▶ 35	Betamethasone (see also Corticosteroids)							Oral Clefts		MA	4–11
36	Betaxolol (see Atenolol)										
37	Bismuth subsalicylate	Intracranial hemorrhage							IUGR	CPP, CS	4–11
38	Bisoprolol (see Atenolol)			Hypertelorism, frontal bossing	Hypoplasia of toes			Rudimentary skull ossification, oral clefts		CR, CS	44–45
39	Bretylium		Bradycardia							PI	4–11
40	Bromides	Macrocephaly, microcephaly	Cardiac defects		Clubfoot, polydactyly	Gastrointestinal anomalies			IUGR	CPP, CR	4–11
41	Bromocriptine	Hydrocephaly, microcephaly	Cardiac defects		Limb-reduction defects		Renal agenisis, hypospadias	Oral cleft	Single umbilical artery	RS	4–11
42	Budesonide	Transposition of great vessels, NTD, microcephaly, hydrocephaly	VSD, ASD, Tricuspidal atresia	Spine malformation	Bowed long bones in limbs, varus deformity of foot, syndactyly/ polydactyly	Esophageal atresia	Male genital malformation, cystic kidney with ureter malformation, hydronephrosis	Cleft lip, ear dysplasia		RS, pop PS	46–47
43	Bumetanide		Cardiac defects							SS	4–11

44	Buprenorphine		VSD						IUGR	CR, RS	48, 16
45	Busulfan	Myeloschisis				Hepatic subscapular calcification	Absent kidney, hydronephrosis, hydroureter	Oral clefts, microphthalmia	IUGR	CR, CS	4–11
46	Butoconazole	NTD								SS	4–11
47	Butriptyline (see Imipramine)										
48	Caffeine		Tachyarryhthmias	Deformational plagiocephaly, musculoskeletal defects			Hydronephrosis		IUGR, tumors	CCS, RS, PS, CPP, CR,CS	4–11, 49–51
49	Calcitriol			Premature closure of the frontal fontanelle			Kidney malformation	Malformation of palate	Stillbirth	CS	52
50	Candesartan	Exencephaly						Rudimentary skull ossification		CS	45
51	Candesartan Cilexetil								Plexus paresis, left-sided facial palsy	CR	53
52	Captopril	Microcephaly, NTD	Cardiac defects, pulmonary hypoplasia	Acrania	Clinodactyly, limb-reduction defects, polydactyly	omphalocele	Hypospadias, renal defects	Low-set ears	IUGR, oligohydramnios	CR, SS	4–11
▶ 53	Carbamazepine	NTD, microcephaly, caudal regression, lissencephaly	VSD, ASD, congenital ventricular hypertrophy, thick mitral valve, hypoplastic left heart, coarctation, SVT, pulmonary stenosis, dextrocardia, cardiomegaly, Tetralogy of Fallot	Hip dysplasia, micrognathia, hypertelorism	Limb reduction defects, midface/ digit hypoplasia, polydactyly, talipes	Inguinal hernia	Hypospadias, hydronephrosis, undescended testes, inguinal hernia	Oral clefts, malformed ears	IUGR, lung hypoplasia, oesophageal atresia	CR, PS, PS, PS, PS, PS, pop PS, pop RS, PS, PS, RS, RS, RS	4–11, 54–67
54	Carbenicillin		Cardiac defects							SS	4–11
55	Carbimazole (see also Methimazole)	Exencephaly, NTD	VSD	Craniosynostosis hypospadias						CS, PS	45, 68
▶ 56	Carbon Monoxide	Cerebral atrophy, hydrocephaly, microcephaly	Bradycardia							CR, PS	4–11
57	Carisoprodol								Oral clefts	SS	4–11
58	Cartelol (see Atenolol)										

(Continued)

Table 6-1
Common Drugs (*Continued*)

▶ #	MEDICATION NAME	CENTRAL NERVOUS SYSTEM	CARDIOVASCULAR	SKELETON	EXTREMITIES	GASTROINTESTINAL	GENITOURINARY	CRANIOFACIAL	MISCELLANEOUS	DESIGN	REF#
59	Casanthranol	NTD	Cardiac defects		Polydactyly					SS	4–11
60	Cefaclor	NTD	Cardiac defects						Oral clefts	SS	4–11
61	Cefadroxil				Limb-reduction defects					SS	4–11
62	Ceftazidime								neonatal death	RCC	29
63	Ceftriaxone		Cardiac defects							SS	4–11
64	Celiprolol (see Atenolol)		Cardiac defects								
65	Cephalexin	NTD	Cardiac defects						Oral clefts	SS	4–11
66	Cephradine									SS	4–11
67	Cerivastatin	Holoprosen-cephaly								CS	35
68	Cetirizine						Renal dysplasia			PS	24
69	Chlorambucil		Cardiac defects				Agenesis of kidney and ureter (in male fetuses)		IUGR	CR, PS, RS	4–11
70	Chlordiazepoxide	Microcephaly	Cardiac defects		Polydactyly	Duodenal atresia			Oral clefts	CCS, SS	4–11
71	Chloroquine		Cardiac defects						Wilms' tumor	CR, CS	4–11
72	Chlorothiazide (see also Hydrochoroth-iazide)						Hypospadias			SS	4–11
73	Chlorphenir-amine	Hydrocephaly			Polydactyly	Gastrointestinal anomalies	Malformation of female genitalia	Eye and ear anomalies		CPP, SS	4–11
74	Chlorpromazine	Microcephaly			Brachymeso-phalangy, clinodactyly, clubfoot/hand, syndactyly	Abdominal wall defect				CPP	4–11
75	Chlorpropamide	Microcephaly	Cardiac defects	Vertebral anomalies	Limb anomalies	Bowel obstruction		Facial and auricular anomalies		CR, CS	4–11
76	Chlorprothixen								Lung hypoplasia	PS	71
77	Chlortetracycline (see tetracycline)										
78	Chlorzoxazone		Cardiac defects							SS	4–11
79	Cholestyramine	Hydrocephaly, intracranial hemorrhage								CR	4–11
80	Cimetidine		Cardiac defects				Renal dysplasia			PS, SS	4–11, 24

81	Ciprofloxacin	Cerebellar hypoplasia	Cardiac defects	Skeletal defects	Amputation of right forearm, femur aplasia		Urethral atresia/stenosis			PS, RS	4–11
82	Citalopram		Cardiac defect, PDA			Duodenal atresia	Hypospadia, undescended testicle, hydronephrosis	Oral clefts	Laryngeal/ bronchial anomaly	pop PS	69
83	Clarithromycin	NTD	VSD, ASD, ventricular hypertrophy, tricuspid dysplasia	Spine and rib anomalies, absent clavicles	Clubfoot	Anal atresia	Undescended testes	Craniofacial anomalies, oral clefts	IUGR	RC, CR	4–11, 40
84	Clavulanate Potassium	NTD							Oral Clefts	SS	4–11
85	Clavulanic Acid		Pulmonic stenosis			hydronephrosis				PC	15
86	Clemastine	NTD			Limb-reduction defects, limb abnormalities					SS	4–11
87	Clindamycin	NTD	VSD						IUGR	CR, RS, RCT, SS	4–11, 46, 70–71
88	Clobazam	NTD								PS, RS	58, 67
89	Clomiphene	Hydrocephaly, microcephaly, NTD	Cardiac defects		Clubfoot, polydactyly, syndactyly		Hypospadias, absent kidney	Oral clefts		CCS, CR, SS	4–11, 72
90	Clomiphene Citrate	Anencephaly, spina bifida								CCS	73
91	Clomipramine		Ebstein's anomaly							RS	16
92	Clomocycline (see Tetracycline)										
93	Clonazepam		Cardiac defects, cardiomegaly					Oral clefts	Dysmorphic features, IUGR	RS, RS, MA, SS	4–11, 64, 74
94	Clonidine		Cardiac defects							SS	4–11
95	Clorazepate		Cardiac defects	Deformities of the lumbosacral vertebrae	Adactyly, shortened thigh, underdeveloped femur		Genital abnormalities			CR	4–11
96	Clotrimazole	NTD	Cardiac defects		Polydactyly					SS	4–11
97	Cloxacillin		Cardiac defects				Hypospadias			SS	4–11
▶ 98	Cocaine	Microcephaly, ocephaly, brain lesions, cerebral hemorrhage, hydrocephaly	Bradycardia, cardiac defects, tachycardia	Hypoplasia of clavicle and scapula, hypertelorism	Amelia, humero-radial synostosis, arm absent, phocomelia, ulnar aplasia, right upper limb reduction defect, adactyly, clubfoot, polydactyly	Intestinal defects	Renal agenesis, genitourinary abnormalities, hydronephrosis, hypospadias	Overlapping sutures, occipital bone prominence, scalp rugae, absence of septum pellucidum, oral clefts	IUGR, oligohydramnios	CR, PS, CR, PS, CR, PS, PS, RC, CR, PS, RS	4–11, 19–20, 75–81

(*Continued*)

Table 6-1
Common Drugs (*Continued*)

▶ #	MEDICATION NAME	CENTRAL NERVOUS SYSTEM	CARDIOVASCULAR	SKELETON	EXTREMITIES	GASTROINTESTINAL	GENITOURINARY	CRANIOFACIAL	MISCELLANEOUS	DESIGN	REF#
99	Cocaine (crack)					Microcolon	Megacystis, Hydronephrosis, enlaged bladder			CR	82
100	Codeine	Hydrocephaly	Cardiac defects	Musculoskeletal malformations	Limb reduction, polydactyly		Genitourinary abnormality		Oral clefts, tumors	CPP, RS, SS	4–11
101	Contraceptive pills				Congenital Limb Defects					RC	83
102	Corticosteroids	Microcephaly, abnormal cerebral ventricles						Oral clefts	Intrauterine death, Dandy Walker malformations, IUGR	RS, PS, RS, RCT, PS	24, 65, 84–86
▶ 103	Cortisone/ Corticotropin	Cyclopia, hydrocephaly	Cardiac defects		Clubfoot	Gastroschisis		Oral clefts	Oral clefts	CPP	4–11
▶ 104	Coumarin Derivatives	Brain structural defects	Cardiac defects	Scoliosis, stippled epiphyses	Bradydactyly, finger hypoplasia, hypoplasia of extremities, polydactyly		Single kidney	Absence of nasal septum, eye defects	Agenesis of diaphragm, IUGR	CR, CS, RS, SS	4–11
▶ 105	Cromolyn Sodium				Polydactyly				Oral clefts	SS	4–11
106	Cyclacillin		Cardiac defects							SS	4–11
107	Cyclophosphamide	Hydrocephalus, small posterior fossa, agenesis of the corpus callosum, microbrachycephaly, microcephaly	Cardiac defects	Hypoplastic Tibiae, absent fibulae, micrognathia	Radial aplasia, ulnar hypoplasia, adactyly, absent phalanges, camptodactly of all digits, hypoplastic thumbs, hypoplastic finger, syndactyly			Low-set ears, rotated and crumpled ears, ear lacking opening, microstomia, high-arched palate, eye defects, oral clefts	IUGR	CR, CR, CR	4–11, 25, 87–88
108	Cyclosporin		Peripheral pulmonic stenosis	Osseous malformation	Rudimentary thumb left hand, bilateral clubfeet, hypoplasia of leg	Jejunal atresia, agenesis of bile conducts	Hypospadias, other urinary tract abnormalities		Intrauterine death, IUGR	CS, PS, CS, RS, RS/PS, CR	4–11, 36–39, 89
109	Cyclothiazide (see Chlorothiazide, Hydrochlorothiazide)										

110	Cyproheptadine					Hypospadias	Oral clefts		SS	4–11
111	Cytarabine	Anencephaly, (paternal use)	Cardiac defects (paternal use)	Ectrodactyly, lower limb abnormalities, adactyly, syndactyly (paternal use)			Ear abnormalities (paternal use)	IUGR (paternal use)	CR	4–11
112	Danazol					Ambiguous genitalia			CR, RS	4–11
▶ 113	Daunorubicin	Anencephaly	Cardiac defects	Sydactyly					CR, CS	4–11
114	Debendox						Oral clefts		CCS	90
115	Demeclocycline (see Tetracycline)									
116	Depakine							Aplasia of lip muscle	CS	91
▶ 117	Dexamethasone (see also Corticosteroids)		Bronchopulmonary dysplasia, VSD				Oral clefts	IUGR	PS, PS, RS, RCT, PS, MA	4–11, 24, 42, 92–94
118	Dextroamph-etamine (see Amphetamine)									
119	Dextrometh-orphan	NTD, Central nervous system defects, Hydrocephaly	Cardiac defects		Small intestinal atresia, gastroschisis		Oral clefts		CCS, CCS	12, 95
▶ 120	Diazepam	CNS abnormalities, microcephaly, NTD	VSD, cardiac defects, hypertelorism	Limb deformity		Urogenital abnormalities	Scalp aplasia cutis congenita, skull defect, craniofacial defects, hypoplastic mandible, oral clefts	IUGR	RS, CR, CR, MA, PS, RS	4–11, 16, 96
121	Diazepam (in over-dose)							IUGR	pop RS	97
122	Dibenzepin (see Imipramine)									
123	Diclofenac		Double outlet right ventricle, premature closure of ductus arteriosus, ASD, VSD						RS, CR, CR, PS	16, 24, 98–99
124	Dicumarol (see Coumarin derivatives)									
125	Dicyclomine	Macrocephaly		Clubfoot, polydactyly				Diphragmatic hernia	CPP, SS	4–11

(Continued)

Table 6-1
Common Drugs (*Continued*)

#	MEDICATION NAME	CENTRAL NERVOUS SYSTEM	CARDIOVASCULAR	SKELETON	EXTREMITIES	GASTROINTESTINAL	GENITOURINARY	CRANIOFACIAL	MISCELLANEOUS	DESIGN	REF#
126	Dienestrol (see Estrogen)										
127	Diethylstilbestrol						Testicular tumors			CR	4–11
128	Diflunisal							Oral clefts		SS	4–11
129	Digoxin								Intrauterine death, IUGR	RS, CR	100–101
130	Dihydroergot-amine						Undescended testicle			CS	102
131	Diltiazem		Cardiac defects							SS	4–11
132	Dimenhydrinate		Cardiac defects							CPP	4–11
133	Diphenadione (see Coumarin Derivatives)										4–11
134	Diphenhydr-amine	Hydrocephaly, hypoplasia of cerebral hemisphere	Cardiac defects		Clubfoot, polydactyly		Hypospadias and other genitourinary abnormalities		Eye and ear anomalies, oral clefts	CPP, CR, PS, SS	4–11
135	Diphenoxylate	NTD	Cardiac defects	Hypertelorism	Limb-reduction defects, polydactyly		Hypospadias			CR	4–11
136	Disulfiram			Vertebral fusion	Clubfoot, phocomelia of lower extremities, radial aplasia					CR	4–11
137	Domperidone		Cardiac defects		Limb-reduction defects					PS	26
138	Dothiepin (see Imipramine)										
139	Doxepin		Cardiac defects		Polydactyly	Bowel obstruction			Oral clefts	CR, SS	4–11
140	Doxorubicin	Microcephaly								CR	4–11
141	Doxycycline (see also Tetracycline)	NTD								CR, PS	4–11
142	Doxylamine-Pyridoxine therapy	Anencephaly	VSD							PS	103
143	Droperidol	Brain hypoplasia, hydrocephaly								CR	4–11
144	Drotaverine				Limb Defects					RS	83
145	Dyphylline		Cardiac defects		Polydactyly					SS	4–11

146	Echinacea				Syndactyly	Inguinal hernia	Hydronephrosis, duplicate renal pelvis		Laryngotrachio-malacia	PS	104
147	Ecstacy (MDMA)	Plagiocephaly	VSD, cardiac defects	Hypoplastic ribs, absent scapula/ clavicle	Clinodactyly, 4th toe underlying 3rd, absent upper limbs, clubfoot	Pyloric stenosis	Hydronephrosis, ambiguous genitalia		IUGR	PS, CCS	22, 105
148	Enalapril	Hydrocephalus with widely open sutures, agenesis of the corpus callosum, other abnormalities of the CNS	Pulmonary cardiac defects		Adactyly, absent phalanges, camptodactly of all digits, polydactyly, limb-reduction defects	Gastrointestinal malformation	Genitourinary malformation, renal pathology, kidney defects	Small posterior fossa, skull ossification deficits, calvarial hypoplasia, craniofacial defects, low-set ears, rotated and crumpled ears, ear lacking opening	IUGR, oligohydramnios	CR, CS, CR, SS	4–11, 25, 106
149	Enoxacin (see Ciprofloxacin)										
150	Ephedrine		Bradycardia		Clubfoot					CPP, CS	4–11
151	Epinepherine	Intracranial hemorrhage								SS	4–11
152	Epoetin alfa								IUGR	CR	4–11
153	Ergotamine	Hydrocephaly, lisencephaly, microcephaly, NTD, ventriculomegaly	VSD, Cardiac defects	Sacral or coccygeal agenesis	Clubfoot, digital and limb hypoplasia, polydactyly	Bowel obstruction	Hypospadias, genital abnormalities, multicycstic dysplastic kidneys	Unspecified skull malformation, unspecified facial anomaly, oral clefts	Tongue tie	CS, CR, RS, SS	4–11, 102
154	Erythromycin	NTD, hydrocephalus	Cardiovascular anomaly, situs inversus	Sacral teratoma	Clubfoot, limb-reduction defect, polydactyly, absence of tibia	Intestinal atresia, congenital genu recurratum	Undescended testes, urinary tract anomalies, hypospadias	Cleft palate, cleft lip	Congenital cataract, webbing of neck, oesophageal atresia, IUGR	RS, PS, pop CCS, CS, SS	4–11, 40, 24, 107
155	Esmolol (see Atenolol)										
156	Estradiol		Cardiac defects				Hypospadias	Eye and ear anomalies		CPP, SS	4–11
157	Estrogens, conjugated		Cardiac defects		Absence of tibia, bowed fibulae, polydactyly		Hypospadias	Eye and ear anomalies, oral clefts		CPP	4–11
▶ 158	Ethanol (see also Alcohol)	Agenesis of corpus callosum, microcephaly, NTD	Cardiac defects	Vertebral and chest abnormalities	Limb and finger abnormalities		Kidney and urinary defects	Eye and ear anomalies	IUGR	CR, CS, PS, RS	4–11

(*Continued*)

Table 6-1
Common Drugs (*Continued*)

▶	#	MEDICATION NAME	CENTRAL NERVOUS SYSTEM	CARDIOVASCULAR	SKELETON	EXTREMITIES	GASTROINTESTINAL	GENITOURINARY	CRANIOFACIAL	MISCELLANEOUS	DESIGN	REF#
	159	Ethinyl Estradiol		Cardiac defects					Eye and ear		CPP	4–11
	160	Ethisterone (see Hydroxyprog-esterone)										
	161	Ethoheptazine								Umbilical hernia	CPP	4–11
▶	162	Ethosuximide	Hydrocephaly						Oral clefts		CR	4–11
	163	Ethotoin							Oral clefts		CR	4–11
	164	Ethyl Biscoumacetate (see Derivatives)										4–11
	165	Ethynodiol (see Oral Contraceptives)										4–11
	166	Etodolac (see Indomethacin)										4–11
	167	Etoposide								IUGR	CR	4–11
▶	168	Etretinate	Cerebral abnormalities, microcephaly, NTD	Cardiac defects	Abnormalities of cervical vertebrae, skeletal anomalies	Absence of terminal phalanges, limb-reduction defects, sydactyly			Skull and face defects, low-set ears, oral clefts		CR	4–11
	169	Famotidine (see also Cimetidine)	NTD, hydrocephaly, Anencephaly	Double outlet right ventricle		Hypoplastic hand					RS, PS	16, 24
	170	Felodipine		PDA		Varus of the left foot, clubbed right foot, fixed external rotation of right knee		Hyperechogenic kidneys			CR	53
	171	Fenfluramine		Cardiomyopathy, VSD		Clubfoot, limb abnormalities	Inguinal hernias				PS, CR, WHO	4–11, 108
	172	Flucloxacillin		VSD							RS	46
	173	Fluconazole	Hydrocephaly	VSD, Cardiac defects	Congenital dislocation of the hip, thin clavicles and ribs	Partial syndactyly, upper and lower limb			Craniofacial abnormalities, low-set ears, oral clefts		CS, RS, CR	4–11, 109–110
	174	Flucytosine (see Fluorouracil)										

175	Flunitrazepam (see Diazepam)										
176	Fluorouracil	Anencephaly, hydrocephaly	Cardiac defects		Absence of thumbs and fingers, radial aplasia	Duodenal atresia			Single umbilical artery	CR	4–11
177	Fluoxetine		VSD, unspecified cardiac defect, left brachial plexus lesion	Spine malformation, unstable hip	Polydactyly	Gastroschisis, abdominal wall defect	Malformation of kidney, cystic kidney, hydronephrosis, undescended testicle, hypospadias	Palate malformation	Branchial vestiga, esophageal atresia, congenital laryngeal stridor, intrauterine death, deformity of sterno-cleidomastoid muscle, nuchal cord	CS, RS, CCS, RS, CR	4–11, 52, 46, 111–112
178	Fluphenazine	Enlarged ventricles	Cardiac defects	Hypertelorism			Hypospadias	Poor ossification of skull bone	IUGR, oral clefts	CR, SS	4–11
179	Flurazepam (see Diazepam)				Polydactyly					SS	4–11
180	Flurbiprofen (see Indomethacin)								IUGR	CR	4–11
181	Fluvoxamine maleate								IUGR	CR	48
▶ 182	Folic Acid Deficiency	NTD							IUGR, placental abruption, placenta previa	CR, PS, RS	4–11
183	Fosinopril (see Captopril)										
184	Furosemide						Hypospadias		Macrosomia	pop RCC, SS	4–11, 113
185	Gabapentin	Holoprosence-phaly				One kidney	Hypospadias	Ear defects	Cyclopia	PS/RS, RS, CR	67, 114
186	Gamma Hydroxybutyric Acid		VSD		Clinodactyly		Hydronephrosis			PS	22
187	Gemfibrozil								Oral clefts	SS	4–11
188	Gentamicin	NTD	Cardiovascular anomaly		Clubfoot	Anal atresia	Hypospadias, undescended testis	Oral clefts		pop CCS	29, 115
189	Ginger (Zingiber officinale)		VSD				Kidney abnormality (pelviectasis)		Lung abnormality	PS	116
190	Glutathione (lack of)					Gastroschisis				RS	23
191	Glyburide		Cardiac defects					Ear defects	Macrosomia	RCT, CS, SS	4–11, 117
192	Gold Sodium Thiomalate								IUGR	CR, CS	4–11

(*Continued*)

Table 6-1
Common Drugs (*Continued*)

▶ #	MEDICATION NAME	CENTRAL NERVOUS SYSTEM	CARDIOVASCULAR	SKELETON	EXTREMITIES	GASTROINTESTINAL	GENITOURINARY	CRANIOFACIAL	MISCELLANEOUS	DESIGN	REF#
193	Griseofulvin		Cardiac defects		Polydactyly/ syndactyly	Pyloric stenosis	Hypospadias, undescended testis		Conjoined twins	pop CCS, CCS, CR	4–11, 118
194	Guaifenesin		Cardiac defects		Polydactyly	Gastroschisis				CCS, CPP, SS	4–11, 12
195	Haloperidol		Cardiac defects, VSD		Adactyly, limb abnormalities, limb-reduction defects	Abdominal wall defect		Full-thickness defect of the parietal scalp	Genu varum	PS, CS, CR, SS	4–11, 66, 119
▶ 196	Heparin		Cardiac defects		Polydactyly		Hypospadias		IUGR	RS, CR, SS	4–11, 120
197	Hepatitis C Vaccine (HCV)					Hepatoblastoma			LBW	RS	121
198	Heroin				Limb-reduction defect, adactyly		Renal agenesis		IUGR	CR, CR, CS	4–11, 20
199	Hexachlorophene	NTD	Cardiac defects		Foot anomalies, limb-reduction defect, polydactyly		Hypospadias, kidney defects	Oral clefts	Microphthalmia	CS	4–11
200	Hexamethonium					Bowel obstruction				CR	4–11
201	Hydralazine Hydrochloride					Hepatoblastoma			LBW	RS	121
202	Hydrochlorothiazide (see also Chlorothiazide)	Exencephaly	PDA, cardiac defects		Varus of the foot, clubfoot, fixed external rotation of right knee		Hyperechogenic kidneys, bowel obstruction		Potter's facies, IUGR	CS, CR, SS	4–11, 45, 53
203	Hydrocodone		Cardiac defects							SS	4–11
204	Hydroflumethiazide (see Chlorothiazide, Hydrochlorthiazide)		Cardiac defects							SS	4–11
205	Hydroxychloroquine (see also Chloroquine)	Hydrocephalus with widely open sutures, agenesis of the corpus callosum, transposition of the great arteries		Pulmonary hypoplasia, interventricular communication, pulmonary stenosis, PDA, VSD		Adactyly, absent phalanges, camptodactly		Hypospadias	Small posterior fossa, craniostenosis, low-set ears, rotated and crumpled ears, ear lacking opening	CR, PS, PS	25, 122–123

206	Hydroxyprogesterone	Hydrocephaly, NTD	Cardiac defects		Absence of thumbs		Ambiguous genitalia, hypospadias			CPP, CS, CSr	4–11
207	Hydroxyzine	Hydrocephaly, NTD	Cardiac defects		Limb-reduction defects		Cystic kidney, hydronephrosis	Oral clefts		RS, CPP, CS	4–11, 46
208	Ibuprofen	Transposition of great vessels, NTD	VSD, ASD, cardiac defects		Polydactyly	Gastroschisis		Oral clefts	Oligohydramnios, micropthalmia	RS, CCS, CR, SS, VR	4–11, 12,16
209	Imipramine	NTD	Cardiac defects		Amelia		Hypospadias, renal cystic dysplasia	Oral clefts	Adrenal hypoplasia	CR, CS, SS	4–11
210	Indigo Carmine	Hydrocephaly			Clubfoot, syndactyly	Intestinal atresia	Urethral obstruction sequence			CR, CS	4–11
211	Indomethacin	Intraventricular hemorrhage	PDA, Periventricular Leukomalacia, bronchopulmonary dysplasia		Limb-reduction defects			Oral clefts	Hydrops, oligohydramnios	RS, RS, PS, CCS, CCS, CR, SS	4–11, 43, 124–127
212	Insulin	Anencephaly, NTD, vertebral anomalies	ASD, atresia of the pulmonary veins, double outlet rightventricle, cardiac defects, Tetralogy of Fallot		Malformation of antebrachium and hand, clubfoot		Hydronephrosis, urogenital anomalies, hypospadias, ambiguous genitalia		Situs inversus, macrosomia	PS, PS, pop PS, PS, PS	128–132
213	Insulin (lispro)	Meningomyelocele	Cardiac defects							PS, PS	131–132
214	Interferon Alpha			Hemivertebrae D6 to D10, 11 pairs of ribs, secondary scoliosis			Ambiguous genitalia, incomplete double pelvis and ureter		IUGR, intrauterine death	CS, CR, CS	133–136
215	Interferon Beta	Hydrocephalus, microcephaly, encephalomalacia with parenchymal destruction				Hepatosplenomegaly			IUGR	CR	137
216	Interferon Gamma								LBW	PS	138
217	Iodinated glycerol				Polydactyly					SS	4–11
218	Iodine (insufficiency)								Goiter	PS	139
219	Iodine (see Potassium Iodide)										
220	Ipratropium						Urinary tract obstruction			CR, SS	4–11

(*Continued*)

Table 6-1
Common Drugs (*Continued*)

▶ #	MEDICATION NAME	CENTRAL NERVOUS SYSTEM	CARDIOVASCULAR	SKELETON	EXTREMITIES	GASTROINTESTINAL	GENITOURINARY	CRANIOFACIAL	MISCELLANEOUS	DESIGN	REF#
221	Iprindole (see Imipramine)										
222	Isoniazid	NTD			Polydactyly		Hypospadias			CPP, CR, RS, SS	4–11
223	Isoproterenol				Clubfoot				Oral clefts	CR, CPP, SS	4–11
▶ 224	Isotretinoin	Hydrocephalus, brain structural abnormalities, microcephaly, NTD	Taussig-Bing malformation, Cardiac defects	Absence of clavicle and scapula, hypertelorism	Limb-reduction defects, syndactyly		Hydroureter, hypospadias, multicystic dysplastic kidneys	Hypoplasia of the facial nerve, absence of the chorda tympani nerve and the stapedius muscle, ear anomalies, inner ear malformation, low-set ears, oral clefts	Anotia, microphthalmia, microtia, single umbilical artery	CR, CR, PS, CS, CR, RS, SS	4–11, 140–143
225	Itraconazole			Hip joint dysplasia	Hand dysplasia, limb abnormalities	Pyloric stenosis			Microphthalmia	PS, CR	4–11, 144
226	Ketoconazole				Finger agenesis, limb abnormalities					CR, CR	4–11, 145
227	Ketoprofen		Aortic stenosis		Polydactyly					RS, SS	4–11, 146
228	Ketorolac (see Indomethacin)										
229	Labetolol		Bradycardia						IUGR	CS, SS	4–11
230	Lamictal			Abduction of the hips						CS	91
231	Lamotrigine	NTD, myelomeningocele, microcephaly, abnormal posterior fossa, encephalocele, Chiari II malformation, transposition of great vessels, anencephaly, hydrocephaly	PDA, ASD, pulmonary stenosis, polyorostenosis, VSD	Hypertelorism, micrognathia	Polydactyly, limb deformaties, clubfoot, arachnodactyly, camptodactyly, hammer toes, decreased creases on the soles		Hydronephrosis with megaureter, atresia of anus, absent right kidney	Minor malformation of external ear canal, absent ear canal opening, cleft palate, low-set malformed auriculas, retrognatia	Esophageal malformation, IUGR, oligohydramnios	PS/RS, RS, PS, CR, VR	4–11, 114, 67, 147–148

232	Lansoprazole		Cardiac defects		Limb-reduction defects					PS	26
233	Levofloxacin (see Ciprofloxacin)										
234	Levothyroxine		Cardiac defects		Polydactyly				Branchial vestiga, IUGR, goiter	RS, CR, CR, CS, PS, SS	4–11, 46, 149–150
235	L-hyoscyamine				Limb-reduction defects, polydactyly					SS	4–11
236	Lidocaine								Respiratory tract anomalies, tumors	CPP, CS, SS	4–11
237	Lindane		Cardiac defects	Acrania			Hypospadias	Oral clefts		SS	4–11
238	Liotrix (see Levothyroxine)										
239	Lisinopril (see Captopril)										
▶ 240	Lithium	Anencephaly, aqueduct stenosis, hydrocephaly, NTD	Bradycardia, cardiac defects	Hypoplasia of maxilla	Clubfoot, polydactyly		Bilateral renal agenisis		Retroplacental hematoma, microtia, polyhydramnios, single umbilical artery	CR, CR, PS, RS	4–11, 151
241	Lomefloxacin (see Ciprofloxacin)										
242	Loperamide		Cardiac anomalies			Oxalosis				PS, RS	152–153
243	Loratadine		VSD, aortic valve stenosis	Congenital hip dislocation		Inguinal hernia, diaphragmatic hernia	Kidney defect, hypospadias		Microphthalmia, oral clefts	PS, PS, CCS, CR	4–11, 154–156
▶ 244	Lorazepam (see also Diazepam)					Anal atresia		Scalp aplasia cutis congenita, skull defect		CR, pop CCS, RS	96, 157–158
245	Losartan		PDA, pulmonary hypoplasia		Varus left foot, clubbed right foot, fixed external rotation of right knee		Hyperechogenic kidneys, large multicystic kidneys	Rudimentary ossification of the occipital and parietal bones, Hypoplastic skull bones with wide sutures	IUGR, intrauterine death, oligoamnios, anhydramnios	CR, CS, CR, CR	45, 53, 159–160
246	Lovastatin	Hydrocephalus, NTD, myelolocele, duplication of spinal cord, cerebellar herniation	ASD, VSD, aortic hypoplasia	Vertebral anomalies	Limb abnormalities		Renal dysplasia	Absent auditory canal	Microtia, intrauterine death	CS, CR, RS	4–11, 35

(*Continued*)

Table 6-1
Common Drugs (*Continued*)

#	MEDICATION NAME	CENTRAL NERVOUS SYSTEM	CARDIOVASCULAR	SKELETON	EXTREMITIES	GASTROINTESTINAL	GENITOURINARY	CRANIOFACIAL	MISCELLANEOUS	DESIGN	REF#
247	Lysergic Acid Diethylamide	Bradycephaly, hydrocephaly, NTD	Cardiac defects		Limb deformities, limb-reduction defects		Urinary tract defects	Oral clefts, ocular defects	Neuroblastoma	CR, CS	4–11
248	Magnesium Sulfate		PDA, intraventricular hemorrhage, periventricular leukomalacia	Rib and bone defects					IUGR, oesophageal atresia	CCS, RCT, CS, RS, RS, CS	43, 161–165
249	Maprotiline							Oral clefts		SS	4–11
250	Marijuana	Porencephaly	Cardiac defects		Syndactyly				LBW, IUGR	RS, CR, CS	4–11, 166
251	Mebendazole		VSD		Limb-reduction defects		Hydronephrosis, hypospadias, undescended testes, genital defects, cyst of hydrocele		Lung hypoplasia, thoracic dystrophy	PS, PS, SS	4–11, 167–168
252	Mechlorethamine	Intracranial hemorrhage			Limb abnormalities		Renal hypoplasia		IUGR	CR	4–11
253	Meclizine	CNS malformation	VSD, ASD, hypoplastic left heart sequence		Polydactyly, sydactyly, limb reduction defect, clubfoot	Diaphragmatic hernia, body wall defect	Hypospadias	Ear malformation, oral clefts, eye anomalies	Oesophagial atresia	CCS, RS, CPP, PS	4–11, 46, 169
254	Meclofenamate (see Indomethacin)										
255	Medroxyproges-terone		Cardiac defects				Hypospadias			CPP, CR, SS	4–11
256	Mefenamic Acid (see Indomethacin)										
257	Mefloquine	Meningocele, other abnormalities of the CNS	Cardiac abnormalities			Gastrointestinal anomaly		Cleft palate	Stillbirth, IUGR	PS, RS, RS, PS/RS	170–173
258	Melphalan								IUGR	CR	4–11
259	Meningococcal Vaccine								Umbilical Hernia, IUGR	RS	174
260	Meperidine				Polydactyly		Hypospadias			CPP, SS	4–11
▶ 261	Mephenytoin (see Phenytoin)										

262	Mepindolol (see Atenolol)										
263	Meprobamate		Cardiac defects, ectopia cordis		Deformed elbows and joints, polydactyly			Oral clefts		CPP, CS, SS	4–11
264	Mercaptopurine (6-MP)	Hydrocephalus, NTD	Cardiac defects					Oral clefts	IUGR, microphthalmia	RS, CR	4–11, 174
265	Mesalamine				Polydactyly		Hypospadias, hydrocele	Laryngotracheal malformations	Umbilical hernia, CDH, IUGR	PS	176
266	Mesalazine					Pyloric stenosis				RS	153
267	Mestranol (see Estrogen, Estradiol)				Polydactyly					SS	4–11
268	Metformin								Periauricular adnex	PS	177
269	Methacycline (see Tetracycline)										
270	Methadone								IUGR, intrauterine death	PS	188
271	Methamphetamine (see Amphetamine)										
272	Methazolamide (see Acetazolamide)										
273	Methenamine				Limb-reduction defects			Oral clefts		SS	4–11
274	Methimazole	NTD	Atrioventricular canal, cardiac defects, trachycardia		Adactyly, polydactyly	Abdominal wall defect, kidney agenesias	Scrotal hypospadias	Full-thickness defect of the parietal scalp, broad forehead, high palate	Aplasia cutis congenita, umbilical hernia, esophageal atresia, micrognathia, polyhydramnios, anhydramnios, goiter	CS, CR, CR, CS, CR, PS, CR, CS, SS	4–11, 68, 119, 179–182
275	Methocarbamol				Clubfoot					CPP, CS, SS	4–11
▶ 276	Methotrexate	NTD	ASD, Tetralogy of Fallot, ventriculomegaly, cardiac defects, tachycardia	Large fontanelles, pectus excavatum, shortened clavicles, micrognathia, absent ribs, gracile ribs, hemivertebrae, Fusion of vertebral bodies	Finger-toe malformations, single bone in lower leg, absent radius, limb-reduction defects, bony abnormalities, foot clubfoot	Diaphragmatic hernias	Hypospadias, undescended testicle, duodenal atresia, enlarged left liver	Hypoplastic scapulae, undermineralization of the skull, cleft palate, low-set and poorly formed ears	Hypoplastic lungs, oligohydramnios, nuchal neck fold, tracheal atresia, hypoplastic lungs, two-vessel umbilical cord, IUGR	CR, CR, CS, CS, CR, CR, CS	4–11, 183–187

(Continued)

Table 6-1
Common Drugs (*Continued*)

▶ #	MEDICATION NAME	CENTRAL NERVOUS SYSTEM	CARDIOVASCULAR	SKELETON	EXTREMITIES	GASTROINTESTINAL	GENITOURINARY	CRANIOFACIAL	MISCELLANEOUS	DESIGN	REF#
277	Methotrexate (low dose)				Metatarsus varus			Eyelid angioma		PS	188
278	Methotrimepr-azine	Hydrocephaly	Cardiac defects							PS	4–11
279	Methyclothiazide (see Chlorothiazide, Hydrochloroth-iazide)										
▶ 280	Methyl Mercury	Microcephaly								CR	4–11
281	Methyldopa	Microcephaly	Cardiac defects			Hepatoblastoma	Hypospadias, renal agenesis	Oral clefts	IUGR	RS, CPP, CR, SS	4–11, 121
282	Methylene blue					Bowel obstruction				CR, CS	4–11
283	Methylphenidate		Cardiac defects							SS	4–11
284	Metoclopramide	Hydrocephalus, brain hypoplasia	VSD, valvular pulmonary stenosis, ASD	Congenital dislocation of hip	Contracture of hand		Undescended testis, hypospadias			PS, RS, CR	4–11, 15, 189
285	Metolazone (see Chlorothiazide, Hydrochloroth-iazide)										
286	Metoprolol (see also Atenolol)		PDA		Varus of the left foot, clubbed right foot, fixed external rotation of right knee	Hyperechogenic kidneys			IUGR	CR	53
287	Metronidazole	Brain defects	VSD, transposition of the great arteries	Micrognatia	Polydactyly, syndactyly, limb abnormalities	Rectal/anal atresia/ stenosis, multicystic kidney	Genital defects, hypospadias, obstructive uropathy	Oral clefts, low-set ears, craniostenosis, midline facial defects	IUGR, short neck, hyperteleorism	pop CCS, RCT, PS, RS, CPP, CR, SS	4–11, 190–193
288	Miconazole		Cardiovascular abnormalities		Polydactyly, syndactyly, clubfoot	Anal atresia	Hypospadias, undescended testis	Oral clefts		pop CCS, pop CCS, SS	4–11, 190, 194
289	Mifepristone			Fused lower limbs		Absence of stomach	Renal agenisis	Oral clefts		CR	4–11
290	Minocycline (see Tetracycline)										

291	Minoxidil (topical)	Brain defects	Cardiac enlargement, cardiac defects	Hypotrophy of the caudal body pole, aplasia of the lower spine	Polydactyly, clinodactyly	Omphalocele	Renal agenesis	Low-set ears		CR, CR, CR	4–11, 195–196
▶292	Misoprostol	Large fontanelles	Teratology of Fallot, Cardiac defects	Pectus excavatum, shortened clavicles, hypertelorism	Syndactyly, bone reductions, adactyly, limb-reduction defects, clubfoot, clynodactyly, limb abnormalities		Hypospadias, undescended testicle	Hypoplastic scapulae, anomalies of cranium, oral clefts	IUGR, oligohydramnios	CS, CR, LACS, PS, SS	4–11, 185
293	MMI [for grave's disease]								IUGR	CR	150
294	Nabumetone (see Indomethacin)										
295	Nadolol (see Atenolol)										
296	Nalidixic Acid	Hydrocephaly								CR	4–11
297	Naproxen	Transposition of the great vessels	Ebstein's anomaly, ASD, VSD, coarctation of aorta	Hypertelorism, frontal bossing	Hypoplasia of toes			Oral clefts		CR, RS	45, 16
298	Neomycin	NTD, Hydrocephaly	Cardiac defects		Clubfoot	Gastroschisis, rectal-anal atresia	Hypospadias		Cleft palate	pop CCS	115
299	Nicoumalone (see Coumarin derivatives)										
300	Nifedipine		Cardiac defects						IUGR	CR, SS	4–11
301	Nimesulide		Constricted ductus arteriosus, ventricle dilated							CR	197
302	Nitrofurantoin	Hydrocephaly				Rectal/anal atresia/ stenosis	Genital abnormalities, renal agenesis	Ocular defects	Oesophageal atresia	pop CCS	198
303	Nitrosamines (high amount)					Gastroschisis				RS	23
304	Nonoxynol-9/ Octoxynol-9				Limb-reduction defects					CCS	4–11
305	Norethindrone	Hydrocephaly, NTD	Cardiac defects				Hypospadias	Oral clefts		CPP, SS	4–11
306	Norethynodrel		Cardiac defects				Hypospadias			CPP	4–11
307	Nortriptyline		Cardiac defects							SS	4–11
308	Norfloxacin	CNS calcification, NTD	Cardiac defects			Abdominal wall defect	Hypospadias, renal agenesis		Dwarfism ectopia cardis	PS, RS	4–11
309	Norgestrel (see Oral Contraceptives)										
310	Nystatin						Hypospadias			pop RCC	199

(*Continued*)

Table 6-1
Common Drugs (*Continued*)

▶ #	MEDICATION NAME	CENTRAL NERVOUS SYSTEM	CARDIOVASCULAR	SKELETON	EXTREMITIES	GASTROINTESTINAL	GENITOURINARY	CRANIOFACIAL	MISCELLANEOUS	DESIGN	REF#
311	Ofloxacin	Hydrocephaly, NTD	Cardiac defects				Hypospadias		IUGR	PS, RS	4–11
312	Olanzapine	Encephalocele						Cleft lip		PS	200
313	Olsalazine (see Para-amino Salycilic Acid)										
314	Omeprazole	Hydranencephaly, NTD	VSD		Clubfoot	Exomphalos	Hypospadias	Ear canal atresia	Esophageal atresia, rectal atresia	PS, RS, PS, CR	4–11, 15, 46, 26
315	Opipramol (see Imipramine)										
316	Oral contraceptives		Cardiac defects	Vertebral malformations	Limb-reduction defects		Renal malformations			CR, CS	4–11
317	Oxacarbamaz-epine		PDA, ASD							RS	67
▶ 318	Oxazepam (see Diazepam)										
319	Oxcarbazepine		Cardiac abnormality, VSD							PS, PS	58, 146
320	Oxprenolol (see Atenolol)										
321	Oxyphenbutazone (see Phenylbutazone)										
322	Oxytetracycline (see also Tetracycline)	NTD				Rectal-anal atresia, gastroschisis, pyloric stenosis		Cleft palate		pop CCS	201
323	Pantoprazole									PS	26
324	Papaverine		VSD		clubfoot					PS	24
325	Para-Amino Salicylic Acid				Limb-reduction defects		Hypospadias			CPP	4–11
326	Paracetamol	Transposition of the great vessels	Cardiac defect, VSD							RS, RS	46, 16
327	Paramethadione (see also Trimethadione)		Cardiac defects							CR, CS	4–11
328	Paramethasone		VSD							PS	24
329	Paraoxonase							Microcephaly		PS	202
330	Paroxetine				Clubfoot		Undescended testicle			RS, PS, CR	4–11, 46, 199

331	Penbutolol (see Atenolol)										
332	Penfluridol				Upper limb reduction, foot deformity					PS	66
333	Penicillamine	Intracranial hemorrhage, hydrocephaly			Clubfoot				IUGR	CR	4–11
334	Penicillamine, D			Limb defects, shoulder defects	Arthrogryposis, bridged palmar creases, camptodactyly, clubfoot, bowed femurs		Undescended testes	Flat and posteriorly rotated ears, micrognathia	Oligohydramnios, single umbilical artery, cutis laxa	CR	204
335	Penicillin V	NTD			Polydactyly					SS	4–11
336	Pentamide								IUGR	CR	4–11
337	Pentazocine		Cardiac defects		Polydactyly				IUGR	CS	4–11
338	Pentoxifylline	NTD	Cardiac defects							SS	4–11
339	Perphenazine	Microcephaly	VSD, cardiac defects		Foot deformaties			Oral clefts		PS, CPP, CR, SS	4–11, 66
340	Phenacetin		Cardiac defects	Musculoskeletal defects			Hydronephrosis, hypospadias	Craniosynostosis		CPP, SS	4–11
341	Phenazopyridine		Cardiac defects							SS	4–11
342	Phendimetrazine (see Amphetamine)										
343	Phenindione (see Coumarin Derivatives)										
344	Pheniramine							Eye and ear anomalies	Respiratory tract malformations	CPP	4–11
▶345	Phenobarbital	Microcephaly, transposition great arteries, anencephaly, NTD	Pulmonary atresia, VSD, coarctation of the aorta with abnormal valves, cardiac defect, Tetralogy of Fallot	Trigonocephaly	Dermal ridge patterns, hypoplasia of phalanges and presence of coned epiphyses in feet, digit hypoplasia, polydactyly	One kidney	Undescended testicle, hypospadias	Oral clefts, midface hypoplasia	Smaller head circumference, IUGR	CR, RS, RS, RS, PS, RS, CCS, PS, pop RS, PS/RS, PS, RS, CPP, CR, SS	4–11, 57–58, 61, 63, 114, 205–211
346	Phenprocoumon (see Coumarin Derivatives)										
347	Phentermine		VSD			Inguinal hernias				PS	108
348	Phenylbutazone	NTD	Cardiac defects							SS	4–11
349	Phenylephrine			Musculoskeletal defects	Clubfoot, syndactyly			Eye and ear anomalies		CPP	4–11
350	Phenylpropanol-amine				Polydactyly	Small intestinal atresia, gastroschisis	Hypospadias	Eye and ear anomalies		CCS, CPP	4–11, 12

(*Continued*)

Table 6-1
Common Drugs (*Continued*)

▶ #	MEDICATION NAME	CENTRAL NERVOUS SYSTEM	CARDIOVASCULAR	SKELETON	EXTREMITIES	GASTROINTESTINAL	GENITOURINARY	CRANIOFACIAL	MISCELLANEOUS	DESIGN	REF#
▶ 351	Phenytoin	NTD, microcephaly	VSD, patent foramen ovale, unspecified abnormality requiring pulmonary artery banding, dextrocardia	Sacrum defect, hypertelorism	Limb-reduction defects, dermal ridge patterns, hypoplasia of phalanges and presence of coned epiphyses in feet, digit hypoplasia, clinodactyly, polydactyly		Undescended testicle, hypospadias	Craniofacial malformations, hypoplastic midface, small and low-set ears, prominent forehead, cleft lip, hypotelorism	IUGR, micrognathia, nail hypoplasia, oesophageal atresia, stiff joints	CR, RS, RS, RS, RS, PS, PS, RS, RS, pop PS, RS, CR, PS, RS, SS	4–11, 54–57, 60, 63–64, 67, 206–208, 212
352	Phytonadione	NTD	Cardiac defects							SS	4–11
353	Pindolol (see Atenolol)										
354	Piperazine				Limb abnormalities			Oral clefts	Anophthalmia	CR	4–11
355	Piroxicam	NTD	Premature closure of ductus arteriosus		Polydactyly				Oral clefts	SS	4–11
356	Pizotifen				Clubfoot					CS	102
357	Podophyllum		Cardiac defects		Absent thumb or toe reduction					CR	4–11
▶ 358	Polychlorinated Biphenyl	Microcephaly							IUGR	PS	4–11
359	Polythiazide (see Chlorothiazide, Hydrochlorothiazide)										
360	Potassium Iodide		Cardiomegaly						IUGR, goiter	CR, CR	4–11, 150
361	Povidone-Iodine (see Potassium Iodide)										
362	Prazepam	NTD								RS	158
363	Prednisolone (see also Corticosteroids)		Cardiac defects				Urinary tract abnormalities, hypospadias	Oral clefts	IUGR, epibulbar dermoid, lipodermoids	RS/PS, CR, MA, SS	4–11, 39, 213
▶ 364	Prednisone (see also Prednisolone)	Hydrocephalus, small posterior fossa, agenesis of the corpus callosum, NTD	Peripheral pulmonic stenosis, pulmonary hypoplasia	Hypoplastic tibiae, absent fibulae, micrognathia	Radial aplasia, ulnar hypoplasia, limb-finger and toe reductions, clubfeet	Hypotrophia	Hypospadia, agenesia of bile conducts	Abnormal and low-set ears, absent external ear opening, oral clefts	Imperforate anus, subcoronal hypospadias, IUGR, single umbilical artery, umbilical hernia	CR, CR, RS, PS, PS, CS, CS	24–25, 36–38, 87, 214

365	Primatene (ephedrine, theophylline, phenobarbital)				Oligoectrosyndactyly					CS	215
▶ 366	Primidone (see also Phenobarbital)										
367	Probenecid		Cardiac defects							SS	4–11
▶ 368	Procarbazine	Intracranial hemorrhage	Cardiac defects		Limb abnormalities, oligodactyly		Malformed kidneys		IUGR	CR	4–11
369	Prochlorperazine		Cardiac defects	Skeletal defects	Limb abnormalities, limb-reduction defects			Oral clefts		CPP, CR	4–11
370	Progestagen		VSD		Clubfoot					PS	24
371	Progesterone (see Hydroxyprogesterone)										
372	Promethazine		Cardiac defects		Polydactyly					CPP, SS	4–11
373	Propiomazine		Cardiac defects				Hypospadias			RS	46
374	Propoxyphene	Microcephaly	Cardiac defects	Arthrogryposis	Limb-reduction defects, limb abnormalities	Omphalocele			Anophthalmia, microphthalmia	CPP, CR, SS	4–11
375	Propranolol (see Atenolol)					Abdominal wall defect		Full-thickness defect of the parietal scalp		CS	119
376	Propylthiouracil		Cardiac defects		Claw-like fingers with a low-set fifth finger, toe abnormalities		Hypospadias	Flat face, low-set ears, upper lip retraction, aplasia cutis congenita	Xiphoid funnel, goiter	CR, CR, CR, SS	4–11, 179, 216
377	Pseudoephedrine				Clubfoot	Small intestinal atresia, gastroschisis				CCS, CPP, SS	4–11, 12
378	Pyridostigmine		Pulmonary hypoplasia, hydrops					Oral clefts	Oesophageal atresia, hydramnios	CS	214
379	Pyridoxine				Phocomelia/amelia					CR	4–11
380	Quazepam							Oral clefts		MA	4–11
381	Quetiapine									CCS	111
382	Quinacrine	Hydrocephaly, NTD				Megacolon	Hydronephrosis, renal agenesis			CR	4–11
383	Quinapril (see Captopril)										
384	Quinethazone (see Chlorothiazide, Hydrochlorothiazide)										

(Continued)

Table 6-1
Common Drugs (*Continued*)

▶ #	MEDICATION NAME	CENTRAL NERVOUS SYSTEM	CARDIOVASCULAR	SKELETON	EXTREMITIES	GASTROINTESTINAL	GENITOURINARY	CRANIOFACIAL	MISCELLANEOUS	DESIGN	REF#
385	Quinidine	Meningocele, NTD, other abnormality of CNS			Phocomelia				IUGR	CR, RS	101, 172
386	Quinine	CNS anomalies, hydrocephaly	Cardiac defects	Vertebral anomaly	Limb deformaties	Gastrointestinal anomalies	Genitourinary abnormalities			CR, SS	4–11
387	Ramipril (see Captopril)										
388	Ranitidine	NTD	VSD, Cardiac defects		Syndactyly, clubfoot			Cleft palate		PS, SS	4–11, 24
389	Resperine	Microcephaly					Hydronephrosis, hydroureter			CPP	4–11
▶ 390	Retinoic Acid	Brain defects, hydrocephaly, microcephaly	Cardiac defects	Malformations of ribs				Malformations of cranium and ear	Microphthalmia	PS, RS	4–11
391	Rifampin	Hydrocephaly, NTD			Limb abnormalities		Renal defects			CR	4–11
392	Secobarbital (see Phenobarbital)										
393	Sertraline	NTD				Abdominal wall defect				CR	4–11
394	Silicone Breast Implants								Lower birthweight (than control babies)	RS	217
395	Simethicone		Cardiac defects		Polydactyly		Hypospadias			SS	4–11
396	Simvastatin				Polydactyly, clubfoot	Duodenal atresia	Balanic hypospadias, constriction of pyeloureteral junction	Cleft lip	IUGR, intrauterine death	CS	35
397	Sodium iodide (see Potassium Iodide)										
398	Sotalol (see Atenolol)										
399	Sparfloxacin (see Ciprofloxacin)										
400	Spermicides				Limb abnormalities, limb-reduction defects		Hypospadias			CR, PS, RS	4–11
401	Spironolactone							Oral clefts		SS	4–11
402	Streptomycin	NTD			Poly/syndactyly, Clubfoot			Cleft palate		pop CCS	115

403	Sucralfate	NTD, hydrocephaly			Polydactyly			Oral clefts		PS, SS	4–11, 24
404	Sulbactam			Pectus excavatum			Hypospadias	Oral clefts	Esophageal atresia	pop CCS	27
405	Sulfacetamide			Congenital hip dislocation						PS	15
406	Sulfadoxine-Pyrimethamine	CNS anomaly	Cardiac defects	Musculoskeletal problem		Gastrointestinal defects			IUGR, respiratory anomaly	PS/RS	173
407	Sulfasalazine	Hydrocephaly, macrocephaly	Cardiac defects		Metatarsus varus, clubfoot		Polycystic or absent kidney	Oral clefts		PS, CR	4–11, 188
408	Sulfonamides: sulfisoxazole and sulfabenzamide		Cardiac defects		Clubfoot, limb reduction, miscellaneous foot defects		Urethral obsturctions	Oral clefts		CR, CPP, PS, SS	4–11
409	Sulindac	Premature closure of ductus arteriosus								CR, SS	4–11
410	Sulphasalazine	NTD, hydrocephaly, macrocephaly	Cardiac defects		Limb deficiencies, poly/syndantyly, clubfoot		Hypospadias, undescended testis, polycystic or absent kidneys	Oral clefts		RS, CCS, CR	4–11, 153, 218
411	Sumatriptan	NTD, absent corpus callosum, holoprocephaly	ASD, VSD, pulmonary artery malformation	Hypertelorism, frontal bossing, unstable hip	Hypoplasia of toes, polydactyly, absence of hands, clubfoot, phocomelia, reduction of lower limbs		Cystic kidney, hypospadias, absent kidney	Craniostenosis, oral cleft	Branchial fistula, diaphragmatic hernia	CR, CS, PS, RS, SS	4–11, 44, 102
412	Tachipirina (Paracetamol or acetaminophen 500 mg)		Constricted ductus arteriosus, ventricle dilated, intraventricular septum bowing to the left							CR	197
413	Tacrolimus	Meningocele	Cardiac anomalies				Nonfunctional cystic kidney, urogenital defects, hypospadia, multicystic dysplastic kidney	Cleft palate	Umbilical hernia, tracheoesophageal fistula, IUGR, macrosomia	PS, RS, RS	219–221
414	Tamoxifen						Ambiguous genitalia			CR	4–11
415	Tedral (theophylline, ephedrine, phenobarbital)		Truncus arteriosus							CR	222
416	Temazepam							Oral clefts		SS	4–11
417	Tenoxicam		ASD, VSD							RS	16

(*Continued*)

Table 6-1
Common Drugs (*Continued*)

▶ #	MEDICATION NAME	CENTRAL NERVOUS SYSTEM	CARDIOVASCULAR	SKELETON	EXTREMITIES	GASTROINTESTINAL	GENITOURINARY	CRANIOFACIAL	MISCELLANEOUS	DESIGN	REF#
418	Terbinafine (topical)		ASD							RS	16
419	Terbutaline	Spine malformation	Cardiac defects							RS	46
420	Terconazole									SS	4–11
421	Terfenadine		Cardiac defects		Limb-reduction defects, polydactyly				small for gestational age	PC, SS	4–11, 223
422	Terpin hydrate				Clubfoot				Benign tumors	CPP	4–11
423	Tetanus Toxoid			Polydactyly				Oral cleft		pop CCS	224
424	Tetracycline		Cardiac defects		Clubfoot, hypoplasia of limbs, limb-reduction defects, polydactyly		Hypospadias			CPP, CR, CS, SS	4–11
▶ 425	Thalidomide		Cardiac defects	Spine defects	Limb-reduction defects, limb abnormalities		Hypospadias			CR, PS	4–11
426	Thiopropazate (see Chloropromazine)										
427	Thiothixene		Cardiac defects							SS	4–11
428	Thyroid		Cardiac defects							SS	4–11
429	Timolol (see Atenolol, Propanolol)										
430	Tobacco (smoking)								IUGR, generalized hypertonia	CS, PS, PS, RS	45, 19, 166, 225
431	Tobramycin	NTD						Cleft lip/palate		pop CCS	115
432	Tolazamide							Ear defect		CR	4–11
433	Tolbutamide		Cardiac defects		Hand and foot anomalies, clubfoot	Gastrointestinal anomalies	Renal anomalies	External ear defect		CR, CS, SS	4–11
434	Tolmetin		Premature closure of ductus arteriosus		Polydactyly					SS	4–11
▶ 435	Tretinoin (see Etretinate, Isotretinoin)										
▶ 436	Tretinoin (topical)	Holoprosencephaly, microcephaly	Cardiac defects		Upper limb reduction	Supraumbilical exomphalos		Abnormal ear	IUGR	CR	4–11

437	Triamcinolone							Oral clefts	IUGR	CR, MA	4–11
438	Triaminic (pseudoephedrine, phenylephrine, phenylpropanol-amine)				Distal limb defects					CS	215
439	Triazolam	Hydrocephaly	Cardiac defects		Polydactyly		Kidney malformations	Oral clefts	IUGR	SS, VR	4–11
440	Trichlormethiazide (see Chlorothiazide, Hydrochloroth-iazide)										
441	Trifluoperazine		Cardiac defects		Limb-reduction defects					CR, SS	4–11
442	Trimethadione	Microcephaly	Cardiac defects		Clubfoot, malformed hand		Genitourinary abnormalities	Abnormal ears, oral clefts	IUGR	CS	4–11
443	Trimethoprim-Sulfamethoxazole	Holopresencephaly	Cardiac defects	Hypotrophy of the caudal body pole, aplasia of the lower spine			Hypospadias	Oral clefts		CR, CR, SS	4–11, 195
444	Triprolidine		Cardiac defects							SS	4–11
445	Ursodeoxycholic Acid			Congenital hip dislocation		Pyloric stenosis			IUGR	RS	153
▶ 446	Valproic Acid	NTD, microcephaly, abnormal posterior fossa, right occipital encephalocele, Chiari II malformation, retrognatia, transposition of great vessels, trigonocephaly, hydrocephalus	Patent foramen ovale, ductus arteriosus, ASD, cardiomegaly, cardiac malformation, VSD, ventriculomegaly, pulmonary artery defects	Subluxation of hip, trigonocephaly, micrognathia, rib anomalies, hip dislocation	finger/toe malformations, hammer toes, decreased creases on the soles, phocomelia, limb deficiency, hypoplastic hand, forearm defect, hypoplastic phalanges, club foot/hands, annular constrictions of leg	Diaphragmatic hernia, Bilateral inguinal hernia	Hypospadias, urinary tract malformation, undescended testis	Craniosynostosis, upturned nose, long philtrum, cleft palate, flattened nasal bridge, low set malformed auriculas, very small and bow-shaped mouth with thin upper lip, facial asymmetry, coarse face	Chest wall cyst, intrauterine death, IUGR, retrognathia	CS, CS, CR, CCS, PS/RS, RS, RS, CCS, pop PS, PS, PS, CR, CCS, PS, CS, CS, CR, CCS, CR, CR, CR	56, 60, 61, 63–64, 67, 111, 114, 147, 148, 205, 226–237
447	Valsartan		Patent ductus arteriosus, coarctation of the aorta				Enlarged hyperechogenic kidneys	Cleft palate	Broadly spaced calvaria, IUGR, anhydramnios	CS	45
448	Varicella Vaccine	Holoprosencephaly	Tetralogy of Fallot		Polydactyly			Preauricular sinuses	Cystic hygroma and anasarca	PS/RS	238
449	Vinblastine (see Vincristine)										

(*Continued*)

Table 6-1
Common Drugs (*Continued*)

▶ #	MEDICATION NAME	CENTRAL NERVOUS SYSTEM	CARDIOVASCULAR	SKELETON	EXTREMITIES	GASTROINTESTINAL	GENITOURINARY	CRANIOFACIAL	MISCELLANEOUS	DESIGN	REF#
450	Vincristine (during gestation or up to one year after treatment)	NTD	Cardiac defects		Clubfoot		Malformed kidneys (reduced size and malpositioned)		IUGR	CR, CS	4–11
451	Vitamin A (retinol)	Transposition of great arteries	Cardiac defects		Limb-reduction defects			Oral clefts	Micro/anophthalmia	CCS, CR	4–11, 239
452	Vitamin E supplement (400 to 1200 IU/day)					Omphalocele			Lower birthweight (than control babies)	PS	240
▶ 453	Warfarin (see also Coumarin Derivatives)	Hydrocephalus, NTD	Coarctation of the aorta, VSD, PDA, ventriculomegaly	Chondrodysplasia, cartilage maldevelopment, pectus carinatum	Telebrachydactyly	Gastrochisis	Pyeloureteral junction syndrome	Nose/stippling/ rhizomelia, nasal hypoplasia, earfold atresia, facial dysmorphism, depressed nasal bridge	IUGR, bilobed lungs, laryngomalacia	CR, CR, CR, RS	120, 241–243
454	Yellow Fever Vaccine		VSD		Pes varus (vaccination 10 days before conception), triphalangeal hallux					PS	244
455	Zidovudine		Cardiac defects		Clubfoot, polydactyly		Hydronephrosis, polycystic kidney, renal agenesis	Oral clefts	Diaphragmatic hernia, IUGR, microphthalmia	PS, RS	4–11
456	Zuclopenthixol (see Chlorpromazine)										

CNS: central nervous system
HCS: historic cohort study
CPP: collaborative perinatal project
NTD: neural tube defect
WHO: World Health Organization
CSr: case series reports
ASD: atrial septal defect
VR: voluntary reports
CCS: case control study
SS: surveillance study
CR: case report
MA: meta-analysis
LACS: Latin-American Collaborative Study
VSD: ventral septal defect
PDA: patent ductus arteriosus
PS: prospective study
RS: retrospective study
SR: sporadic reports
CS: cohort study
M: Manufacturer
IUGR: intrauterine growth retardation
pop: population-based study

REFERENCES

1. Koren G, Brill Edwards M, Miskin M. Fetal malformations associated with drugs and chemicals: Visualization by sonography. In Maternal-Fetal Toxicology, 1st ed (Koren G, ed). Marcel Dekker, New York, 1990, pp 297–307.
2. Norgard B, Fonager K, Pedersen L, et al. Birth outcome in women exposed to 5-aminosalicylic acid during pregnancy: a Danish cohort stydy. *Gut.* 2003;52:243–247.
3. Norgard B, Pedersen L, Fonager K, et al. Azathioprine, mercaptopurine and birth outcome: a population-based cohort study. *Aliment Pharmacol Ther.* 2003;17:827–834.
4. Schardein J. Chemically Induced Birth Defects. Marcel Dekker, New York, 1985.
5. Fabro S. Reproductive Toxicology. A medical Letter. Reproductive Toxicology Center, Washington, DC, 1984.
6. Mattison DR. Reproductive Toxicology. Alan R Liss, New York, 1983.
7. Briggs GG, Freeman RK, Sumner JY. Drugs in Pregnancy and Lactation, 7th ed. Lippincott Williams & Wilkins, Baltimore, 2005.
8. Heinonen OP, Slone D, Shapiro S. Birth Defects and Drugs in Pregnancy. PSG Publishing, Littleton, MA, 1977.
9. Shepard TH. Catalog of Teratogenic Agents, 6th ed. John Hopkins University Press, Baltimore, 1989.
10. Onnis A, Grella P. The Biochemical Effects of Drugs in Pregnancy. Ellis Horwood, Chichester, 1984.
11. Berglund F, Flodh H, Lundborg P, et al. Drug use during pregnancy and breast-feeding. A classification system for drug information. *Acta Obstet Gynecol Scand Suppl.* 1984; A medical letter "Ultrasound in Industry and Medicine" 126:1–55.
12. Werler MM, Sheehan JE, Mitchell AA. Maternal medication use and risks of gastroschisis and small intestinal atresia. *Am J Epidemiol.* 2002;155:26–31.
13. Werler MM, Louik C, Mitchell AA. Epidemiologic analysis of maternal factors and amniotic band defects. *Birth Defects Res.* 2003;67:68–72.
14. Perez-Molina JJ, Alfaro-Alfaro N, Ochoa-Ponce C. Upper and lower neural tube defects: prevalence and association with illnesses and drugs. *Ginecol Obstet Mex.* 2002;70:443–450.
15. Berkovitch M, Diav-Citrin O, Greenberg R, et al. First-trimester exposure to amoxycillin/clavulanic acid: A prospective, controlled study. *Br J Clin Pharmacol.* 2004;58:298–302.
16. Ericson A, Kallen BA. Nonsteroidal anti-inflammatory drugs in early pregnancy. *Reprod Toxicol.* 2001;15:371–375.
17. Stone KM, Reiff-Eldridge R, White AD, et al. Pregnancy Outcomes following Systemic Prenatal Acyclovir Exposure: Conclusions from the International Acyclovir Pregnancy Registry, 1984–1999. *Birth Defects Res Part A Clin Mol Teratol.* 2004;70:201–207.
18. Aktas D, Tuncbilek E, Onderoglu L. Chromosomal mosaicism in a pregnant woman treated with acyclovir for herpes simplex encephalitis. *Am J Perinatol.* 2001;18:179–183.
19. Bada HS, Das A, Bauer CR, et al. Gestational cocaine exposure and intrauterine growth: Maternal lifestyle study. *Obstet Gynecol.* 2002;100(5 Pt 1):916–924.
20. Kashiwagi M, Chaoui R, Stallmach T, et al. Fetal Bilateral Renal Agenesis, Phocomelia, and Single Umbilical Artery Associated with Cocaine Abuse in Early Pregnancy. *Birth Defects Res Part A Clin Mol Teratol.* 2003;67:951–952.
21. Kesrouani A, Fallet C, Vuillard E, et al. Pathologic and laboratory correlation in microcephaly associated with prenatal cocaine exposure. *Early Hum Dev.* 2001;63:79–81.
22. McElhatton PR, Bateman DN, Evans C, et al. Congenital anomalies after prenatal ecstasy exposure. *Lancet.* 1999;354:1441–1442.
23. Torfs CP, Lam PK, Schaffer DM, et al. Association between mothers' nutrient intake and their offspring's risk of gastroschisis. *Teratology.* 1998;58:241–250.
24. Garbis H, Elefant E, Diav-Citrin O, et al. Pregnancy outcome after exposure to ranitidine and other H2-blockers: A collaborative study of the European Network of Teratology Information Services. *Reprod Toxicol.* 2005;19:453–458.
25. Vaux KK, Kahole NCO, Jones KL. Cyclophosphamide, Methotre-xate, and Cytarabine Embropathy: Is Apoptosis the Common Pathway? *Birth Defects Res Part A Clin Mol Teratol.* 2003;67:403–408.
26. Diav-Citrin O, Arnon J, Shechtman S, et al. The safety of proton pump inhibitors in pregnancy: A multicentre prospective controlled study. *Aliment Pharmacol Ther.* 2005;21:269–275.
27. Czeizel AE, Rockenbauer M, Sorensen HT, et al. A population-based case-control teratologic study of ampicillin treatment during pregnancy. *Am J Obstet Gynecol.* 2001;185:140–147.
28. Terrone DA, Rinehart BK, Einstein MH, et al. Neonatal sepsis and death caused by resistant Escherichia coli: possible consequences of extended maternal ampicillin administration. *Am J Obstet Gynecol.* 1999;180:1345–1348.
29. Orrett FA, Shurland SM. Neonatal sepsis and mortality in a region hospital in Trinidad: Aetiology and risk factors. *Ann Trop Paediatr.* 2001;21:20–25.
30. Butters L, Kennedy S, Rubin PC. Atenolol in essential hypertension during pregnancy. *BMJ.* 1990;301:587–589.
31. Lip GYH, Beevers M, Churchill D, et al. Effect of atenolol on birth weight. *Am J Cardiol.* 1997;79:1436–1438.
32. Lydakis C, Lip GYH, Beevers M, et al. Atenolol and fetal growth in pregnancies complicated by hypertension. *Am J Hypertens.* 1999;12:541–547.
33. Bayliss H, Churchill D, Beevers M, Beevers DG. Anti-hypertensive drugs in pregnancy and fetal growth: evidence for "pharmacological programming" in the first trimester? *Hypertens Pregnancy.* 2002;21:161–174.
34. Easterling TR, Carr DB, Brateng D, et al. Treatment of hypertension in pregnancy: effect of atenolol on maternal disease, preterm delivery, and fetal growth. *Obstet Gynecol.* 2001;98:427–433.
35. Edison RJ, Muenke M. Mechanistic and epidemiologic considerations in the evaluation of adverse birth outcomes following gestational exposure to statins. *Am J Med Genet.* 2004;Part A. 131:287–298.
36. Bar J, Stahl B, Hod M, et al. Is immunosuppression therapy in renal allograft recipients teratogenic? A single-center experience. *Am J Med Genet.* 2003;Part A. 116:31–36.
37. Moon JI, Park SG, Cheon KO, et al. Pregnancy in renal transplant patients. *Transplant Proc.* 2000;32:1869–1870.
38. Sgro MD, Barozzino T, Mirghani HM, et al. Pregnancy outcome post renal transplantation. *Teratology.* 2002;65:5–9.
39. Willis FR, Findlay CA, Gorrie MJ, et al. Children of renal transplant recipient mothers. *Paediatr Child Health.* 2000;36(3):230–235.
40. Mahon BE, Rosenman MB, Kleiman MB. Maternal and infant use of erythromycin and other macrolide antibiotics as risk factors for infantile hypertrophic pyloric stenosis. *J Pediatr.* 2001;139:380–384.
41. Cox RM, Anderson JM, Cox P. Defective embryogenesis with angiotensin II receptor antagonists in pregnancy. *BJOG.* 2003;110:1038.
42. Subtil D, Tiberghien P, Devos P, et al. Immediate and delayed effects of antenatal corticosteroids on fetal heart rate: a randomized trial that compares betamethasone acetate and phosphate, betamethasone phosphate, and dexamethasone. *American Am J Obstet Gynecol.* 2003;188:524–531.
43. Suarez RD, Grobman WA, Parilla BV. Indomethacin tocolysis and intraventricular hemorrhage. *Obstet Gynecol.* 2001;97:921–925.
44. Kajantie E, Somer M. Bilateral cleft lip and palate, hypertelorism and hypoplastic toes. *Clin Dysmorphol.* 2004;13:195–196.
45. Schaefer C. Angiotensin II-receptor-antagonists: Further evidence of fetotoxicity but not teratogenicity. *Birth Defects Res Part A Clin Mol Teratol.* 2003;67:591–594.
46. Kallen B. Fluoxetine use in early pregnancy. *Birth Defects Res Part B Dev Reprod Toxicol.* 2004;71:395–396.

47. Kallen B, Rydhstroem H, Aberg A. Congenital malformations after the use of inhaled budesonide in early pregnancy. *Obstet Gynecol.* 1999;93:392–395.
48. Ross D. High dose buprenorphine in pregnancy. *Aust N Z J Obstet Gynaecol.* 2004;44:80.
49. Habal MB, Castelano C, Hemkes N, et al. In search of causative factors of deformational plagiocephaly. *J Craniofac Surg.* 2004; 15:835–841.
50. Eskenazi B, Stapleton AL, Kharrazi M, et al. Associations between maternal decaffeinated and caffeinated coffee consumption and fetal growth and gestational duration. *Epidemiology.* 1999;10:242–249.
51. Cook DG, Peacock JL, Feyerabend C, et al. Relation of caffeine intake and blood caffeine concentrations during pregnancy to fetal growth: prospective population based study. *BMJ.* 1996;313: 1358–1362.
52. Callies F, Arlt W, Scholz HJ, et al. Management of hypoparathyroidism during pregnancy—Report of twelve cases. *Eur J Endicronol.* 1998;139:284–289.
53. Lambot MA, Vermeylen D, Noel JC. Angiotensin-II-receptor inhibitors in pregnancy. *Lancet.* 2001;357:1619–1620.
54. Wester U, Brandberg G, Larsson M, et al. Chondrodysplasia punctata (CDP) with features of the tibia-metacarpal type and maternal phenytoin treatment during pregnancy. *Prenat Diagn.* 2002;22: 663–668.
55. Wide K, Winbladh B, Tomson T, et al. Psychomotor development and minor anomalies in children exposed to antiepileptic drugs in utero: A prospective population-based study. *Dev Med Child Neurol.* 2000;42:87–92.
56. Kaaja E, Kaaja R, Hiilesmaa V. Major malformations in offspring of women with epilepsy. *Neurology*;60:575–579.
57. Holmes LB, Coull BA, Dorfman J, et al. The correlation of deficits in IQ with midface and digit hypoplasia in children exposed in utero to anticonvulsant drugs. *J Pediatr.* 2005;146:118–122.
58. Meischenguiser R, D'Giano CH, Ferraro SM. Oxcarbazepine in pregnancy: clinical experience in Argentina. *Epilepsy Behav.* 2004;5:163–167.
59. Diav-Citrin O, Shechtman S, Arnon J, et al. Is carbamazepine teratogenic? A prospective controlled study of 210 pregnancies. *Neurology.* 2001;57:321–324.
60. Holmes LB, Harvey EA, Coull BA, et al. The teratogenicity of anticonvulsant drugs. *N Engl J Med.* 2001;344:1132–1138.
61. Fairgrieve SD, Jackson M, Jonas P, et al. Population based, prospective study of the care of women with epilepsy in pregnancy. *BMJ.* 2000;321:674–675.
62. Kaaja E, Kaaja R, Hiilesmaa V. Major malformations in offspring of women with epilepsy. *Neurology.* 2003;60:575–579.
63. Samren EB, Van Duijn CM, Christiaens GCML, et al. Antiepileptic drug regimens and major congenital abnormalities in the offspring. *Ann Neurol.* 1999;46:739–746.
64. Al Bunyan M, Abo-Talib Z. Outcome of pregnancies in epileptic women: A study in Saudi Arabia. *Seizure.* 1999;8:26–29.
65. Werler MM, Bower C, Payne J, et al. Findings on potential teratogens from a case-control study in Western Australia. *Aust N Z J Obstet Gynaecol.* 2003;43:443–447.
66. Diav-Citrin O, Shechtman S, Ornoy S, et al. Safety of haloperidol and penfluridol in pregnancy: a multicenter, prospective, controlled study. *J Clin Psychiatry.* 2005;66:317–322.
67. Cunnington M, Tennis P. Lamotrigine and the risk of malformations in pregnancy. *Neurology.* 2005;64:955–960.
68. Di Gianantonio E, Schaefer C, Mastroiacovo PP, et al. Adverse effects of prenatal methimazole exposure. *Teratology.* 2001;64:262–266.
69. Ericson A, Kallen B, Wilholm BE. Delivery outcome after the use of antidepressants in early pregnancy. *Eur J Clin Pharmacol.* 1999; 55:503–508.
70. Nishijima K, Shukunami K, Kotsuji F. Natural history of bacterial vaginosis and intermediate flora in pregnancy and effect of oral clindamycin. *Obstet Gynecol.* 2004;104:1106–1107.
71. Joesoef MR, Hillier SL, Wiknjosastro G, et al. Intravaginal clindamycin treatment for bacterial vaginosis: effects on preterm delivery and low birth weight. *Am J Obstet Gynecol.* 1995;173: 1527–1531.
72. Sorensen HT, Pedersen L, Skriver MV, et al. Use of clomifene during early pregnancy and risk of hypospadias: Population based case-control study. *BMJ.* 2005;330(7483):126–127.
73. Sorensen HT, Pedersen L, Skriver MV, et al. Use of clomifene during early pregnancy and risk of hypospadias: population based case-control study. *BMJ.* 2005;330:126–127.
74. Lin AE, Peller AJ, Westgate MN, et al. Clonazepam use in pregnancy and the risk of malformations. *Birth Defects Res A Clin Mol Teratol.* 2004;70:534–536.
75. Marles SL, Reed M, Evans JA. Humeroradial synostosis, ulnar aplasia and oligodactyly, with contralateral amelia, in a child with prenatal cocaine exposure. *Am J Med Genet A.* 2003;116:85–89.
76. Singer LT, Salvator A, Arendt R, et al. Effects of cocaine/polydrug exposure and maternal psychological distress on infant birth outcomes. *Neurotoxicol Teratol.* 2002;24:127–135.
77. Bandstra ES, Morrow CE, Anthony JC, et al. Intrauterine growth of full-term infants: Impact of prenatal cocaine exposure. *Pediatrics.* 2001;108:1309–1319.
78. Bellini C, Massocco D, Serra G. Prenatal cocaine exposure and the expanding spectrum of brain malformations. *Arch Intern Med.* 2000;160:2393.
79. Kuhn L, Kline J, Ng S, et al. Cocaine use during pregnancy and intrauterine growth retardation: New insights based on maternal hair tests. *Am J Epidemiol.* 2000;152:112–119.
80. Bateman DA, Chiriboga CA. Dose-response effect of cocaine on newborn head circumference. *Pediatrics.* 2000;106:E33.
81. Messner U, Gunkel C, Dressler F, et al. Maternal and fetal outcome in pregnancies of opioid-dependent women. *Zentralblatt fur Gynakologie.* 1999;121:281–286.
82. Lorenzo AJ, Twickler DM, Baker LA. Megacystis microcolon intestinal hypoperistalsis syndrome with bilateral duplicated systems. *Urology.* 2003,62:144.
83. Czeizel AE, Petik D, Vargha P. Validation studies of drug exposures in pregnant women. *Pharmacoepidemiol Drug Saf.* 2003;12: 409–416.
84. Gur C, Diav-Citrin O, Shechtman S, et al. Pregnancy outcome after first trimester exposure to corticosteroids: A prospective controlled study. *Reprod Toxicol.* 2004;18:93–101.
85. Murphy DJ. Effect of antenatal corticosteroids on postmortem brain weight of preterm babies. *Early Hum Dev.* 2001;63:113–122.
86. Yost NP, McIntire DD, Wians Jr FH, et al. A randomized, placebo-controlled trial of corticosteroids for hyperemesis due to pregnancy. *Obstet Gynecol.* 2003;102:1250–1254.
87. Paladini D, Vassallo M, D'Armiento MR, et al. Prenatal detection of multiple fetal anomalies following inadvertent exposure to cyclophosphamide in the first trimester of pregnancy. *Birth Defects Res Part A Clin Mol Teratol.* 2004;70:99–100.
88. Enns GM, Roeder E, Chan RT, et al. Apparent cyclophosphamide (cytoxan) embryopathy: a distinct phenotype?. *Am J Med Genet.* 1999;86:237–241.
89. Choudhry VP, Gupta S, Gupta M, et al. Pregnancy associated aplastic anemia—a series of 10 cases with review of literature. *Hematology.* 2002;7:233–238.
90. Golding J, Vivian S, Baldwin JA. Maternal anti-nauseants and clefts of lip and palate. *Hum Toxicol.* 1983;2:63–73.
91. Cissoko H, Jonville-Bera AP, Autret-Leca E. New antiepileptic drugs in pregnancy: Outcome series of 12 exposed pregnancies. *Therapie.* 2002;57:397–401.
92. LeFlore JL, Salhab WA, Sue BR, et al. Association of antenatal and postnatal dexamethasone exposure with outcomes in extremely low birth weight neonates. *Pediatrics.* 2002;110(2 Pt 1):275–279.
93. Bloom SL, Sheffield JS, McIntire DD, et al. Antenatal dexamethasone and decreased birth weight. *Obstet Gynecol.* 2001;97(4):485–490.

94. Franckart G, Kurz X, Adam E, et al. Multiple benefit of antenatal corticotherapy. Current status in the Belgian French Community. *Rev Med Liege.* 1999;54:157–165.
95. Martinez-Frias ML, Rodriguez-Pinilla E. Epidemiologic analysis of prenatal exposure to cough medicines containing dextromethorphan: No evidence of human teratogenicity. *Teratology.* 2001;63:38–41.
96. Martinez-Lage JF, Almagro MJ, Lopez HF, et al. Aplasia cutis congenita of the scalp. *Childs Nerv Syst.* 2002;18:634–637.
97. Flint C, Larsen H, Nielsen GL, et al. Pregnancy outcome after suicide attempt by drug use: a Danish population-based study. *Acta Obstet Gynecol Scand.* 2002;81:516–522.
98. Auer M, Brezinka C, Eller P, et al. Prenatal diagnosis of intrauterine premature closure of the ductus arteriosus following maternal diclofenac application. *Ultrasound Obstet Gynecol.* 2004;23:513–516.
99. Porta RR, Cespedes MC, Molina V, et al. Premature closure of the fetal ductus arterious after maternal treatment with diclofenac. *Pediatria Catalana.* 2003;63:177–180.
100. Jouannic JM, Delahaye S, Le Bidois J, et al. Results of prenatal management of fetuses with supraventricular tachycardia. A series of 66 cases. *J Gynecol Obstet Biol Reprod.* (Paris) 2003;32:338–344.
101. Yu HT, Chang YL, Chao AS, et al. Prenatal diagnosis and management of fetal atrial flutter: A case report. *Journal of Medical Ultrasound.* 2003;11:160–162.
102. Kallen B, Lygner E. Delivery outcome in women who used drugs for migraine during pregnancy with special reference to sumatriptan. *Headache.* 2001;41:351–356.
103. Boskovic R, Rudic N, Danieliewska-Nikiel B, et al. Is lack of morning sickness teratogenic? A prospective controlled study. *Birth Defects Res A Clin Mol Teratol.* 2004;70(8):528–530.
104. Gallo M, Sarkar M, Au W, et al. Pregnancy outcome following gestational exposure to echinacea: a prospective controlled study. *Arch Intern Med.* 2000;160:3141–3143.
105. Bateman DN, McElhatton PR, Dickinson D, et al. A case control study to examine the pharmacological factors underlying ventricular septal defects in the North of England. *European J Clin Pharmacol.* 2004;60:635–641.
106. Tabacova S, Little R, Tsong Y, et al. Adverse pregnancy outcomes associated with maternal enalapril antihypertensive treatment. *Pharmacoepidemiol Drug Saf.* 2003;12:633–646.
107. Czeizel AE, Rockenbauer M, Sorensen HT, et al. A population-based case-control teratologic study of oral erythromycin treatment during pregnancy. *Reprod Toxicol.* 1999;13:531–536.
108. Jones KL, Johnson KA, Dick LM, et al. Pregnancy outcomes after first trimester exposure to phentermine/fenfluramine. *Teratology.* 2002;65:125–130.
109. Rodriguez-Pinilla E, Mejias C, Pavon MT, et al. Imidazole antifungal agents and pregnancy. *Progresos de Obstetricia y Ginecologia.* 1999;42:359–364.
110. Sorensen HT, Nielsen GL, Olesen C, et al. Risk of malformations and other outcomes in children exposed to fluconazole in utero. *Br J Clin Pharmacol.* 1999;48:234–238.
111. Yaris F, Ulku C, Kesim M, Kadioglu M, Unsal M, Dikici MF et al. Psychotropic drugs in pregnancy: A case-control study. *Prog Neuropsychopharmacol Biol Psychiatry.* 2005;29:333–338.
112. Cohen LS, Heller VL, Bailey JW, et al. Birth outcomes following prenatal exposure to fluoxetine. *Biol Psychiatry.* 2000;48:996–1000.
113. Czeizel AE, Rockenbauer M, Mosonyi A. Furosemide as a fetal growth promoter. *Clinical Drug Investigation.* 2000;20:53–60.
114. Montouris G. Gabapentin exposure in human pregnancy: Results from the gabapentin pregnancy registry. *Epilepsy Behav.* 2003; 4:310–317.
115. Czeizel AE, Rockenbauer M, Olsen J, et al. A teratological study of aminoglycoside antibiotic treatment during pregnancy. *Scand J Infect Dis.* 2000;32:309–313.
116. Portnoi G, Chng LA, Karimi-Tabesh L, et al. Prospective comparative study of the safety and effectiveness of ginger for the treatment of nausea and vomiting in pregnancy. *Am J Obstet Gynecol.* 2003;189:1374–1377.
117. Langer O, Conway DL, Berkus MD, et al. A comparison of glyburide and insulin in women with gestational diabetes mellitus. *N Engl J Med.* 2000;343:1134–1138.
118. Czeizel AE, Metneki J, Kazy Z, et al. A population-based case-control study of oral griseofulvin treatment during pregnancy. *Acta Obstet Gynecol Scand.* 2004;83:827–831.
119. Ferraris S, Valenzise M, Lerone M, et al. Malformations following methimazole exposure in utero: an open issue. *Birth Defects Res Part A Clin Mol Teratol.* 2003;67:989–992.
120. Nassar AH, Hobeika EM, Abd Essamad HM, et al. Pregnancy outcome in women with prosthetic heart valves. *Am J Obstet Gynecol.* 2004;191:1009–1013.
121. Maruyama K, Ikeda H, Koizumi T, et al. Prenatal and postnatal histories of very low birthweight infants who developed hepatoblastoma. *Pediatr Int.* 1999;41:82–89.
122. Costedoat-Chalumeau N, Amoura Z, Duhaut P, et al. Safety of Hydroxychloroquine in Pregnant Patients With Connective Tissue Diseases: A Study of One Hundred Thirty-Three Cases Compared With a Control Group. *Arthritis Rheum.* 2003;48:3207–3211.
123. Klinger G, Morad Y, Westall CA, et al. Ocular toxicity and antenatal exposure to chloroquine or hydroxychloroquine for rheumatic diseases. *Lancet.* 2001;358:813–814.
124. Abbasi S, Gerdes JS, Sehdev HM, et al. Neonatal outcome after exposure to indomethacin in utero: A retrospective case cohort study. *Am J Obstet Gynecol.* 2003;189:782–785.
125. Butler-O'Hara M, D'Angio CT. Risk of persistent renal insufficiency in premature infants following the prenatal use of indomethacin for suppression of preterm labor. *J Perinatol.* 2002;22:541–546.
126. Rasanen J, Debbs RH, Wood DC, et al. The effects of maternal indomethacin therapy on human fetal branch pulmonary arterial vascular impedance. *Ultrasound Obstet Gynecol.* 1999;13: 112–126.
127. Vermillion ST, Newman RB. Recent indomethacin tocolysis is not associated with neonatal complications in preterm infants. *Am J Obstet Gynecol.* 1999;181:1083–1086.
128. Howorka K, Pumprla J, Gabriel M, et al. Normalization of pregnancy outcome in pregestational diabetes through functional insulin treatment and modular out-patient education adapted for pregnancy. *Diabet Med.* 2001;18:965–972.
129. Hellmuth E, Damm P, Molsted-Pedersen L, et al. Prevalence of nocturnal hypoglycemia in first trimester of pregnancy in patients with insulin treated diabetes mellitus. *Acta Obstet Gynecol Scand.* 2000;79:958–962.
130. Evers IM, de Valk HW, Visser GH. Risk of complications of pregnancy in women with type 1 diabetes: nationwide prospective study in the Netherlands. *BMJ.* 2004;328:915.
131. Scherbaum WA, Lankisch MR, Pawlowski B, et al. Insulin Lispro in pregnancy—retrospective analysis of 33 cases and matched controls. *Exp Clin Endocrinol Diabetes.* 2002;110:6–9.
132. Bhattacharyya A, Brown S, Hughes S, et al. Insulin lispro and regular insulin in pregnancy. *Qjm.* 2001;94:255–260.
133. Hiratsuka M, Minakami H, Koshizuka S, et al. Administration of interferon-a during pregnancy: Effects on fetus. *J Perinat Med.* 2000;28:372–376.
134. Watanabe M, Kohge N, Akagi S, et al. Congenital anomalies in a child born from a mother with interferon-treated chronic hepatitis B. *Am J Gastroenterol.* 2001;96:1668–1669.
135. Martinelli P, Martinelli V, Agangi A, et al. Interferon alfa treatment for pregnant women affected by essential thrombocythemia: case reports and a review. *Am J Obstet Gynecol.* 2004;191:2016–2020.
136. Mubarak AA, Kakil IR, Awidi A, et al. Normal outcome of pregnancy in chronic myeloid leukemia treated with interferon-alpha in 1st trimester: report of 3 cases and review of the literature. *Am J Hematol.* 2002;69:115–118.
137. Hoppen T, Eis-Hubinger AM, Schild RL, et al. Intrauterine herpes simplex virus infection. *Klin Padiatr.* 2001;213:63–68.

138. Fried M, Muga RO, Misore AO, et al. Malaria elicits type 1 cytokines in the human placenta: IFN-gamma and TNF- alpha associated with pregnancy outcomes. *J Immunol.* 1998;160:2523–2530.
139. Fadeyev V, Lesnikova S, Melnichenko G. Prevalence of thyroid disorders in pregnant women with mild iodine deficiency. *Gynecol Endocrinol.* 2003;17:413–418.
140. Ishijima K, Sando I. Multiple temporal bone anomalies in isotretinoin syndrome: a temporal bone histopathologic case report. *Arch Otolaryngol Head Neck Surg.* 1999;125:1385–1388.
141. Ceviz N, Ozkan B, Eren S, et al. A case of isotretinoin embryopathy with bilateral anotia and Taussig-Bing malformation. *Turk J Pediatr.* 2000;42:239–241.
142. Honein MA, Paulozzi LJ, Erickson JD. Continued occurrence of Accutane-exposed pregnancies. *Teratology.* 2001;64:142–147.
143. Moerike S, Pantzar JT, De Sa D. Temporal bone pathology in fetuses exposed to isotretinoin. *Pediatr Dev Pathol.* 2002;5:405–409.
144. Bar-Oz B, Moretti ME, Bishai R, et al. Pregnancy outcome after in utero exposure to itraconazole: a prospective cohort study. *Am J Obstet Gynecol.* 2000;183:617–620.
145. Cabou C, Lacroix I, Rista C, et al. Finger agenesis after in utero exposure to ketoconazole: A case report. *Therapie.* 2003;58:172–174.
146. Diket AL, Nolan TE. Anxiety and depression diagnosis amd treatment during pregnancy. *Obstet Gynecol Clin North Am.* 1997;24: 535–557.
147. Sabers A, Dam M, Rogvi-Hansen B, et al. Epilepsy and pregnancy: lamotrigine as main drug used. *Acta Neurol Scand.* 2004;109:9–13.
148. Ozkinay F, Cogulu O, Gunduz C, et al. Valproic acid and lamotrigine treatment during pregnancy: The risk of chromosomal abnormality. *Mutat Res.* 2003;534:197–199.
149. Rotondi M, Caccavale C, Di Serio C, et al. Successful outcome of pregnancy in a thyroidectomized-parathyroidectomized young woman affected by severe hypothyroidism. *Thyroid.* 1999; 9:1037–1040.
150. Yamashita Y, Yamane K, Fujikawa R, et al. A successful pregnancy and delivery case of Graves' disease with myeloperoxidase antineutrophil cytoplasmic antibody induced by propylthiouracil. *Endocr J.* 2002;49:555–559.
151. Grover S, Gupta N. Lithium-associated anencephaly. *Can J Psychiatry.* 2005;50:185–186.
152. Einarson A, Mastroiacovo P, Arnon J, et al. Prospective, controlled, multicentre study of loperamide in pregnancy. *Can J Gastroenterol.* 2000;14:185–187.
153. Marteau P, Tennenbaum R, Elefant E, et al. Foetal outcome in women with inflammatory bowel disease treated during pregnancy with oral mesalazine microgranules. *Aliment Pharmacol Ther.* 1998;12:1101–1108.
154. Diav-Citrin O, Shechtman S, Aharonovich A, et al. Pregnancy outcome after gestational exposure to loratadine or antihistamines: A prospective controlled cohort study. *J Allergy Clin Immunol.* 2003;1239–1243.
155. Moretti ME, Caprara D, Coutinho CJ, et al. Fetal safety of loratadine use in the first trimester of pregnancy: a multicenter study. *J Allergy Clin Immunol.* 2003;111:479–483.
156. Centers for Disease Control and Prevention (CDC). Evaluation of an association between loratadine and hypospadias—United States, 1997–2001. *MMWR Morb Mortal Wkly Rep.* 2004;53:219–221.
157. Bonnot O, Vollset SE, Godet PF, et al. In utero exposure to benzodiazepine. Is there a risk for anal atresia with lorazepam? *Encephale.* 2003;29:553–559.
158. Bonnot O, Vollset SE, Godet PF, et al. Maternal exposure to lorazepam and anal atresia in newborns: results from a hypothesis-generating study of benzodiazepines and malformations. *J Clin Psychopharmacol.* 2001;21:456–458.
159. Saji H, Yamanaka M, Hagiwara A, et al. Losartan and fetal toxic effects. *Lancet.* 2001;357:363.
160. Nayar B, Singhal A, Aggarwal R, et al. Losartan induced fetal toxicity. *Indian J Pediatr.* 2003;70:923–924.
161. Mittendorf R, Dambrosia J, Pryde PG, et al. Association between the use of antenatal magnesium sulfate in preterm labor and adverse health outcomes in infants. *Am J Obstet Gynecol.* 2002;186:1111–1118.
162. Malaeb SN, Rassi AI, Haddad MC, et al. Bone mineralization in newborns whose mothers received magnesium sulphate for tocolysis of premature labour. *Pediatr Radiol.* 2004;34:384–386.
163. Elimian A, Verma R, Ogburn P, et al. Magnesium sulfate and neonatal outcomes of preterm neonates. *J Matern Fetal Neonatal Med.* 2002;12:118–122.
164. Matsuda Y, Maeda Y, Ito M, et al. Effect of magnesium sulfate treatment on neonatal bone abnormalities. *Gynecol Obstet Invest.* 1997;44:82–88.
165. Santi MD, Henry GW, Douglas GL. Magnesium sulfate treatment of preterm labor as a cause of abnormal neonatal bone mineralization. *J Pediatr Orthop.* 1994;14:249–253.
166. Sherwood RA, Keating J, Kavvadia V, et al. Substance misuse in early pregnancy and relationship to fetal outcome. *Eur J Pediatr.* 1999;158:488–492.
167. Diav-Citrin O, Shechtman S, Arnon J, et al. Pregnancy outcome after gestational exposure to mebendazole: a prospective controlled cohort study. *Am J Obstet Gynecol.* 2003;188:282–285.
168. de Silva NR, Sirisena JL, Gunasekera DP, et al. Effect of mebendazole therapy during pregnancy on birth outcome. *Lancet.* 1999; 353:1145–1149.
169. Kallen B, Mottet I. Delivery outcome after the use of meclozine in early pregnancy. *Eur J Epidemiol.* 2003;18:665–669.
170. Adam I, Ali DA, Alwaseila A, et al. Mefloquine in the treatment of falciparum malaria during pregnancy in Eastern Sudan. *Saudi Med J.* 2004;25:1400–1402.
171. Smoak BL, Writer JV, Keep LW, et al. The effects of inadvertent exposure of mefloquine chemoprophylaxis on pregnancy outcomes and infants of US army servicewomen. *J Infect Dis.* 1997; 176:831–833.
172. Nosten F, Vincenti M, Simpson J, et al. The effects of mefloquine treatment in pregnancy. *Clin Infect Dis.* 1999;28:808–815.
173. Phillips-Howard PA, Steffen R, et al. Safety of mefloquine and other antimalarial agents in the first trimester of pregnancy. *J Travel Med.* 1998;5:121–126.
174. Letson GW, Little JR, Ottman J, et al. Meningoccal vaccine in pregnancy: An assessment of infant risk. *Pediatr Infect Dis J.* 1998;17:261–263.
175. Francella A, Dyan A, Bodian C, et al. The safety of 6-mercaptopurine for childbearing patients with inflammatory bowel disease: a retrospective cohort study. *Gastroenterology.* 2003;124:9–17.
176. Diav-Citrin O, Park YH, Veerasuntharam G, et al. The safety of mesalamine in human pregnancy: A prospective controlled cohort study. *Gastroenterology.* 1998;114:23–28.
177. Vanky E, Salvesen KA, Heimstad R, et al. Metformin reduces pregnancy complications without affecting androgen levels in pregnant polycystic ovary syndrome women: results of a randomized study. *Hum Reprod.* 2004;19:1734–1740.
178. Kashiwagi M, Arlettaz R, Lauper U, et al. Methadone maintenance program in a Swiss perinatal center: (I): Management and outcome of 89 pregnancies. *Acta Obstet Gynecol Scand.* 2005;84:140–144.
179. Karg E, Bereg E, Gaspar L, et al. Aplasia cutis congenita after methimazole exposure in utero. Pediatr Dermatol 2004;21:491–494.
180. Barbero P, Ricagni C, Mercado G, et al. Choanal atresia associated with prenatal methimazole exposure: Three new patients. *Am J Med Genet A.* 2004;129:83–86.
181. Rodriguez-Garcia R. Bilateral renal agenesis (Potter syndrome) in a newborn of a hyperthyroid woman receiving methimazole during early pregnancy. *Ginecologia y Obstetricia de Mexico.* 1999; 67:587–589.
182. Clementi M, Di Gianantonio E, Pelo E, et al. Methimazole embryopathy: Delineation of the phenotype. *Am J Med Genet.* 1999;83:43–46.
183. Krahenmann F, OStensen M, Stallmach T, et al. In utero first trimester exposure to low-dose methotrexate with increased fetal

nuchal translucency and associated malformations. *Prenat Diagn.* 2002;22:489–490.
184. Granzow JW, Thaller SR, Panthaki Z. Cleft palate and toe malformations in a child with fetal methotrexate exposure. *J Craniofac Surg.* 2003;14:747–748.
185. Adam MP, Manning MA, Beck AE, et al. Methotrexate/misoprostol embryopathy: report of four cases resulting from failed medical abortion. *Am J Med Genet.* 2003;Part A. 123:72–78.
186. Yedlinsky NT, Morgan FC, Whitecar PW. Anomalies associated with failed methotrexate and misoprostol termination. *Obstet Gynecol.* 2005;105:1203–1205.
187. Nguyen C, Duhl AJ, Escallon CS, et al. Multiple anomalies in a fetus exposed to low-dose methotrexate in the first trimester. *Obstet Gynecol.* 2002;99:599–602.
188. Lewden B, Vial T, Elefant E, et al. Low dose methotrexate in the first trimester of pregnancy: results of a French collaborative study. *J Rheumatol.* 2004;31:2360–2365.
189. Sorensen HT, Nielsen GL, Christensen K, et al. Birth outcome following maternal use of metoclopramide. *Br J Clin Pharmacol.* 2000;49:264–268.
190. Kazy Z, Puho E, Czeizel AE. The possible association between the combination of vaginal metronidazole and miconazole treatment and poly-syndactyly: Population-based case-control teratologic study. *Reprod Toxicol.* 2005;20:89–94.
191. Kigozi GG, Brahmbhatt H, Wabwire-Mangen F, et al. Treatment of Trichomonas in pregnancy and adverse outcomes of pregnancy: A subanalysis of a randomized trial in Rakai, Uganda. *Am J Obstet Gynecol.* 2003;189:1398–13400.
192. Diav-Citrin O, Shechtman S, Gotteiner T, et al. Pregnancy outcome after gestational exposure to metronidazole: a prospective controlled cohort study. *Teratology.* 2001;63:186–192.
193. Sorensen HT, Larsen H, Jensen ES, et al. Safety of metronidazole during pregnancy: a cohort study of risk of congenital abnormalities, preterm delivery and low birth weight in 124 women. *J Antimicrob Chemother.* 1999;44:854–856.
194. Czeizel AE, Kazy Z, Puho E. Population-based case-control teratologic study of topical miconazole. *Congenit Anom (Kyoto).* 2004; 44:41–45.
195. Rojansky N, Fasouliotis SJ, Ariel I, et al. Extreme caudal agenesis. Possible drug-related etiology? *J Reprod Med.* 2002;47:241–245.
196. Smorlesi C, Caldarella A, Caramelli L, et al. Topically applied minoxidil may cause fetal malformation: a case report. *Birth Defects Res A Clin Mol Teratol.* 2003;67:997–1001.
197. Simbi KA, Secchieri S, Rinaldo M, et al. In utero ductal closure following near-term maternal self-medication with nimesulide and acetaminophen. *Journal Obstet Gynaecol.* 2002;22:440–441.
198. Czeizel AE, Rockenbauer M, Sorensen HT, et al. Nitrofurantoin and congenital abnormalities. *Eur J Obstet Gynecol Reprod Biol.* 2001;95:119–126.
199. Czeizel AE, Kazy Z, Puho E. A population-based case-control teratological study of oral nystatin treatment during pregnancy. *Scand J Infect Dis.* 2003;35:830–835.
200. McKenna K, Koren G, Tetelbaum M, et al. Pregnancy outcome of women using atypical antipsychotic drugs: A prospective comparative study. *J Clin Psychiatry.* 2005;66:444–449.
201. Czeizel AE, Rockenbauer M. A population-based case-control teratologic study of oral oxytetracycline treatment during pregnancy. *Eur J Obstet Gynecol Reprod Biol.* 2000;88:27–33.
202. Berkowitz GS, Wetmur JG, Birman-Deych E, et al. In utero pesticide exposure, maternal paraoxonase activity, and head circumference. *Environ Health Perspect.* 2004;112:388–391.
203. Hendrick V, Smith LM, Suri R, et al. Birth outcomes after prenatal exposure to antidepressant medication. *Am J Obstet Gynecol.* 2003;188:812–815.
204. Pinter R. Hogge WA. McPherson E. Infant with severe penicillamine embryopathy born to a woman with Wilson disease. *Am J Med Genet A.* 2004;128:294–298.
205. Assencio-Ferreira VJ, Abraham R, Veiga JCE, et al. Metopic suture craniosynostosis: Sodium valproate teratogenic effect. Case report. *Arq Neuropsiquiatr.* 2001;59:417–420.
206. Dessens AB, Cohen-Kettenis PT, Mellenbergh GJ, et al. Association of prenatal phenobarbital and phenytoin exposure with genital anomalies and menstrual disorders. *Teratology.* 2001;64:181–188.
207. Bokhari A, Coull BA, Holmes LB. Effect of prenatal exposure to anticonvulsant drugs on dermal ridge patterns of fingers. *Teratology.* 2002;66:19–23.
208. Bokhari A, Connolly S, Coull BA, et al. Effects on toes from prenatal exposure to anticonvulsants. *Teratology.* 2002;66:122–126.
209. Holmes LB, Wyszynski DF, Lieberman E. The AED (antiepileptic drug) pregnancy registry: a 6-year experience. *Arch Neurol.* 2004;61:673–678.
210. Dessens AB, Cohen-Kettenis PT, Mellenbergh GJ, et al. Association of prenatal phenobarbital and phenytoin exposure with small head size at birth and with learning problems. *Acta Paediatr.* 2000;89:533–541.
211. Arpino C, Brescianini S, Robert E, et al. Teratogenic effects of antiepileptic drugs: Use of an international database on Malformations and Drug Exposure (MADRE). *Epilepsia.* 2000;41:1436–1443.
212. Orup HI, Jr., Holmes LB, Keith DA, et al. Craniofacial skeletal deviations following in utero exposure to the anticonvulsant phenytoin: monotherapy and polytherapy. *Orthod Craniofac Res.* 2003;6:2–19.
213. Doi M, Matsubara H, Uji Y. Vogt-Koyanagi-Harada syndrome in a pregnant patient treated with high-dose systemic corticosteroids. *Acta Ophthalmol Scand.* 2000;78:93–96.
214. Daskalakis GJ, Papageorgiou IS, Petrogiannis ND,et al. Myasthenia gravis and pregnancy. *Eur J Obstet Gynecol Reprod Biol.* 2000;89:201–204.
215. Gilbert-Barness E, Drut RM. Association of sympathomimetic drugs with malformations. *Vet Hum Toxicol.* 2000;42:168–171.
216. Bihan H, Vazquez MP, Krivitzky A, et al. Aplasia cutis congenita and dysmorphic syndrome after antithyroid therapy during pregnancy. *Endocrinologist.* 2002;12:87–91.
217. Hemminki E. Hovi SL. Sevon T. Asko-Seljavaara S. Births and perinatal health of infants among women who have had silicone breast implantation in Finland, 1967–2000. *Acta Obstet Gynecol Scand.* 2004;83:1135–1140.
218. Norgard B, Puho E, Pedersen L, et al. Risk of congenital abnormalities in children born to women with ulcerative colitis: A population-based, case-control study. *Am J Gastroenterol.* 2003;98:2006–2010.
219. Jain AB, Reyes J, Marcos A, et al. Pregnancy after liver transplantation with tacrolimus immunosuppression: a single center's experience update at 13 years. *Transplantation.* 2003;76:827–832.
220. Rayes N, David M, Neuhaus R, et al. Experience with 20 pregnancies under cyclosporine and tacrolimus following liver transplantation. *Transplantationsmedizin: Organ der Deutschen Transplantationsgesellschaft.* 1999;11:89–93.
221. Kainz A, Harabacz I, Cowlrick IS, et al. Analysis of 100 pregnancy outcomes in women treated systemically with tacrolimus. *Transpl Int.* 2000;13 Suppl 1:S299–S300.
222. Matsuoka R, Gilbert EF, Bruyers JH, et al. An aborted human fetus with truncus arteriosus communis—Possible teratogenic effect of Tedral. *Heart Vessels.* 1985;1:176–178.
223. Loebstein R, Lalkin A, Addis A, et al. Pregnancy outcome after gestational exposure to terfenadine: A multicenter, prospective controlled study. *J Allergy Clin Immunol.* 1999;104:953–956.
224. Silveira CM, Caceres VM, Dutra MG, et al. Safety of tetanus toxoid in pregnant women: A hospital-based case-control study of congenital anomalies. *Bull World Health Organ.* 1995;73:605–608.
225. Dempsey DA, Hajnal BL, Partridge JC, et al. Tone abnormalities are associated with maternal cigarette smoking during pregnancy in utero cocaine-exposed infants. *Pediatrics.* 2000;106:79–85.
226. Kozma C. Valproic acid embryopathy: Report of two siblings with further expansion of the phenotypic abnormalities and a review of the literature. *Am J Med Genet.* 2001;98:168–175.

227. Duncan S, Mercho S, Lopes-Cendes I, et al. Repeated neural tube defects and valproate monotherapy suggest a pharmacogenetic abnormality. *Epilepsia.* 2001;42:750–753.
228. Glover SJ, Quinn AG, Barter P, et al. Ophthalmic findings in fetal anticonvulsant syndrome(s). *Ophthalmology.* 2002;109:942–947.
229. Rodriguez-Pinilla E, Arroyo I, Fondevilla J, et al. Prenatal exposure to valproic acid during pregnancy and limb deficiencies: A case-control study. *Am J Med Genet.* 2000;90:376–381.
230. Stoll C, Audeoud F, Gaugler C, et al. Multiple congenital malformations including generalized hypertrichosis with gum hypertrophy in a child exposed to valproic acid in utero. *Genet Couns.* 2003; 14:289–298.
231. Mawer G, Clayton-Smith J, Coyle H, et al. Outcome of pregnancy in women attending an outpatient epilepsy clinic: adverse features associated with higher doses of sodium valproate. *Seizure.* 2002; 11(8):512–518.
232. Malm H, Kajantie E, Kivirikko S, et al. Valproate embryopathy in three sets of siblings: further proof of hereditary susceptibility. *Neurology.* 2002;59:630–633.
233. Chabrolle JP, Bensouda B, Bruel H, et al. Metopic craniosynostosis, probable effect of intrauterine exposure to maternal valproate treatment. *Arch Pediatr.* 2001;8:1333–1336.
234. Sodhi P, Poddar B, Parmar V. Fatal cardiac malformation in fetal valproate syndrome. *Indian J Pediatr.* 2001;68:989–990.
235. Lajeunie E, Barcik U, Thorne JA, et al. Craniosynostosis and fetal exposure to sodium valproate. *J Neurosurg.* 2001;95:778–782.
236. Craig J, Morrison P, Morrow J, et al. Failure of periconceptual folic acid to prevent a neural tube defect in the offspring of a mother taking sodium valproate. *Seizure.* 1999;8:253–254.
237. Mo CN, Ladusans EJ. Anomalous right pulmonary artery origins in association with the fetal valproate syndrome. *J Med Genet.* 1999;36:83–84.
238. Shields KE, Galil K, Seward J, et al. Varicella vaccine exposure during pregnancy: Data from the first 5 years of the pregnancy registry. *Obstet Gynecol.* 2001;98:14–19.
239. Botto LD, Loffredo C, Scanlon KS, et al. Vitamin A and cardiac outflow tract defects. *Epidemiology.* 2001;12:491–496.
240. Boskovic R, Gargaun L, Oren D, et al. Pregnancy outcome following high doses of Vitamin E supplementation. *Reprod Toxicol.* 2005;20:85–88.
241. Vitale N, De Feo M, De Santo LS, et al. Dose-dependent fetal complications of warfarin in pregnant women with mechanical heart valves. *J Am Coll Cardiol.* 1999;33:1637–1641.
242. Bony C, Zyka F, Tiran-Rajaofera I, et al. Warfarin fetopathy. *Arch Pediatr.* 2002;9:705–708.
243. Tongsong T, Wanapirak C, Piyamongkol W. Prenatal ultrasonographic findings consistent with fetal warfarin syndrome. *J Ultrasound Med.* 1999;18:577–580.
244. Robert E, Vial T, Schaefer C, et al. Exposure to yellow fever vaccine in early pregnancy. *Vaccine.* 1999;17:283–285.

CHAPTER 7

DRUGS AND CHEMICALS MOST COMMONLY USED BY PREGNANT WOMEN

Doreen Matsui and David Knoppert

INTRODUCTION

The thalidomide tragedy of the late 1950s lead to a heightened awareness of the potential risks of in utero exposure to drugs. However, use of medication during pregnancy is often necessary and unavoidable. Recent studies have suggested that between 64% and 83% of women use at least one medication during pregnancy.[1,2,3] Although there is a lack of knowledge regarding the effects of a number of drugs during pregnancy, for many of the more commonly prescribed medications there is data available upon which to make an informed decision regarding therapy. It is crucial that physicians provide women with balanced, evidence-based information concerning drug exposures during pregnancy as misinformation and unrealistic perception of the teratogenic risk of medications may lead to inadequate treatment of maternal disease or unnecessary termination of pregnancies.[4,5]

For the majority of exposures reviewed in this chapter, a few representative articles are referenced. For more information, the reader may refer to one of several textbooks or computer databases.[6,7]

The Motherisk Program is a counseling service that provides pregnant women and health care providers with information on the safety and risks of exposures to medications, chemicals, and radiation. The topics covered in this chapter are based on the drugs Canadian family physicians ask this teratogen information service about most frequently,[8] with the addition of a few other common exposures. Herbal products are not discussed, as they are the focus of another chapter.

ANTIDEPRESSANTS

Questions regarding the use of antidepressants, in particular the newer selective serotonin reuptake inhibitors (SSRIs) and related drugs, are among the most common, which is not surprising given the frequency with which depression is reported during pregnancy. Twenty percent of pregnant women screened in obstetric clinics showed elevated depressive symptomatology as measured by the Center for Epidemiological Studies-Depression scale (CES-D)[9] Fortunately, SSRIs including fluoxetine,[10] paroxetine,[12] sertraline,[11] citalopram,[12] as well as venlafaxine[13] and bupropion[14] have not been shown to be major teratogens. Recently it has been suggested that exposure to paroxetine in pregnancy may be associated with an increased risk of infant cardiovascular defects (ventricular and atrial septal defects).[15]

More recently concern has been raised regarding transient symptoms reported in some newborns after exposure to SSRIs during the third trimester. Based on available studies late SSRI in utero exposure carries an overall risk ratio of 3.0 (95% CI = 2.0–4.4) for neonatal behavioral syndrome. Neonates display central nervous system, motor, respiratory and gastrointestinal signs that are usually mild and require supportive care only.[16] The debate regarding the underlying mechanism of this "poor neonatal adaptation" continues with both neonatal withdrawal and toxicity having been suggested as possible etiologies.

Whether there are effects of in utero exposure to antidepressants on long-term neurodevelopmental outcome also remains unresolved. Although subtle effects have been found with some SSRIs on testing infants,[17,18,19] there are also several studies that demonstrate no impairment of infant neurodevelopment.[20] It is important to balance these concerns with the risks both to the mother and fetus of untreated depression during pregnancy.

ANTIEPILEPTICS

Pregnancy for the woman who suffers from epilepsy poses a dilemma. It is well established that the risk of a major congenital malformation in offspring of mothers who take older antiepileptic drugs (AEDs) (i.e., phenobarbital, phenytoin, primidone, carbamazepine, and valproic acid) ranges from 4 to 8% compared to 2 to 4% in the general population.[21,22] The teratogenic potential of these agents has been well described: congenital heart defects and cleft palate with phenobarbital, phenytoin, and primidone; neural tube defects with carbamazepine and valproic acid.[21,22] There is much less information available for newer AEDs such as gabapentin, vigabatrin, lamotrigine, and topiramate. During the last decade pregnancy registries in epilepsy have been developed by collaborative groups of physicians in Europe, North America, Australia, and Europe with the purpose of prospectively monitoring women who are taking these newer AEDs.[21,23,24,25] Pharmaceutical companies that market these agents have also initiated pregnancy registries.

A gabapentin registry reported on the pregnancy outcomes of 39 women who were taking gabapentin for epilepsy and other conditions. In this small group of women there were no differences in rates of maternal complication, miscarriage, low birth weight, or malformations compared to the general population.[26] The outcomes of many more gabapentin-exposed pregnancies are needed, however, before the safety of this agent can be established.

A recent publication describes the experience of the United Kingdom Epilepsy and Pregnancy Register. Pregnant women with epilepsy, whether or not they were taking an AED and receiving monotherapy or polytherapy, were included provided that they were referred to the register before the outcome of the pregnancy was known. The number of reported outcomes with each AED is as follows: carbamazepine (900), valproate (715), lamotrigine (647), phenytoin (82), gabapentin (31), topiramate (28), and levetiracetam (22). Outcome data were collected at 3 months after the expected date of delivery by sending a questionnaire to the family doctor. A major congenital malformation (MCM) was defined as "an abnormality of an essential embryonic structure requiring significant therapy and present at birth or discovered during the first 6 weeks of life". Of 4414 pregnancies that had been registered over a 9 year period, 3607 had full outcome data. There were 72% of women exposed to a single AED, 21.3% to more than a single AED, and

6.7% who had epilepsy but were not exposed to an AED during their pregnancy. The MCM rate for all AED exposed pregnancies was 4.2% (95% CI = 3.6–5.0%). In the group of women who had epilepsy, but who did not receive any AED during pregnancy, the MCM rate was 3.5% (95% CI = 1.8–6.8%). There appeared to be a possible dose response relationship between the daily lamotrigine dose and the MCM rate, which increased from about 1% for doses <100 mg daily to over 5% for doses >200 mg daily. Polytherapy resulted in higher MCM rates, as might be expected. Valproate, as part of polytherapy, was particularly significant. Polytherapy combinations that contained valproate in any combination had a significantly higher risk of MCM than polytherapy that did not contain valproate (OR 2.49; 95% CI = 1.31–4.70). Some of the limitations of this report, as acknowledged by the authors, include the fact that this was an observational study, less than one-half of all eligible cases in the United Kingdom were recruited, MCMs were only looked for up to 3 months of life, and the relatively small numbers of patients on the newer AEDs[22] Nonetheless, it does provide additional information for the newer AEDs, looks at the effect of epilepsy itself on pregnancy outcomes, and provides insight into the importance of dose and polytherapy in the development of MCMs.

A recent report of the Lamotrigine Pregnancy Registry was published. Outcomes for 414 women who took lamotrigine in the first trimester as monotherapy demonstrated major birth defects in 2.9% (95% CI = 1.6–5.1%). In 88 women whose polytherapy included lamotrigine, and at least valproic acid, the rate of major birth defects was 12.5% (95% CI = 6.7–21.7%). In 182 women who received lamotrigine and at least 1 other AED (*not* valproic acid), the rate of major birth defects was 2.7% (95% CI = 1.0–6.6%).[27] A high rate (10.7%, 95% CI = 6.3–16.9%) of major birth defects due to monotherapy with valproic acid has also been reported in 149 exposures from the North American AED Pregnancy Registry.[28] Preliminary data from this Registry also suggest a possible relation between lamotrigine exposure during the first trimester and the development of cleft lip and/or cleft palate.[29] A recent case report[30] suggests an association between lamotrigine exposure and elevated gamma-glutamyl transpeptidase levels in a newborn. The authors recommend routine monitoring of liver function in exposed infants. The Australian AED Registry has also reported a high rate of malformations (16%) with valproic acid exposure, which also appeared to be dose–related.[25]

ANTIHISTAMINES

In a recent study using data from the Swedish Medical Birth Registry the malformation rate after antihistamine use (3.17%) for nausea and vomiting (12,934 women) or allergy (5041 women) was similar to that found in the general population (3.16%)[31] As there is considerable experience with the older antihistamines such as chlorpheniramine, the oral first generation agents are often preferred for use during pregnancy, especially during the first trimester; however, these drugs may not be tolerated due to their sedating effects. Although there is less information available regarding the effects of the newer less sedating antihistamines during pregnancy studies do exist for some of the more popular medications.

In a prospective study of 120 pregnant women who were followed after exposure to cetirizine or hydroxyzine during pregnancy (75% during organogenesis), no significant differences in the rates of major or minor anomalies were demonstrated between study and control groups.[32] As cetirizine is metabolite of hydroxyzine, it is reassuring that the latter medication, which has been on the market for much longer, has not been shown to be teratogenic[33,34] although neonatal withdrawal has been reported.[35,36]

If a second-generation antihistamine is chosen, the other antihistamine that has been recommended is loratadine.[37] In a multicenter study of loratadine use during pregnancy, there were 161 exposed pregnancies with no significant differences in the rates of major malformations between the study (3.5%) and control (4%) group.[38] Similarly, in a study conducted of 210 pregnancies with exposure to loratadine during pregnancy (78% during the first trimester) the rate of congenital anomalies did not differ between the loratadine group (2.3%) and two control groups [other antihistamines (4%) and non-teratogenic exposures (3%)].[39] The Swedish Medical Birth Registry study on antihistamines raised the possibility of an association between in utero exposure to loratadine and hypospadias as this defect was noted in 7 of 1796, twice the rate they found in the general population.[31] The Centers for Disease Control and Prevention (CDC) subsequently analyzed data from the National Birth Defects Prevention Study with 563 male infants with hypospadias and 1444 male infant controls. No association was shown between use of loratidine (from 1 month before pregnancy through the first trimester) and second- or third-degree hypospadias.[40]

VACCINES

Vaccination of pregnant women provides important health benefits to both mother and infant[41]; however, vaccine exposure is often avoided during pregnancy, especially live virus vaccines, which are generally contraindicated for pregnant women. However, inadvertent exposure is not uncommon and there are circumstances when immunization is recommended even during pregnancy due to high risk of infection or the severity of the potential consequences of the disease.

As rubella virus is a known human teratogen, much concern has been raised about the potential fetal effects of exposure to rubella vaccination during pregnancy. However, in 2001 the Advisory Committee on Immunization Practices (ACIP) reviewed data from several sources indicating that no cases of congenital rubella syndrome (CRS) had been identified among infants born to women who were vaccinated inadvertently against rubella within 3 months or early in pregnancy. Data were available on 680 live births to susceptible women who were vaccinated 3 months before or during pregnancy and none of the infants were born with CRS, although a small theoretic risk of 0.5% could not be ruled out.[42] In a recent prospective controlled study, 94 women exposed to the rubella (or MMR) vaccine, 56 prior to conception and 38 during the first trimester, were followed. None of the children exhibited signs of congenital rubella syndrome and rates of major malformations were similar in the exposed and control groups.[43] Receipt of rubella vaccination during pregnancy is not considered an indication for interruption of that pregnancy.[44]

Influenza-associated excess deaths among pregnant women were documented during pandemics and case reports and limited studies have indicated that pregnancy can increase the risk of serious medical complications of influenza.[45] It is recommended that pregnant women be immunized if they are expected to deliver during influenza season.[45,46] Safe use of influenza vaccine during pregnancy without adverse fetal effects has been demonstrated with most experience involving exposure during the second and third trimesters.[45–49]

Data on exposure to hepatitis A vaccine during pregnancy is lacking; however because hepatitis A vaccine is produced from inactivated hepatitis A virus, the theoretical risk to the developing fetus is expected to be low.[50] Similarly, hepatitis B vaccine contains noninfectious HbsAg particles and pregnancy is not considered a contraindication to vaccination in women at high risk.[51] Reports have examined the safety of hepatitis B immunization during the last trimester of pregnancy.[52,53] With respect to exposure earlier in pregnancy, no congenital abnormalities were observed among the infants born to 10 women who received the vaccine during the first trimester of pregnancy.[54]

ANTIBIOTICS AND ANTIVIRALS

Questions regarding the effects of antibiotics during pregnancy remain common although they have shifted from the penicillins and erythromycin to some of the newer agents. The risk of yellow-brown discoloration of teeth with in utero exposure to tetracycline after the 5th or 6th month of gestation is well–known. More recently, an association between use of trimethoprim-sulfonamide combinations in pregnancy and neural tube defects[55] and cardiovascular malformations[56,57] has been described.

Concern has been raised about possible fetal effects of intrauterine exposure to ciprofloxacin and other fluoroquinolones based on lesions demonstrated in the cartilage of young dogs given these medications.[58] However, subsequent studies in humans have not found major problems with the use of this group of antibiotics during pregnancy, although they are generally not considered first-line therapy when other alternatives are available. In a small study, no malformations were noted in 38 pregnant women who were treated with quinolones during pregnancy.[59] The European Network of Teratology Information Services prospectively followed 549 pregnancies and found a malformation rate of 4.9%, which was interpreted as not exceeding published background rates.[60] In a prospective controlled study conducted by the Motherisk Program of 200 women exposed to fluoroquinolones during pregnancy, the rates of major congenital abnormalities did not differ between the group exposed during the first trimester (2.2%) and the control group (2.6%). Gross motor developmental milestone achievements also did not differ between the children of the mothers in the two groups.[61]

Clarithromycin is a newer macrolide structurally related to erythromycin, which has previously been one of the drugs of choice to use during pregnancy. There were no differences found in the rates of major malformations between the exposed group (2.3%) and control groups (1.4%) in a prospective controlled study of 157 pregnant women exposed to clarithromycin, 122 during the first trimester.[62] In a retrospective postmarketing surveillance study using claims data, the observed rate of 3.4% for major malformations in infants born to women who had a delivery claim within 270 days of a clarithromycin prescription was not significantly different compared to the expected rate.[63]

Metronidazole remains widely used for infections in women of reproductive age. Controversy remains among some health care providers regarding its use during pregnancy. However, two previous meta-analyses on the teratogenic risk of metronidazole did not find an association between its use during the first trimester and birth defects.[64,65] Subsequent studies including a prospective controlled study did not show an increased risk of congenital abnormalities.[66,67] Although a possible association with cleft lip with or without cleft palate was raised in a study based on the Hungarian Case-Control Surveillance of Congenital Abnormalities dataset, it was not possible to exclude recall bias and the finding was not confirmed by the comparison of the cases and the total group control group.[68]

As it is a nucleoside analogue, questions have been raised about the teratogenic potential of acyclovir; however, most human experience to date has been relatively reassuring. Information on pregnancy outcomes following systemic acyclovir exposure is available from the Acyclovir in Pregnancy Registry. Of 1695 cases registered prospectively between June 1, 1984 and June 30, 1998, 1246 outcomes (61% first trimester) are known. The risk of birth defects among live births exposed to acyclovir in the first trimester was 19 of 596 (3.2%; 95% CI = 2–5%). No unusual defect or pattern of defects was apparent.[69] Of 90 pregnant women who redeemed a prescription for systemic acyclovir during pregnancy or 30 days before conception, as identified from the North Jutland Pharmacoepidemiological Prescription Database in Denmark, one case with a defect of the atrial septum and unspecified congenital malformation of the heart was found among the exposed women (OR 0.69; 95% CI = 0.17–2.82).[70] More limited data is available regarding valacyclovir, a prodrug of acyclovir. The Acyclovir in Pregnancy Registry documented the pregnancy outcomes in 111 women exposed to valacyclovir and there was no increase in birth defects compared with the general population.[71] Published information on the use of ganciclovir during human pregnancy is limited to isolated case reports.[72,73]

H2-BLOCKERS AND PROTON PUMP INHIBITORS

Early reports of H2 receptor antagonist use in over 450 pregnancies suggested that these agents do not cause an increase in major malformations.[74–75] These results have been confirmed in a recent publication from the European Network of Teratology Information Services, which reported on the outcome of 553 pregnancies with exposure to an H2 blocker (ranitidine 335, cimetidine 113, famotidine 75, nizatidine 15 and roxatidine 15). Most of the exposures were at least in the first trimester. The major malformation rate in the exposed group was 2.7% versus 3.5% in 1390 pregnant women who served as controls (RR 0.78, 95% CI = 0.42–1.44).[77] Thus, H2 receptor antagonists do not appear to be a major teratogenic risk in humans.

A meta-analysis, published in 2002, represented outcomes in almost 600 infants who had been exposed to either omeprazole, pantoprazole, or lansoprazole in utero. The summary relative risk for major malformations was 1.18 (95% CI = 0.72–1.94).[78] The results of this study, suggesting that exposure to a PPI during pregnancy does not represent a major teratogenic risk, were further supported by a recent multicenter study that examined over 300 pregnancies exposed to omeprazole, lansoprazole, or pantoprazole. The rate of major congenital anomalies for any of the three PPIs was not different from control groups.[79]

ANTIFUNGALS

A recent population based, case control study examined the effect of oral ketoconazole that was used in the second to third month of pregnancy. Use of ketoconazole in over 22,800 infants with congenital anomalies (CAs) and over 38,100 controls was studied. Results were adjusted for potential confounders. Six infants (0.03%) with CAs and 12 controls (0.03%) had mothers who had received oral ketoconazole (prevalence OR 0.8, 95% CI = 0.3–2.2). This epidemiologic study with a huge database did not demonstrate a higher rate of CAs in babies born to mothers who had taken oral ketoconazole during the first 2–3 months of pregnancy. The author's caution, however, that a larger data set is needed before final judgment is made regarding ketoconazole use during pregnancy, given the fact that it is teratogenic and embryotoxic in animals.[80]

Fluconazole is teratogenic in animals. Developmental phase specificity was determined in mice using single oral doses of 700 mg/kg. Specific gestational days were identified as the phase of maximal sensitivity for induction of cleft palate and skeletal and limb anomalies. A dose-response relationship was also demonstrated.[81] In vitro work suggests a common intrinsic teratogenic pathway for the azole compounds.[82]

Three case reports (two siblings) described congenital anomalies (craniofacial, skeletal, and cardiac) in newborns whose mothers had taken 400–800 mg of fluconazole daily for the first 7–24 weeks of gestation. The women received chronic fluconazole therapy to prevent, in 1 case, and to treat, in the other case, coccidioidal meningitis.[83]

A retrospective study, based on returned questionnaires from general practitioners, identified 289 women who had taken fluconazole for vaginal candidiasis, before or during pregnancy. Most women (275) took a single 150 mg dose. There were multiple 50 mg doses (3 women) and 150 mg doses (11 women). There were no congenital anomalies in the newborns whose mothers took fluconazole during the pregnancy.[84] A prospective, case control study assessed pregnancy outcomes in 226 women (and a reference group of 452 women) who were exposed to fluconazole during the first 12 weeks of gestation. The primary indication (92% of women) was vaginal candidiasis. A single 150 mg dose was taken by 46.5% of the women; multiple doses of 150 mg were taken by 35.8% of the women. The remaining women were exposed to 50 mg or 100 mg in single or multiple doses. There was no difference in the prevalence of congenital anomalies between the two groups (4.0% vs. 4.2% in the fluconazole and reference groups, respectively).[85] A case control study that involved 234 women who received fluconazole (92% of whom received a single 150 mg tablet) in the first trimester of pregnancy did not show an increase in congenital anomalies compared to a group of 1629 control women (RR 1.1, 95% CI = 0.4–3.30).[86] A case control study from Denmark identified 165 women from a prescription database who had taken a single 150 mg dose of fluconazole during pregnancy (121 during the first trimester) for vaginal candidiasis. Birth outcomes (malformations, low birth weight and preterm delivery) were compared with those from 13,327 women who served as controls. No elevated risk of malformation was found (OR 0.65, 95% CI = 0.24–1.77) in the offspring of women who had taken fluconazole.[87]

A review of the literature did not reveal any recent reports of Amphotericin B teratogenicity. An earlier review also did not find any reports of teratogenicity with the use of Amphotericin B.[88]

An epidemiological case control study, based on the population-based Hungarian Surveillance of Congenital Abnormalities, did not show an increase in congenital abnormalities with nystatin exposure during pregnancy.[89] This is not unexpected since nystatin is poorly absorbed. A different statistical approach suggested a possible association between nystatin use and hypospadias.

ANTIHELMINTICS

Although many of the commonly used antihelmintics have been in use for years, there is a paucity of data regarding safety of exposure to these agents during pregnancy. However, the lack of reported difficulties with time is somewhat reassuring.

The effect of mebendazole therapy during pregnancy was studied in Sri Lanka where prescription of this drug to women in the second trimester of pregnancy was recommended for endemic hookworm infection. The rate of major congenital defects was not significantly higher in the mebendazole group (97/5275, 1.8%) than in the control group (26/1737, 1.5%). Among the babies of 407 women who had taken mebendazole during the first trimester, 10 (2.5%) had major congenital defects.[90] The Israel Teratogen Information Service prospectively followed 192 pregnancies with exposure to mebendazole (71.5% during the first trimester). The rate of major anomalies in the mebendazole group (3.3%) was not significantly different compared with the rate in a control group who were counseled for nonteratogenic exposures (1.7%).[91]

Data on the use of piperazine, pyrantel pamoate, and pyrvinium pamoate during pregnancy is lacking.

ANALGESICS

The treatment of pain, both acute and chronic during pregnancy is a common dilemma for pregnant women and their physicians. Acetaminophen is often recommended as the drug of choice; however, may not provide adequate pain control in all circumstances. Nonsteroidal anti-inflammatory drugs are covered in a subsequent section of this chapter.

In general, narcotics are not considered major teratogens. Although associations between first trimester use of codeine and various congenital anomalies have been observed,[92,93] other studies have not found an increased risk.[94] Use in late pregnancy may result in neonatal withdrawal.[95,96]

Respiratory depression[97–99] and impaired behavioral response in the newborn[100–102] have been observed with use of meperidine during labor.

A review of studies of the treatment of migraine headaches with sumatriptan in pregnancy has been published. The available literature failed to note an increased risk of birth defects with sumatriptan use compared to the general population. However, the authors do state that the number of reports is insufficient to reach a definitive conclusion concerning treating migraines in pregnancy with sumatriptan although the currently available evidence is reassuring for accidental exposure.[103] In a Motherisk study, outcome was determined in 96 pregnant women exposed to sumatriptan, 95 during the first trimester, with 38 reporting multiple use. There were two control groups, a disease-matched one and a group exposed to known nonteratogens. The incidence of major birth defects did not differ among groups.[104] GlaxoSmithKline, the manufacturer of this drug, maintains a registry for sumatriptan exposures during pregnancy. In published data as of October 31, 1998 there were 7 birth defects among 208 pregnancies involving earliest exposure to sumatriptan in the first trimester.[105] More recent interim data is available by contacting the company registry office.

ASPIRIN, NSAIDs AND COX-2 INHIBITORS

A recent population-based case-control study that included over 3400 children with 4 selected and isolated congenital abnormalities (neural tube defects, exomphalos/gastroschisis, cleft lip ± palate, and posterior cleft palate) suggested that the maternal use of aspirin during 5–12 weeks of gestation is not associated with an increased risk of these abnormalities.[106] The data from this study, originally published in 2000,[107] was not included in a previously conducted meta-analysis,[108] which found no evidence of an overall risk of congenital malformations, but a significantly increased risk of gastroschisis, in babies who were exposed to aspirin during the first trimester. Another recent meta-analysis[109] found that women who took aspirin had a significantly lower risk of preterm delivery. However, routine administration of aspirin during every pregnancy is not recommended at this time. There were no other differences in the offspring of women who had taken aspirin during pregnancy.

A prospective cohort study that examined the use of ibuprofen and naproxen around the time of conception or during pregnancy provided evidence of an association between NSAID use and miscarriage. The risk of miscarriage increased when NSAID use was around the time of conception or when NSAID use was longer than a week.[110] Prostaglandins are important for the successful implantation of the embryo into the uterus wall. Inhibition of prostaglandin synthesis by NSAIDs may explain, in part at least, an association of miscarriage with NSAID use.

A report from Denmark identified 2557 infants born to women who reported the use of an NSAID early in pregnancy (first trimester). There was no increased rate of any congenital malformation (OR 1.04; 95% CI = 0.84–1.29), but the number of cardiac defects was high (OR 1.86; 95% CI = 1.32–1.62). These were relatively mild conditions and were not attributed to one particular NSAID.[111]

The use of cyclooxygenase inhibitors during pregnancy can also cause premature closure of the ductus arteriosus and neonatal renal failure.[112,113]

Experience with the use of COX-2 inhibitors during pregnancy is limited. Given that studies in fetal lambs demonstrated that celecoxib constricted the isolated ductus arteriosus in vitro and produced both an increase in pressure gradient and resistance across the ductus in vivo, use of these drug during the 3rd trimester of pregnancy is best avoided.[114] COX-2 inhibitors have also been shown to exert relaxant effects on contractility in pregnant human myometrial strips in vitro.[115]

ATYPICAL ANTIPSYCHOTICS

A recent, prospective cohort study reported on the pregnancy outcomes of 151 women in 3 different centers who took an atypical antipsychotic during the first trimester. Women were exposed to olanzapine (60), risperidone (49), quetiapine (36), and clozapine (6). Only 105 of the exposed women were matched with controls. The women who took one of these atypical antipsychotic agents also took other medication, including antidepressants, antiepileptics, and benzodiazepines. There was no difference in the rate of major malformations between the two groups. The major limitation of this study is the small sample size. The authors indicated that 800 women per group would be required to detect a twofold increase in relatively common malformations.[116] However, it does provide hope for women who require these medications. Much additional work is required to provide a better estimation of the true effect of these drugs on pregnancy outcomes.

ORAL CONTRACEPTIVES

Given their indication, it is not surprising that oral contraceptives may be taken early in pregnancy prior to the woman realizing that she is pregnant at which time the medication is discontinued. Lack of association between oral contraceptives and birth defects was observed in a meta-analysis of prospective studies of oral contraceptive exposure early in pregnancy. Relative risks for all malformations, congenital heart defects and limb reduction defects were 0.99 (95% CI = 0.83–1.19), 1.06 (0.72–1.56) and 1.04 (0.30–3.55), respectively.[117] Similarly a meta-analysis of cohort and case-control studies found no significant association between first trimester exposure to sex hormones generally (or to oral contraceptives specifically) and external genital malformations.[118]

Despite the findings of these meta-analyses, the safety of oral contraceptives during pregnancy remains controversial. In a subsequent case-control study, Luisa Martinez-Frias, et al. found an odds ratio for congenital defects associated with oral contraceptive exposure during the first trimester of pregnancy of 1.38 (95% CI = 1.04–1.84). They concluded that the results of their study did not support the suspicion of a teratogenic effect after prenatal exposure to sex hormones and that the risk should be small if it exists.[119] However, their findings were also interpreted as showing that prenatal exposure to oral contraceptives and estrogens increases the risk of overall birth defects.[120]

ORAL HYPOGLYCEMICS

Oral hypoglycemic drugs have traditionally been avoided during pregnancy although more recent reports have examined their use in pregnant women. No significant difference was found in the rate of major malformations between those exposed to oral hypoglycemic agents and those not exposed (OR 1.05, 95% CI = 0.65–1.70) in a meta-analysis of 10 studies that reported on first-trimester exposure to an oral hypoglycemic agent.[121] Metformin has not been implicated as a teratogen over and above the confounding factor of poorly controlled diabetes.[122] A meta-analysis on the use of metformin during pregnancy found an overall malformation rate of just 1.01% in 496 first trimester exposures.[123] Glyburide does not cross the placenta and has not been associated with increased risk of adverse fetal effects.[124] A recent case report describes the successful pregnancy outcome of a woman who had been taking a multidrug regimen, including rosiglitazone and gliclazide, for the first 7 weeks of pregnancy.[125] Questions have, however, been raised about the adequacy of control of maternal diabetes during pregnancy with oral hypoglycemic agents and their role remains to be defined.

CHOLESTEROL-LOWERING AGENTS

A recent uncontrolled case series of statin exposures during the first trimester suggests an association between statins and structural defects in the newborn, specifically CNS and limb deficiencies. All first trimester exposures to statins that had been reported to the FDA, 2 cases from the literature, and 42 cases obtained from the manufacturers comprised the database. Of 70 exposures that were evaluable there were 22 cases of structural anomaly, 4 cases of intrauterine growth restriction, 5 cases of intrauterine fetal demise and 40 normal babies. Among the cases of limb deficiency were 2 cases of multiple malformations that met the criteria for the VACTERL association (anomalies of 3 or more among the following: vertebral, anal, cardiac, tracheo-esophageal, renal structures and limb deficiency).[126] The plausible biological mechanism for the teratogenicity is a down regulation of cholesterol biosynthesis in the developing embryo. All statins may not be equal in their teratogenic potential. Pravastatin, which unlike the other statins is hydrophilic, was not associated with any evaluatable reports of abnormal pregnancy outcome.

DECONGESTANTS

It has been suggested that gastroschisis and small intestinal atresia may be associated with disruption of vascular flow caused by certain vasoconstrictive medications.[127] A case control study of gastroschisis suggested a possible association with decongestants: pseudoephedrine (OR 2.1, 95% CI = 0.8–5.5) and phenylpropanolamine (OR 10.0, 95% CI = 1.2–85.6) although the 95% confidence intervals for the ORs either crossed or approach unity.[128] A subsequent retrospective case control study looked at 205 cases of gastroschisis and 127 cases of small intestinal atresia. Combined exposure to vasoconstrictive drugs (which included mostly pseudoephedrine, and phenylpropanolamine) and cigarette smoking was reported in 9% of both gastroschisis and small intestinal atresia cases, but only in 4% of controls. Adjusted ORs with combined exposure were 2.1 (95% CI = 1.0–4.4) for gastroschisis and 2.8 (95% CI = 1.1–6.9) for small intestinal atresias The OR increased significantly more when daily cigarette consumption was more than 20 cigarettes per day.[129] The role of the underlying maternal illness for which these drugs are taken (and other concomitant exposures such as cigarette smoking) must also be taken into account. Indiscriminate use of decongestants during pregnancy should be avoided.

DEXTROMETHORPHAN

In a Motherisk study outcomes were available in 184 women who took dextromethorphan during pregnancy (128 during the 1st trimester). Three (2.3%) major malformations were found among the babies of women who used this drug in the first trimester, which was not significantly different from the control group.[130]

CORTICOSTEROIDS

Cortiocosteroids are commonly prescribed to pregnant women for the treatment of autoimmune disease, inflammatory bowel disease, asthma, and other chronic disorders. Although attempts may be made to minimize the dose given, it is often not possible to discontinue corticosteroid therapy. In a prospective study of 184 women exposed to prednisone during pregnancy, the rate of major anomalies (4/111) was no different than the rate in a control group. A meta-analysis of studies of first trimester exposure to corticosteroids was also conducted. The summary odds ratio for case-control studies examining oral clefts was significant (OR 3.35, 95% CI = 1.97–5.69). This finding is consistent with previous animal studies. The investigators do, however, note that since oral clefts occur in about 1 in 1000 births, the increased risk will have minimal effect on the overall malformation rate in newborn infants.[131] A more recently published case-control study using the MADRE database confirmed the association between systemic exposure to corticosteroids and the occurrence of cleft lip with or without cleft palate (OR 2.59, 95% CI = 1.18–5.67).[132]

PAINTS

Pregnant women may be exposed to paint either at home or at work. The toxic potential of paint depends on which pigments, vehicles, and other components are present in the paint.[133] Latex or water-based paints are the safest choice.[134] Concern has arisen regarding exposure to organic solvents during pregnancy[135] and minimization of exposure to these paints is prudent. For home use it may be advisable to have someone else paint, while in the occupational setting, exposure should be limited by adequate ventilation and protective clothing.[133] Lead-containing paint should be avoided based on the suspected harmful neurotoxic effects of lead exposure during pregnancy.[136]

HAIR DYES

Although hair coloring is a common practice in women of childbearing age, there is a paucity of studies related to the safety of hair dye use during pregnancy. In teratology studies of pregnant rats following topical application of 12 hair dye formulations, no significant soft tissue or skeletal changes were noted.[137] There was no evidence of teratogenic effect in rats[138] or rabbits[139] after administration of hair dye by gavage. Only a small amount of the dye applied to the scalp is absorbed into the system and very little is available to the fetus.[134] It is likely that the occasional use of these products is not harmful; however, the cautious approach would be to limit their application. Studies of childhood cancers and maternal hair dye use have yielded inconsistent results. An association between use of hair dye in the month before and/or during pregnancy and increased risk of neuroblastoma has been described (odds ratio 1.6, 95% CI = 1.2–2.2) although recall bias may have affected the results of this study.[140] A recent case-control study found no evidence of an association between risk for childhood brain tumors and use of hair dyes during pregnancy.[141]

In a study examining reproductive outcomes among hairdressers using data from the Swedish Medical Birth Register, there was no indication of an increased risk of major malformations although birth weight was significantly lower compared with women working full-time in other occupations.[142]

REFERENCES

1. Andrade SE, Gurwitz JH, Davis RL, et al. Prescription drug use in pregnancy. *Am J Obstet Gynecol.* 2004;191:398–407.
2. Donati S, Baglio G, Spinelli A, et al. Drug use in pregnancy among Italian women. *Eur J Clin Pharmacol.* 2000;56:323–328.
3. Headley J, Northstone K, Simmons H, et al. Medication use during pregnancy: data from the Avon Longitudinal Study of Parents and Children. *Eur J Clin Pharmacol.* 2004;60:355–361.
4. Sanz E, Gomez-Lopez T, Martinez-Quintas MJ. Perception of teratogenic risk of common medicines. *Eur J Obstet Gynecol Reprod Biol.* 2001;95:127–131.
5. Koren G, Bologa M, Long D, et al. Perception of teratogenic risk by pregnant women exposed to drugs and chemical during the first trimester. *Am J Obstet Gynecol.* 1989;160:1190–1194.
6. Briggs GG, Freeman RK, Yaffe SJ. Drugs in Pregnancy and Lactation, 7th ed. Philadelphia: Lippincott Williams & Wilkins, 2005.
7. REPRORISK®System. Thomson micromedex, http://www.thomsonhc.com
8. Einarson A, Portnoi G, Koren G. Update on Motherisk Updates—Seven years of questions and answers. *Can Fam Physician.* 2002;48:1301–1304.

9. Marcus SM, Flynn HA, Blow FC, et al. Depressive Symptoms among Pregnant Women Screened in Obstetrics Settings. *J Women's Health.* 2003;12:373–380.
10. Addis A, Koren G. Safety of fluoxetine during the first trimester of pregnancy: a meta-analytical review of epidemiological studies. *Psychol Med.* 2000;30:89–94.
11. Kulin NA, Pastuszak A, Sage SR, et al. Pregnancy outcome following maternal use of the new selective serotonin reuptake inhibitors: a prospective controlled multicenter study. *JAMA.* 1998;279:609–610.
12. Sivojelezova A, Snuhaiber S, Sarkission L, et al. Citalopram use in pregnancy: Prospective comparative evaluation of pregnancy and fetal outcome. *Am J Obstet Gynecol.* 2005;193:2004–2009.
13. Einarson A, Fatoye B, Sarkar M, et al. Pregnancy outcome following gestational exposure to venlafaxine: a multicenter prospective controlled study. *Am J Psychiatry.* 2001;158:1728–1730.
14. Chun-Fai-Chan B, Koren G, Fayez I, et al. Pregnancy outcome of women exposed to bupropion during pregnancy: a prospective comparative study. *Am J Obstet Gynecol.* 2005;192:932–936.
15. Kallen BAJ, Otterblad Olausson P. Maternal use of selective serotonin re-uptake inhibitors in early pregnancy and infant congenital malformations. *Birth Defects Res A Clin Mol Teratol.* 2007 Jan10; [EQub ahead of print].
16. Moses-Kolko EL, Bogen D, Perel J, et al. Neonatal signs after late in utero exposure to serotonin reuptake inhibitors. *JAMA.* 2005;293:2372–2383.
17. Zeskind PS, Stephens LE. Maternal Selective Serotonin Reuptake Inhibitor Use During Pregnancy and Newborn Neurobehavior. *Pediatrics.* 2004;113:368–375.
18. Oberlander T, Eckstein Grunau R, Fitzgerald C, et al. Pain Reactivity in 2-Month-Old Infants after Prenatal and Postnatal Serotonin Reuptake Inhibitor Medication Exposure. *Pediatrics.* 2005;115:411–425.
19. Casper RC, Fleisher BE, Lee-Ancajas JC, et al. Follow-up of children of depressed mothers exposed or not exposed to antidepressant drugs during pregnancy. *J Pediatr.* 2003;142:402–408.
20. Gentile S. SSRIs in pregnancy and lactation—Emphasis on neurodevelopmental outcome. *CNS Drugs.* 2005;19:623–633.
21. Beghi E, Annegers JF. Pregnancy registries in epilepsy. *Epilepsia.* 2001;42:1422–1425.
22. Morrow JI, Russell A, Gutherie E, et al. Malformation risks of antiepileptic drugs in pregnancy: a prospective study from the UK Epilepsy and Pregnancy Register. *J Neurol Neurosurg Psychiatry.* Published online 12 Sep 2005; doi:10.1136/jnnp.2005.074203.
23. Holmes LB, Wyszynski DF. North American antiepileptic drug pregnancy registry. *Epilepsia.* 2004;45:1465.
24. Russell AJ, Craig JJ, Morrison P. UK epilepsy and pregnancy group. *Epilepsia.* 2004;45:1467.
25. Vajda F, Lander C, O'Brien T. Australian pregnancy registry of women taking antiepileptic drugs. *Epilepsia.* 2004;45:1466.
26. Montouris G. Gabapentin exposure in human pregnancy: results from the gabapentin pregnancy registry. *Epilepsy and Behavior.* 2003;4:310–317.
27. Cunnington M, Tennis P and the International Pregnancy Registry Scientific Advisory Committee. Lamotrigine and the risk of malformations in pregnancy. *Neurology.* 2005;64:1161–1167.
28. Wyszynski D, Nambisan M, Surve T, et al. Increased risk of major malformations in offspring exposed to valproate during pregnancy. *Neurology.* 2005;64:961–965.
29. Lamictal® (lamotrigine). Information for Health Care Professionals (Sep 28, 2006). *Accessed at*: www.fda.gov/cder/drug/InfoSheets/HCP/lamotrigineHCP.htm (on Feb 15, 2007.)
30. Dubnov-Raz G, Shapiro R, Merlob P. Maternal lamotrigine treatment and elevated neonatal gamma-glutamyl transpeptidase. *Pediatr Neurol.* 2006;35:220–222.
31. Kallen B. Use of antihistamine drugs in early pregnancy and delivery outcome. *J Matern Fetal Neonatal Med.* 2002;11:146–152.
32. Einarson A, Bailey B, Jung G, et al. Prospective controlled study of hydroxyzine and cetirizine in pregnancy. *Ann Allergy Asthma Immunol.* 1997;78:183–186.
33. Erez S, Schifrin BS, Dirim O. Double-blind evaluation of hydroxyzine as an antiemetic in pregnancy. *J Reprod Med.* 1977;7:35–37.
34. Schatz M. H1-Antihistamines in pregnancy and lactation. *Clin Allergy Immunol.* 2002;17:421–436.
35. Serreau R, Komiha M, Blanc F, et al. Neonatal seizures associated with maternal hydroxyzine hydrochloride in late pregnancy. *Reprod Toxicol.* 2005;20:573–574.
36. Prenner BM. Neonatal withdrawal syndrome associated with hydroxyzine hydrochloride. *Am J Dis Child.* 1977;131:529–530.
37. National Heart, Lung and Blood Institute, National Asthma Education and Prevention Program Asthma and Pregnancy Working Group. NAEPP Expert Panel Report Managing Asthma during Pregnancy: Recommendations for Pharmacologic Treatment—2004 Update. *J Allergy Clin Immunol.* 2005;115:34–46.
38. Moretti ME, Caprara D, Coutinho CJ, et al. Fetal safety of loratidine use in the first trimester of pregnancy: a multicenter study. *J Allergy Clin Immunol.* 2003;111:479–483.
39. Diav-Citrin O, Shechtman S, Aharonovich A, et al. Pregnancy outcome after gestational exposure to loratidine or antihistamines: A prospective controlled cohort study. *J Allergy Clin Immunol.* 2003;111:1239–1243.
40. Werler M, McCloskey C, Edmonds LD, et al. Evaluation of an association between loratidine and hypospadius—United States, 1997–2001. *MMWR.* 2004;53:219–221.
41. Gruber MR. Maternal immunization: US FDA regulatory considerations. *Vaccine.* 2003;21:3487–3491.
42. CDC. Notice to Readers: Revised ACIP recommendation for avoiding pregnancy after receiving a rubella-containing vaccine. *MMWR Morb Mortal Wkly Rep.* 2001;50:1117.
43. Bar-Oz B, Levichek Z, Moretti ME, et al. Pregnancy outcome following rubella vaccination. *Am J Med Genet.* 2004;130A:52–54.
44. ACOG committee opinion, The American College of Obstetricians and Gynecologists. Rubella Vaccination. *Int J Gynecol Obstet.* 2003;81:241.
45. CDC. Prevention and Control of Influenza. *MMWR Morb Mortal Wkly Rep.* 2005;54:1–40.
46. National Advisory Committee on Immunization. Statement on influenza vaccination for the 2005–2006 season. *Can Commun Dis Rep.* 2005;31:1–30.
47. Munoz FM, Greisinger AJ, Wehmanen OA, et al. Safety of influenza vaccination during pregnancy. *Am J Obstet Gynecol.* 2005;192: 1098–1106.
48. Deinard AS, Ogburn P. A/NJ/8/76 influenza vaccination program: effects on maternal health and pregnancy outcome. *Am J Obstet Gynecol.* 1981;140:240–245.
49. Sumaya CV, Gibbs RS. Immunization of pregnant women with influenza A/New Jersey/76 virus vaccine: reactogenicity and immunogenicity in mother and infant. *J Infect Dis.* 1979;140:141–146.
50. CDC. Prevention of Hepatitis A through active or passive immunization: recommendations of the advisory committee on immunization practices (ACIP). *MMWR Morb Mortal Wkly Rep.* 1999;48:1–37.
51. CDC. Hepatitis B virus: a comprehensive strategy for eliminating transmission in the United States through universal childhood vaccination: recommendations of the immunization practices advisory committee (ACIP). *MMWR Morb Mortal Wkly Rep.* 1991;40:1–19.
52. Gupta I, Ratho RK. Immunogenicity and safety of two schedules of Hepatitis B vaccination during pregnancy. *J Obstet Gynaecol Res.* 2003;29:84–86.
53. Ayoola EA, Johnson AOK. Hepatitis B vaccine in pregnancy: immunogenicity, safety and transfer of antibodies to infants. *Int J Gynaecol Obstet.* 1987;25:297–301.
54. Levy M, Koren G. Hepatitis B vaccine in pregnancy: maternal and fetal safety. *Am J Perinatol.* 1991;8:227–232.
55. Hernandez-Diaz S, Werler MM, Walker AM, et al. Neural tube defects in relation to use of folic acid antagonists during pregnancy. *Am J Epidemiol.* 2001;153:961–968.
56. Hernandez-Diaz S, Werler MM, Walker AM, et al. Folic acid antagonists during pregnancy and the risk of birth defects. *N Engl J Med.* 2000;343:1608–1614.

57. Czeizel AD, Rockenbauer M, Sorensen HT, et al. The teratogenic risk of trimethoprim-sulfonamides: a population based case-control study. *Reprod Toxicol.* 2001;15:637–646.
58. Gough AW, Kasali OB, Sigler RE, et al. Quinolone Arthropathy—Acute Toxicity to Immature Articular Cartilage. *Toxicol Pathol.* 1992;20:436–449.
59. Berkovitch M, Pastuszak A, Gazarian M, Lewis M, Koren G. Safety of the new quinolones in pregnancy. *Obstet Gynecol.* 1994;84:535–538.
60. Schaefer C, Amoura-Elefant E, Vial T, et al. Pregnancy outcome after prenatal quinolone exposure. Evaluation of a case registry of the European Network of Teratology Information Services (ENTIS). *Eur J Obstet Gynecol Reprod Biol.* 1996;69:83–89.
61. Loebstein LR, Addis A, Ho E, et al. Pregnancy outcome following gestational exposure to fluoroquinolones: a multicenter prospective controlled study. *Antimicrob Agents Chemother.* 1998;42:1336–1339.
62. Einarson A, Phillips E, Mawji F, et al. A prospective controlled multicentre study of clarithromycin in pregnancy. *Am J Perinatol.* 1998;15:523–525.
63. Drinkard CR, Shatin D, Clouse J. Postmarketing surveillance of medications and pregnancy outcomes: clarithromycin and birth malformations. *Pharmacoepidemiol Drug Saf.* 2000;9:549–556.
64. Caro-Paton T, Carvajal A, Martin de Diego I, et al. Is metronidazole teratogenic? A meta-analysis. *Br J Clin Pharmacol.* 1997;44:179–182.
65. Burtin P, Taddio A, Ariburnu O, et al. Safety of metronidazole in pregnancy: a meta-analysis. *Am J Obstet Gynecol.* 1995;172:525–529.
66. Diav-Citrin O, Shechtman S, Gotteiner T, et al. Pregnancy outcome after gestational exposure to metronidazole: a prospective controlled cohort study. *Teratology.* 2001;63:186–192.
67. Sorensen HT, Larsen H, Jensen ES, et al. Safety of metronidazole during pregnancy: a cohort study of risk of congenital abnormalities, preterm delivery and low birth weight in 124 women. *J Antimicrob Chemother.* 1999;44:847–855.
68. Czeizel AE, Rockenbauer M. A population based case-control teratologic study of oral metronidazole treatment during pregnancy. *Br J Obstet Gynaecol.* 1998;105:322–327.
69. Stone KM, Reiff-Eldridge R, White AD. Pregnancy outcomes following systemic prenatal acyclovir exposure: conclusions from the International Acyclovir Pregnancy Registry, 1984–1999. *Birth Defects Res A Clin Mol Teratol.* 2004;70:201–207.
70. Ratanajamit C, Skriver MV, Jepsen P, et al. Adverse pregnancy outcome in women exposed to acyclovir during pregnancy: a population-based observational study. *Scand J Infect Dis.* 2003;35:255–259.
71. Tyring SK, Baker D, Snowden W. Valacyclovir for herpes simplex virus infection: long-term safety and sustained efficacy after 20 years' experience with acyclovir. *J Infect Dis.* 2002;186(Suppl 1):S40–S46.
72. Miller BW, Howard TK, Goss JA, et al. Renal transplantation one week after conception. *Transplantation.* 1995;60:1353–1354.
73. Pescovitz MD. Absence of teratogenicity of oral ganciclovir used during early pregnancy in a liver transplant recipient. *Transplantation.* 1999;67:758–759.
74. Koren G, Zemlickis DM. Outcome of pregnancy after first trimester exposure to H2 receptor antagonists. *Am J Perinatol.* 1991;8:37–38.
75. Magee LA, Inocencion G, Kamboj L, et al. Safety of first trimester exposure to histamine H blockers. *Dig Dis Sci.* 1996;41:1145–1149.
76. Kallen B. Delivery outcome after the use of acid-suppressing drugs in early pregnancy with special reference to omeprazole. *Br J Obstet Gynaecol.* 1998;105:877–881.
77. Garbis H, Elefant E, Diav-Citrin O, et al. Pregnancy outcome after exposure to ranitidine and other H_2 blockers. A collaborative study of the European Network of Teratology Information Services. *Reprod Toxicol.* 2005;19:453–458.
78. Nifkar S, Abdollahi M, Moretti M, et al. Use of proton pump inhibitors during pregnancy and rates of major malformations: a meta-analysis. *Dig Dis Sci.* 2002;47:1526–1529.
79. Diav-Citrin O, Arnon J, Shechtman S, et al. The safety of proton pump inhibitors in pregnancy: a multicentre prospective controlled study. *Aliment Pharmacol Ther.* 2005;21:269–275.
80. Kazy Z, Czeizel AE. Population-based case-control study of oral ketoconazole treatment for birth outcomes. *Congenit Anom.* 2005;45:5–8.
81. Tiboni GM, Giampietro F. Murine teratology of fluconazole: evaluation of developmental phase specificity and dose dependence. *Pediatr Res.* 2005;58:94–99.
82. Menegola E, Broccia ML, Di Renzo F, et al. Study on the common teratogenic pathway elicited by the fungicides triazole-derivatives. *Toxicol In Vitro.* 2005;19:737–748.
83. Pursley TJ, Blomquist IK, Abraham J, et al. Fluconazole-induced congenital anomalies in three infants. *Clin Infect Dis.* 1996; 22:336–340.
84. Inman W, Pearce G, Wilton L. Safety of fluconazole in the treatment of vaginal candidiasis. A prescription—event monitoring study, with special reference to the outcome of pregnancy. *Eur J Clin Pharmacol.* 1994;46:115–118.
85. Mastroiacovo P, Mazzone T, Botto LD, et al. Prospective assessment of pregnancy outcomes after first trimester exposure to fluconazole. *Am J Obstet Gynecol.* 1996;175:1645–1650.
86. Jick SS. Pregnancy outcomes after maternal exposure to fluconazole. *Pharmacotherapy.* 1999;19:221–222.
87. Sorensen HT, Nielsen GL, Olesen C, et al. Risk of malformations and other outcomes in children exposed to fluconazole in utero. *Br J Clin Pharmacol.* 1999;48:234–238.
88. King CT, Rogers PD, Cleary JD, et al. Antifungal therapy during pregnancy. *Clin Infect Dis.* 1998;27:1151–1160.
89. Czeizel AE, Kazy Z, Puho E. A population based, case control teratological study of oral nystatin treatment during pregnancy. *Scand J Infect Dis.* 2003;35:830–835.
90. de Silva NR, Sirisena JLGJ, Gunasekera DPS, et al. Effect of mebendazole therapy during pregnancy on birth outcome. *Lancet.* 1999;353:1145–1149.
91. Diav-Citrin O, Shechtman S, Arnon J, et al. Pregnancy outcome after gestational exposure to mebendazole: A prospective controlled cohort study. *Am J Obstet Gynecol.* 2003;188:282–285.
92. Bracken MB, Holford TR. Exposure to Prescribed Drugs in Pregnancy and Association with Congenital Malformations. *Obstet Gynecol.* 1981;58:336–344.
93. Aselton P, Jick J, Milunsky A, et al. First-Trimester Drug Use and Congenital Disorders. *Obstet Gynecol.* 1985;65:451–455.
94. Jick H, Holmes LB, Hunter JR, et al. First Trimester Drug Use and Congenital Disorders. *JAMA.* 1981;246:343–346.
95. Khan K, Chang J. Neonatal abstinence syndrome due to codeine. *Arch Dis Child.* 1997;76:F59–F60.
96. Mangurten HH, Benawra R. Neonatal Codeine Withdrawal in Infants of Nonaddicted Mothers. *Pediatrics.* 1980;65:159–160.
97. Refstad SO, Lindbaek E. Ventilatory depression of the newborn of women receiving pethidine or pentazocine. *Br J Anaesth.* 1980;52:265–271.
98. Morrison JC, Wiser WL, Rosser SI, et al. Metabolites of meperidine related to fetal depression. *Am J Obstet Gynecol.* 1973;115:1132–1137.
99. Shnider SM, Moya F. Effects of meperidine on the newborn infant. *Am J Obstet Gynecol.* 1964;89:1009–1015.
100. Hafstrom M, Kjellmer I. Non-nutritive sucking by infants exposed to pethidine in utero. *Acta Paediatr.* 2000;1196–1200.
101. Hodgkinson R, Bhatt M, Wang CN. Double-blind comparison of the neurobehaviour of neonates following the administration of different doses of meperidine to the mother. *Can Anaesth Soc J.* 1978;25: 405–411.
102. Hodgkinson R, Bhatt M, Grewal G, et al. Neonatal Neurobehavior in the First 48 Hours of Life: Effect of the Administration of Meperidine With and Without Naloxone in the Mother. *Pediatrics.* 1978;62:294–298.
103. Hilaire ML, Cross LB, Eichner SF. Treatment of Migraine Headaches with Sumatriptan in Pregnancy. *Ann Pharmacother.* 2004;38:1726–1730.
104. Shuhaiber S, Pastuszak A, Schick B, et al. Pregnancy outcome following first trimester exposure to sumatriptan. *Neurology.* 1998;51:581–583.

105. Reiff-Eldridge R, Heffner CR, Ephross SA, et al. Monitoring pregnancy outcomes after prenatal drug exposure through prospective pregnancy registries: a pharmaceutical company commitment. *Am J Obstet Gynecol.* 2000;182:159–163.
106. Norgard B, Puho E, Czeizel AE, et al. Aspirin use during early pregnancy and the risk of congenital abnormalities: A population-based case-control study. *Amer J Obstet Gynecol.* 2005;192:922–923.
107. Czeizel AE, Rockenbauer M, Mosonyi A. A population-based case-control teratologic study of acetylsalicylic acid treatments during pregnancy. *Pharmacoepidemiol Drug Saf.* 2000;9:193–205.
108. Kozer E, Nifkar S, Costei A, et al. Aspirin consumption during the first trimester of pregnancy and congenital anomalies: A meta-analysis. *Amer J Obstet Gynecol.* 2002;187:1623–1630.
109. Kozer E, Costei AM, Boskovic R, et al. Effects of aspirin consumption during pregnancy on pregnancy outcomes : meta-analysis. *Birth Defects Research (Part B).* 2003;68:70–74.
110. Li D, Liu L, Odouli R. Exposure to non-steroidal anti-inflammatory drugs during pregnancy and risk of miscarriage: population based cohort study. *BMJ.* 2003;327:368–372.
111. Ericson A, Kallen BAJ. Nonsteroidal anti-inflammatory drugs in early pregnancy. *Reprod Toxicol.* 2001;15:371–375.
112. Adverse Drug Reactions Advisory Committee. Premature closure of the fetal ductus arteriosus after maternal use of non-steroidal anti-inflammatory drugs. *Med J Aust.* 1998:169:270–271.
113. Benini D, Fanos V, Cuzzolin L, et al. In utero exposure to nonsteroidal anti-inflammatory drugs:neonatal renal failure. *Pediatr Nephrol.* 2004;19:232–234.
114. Takahashi Y, Roman C, Chemtob S, et al. Cyclooxygenase-2 inhibitors constrict the fetal lamb ductus arteriosus both in vitro and in vivo. *Am J Physiol Regul Integr Comp Physiol.* 2000;278: R1496–R1505.
115. Slattery MM, Friel AM, Healy DG, et al. Uterine relaxant effects of cyclooxygenase-2 inhibitors in vitro. *Obstet Gynecol.* 2001;98: 563–569.
116. McKenna K, Koren G, Tetelbaum M, et al. Pregnancy outcome of women using atypical antipsychotic drugs: a prospective comparative study. *J Clin Psychiatry.* 2005:66:444–449.
117. Bracken MB. Oral contraception and congenital malformations in offspring: a review and meta-analysis of the prospective studies. *Obstet Gynecol.* 1990;76:552–557.
118. Raman-Wilms L, Lin-in Tseng A, Wighardt S, et al. Fetal Genital Effects of First-Trimester Sex Hormone Exposure: A Meta-analysis. *Obstet Gynecol.* 1995;85:141–149.
119. Luisa Martinez-Frias M, Rodriguez-Pinilla E, Bermejo E, et al. Prenatal Exposure to Sex Hormones: A Case-Control Study. *Teratology.* 1998;57:8–12.
120. Li D. Reply to "Prenatal Exposure to Sex Hormones: A Case-Control Study." *Teratology.* 1998;58:1.
121. Gutzin SJ, Kozer E, Magee L, et al. The safety of oral hypoglycemic agents in the first trimester of pregnancy: A meta-analysis. *Can J Clin Pharmacol.* 2003;179–183.
122. McCarthy EA, Walker SP, McLachlan K, et al. Metformin in Obstetric and Gynecologic Practice: A Review. *Obstet Gynecol Survey.* 2004;59:118–127.
123. Gilbert CJ, Koren G. Safety of metformin use during the first trimester (Letter). *Canadian Family Physician.* 2005;51:1070.
124. Saade G. Gestational Diabetes Mellitus: A Pill or a Shot? *Obstet Gynecol.* 2005;105:456–457.
125. Yaris F, Yaris E, Kadioglu M, et al. Normal pregnancy outcome following inadvertent exposure to rosiglitazone, gliclazide, and atorvastatin in a diabetic and hypertensive woman. *Reprod Toxicol.* 2004;18:619–621.
126. Edison RJ, Muenke M. Mechanical and epidemiologic considerations in the evaluation of adverse birth outcomes following gestational exposure to statins. *Am J Med Genet.* 2004;131A:287–298.
127. Werler MM, Mitchell AA, Shapiro S. First trimester maternal medication use in relation to gastroschisis. *Teratology.* 1992;45:361–367.
128. Torfs CP, Katz EA, Bateson TF, et al. Maternal medications and environmental exposures as risk factors for gastroschisis. *Teratology.* 1996;54:84–92.
129. Werler MM, Sheehan JE, Mitchell AA. Association of Vasoconstrictive Exposures with Risks of Gastroschisis and Small Intestinal Atresia. *Epidemiology.* 2003;14:349–354.
130. Einarson A, Lyszkiewicz D, Koren G. The safety of dextromethorphan in pregnancy: results of a controlled study. *Chest.* 2001;119:466–469.
131. Park-Wyllie L, Mazzotta P, Pastuszak A, et al. Birth Defects after Maternal Exposure to Corticosteroids: Prospective Cohort Study and Meta-Analysis of Epidemiological Studies. *Teratology.* 2000; 62:385–392.
132. Pradat P, Robert-Gnansia E, Luca Di Tanna G, et al. First Trimester Exposure to Corticosteroids and Oral Clefts. *Birth Defects Res A Clin Mol Teratol.* 2003;67:968–970.
133. Scialli AR. Who should paint the nursery? *Reprod Toxicol.* 1989;3:159–164.
134. Koren G. The Complete Guide to Everyday Risks in Pregnancy & Breastfeeding. Toronto: Robert Rose Inc., 2004:141.
135. Khattak S, Moghtader GK, McMartin K, et al. Pregnancy Outcome Following Gestational Exposure to Organic Solvents—A Prospective Controlled Study. *JAMA.* 1999;281:1106–1109.
136. Bellinger DC. Teratogen Update: Lead and Pregnancy. *Birth Defects Res A Clin Mol Teratol.* 2005;73:409–420.
137. Burnett C, Goldenthal EI, Harris SB, et al. Teratology and percutaneous toxicity studies on hair dyes. *J Toxicol Environ Health.* 1976;1:1027–1040.
138. DiNardo JC, Picciano JC, Schnetzinger RW, Morris WE, Wolf BA. Teratological assessment of five oxidative hair dyes in the rat. *Toxicol Appl Pharmacol.* 1985;78:163–166.
139. Wernick T, Lanman BM, Fraux JL. Chronic Toxicity, Teratologic, and Reproduction Studies with Hair Dyes. *Toxicol Appl Pharmacol.* 1975;32:450–460.
140. MCcCall EE, Olshan AF, Daniels JL. Maternal hair dye use and risk of neuroblastoma in offspring. *Cancer Causes Control.* 2005;16:743–748.
141. Holly EA, Bracci PM, Hong M, et al. West Coast study of childhood brain tumours and maternal use of hair-colouring products. *Paediatr Perinat Epidemiol.* 2002;16:226–235.
142. Rylander L, Kallen B. Reproductive outcomes among hairdressers. *Scand J Work Environ Health.* 2005;31:212–217.

CHAPTER 8

DIRECT DRUG TOXICITY TO THE FETUS

Orna Diav-Citrin and Gideon Koren

The fetal phase, from the end of the embryonic stage to term, is the period when growth and functional maturation of organs and systems already formed occur. Teratogen exposure in this period may adversely affect fetal growth (e.g., intrauterine growth restriction), the size of a specific organ, or the function of the organ, rather than cause gross structural anomalies. The term fetal toxicity, rather than teratogenicity, is commonly used to describe such an effect. Fetal toxicity, unlike teratogenicity, is often predicted from the known pharmacological profile and toxicological effects of the agents involved. Fetal toxic effects may have a major impact on the morbidity and mortality of the neonate. In counseling pregnant women regarding drug exposure during pregnancy, it is important to address fetal toxic effects and estimate their risk.

Table 8-1 reviews medicinal drugs that may cause direct fetal toxicity in humans, and summarizes the evidence for the fetal toxic effect with an attempt to estimate the rate of its occurrence. Whenever fetal toxic effects are based on case reports, they are used as a warning signal. In such cases, it is virtually impossible to give a true risk estimate, because the denominator of the total number of exposed fetuses is unknown. Other chapters deal with drugs and substances of abuse and with neonatal withdrawal syndromes. The potential effect of psychoactive agents on the developing central nervous system, which belongs to the evolving field of behavioral teratology, is beyond the scope of this chapter.

Table 8-1
Direct Drug Toxicity to the Fetus

NO.	DRUG	FETAL/NEONATAL TOXIC EFFECTS	REPORTED RATE OF OCCURRENCE*	COMMENTS/RECOMMENDATIONS	REFERENCE
1.	Acebutolol	Lower mean birth weight than in neonates exposed, to pindolol; (higher than in those exposed to atenolol)	C/R	Not known whether due to the degree of maternal hypertension or, the potency of the drug or a combination of these and other factors	1
		Transient hypoglycemia			2
		Lower blood pressure and heart rate than of similar infants exposed to methyldopa		Neonates should be closely observed for signs of β-blockade	3
2.	Acetaminophen	Polyhydramnios and fatal neonatal kidney disease in the newborn	C/R	Continuous maternal high daily dose	4
		Fetal death with hepatic and renal toxicity	C/R	In an overdose situation	5
		Severe fetal distress, neonatal death with hepatorenal toxicity	C/R	In an overdose situation	6
		Stillbirth with massive centrilobular heaptic necrosis	1/60	In overdose situations	7
3.	Acetazolamide	Asymptomatic hypocalcemia, hypomagnesemia, and metabolic acidosis in the newborn	1/3	Resolved after treatment	8
4.	Acetohexamide	Prolonged symptomatic hypoglycemia in the newborn	C/R	Oral hypoglycemics generally not recommended	9
		Prolonged hypoglycemia and convulsions in the newborn	C/R	in pregnancy because of concerns regarding insufficient glycemic control	10
5.	Albuterol	Fetal tachycardia transient fetal atrial flutter	C/R	Adverse reactions secondary to the cardiovascular and metabolic effects of the drug	11–16
		Transient fetal hyperglycemia followed by hyperinsulinemia		Effects more pronounced in diabetic patients	17–21
				Neonatal hypoglycemia should be prevented with adequate intake of glucose	22, 23
		Higher growth hormone levels in cord blood		Direct adrenergic stimulation of the pituitary	24
6.	Alfentanil	Neonatal apnea and hypotonia		Can be reversed with naloxone	25, 26
7.	Alphaprodine	Respiratory depression			27–34
		Transient sinusoidal fetal heart rate pattern	17/40 (42.5%)	No short-term neonatal adverse effects were observed	35
		Suppression of collagen induced platelet aggregation		Abnormal bleeding not reported	36
8.	Ambenonium	Transient muscular weakness	20% of newborns whose mothers were treated with cholineesterase inhibitors during pregnany	Neonatal myasthenia may be caused by transplacentsl passage of antiacetylcholine receptor immunoglobulin G antibodies, rather than a drug effect	37, 38
9.	Aminoglutethimide	Virilization		May be caused by inhibition of adrenocortical function	39, 40

10.	Amiodarone	Prolonged QT interval	C/R	Not clinically significant	41, 42
		Transient bradycardia			43, 44
		Transient hypothyroidism		Thyroid function tests recommended for newborns exposed to amiodarone in utero because of the high iodine content of the drug	45–47
		Congenital hypothyroidism with goiter			48
		Transient asymptomatic hyperthyroidism			43
		Elevated serum iodine level			49
		IUGR		May be an effect of amiodarone, a result of the maternal disease, concurrent medications, or a combination of the above	50, 48
		Transient asympomatic hyperthyroidism	1/11		51
		Hypothyroidism	1/11		
		Fetal bradycardia	3/11	Two of whom also exposed to β-blockers (acebutolol and propranolol)	
		SGA	4/11	Three also exposed to β-blockers	
11.	Ammonium chloride	Fetal acidosis		In large amounts near term	52, 53
12.	Amphetamine	IUGR		Multifactorial: multidrug abuse, lifestyle, poor maternal health, and antenatal care	54
		Prematurity	6/17		55, 56
		Cerebral injuries		Due to the vasoconstrictive properties of the drug	57
		Intrauterine death	C/R	In an acute poisoning	58
13.	Ampicillin	Severe neonatal distress with neorologic sequelae	C/R	Maternal anaphylaxis	59
14.	Antihistamines	Increased risk of retrolental fibroplasia in premature infants	22% vs. 11% in not exposed	During the last 2 weeks of pregnancy, specific agents and doses not reported	60
15.	Aprotinin	Decreased fibrinolytic activity			61
16.	Asparaginase	Transient bone marrow hypoplasia in the newborn	2 C/Rs	In combination with other antineoplastic agents	62, 63
		Chromosomal damage	C/R	Clinical significance- not clear	64
17.	Aspirin	IUGR			
		Increased perinatal mortality (stillbirths more than neonatal)		Some associated with antepartum hemorrhage, others may have been caused by closure of the ductus	65, 67
		Premature closure of the ductus arteriosus			68
		Decreased clotting ability		Depressed platelet function	69–76
		Increased incidence of intracranial hemorrhage		In premature or low-birth-weight infants after full dose given near term	77–80
		Toxic effects		Large doses	81, 82
		Congenital salicylate intoxication			83, 84
		Depressed albumin binding capacity		No increase in the incidence of jaundice	85
18.	Atenolol	IUGR		May be related to increased vascular resistance and is a function of length of drug exposure	86–88
		Lower birth weight			
		Persistent β-blockade		Newborns exposed near delivery should be closely observed during the first 24–48 hours for signs and symptoms of β-blockade	89–94

(*Continued*)

Table 8-1
Direct Drug Toxicity to the Fetus (*Continued*)

NO.	DRUG	FETAL/NEONATAL TOXIC EFFECTS	REPORTED RATE OF OCCURRENCE*	COMMENTS/RECOMMENDATIONS	REFERENCE
19.	Azathioprine	Immunosuppression		Dose reduction is recommended according to maternal leukocyte count at 32 weeks' gestation to avoid neonatal leukopenia and thrombocytopenia	95–97
		IUGR	Incidence of SGA: 20–40%	Other potential contributors: underlying disease, (hypertension, vascular disease, and renal impairment), multiple medications	98–102
		Chromosomal abberations		Clinical significance unknown	103
20.	Benztropine	Paralytic ileus	Two newborns	Exposure at term to chlorpromazine as well	104
21.	Betamethasone	Hypoglycemia			105
		Leukocytosis	C/Rs		106, 107
		Transient constriction of the ductus arteriosus	2/11	Clinical significance not clear	108
		Transient decrease in glucocorticoid activity in the neonate		Rebounded to above normal when the newborns were 2 hours of age, then returned to normal values	109
		Adrenal suppression with cushingoid features		After multiple courses	110, 111
		Lower birth weight and reduced head circumference		After multiple courses	111–113
		Decreased fetal heart rate variability			114, 115
22.	Bleomycin	Profound transient leukopenia with neutropenia and alopecia	C/R	Other chemotherapeutic agents involved, by 12 weeks of age hair regrowth, at 1 year normal development except for moderate hearing loss	116
		Chromosomal aberrations		In human marrow cells, significance to the fetus unknown	117
23.	Bromides	IUGR			118, 119
		Neonatal bromide intoxication (poor suck, weak cry, diminished Moro reflex, lethargy and hypotonia)	3 C/Rs	Normal growth and development after several months	120–122
24.	Busulfan	IUGR			123, 124
		Chromosomal aberrations		Clinical significance unknown	125
25.	Butorphanol	Depressant effect			126–128
		Sinusoidal fetal heart rate pattern	75% (38/51) vs. 13% (7/55)	Clinical significance unknown	129, 130
26.	Caffeine	Low birth weight		High consumption	131
		Tachyarrhythmias	25% vs. 1.7%	Associated with maternal caffeine consumption of more than 500 mg/day (n = 16) in comparison to offspring of women who used less than 250 mg/day (n = 56) of caffeine	132
		Premature atrial contraction	12.5% vs. 0		
		Fine tremors	100% vs. 10.7%		
		Tachypnea	25% vs. 3.5%		
		Fetal behavioral and sleep pattern changes		In high amounts of caffeine consumption (>500mg/day)	133
27.	Calcitonin	Marked increase of calcitonin concentrations in fetal serum at term		Clinical significance unknown	134

28.	Calcitriol	Mild transient hypercalcemia in the first 2 days of life	C/R	After exposure to a maternal dose of 17–36 μg/day (approximately 17–36 times the maximum recommended dose	135
29.	Camphor	Fetal toxicity and neonatal respiratory failure	5 C/Rs	Accidental ingestion, camphor poisoning	136–140
30.	Candesartan	Oligohydramnios, anuria, skull hypoplasia, and abnormal sonographic appearance of the kidneys	3 C/Rs	Similar mechanism as in angiotensin-converting enzyme inhibitor fetopathy	141–143
31.	Captopril	Oligohydramnios IUGR Renal dysplasia Intrauterine fetal death Fetal hypotension Neonatal anuria Renal failure Craniofacial deformations: hypocalvaria/acalvaria Pulmonary hypoplsia Limb contractures Neonatal death	Cluster of C/Rs	When used in the second and third trimesters of pregnancy risk of angiotensin-converting enzyme inhibitor fetopathy. Speculated mechanism related to drug-induced oligohydramnios, causing a mechanical insult, combined with drug-induced fetal hypotension and decreased renal blood flow. In cases in which maternal disease requires captopril in late pregnancy, monitoring of amniotic fluid volume is advised during gestation, as well as close observation of blood pressure and renal function in the neonate	144
32.	Carbamazepine	Lower cord serum vitamin D levels compared to normal controls		The levels were still within normal limits, questionable clinical significance	145
		Neonatal vitamin K deficiency associated with early hemorrhagic disease of the newborn		Vitamin K prophylaxis advised to the mother before the expected time of delivery	146–148
		Transient cholestatic hepatitis	3 C/Rs	Exposure during pregnancy and breastfeeding	149–151
33.	Carbimazole	See methimazole		Converted in vivo to methimazole	
34.	Celecoxib	Transient decrease in amniotic fluid volume	n = 12	Less than with indomethacin	152
35.	Chlorambucil	Mutagenicity and carcinogenicity		Not reported in newborns following in utero exposure	153–157
		Low birth weight	40%		123
36.	Chloramphenicol	Cardiovascular collapse ("gray baby syndrome")		During the final stage of pregnancy	158
37.	Chlordiazepoxide	Marked deppression of the infants (they were unresponsive, hypotonic, hypothermic, and fed poorly)	3 infants	Exposure within hours of delivery Hypotonicity persisted for up to a week	159
38.	Chloroquine	Cochleovestibular paresis	2 siblings	Concern regarding cumulative ocular toxicity of high doses used for rheumatological conditions if used for prolonged periods during pregnancy	160
39.	Chlorothiazide	Neonatal hypoglycemia	0.1% (14/13725) vs. 0.02% in controls	Newborns exposed to thiazide diuretics near term should be observed for hypoglycemia as a result of maternal hyperglycemia	161
		Neonatal thrombocytopenia		Transfer of antiplatelet antibody demonstrated	162–169
		Hemolytic anemia			164
		Hyponatremia	2 cases		170
		Hypokalemia	2 cases		171–172
		Fetal death attributed to matrenal hemorrhagic pancreatitis	2 cases		173

(*Continued*)

Table 8-1
Direct Drug Toxicity to the Fetus ***(Continued)***

NO.	DRUG	FETAL/NEONATAL TOXIC EFFECTS	REPORTED RATE OF OCCURRENCE*	COMMENTS/RECOMMENDATIONS	REFERENCE
40.	Chlorpromazine	Neonatal hopotonia, lethargy, depressed reflexes, and jaundice	C/R	High doses, resolved within 3 weeks	174
		Paralytic lieus	2 cases	Doxepin coadministered in one case	104
		An extrapyramidal syndrome (tremors, hypertonia, spasticity, hyperactive reflexes)		Near term, may persist for months	175–179
41.	Chlorpropamide	Prolonged neonatal symptomatic hypoglycemia secondary to hyperinsulinism	4 cases	Near term, lasted for 4–6 days	180–182
		Severe hypoglycemia	3 cases	Generally, insulin provides better glycemic control and is the drug of choice for diabetes in pregnancy	183
		Hyperbilirubinemia	10/15 (67%) vs. 13/36 (36%)		
		Polycythemia and hyperviscosity	4/15 (27%) vs. 1/36 (3.0%)		
42.	Cholestyramine	Fatal fetal subdural hematomas	C/R	Possible result of vitamin K deficiency caused by long-term use in of high-dose cholestyramine, cholestasis, or both	184
43.	Cimetidine	Transient neonatal liver impairment	C/R	Exposure at term	185
44.	Cisplatin	Profound transient leukopenia with neutropenia and alopecia	C/R	Other chemotherapeutic agents involved, by 12 weeks of age hair regrowth, at 1 year normal development except for moderate hearing loss (thought to be gentamicin or cisplatin related)	116
45.	Clofazimine	Skin pigmentation at birth		In at least 3 infants, gradually resolved during a 1-year period	186–187
46.	Clonazepam	Neonatal apneic episodes with hypotonia and lethargy	C/R	Exposure throughout pregnancy and in braestfeeding	188
				Hypotonia resolved within 5 days, clinical apnea persisted for 10 days, for 10 weeks by follow-up pneumograms	
		Paralytic ileus	C/R	Normal bowel movements started after 3 Gastrografin enemas	189
47.	Codeine	Neonatal respiratory depression		Use during labor	190
48.	Coumarin derivatives	CNS damage Hemorrhage IUGR Miscarriage Prematurity Stillbirth/neonatal death		Exposure in the second and/or third trimesters, probably caused by fetal or neonatal hemorrhage	191

49.	Cyclophosphamide	Pancytopenia		Exposure to five other antineoplastics in the third trimester	192
		Transient neonatal severe bone marrow hypoplasia	C/R	Combination chemotherapy including mercaptopurine and radiation	62
		Transient anemia	C/R	Initially received vinorelbine and fluorouracil, then six courses of epidoxorubicin and cyclophoshamide	193
		Transient leukopenia			
		IUGR		In combination with various other agents	194
		Stillbirth	40%		
		Neonatal death			
		Low birth weight		Following administration of anticancer drugs during pregnancy	123
		Chromosomal aberrations		Clinical significance unknown	64, 195
50.	Cyclosporine	Neonatal thrombocytopenia	C/R	May have been related to hydralazine concurrently administered to the mother	196
		Neonatal leukopenia	C/R		197
		Neonatal hypoglycemia and mild DIC	C/R	Resolved spontaneously	198
		IUGR	8–45%	In the offspring of renal transplant patients, potentially multifactorial (maternal hypertension, renal function, immunosuppressive drugs, or a combination of the above)	199
51.	Cytarabine	Chromosomal aberrations		Clinical significance unknown	64, 200
		Pancytopenia	C/R	Exposure in the third trimester, other antineoplastics involved	192
		Low birth weight	40%	Following administration of anticancer drugs during pregnancy	123
		Intrauterine fetal death	C/R		201
52.	Dactinomycin	Low birth weight	40%	Following administration of anticancer drugs during pregnancy	123
53.	Danazol	Female pseudohermaphrositism	~30–67% of female fetuses	Exposure beyond 8 weeks' gestation	202–211
54.	Dapsone	Neonatal hemolytic anemia	C/R	Spontaneously resolved within 10 days	212
		Neonatal hyperbilirubinemia	C/R		213
55.	Daunorubicin	Anemia, hypoglycemia, and electrolyte abnormalities	1 case		214
		Transient neutropenia at 2 months	2 cases		215
		Severe transient bone marrow hypoplasia	C/R	Five other antineoplastic agents involved, thought to be secondary to mercaptopurine	62
		Low birth weight	40%	Following administration of anticancer drugs during pregnancy	123
		Chromosomal aberrations		Clinical significance unknown	64

(*Continued*)

Table 8-1
Direct Drug Toxicity to the Fetus (*Continued*)

NO.	DRUG	FETAL/NEONATAL TOXIC EFFECTS	REPORTED RATE OF OCCURRENCE*	COMMENTS/RECOMMENDATIONS	REFERENCE
56.	Deferoxamine	Low neonatal iron levels	C/R	In acute iron overdose at 34 weeks' gestation	216
57.	Dexamethasone	Neonatal leukocytosis		White cell counts returned to normal in ~1 week	217–218
58.	Diatrizoate	Clinical neonatal hypothyroidism	3/7	When administered by intra-amniotic injection with ethiodized oil	219
		Biochemical neonatal hypothyroidism	6/7	Greater thyroid suppression, the longer the time interval between injection and delivery	
59.	Diazepam	"Floppy infant" syndrome (hypotonia, lethargy, and sucking difficulties)		The frequency of newborn complications increases when doses exceed 30–40 mg or when diazepam is taken for long periods	220–223
		Altered neonatal thermogenesis		When administered in labor	224–227
		Loss of beat-to-beat variability in fetal heart rate			228
		Decreased fetal movements			229
60.	Diazoxide	Transient fetal bradycardia		After rapid drop in maternal blood pressure following intravenous bolus administration	230, 231
		Newborn hyperglycemia		Following intravenous administration	232, 233
		Newborn alopecia, hypertrichosis lanuginosa, and decreased ossification of the wrist		Following oral treatment during the last 19–69 days of pregnancy	234
61.	Diclofenac	Premature closure of the fetal ductus arteriosus	C/R	Exposed to 50 mg twice daily for 2 weeks from the 34th week of gestation	235
		Severe pulmonary hypertension secondary to intrauterine ductal closure	3 C/Rs	Exposed after the 34th gestational week	236–238
		Transient constriction of the fetal ductus	C/R	After a single 75 mg IM dose of diclofenac at 36 weeks' gestation	239
62.	Diethylstilbestrol	Cervical or vaginal structural changes in the exposed female and genitourinary abnormalities in the exposed male offspring	22–58%		198, 240–242
		Masculinization of the female infant			
		Benign and malignant tumors of female and male reproductive system			
63.	Digitalis	Fetal intoxication and neonatal death	C/R	Following maternal acute digitoxin overdose	243
64.	Dihydrocodeine bitartrate	Newborn respiratory depression			144–244, 245, 190
65.	Dihydroergotamine	Stillbirth	4/20	After 1 mg in 500 mL water IV over a period of 2–4 hours to induce labor	246
		Neonatal death	1/20		
		Severe depression with seizures	1/20		
66.	Dimenhydrinate	Fetal distress (e.g., bradycardia, and loss of beat-to-beat variability)		Possible result of uterine hyperstimulation	247
67.	Diphenhydramine	Stillbirth	C/S	Potential drug interaction with temazepam	248

68.	Docusate sodium	Neonatal hypomagnesemia	C/R	Chronic maternal overuse Resolved spontaneously	249
69.	Doxepin	Paralytic ileus in a neonate	C/R	Thought to be caused primarily by coadministered chlorpromazine	104
70.	Enalapril	Oligohydramnios IUGR Renal dysplasia Intrauterine fetal death Fetal hypotension Neonatal anuria Renal failure Craniofacial deformations: hypocalvaria/acalvaria Pulmonary hypoplsia Limb contractures Neonatal death	Cluster of C/Rs	When used in the second and third trimesters of pregnancy. Speculated mechanism related to drug-induced oligohydramnios, causing a mechanical insult, combined with drug-induced fetal hypotension and decreased renal blood flow. In cases in which maternal disease requires enalapril in late pregnancy, monitoring of amniotic fluid volume is advised during gestation, as well as close observation of blood pressure and renal function in the neonate	198
71.	Ephedrine	Increase in fetal heart rate and beat-to-beat variability		When used to treat or prevent maternal hypotension following spinal anesthesia	250–252
72.	Epinephrine	Decrease in uterine blood flow and contribution to intrauterine anoxic insult resulting in neonatal death	C/R	Following a large intravenous dose to reverse severe maternal hypotension secondary to anaphylaxis	253
73.	Epirubicin	Stillbirth Neonatal death Transient leukopenia		Other antineoplastic agents involved	194
74.	Epoetin-α	Abruptio placentae with resulting fetal death at 23 weeks	C/R	Erythropoietin could not be excluded as a contributing factor in a woman with severe hypertension and chronic renal failure	254
75.	Ergotamine	Fetal death	C/R	Following acute overdose, in a suicide attempt at 35 weeks	255
		Fetal distress	C/R	Accidental use of ergotamine and caffeine at 38 weeks	256
76.	Esmolol	Fetal bradycardia	C/R		257
		β-blaockade in the fetus and infant	2 cases	Resolved spontaneously by 60 hours of age Newborns exposed near delivery should be closely observed during the first 24–48 hours for signs and symptoms of β-blockade	258, 259
77.	Ethacrynic acid	Ototoxicity observed in the newborn and mother	C/R	Following the use during the third trimester Concomitant exposure to kanamycin	260
78.	Ethosuximide	Spontaneous hemorrhage in the neonate	C/R	Rarely used today	261

(*Continued*)

Table 8-1
Direct Drug Toxicity to the Fetus (*Continued*)

NO.	DRUG	FETAL/NEONATAL TOXIC EFFECTS	REPORTED RATE OF OCCURRENCE*	COMMENTS/RECOMMENDATIONS	REFERENCE
79.	Etoposide	Oligohydramnios, IUGR	C/R	Four cycles of chemotherapy consisting of etoposide and cisplatin given from 27 weeks' gestation for dysgerminoma, initially treated surgically Normal hematological profile in the newborn	262
		Anemia, leukopenia, and profound neutropenia and thrombocytopenia in the neonate	C/R	Following combination chemotherapy consisting of two courses of etoposide, cytarabine, and daunorubicin given from 25 weeks' gestation for acute myeloid leukemia Treated successfully, at 1 year of age normal blood counts no longer treated	263
		Marked leukopenia with neutropenia in the neonate on day 3 (10 days after in utero exposure to the chemotherapy), scalp hair loss and loss of lanugo at 10 days of age, moderate bilateral sensorineural hearing loss at 1 year follow-up	C/R	Combination chemotherapy consisting of etoposide, cisplatin, and bleomycin given from 26 weeks' gestation, the patient became profoundly neutropenic and developed septicemia By 12 weeks of age the infant had hair growth Aminoglycoside therapy also given to the mother and neonate	116
80.	Etretinate	Transient pronounced jaundice with elevated transaminases in the newborn	C/R	Following in utero exposure to etretinate, no other anomalies observed, resolved at 5 months' follow-up	264
81.	Fentanyl	Respiratory depression in the neonate	C/R	Following epidural fentanyl during labor	265
		Loss of fetal heart rate variability without causing fetal hypoxia		Was the only effect in a prospective study of 137 women receiving fentanyl in labor	266, 267
		Respiratory muscle rigidity	C/R		268
82.	Flecainide	Loss of fetal heart rate variability and accelerations	C/R	Following treatment of fetal supraventricular tachycardia during the third trimester Fetal heart rate returned to a reactive pattern 5 days after delivery	269
		Transient conjugated hyperbilirubinemia in the neonate	C/R	Following successful treatment of fetal supraventricular tachycardia at 28 weeks' gestation after a trial of digoxin and adenosine had failed Resolved at 2 months' follow-up	270
83.	Fluorouracil	Cyanosis and jerking extremities in the newborn	C/R	Following third trimester exposure	271
		Neonatal death			194
		Transient leukopenia			
		IUGR			

84.	Fluoxetine	Poor neonatal adaptation		Overall very safe	272
		Lower mean birth weight			
		Persistent pulmonary hypertension	2.7%		
		Hypoglycemia, acrocyanosis, jitteriness, tachypnea, tremor, hypertonicity, hyperactive Moro reflex, and emesis	C/Rs		273, 274
85.	Fluphenazine	Minor extrapyramidal symptoms in the infant at 4 weeks of age	C/R	Following treatment in pregnancy with fluphenazine decanoate injections every 3 weeks, readily responded to diphenhydramine, resolved at 2 months of age	275
		Severe rinorrhea and upper respiratory distress at 8 hours of age, poor feeding, periodic vomiting choreoathetoid movements, and intermittent arching of the body	C/R	Following treatment with fluphenazine throughout pregnancy for schizophrenia, symptoms improved with pseudoephedrine solution, rinorrhea and nasal congestion persisted for 3 months	276
86.	Flurazepam	Sleepiness and lethargy	C/R	In the first 4 days of life	277
87.	Gabapentin	Jaundice and intermittent tremors that occurred for about 5 days after birth	C/R	Following first trimester exposure to lamotrigine in addition to administration of gabapentin before and throughout pregnancy, skin tags and ear anomalies also noted in the infant	278
88.	Glyburide	Neonatal hypoglycemia (blood glucose <25 mg/dL)	4/15 (27%)	3.5 times more often than observed in newborns whose mothers were treated with insulin, in 1 newborn, the hypoglycemia persisted for more than 48 hours, insulin recommended when drug therapy indicated for diabetes	279, 280
		Hypoglycemia Hyperbilirubinemia Polycythemia			281
89.	Haloperidol	Tardive dyskinesia	2 C/Rs		282, 283
90.	Hexamethonium	Paralytic ileus	3 cases	The drug had been used in the treatment of preeclampsia and essential hypertension	284, 285
91.	Hydralazine	Neonatal thrombocytopenia and bleeding	3 infants	Daily exposure throughout the third trimester, may be related to severe maternal hypertension rather than to the drug	286–288
		Fetal premature atrial contractions	C/R	Noted at 36 weeks' gestational age, a week following the addition of hydralazine to the woman's treatment with methyldapa, tacchyarrhythmias not observed, the fetal arrhythmia resolved 24 hours after stopping hydralazine	289

(Continued)

Table 8-1
Direct Drug Toxicity to the Fetus (*Continued*)

NO.	DRUG	FETAL/NEONATAL TOXIC EFFECTS	REPORTED RATE OF OCCURRENCE*	COMMENTS/RECOMMENDATIONS	REFERENCE
		Lupus-like syndrome in the newborn who died at 36 hours of age due to cardiac tamponade induced by pericardial effusion	C/R	Treated with IV hydralazine during a 6-day period in the 28th week of gestation for hypertension, IV methyldopa was administered on the 6th day of therapy, lupus-like syndrome developed in the mother on the 5th day of therapy and gradually resolved following discontinuation of hydralazine and delivery	290
		Fetal distress	5/7 (71%)	Associated with rapid uncontrolled decline in maternal blood pressure when given IV for hypertension	291
92.	Hydroxy-progesterone	Masculinization of the female fetus			292–294
93.	Hydroxyzine	Decrease in fetal heart rate variability	10/16	Maximal effect within 25 minutes	295
		Reduced platelet aggregation		Clinical significance unknown	296
94.	Ibuprofen	Decreased amniotic fluid volume	3/4 (75%)	Used as a tocolytic agent	297
			C/R of triplets		298
		Oligohydramnios	8/30 (27%)	In temporal relationship to therapy with ibuprofen	299
			3/61 (4.9%)	Resolved on discontinuation of treatment, less than with indomethacin	300
		Low-normal amniotic fluid volume	4/61 (6.6%)	Resolved after discontinuation of ibuprofen, true oligohydramnios not observed	300
		Mild constriction of the ductus arteriosus (non-dose-related)		Normal echocardiograms in all 4 cases within 1 week of discontinuing therapy	300
95.	Idarubicin	Fetal death	C/R	Concomitant treatment with cytarabine for acute myeloblastic leukemia during the second trimester	301
		IUGR and decreased fetal movements, neonatal hyperbilirubinemia	C/R	Concomitant treatment with cytarabine during the second trimester	302
		Diffuse cardiomyopathy of both ventricles and the interventricular septum	C/R	Cardiac function returned to normal within 3 days with supportive care	303
96.	Ifosfamide	Anhydramnios, cessation of fetal growth, acute fetal hypoxia, and eventual neonatal death	C/R	Suspected ifosphamide-induced renal toxicity	304
		IUGR	C/R		305
97.	Indomethacin	Reduction in the amniotic fluid volume	6/52 (11.5%)–26/37 (73%)	In preterm labor with intact membranes at gestational age of 32 weeks or less	297, 299, 306–308
		Reduced fetal urine output		Usually transient	309
		Impaired renal function in preterm neonates			310

		Constriction of the fetal ductus arteriosus with or without tricuspid regurgitation		Ductal constriction is dependent on the gestational age of the fetus, starting as early as 27 weeks and increasing markedly at 27–32 weeks, independent of fetal serum indomethacin levels, usually transient and reversible if therapy is stopped an adequate time prior to delivery	311–340
		Premature closure of the ductus arteriosus			
		Primary pulmonary hypertension of the newborn, persistent fetal circulation after birth, and in severe cases, fetal or neonatal death		Most likely due to ductal constriction and shunting of the right ventricular outflow into the pulmonary vessels, results in pulmonary arterial hypertrophy	
		Unilateral pleural effusion	C/R	In one twin fetus after 28 days of indomethacin treatment, possibly due to ductal constriction, resolved completely within 48 hours of stopping the drug	341
		Periventricular leukomalacia in preterm neonates	26/76 (34%)		342
		Edema or hydrops, oliguric renal failure, gastrointestinal bleeding, subcutaneous bruising, intraventricular hemorrhage, absent platelet aggregation, and perforation of the terminal ileum	3 preterm infants		339
98.	Insulin (bovine or porcine)	Fetal macrosomia	21/46 (47%)	Crosses the placenta as an insulin-antibody complex, the amount of transfer correlated with the amount of anti-insulin antibodies in the mother, high concentrations of animal insulin in cord blood were significantly associated with the development of fetal macrosomia. It is difficult to separate the effect of insulin from the mother's glycemic control. Human insulin is the drug of choice for the control of diabetes mellitus in women who may become pregnant.	343
99.	Iodides:				
	Iodide or iodine containing products	Hypothyroidism and goiter in the fetus and newborn, cardiomegaly		When used for prolonged periods or close to term. Goiter may be large enough to cause tracheal compression and death	344–349
	Radioiodine	Partial or complete ablation of the fetal thyroid gland	Several C/Rs	The effect is dose-dependent (in the pregnancies terminating with a hypothyroid infant ^{131}I doses ranged from 10 to 225 mCi) and may occur only after 10 weeks' gestation when the fetal thyroid begins concentrating iodine	350–356
		Combined hypothyroidism and hypoparathyroidism	C/R		357

(*Continued*)

Table 8-1
Direct Drug Toxicity to the Fetus (*Continued*)

NO.	DRUG	FETAL/NEONATAL TOXIC EFFECTS	REPORTED RATE OF OCCURRENCE*	COMMENTS/RECOMMENDATIONS	REFERENCE
100.	Isoniazid	Hemorrhagic disease of the newborn	2 cases	The mothers were also treated with rifampin and ethambutol	358
				Vitamin K supplementation of women taking the drug near term recommended prior to delivery for prevention	
101.	Isoproterenol	An isolated 5 beats/min late decelaration in a fetus	C/R	Two minutes after the mother received 0.25 μg of the drug	359
102.	Isoxsuprine	Severe neonatal toxicity with respiratory depression and hypotension		Rare if cord levels are less than 2 ng/mL, increased if cord blood serum levels exceeded 10 ng/mL	360, 361
		Hypotension	89%	When cord levels exceeded 10 ng/mL	360
		Hypocalcemia	100%	Not related to cord concentrations	362
		Paralytic ileus	33%		
		Tachycardia			
		Hypoglycemia			
		Death	16%		
		ECG changes suggesting myocardial ischemia	6/9	Transient	363
103.	Kanamycin	Ototoxicity:			
		Deafness	C/R	The mother also experienced ototoxicity, ethacrinic acid also given during pregnancy	260
		Hearing impairment	9/391 (2.3%)	In women who had received kanamycin, 50 mg/kg, for prolonged periods during pregnancy	364
104.	Ketamine	Depression of the newborn Excessive neonatal muscle tone sometimes with apnea		When used close to delivery for obstetrical anesthesia, transient dose-related toxicity, usually avoided with lower doses	365–375
105.	Labetalol	Newborn bradycardia	5 infants	Bradycardia marked and persistent in one infant, all survived	376–381
		Hypotension	1 infant	Delivered by C/S at 28 weeks' gestation	
		Mild transient hypotension in term newborns	11 infants	Other measures of β-blockade did not differ when compared to matched controls	
		Neonatal hypoglycemia	C/R	The woman was also taking a thiazide diuretic	
		Significantly more with IUGR after exposure to labetolol plus hospitalization compared with hospitalization alone	18/94 (19.1%) vs. 9/97 (9.3%)	Women were treated for mild preeclampsia presenting at 26–35 weeks' gestation	
				Newborns should be closely observed during the first 24–48 hours for signs and symptoms of α/β-blockade if exposed close to delivery	

106.	Lamivudine	Mitochondrial dysfunction	4 cases	In combination with zidovudine	382
		Transient mitochondrial and peroxisomal dysfunction, anemia, hyocalcemia, ventricular extrasystoles, prolonged metabolic acidosis, lactic acidemia, mild elevation of long chain fatty acids and neutropenia	C/R	After exposure to lamivudine and zidovudine combined with ritonavir and saquinavir	383
107.	Lidocaine	Abnormal fetal rhythm (tachycardia or bradycardia)	6/12 (50%)	Following paracervical block with lidocaine in 12 laboring women	384
		Lower scores on tests of muscle strength and tone in newborns compared to controls		After continuous lumbar epidural blocks	385
		Central nervous system depression in the newborn (low Apgar scores)		With high serum levels	386
108.	Lisinopril	Chronic renal failure in the newborn	2 cases		387–390
		Fatal hypocalvaria and chronic renal failure in the premature newborn	C/R	Fetal calvarial hypoplasia, open biopsy at 11 weeks of age showed extensive atrophy and loss of tubules with interstitial fibrosis	
		Severe oligohydramnios, IUGR, fetal distress, hypocalvaria, and persistent renal insufficiency	C/R		
		Fetal calvarial hypoplasia	C/R		
		ACE inhibitor fetopathy		See captopril and enalapril for further details	
109.	Lithium	Hypotonia		Most of the toxic effects self limited, (returning to normal within 2 weeks)	198, 391–408
		Cyanosis			
		Bradycardia			
		Atrial flutter			
		T-wave inversion on ECG			
		Cardiomegaly			
		Thyroid depression with goiter			
		Nephrogenic diabetes insipidus		Two of the reported cases of nephrogenic diabetes insipidus persisted for 2 months or longer	
		Polyhydramnios			
		Shock			
		Seizures			
		Gastrointestinal bleeding			
		Hepatomegaly			
		Neonatal jaundice			
		Stillbirth			
		Fetal and newborn lithium intoxication			
110.	Lorazepam	"Floppy infant" syndrome		With high IV maternal doses	409, 410
		Transient mild "floppy infant" syndrome	C/R	The woman was also taking clozapine, resoved at 5 days of age	
111.	Losartan	Oligohydramnios, neonatal anuria, pulmonary hypoplasia, skull hypoplasia, limb contractures, IUGR, stillbirth, neonatal death	7 C/Rs	Similar mechanism as in angiotensin converting enzyme inhibitor fetopathy	142, 411–414

(Continued)

Table 8-1
Direct Drug Toxicity to the Fetus (*Continued*)

NO.	DRUG	FETAL/NEONATAL TOXIC EFFECTS	REPORTED RATE OF OCCURRENCE*	COMMENTS/RECOMMENDATIONS	REFERENCE
112.	Magnesium sulfate	Newborn depression and hypotonia	series	Intrauterine hypoxia could not be ruled out as a potential cause or contributing factor	415–421
		Severe depression at birth	2 cases	Spontaneous remission in 1 infant, residual effects of anoxic encephalopathy in the second	422
		Muscle contraction impairement		Up to 48 hours after birth	423
		Newborn depression without spontaneous respirations, movement, or reflexes	C/R	An exchange transfusion reversed the condition	424
		Decreased gastrointestinal motility, ileus, hypotonia		Other drugs or maternal severe hypertension could have been the causes	425
		Cogenital rickets	2/5		418
		Wide spaced fontanelles and parietal bone thinning	2/22	With long-term infusions of magnesium, probably due to sustained fetal hypocalcemia	420
		Adverse effects on fetal bone mineralization		Effects returned to normal with time	426–430
		Fetal bradycardia	C/R	Maternal hypothermia with maternal bradycardia	431
113.	Medroxy-progesterone	Ambiguous genitalia			432
114.	Mefenamic acid	Premature closure of the ductus arteriosus	C/R	The drug used in an attempt to prevent premature delivery	433
115.	Melphalan	IUGR			123
116.	Menadione	Marked hyperbilirubinemia and kernicterus in the newborn		Especially in premature infants, phytonadione is considered the vitamin K of choice for administration during pregnancy	434–437
117.	Meperidine	Respiratory depression in the newborn		Following exposure during labor, time and dose dependent	438–439
		Impaired behavioural response and EEG changes in the neonate		Persisting for several days	440–441
		Transient decrease in oxygenation		Mean decline in $TcPO_2$ 11.7 torr mean duration 4.6 minutes after injection	442
118.	Mepivacaine	Fetal bradycardia		Correlated with high fetal mepivacaine blood levels after paracervical block	443
119.	Mercaptopurine	Myelosuppression	2 cases		62, 192
		Microangiopathic hemolytic anemia	C/R	} After combination chemotherapy	444
		IUGR	40%	Clinical significance unknown	123
		Chromosomal aberrations	C/R		64
120.	Methadone	Neonatal hyperbilirubinemia			445
		Thrombocytosis		In polydrug users	446

121.	Methimazole/ Carbimazole	Mild fetal hypothyroidism	C/R	Usually resolves spontaneously within a few days	447
		Hypothyroidism evident at 2 months of age	C/R	With subsequent mental retardation	448
		Neonatal hypothyroidism with goiter	2 cases		449
		Small goiters in the newborn	2 cases	In carbimazole-exposed newborns	450
122.	Methotrexate	Severe newborn myelosuppression	2 cases	Concomitant administration of other antineoplastic agents	62, 192
		IUGR	40%		123
		Chromosomal aberrations	C/R	Clinical significance unknown	64
123.	Methyldopa	Mild reduction in neonatal systolic blood pressure in the first two days of life	24 infants	Reduction not clinically significant	451
		Transient neonatal nasal obstruction			452
124.	Methylene blue	Newborn complications: Hemolytic anemia, Hyperbilirubinemia, Methemoglobinemia, Deep blue staining, Intestinal obstruction		Following intra-amniotic injection of methylene blue	453–463
		Jejunal atresia	In 19% (17/89) of twin pregnancies	When used in genetic amniocentesis in twins, possible mechanism: mesenteric vasoconstriction	464, 465
125.	Methylergonovine	Fetal bradycardia	2 C/Rs	Accidental administration resulting in uterine hypertonus	466, 467
126.	Metoprolol	IUGR	C/R		468
127.	Midazolam	Newborn respiratory depression	5/26 (19%)	When used in combination with succinylcholine for rapid sequence anesthetic induction before cesarean section, higher proportion than the one found with thiopenthal	469
		Respiratory depression on the day 1, hypoglycemia and jaundice on day 3		When used before elective cesarean section	470
128.	Minoxidil	Hypertrichosis	2 cases	Less prominent at 2 months of age	471, 472
129.	Misoprostol	Fetal death	C/R	Following maternal poisoning in a suicide attempt at 31 weeks' gestation	473
130.	Morphine	Respiratory newborn depression		When used in labor, more common than with meperidine	474, 475
131.	Nadolol	IUGR, tachypnea, hypoglycemia, hypothermia, cardiorespiratory depression	C/R	Other possible contributing factors to some of the effects: concomitant administration of hydrochlorothiazide and maternal disease	476
132.	Nalbuphine	Sinusoidal fetal heart rate pattern	C/R		477
		Fetal distress and neonatal respiratory depression			478–482
133.	Naloxone	Fatal respiratory failure in the newborn	C/R	When used at term to treat fetal heart rate baseline with low beat-to-beat variability	483
134.	Naproxen	Primary pulmonary hyepertension of the newborn with severe hypoxemia, coagulopathy, hyperbilirubinemia, and impaired renal function	3 cases	Following exposure at 30 weeks for 2–6 days, attributed to prostaglandin inhibition, one infant died at 4 days of age and autopsy revealed a short and constricted ductus arteriosus	484
		Primary pulmonary hypertension	C/R	After exposure 4 days before delivery	485

(*Continued*)

Table 8-1
Direct Drug Toxicity to the Fetus (*Continued*)

NO.	DRUG	FETAL/NEONATAL TOXIC EFFECTS	REPORTED RATE OF OCCURRENCE*	COMMENTS/RECOMMENDATIONS	REFERENCE
135	Nitrofurantoin	Neonatal hemolytic anemia	10 cases	After exposure close to delivery	486, 487
136.	Nitroglycerin	Fetal heart changes (loss of beat-to-beat variability, late decelarations, and bradycardia)		Dose dependent, following maternal IV treatment with nitroglycerin without volume expansion for severe pregnancy-induced hypertension	488, 489
137.	Nitroprusside	Transient fetal bradycardia	C/R	Follow-up of neonatal cardiovascular system	490
138.	Norethindrone	Masculinization of the female fetus	0.3–18.3%		491–494
139.	Norethynodrel	Masculinization of the female fetus	1/4 (25%)		491, 493
140.	Nortriptyline	Neonatal urinary retention	C/R		495
141.	Oral contraceptives	Neonatal hyperbilirubinemia ± clinically significant jaundice		Quite safe	496
		Transient choreoathetosis	C/R	Resolved spontaneously	497
142.	Oxymetazoline	Fetal heart rate changes	C/R	The woman used the nasal spray more frequently than the recommended dosage interval, speculated mechanism: α-adrenergic effect on the uterine vessels reducing the uterine blood flow and causing fetal hypoxia and bradycardia	498
143.	Pancuronium	Transient fetal heart rate changes, such as decreased accelerations and beat-to-beat variability, and an occasional sinusoidal pattern		After direct fetal administration, no indication of fetal compromise	499–502
144.	Paroxetine	Perinatal complications, respiratory distress, hypoglycemia, and jaundice			503
		Lethargy, absence of cry, and EEG changes	C/R	Follow-up for discontinuation syndrome	504
145.	Pentazocine	Neonatal respiratory depression		Following use during labor	505, 506
146.	Phenazocine	Neonatal respiratory depression		Following use during labor	507, 508
147.	Phenobarbital	Early hemorrhagic disease of the newborn	C/Rs	Probably as a result of induction of fetal microsomal enzymes that deplete the already low reserves of vitamin K, resulting in suppression of the vitamin K-dependent coagulation factors II, VII, IX, and X, vitamin K prophylaxis recommended prior to delivery	509–518
148.	Phenytoin	Early hemorrhagic disease of the newborn	C/Rs	Probably as a result of induction of fetal microsomal enzymes that deplete the already low reserves of vitamin K, resulting in suppression of the vitamin K-dependent coagulation factors II, VII, IX, and X, vitamin K prophylaxis recommended prior to delivery	509–512, 514, 516–525
		Neonatal hemorrhage seconday to throbmocytopenia	C/R		526
149.	Pindolol	Decrease in fetal heart rate		When compared before and after therapy in women with pregnancy induced hypertension in the third trimester	527

150.	Podophyllum	Stillbirth	C/R	Podophyllum poisoning following topical administration of 7.5 mL of 25% podophyllum resin to florid vulval warts	528
151.	Prednisone/ prednisolone	Immunosuppression in the newborn	C/R	Following exposure to high doses of prednisone and azathioprine throughout gestation, resolved at 15 weeks of age	95
		Stillbirth	8/34 (23.5%) vs. 1/34 (3%) in controls	Attributed to failure of placental function, controls had similar diagnoses	529
152.	Primidone	Overactivity, tremors, jitteriness	C/R	Malformed newbon, died at 3 weeks of age	530, 531
		Hemorrhagic disease of the newborn	C/Rs	Probably as a result of induction of fetal microsomal enzymes that deplete the already low reserves of vitamin K, resulting in suppression of the vitamin K-dependent coagulation factors II, VII, IX, and X, vitamin K prophylaxis recommended prior to delivery	510, 512–515
153.	Promazine	Neonatal hyperbilirubinemia		From exposure to 100 mg or more during labor, mean bilirubin significantly higher in 317 exposed neonates compared to 272 controls	532
154.	Promethazine	Neonatal respiratory depression	Small case series		533
		Transient and behavioral and EEG changes	28/28 (100%)	Most women (27/28) received a combination of meperidine with promethazine or phenobarbital, persisted for less than 3 days	440
		Impaired platelet aggregation in the newborn	16/18 (88.9%)		534, 535
155.	Propofol	Neonatal changes:		Following use in cesarean section	536
		Low Apgar scores			
		Hypotonia	5/20		
		Somnolence	1/20		
		Irritability	5/20		
156.	Propranolol	Fetal and Neonatal effects:	14%	From analysis of 23 reports involving 167 liveborn infants exposed chronically to propranolol in utero. Other possible factors that may have caused these effects or contributed are maternal disease, concomitant medications or a combination of those factors. Newborn exposed to propranolol near delivery should be closely observed in the first 24–48 hours for signs and symptoms of β-blockade	198, 537–558
		IUGR	10%		
		Hypoglycemia	7%		
		Bradycardia	4%		
		Respiratory depression	4%		
		Hyperbilirubinemia	1%		
		Polycythemia	0.6%		
		Thrombocytopenia	0.6%		
		Hyperirritabilty	0.6%		
		Hypocalcemia with convulsions	0.6%		
		Coagulopathy			
		Respiratory depression	4/5 (80%)	When given IV prior to cesarean section	559
		Prematurity	3/9 (33%)	When administered for pregnancy-induced hypertension	560
		Transient fetal bradycardia	2/10 (20%)	For dysfunctional labor	561

(Continued)

Table 8-1
Direct Drug Toxicity to the Fetus (*Continued*)

NO.	DRUG	FETAL/NEONATAL TOXIC EFFECTS	REPORTED RATE OF OCCURRENCE*	COMMENTS/RECOMMENDATIONS	REFERENCE
157.	Propylthiouracil	Mild fetal hypothyroidism		When used close to term, resolves spontaneously within a few days	562
		Fetal goiter	(29/241) (12%)	Usually smaller than iodide-induced goiters	198
		Newborn goiter with tracheal compression	2 cases	Resulted in death in one case and moderate respiratory distress in the second	563, 564
		Clinical hypothyroidism with mental and physical delay in development	2 cases	One of the infants also exposed to high doses of iodide during gestation	565, 566
		Neonatal hepatitis	C/R	Resolved spontaneously	567
158.	Pyridoxine	Intrauterine and infantile convulsions		High doses of pyridoxine early in gestation presumably altered the normal metabolism of pyridoxine leading to intractable seizures in the newborn	568–571
159.	Quinidine	Neonatal thrombocytopenia	2/234 (0.9%)		572
160.	Quinine	Auditory and optic nerve damage		Usually in potentially toxic doses as an abortifacient	573–577
		Neonatal thrombocytopenic purpura			578
		Neonatal hemolytic anemia		In G6PD deficient newborns	579
161.	Reserpine	Nasal discharge, cyanosis, lethrgy, and poor feeding in the newborn	n = 12	From use near term	580
162.	Rifampicin	Hemorrhagic disease of the newborn	3 cases	Prophylacic vitamin K is recommended prior to delivery	358
163.	Ritodrine	Fetal and neonatal complications:			581–592
		Tachycardia			
		Neonatal cardiac arrhthmias			
		Disproportionate septal hypertrophy		Following in utero exposure to ritodrine for 2 weeks or longer	
		Newborn hypoglycemia		As a result of transient fetal hyperglycemia followed by hyperinsulinemia, more common following intravenous administration	
		Fetal death		Following severe maternal ketoacidosis	
		Neonatal hyperbilirubinemia			
		Transient decrease in the glomerular filtration rate in the newborn		Noted between 12 and 36 hours of age, clinical significance—unknown	
164.	Scopolamine	Fetal tachycardia, decreased heart rate variability, and decreased heart rate deceleration		When administered at term	593–595
		Newborn toxicity (fever, tachycardia, lethrgy)	C/R	Reversed following treatment with physostigmine	596

165.	Sotalol	Fetal bradycardia	5/6	Lasting up to 24 hours, newborns exposed near delivery should be closely observed during the first 24–48 hours for signs and symptoms of β-blockade	597
166.	Streptomycin	Ototoxicity (cochlear and vestibular)	3 C/Rs	From exposure to long-term high doses in late pregnancy	598–600
167.	Sulfonamides	Jaundice		When given close to delivery	601–606
		Hemolytic anemia	3 cases (2 newbors and 1 fetus)	In the 1 case involving the fetus, resulting in hydrops fetalis and stillbirth	601, 602, 606
168.	Sulindac	Transient constriction of the fetal ductus arteriosus			607, 608
169.	Tacrolimus	Hyperkalemia			609–612
		Renal toxicity			
		IUGR			
		Cardionyopathy	C/R of twins		613
170.	Tamoxifen	Ambiguous genitalia in a female newborn	C/R	Following exposure during the first 20 weeks of pregnancy	614
171.	Telmisartan	Oligohydramnios, transient renal failure	C/R	Similar mechanism as in angiotensin converting enzyme inhibitor fetopathy	615
172.	Terbutaline	Transient fetal tachycardia			616–619
		Neonatal hypoglycemia	C/R		620, 621
		Myocardial necrosis in a newborn			622
		Cardiovascular decompensation	In 3 of a quadruplet pregnancy	Possibly due to downregulation of fetal β-adrenergic receptors leading to decreased myocardial function and reduced cardiac output	623
173.	Testosterone	Masculinization of the female fetus			624
174.	Tetracyclines	Yellow-gold fluorescence in the mineralized structures of a fetal skeleton	C/R	Following exposure prior to delivery	625
		Permanent yellow-brown discoloration of teeth		Due to the chelating ability of the drug forms a complex with calcium orthophosphate and becomes incorporated into bones and teeth undergoing calcification, effect on deciduous or permanent teeth depends on timing of exposure in pregnancy	626–641
175.	Theophylline	Transient tachycardia, irritability, and vomiting in the newborn	3 cases	More likely to occur when maternal serum levels at term are in the high therapeutic range or above	642–644
176.	Thioguanine	Intrauterine fetal death	2 cases	After antineoplastic therapy with thioguanine and other agents at 15 weeks' gestation	645, 646
		IUGR	40%		123
177.	Tolbutamide	Neonatal thrombocytopenia	C/R	Persisted for ~2 weeks	647

(*Continued*)

Table 8-1
Direct Drug Toxicity to the Fetus (*Continued*)

NO.	DRUG	FETAL/NEONATAL TOXIC EFFECTS	REPORTED RATE OF OCCURRENCE*	COMMENTS/RECOMMENDATIONS	REFERENCE
178.	Valproic acid	IUGR			198
		Neonatal hyperbilirubinemia	3 cases	Causal relationship uncertain	648–650
		Liver toxicity	3 cases	May be fatal	650, 651
		Neonatal afibrinogenemia with fatal hemorrhage	C/R		652
		Transient hyperglycinemia	2 cases	No adverse effects seen in the newborns	653
		Fetal and neonatal disteress	6/14 (43%)		654
179.	Valsartan	Oligohydramnios Neonatal anuria Skull hypolplasia Pulmonary hypoplasia Limb contractures	5 C/Rs	Similar mechanism as in angiotensin-converting enzyme inhibitor fetopathy	413, 142, 655
180.	Vancomycin	Transient fetal bradycardia	C/R	1 g IV dose was given in 3 min/hour before delivery causing maternal hypotension	656
181.	Vinblastine	IUGR	40%		123
182.	Vincristine	Pancytopenia	C/R	With other antineoplastic agents	192
		Transient severe bone marrow hypoplasia	C/R	After combination chemotherapy with	62
		Chromosomal abberations	C/R	mercaptopurine	64
		IUGR	40%		123
183.	Zidovudine	IUGR	2/45 (4%)		657
		Anemia	6/31 (19%)	Difference in hemoglobin between exposed and unexposed infants was 1 g/dL, occurring at 3 weeks of age, with similar values by 12 weeks of age	657, 658
		Profound anemia	C/R	Following exposure to antiretroviral agents	659
		Mitochondrial dysfunction	8 cases	Four in combination with lamivudine	382
		Transient mitochondrial and peroxisomal dysfunction, anemia, hyocalcemia, ventricular extrasystoles, prolonged metabolic acidosis, lactic acidemia, mild elevation of long chain fatty acids and neutropenia	C/R	After exposure to lamivudine and zidovudine combined with ritonavir and saquinavir	383

* Rates are given when available.

REFERENCES

1. Dubois D, Petitcolas J, Temperville B, et al. Treatment of hypertension in pregnancy with β-adrenoceptor antagonists. *Br J Clin Pharmacol.* 1982;13(suppl):375S–378S.
2. Williams ER, Morrissey JR. A comparison with methyldopa in hypertensive pregnancy. *Pharmatherapeutica.* 1983;3:487–491.
3. Dumez Y, Tchobroutsky C, Hornych H, et al. Neonatal effects of maternal administration of acebutolol. *Br Med J.* 1981;283:1077–1079.
4. Char VC, Chandra R, Fletcher AB, et al. Polyhydramnios and neonatal renal failure: a possible association with maternal acetaminophen ingestion. *J Pediatr.* 1975;86:638–639.
5. Haibach H, Akhter JE, Muscato MS, et al. Acetaminophen overdose with fetal demise. *Am J Clin Pathol.* 1984;82:240–242.
6. Wang PH, Yang MJ, Lee WL, et al. Acetaminophen poisoning in late pregnancy: a case report. *J Reprod Med.* 1997;42:367–371.
7. Riggs BS, Bronstein AC, Kulig K, et al. Acute acetaminophen overdose during pregnancy. *Obstet Gynecol.* 1989;74:247–253.
8. Merlob P, Litwin A, Mor N. Possible association between acetazolamide administration during pregnancy and metabolic disorders in the newborn. *E J Obstet Gynecol Reprod Biol.* 1990;35:85–88.
9. Kemball ML, McIver C, Milnar RDG, et al. Neonatal hypoglycaemia in infants with diabetic mothers given sulphonylurea drugs in pregnancy. *Arch Dis Child.* 1970;45:696–701.
10. Harris EL. Adverse reactions to oral antidiabetic agents. *Br Med J.* 1971;3:29–30.
11. Liggins GC, Vaughan GS. Intravenous infusion of salbutamol in the management of premature labor. *J Obstet Gynaecol Br Commonw.* 1973;80:29–33.
12. Korda AR, Lynerum RC, Jones WR. The treament of premature labor with intravenous administered salbutamol. *Med J Austr.* 1974;1:744–746.
13. Hastwell G. Salbutamol aerosol in premature labour. *Lancet.* 1975;2:1212–1213.
14. Eggers TR, Doyle LW, Pepperell RJ. Premature labour. *Med J Austr.* 1979;1:213–216.
15. Wager J, Fredholm B, Lunell NO, et al. Metabolic and circulatory effects of intravenous and oral salbutemol in late pregnancy in diabetic and non-diabetic women. *Acta Obstet Gynecol Scand.* 1982;108(suppl):41–46.
16. Baker ER, Flanagan MF. Fetal atrial flutter associated with maternal beta-sympathomimetic drug exposure. *Obstet Gynecol.* 1997;89:861.
17. Hastwell GB, Halloway CP, Taylor TLY. A study of 208 patients in premature labor treated with orally administered salbutamol. *Med J Austr.* 1978;1:465–469.
18. Thomas DJB, Dove AF, Alberti KGMM. Metabolic effects of salbutamol infusion during premature labour. *Br J Obstet Gynaecol.* 1977;84:497–499.
19. Wager J, Lunell NO, Nadal M, et al. Glucose tolerance following oral salbutamol treatment in late pregnancy. *Acta Obstet Gynecol Scand.* 1981;60:291–294.
20. Lunell NO, Joelsson I, Larsson A, et al. The immediate effect of β-adrenergic agonist (salbutamol) on carbohydrate and lipid metabolism during the third trimester of pregnancy. *Acta Obstet Gynecol Scand.* 1977;56:475–478.
21. Procianoy RS, Pinheiro CEA. Neonatal hyperinsulinism after short-term maternal beta sympathomimetic therapy. *J Pediatr.* 1982;101:612–614.
22. Barnett AH, Stubbs SM, Mander AM. Management of premature labour in diabetic pregnancy. *Diabetologia.* 1980;18:365–368.
23. Wager J, Fredholm BB, Lunell NO, et al. Metabolic and circulatory effects of oral salbutamol in the third trimester of pregnancy in diabetic and non diabetic women. *Br J Obstet Gynaecol.* 1981;88:352–361.
24. Desgranges MF, Moutquin JM, Peloquin A. Effects of maternal oral salbutamol therapy on neonatal endocrine status at birth. *Obstet Gynecol.* 1987;69:582–584.
25. Redfern N, Bower S, Bullock RE, et al. Alfentanil for caesaean section complicated by severe aortic stenosis: a case report. *Br J Anaesth.* 1987;59:1309–1312.
26. Heytens L, Cammu H, Camu F. Extradural analgesia during labour using alfentanil. *Br J Anaesth.* 1987;59:331–337.
27. Smith EJ, Nagyfy SF. A report on comparative studies of new drugs used for obstetrical analgesia. *Am J Obstet Gynecol.* 1949;58:695–702.
28. Hapke FB, Barnes AC. The obstetric use and effect on fetal respiration of nisentil. *Am J Obstet Gynecol.* 1949;58:799–801.
29. Kane WM. The results of nisentil in 1,000 obstetrical cases. *Am J Obstet Gynecol.* 1953;65:1020–1026.
30. Backner DD, Foldes FF, Gordon EH. The combined use of alphaprodine (nisentil) hydrochloride and levallorphan (lorifan) tartate for analgesia in obstetrics. *Am J Obstet Gynecol.* 1957;74:271–282.
31. Gillan JS, Hunter GW, Dorner CB, et al. Meperidine hydrochloride and alphaprodine as obstetric analgesic agents; a double blind study. *Am J Obstet Gynecol.* 1958;75:1105–1110.
32. Roberts H, Kuck MAC. Use of alphaprodine and levallorphan during labor. *Can Med Assoc J.* 1960;83:1088–1093.
33. Burnett RG, White CA. Alphaprodine for continuous intravenous obstetric analgesia. *Obstet Gynecol.* 1966;27:472–477.
34. Anthinarayanan PR, Mangurthen HH. Unusually prolonged action of maternal alphaprodine causing fetal depression. *Q Pediatr Bull.* 1977;3:14–16.
35. Gray JH, Cudmore DW, Luther ER, et al. Sinusoidal fetal heart rate pattern associated with alphaprodine administration. *Obstet Gynecol.* 1978;52:678–681.
36. Corby DG, Schulman I. The effects of antenatal drug administration on aggregation of platelets of newborn infants. *J Pediatr.* 1971;79:307–313.
37. McNall PG, Jafarnia MR. Management of myasthenia gravis in the obstetrical patient. *Am J Obstet Gynecol.* 1965;92:518–525.
38. Plauche WC. Myasthenia gravis in pregnancy: an update. *Am J Obstet Gynecol.* 1979;135:691–697.
39. Iffy L, Ansell JS, Bryant FS, et al. Nonadrenal female pseudohermaphroditism: an unusual case of masculinization. *Obstet Gynecol.* 1965;26:59–65.
40. Marek J, Horky K. Aminoglutethimide administration in pregnancy. *Lancet.* 1970;2:1312–1313.
41. Candlepergher G, Buchberger R, Suzzi GL, et al. Trans-placental passage of aniodarone: electrocardiographic and pharmacologic evidence in the newborn. *G Ital Cardiol.* 1982;12:79–82.
42. Penn IM, Barrett PA, Pannikote V, et al. Amiodarone in pregnancy. *Am J Cardiol.* 1985;56:196–197.
43. McKanna WJ, Harris L, Rowland E, et al. Amiodarone therapy during pregnancy. *Am J Cardiol.* 1983;51:1231–1233.
44. Robson DJ, Jeeva Raj MV, Storey GAC, et al. Use of amiodarone during pregnancy. *Postgrad Med J.* 1985;61:75–77.
45. Plomp TA, Vulsma T, de Vijlder JJM. Use of amiodarone during pregnancy. *Eur J Obstet Gynecol Repro Biol.* 1992;43:201–207.
46. Laurent M, Betremieux P, Biron Y, et al. Neonatal hypothyroidism after treatment by amiodarone during pregnancy (letter). *Am J Cardiol.* 1987;60:942.
47. De Catte L, De Wolf D, Smitz J, et al. Fetal hypothyroidism as a complication of amiodarone treament for persistent fetal supraventricular tachycardia. *Prenatal Diagn.* 1994;14:762–765.
48. De Wolf D, De Schepper J, Verhaaren H, et al. Congenital hypothyroid goiter and amiodarone. *Acta Paediatr Scan.* 1988;77:616–618.
49. Rey E, Bachrach LK, Burrow GN. Effects of amiodarone during pregnancy. *Can Med Assoc J.* 1987;136:959–960.
50. Widerhorn J, Bhandari AK, Bughi S, et al. Fetal and neonatal adverse effects profile of amiodarone treatment during pregnancy. *Am Heart J.* 1991;122:1162–1168.

51. Magee LA, Downar E, Sermer M, et al. Pregnancy outcome after gestational exposure to amiodarone in Canada. *Am J Obstet Gynecol.* 1995;172:1307–1311.
52. Goodlin RC, Kaiser IH. The effect of ammonium chloride induced maternal acidosis on the human fetus at term. I pH, hemoglobin, blood gases. *Am J Med Sci* 1957;233:666–674.
53. Kaiser IH, Goodlin RC. The effect of ammonium chloride induced maternal acidosis on the human fetus at term. II Electrolites. *Am J Med Sci.* 1958;235:549–554.
54. Larsson G. The amphetamine addicted mother and her child. *Acta Paediatr Scan.* 1980;278(suppl):7–24.
55. Little BB, Snell LM, Gilstrap LC III. Metamphetamine abuse during pregnancy: outcome and fetal effects. *Obstet Gynecol.* 1988;72: 541–544.
56. Eriksson M, Larsson G, Winbladh B, et al. The influence of amphetamine addiction on pregnancy and the newborn infant. *Acta Paediatr Scan.* 1978;67:95–99.
57. Dixon SD, Bejar R. Echoencephalographic findings in neonates associated with maternal cocaine and methamphetamine use: incidence and clinical correlates. *J Pediatr.* 1989;115:770–778.
58. Dearlove JC, Betteridge T. Stillbirth due to intravenous amphetamine. *Br Med J.* 1992;304:548.
59. Heim K, Alge A, Marth C. Anaphylactic reaction to ampicillin and severe complication in the fetus. *Lancet.* 1991;337:859.
60. Zierler S, Purohit D. Prenatal antihistamine exposure and retrolental fibroplasia. *Am J Epidemiol.* 1986;123:192–196.
61. Hoffhauer H, Dobbeck P. Untersuchungen uber die plactapassage des kallikrein inhibitors. *Klin Wochenschr.* 1970;48:183–184.
62. Okun DB, Groncy PK, Sieger L, et al. Acute leukemia in pregnancy: transient neonatal myelosuppression after combination chemotherapy in the mother. *Med Pediatr Oncol.* 1979;7: 315–319.
63. Khurshid M, Saleem M. Acute leukaemia in pregnancy. *Lancet.* 1978;2:534–535.
64. Schleuning M, Clemm C. Chromosomal aberrations in a newborn whose mother received cytotoxic treament during pregnancy. *N Eng J Med.* 1987;317:1666–1667.
65. Collins E, Turner G. Maternal effects of regular salicylate ingestion in pregnancy. *Lancet.* 1975;2:335–337.
66. Turner G, Collins E. Fetal effects of regular salicylate ingestion in pregnancy. *Lancet.* 1975;2:338–339.
67. Shapiro S, Monson RR, Kaufman DW, et al. Perinatal mortality in relation to aspirin taken during pregnancy. *Lancet.* 1976;1:1375–1376.
68. Arcilla RA, Thilenius OG, Ranniger K. Congestive heart failure from suspected ductal closure in utero. *J Pediatr.* 1969;75:74–78.
69. Bleyer WA, Breckenridge RJ. Studies on the detection of adverse drug reactions in the newborn. II. The effects of prenatal aspirin on newborn hemostasis. *JAMA.* 1970;213:2049–2053.
70. Corby DG, Schulman I. The effects of antenatal drug administration on aggregation of platelets of newborn infants. *J Pediatr.* 1971;79: 307–313.
71. Casteels-Van Daele M, de Gaetano G, Vermijlen J. More on the effects of antenatally adminitered aspirin on aggregation of platelets of neonates. *J Pediatr.* 1972;80:685–686.
72. Haslam RR, Ekert H, Gillam GL. Hemorrhage in a neonate possibly due to maternal ingestion of salicilate. *J Pediatr.* 1974;84:556–557.
73. Ekert H, Haslam RR. Maternal ingested salicylate as a cause of neonatal hemorrhage. Reply. *J Pediatr.* 1974;85:738.
74. Pearson H. Comparative effects of aspirin and acetaminophen on hemostasis. *Pediatrics.* 1978;62(suppl):962–969.
75. Haslam RR. Neonatal purpura secondary to maternal salicylism. *J Pediatr.* 1975;86:653.
76. Stuart MJ, Gross SJ, Elrad H, et al. Effects of acetylsalicylic acid ingestion on maternal and neonatal hemostasis. *N Eng J Med.* 1982;307:909–912.
77. Stuart MJ. Aspirin and maternal or neonatal hemostasis. *N Eng J Med.* 1983;308:281.
78. Rumack CM, Guggenheim MA, Rumack BH, et al. Neonatal intracranial hemorrhage and maternal use of aspirin. *Obstet Gynecol.* 1981;58(suppl):52S–56S.
79. Soller RW, Stander H. Maternal drug exposure and perinatal intracranial hemorrhage. *Obstet Gynecol.* 1981;58:735–737.
80. Corby DG. Editorial comment. *Obstet Gynecol.* 1981;58:737–740.
81. Jackson AV. Toxic effects of salicylate on the foetus and mother. *J Pathol Bacteriol.* 1948;60:587–593.
82. Aterman K, Holzbecker M, Ellenberger HA. Salicylate levels in a stillborn to a drug-addicted mother, with comments on pathology and analytical methodology. *Clin Toxicol.* 1980;16:263–268.
83. Earle R Jr. Congenital salicylate intoxication-report of a case. *N Eng J Med.* 1961;265:1003–1004.
84. Lynd PA, Andeasen AC, Wyatt RJ. Intrauterine salicilate intoxication in a newborn: a case report. *Clin Pediatr (Phila).* 1976;15:912–913.
85. Palmisano PA, Cassady G. Salicylate exposure in the perinate. *JAMA.* 1969;209:556–558.
86. Dubois D, Petitcolas J, Temperville B, et al. Treatment with atenolol of hypertension in pregnancy. *Drugs.* 1983;25(suppl 2):215–218.
87. Butters L, Kennedy S, Rubin PC. Atenolol in essential hypertension during pregnancy. *Br Med J.* 1990;301:587–589.
88. Lip GYH, Beevers M, Churchill D, et al. Effect of atenolol on birth weight. *Am J Cardiol.* 1997;79:1436–1438.
89. Al Kasab SM, Sabag T, Al Zaibag M, et al. β-Adrenergic receptor blockade in the management of pregnant women wuth mitral stenosis. *Am J Obstet Gynecol.* 1990;163:37–40.
90. Lardoux H, Gerard J, Blazquez G, et al. Hypertension in pregnancy: evaluation of two beta blockers atenolol and labetolol. *Eur Heart J.* 1983;4(suppl G):35–40.
91. Tuimala R, Hartikainen Sorri AL. Randomised comparison of atenolol and pindolol for treatment of hypertension in pregnancy. *Curr Ther Res.* 1988;44:579–584.
92. Ingemarsson I, Liedholm H, Montan S, et al. Fetal heart rate during treatment of maternal hypertension with beta adrenergic antagonists. *Acta Obstet Gynecol Scand.* 1984;118(suppl):95–97.
93. Woods DL, Morrell DF. Atenolol: side effects in a newborn infant. *Br Med J.* 1982;285:691–692.
94. Rubin PC, Butters L, Clark DM, et al. Placebo controlled trial of atenolol in treatment of pregnancy associated hypertension. *Lancet.* 1983;1:431–434.
95. Cote CJ, Meuwissen HJ, Povkering RJ. Effects on the neonate of prednisone and azathioprine administered to the mother during pregnancy. *J Pediatr.* 1974;85:324–328.
96. DeWitte DB, Buick MK, Cyran SE, et al. Neonatal pancytopenia and severe combined immunodeficiency associated with antenatal administration of azathioprine and prednisone. *J Pediatr.* 1984;105:625–628.
97. Davison JM, Dellagrammatikas H, Parkin JM. Maternal azathioprine therapy and depressed haemopoiesis in the babies of renal allograft patients. *Br J Obstet Gynaecol.* 1985;92:233–239.
98. Scott JR. Fetal growth retardation associated with maternal administration of immunosuppressive drugs. *Am J Obstet Gynecol.* 1977;128:668–676.
99. Pirson Y, Van Lierde M, Ghysen J, et al. Retardation of fetal growth in patients receiving immunosuppressive therapy. *N Eng J Med.* 1985;313:328.
100. Marushak A, Weber T, Bock J, et al. Pregnancy following kidney transplantation. *Acta Obstet Gynecol Scand.* 1986;65:557–559.
101. Davison JM, Lindheimer MD. Pregnancy in renal trasplant recipients. *J Reprod Med.* 1982;27:613–621.
102. The Registration Committee of the European Dialysis and Transplant association. Successful pregnancies in women treated by dialysis and kidney transplantation. *Br J Obstet Gynaecol.* 1980;87:839–845.
103. Leb DE, Weisskopf B, Kanovitz BS. Chromosome abberations in a child of a kidney transplant recipient. *Arch Intern Med.* 1971; 128:441–444.

104. Falterman CG, Richardson CJ. Small left colon syndrome associated with maternal ingestion of psychotropic drugs. *J Pediatr.* 1980;97:308–310.
105. Papageorgiou AN, Desgranges MF, Masson M, et al. The antenatal use of betamethasone in the prevention of respiratory distress syndrome: a controlled double blind study. *Pediatrics.* 1979;63:73–79.
106. Bielawski D, Hiatt IM, Hegyi T. Betamethasone induced leukemoid reaction in preterm infant. *Lancet.* 1978;1:218–219.
107. Hoff DS, Mammel MC. Suspected betamethasone-induced leukemoid reaction in a premature infant. *Pharmacotherapy.* 1997;17: 1031–1034.
108. Wasserstrum N, Huhta JC, Mari G, et al. Betamethasone and the human fetal ductus arteriosus. *Obstet Gynecol.* 1989;74:897–900.
109. Dorr HG, Versmold HT, Sippell WG, et al. Antenatal betamethasone therapy: effects on maternal, fetal, and mineralocorticoids, glucocorticoids, and progestins. *J Pediatr.* 1986;108:990–993.
110. Bradley BS, Kumar SP, Mehta PN, et al. Neonatal cushingoid syndrome resulting from serial courses of antenatal betamethasone. *Obstet Gynecol.* 1994;83:869–872.
111. Banks BA, Cnaan A, Morgan MA, and the North American Thyrotropin-Releasing Hormone Study Group. Multiple courses of antenatal corticosterods and outcome of premature neonates. *Am J Obstet Gynecol.* 1999;181:709–717.
112. French NP, Hagan R, Evans SF, et al. Repeated antenatal corticosteroids: size at birth and subsequent development. *Am J Obstet Gynecol.* 1999;180:114–121.
113. Abbasi S, Hirsch D, Davis J, et al. Effect of single versus multiple courses of antenatal corticosteroids on maternal and neonatal outcome. *Am J Obstet Gynecol.* 2000;182:1243–1249.
114. Ville Y, Vincent Y, Tordjman N, et al. Effect of betamethasone on the fetal heart rate pattern assessed by computerized cardiotocography in normal twin pregnancies. *Fetal Diagn Ther.* 1995;10: 301–306.
115. Senat MV, Minoui S, Multon O, et al. Effect of dexamethasone on fetal heart rate variability in preterm labour: a randomised study. *Br J Obstet Gynaecol.* 1998;105:749–755.
116. Raffles A, Williams J, Costeloe K, et al. Transplacental effects of maternal cancer chemotherapy: case report. *Br J Obstet Gynaecol.* 1989;96:1099–1100.
117. Bornstein RS, Hungerford DA, Haller G, et al. Cytogenic effects of bleomycin therapy in man. *Cancer Res.* 1971;31:2004–2007.
118. Opitz JM, Grosse RF, HanebergB. Congenital effects of bromism? *Lancet.* 1972;1:91–92.
119. Rossiter EJR, Rendel Short TJ. Congenital effects of bromism? *Lancet.* 1972;2:705.
120. Finken RL, Robertson WO. Transplacental bromism. *Am J Dis Child.* 1963;106:224–226.
121. Mangurten HH, Ban R. Neonatal hypotonia secondary to transplacental bromism. *J Pediatr.* 1974;85:426–428.
122. Pleasure JR, Blackburn MG. Neonatal bromide intoxication: prenatal ingestion of a large quantity of bromides with transplacental accumulation in the fetus. *Pediatrics.* 1975;55:503–506.
123. Nicholson HO. Cytotoxic drugs in pregnancy: review of reported cases. *J Obstet Gynaecol Br Commonw.* 1968;75:307–312.
124. Boros SJ, Reynolds JW. Intrauterine growth retardation following third trimester exposure to busulfan. *Am J Obstet Gynecol.* 1977;129:111–112.
125. Gebhart E, Schwanitz G, Hartwich G. Chromosomal abberations during busulfan therapy. *Dtsch Med Wochenschr.* 1974;99:52–56.
126. Maduska AL, Hajghassemali M. A double blind comparison of butorphanol and meperidine in labour: maternal pain relief and effect on the newborn. *Can Anaesth Soc J.* 1978;25:398–404.
127. Pittman KA, Smyth RD, Losada M, et al. Human perinatal distribution of butorphanol. *Am J Obstet Gynecol.* 1980;138:797–800.
128. Quilligan EJ, Keegan KA, Donahue MJ. Double blind comparison of intravenously injected butorphanol and meperidine in parturients. *Int J Gynaecol Obstet.* 1980;18:363–367.
129. Angel JL, Knuppel RA, Lake M. Sinusoidal fetal heart rate pattern associated with intravenous butorphanol administration: a case report. *Am J Obstet Gynecol.* 1984;149:465–467.
130. Hatjis CG, Meis PJ. Sinusoidal fetal heart rate pattern associated with intravenous butorphanol administration. *Obstet Gynecol.* 1986; 67:377–380.
131. Mau G, Netter P. Kaffee- und alkoholkonsum-riskofaktoren in der schwangerschaft? *Geburtshilfe Frauenheilkd.* 1974;34:1018–1022.
132. Hadeed A, Siegel S. Newborn cardiac arrhythmias associated with maternal caffeine use during pregnancy. *Clin Pediatr.* 1993;32:45–47.
133. Devoe LD, Murray C, Youssif A, et al. Maternal caffeine consumption and fetal behavior in normal third trimester pregnancy. *Am J Obstet Gynecol.* 1993;168:1105–1112.
134. Kovarik J, Woloszczuk W, Linkesch W, et al. Calcitonin in pregnancy. *Lancet.* 1980;1:199–200.
135. Product information. Rocatrol. Roche Laboratories, 2000.
136. Figgs J, Hamilton R, Homel S, et al. Camphorated oil intoxication in pregnancy: report of a case. *Obstet Gynecol.* 1965;25:255–258.
137. Weiss J, Catalano P. Camphorated oil intoxication during pregnancy. *Pediatrics.* 1973;52:713–714.
138. Blackman WB, Curry HB. Camphor poisoning: report of case occurring during pregnancy. *J Fla Med Assoc.* 1957;43:99.
139. Jacobziner H, Raybin HW. Camphor poisoning. *Arch Pediatr.* 1962;79:28.
140. Rabl W, Katzgraber F, Steinlechner M. Camphor ingestion for abortion (case report). *Forensic Sci Int.* 1997;89:137–140.
141. Hinsberger A, Wingen AM, Hoyer PF. Angiotensin-II-receptor inhibitors in pregnancy. *Lancet.* 2001;357:1620.
142. Schaefer C. Angiotensin II-receptor antagonists: further evidence of fetotoxicity but not teratogenicity. *Birth Defects Res A Clin Mol Teratol.* 2003;67:591–594.
143. Cox RM, Anderson JM, Cox P. Defective embryogenesis with angiotensin II receptor antagonists in pregnancy. *Br J Obstet Gynaecol.* 2003;110:1038.
144. Hanssens M, Keirse MJNC, Vankelecom F, et al. Fetal and neonatal effects of treatment with angiotensin converting enzyme inhibitors in pregnancy. *Obstet Gynecol.* 1991;78:128–135.
145. Markestad T, Ulstein M, Strandjord RE, et al. Anticonvulsant drug therapy in human pregnancy: effects on serum concentrations of vitamin D metabolites in maternal and cord blood. *Am J Obstet Gynecol.* 1984;150:245–258.
146. Mountain KR, Hirsh J, Gallus AS. Neonatal coagulation defect due to anticonvulsant drug treatment in pregnancy. *Lancet.* 1970;1: 265–268.
147. Cornelissen M, Steegers-Theunissen R, Kollee L, et al. Increased incidence of neonatal vitamin K deficiency resulting from maternal anticonvulsant therapy. *Am J Obstet Gynecol.* 1993;168:923–928.
148. Cornelissen M, Steegers-Theunissen R, Kollee L, et al. Supplementation of vitamin K in pregnant women receiving anticonvulsant therapy prevents neonatal vitamin K deficiency. *Am J Obstet Gynecol.* 1993;168:884–888.
149. Frey B, Schuigr G, Musy JP. Transient cholestatic hepatitis in a neonate associated with carbamazepine exposure during pregnancy and breast feeding. *Eur J Pediatr.* 1990;150:136–138.
150. Merlob P, Mor N, Litwin A. transient hepatic dysfunction in an infant of an epileptic mother treated with carbamazepine during pregnancy and breastfeeding. *Ann Pharmacother.* 1992;26:1563–1565.
151. Frey B, Braegger CP, Ghelfi D. Neonatal cholestatic hepatitis from carbamazepine exposure during pregnancy and breast feeding. *Ann Pharmacother.* 2002;36:644–647.
152. Stika CS, Gross GA, Leguizamon G, et al. A prospective randomized safety trial of celecoxib for treatment of preterm labor. *Am J Obstet Gynecol.* 2002;187:653–660.
153. Lawler SD, Lele KP. Chromosomal damage induced by chlorambucil and lymphocytic leukemia. *Scand J Haematol.* 1972;9:603–612.
154. Westin J. Chromosome abnormalities after chlorambucil therapy of polycythemia vera. *Scand J Haematol.* 1976;17:197–204.

155. Catovsky D, Galton DAG. Myelomonocytic leukaemia supervening on chronic lymphocytic leukemia. *Lancet.* 1971;1:478–479.
156. Rosner R. Acute leukemia as a delayed consequence of cancer chemotherapy. *Cancer.* 1976;37:1033–1036.
157. Reimer RR, Hover R, Fraumeni JF, et al. Acute leukemia after alkylating agent therapy of ovarian cancer. *N Eng J Med.* 1977;297: 177–181.
158. Oberheuser F. Praktische Erfahrungen mit Medikamenten in der Schwangerschaft. Therapiewoche 1971;31:2200. As reported in Manten A. Antibiotic drugs. In Dukes MNG, ed. Meyler's Side Effects of Drugs, Vol VIII. New York: American Elsevier, 1975:604.
159. Stirrat GM, Edinston PT, Berry DJ. Transplacental passage of chlordiazepoxide. *Br Med J.* 1974;2:729.
160. Hart CW, Naunton RF. The ototoxicity of chloroquine phosphate. *Arch Otolarygol.* 1964;80:407–412.
161. Senior B, Slone D, Shapiro S, et al. Benzothiadiazides and neonatal hypoglycaemia. *Lancet.* 1976;2:377.
162. Gray MJ. Use and abuse of thiazides in pregnancy. *Clin Obstet Gynecol.* 1968;11:568–578.
163. Menzies DN. Controlled trial of chlorothiazide in treatment of early pre-eclampsia. *Br Med J.* 1964;1:739–742.
164. Harley JD, Robin H, Robertson SEJ. Thiazide induced neonatal haemolysis? *Br Med J.* 1964;1:696–697.
165. Rodriguez SU, Leikin SL, Hiller MC. Neonatal thrombocytopenia associated with ante-partum administration of thiazide drugs. *N Engl J Med.* 1964;270:881–884.
166. Leikin SL. Thiazide and neonatal thrombocytopenia. *N Eng J Med.* 1964;271:161.
167. Prescott LF. Neonatal thrombocytopenia and thiazide drugs. *Br Med J.* 1964;1:1438.
168. Jones JE, Reed JF Jr. Renal vein thrombosis and thrombocytopenia in the newborn infant. *J Pediatr.* 1965;67:681–682.
169. Karpatkin S, Strick N, Karpatkin MB, et al. Cumulative experience in the detection of antiplatelet antibody in 234 patients with idiopathic thrombocytopenic purpura, systemic lupus erythematosus and other clinical disorders. *Am J Med.* 1972;52:776–785.
170. Alstatt LB. Transplacental hyponatremia in the newborn infant. *J Pediatr.* 1965;66:985–988.
171. Pritchard JA, Walley PJ. Severe hypokalemia due to prolonged administration of chlorothiazide during pregnancy. *Am J Obstet Gynecol.* 1961;81:1241–1244.
172. Anderson GG, Hanson TM. Chronic fetal bradycardia: possible association with hypokalemia. *Obstet Gynecol.* 1974;44:896–898.
173. Minkowitz S, Soloway HB, Hall JE, et al. Fatal hemorrhagic pancreatitis following chlorothiazide administration in pregnancy. *Obstet Gynecol.* 1964;24:337–342.
174. Hammond JE, Toseland PA. Placental transfer of chlorpromazine. *Arch Dis Child.* 1970;45:139–140.
175. Hill RM, Desmond MM, Kay JL. Extrapyramidal dysfunction in newborn infant of a schizophrenic mother. *J Pediatr.* 1966;69:589–595.
176. Ayd FJ Jr, ed. Phenothiazine therapy during pregnancy-effects on the newborn infant. *Int Drug Ther Newslett.* 1968;3:39–40.
177. Tamer A, McKay R, Arias D, et al. Phenothiazine-induced extrapyramidal dysfunction in the neonate. *J Pediatr.* 1969;75:479–480.
178. Levy W, Wisniewski K. Chlorpromazine causing extrapyramidal dysfunction in newborn infant of psychotic mother. *NY State J Med.* 1974;74:684–685.
179. O'Connor M, Johnson GH, James DI. Intrauterine effect of phenothiazines. *Med J Austr.* 1981;1:416–417.
180. Zucker P, Simon G. Prolonged symptomatic neonatal hypoglycemia associated with maternal chlorpropamide therapy. *Pediatrics.* 1968;42:824–825.
181. Kemball ML, McIver C, Milnar RDG, et al. Neonatal hypoglycemia in infants of diabetic mothers given sulphonylurea drugs in pregnancy. *Arch Dis Child.* 1970;45:696–701.
182. Harris EL. Adverse reactions to oral antidiabetic agents. *Br Med J.* 1971;3:29–30.
183. Piacquadio K, Hollingworth DR, Murphy H. Effects of in-utero exposure to oral hypoglycemic drugs. *Lancet.* 1991;338:866–869.
184. Sadler LC, Lane M, North R. Severe fetal intracranial haemorrhage during treatment with cholestyramine for intrahepatic cholestasis of pregnancy. *Br J Obstet Gynecol.* 1995;102:169–170.
185. Glade G, Saccar CL, Pereira GR. Cimetidine in pregnancy: apparent transient liver impairment in the newborn. *Am J Dis Child.* 1980; 134:87–88.
186. Karat AB. Long-term follow up of clofazimine (Lamprene) in the management of reactive phases of leprosy. *Lepr Rev.* 1975;46 (suppl):105–109.
187. Farb H, West DP, Pedvis-Leftick A. Clofazimine in pregnancy complicated by leprosy. *Obstet Gynecol.* 1982;59:122–123.
188. Fisher JB, Edgren BE, Mammel MC, et al. Neonatal apnea associated with maternal clonazepam therapy: a case-report. *Obstet Gynecol.* 1985;66(suppl):34S–35S.
189. Haeusler MC, Hoellwarth ME, Holzer P. Paralytic ileus in a fetus-neonate after maternal intake of benzodiazepine. *Prenat Diagn.* 1995;15:1165–1167.
190. Bonica JJ. *Principles and Practice of Obstetric Analgesia and Anesthesia.* Philadelphia, PA: FA Davis, 1967:245.
191. Hall JG, Pauli RM, Wilson KM. Maternal and fetal sequelae of anticoagulation during pregnancy. *Am J Med.* 1980;68:122–140.
192. Pizzuto J, Aviles A, Noriega L, et al. Treatment of acute leukemia during pregnancy: presentation of nine cases. *Cancer Treat Rep.* 1980;64:697–683.
193. Cuvier C, Espie M, Extra JM, et al. Vinorelbine in pregnancy. *Eur J Cancer.* 1997;33:168–169.
194. Giacalone PL, Laffargue F, Benos P. Chemotherapy for breast carcinoma during pregnancy. *Cancer.* 1999;86:2266–2272.
195. Tolchin SF, Winkelstein A, Rodnan GP, et al. Chromosome abnormalities from cyclophosphamide therapy in rheumatoid arthritis and progressive systemic sclerosis (scleroderma). *Arthritis Rheum.* 1974;17:375–382.
196. Klintmalm G, Althoff P, Appleby G, et al. Renal function in a newborn baby delivered of a renal transplant patient taking cyclosporine. *Transplantation.* 1984;38:198–199.
197. Burrows DA, O'Neil TJ, Sorrells TL. Successful twin pregnancy after renal transplant maintained on cyclosporine A immunosuppression. *Obstet Gynecol.* 1988:72:459–461.
198. Briggs GG, Freeman Rk, Yaffe SJ. *Drugs in Pregnancy and Lactation.* 7th ed. Baltimore, MD; Williams & Wilkins, 2005.
199. Lau RJ, Scott JR. Pregnancy folowing renal transplantation. *Clin Obstet Gynecol.* 1985;28:339–350.
200. Maurer LH, Forcier RJ, McIntyre OR, et al. Fetal group C trisomy after cytosine arabinoside and thioguanine. *Ann Intern Med.* 1871;75:809–810.
201. Volkenandt M, Buchner T, Hiddemann W, et al. Acute leukemia during pregnancy. *Lancet.* 1987;2:1521–1522.
202. Duck SC, Katayama KP. Danazol may cause female pseudohermaphroditism. *Fertil Steril.* 1981;35:230–231.
203. Castro-Magana M, Cheruvanky T, Collipp PJ, et al. Transient adrenogenital syndrome due to exposure to danazol in utero. *Am J Dis Child.* 1981;135:1032–1034.
204. Peress MR, Kreutner AK, Mathur RS, et al. Female pseudohermaphroditism with somatic chromosomal anomaly in association with in utero exposure to danasol. *Am J Obstet Gynecol.* 1982;142: 708–709.
205. Schwartz RP. Ambiguous genitalia in a term female infant due to exposure to danazol in utero. *Am J Dis Child.* 1982;136:474.
206. Wentz AC. Adverse effects of danazol in pregnancy. *Ann Intern Med.* 1982;96:672–673.
207. Shaw RW, Farquar JW. Female pseudohermaphroditism associated with danazol exposure in utero: case report. *Br J Obstet Gynaecol.* 1984;91:386–389.
208. Rosa FW. Virilization of the female fetus with maternal danazol exposure. *Am J Obstet Gynecol.* 1984;149:99–100.

209. Kingsbury AC. Danazol and fetal masculinization: a warning. *Med J Aust.* 1985;143:410–411.
210. Quagliarello J, Greco MA. Danazol and urogenital sinus formation in pregnancy. *Fertil Steril.* 1985;43:939–942.
211. Brunskill PJ. The effects of fetal exposure to danazol. *Br J Obstet Gynaecol.* 1992;99:212–215.
212. Hocking DR. Neonatal haemolytic disease due to dapsone. *Med J Aust.* 1968;1:1130–1131.
213. Thornton YS, Bowe ET. Neonatal hyperbilirubinemia after treatment of maternal leprosy. *South Med J.* 1989;82:668.
214. Gililland J, Weinstein L. The effects of cancer chemotherapeutic agents on the developing fetus. *Obstet Gynecol Surv.* 1983;38:6–13.
215. Colbert N, Najman A, Gorin NC, et al. Acute leukaemia during pregnancy: favourable course of pregnancy in two patients treated with cytosine arabinoside and anthracyclines. *Nouv Presse Med.* 1980;9:175–178.
216. Rayburn WF, Donn SM, Wulf ME. Iron overdose during pregnancy: successful therapy with deferoxamine. *Am J Obstet Gynecol.* 1983;147:717–718.
217. Otero L, Conlon C, Reynolds P, et al. Neonatal leukocytosis associated with prenatal administration of dexamethasone. *Pediatrics.* 1981;68:778–780.
218. Anday EK, Harris MC. Leukemoid reaction associated with antenatal dexamethasone administration. *J Pediatr.* 1982;101:614–616.
219. Rodesch F, Camus M, Ermans AM, et al. Adverse effect of amniofetography on fetal thyroid function. *Am J Obstet Gynecol.* 1976;126: 723–726.
220. Scanlon JW. Effect of benzodiazepines in neonates. *N Eng J Med.* 1975;292:649.
221. Gillberg C. "Floppy infant syndrome" and maternal diazepam. *Lancet.* 1977;2:244.
222. Haram K. "Floppy infant syndrome" and maternal diazepam. *Lancet.* 1977;2:612–613.
223. Speight AN. Floppy-infant syndrome and maternal diazepam and/or nitrazepam. *Lancet.* 1977;1:878.
224. Cree JE, Meyer J, Haily DM. Diazepam in labour: its metabolism and effect on the clinical condition and thermogenesis of the newborn. *Br Med J.* 1973;4:251–255.
225. McAllister CB. Placental transfer and neonatal effects of diazepam when administered to women just before delivery. *Br J Anaesth.* 1980;52:423–427.
226. Owen JR, Irani SF, Blair AW. Effect of diazepam administered to mothers during labour on temperature regulation of the neonate. *Arch Dis Child.* 1972;47:107–110.
227. Scher J, Hailey DM, Beard RW. The effects of diazepam on the fetus. *J Obstet Gynaecol Br Commonw.* 1972;79:635–638.
228. Van Geijn HP, Jongsma HW, Doesberg WH, et al. The effect of diazepam administration during pregnancy or labor on the heart rate variability of the newborn infant. *Eur J Obstet Gynaecol Reprod Biol.* 1980;10:187–201.
229. Birger M, Homberg R, Insler V. Clinical evaluation of fetal movements. *Int J Gynaecol Obstet.* 1980;183:377–382.
230. Morris JA, Arce JJ, Hamilton CJ, et al. The management of severe preeclampsia and eclampsia with intravenous diazoxide. *Obstet Gynecol.* 1977;49:675–680.
231. Michael CA. Intravenous diazoxide in the treatment of severe preeclamptic toxaemia and eclampsia. *Aust NZ J Obstet Gynaecol.* 1973;13:143–146.
232. Neuman J, Weisss B, Rabello Y, et al. Diazoxide for acute control of severe hypertension complicating pregnancy: a pilot study. *Obstet Gynecol.* 1979;53(suppl.):50S–55S.
233. Milsap RL, Auld PAM. Neonatal hyperglycemia following maternal diazoxide administration. *JAMA.* 1980;243:144–145.
234. Milner RDG, Chouksey SK. Effects of fetal exposure to diazoxide in man. *Arch Dis Child.* 1972;47:537–543.
235. Adverse Drug Reactions Advisory Committee. Premature closure of the fetal ductus arteriosus after maternal use of non-steroidal anti-inflammtory drugs. *Med J Aust.* 1998;169:270–271.
236. Zenker M, Klinge J, Kruger C, et al. Severe pulmonary hypertension in a neonate caused by premature closure of the ductus arteriosus following maternal treatment with diclofenac: a case report. *J Perinat Med.* 1998;26:231–234.
237. Mas C, Menahem S. Premature in utero closure of the ductus following maternal ingestion of sodium diclofenac. *Aust N Z J Obstet Gynaecol.* 1999;39:106–107.
238. Siu KL, Lee WH. Maternal diclofenac sodium ingestion and severe neonatal pulmonary hypertension. *J Paediatr Child Health.* 2004;40:152–153.
239. Rein AJJT, Nadjari M, Elchalal U, et al. Contraction of the fetal ductus arteriosus induced by diclofenac. *Fetal Diagn Ther.* 1999;14:24–25.
240. Jefferies JA, Robboy SJ, O'Brien PC, et al. Structural anomalies of the cervix and vagina in women enrolled in the Diethylstilbestrol Adenosis ((DESAD) Project. *Am J Obstet Gynecol.* 1984;148:59–66.
241. Peress MR, Tsai CC, Mathur RS, et al. Hirsutism amd menstrual patterns in women exposed to diethylstilbestrol in utero. *Am J Obstet Gynecol.* 1982;144:135–140.
242. Vessey MP, Fairweather DVI, Norman-Smith B, et al. A randomized double-blind controlled trial of the value of stilboestrol therapy in pregnancy: long-term follow-up of mothers and their offspring. *Br J Obstet Gynaecol.* 1983;90:1007–1017.
243. Sherman JL Jr, Locke RV. Transplacental neonatal digitalis intoxication. *Am J Cardiol.* 1960;6:834–837.
244. Ruch WA, Ruch RM. A preliminary report on dihydrocodeine-scopolamine in obstetrics. *Am J Obstet Gynacol.* 1957;74:1125–1127.
245. Myers JD. A preliminary clinical evaluation of dihydrocodeine bitartrate in normal parturition. *Am J Obstet Gynecol.* 1958;75:1096–1100.
246. Altman SG, Waltman R, Lubin S, et al. Oxytocic and toxic actions of dihydroergotamine-45. *Am J Obstet Gynecol.* 1852;64:101–109.
247. Hara GS, Carter RP, Kranz KE. Dramamine in labor: potential boon or a possible bomb? *J Kans Med Soc.* 1980;81:134–136, 155.
248. Kargas GA, Kargas SA, Bruyere HJ Jr, et al. Perinatal mortality due to interaction of diphenhydramine and temazepam. *N Eng J Med.* 1985;313:1417.
249. Schindler AM. Isolated neonatal hypomagnesaemia associated with maternal overuse of stool softener. *Lancet.* 1984;2:822.
250. Wright RG, Scnider SM, Levinson G, et al. The effect of maternal administration of ephedrine on fetal heart rate and variability. *Obstet Gynecol.* 1981;57:734–738.
251. Antoine C, Young BK. Fetal lactic acidosis with epidural anesthesia. *Am J Obstet Gynecol.* 1982;142:55–59.
252. Datta S, Alper MH, Ostheimer GW, et al. Method of ephedrine administration and nausea and hypotension during spinal anesthesia for cesarean section. *Anesthesiology.* 1982;56:68–70.
253. Entman SS, Moise KJ. Anaphylaxis in pregnancy. *South Med J.* 1984;77:402.
254. Braga J, Marques R, Branco A, et al. Maternal and perinatal implications of the use of human recombinant erythropoeitin. *Acta Obstet Gynecol Scand.* 1996;75:449–453.
255. Au KL, Woo JSK, Wong VCW. Intrauterine death from ergotamine overdosage. *Eur J Obstet Gynecol Reprod Biol.* 1985;19:313–315.
256. de Groot ANJA, van Dongen PWJ, van Roosmalen J, et al. Ergotamine-induced fetal stress: review of side effects of ergot alkaloids during pregnancy. *Eur J Obstet Gynecol Reprod Biol.* 1993;51: 73–77.
257. Ducey JP, Knape KG. Maternal esmolol administration resulting in fetal distress and cesarean section in a term pregnancy. *Anesthesiology.* 1992;77:829–832.
258. Gilson GJ, Knieriem KJ, Smith JF, et al. Short-acting beta-adrenergic blockade and the fetus: a case report. *J Reprod Med.* 1992;37: 277–279.
259. Fairly CJ, Clarke JT. Use of esmolol in a parturient with hpertrophic obstructive cardiomyopathy. *Br J Anaesth.* 1995;75:801–804.
260. Jones HC. Intrauterine ototoxicity: a case report and review of literature. *J Natl Med Assoc.* 1973;65:201–203.
261. Speidel BD, Meadow SR. Epilepsy, anticonvulsants and congenital malformations. *Drugs.* 1974;8:354–365.

262. Buller RE, Darrow V, Manetta A, et al. Conservative surgical management of dysgerminoma concomitant with pregnancy. *Obstet Gynecol.* 1992;79:887–890.
263. Murray NA, Acolet D, Deane M, et al. Fetal marrow suppression after maternal chemotherapy for leukemia. *Arch Dis Child.* 1994;71:F209–F210.
264. Jager K, Schiller F, Stech P. Congenital ichthyosiforme erythroderma, pregnancy under aromatic retinoid treatment. *Hautarzt.* 1985;36:150–153.
265. Carrie LES, O'Sullivan GM, Seegobin R. Epidural fentanyl in labour. *Anaesthesia.* 1981;36:965–969.
266. Rayburn W, Rathke A, Leuschen MP, et al. Fentanyl citrate analgesia during labor. *Am J Obstet Gynecol.* 1989;161:202–206.
267. Johnson ES, Colley PS. Effects of nitrous oxide and fentanyl anesthesia on fetal heart-rate variability intra- and postoperatively. *Anesthesiology.* 1980;52:429–430.
268. Lindemann R. Respiratory muscle rigidity in a preterm infant after use of fentanyl during caesarean section. *Eur J Pediatr.* 1998;157:1012–1013.
269. van Gelder-Hasker MR, de Jong CLD, de Vries JIP, et al. The effect of flecainide acetate on fetal heart rate variability: a case report. *Obstet Gynecol.* 1995;86:667–669.
270. Vanderhal AL, Cocjin J, Santulli TV, et al. Conjugated hyperbilirubinemia in a newborn infant after maternal (transplacental) treatment with flecainide acetate for fetal tachycardia and fetal hydrops. *J Pediatr.* 1995;126:988–990.
271. Stadler HE, Knowles J. Fluorouracil in pregnancy: effect on the neonate. *JAMA.* 1971;217:214–215.
272. Chambers CD, Johnson KA, Dick LM, et al. Birth outcoms in pregnant women taking fluoxetine. *N Eng J Med.* 1996;335:1010–1015.
273. Spencer MJ. Fluoxetine hydrochloride (Prozac) toxicity in a neonate. *Pediatrics.* 1993;92:721–722.
274. Mhanna MJ, Bennet JB II, Izatt SD. Potential fluoxetine chloride (Prozac) toxicity in a newborn. *Pediatrics.* 1997;100:158–159.
275. Cleary MF. Fluphenazine decanoate during pregnancy. *Am J Psychiatry.* 1977;134:815–816.
276. Nath SP, Miller DA, Muraskas JK. Severe rinorrhea and respiratory distress in a neonate exposed to fluphenazine hydrochloride prenatally. *Ann Pharmacother.* 1996;30:35–37.
277. Product information. Dalmane. Roche Laboratories, 1993.
278. Lamotrigine Pregnancy Registry. Interim Report. 1 September 1992 through 30 September 1996. Glaxo Wellcome Inc., 1997.
279. Coetzee EJ, Jackson WPU. Pregnancy in established non-insulin-dependent diabetics; a five-and-a-half year study at Groote Schuur Hospital. *S Afr Med J.* 1980;58:795–802.
280. Coetzee EJ, Jackson WPU. Oral hypoglycemics in the first trimester and fetal outcome. *S Afr Med J.* 1984;65:635–637.
281. Piacquadio K, Hollingsworth DR, Murphy H. Effects of in utero exposure to oral hypoglycaemic drugs. *Lancet.* 1991;338:866–869.
282. Sexon WR, Barak Y. Withdrawal emergent syndrome in an infant associated with maternal haloperidol therapy. *J Perinatol.* 1989;9:170–172.
283. Collins KO, Comer JB. Maternal haloperidol therapy associated with dyskinesia in a newborn. *Am J Health Syst Pharm.* 2003;60:2253–2255.
284. Morris N. Hexamethonium in the treatment of pre-eclampsia and essential hypertension during pregnancy. *Lancet.* 1953;1:322–324.
285. Hallum JL, Hatchuel WLF. Congenital paralytic ileus in a premature baby as a complication of hexamethonium bromide therapy for toxemia of pregnancy. *Arch Dis Child.* 1954;29:354–356.
286. Widerlov E, Karlman I, Storsater J. Hydralazine-induced neonatal thrombocytopenia. *N Eng J Med.* 1980;303:1235–1238.
287. Brazy JE, Grimm JK, Litte VA. Neonatal manifestations of severe maternal hypertension occurring before the thirty-sixth week of pregnancy. *J Pediatr.* 1982;100:265–271.
288. Sibai BM, Anderson GD. Pregnancy outcome of intensive therapy in severe hypertension in first trimester. *Obstet Gynecol.* 1986;67:517–522.
289. Lodeiro JG, Feinstein SJ, Lodeiro SB. Fetal premature atrial contractions associated with hydralazine. *Am J Obstet Gynecol.* 1989;160:105–107.
290. Yemini M, Shoham (Schwartz) Z, Dgani R, et al. Lupus-like syndrome in a mother and newborn following administration of hydralazine: a case report. *Eur J Obstet Gynecol Reprod Biol.* 1989;30:193–197.
291. Kirshon S, Wasserstrum N, Cotton DB. Should continuous hydralazine infusions be utilized in severe pregnancy-induced hypertension? *Am J Perinatol.* 1991;8:206–208.
292. Wilkins L. Masculinization of female fetus due to use of orally given progestins. *JAMA.* 1960;172:1028–1032.
293. Wilkins L, Jones HW, Holman GH, et al. Masculinization of the female fetus associated with administration of oral and intramuscular progestins during gestation: non-adrenal female pseudohermaphrodism. *J Clin Endocrinol Metab.* 1958;68:559–585.
294. Dayan E, Rosa FW. Fetal ambiguous genitalia associated with sex hormone use early in pregnancy. ADR Highlights 1981:1–14. Food and Drug Administration, Division of Drug Experience.
295. Petrie RH, Yeh SY, Murata Y, et al. The effects of drugs on fetal heart rate variability. *Am J Obstet Gynecol.* 1978;130:294–299.
296. Whaun JM, Smith GR, Sochor VA. Effect of prenatal drug administration on maternal and neonatal platelet aggregation and PF_4 release. *Haemostasis.* 1980;9:226–237.
297. Hickok DE, Hollenbach KA, Reilley SF, et al. The association between decreased amniotic fluid volume and treatment with nonsteroidal anti-inflammatory agents for preterm labor. *Am J Obstet Gynecol.* 1989;160:1525–1531.
298. Wiggins DA, Elliott JP. Oligohydramnios in each sac of a triplet gestation caused by Motrin-fulfilling Kock's postulates. *Am J Obstet Gynecol.* 1990;162:460-461.
299. Hendricks SK, Smith JR, Moore DE, et al. Oligohydramnios associated with prostaglandin synthetase inhibitors in preterm labour. *Br J Obstet Gynaecol.* 1990;97:312–316.
300. Hennessy MD, Livingston EC, Papagianos J, et al. The incidence of ductal constriction and oligohydramnios during tocolytic therapy with ibuprofen (abstract). *Am J Obstet Gynecol.* 1992;166:324.
301. Reynoso EE, Huerta F. Acute leukemia and pregnancy—fatal fetal outcome after exposure to idarubicin during the second trimester. *Acta Oncol.* 1994;33:703–716.
302. Claahsen HL, Semmekrot BA, van Dongen PWJ, et al. Successful fetal outcome after exposure to idarubicin and cytosine-arabinoside during the second trimester of pregnancy—a case report. *Am J Perinatol.* 1998;15:295–297.
303. Achtari C, Hohfeld P. Cardiotoxic transplacental effect of idarubicin administered during the second trimester of pregnancy. *Am J Obstet Gynecol.* 2000;183:511–512.
304. Fernandez H, Diallo A, Baume D, et al. Anhydramnios and cessation of fetal growth in a pregnant mother with polychemotherapy during the second trimester. *Prenat Diag.* 1989;9:681–682.
305. Merimsky O, Chevalier TL, Missenard G, et al. Management of cancer in pregnancy: a case of Ewing's sarcoma of the pelvis in the third trimester. *Ann Oncol.* 1999;10:345–350.
306. Morales WJ, Smith SG, Angel JL, et al. Efficacy and safety of indomethacin compared versus ritodrine in the management of preterm labor: a randomized study. *Obstet Gynecol.* 1989;74:567–572.
307. De Wit W, Van Mourik I, Wiesenhaan PF. Prolonged maternal indomethacin therapy associated with oligohydramnios: case reports. *Br J Obstet Gynaecol.* 1988;95:303–305.
308. Goldenberg RL, Davis RO, Baker RC. Indomethacin-induced oligohydramnios. *Am J Obstet Gynecol.* 1989;160:1196–1197.
309. Kirshon B, Moise KJ Jr, Wasserstrum N, et al. Influence of short-term indomethacin therapy on fetal urine output. *Obstet Gynecol.* 1988;72:51–53.
310. Heijden AJ, Provost AP, Nauta J, et al. Renal functional impairment in preterm neonates related to intrauterine indomethacin exposure. *Pediatr Res.* 1988;24:644–648.

311. Atad J, David A, Moise J, et al. Classification of threatened premature labor related to treatment with a prostastaglandin inhibitor: indomethacin. *Biol Neonate.* 1980;37:291–296.
312. Sureau C, Piovani P. Clinical study of indomethacin for prevention of prematurity. *Eur J Obstet Gynecol Reprod Biol.* 1983;46:400–402.
313. Van Kets H, Thiery M, Derom R, et al. Perinatal hazards of chronic antenatal tocolysis with indomethacin. *Prostaglandins.* 1979;18:893–907.
314. Van Kets H, Thiery M, Derom R, et al. Prostaglandin synthase inhibitors in preterm labor. *Lancet.* 1980;2:693.
315. Leonardi MR, Hankins GDV. What's new in tocolytics. *Clin Perinatol.* 1992;19:367–384.
316. Higby K, Xenakis EM-J, PauersteinCJ. Do tocolytic agents stop preterm labor? A critical and comprehensive review of efficacy and safety. *Am J Obstet Gynecol.* 1993;168:1247–1259.
317. Levin DL. Effects of inhibition of prostaglandin synthesis on fetal development, oxygenation, and the fetal circulation. *Semin Perinatol.* 1980;4:35–44.
318. Csaba IF, Sulyok E, Ertl T. Relationship of maternal treatment with indomethacin to persistance of fetal circulation syndrome. *J Pediatr.* 1978;92:484.
319. Levin DL, Fixler DE, Morriss FC, et al. Morphologic analysis of the pulmonary vascular bed in infants exposed in utero to prostaglandin synthetase inhibitors. *J Pediatr.* 1978;92:478–483.
320. Rubaltelli FF, Chiozza ML, Zanardo V, et al. Effect on neonate of maternal treatment with indomethacin. *J Pediatr.* 1979;94:161.
321. Manchester D, Margolis HS, Sheldon RE. Possible association between maternal indomethacin therapy and primary pulmonary hypertension of the newborn. *Am J Obstet Gynecol.* 1976;126:467–469.
322. Besinger RE, Niebyl JR, Keyes WG, et al. Randomized comparative trial of indomethacin and ritodrine for the long-term treatment of preterm labor. *Am J Obstet Gynecol.* 1991;164:981–988.
323. Demandt E, Legius E, Devlieger H, et al. Prenatal indomethacin toxicity in one member of monozygous twins: a case report. *Eur J Obstet Gynecol Reprod Biol.* 1990;35:267–269.
324. Goudie BM, Dossetor JFB. Effect on the fetus of indomethacin given to suppress labour. *Lancet.* 1979;2:1187–1188.
325. Mogilner BM, Ashkenazy M, Borenstein R, et al. Hydrops fetalis caused by maternal indomethacin treatment. *Acta Obstet Gynecol Scand.* 1982;61:183–185.
326. Moise KJ Jr, Huhta JC, Sharif DS, et al. Indomethacin in the treatment of premature labor: effects on the fetal ductus arteriosus. *N Eng J Med.* 1988;319:327–331.
327. Van Den Veyver I, Moise K Jr, Ou C-N, et al. The effect of gestational age and fetal indomethacin levels on the incidence of constriction of the fetal ductus arteriosus (abstract). *Am J Obstet Gynecol.* 1993;168:373.
328. Van Den Veyver IB, Moise K Jr, Ou C-N, et al. The effect of gestational age and fetal indomethacin levels on the incidence of constriction of the fetal ductus arteriosus. *Obstet Gynecol.* 1993;82:500–503.
329. Moise KJ Jr. Effect of advancing gestational age on the frequency of fetal ductal constriction in association with maternal indomethacin use. *Am J Obstet Gynecol.* 1993;168:1350–1353.
330. Evans DJ, Kofinas AD, King K. Intraoperative amniocentesis and indomethacin treatment in the management of an immature pregnancy with completely dialated cervix. *Obstet Gynecol.* 1992;79:881–882.
331. Eronen M, Pesonen E, Kurki T, et al. The effects of indomethacin and a β-sympathomimetic agent on the fetal ductus arteriosus during treatment of premature labor: a randomized double-blind dtudy. *Am J Obstet Gynecol.* 1991;164:141–146.
332. Hallak M, Reiter AA, Ayres NA, et al. Indomethacin for preterm labor: fetal toxicity in a dizygotic twin gestation. *Obstet Gynecol.* 1991;78:911–913.
333. Rosemond RL, Boehm FH, Moreau G, et al. Tricuspid regurgitation: a method of monitoring patients treated with indomethacin (abstract). *Am J Obstet Gynecol.* 1992;166;336.
334. Bivins HA Jr, Newman RB, Fyfe DA, et al. Randomized comparative trial of indomethacin and terbutaline for the long term treatment of preterm labor (abstract). *Am J Obstet Gynecol.* 1993;168:375.
335. Mari G, Moise KJ Jr, Deter RL, et al. Doppler assessment of the renal blood flow velocity waveform during indomethacin therapy for preterm labor and polyhydramnios. *Obstet Gynecol.* 1990;75:199–201.
336. Kirshon B, Mari G, Moise KJ Jr, et al. Effect of indomethacin on the fetal ductus arteriosus during treatment of symptomatic polyhydramnios. *J Reprod Med.* 1990;35:529–532.
337. Buderus S, Thomas B, Fahneestich H, et al. Renal failure in two preterm infants: toxic effect of prenatal maternal indomethacin treatment? *Br J Obstet Gynaecol.* 1993;100:97–98.
338. Veersema D, de Jong PA, van Wijck JAM. Indomethacin and the fetal renal nonfunction syndrome. *Eur J Obstet Gynecol Reprod Biol.* 1983;16:113–121.
339. Vanhaesebrouck P, Thiery M, Leroy GJ, et al. Oligohydramnios, renal insufficiency, and ileal perforation in preterm infants after intrauterine exposure to indomethacin. *J Pediatr.* 1988;113:738–743.
340. Itskovitz J, Abramovici H, Brandes JM. Oligohydramnion, meconium and perinatal death concurrent with indomethacin treatment in human pregnancy. *J Reprod Med.* 1980;24:137–140.
341. Murray HG, Stone PR, Strand L, et al. Fetal pleural effusion following maternal indomethacin therapy. *Br J Obstet Gynaecol.* 1993;100:277–282.
342. Baerts W, Fetter WPF, Hop WCJ, et al. Cerebral lesions in preterm infants after tocolytic indomethacin. *Dev Med Child Neurol.* 1990;32:910–918.
343. Menon RK, Cohen RM, Sperling MA, et al. Transpacental passage of insulin in pregnant women with insulin-dependent diabetes-mellitus: Its role in fetL Mcrosomia. *N Eng J Med.* 1990;323:309–315.
344. Mehta PS, Mehta SJ, Virherr H. Congenital iodide goiter and hypothyroidism: a review. *Obstet Gynecol Surv.* 1983;38:237–247.
345. I'Allemand D, Gruters A, Heidemann P, et al. Iodine-induced alterations of thyroid function in newborn infants after prenatal and perinatal exposure to povidone iodide. *J Pediatr.* 1983;102:935–938.
346. Bachrach LK, Burrow GN, Gare DJ. Maternal-fetal absorption of povidone-iodide. *J Pediatr.* 1984;102:158–189.
347. Jacobson JM, Hankins GV, Young RL, et al. Changes in thyroid function and serum iodine levels after prepartum use of a povidone-iodine vaginal lubricant. *J Reprod Med.* 1984;29:98–100.
348. Danziger Y, Perzelan A, Mimouni M. Transient congenital hypothyroidism after topical iodine in pregnancy and lactation. *Arch Dis Child.* 1987;62:295–296.
349. Wolff J. Iodide goiter and the pharmacologic effects of excess iodide. *Am J Med.* 1969;47:101–124.
350. Russell KP, Rose H, Starr P. The effects of radioactive iodine on maternal and fetal thyroid function during pregnancy. *Surg Gynecol Obstet.* 1957;104:560–564.
351. Ray EW, Sterling K, Gardner LI. Congenital cretinism associated with I^{131} therapy of the mother. *Am J Dis Child.* 1959;98:506–507.
352. Hamill GC, Jarman JA, Wynne MD. Fetal effects of radioactive iodine therapy in a pregnant woman with thyroid cancer. *Am J Obstet Gynecol.* 1961;81:1018–1023.
353. Fisher WD, Voorhess ML, Gardner LI. Congenital hypothyroidism in infant following maternal I^{131} therapy. *J Pediatr.* 1963;62:132–146.
354. Green HG, Garies FJ, Shepard TH, et al. Cretinism associated with maternal sodium iodide I^{131} therapy during pregnancy. *Am J Dis Child.* 1971;122:247–249.
355. Jafek BW, Small R, Lillian DL. Congenital radioactive iodine-induced stridor and hypothyroidism. *Arch Otolaryngol.* 1974;99:369–371.
356. Exss R, Graewe B. Congenital athyroidism in the newborn infant frrom intra-uterine radioiodine action. *Biol Neonate.* 1974;24:289–291.
357. Richards GE, Brewer ED, Conley SB, et al. Combined hypothyroidism and hypoparathyoidism in an infant after maternal ^{131}I administration. *J Pediatr.* 1981;99:141–143.

358. Eggermont E, Logghe N, Van De Casseye W, et al. Haemorrhagic disease of the newborn in the offspring of rifampicin and isoniazid treated mothers. *Acta Paediatr Belg.* 1976;29:87–90.
359. DeSimone CA, Leighton BL, Norris MC, et al. The chronotropic effect of isoproterenol is reduced in term pregnant women. *Anesthesiology.* 1988;69:626–628.
360. Brazy JE, Little V, Grimm J, et al. Risk:benefit considerations for the use of isoxsuprine in the treatment of premature labor. *Obstet Gynecol.* 1981;58:297–303.
361. Brazy JE, Pupkin MJ. Effects of maternal isoxsuprine administration on preterm infants. *J Pediatr.* 1979;94:444–448.
362. Brazy JE, Little V, Grimm J. Isoxsuprine in the perinatal period. II. Relationships between neonatal symptoms, drug exposure, and drug concentration at the time of birth. *J Pediatr.* 1981;98: 146–151.
363. Gemelli M, De Luca F, Manganaro R, et al. Transient electrocardiographic changes suggesting myocardial ischemia in newborn infants following tocolysis with beta-sympathomimetics. *Eur J Pediatr.* 1990;149:730–733.
364. Nishimura H, Tanimura T. Clinical Aspects of Teratogenicity of Drugs. Experta Medica, 1976; pp 131–145.
365. Little B, Chang T, Chucot L, et al. Study of ketamine as an obstetric anesthetic agent. *Am J Obstet Gynecol.* 1972;113:247–260.
366. Meer FM, Downing JW, Coleman AJ. An intravenous method of anaesthesia for caesarean section. Part II: Ketamine. *Br J Anaesth.* 1973;45:191–196.
367. Galbert MW, Gardner AE. Ketamine for obstetrical anesthesia. *Anesth Analg.* 1973;52:926–930.
368. Corssen G. Ketamine in obstetric anesthesia. *Clin Obstet Gynecol.* 1974;17:249–258.
369. Janeczko GF, El-Etr AA, Younes S. Low-dose ketamine anesthesia for obstetrical delivery. *Anesth Analg.* 1974;53:828–831.
370. Downing JW, Mahomedy MC, Jeal DE, et al. Anaesthesia for caesarean section with ketamine. *Anaesthesia.* 1976;31:883–892.
371. Ellingson A, Haram K, Sagen N. Ketamine and diazepam as anaesthesia for forceps delivery. A comparative study. *Acta Anaesth Scand.* 1977;21:37–40.
372. White PF, Way WL, Trevor AJ. Ketamine-its pharmacology and therapeutic uses. *Anesthesiology.* 1982;56:119–136.
373. Baraka A, Louis F, Dalleh R. Maternal awareness and neonatal outcome after ketamine induction of anaesthesia for caesarean section. *Can J Anaesth.* 1990;37:641–644.
374. Bovill JG, Coppel DL, Dundee JW, et al. Current status of ketamine anaesthesia. *Lancet.* 1971;1:1285–1288.
375. Moore J, McNabb TG, Dundee Jw. Preliminary report on ketamine in obstetrics. *Br J Anaesth.* 1971;43:779–782.
376. Michael CA, Potter JM. A comparison of labetolol with other antihypertensive drugs in the treatment of hypertensive disease of pregnancy. In: Riley A, Symonds EM. Eds. *The Investigation of Labetolol in the Management of Hypertension in Pregnancy.* Amsterdam: Excerpta Medica, 1982:111–122.
377. Davey DA, Dommisse J, Garden A. Intravenous labetolol and intravenous dihydralazine in severe hypertension in pregnancy. In: Riley A, Symonds EM, eds. *The Investigation of Labetolol in the Management of Hypertension in Pregnancy.* Amsterdam: Excerpta Medica, 1982:52–61.
378. Michael CA. Use of labetolol in the treatment of severe hypertension during pregnancy. *Br J Clin Pharmacol.* 1979;8(Suppl 2):211S–215S.
379. MacPherson M, Broughton Pipkin F, Rutter N. The effect of maternal labetolol on the newborn infant. *Br J Obstet Gynaecol.* 1986;93:539–542.
380. Riley AJ. Clinical pharmacology of labetolol in pregnancy. *J Cardiovasc Pharmacol.* 1981;3(Suppl 1):S53–S59.
381. Sibai BM, Gonzalez AR, Mabie WC, et al. A comparison of labetolol plus hospitalization versus hospitalization alone in the management of preeclampsia remote from term. *Obstet Gynecol.* 1987;70:323–327.
382. Blanche S, Tardieu M, Rustin P, et al. Persistent mitochondrial dysfunction and perinatal exposure to antiretroviral nucleoside analogues. *Lancet.* 1999;354:1084–1089.
383. Stojanov S, Wintergerst U, Belohradsky BH. Mitochondrial and perioxisomal dysfunction following perinatal exposure to antiretroviral drugs. *AIDS.* 2000;14:1669.
384. Liston WA, Adjepon-Yamoah KK, Scott DB. Foetal and maternal lignocaine levels after paracervical block. *Br J Anaesth.* 1973;45:750–754.
385. Scanlon JW, Brown WU Jr, Weiss JB, et al. Neurobehavioral responses of newborn infants after maternal epidural anesthesia. *Anesthesiology.* 1974;40:121–128.
386. Shnider SM, Way EL. Plasma levels of lidocaine (Xylocaine) in mother and newborn following obstetrical conduction anesthesia: clinical applications. *Anesthesiology.* 1968;29:951–958.
387. Rosa F, Bosco L. Infant renal failure with maternal ACE inhibition (abstract). *Am J Obstet Gynecol.* 1991;164:273.
388. Bhatt-Mehta V, Deluga KS. Chronic renal failure (CRF) in a neonate due to in-utero exposure to lisinopril. Presented at the 12th Annual Meeting of the American College of Clinical Pharmacy, Minneapolis, MN, August 20, 1991, abstract No. 43.
389. Pryde PG, Nugent CE, Sedman AB, et al. ACE inhibitor fetopathy (abstract). *Am J Obstet Gynecol.* 1992;166:348.
390. Barr M Jr, Cohen MM Jr. ACE inhibitor fetopathy and hypocalvaria: the kidney-skull connection. *Teratology.* 1991;44:485–495.
391. Mizrahi EM, Hobbs JF, Goldsmith DI. Nephrogenic diabetes incipidus in transplacental lithium intoxication. *J Pediatr.* 1979;94:493–495.
392. Rane A, Tomson G, Bjarke B. Effects of maternal lithium therapy in a newborn infant. *J Pediatr.* 1978;93:296–297.
393. Woody JN, London WL, Wilbanks GD Jr. Lithium toxicity in a newborn. *Pediatrics.* 1971;47:94–96.
394. Tunnessen WW Jr, Hertz CG. Toxic effects of lithium in newborn infants: a commentary. *J Pedaitr.* 1972;81:804–807.
395. Piton M, Barthe ML, Laloum D, et al. Acute lithium intoxication. Report of two cases: mother and her newborn. *Therapie.* 1973;28:1123–1144.
396. Wilbanks GD, Bressler B, Peete CH Jr, et al. Toxic effects of lithium carbonate in a mother and newborn infant. *JAMA.* 1970;213: 865–867.
397. Morrell P, Sutherland GR, Baumah PK, et al. Lithium toxicity in a neonate. *Arch Dis Child.* 1982;58:539–541.
398. Schou M, Goldfield MD, Weinstein MR, et al. Lithium and pregnancy. I. Report from the register of lithium babies. *Br Med J.* 1973;2:135–136.
399. Silverman JA, Winters RW, Strande C. Lithium carbonate therapy during pregnancy: apparent lack of effect upon the fetus. *Am J Obstet Gynecol.* 1971;109:934–936.
400. Strothers JK, Wilson DW, Royston N. Lithium toxicity in the newborn. *Br Med J.* 1973;3:233–234.
401. Karlsson K, Lindstedt G, Lundberg PA, et al. Transplacental lithium poisoning: reversible inhibition of fetal thyroid. *Lancet.* 1975;1:1295.
402. Krause S, Ebbesen F, Lange AP. Polyhydramnios with maternal lithium treatment. *Obstet Gynecol.* 1990;75:504–506.
403. Stevens D, Burman D, Midwinter A. Transplacental lithium poisoning. *Lancet.* 1974;2:595.
404. Wilson N, Forfar JC, Goodman MJ. Atrial flutter in the newborn resulting from maternal lithium intoxication. *Arch Dis Child.* 1983;58:538–539.
405. Ang MS, Thorp JA, Parisi VM. Maternal lithium therapy and polyhydramnios. *Obstet Gynecol.* 1990;76:517–519.
406. Connoley G, Menahem S. A possible association between neonatal jaundice and long-term maternal lithium ingestion. *Med J Aust.* 1990;152:272.
407. Khandelwal SK, Sagar RS, Saxena S. Lithium in pregnancy and stillbirth: a case report. *Br J Psychiatry.* 1989;154:114–116.

408. Nishiwaki T, Tanaka K, Sekiya S. Acute lithium intoxication in pregnancy. *Int J Gynecol Obstet.* 1996;52:191–192.
409. McBride RJ, Dundee JW, Moore J, et al. A study of the plasma concentrations of lorazepam in mother and neonate. *Br J Anaesth.* 1979;51:971–978.
410. Di Michele V, Ramenghi LA, Sabatino G. Clozapine and lorazepam administration in pregnancy. *Eur Psychiatry.* 1996;11:214.
411. Saji H, Yamanaka M, Hagiwara A, et al. Losartan and fetal toxic effects. *Lancet.* 2001;357:363.
412. Lambot MA, Vermeylen D, Noel JC. Angiotensin-II-receptor inhibitors in pregnancy. *Lancet.* 2001;357:1619–1620.
413. Martinovic J, Benachi A, Laurent N, et al. Fetal toxic effects and angiotensin-II-receptor antagonists. *Lancet.* 2001;358:241–242.
414. Nayar B, Singhal A, Aggarwal R, et al. Losartan induced fetal toxicity. *Indian J Pediatr.* 2003;70:923–924.
415. Dangman BC, Rosen TS. Magnesium levels in infants of mothers treated with $MgSO_4$ (abstract #262). *Pediatr Res.* 1977;11:415.
416. Lipsitz PJ, English IC. Hypermagnesemia in the newborn infant. *Pediatrics.* 1967;40:856–862.
417. Lipsitz PJ. The clinical and biochemical effects of excess magnesium in the newborn. *Pediatrics.* 1971;47:501–509.
418. Lamm CI, Norton KI, Murphy RJC, et al. Congenital rickets associated with magnesium sulfate infusion for tocolysis. *J Pediatr.* 1988;113:1078–1082.
419. Wilkins IA, Goldberg JD, Phillips RN, et al. Long-term use of magnesium sulfate as a tocolytic agent. *Obstet Gynecol* 1986;67:38S–40S.
420. Dudley D, Gagnon D, Varner M. Long-term tocolysis with intravenous magnesium sulfate. *Obstet Gynecol.* 1989;73:373–378.
421. Pruett KM, Kirshon B, Cotton DB, et al. The effects of magnesium sulfate therapy on Apgar scores. *Am J Obste Gynecol.* 1988;159:1047–1048.
422. Savory J, Monif GRG. Sreum calcium levels in cord sera of the progeny of mothers treated with magnesium for toxemia. *Am J Obstet Gynecol.* 1971;110:556–559.
423. Rasch DK, Huber PA, Richardson CJ, et al. Neurobehavioural effects of neonatal hypermagnesemia. *J Pediatr.* 1982;100:272–276.
424. Brady JP, Williams HC. Magnesium intoxication in a premature infant. *Pediatrics.* 1967;40:100–103.
425. Brazy JE, Grimm JK, Little VA. Neonatal manifestations of severe maternal hypertension occurring before the thirty-sixth week of pregnancy. *J Pediatr.* 1982;100;265–271.
426. Holocomb WL Jr, Shackelford GD, Petrie RH. Prolonged magnesium therapy affects fetal bone (abstract). *Am J Obstet Gynecol.* 1991;164:386.
427. Smith LG Jr, Schanler RJ, Burns P, et al. Effect of magnesium sulfate therapy ($MgSO_4$) on the bone mineral content of women and their newborns (abstract). *Am J Obstet Gynecol.* 1991;164:427.
428. Holocomb WL Jr, Shackelford GD, Petrie RH. Magnesium tocolysis and neonatal bone abnormalities: a controlled study. *Obstet Gynecol.* 1991;78:611–614.
429. Smith LG Jr, Burnes PA, Schanler RJ. Calcium homeostasis in pregnant women receiving long-term magnesium sulfate therapy for preterm labor. *Am J Obstet Gynecol* 1992;167:45–51.
430. Cruishank DP, Chan GM, Doerrfeld D. Alterations in vitamin D and calcium metabolism with magnesium sulfate treatment of preeclampsia. *Am J Obstet Gynecol.* 1993;168:1170–1177.
431. Rodis JF, Vinzileos AM, Campbell WA, et al. Maternal hypothermia: an unusual complication of magnesium sulfate therapy. *Am J Obstet Gynecol.* 1987;156:435–436.
432. Dayan E, Rosa FW. Fetal ambiguous genitalia associated with sex hormones use early in pregnancy. Food and Drug Administration, Division of Drug Experience. ADR Highlights 1981;1–14.
433. Menahem S. Administration of prostaglandin inhibitors to the mother; the potential risk to the fetus and neonate with duct-dependent circulation. *Reprod Fertil Dev.* 1991;3:489–494.
434. Lane PA, Hathaway WE. Vitamin K in infancy. *J Pediatr.* 1985;106: 351–359.
435. Payne NR, Hasegawa DK. Vitamin K deficiency in newborns: a case report in α-1-antitrypsin deficiency and a review of factors predisposing to hemorrhage. *Pediatrics.* 1984;73:712–716.
436. Wynn RM. The obstetric significance of factors affecting the metabolism of bilirubin, with particular reference to the role of vitamin K. *Obstet Gynecol Surv.* 1963;18:333–354.
437. Finkel MJ. Vitamin K_1 and vitamin K analogues. *Clin Pharmacol Ther.* 1961;2:795–814.
438. Morrison JC, Wiser WL, Rosser SI, et al. Metabolites of meperidine related to fetal depression. *Am J Obstet Gynecol.* 1973;115: 1132–1137.
439. Belfrage P, Boreus LO, Hartvig P, et al. Neonatal depression after obstetrical analgesia with pethidine. The role of the injection-delivery time interval and the plasma concentrations of pethidine and norpethidine. *Acta Obstet Gynecol Scand.* 1981;60:43–49.
440. Borgstedt AD, Rosen MG. Medication during labor correlated with behavior and EEG of the newborn. *Am J Dis Child.* 1968;115:21–24.
441. Hodgkinson R, Bhatt M, Wang CN. Double-blind comparison of the neurobehavior of neonates following the administration of different doses of meperidine to the mother. *Can Anaesth Soc J.* 1978;25:405–411.
442. Baxi LV, Petrie RH, James LS. Human fetal oxygenation ($TcPO_2$), heart rate and uterineactivity following maternal administration of meperidine. *J Perinat Med.* 1988;16:23–30.
443. Gordon HR. Fetal bradycardia after paracervical block: correlation with fetal and maternal blood levels of local anesthetic (mepivacaine). *N Eng J Med.* 1968;279:910–914.
444. McConnell JF, Bhoola R. A neonatal complication of maternal leukemia treated with 6-mercaptopurine. *Postgrad Med.* 1973;49: 211–213.
445. Zelson C, Lee SJ, Casalino M. Neonatal narcotic addiction. *N Eng J Med.* 1973;289:1216–1220.
446. Burstein Y, Giardina PJV, Rausen AR, et al. Thrombocytosis and increased circulating platelet aggregates in newborn infants of polydrug users. *J Pediatr.* 1979;94:895–899.
447. Low L, Ratcliffe W, Alexander W. Intrauterine hypothyroidism due to antithyroid-drug therapy for thyrotoxicosis during pregnancy. *Lancet.* 1978;2:370–371.
448. Hawe P, Francis HH. Pregnancy and thyrotoxicosis. *Br Med J.* 1962;2:817–822.
449. Refetoff S, Ochi Y, Selenkow HA, et al. Neonatal hypothyroidism and goiter in one infant of each of two sets of twins due to maternal therapy with antithyroid drugs. *J Pediatr.* 1974;85:240–244.
450. Sugrue D, Drury MI. Hyperthyroidism complicating pregnancy: results of treatment by antithyroid drugs in 77 pregnancies. *Br J Obstet Gynaecol.* 1980;87:970–975.
451. Whitelaw A. Maternal methyldopa and neonatal blood pressure. *Br Med J.* 1981;283:471.
452. Le Grass MD, Seifert B, Casiro O. Neonatal nasal obstruction associated with methyldopa treatment during pregnancy [letter]. *Am J Dis Child.* 1990;144:143–144.
453. Plunkett GD. Neonatal complications. *Obstet Gynecol.* 1973;41: 476–477.
454. Cowett RM, Hakanson DO, Kocon RW, et al. Untoward neonatal effect of intraamniotic administration of methylene blue. *Obstet Gynecol.* 1976;48:74S–75S.
455. Kirsch IR, Cohen HJ. Heintz body hemolytic anemia from the use of methylene blue in neonates. *J Pediatr.* 1980;96:276–278.
456. Crooks J. Haemolytic jaundice in a neonate after intra-amniotic injection of methylene blue. *Arch Dis Child.* 1982;57:872–873.
457. McEnerney JK, McEnerney LN. Unfaorable neonatal outcome after intraamniotic injection of methylene blue. *Obstet Gynecol.* 1983;61:35S–36S.
458. Serota FT, Bernbaum JC, Schwartz E. The methylene-blue baby. *Lancet.* 1979;2:1142–1143.
459. Vincer MJ, Allen AC, Evans JR, et al. Methylene-blue-induced hemolytic anemia in a neonate. *Can Med Assoc J.* 1987;136:503–504.

460. Spahr RC, Salbburey DJ, Krissberg A, et al. intraamniotic injection of methylene blue leading to methemoglobinemia in one of twins. *Int J Gynaecol Obstet.* 1980;17:477–478.
461. Poinsot J, Guillois B, Margis D, et al. Neonatal hemolytic anemia after intraamniotic injection of methylene blue. *Arch Fr Pediatr.* 1988;45:657–660.
462. Fish WH, Chazen EM. Toxic effects of methylene blue on the fetus. *Am J Dis Child.* 1992;146:1412–1413.
463. Troche BI. The methylene-blue baby. *N Eng J Med.* 1989;320: 1756–1757.
464. Nicolini U, Monni G. Intestinal obstruction in babies exposed in utero to methylene blue. *Lancet.* 1990;336:1258–1259.
465. Van Der Pol JG, Wolf H, Boer K, et al. Jejunal atresia related to the use of methylene blue in genetic amniocentesis in twins. *Br J Obstet Gynaecol.* 1992;99:141–143.
466. Wong R, Paul RH. Methergine-induced uterine tetany treated with epinephreine: case report. *Am J Obstet Gynecol.* 1979;134:602–603.
467. Moise KJ Jr, Carpenter RJ Jr. Methylergonovine-induced hypertonus in term pregnancy: a case report. *J Reprod Med.* 1988;33: 771–773.
468. Braverman AC, Bromley BS, Rutherford JD. New onset ventricular tachycardia during pregnancy. *Int J Cardiol.* 1991;33:409–412.
469. Bland BAR, Lawes EG, Duncan PW, et al. Comparison of midazolam and thiopental for rapid sequence anesthetic induction for elective cesarean section. *Anesth Analg.* 1987;66:1165–1168.
470. Ravlo O, Carl P, Crawford ME, et al. A randomized comparison between midazolam and thiopental for elective cesarean section anesthesia: II. Neonates. *Anesth Analg.* 1989;68:234–237.
471. Kaler SG, Patrinos ME, Lambert GH, et al. Hypertrichosis and congenital anomalies associated with maternal use of minoxidil. *Pedaitrics.* 1987;79:434–436.
472. Rosa FW, Idanpaan-Heikkila J, Asanti R. Fetal minoxidil exposure. *Pedaitrics.* 1987;80:120.
473. Bond GR, Zee AV. Ovedosage of misoprostol in pregnancy. *Am J Obstet Gynecol.* 1994;171:561–562.
474. Gilbert G, Dixon AB. Observations on Demerol as an obstetric analgesic. *Am J Obstet Gynecol.* 1943;45:320–326.
475. Way WL, Costley EC, Way EL. Respiratory sensitivity of the newborn infant to meperidine and morphine. *Clin Pharmacol Ther.* 1965;6:454–461.
476. Fox RE, Marx C, Stark AR. Neonatal effects of maternal nadolol therapy. *Am J Obstet Gynecol.* 1985;152:1045–1046.
477. Feinstein SJ, Lodeiro JG, Vintzileos AM, et al. Sinusoidal fetal heart rate pattern after administration of nalbuphine hydrochloride: a case report. *Am J Obstet Gynecol.* 1986;154:159–160.
478. Miller RR. Evaluation of nalbuphine hydrochloride. *Am J Hosp Pharm.* 1980;37:942–949.
479. Guillonneau M, Jacqz-Aigrain E, De Grepy A, et al. Perinatal adverse effects of nalbuphine given during parturition. *Lancet.* 1990;335:1588.
480. Sgro C, Escousse A, Tennenbaum D, et al. Perinatal adverse effects of nalbuphine given during labour. *Lancet.* 1990;336:1070.
481. Wilson CM, McClean E, Moore J, et al. A double-blind comparison of intramuscular pethidine and nalbuphine in labour. *Anaesthesia.* 1986;41:1207–1213.
482. Frank M, McAteer EJ, Cattermole R, et al. Nalbuphine for obstetric analgesia. *Anaesthesia.* 1987;42:697–703.
483. Goodlin RC. Naloxone and its possible relationship to fetal endorphin levels and fetal distress. *Am J Obstet Gynecol.* 1981;139:16–19.
484. Wilkinson AR, Aynsley-Green A, Mitchell MD. Persistent pulmonary hypertension and abnormal prostaglandin E levels in preterm infants after maternal treatment with naproxen. *Arch Dis Child.* 1979;54:942–945.
485. Talati AJ, Salim MA, Korones SB. Persistent pulmonary hypertension after maternal naproxen ingestion in a term newborn: a case report. *Am J Perinatol.* 2000;17:69–71.
486. Gait JE. Hemolytic reactions to nitrofurantoin in patients with glucose-6-phosphate dehydrogenase deficiency: theory and practice. *DICP.* 1990;24:1210–1213.
487. Bruel H, Guillemant V, Saladin-Thiron C, et al. Hemolytic anemia in a newborn after maternal treatment with nitrofurantoin at the end of pregnancy. *Arch Pediatr.* 2000;7:745–747.
488. Cotton DB, Longmire S, Jones MM, et al. Cardiovascular alterations in severe pregnancy-induced hypertension: effects of intravenous nitroglycerin coupled with blood volume expansion. *Am J Obstet Gynecol.* 1986;154:1053–1059.
489. Longmire S, Leduc L, Jones MM, et al. The hemodynamic effects of intubation during nitroglycerin infusion in severe preeclampsia. *Am J Obstet Gynecol.* 1991;164:551–556.
490. Donchin Y, Amirav B, Sahar A, et al. Sodium nitroprusside for aneurysm surgery in pregnancy. *Br J Anaesth.* 1978;50:849–851.
491. Hagler S, Schultz A, Hankin H, et al. Fetal effects of steroid therapy during pregnancy. *Am J Dis Child.* 1963;106:586–590.
492. Jacobson BD. Hazards of norethindrone therapy during pregnancy. *Am J Obstet Gynecol.* 1962;84:962–968.
493. Wilson JG, Brent RL. Are female sex hormones teratogenic? *Am J Obstet Gynecol.* 1981;141:567–580.
494. Bongiovanni AM, McFadden AJ. Steroids during pregnancy and possible fetal consequences. *Fertil Steril.* 1960;11:181–184.
495. Shearer WT, Schreiner RL, Marshall RE. Urinary retention in a neonate secondary to maternal ingestion of nortriptyline. *J Pedaitr.* 1972;81:570–572.
496. McConell JB, Glasgow JF, McNair R. Effect on neonatal jaundice of oestogens and progesterons taken before and after conception. *Br Med J.* 1973;3:605–607.
497. Profuno R, Toce S, Kotagal S. Neonatal choreoathetosis following prenatal exposure to oral contraceptives [letter]. *Pediatrics.* 1990;86:648–649.
498. Baxi LV, Gindoff PR, Pregenzer GJ, et al. Fetal heart rate changes following maternal administration of a nasal decongestant. *Am J Obstet Gynecol.* 1985;153:799–800.
499. Pielet BW, Socol ML, MacGregor SN, et al. Fetal heart rate changes after fetal intravascular treatment with pancuronium bromide. *Am J Obstet Gynecol.* 1988;159:640–643.
500. Spencer JAD, Ronderos-Dumit D, Rodeck CH. The effect of neuromuscular blockade on human fetal heart rate and its variation. *Br J Obstet Gynaecol.* 1994;101:121–124.
501. Watson WJ, Atchinson SR, Harlass FE. Comparison of pancuronium and vecuronium for fetal neuromuscular blockade during invasive procedures. *J Matern Fetal Med.* 1996;5:151–154.
502. Tanaka M, Natori M, Ishimoto H, et al. Intravascular pancuronium bromide infusion for prenatal diagnosis of twin-twin transfusion syndrome. *Fetal Diagn Ther.* 1992;7:36–40.
503. Costei AM, Kozer E, Ho T, et al. Perinatal outcome following third trimester exposure to paroxetine. *Arch Pediatr Adolesc Med.* 2002;156:1129–1132.
504. Morag I, Batash D, Keidar R, et al. Paroxetine use throughout pregnancy: does it pose any risk to the neonate? *J Toxicol Clin Toxicol.* 2004;42:97–100.
505. Freedman H, Tafeen CH, Harris H. Parenteral Win 20,228 as analgesic in labor. *NY State J Med.* 1967;67:2849–2851.
506. Refstad SO, Lindbaek E. Ventilatory depression of the newborn of women receiving pethidine or pentazocine. *Br J Anaesth.* 1980;52:165–270.
507. Sadove M, Balagot R, Branion J Jr, et al. Report on the use of a new agent, phenazocine, in obstetric analgesia. *Obstet Gynecol.* 1960;16:448–453.
508. Corbit J, Fisrt S. Clinical comparison of phenazoxine and meperidine in obstetric analgesia. *Obstet Gynecol.* 1961;18:488–491.
509. Spiedel BD, Meadow SR. Maternal epilepsy and abnormalies of the fetus and the newborn. *Lancet.* 1972;2:839–843.
510. Bleyer WA, Skinner AL. Fatal neonatal hemorrhage after maternal anticonvulsant therapy. *JAMA.* 1976;235:826–827.

511. Lawrence A. Anti-epileptic drugs and the foetus. *Br Med J.* 1963;2:1267–1273.
512. Kohler HG. Haemorrhage in the newborn of epileptic mothers. *Lancet.* 1966;1:267.
513. Mountain KR, Hirsh J, Gallus AS. Neonatal coagulation defect due to anticonvulsant drug treatment in pregnancy. *Lancet.* 1970;1:265–268.
514. Evans AR, Forrester RM, Discombe C. Neonatal haemorrhage during anticonvulsant therapy. *Lancet.* 1970;1:517–518.
515. Margolin FG, Kantor NM. Hemorrhagic disease of the newborn. An unusual case related to maternal ingestion of an anti-epileptic drug. *Clin Pediatr (Phila).* 1972;11:59–60.
516. Srinivasan G, Seeler RA, Tiruvury A, et al. Maternal anticonvulsant therapy and hemorrhagic disease of the newborn. *Obstet Gynecol.* 1982;59:250–s252.
517. Payne NR, Hasegawa DK. Vitamin K deficiency in newborns: a case report in α-1-antitrypsin deficiency and a review of factors predisposing to hemorrhage. *Pediatrics.* 1984;73:712–716.
518. Lane PA, Hathaway WE. Vitamin K in infancy. *J Pediatr.* 1985;106:351–359.
519. Allen RW Jr, Ogden B, Bentley FL, et al. Fetal hydantoin syndrome, neuroblastoma, and hemorrhagic disease in a neonate. *JAMA.* 1980;244:1464–1465.
520. Douglas H. Haemorrhage in the newborn. *Lancet.* 1966;1:816–817.
521. Davis PP. Coagulation defect due to anticonvulsant drug treatment in pregnancy. *Lancet.* 1970;1:413.
522. Stevensom MM, Bilbert EF. Anticonvulsants and hemorrhagic diseases of the newborn infant. *J Pediatr.* 1970;77:516.
523. Truog WE, Feusner JH, Baker DL. Association of hemorrhagic disease and the syndrome of persistent fetal circulation with the fetal hydantoin syndrome. *J Pedaitr.* 1980;96:112–114.
524. Solomon GE, Hilgartner MW, Kutt H. Coagulation defects caused by diphenyhydantoin. *Neurology.* 1972;22:1165–1171.
525. Griffiths AD. Neonatal haemorrhage associated with maternal anticonvulsant therapy. *Lancet.* 1981;2:1296–1297.
526. Page TE, Hoyme HM, Markarian M, et al. Neonatal hemorrhage secondary to thrombocytopenia: an occasional effect of prenatal hydantoin exposure. *Birth Defects.* 1982;18:47–50.
527. Montan S, Ingemarsson I, Marsal K, et al. Randomized controlled trial of atenolol and pindolol in human pregnancy: effects on fetal haemodynamics. *Br Med J.* 1992;304:946–949
528. Chamberlain MJ, Reynolds AL, Yeoman WB. Toxic effects of podophyllum application in pregnancy. *Br Med J.* 1972;3:391–392.
529. Warrell DW, Taylor R. Outcome for the foetus of mothers receiving prednisolone during pregnancy. *Lancet.* 1968;1:117–118.
530. Rudd NL, Freedom RM. A possible primidone embryopathy. *J Pediatr.* 1979;94:835–837.
531. Thomas P, Buchanan N. Teratogenic effect of anticonvulsants. *J Pediatr.* 1981;99:163.
532. John E. Promazine and neonatal hyperbilirubinemia. *Med J Aust.* 1975;2:342–344.
533. Crawford JS, as quoted by Moya F, Thorndike V. The effects of drugs used in labor on the fetus and newborn. *Clin Pharmacol Ther.* 1963;4:628–653.
534. Corby DG, Shulman I. The effects of antenatal drug administration on aggregation of platelets of newborn infants. *J Pediatr.* 1971;79:307–313.
535. Whaun JM, Smith GR, Sochor VA. Effect of prenatal drug administration on maternal and neonatal platelet aggregation and PF_4 release. *Haemostasis.* 1980;9:226–237.
536. Celleno D, CapognaG, Tomassetti M, et al. Neurobehavioural effects of propofol on the neonate following elective caesarean section. *Br J Anaesth.* 1989;62:649–654.
537. Jackson GL. Treatment of hyperthyroidism in pregnancy. *Pa Med.* 1973;76:56–57.
538. Langer A, Hung CT, McA'Nulty JA, et al. Adrenergic blockade: a new approach to hyperthyroidism during pregnancy. *Obstet Gynecol.* 1974;44:181–186.
539. Bullock JL, Harris RE, Young R. Treatment of thyrotoxicosis during pregnancy with propranolol. *Am J Obstet Gynecol.* 1975;121:242–245.
540. Lightner ES, Allen HD, Aoughlin G. Neonatal hyperthyroidism and heart failure: a different approach. *Am J Dis Child.* 1977;131:68–70.
541. Habib A, McCarthy JS. Effects on the neonate of propranolol administered during pregnancy. *J Pediatr.* 1977;91:808–811.
542. Pruyn SC, Phelan JP, Buchanan GC. Long-term propranolol therapy in pregnancy: maternal and fetal outcome. *Am J Obstet Gynecol.* 1979;135:485–489.
543. Turner GM, Aukley CM, Dixon HG. Management of pregnancy complicated by hypertrophic obstructive cardiomyopathy. *Br Med J.* 1968;4:281–284.
544. Schroeder JS, Harrison DC. Repeated cardioversion during pregnancy. *Am J Cardiol.* 1971;27:445–446.
545. Levitan AA, Manion JC. Propranolol therapy during pregnancy and lactation. *Am J Cardiol.* 1973;32:247.
546. Reed RL, Cheney CB, Fearon RE, et al. Propranolol therapy throughout pregnancy: a case report. *Anesth Analg (Cleve).* 1974;53:214–218.
547. Fiddler GI. Propranolol in pregnancy. *Lancet.* 1974;2:722–723.
548. Bauer JH, Pape B, Zajicek J, et al. Propranolol in human plasma and breast milk. *Am J Cardiol.* 1979;43:860–862.
549. Teuscher A, Boss E, Imhof P, et al. Effect of propranolol on fetal tachydardia in diabetic pregnancy. *Am J Cardiol.* 1978;42:304–307.
550. Gladstone GR, Hordof A, Gersony WM. Proranolol administration during pregnancy: effects on the fetus. *J Pediatr.* 1975;86:962–964.
551. Tcherdakoff PH, Colliard M, Berrard E, et al. Propranolol in hypertension during pregnancy. *Br Med J.* 1978;2:670.
552. Eliahou HE, Silverberg DS, Reisin E, et al. Propranolol for the treatment of hypertension in pregnancy. *Br J Obstet Gynaecol.* 1978;85:431–436.
553. Bott-Kanner G, Schweitzer A, Schonfeld A, et al. Treatment with propranolol and hydralazine throughout pregnancy in a hypertensive patient: a case report. *Isr J Med Sci.* 1978;14:466–468.
554. Bott-Kanner G, Reisner SH, Rosenfeld JB. Propranolol and hydralazine in the management of essntial hypertension in pregnancy. *Br J Obstet Gynaecol.* 1980;87:110–114.
555. Taylor EA, Turner P. Anti-hypertensive therapy with propranolol during pregnancy and lactation. *Postgrad Med.* 1981;57:427–430.
556. O'Connor PC, Jick H, Hunter JR, et al. Propranolol and pregnancy outcome. *Lancet.* 1981;2:1168.
557. Caldroney RD. Beta-blockers in pregnancy. *N Eng J Med.* 1982;306:810.
558. Livingstone I, Craswell PW, Bevan EB, et al. Propranolol in pregnancy: three year prospective study. *Clin Exp Hypertens (B).* 1983;2:341–350.
559. Tunstall ME. The effect of propranolol on the onset of breathing at birth. *Br J Anaesth.* 1969;41:792–796.
560. Goodlin RC. Beta blocker in pregnancy-induced hypertension. *Am J Obstet Gynecol.* 1982;143:237–241.
561. Mitrani A, Oettinger M, Abinader EG, et al. Use of propranolol in dysfunctional labour. *Br J Obstet Gynaecol.* 1975;82:651–655.
562. Cheron RG, Kaplan MM, Larsen PR, et al. Neonatal thyroid function after propylthiouracil therapy for maternal Graves' disease. *N Eng J Med.* 1981;304:525–528.
563. Aaron HH, Schneierson SJ, Siegel E. Goiter in newborn infant due to mother's ingestion of propylthiouracil. *JAMA.* 1955;159:848–850.
564. Krementz ET, Hooper RG, Kempson RL. The effects on the rabbit fetus of the maternal administration of propylthiouracil. *Surgery.* 1957;41:619–631.
565. Branch LK, Tuthill SW. Goiters in twins resulting from propylthiouracil given during pregnancy. *Ann Int Med.* 1957;46:145–148.
566. Man EB, Shaver BA Jr, Cooke RE. Studies of children born to women with thyroid disease. *Am J Obstet Gynecol.* 1958;75:728–741.
567. Hayashida CY, Duarte AJS, Sato AE, et al. Neonatal hepatitis and lymphocyte sensitization by placental transfer of propythiouracil. *J Endocrinol Invest.* 1990;13:937–941.

568. Scriver CR. Vitamin B6 deficiency and dependency in man. *Am J Dis Child.* 1967;113:109–114.
569. Hunt AD Jr, Stokes J Jr, McCrory WW, et al. Pyridoxine dependency: report of a case of intractable convulsions in an infant controlled by pyridoxine. *Pediatrics.* 1954;13:140–145.
570. Bankier A, Turner M, Hopkins IJ. Pyridoxine dependent seizures—a wider clinical spectrum. *Arch Dis Child.* 1983;58:415–418.
571. Bejsovec MIR, Kulenda Z, Ponca E. Familial intrauterine convulsions in pyridoxine dependency. *Arch Dis Child.* 1967;42:201–207.
572. Domula VM, Weissach G, Lenk H. Uber die auswirkung medicamentoser Behandlung in der Schwangerschaft auf das Gerennungspotential des Neugeborenen. *Zentralbl Gynaekol.* 1977;99:473–479.
573. Nishimura H, Tanimura T. *Clinical Aspects of the Teratogenicity of Drugs.* New York, NY: American Elsevier, 1976:140–143.
574. Robinson GC, Brummitt JR, Miller JR. Hearing loss in infants and preschool children. II. Etiological considerations. *Pediatrics.* 1963;32:115–124.
575. West RA. Effect of quinine upon auditory nerve. *Am J Obstet Gynecol.* 1938;36:241–248.
576. McKinna AJ. Quinine induced hupoplasia of the optic nerve. *Can J Ophthalmol.* 1966;1:261–264.
577. Morgon A, Charachon D, Brinquier N. Disorders of the auditory apparatus caused by embryopathy or fetopathy: prophylaxis and treatment. *Acta Otolaryngol (Stockh).* 1971;291:(Suppl):5.
578. Mauer MA, DeVaux W, Lahey ME. Neonatal and maternal thrombocytopenic purpura due to quinine. *Pediatrics.* 1957;19:84–87.
579. Glass L, Rajegowda BK, Bowne E, et al. Exposure to quinine and jaundice in a glucose-6-phosphate dehydrogenase-deficient newborn infant. *Pediatrics.* 1973;82:734–735.
580. Budnick IS, Leikin S, Hoeck LE. Effect in the newborn infant to reserpine administration ante partum. *Am J Dis Child.* 1955;90:286–289.
581. Barden TP, Peter JB, Merkatz IR. Ritodrine hydrochloride: a betamimetic agent for use in preterm labor. I. Pharmacology, clinical history, administration, side effects, and safety. *Obstet Gynecol* 1980;56:1–6.
582. Anonymous. Ritodrine for inhibition of preterm labor. *Med Lett Drugs Ther.* 1980;22:89–90.
583. Finkelstein BW. Ritodrine (Yutopar, Merrell Dow Pharmaceuticals Inc.). *Drig Intell Clin Pharm.* 1981;15:425–433.
584. Brosset P, Ronayette D, Pierre MC, et al. Cardiac complications of ritodrine in mother and baby. *Lancet.* 1982;1:1468.
585. Hermansen MC, Johnson GL. Neonatal supraventricular tachycardia following prolonged maternal ritodrine administration. *Am J Obstet Gynecol.* 1984;149:798–799.
586. Beitzke A, Winter R, Zach M, et al. Kongenitales vorhofflattern mit hydrops fetalis durch mutterliche tokolytikamedikation. *Klin Paediatr.* 1979;191:410–417.
587. Nuchpuckdee P, Brodsky N, Porat R, et al. Ventricular septal thickness and cardiac function in neonates after in utero ritodrine exposure. *J Pediatr.* 1986;109:687–691.
588. Leake RD, Hobel CJ, Oh W, et al. A controlled, prospective study of the effects of ritodrine hydrochloride for premature labor (abstract). *Clin Res.* 1980;28:90A.
589. Kazzi NJ, Gross TL, Kazzi GM, et al. Neonatal complications following in utero exposure to intravenous ritodrine. *Acta Obstet Gynecol Scand.* 1987;66:65–69.
590. Schilthuis MS, Aarnoudse JG. Fetal death associated with severe ritodrine induced ketoacidosis. *Lancet.* 1980;1:1145.
591. Huisjes HJ, Touwen BCL. Neonatal outcome after treatment with ritodrine: a controlled study. *Am J Obstet Gynecol.* 1983;147:250–253.
592. Hansen NB, Oh W, LaRochelle F, et al. Effects of maternal ritodrine administration on neonatal renal function. *J Pediatr.* 1983;103:774–780.
593. Shenker L. Clinical experience with fetal heart rate monitoring of one thousand patients in labor. *Am J Obstet Gynecol.* 1973;115:1111–1116.
594. Boehm FH, Growdon JH Jr. The effects of scopolamine on fetal heart rate baseline variability. *Am J Obstet Gynecol.* 1974;120:1099–1104.
595. Ayromlooi J, Tobias M, Berg P. The effects of scopolamine and ancillary analgesics upon the fetal heart rate recording. *J Reprod Med.* 1980;25:323–326.
596. Evens RP, Leopold JC. Scopolamine toxicity in a newborn. *Pediatrics.* 1980;56:245–248.
597. O'Hare MF, Murnaghan GA, Russell CJ, et al. Sotalol as a hypotensive agent in pregnancy. *Br J Obstet Gynaecol.* 1980;87:814–820.
598. Leroux M. Existe-t-il une surdite congenitale acquise due a la streptomycine? *Ann Otolaryngol.* 1950;67:194–196.
599. Nishimura H, Tanimura T. *Clinical Aspects of the Teratogenicity of Drugs.* New York, NY: Excerpta Medica, 1976:130.
600. Donald PR, Sellars SL. Streptomycin ototoxicity in the unborn child. *S Afr Med J.* 1981;60:316–318.
601. Heckel GP. Chemotherapy during pregnancy. Danger of fetal injury from sulfanilamide and its derivatives. *JAMA.* 1941;117:1314–1316.
602. Ginzler AM, Cherner C. Toxic manifestations in the newborn infant following placental transmission of sulfanilamide. With a report of 2 cases simulating erythroblastosis fetalis. *Am J Obstet Gynecol.* 1942;44:46–55.
603. Lucey JF, Driscoll TJ Jr. Hazard to newborn infants of administration of long-acting sulfonamides to pregnant women. *Pediatrics.* 1959;24:498–499.
604. Kantor HI, Sutherland DA, Leonard JT, et al. Effect on bilirubin metabolism in the newborn of sulfisoxazole administration to the mother. *Obstet Gynecol.* 1961;17:494–500.
605. Dunn PM. The possible relationship between the maternal administration of sulphamethoxypyridazine and hyperbilirubinaemia in the newborn. *J Obstet Gynaecol Br Commonw.* 1964;71:128–131.
606. Perkins RP. Hydrops fetalis and stillbirth in a male glucose-6-phosphate dehydrogenase-deficient fetus possibly due to maternal ingestion of sulfisoxazole. *Am J Obstet Gynecol.* 1971;111:379–381.
607. Kramer W, Saade G, Belfort M, et al. Randomized double-blind study comparing sulindac to terbutaline: fetal cardiovascular effects (abstract). *Am J Obstet Gynecol.* 1996;174:326.
608. Rasanen J, Jouppila P. Fetal cardiac function and ductus arteriosus during indomethacin and sulindac therapy for threatened preterm labor: a randomized study. *Am J Obstet Gynecol.* 1995;173:20–25.
609. Jain A, Venkataramanan R, Lever J, et al. FK 506 and pregnancy in liver transplant patients. *Transplantation.* 1993;56:751.
610. Jain A, Venkataramanan R, Fung JJ, et al. Pregnancy after liver transplantation under tacrolimus. *Transplantation.* 1997;64:559–565.
611. Yoshimura N, Oka T, Fujiwara Y, et al. A case report of pregnancy in a renal transplant recipient treated with FK 506 (tacrolimus). *Transplantation.* 1996;61:1552–1553.
612. Resch B, Mache CJ, Windhager T, et al. FK 506 and successful pregnancy in a patient after renal transplantation. *Transplant Proc.* 1998;30:163–164.
613. Vyas S, Kumar A, Piecuch S, et al. outcome of twin pregnancy in a renal transplant recipient treated with tacrolimus. *Transplantation.* 1999;67:490–492.
614. Tewari K, Bonebrake RG, Asrat T, et al. Ambiguous genitalia in infant exposed to tamoxifen in utero. *Lancet.* 1997;350:183.
615. Pietrement C, Malot L, Santerne B, et al. Neonatal acute renal failure secondary to maternal exposure to telmisartan, angiotensin II receptor antagonist. *J Perinatol.* 2003;23:254–255.
616. Haller DL. The use of terbutaline for premature labor. *Drug Intell Clin Pharm.* 1980;14:757–764.
617. Andersson KE, Bengtsson LP, Gustafson I, et al. The relaxing effect of terbutaline on the human uterus during term labor. *Am J Obstet Gynecol.* 1975;121:602–609.
618. Ingermarsson I. Effect of terbutaline on premature labor. A double-blind placebo-controlled study. *Am J Obstet Gynecol.* 1976;125:520–524.

619. Ravindran R, Viegas OJ, Padilla LM, et al. Anesthetic considerations in pregnant patients receiving terbutaline therapy. *Anesth Analg (Cleve)* 1980;59:391–392.
620. Epstein MF, Nicholls RN, Stubblefield PG. Neonatal hypoglycemia after beta-sympathomimetic tocolytic therapy. *J Pediatr.* 1979;94:449–453.
621. Westgren M, Carlsson C, Lindholm T, et al. Continuous maternal glucose measurements and fetal glucose and insulin levels after administration of terbutaline in term labor. *Acta Obstet Gynecol Scand.* 1982;108(Suppl):63–65.
622. Fletcher SE, Fyfe DA, Case CL, et al. Myocardial necrosis in a newborn after long-term maternal subcutaneous terbutaline infusion for suppression of preterm labor. *Am J Obstet Gynecol.* 1991;165:1401–1404.
623. Thorkelsson T, Loughead JL. Long-term subcutaneous terbutaline tocolysis: report of possible neonatal toxicity. *J Perinatol.* 1991;11:235–238.
624. Reily WA. Hormone therapy during pregnancy: effects on the fetus and newborn. *Q Rev Pediatr.* 1958;13:198–202.
625. Cohlan SQ, Bevelander G, Bross S. Effect of tetracycline on bone growth in the ptremature infant. *Antimicrob Agents Chemother.* 1961;6:340–347.
626. Harcourt Jk, Johnson NW, Storey E. In vivo incorporation of tetracycline in the teeth of man. *Arch Oral Biol.* 1962;7:431–437.
627. Rendle-Short TJ. Tetracycline in teeth and bone. *Lancet.* 1962;1:1188.
628. Douglas AC. The deposition of tetracycline in human nails and teeth: a complication of long term treatment. *Br J Dis Chest.* 1963;57:44–47.
629. Kutscher AH, Zegarelli EV, Tovell HM, et al. Discoloration of teeth induced by tetracycline. *JAMA.* 1963;184:586–587.
630. Kline AH, Blattner RJ, Lunin M. Transplacental effect of tetracyclines on teeth. *JAMA.* 1964;188:178–180.
631. Macaulay JC, Lestyna JA. Preliminary observations on the prenatla administration of demethylchlortetracycline HCl. *Pediatrics.* 1964;34:423–424.
632. Stewart DJ. The effects of tetracyclines upon the dentition. *Br J Dermatol.* 1964;76:374–378.
633. Swallow JN. Discoloration of primary dentition after maternal tetracycline ingestion in pregnancy. *Lancet.* 1964;2:611–612.
634. Porter PJ, Sweeney EA, Golan H, et al. Controlled study of the effect of prenatal tetracycline on primary dentition. *Antimicrob Agents Chemother.* 1965;10:668–671.
635. Toaff R, Ravid R. Tetracyclines and the teeth. *Lancet.* 1966;2:281–281.
636. Kutscher AH, Zegarelli EV, Tovell HM, et al. Discoloration of deciduous teeth induced by administrations of tetracycline antepartum. *Am J Obstet Gynecol.* 1966;96:291–292.
637. Brearley LJ, Stragis AA, Storey E. Tetracycline-induced tooth changes. Part 1. Prevalence in preschool children. *Med J Austr.* 1968;2:653–658.
638. Brearley LJ, Storey E. Tetracycline-induced tooth changes. Part 2. Prevalence, localization and nature of staining in extracted deciduous teeth. *Med J Austr.* 1968;2:714–719.
639. Baker KL, Storey E. Tetracycline-induced tooth changes. Part 3. Incidence in extracted first permanent molar teeth. *Med J Austr.* 1970;1:109–113.
640. Anthony JR. Effect on deciduous and permanent teeth of tetracycline deposition in utero. *Postgrad Med.* 1970;48:165–168.
641. Genot MT, Golan HP, Porter PJ, et al. Effect of administration of tetracycline in pregnancy on the primary dentition of the offspring. *J Oral Med.* 1970;25:75–79.
642. Arwood LL, Dasta JF, Friedman C. Placental transfer of theophylline: two case reports. *Pediatrics.* 1979;63:844–846.
643. Yeh TF, Pildes RS. Transplacental aminophylline toxicity in a neonate. *Lancet.* 1977;1:910.
644. Labovitz E, Spector S. Placental theophylline transfer in pregnant asthmatics. *JAMA.* 1982;247:786–788.
645. O'Donnell R, Costigan C, O'Connell LG. Two cases of acute leukaemia in pregnancy. *Acta Haematol.* 1979;61:298–300.
646. Volkenandt M, Buchner T, Hiddemann W, et al. Acute leukaemia during pregnancy. *Lancet.* 1987;2:1521–1522.
647. Schiff D, Aranda J, Stern L. Neonatal thrombocytopenia and congenital malformation associated with administartion of tolbutamide to the mother. *J Pediatr.* 1970;77:457–458.
648. Nau H, Rating D, Koch S, et al. Valproic acid and its metabolites: placental transfer, neonatal pharmacokinetics, transfer via mother's milk and clinical status in neonates of epileptic mothers. *J Pharmacol Exp Ther.* 1981;219:768–777.
649. Bantz EW. Valproic acid and congenital malformations: a case report. *Clin Pediar.* 1984;23:353–354.
650. Legius E, Jaeken J, Eggermont E. Sodium valproate, pregnancy, and infantile fatal liver failure. *Lancet.* 1987;2:1518–1519.
651. Felding I, Rane A. Congenital liver damage after treatment of mother with valproic acid and phenytoin? *Acta Paediatr Scand.* 1984;73:656–658.
652. Majer RV, Green PJ. Neonatal afibrinogenaemia due to sodium valproate. *Lancet.* 1987;2:740–741.
653. Simila S, von Wendt L, Hartikainen-Sorri A-L, et al. Sodium valproate, pregnancy, and neonatal hyperglycinaemia. *Arch Dis Child.* 1979;54:985–986.
654. Jager-Roman E, Deichi A, Jakob S, et al. Fetal growth, major malformations, and minor anomalies in infants born to women receiving valproic acid. *J Pediatr.* 1986;108:997–1004.
655. Briggs GG, Nageotte MP. Fatal fetal outcome with the combined use of valsartan and atenolol. *Ann Pharmacother.* 2001;35:859–861.
656. Hill LM. Fetal distress secondary to vancomycin-induced maternal hypotension. *Am J Obstet Gynecol.* 1985;153:74–75.
657. Sperling RS, Stratton P, O'Sullivan MJ, et al. A survey of zidovudine use in pregnant women with human immunodeficiency virus infection. *N Eng J Med.* 1992;326:857–861.
658. Connor EM, Sperling RS, Gelber R, for the Pediatric AIDS Clinical Trials Group Protocol 076 Study Group. Reduction of maternal-infant transmission of human immunodeficiency virus type 1 with zidovudine treatment. *N Eng J Med.* 1994;331:1173–1180.
659. Watson WJ, Stevens TP, Weinberg GA. Profound anemia in a newborn infant of a mother receiving antiretroviral therapy. *Pediatr Infect Dis J.* 1998;17:435–436.

CHAPTER 9

POISONING IN PREGNANCY

Yaron Finkelstein

INTRODUCTION

Acute and chronic poisonings during pregnancy are an important health concern worldwide, with potential short- and long-term implications for both the mother and fetus. Approximately 8000 acute poisoning cases in pregnancy are reported annually in the United States alone.[1] Limited attention has been paid in the medical literature to this important issue, despite the fact that there are two patients at risk involved. Specifically, maternal and fetal outcome (e.g., miscarriage rate, incidence of birth defects, and neurobehavioral development) has not been systematically explored. Delay in the appropriate treatment of the pregnant woman may result in morbidity and mortality of both mother and fetus. Moreover, the fetal and maternal risks are not necessarily equal, and fetal mortality has been reported despite maternal recovery.[2]

Intoxications in pregnancy occur for a number of reasons. Deliberate self-poisoning is the most common method of suicide attempt in pregnancy, and may stem from a desire to terminate pregnancy. Recreational drug abuse is another type of toxic exposure. In addition, accidental or unintentional intoxications in pregnancy (e.g., in a woman unaware of her pregnancy at its initial stages) may occur.

Most poisonings during pregnancy are suicidal gestures. However, in one large series of hospitalized poisoned pregnant patients, 14% of the cases were accidental.[3] In this series of 162 patients, there were 2 maternal and 4 fetal deaths. This cohort consisted of relatively serious cases. The occurrence of only four fetal deaths, a 2.5% rate, would seem to indicate a relative resistance to an acute toxic insult. In a recent population-based study from Denmark, Flint et al.[4] reported on 122 self-poisoned pregnant women. Out of them, 44 had an elective abortion, 17 experienced miscarriage, and 61 exposed mainly to weak analgesics and psychotic drugs gave birth to 62 infants.

Extent of toxin exposure may be different on both sides of the placenta. Although most agents that are absorbed across the gastrointestinal epithelium freely traverse the placenta, some, such as iron, have a specialized transplacental absorptive mechanism. In a massive overdose situation, this mechanism may become a rate-limiting step, thus resulting in a relatively smaller fetal exposure. Conversely, some agents, such as salicylates, are present in higher concentrations in the fetus.[5] Fetal metabolic pathways are often immature, which in some cases (e.g., an acetaminophen overdose in early pregnancy) can protect the fetus from a toxic metabolite.

This chapter reviews the management of the poisoned pregnant woman. We discuss the general management of the overdosed pregnant mother and the risks and management options of the most common and relevant specific poisonings.

GENERAL MANAGEMENT OF THE POISONED PREGNANT PATIENT

At the time of first contact with a poisoned woman, the fact that she is pregnant may not be disclosed by her or may not even be known to her. Jones and colleagues [6] recommended that a pregnancy test should be performed in all women of reproductive age who present with poisoning or drug overdose.

The general approach to the pregnant patient who has taken an acute overdose should not differ from that of the nonpregnant individual. Management includes acute supportive care (airway, breathing, circulation, neurologic status assessment), history, physical examination, prevention of absorption, enhancement of elimination, and specific antidote therapy. Maternal support improves the ability of the fetus to survive a toxic insult. In addition, fetal well-being should be monitored.

However, some modifications may be necessary. For example, treatment of hypotension in the pregnant patient differs from that of the nonpregnant patient. The first step is to move the patient to a lateral decubitus position, and to move the fundus of the gravid uterus off of the inferior vena cava. This may increase central venous pressure, resulting in increased circulatory perfusion.[7] Emergent cesarean section may be necessary if monitoring indicates fetal compromise in the late stages of pregnancy.

Decontamination

Decontamination is tailored specifically for each patient and the specific exposure. Syrup of ipecac is specifically contraindicated in pregnancy, because of increased abdominal and thoracic pressure during protracted emesis. Gastric lavage and activated charcoal have the same indications and contraindication as in the nonpregnant patient. Since activated charcoal is not absorbed, adverse effects on the fetus are not expected. Because gastric motility is slowed in pregnancy, delayed administration of activated charcoal and whole bowel irrigation may still be beneficial.[7]

Enhanced Elimination

Multiple dose-activated charcoal is indicated for the same toxic overdoses as in the nonpregnant patient (e.g., theophylline and phenobarbital). Hemodialysis appears to be safe for the mother and fetus during pregnancy, and the use of chronic hemodialysis has been reported in pregnant patients.[8,9] Premature labor and intrauterine growth retardation in pregnant dialysis patients are usually associated with the underlying renal disease.

Antidotes

The risks to the fetus from the administration of most antidotes are unknown. These risks may manifest as teratogenicity or as an acute fetal toxicity. For example, the administration of a specific dose of atropine for organophosphate poisoning in a pregnant woman may not be similarly reflected in the fetus; the latter may be exposed to either a relative underdose or an overdose of this antidote.[10] Despite these fetal risks, the needs of the mother outweigh the potential fetal harm, and if an antidote is indicated, its administration should not be withheld in the pregnant woman. It is very unlikely that a single exposure to an antidote will have a teratogenic effect on the fetus (especially if beyond the first trimester). Tragic maternal and/or fetal deaths associated with withholding of an antidote because of fears of teratogenicity have been published following iron and organophosphate poisonings.[11,12]

PHARMACEUTICALS

Acetaminophen

The ability of acetaminophen to cross the human placenta is well-documented.[13] Thus, the potential for fetal risk due to significant drug exposure is real. As an agent readily available in most homes and the most common pharmaceutical agent taken by pregnant women, acetaminophen overdose is a frequently reported poisoning in pregnancy.[4,14]

The susceptibility of the fetus to toxicity due to acetaminophen overdose can be largely explained by the differences in adult and fetal drug metabolism, which are markedly different for acetaminophen. In adults, therapeutic doses of acetaminophen are largely excreted as urinary sulfates or glucuronides. A small amount is oxidized by the cytochrome P-450 system (specifically CYP 2E1). This produces a highly reactive metabolite (*N*-acetylbenzoaminoquinoneimine, NAPQI) that binds to the hepatocellular macromolecules, producing hepatotoxicity. This effect can be prevented by complex formation with hepatic glutathione. In an overdose situation, sulfation and glucuronidation become saturated, thus presenting an increased load to the cytochrome P-450 pathway. Hepatotoxicity occurs after glutathione has been depleted. Administration of *N*-acetylcysteine is protective through several mechanisms, mainly because it acts as a glutathione precursor.

Therefore, for hepatotoxicity to occur, the fetal hepatocyte must have an active cytochrome P-450 system. Also, absence or decreased capacity for sulfation, glucuronidation, and glutathione generation would increase the risk of fetal liver damage.

In vitro metabolic studies on human fetal cell lines have been central to describing the metabolic pathways that acetaminophen follows.[15,16] Studies in fetal hepatocytes have indicated that cytochrome P-450 activity was only 10% of adult values, but there were linear increases with advancing gestational age. Hence, the younger the fetus, the less amount of the reactive metabolite that would form in its hepatocytes. Glucuronidation was not observed, but glutathione generation and sulfation were noted. Thus, it appears that the degree of fetal risk from maternal acetaminophen ingestion correlates with gestational age. This has been supported by in vivo observations, in which fetal death following acetaminophen overdose occurred in third trimester gestations.[2,17] Embryonic CYP2E1 (the cytochrome P-450 isoenzyme responsible for acetaminophen metabolism) expression was further confirmed by the reverse transcriptase reaction with RNA from a 19-week gestational fetal liver used as template. Catalytic capabilities of human fetal microsomes were assessed by measurement of the rate of ethanol oxidation to acetaldehyde (also metabolized by CYP 2E1), which were 12–27% of those exhibited by adult liver microsomes, and it varied among xenobiotics and with gestational age.[15]

The earliest reported case of acetaminophen poisoning in pregnancy was published in 1978 and presented limited outcome data; however, it describes a mother with severe hepatotoxicity following an overdose in early pregnancy. She subsequently terminated the pregnancy, and there is no subsequent report of any postmortem examination of the abortus.[18]

Riggs et al.[2] conducted a multicenter study on acetaminophen overdose. Complete data were available in 60 of 113 cases. Of these, 19 women overdosed during the first trimester, 22 during the second trimester, and 19 during the third trimester of pregnancy. Of the 24 patients with acetaminophen levels above the nomogram line, 10 were treated with *N*-acetylcysteine within 10 hours postingestion; 8 delivered normal infants and 2 had elective abortions. Of 10 patients treated with *N*-acetylcysteine 10–16 hours postingestion, 5 delivered viable infants, 2 had elective abortions, and 3 had spontaneous abortions. Of four women treated with *N*-acetylcysteine 16–24 hours postingestion, one mother died, and there was one spontaneous abortion, one stillbirth, one elective abortion, and one delivery. Multiple logistic regression analysis demonstrated a significant correlation between the time to loading dose of *N*-acetylcysteine and pregnancy outcome, with an increase in the incidence of spontaneous abortion or fetal death when treatment began late. Significant maternal toxicity in the third trimester, which is correlated with maturation of the hepatic cytochrome P-450 system in the fetus is a marker for potential fetal demise.[19] Moreover, reports of fetal death prior to or during the development of maternal toxicity are published.[19,20] Use of acetaminophen during the first 20 weeks of pregnancy was not associated with an increased risk of miscarriage over nonuse in a recent population-based study of 1055 women. Use of products containing acetaminophen, such as Tylenol with Codeine was also included in the analysis.[21]

McElhatton et al. conducted a prospective study[22] on pregnancy outcome of 300 women with acetaminophen overdose. Exposure occurred in all trimesters. The majority of the pregnancies had normal outcomes. Over half of the mothers (160 = 53%) required treatment for the overdose, and 33 were treated with *N*-acetylcysteine. None of the mothers died. There were 219 liveborn infants with no malformations (including those born to mothers treated with *N*-acetylcysteine), 61 of whom had been exposed to acetaminophen in the first trimester. Eleven liveborn infants had malformations; none were exposed to acetaminophen in the first trimester. One other infant exposed at 18 weeks had a diaphragmatic hernia; this pregnancy was terminated at 22 weeks. In none of these 12 infants, can the malformations be associated with acetaminophen exposure. There was no obvious relationship between the time of exposure and the time of delivery.

Horowitz et al.[23] were the first to document placental transfer of *N*-acetylcysteine in humans. They studied four pregnant women with acetaminophen toxicity, who delivered their infants while receiving *N*-acetylcysteine. Maternal and cord blood were analyzed for the presence of *N*-acetylcysteine and aminotransferase activities, and autopsy findings on the nonviable infant were used to assess hepatic injury. *N*-Acetylcysteine was detected in the cord blood of three viable infants and in cardiac blood of a fourth. The mean *N*-acetylcysteine concentration in cord blood was 9.4 ± 1.3 µg/mL. This is well within the range associated with therapeutic doses of *N*-acetylcysteine typically administered to adults with acetaminophen poisoning. No adverse sequelae developed in the three viable infants. The fourth infant, delivered at 22 weeks gestational age died 3 hours after birth. All mothers recovered and none of the four infants had evidence of acetaminophen-related toxicity.

Treatment. The management of the pregnant woman with an acetaminophen overdose should not differ from that of the nonpregnant individual, and include supportive care, toxicity assessment using the Mathiew-Rumack monogram, appropriate gastrointestinal decontamination, and early *N*-acetylcysteine therapy (within 10–16 hours after ingestion). In any event, antidote therapy should not be withheld or delayed if the mother is at risk. Some researchers[24] advocate an immediate delivery of a mature fetus for direct *N*-acetylcysteine therapy in a significant third-trimester acetaminophen overdose.

Iron

Iron supplementation during pregnancy has become routine, making this agent readily accessible. Prenatal vitamins and iron have been documented as the second most common drug group overdosed during pregnancy.[14]

Major features of iron poisoning include gastrointestinal hemorrhage, shock, acidosis, hepatic failure, and coagulopathy. Maternal death is usually due to cardiovascular collapse or hepatic failure. The well-being of a fetus presents an additional challenge to the management of an already complex problem.

There are reports of newborns that did well and showed no signs of iron intoxication despite maternal death, that occurred shortly after their delivery.[11,25] A fetal death occurred as a miscarriage in a 17-year-old girl who was seriously ill and subsequently died of iron overdose. The abortus and the placenta were examined for evidence of iron toxicity and the presence of increased iron burden, but neither was found.[26] In the cases of iron poisonings, the available data seem to suggest that, similar to acetaminophen poisoning in early pregnancy, the fetal risks are outweighed by striking maternal risks.

The passage of iron across cellular membranes and its transport throughout the body involve complex processes. Under normal physiologic conditions, the plasma protein, transferrin, is required to move the oxidized (ferric) iron across membranes. Iron is believed to transfer across the human placenta, as it does across most biological membranes. As a result, it is only transferrin-bound iron that can cross. This transport is an active process, which occurs against the concentration gradient, and is facilitated by specific membrane proteins. In the placenta, this process may become saturated, which limits the rate of iron transported through the placenta, and serves as a protective barrier for the fetus. Thus, the main risk to the fetus is not from direct iron burden, but secondary to the pathophysiological alterations induced in the mother.

Deferoxamine is a potent iron chelator, capable of removing intracellular iron and iron from ferritin and hemosiderin. Once deferoxamine binds ferric iron, ferrioxamine complex is formed and the complex is eliminated in the urine.[27] Because deferoxamine is negligibly absorbed across the gastrointestinal tract and is a charged and relatively large molecule, it would not be expected to cross the placenta. In addition, chelation of other micronutrients would be less likely in a hyperferremic state and over a typical short period of chelation therapy. This is supported by several reports of first-trimester treatment with deferoxamine in pregnant thalassemic patients, all with no signs of deferoxamine toxicity and no birth malformations in the offspring.[28–30]

Review of the literature discloses over 40 cases in which deferoxamine was given in various periods of gestation to thalassemic patients without evidence of teratogenic effect. Singer et al.[30] concluded that sufficient documentation exists to suggest that deferoxamine can be considered for use in cases of pregnant women who need iron chelation therapy.

Tran et al.[27] conducted a systematic review of the English literature from 1966 to 1998 reporting on iron poisoning in pregnancy. Their objectives were to determine if peak maternal serum iron level or toxicity stage after intentional overdose is associated with adverse maternal-fetal outcome, and to describe the use of deferoxamine therapy in pregnant patients. Fourteen publications were identified, describing 61 cases of obstetric iron overdose. Compared with women who had lower peak levels, women with peak serum iron levels >400 μg/dL were more frequently symptomatic. Peak iron level >400 μg/dL was not associated with increased risk of spontaneous abortion, preterm delivery, congenital anomalies, or maternal death. However, patients with severe toxicity were more likely to spontaneously abort, deliver preterm babies, or experience maternal death. Only 57% of symptomatic patients were treated with deferoxamine. Of note, the three reported fatal ingestions were characterized by intentional withholding of chelation, delayed initiation of chelation, and chelation with EDTA.[27] No information was provided regarding birth malformations in the offspring of women treated with deferoxamine.

Treatment. Management principles should follow those of the nonpregnant patient.[31,32] Plasma peak iron concentrations drawn 2–6 hours postingestion may guide management decisions. Activated charcoal is of no use as it does not adsorb iron. Whole bowel irrigation may be effective if opacities are seen on an abdominal radiograph. The amount of radiation to the fetus from a single abdominal radiograph is negligible.[7] Deferoxamine is the specific antidote for iron overdose. The teratogenic risk of deferoxamine is overestimated. Moreover, as in all situations, maternal well-being takes precedence over fetal concerns. Withholding of deferoxamine therapy because of concern over teratogenicity or inappropriate use of EDTA resulted in the death of several pregnant women.[11,26,33] Thus, deferoxamine should not be withheld nor administration delayed in pregnant women when indicated.[27]

Salicylates

Salicylate poisoning is associated with significant morbidity and mortality.

Salicylate overdose during pregnancy is relatively common and presents challenging management decisions for the mother and her offspring. Because of major differences between the physiology of the fetus and its mother, and because of aspirin's perinatal pharmacokinetic profile, the risk for the fetus is predictably greater.[5] The increased sensitivity of the fetus relative to its mother is demonstrated by several reported intrauterine deaths following both acute and chronic ingestions.[5,34]

Salicylates freely cross the placenta and accumulate in the fetus.[35] Toxic effects of aspirin include uncoupling of oxidative phosphorylation, interference with acid-base homeostasis, neonatal salicylism, and bleeding diathesis in the newborn, including intracranial hemorrhages. A unique problem of neonatal salicylism is an increased risk of kernicterus due to competition of salicylate for bilirubin binding sites on albumin.[5] Toxic doses of aspirin also produce stimulation of the respiratory center of the medulla oblongata. This is of no concern for the fetus, since its lungs do not have a role in oxygenation.

The increased fetal sensitivity is due to a number of factors. The salicylate concentration is greater on the fetal side of the placenta by as much as 1.5:1. Fetal artery pH is lower than that of the mother. This results in a smaller intravascular to intracellular pH gradient, favoring penetration of this weak acid into the fetal brain. Fetal acidosis lags hours behind maternal acidosis. Therefore, fetal acidosis occurs after sustained maternal acidosis, and its correction would also lag behind normalization of the mother's acid-base status.[5]

Another contributing factor is that the fetus has a decreased capacity to metabolize and excrete this drug. Persistence of salicylate level in the newborn compared to its mother has been observed.[36,37]

Rejent and Baik[34] described a woman in the eighth month of pregnancy who ingested 36.5 g of aspirin. She was symptomatic, but the fetus was not felt to be in distress. However, 20 hours later, the fetus was dead. Postmortem fetal salicylate level was 243 mg/L, with a brain concentration of 200 μg/g.

The fetus in distress secondary to maternal salicylate poisoning is a unique clinical problem. The most likely etiology is fetal acidosis, and maternal hemodialysis or alkali therapy would not be of immediate benefit for the fetus. Therefore, consideration should be given to the expeditious delivery of the distressed fetus, if it is potentially viable.

Treatment. Treatment of salicylate poisoning in pregnancy does not significantly differ from that of the nonpregnant patient and includes stabilization, appropriate gastrointestinal decontamination, administration of fluids, electrolytes and glucose, urinary alkalinization, and when indicated, hemodialysis.

Bicarbonate transfer through the placenta is slow, and correction of metabolic acidosis in the fetus is delayed.[5] Thus, fetal monitoring should persist even when the mother's condition improves.[38]

In pregnancy, it is hoped that the positive effects of these maneuvers will be reflected transplacentally. However, several of the previously described fetal factors (higher serum concentrations, larger proportion of salicylate in the brain, lower buffering capacity, and decreased salicylate metabolism) would somewhat negate such benefits. Therefore, an earlier (at serum levels as low as 25 mg/dL) and more aggressive treatment should be practiced. When the fetus is potentially viable, ex utero consideration should be given to prompt delivery. This provides the opportunity for direct provision of care to the newborn.

Abortifacients

Pregnant women may have different reasons to induce a nonmedical abortion of an unanticipated or undesired pregnancy, including socioeconomical (e.g., unmarried, teen pregnancy), medical and psychiatric issues.

In a recent report[39] of four pregnant women who presented to an emergency department in New Orleans, all four reported limited access to health care due to lack of insurance and resources.

Historically, lead and quinine have been commonly used as chemical abortifacients.[7] The vast majority of modern literature on the use of illegal or nonmedical abortifacients is sparse and focuses on international experiences, where the use of traditional remedies for abortion by native populations is described. Interestingly, in many countries, potent pharmacologically active agents that can serve as abortifacients are sold over the counter without need for prescription.

Presently, over-the-counter preparations such as acetaminophen, aspirin, and iron, as well as potent pharmaceutical agents, such as misoprostol[40,41] and methotrexate[42], are more commonly reported for nonmedical abortion induction. Herbal preparations (e.g., Angelica root, Poison hemlock, Windflower) are also used to terminate pregnancy, and may induce severe toxidromes.[39]

The greatest dangers of abortifacients are the effects of the toxin on the mother, their potential teratogenic effect, and the complications from delaying a physician-assisted abortion. Most attempts to chemically abort a fetus are made in the first trimester. Acetaminophen and multidrug ingestion are the most common exposures, with minor maternal toxicity reported in most cases.[43]

Austin et al.[40] reported on a 25-year-old gravid female who self-administered 6000 μg misoprostol intravaginally and 600 μg orally. She rapidly developed abdominal and extremity cramping, emesis, and confusion. Hyperthermia (41.4°C) and hypotension developed within 4 hours, and no fetal movement or heart function were noted by ultrasound. A nonviable fetus was delivered by emergent cesarean section. Treatment of the mother was supportive and included intravaginal decontamination and mechanical ventilation with paralytic agents to control hyperthermia and agitation. Recovery was complete within 15 hours of drug administration.

As a result of the serious nature of an abortion attempt and the nonspecific clinical manifestations of the ingestion, a high index of suspicion is required. Therefore, every female overdosed patient of child-bearing age should have a pregnancy test. In addition, women who present with significant vaginal bleeding should be historically screened for possible abortifacient use. In fact, this is uncommonly done. Perrone et al.[43] recommended through their poison information center consultation service, to perform pregnancy tests to all female patients aged 12–30 who presented to a health-care facility in Philadelphia over a 5-month period. Pregnancy tests were obtained for only 32% (371/1142) of eligible patients. Forty three (12%) of them were pregnant. Five of the 43 pregnant patients ingested known abortifacients.

Alfaro et al.[42] reported on two female pregnant patients, aged 15 and 24 years old, who presented with mucositis, erythrodermia, pancytopenia, and elevated liver enzymes, typical of acute methotrexate overdose. Plasma methotrexate levels confirmed the clinical diagnosis, and both patients were treated with high leucovorin doses. In one patient, pregnancy continued, giving birth to a newborn with cranial, facial, and limb malformations. The second patient had a late rescue with leucovorin and was discharged with a persistent sensory motor neuropathy.

In conclusion, the use of abortifacients in self-poisoned pregnant women is not an infrequent finding. A pregnancy test should be obtained for all female patients of childbearing age presenting with an intentional overdose.[6]

CHEMICALS AND ENVIRONMENTAL TOXINS

Lead

Lead serves no useful purpose in the body. It produces chronic rather than acute toxicity, and most individuals with increased body burdens are asymptomatic. In October 2005, the American Academy of Pediatrics published a policy statement[44] on lead poisoning in children. Exposure to lead during infancy can result in adverse neurodevelopmental sequelae, and it is speculated that the developing fetal nervous system may have an increased sensitivity. The neurodevelopmental effects of lead exposure are under ongoing investigation. Over the last 25 years, the blood level thought to be associated with toxicity has dropped dramatically, from 60 μg/dL in 1960 to 10 μg/dL today. In fact, a threshold value below which lead has no apparent adverse developmental effects has not been identified.[45] Recent evidence suggests that postnatal blood lead levels <10 μg/dL are associated with enduring adverse neurodevelopment.[46,47] Whether this is true, as well, for prenatal lead levels <10 μg/dL, is unknown.

Lead freely crosses the placenta and the blood lead concentration of the infant is similar or even higher than that of the mother.[48,49] Consequently, gestational lead poisoning is not only harmful to the woman but also to the developing fetus, invariably producing congenital lead poisoning.

Lead accumulates and is stored in bone for decades, and these bone lead stores may pose a threat to women of reproductive age long after their exposure to lead has ended. The source of lead in the infant's blood seems to be a mixture of approximately two-thirds dietary and one-third skeletal lead.[44,50] Others suggest that skeletal lead stores are the dominant contributor to blood lead levels during pregnancy and the postpartum period.[51] Maternal lead exposure as low as 5–9 μg/dL might be associated with a doubling of the risk of miscarriage.[52]

In a Norwegian study, neither maternal nor paternal lead exposure were associated with an increased risk of "serious birth defects."[53]

Gonzalez-Cossio et al.[54] suggested that maternal lead exposure during pregnancy is inversely related to fetal growth, as reflected in duration of pregnancy and infant size.

Sowers et al.[55] correlated blood lead concentrations with Apgar scores, birth weight, gestational age, small-for-gestational age status, and hypertension in pregnancy or toxemia. Data and blood were collected four times during pregnancy from 705 women, aged 12–34. Blood lead concentrations were correlated with pregnancy outcomes. Average blood lead concentrations were 1.2 ± 0.03 μg/dL. Maternal blood lead concentrations were significantly associated with hypertension in pregnancy/toxemia, but were not associated with other pregnancy outcomes.

Shannon et al.[49] have recently characterized the scope and consequences of severe lead poisoning (blood lead level >45 μg/dL) in 15 pregnant women. Among them, 70% were from Hispanic origin, all of whom developed lead poisoning from the ingestion of soil, clay, or pottery. Other sources of lead poisoning were paint chip ingestion, household renovation, and use of an alternative medicine (bone meal). Lead poisoning was discovered in the first trimester in 12 (86%) subjects after they presented with subtle but characteristic findings including malaise, anemia, basophilic stippling on blood smear; one woman was identified when she presented after a generalized seizure with a blood lead level of 104 μg/dL. Five women received chelation therapy during pregnancy with EDTA, dimercaprol, or succimer. At delivery mean maternal blood lead level was 55 μg/dL, whereas mean neonatal lead level was 74 μg/dL. Thirteen neonates underwent chelation, all within the first month of life. No infant had a birth defect. The authors concluded that severe lead poisoning in pregnancy most often occurs because of intentional pica, its presenting symptoms are subtle, and blood lead levels in the neonate are higher than simultaneous maternal lead levels. In another case of EDTA therapy during pregnancy[56], the mother's blood lead level declined from 86 μg/dL to 26 μg/dL, but the cord blood concentration remained elevated at 79 μg/dL.

Treatment. It is unlikely that EDTA is transferred through the placenta in significant amounts. Dimercaprol penetrates the central nervous system making fetal penetration more likely. However, its use in adults is seldom indicated. Since dimercaprol must be given intramuscularly and is associated with several adverse effects, it is a poor candidate for maternal administration for fetal benefit. Few reports on the use of succimer, an orally administered chelator, in pregnancy have been disappointing. Mirkin et al.[57] reported on a 19 days' course of succimer to a woman in the 25th week of pregnancy. Maternal blood lead levels remained unchanged (44 μg/dL before and after chelation). The authors suggested that the ongoing mobilization of maternal blood lead continued or that an unrecognized exposure may have affected succimer's efficacy. Succimer failed to reduce blood lead burden in a preterm infant, whose mother had chronic lead exposure.[58]

Even with a chelator exhibiting good fetal penetration, transplacental chelation would be difficult. Although chelators efficiently clear the blood, this compartment is refilled from tissue stores (mostly bones) during the first few days after administration. Thus, prolonged courses are required. This practice may deny the fetus from getting essential trace elements. Thus, maternal indications would seem to be the only valid reason for the administration of lead chelators during pregnancy.

Organophosphates

Organophosphate agents are used as insecticides and pesticides, and their widespread use poses a potential health hazard. Organophosphates inhibit acetylcholine esterase and cause cholinergic symptoms, ranging in muscarinic, nicotinic, and central properties determined by different compounds.

Despite the widespread use of pesticides and the extensive body of knowledge regarding their toxicity, little is known about adverse effects in utero following exposure of pregnant women to organophosphates.[12] Organophosphates cross the placental barrier in animal models as well as in humans.[59]

Extensive research has been conducted regarding chlorpyrifos, a common ingredient in pesticides, which was reported not to be teratogenic.[60] At high dose, exposure of pregnant mice caused the birth of smaller offspring with an increased incidence of skeletal abnormalities.[61] Chlorpyrifos may be detected in human milk, sperm fluid, and cervical mucous.[62]

In 1993 it was claimed to cause neurological abnormalities following in utero exposure in humans. A family had two babies with similar neurologic problems including cerebral palsy, cataracts, and seizures. It was learned that the parents used a chlorpyrifos-containing pesticide to protect their first baby from Lyme disease.[63]

Weis et al.[10] reported on a 21-year-old female in her 34th week of pregnancy who never admitted to ingesting an organophosphate but had the rapid onset of severe cholinergic syndrome, absence of plasma and erythrocyte cholinesterase activity, and a dramatic response to large doses of atropine, which preclude any other diagnosis. The stress of spontaneous onset of labor early on, along with the atropine therapy, resulted in a fetal heart rate of 200 beats/min. An emergency cesarean section was done resulting in the delivery of a small floppy depressed neonate. As in the mother, assisted ventilation and atropine infusion were required. Curiously, the mother seemed to have been severely affected since she had a long requirement for assisted ventilation and atropine, her cholinesterase levels took longer to return to normal, and her therapeutic atropine dose was a toxic dose for the fetus in utero.

Sarin is an organophosphate with anticholinergic activity. The Tokyo subway Sarin gas attack in 1996 involved about 640 victims, 5 of whom were reported to be pregnant (8–36 weeks of gestation).[64] The clinical effect of the Sarin gas was mild in all pregnant women. Their plasma pseudocholinesterase levels ranged between 70–126 IU/L, and no hypoxic episodes occurred. Therefore, the clinical team decided not to treat them with pralidoxime, since data about its safety in pregnancy are lacking. No fetal malformations were reported in a follow-up of this small group.

Limited data are available on the use of pralidoxime in treating pregnant women with organophosphate poisoning. Presently, eight cases of cholinesterase reactivating agent therapy in pregnant women were published.

In the first case, a woman in her third month of pregnancy was treated with obidoxime, and analog of pralidoxime. This patient opted for a therapeutic abortion. The findings in the abortus are not known.[65]

A second woman, 16 weeks pregnant, and the third, 36 weeks pregnant, were successfully treated with atropine, pralidoxime, and respiratory support, both delivered normal-term infants.[66]

Another case involved a 42-year-old pregnant woman (26 weeks of gestation) who presented with dizziness, blurred vision, and repeated vomiting following the use of an undiluted insecticide as a cleaning liquid. After clinical and laboratory confirmation for organophosphates poisoning (plasma pseudocholinesterase levels of 161 U/I), treatment with atropine and pralidoxime was started. She recovered within 7 days and delivered a healthy baby 12 weeks later. The child showed no signs or symptoms of organophosphate, atropine, or pralidoxime exposure.[67]

Recently, Sebe et al.[12] reported on a suicide attempt of a 23-year-old pregnant woman (19 weeks of gestation), who ingested an extensive amount of chlorpyrifos ethyl insecticide. She could not feel her baby's movement 2 hours after ingestion of the substance, and was diagnosed with in utero death of the fetus by ultrasonography. Autopsy findings of the fetus include normal macroscopic anatomy. Fetal blood samples revealed the presence of high levels of 264 ppb chlorpyrifos. The mother had suppressed serum pseudocholinesterase levels but did not develop severe cholinergic toxicity and was successfully treated with atropine and pralidoxime. The authors concluded that delayed treatment of the mother may be responsible for the fetal death. Sebe et al.[12] also reported of their experience with three other organophosphate poisoning (specific agents unknown) cases during pregnancy (one at 20th week of gestation and two patients near term). All three women were treated with atropine and pralidoxime immediately following admission and all had good outcome with normal babies born. An "Intermediate Syndrome" may occur following organophosphate poisoning. It may arise 48–96 hours after the cholinergic crisis and it is characterized by respiratory paresis with difficulties of weaning from the assisted respiratory, deficit of proximal limbs, neck flexors, and cranial nerves. This syndrome coincides with the prolonged inhibition of the acetylcholinesterase, and is not due to the necrosis of muscular fiber's necrosis. Both clinical and electromyographic features are explained by a combined pre- and postsynaptic dysfunction of the neuromuscular transmission.[68] It may develop despite pralidoxime therapy.[69] The occurrence of this rare syndrome along with its required therapeutic interventions represents a more serious risk to pregnancy and delivery.

Another concern is the possibility of differences in the sensitivity to organophosphates by maternal and fetal cholinesterase systems. Decreased activity of neonatal plasma and red cell cholinesterase ranging from 50% to 70% of adult values have been consistently documented.[70,71] Therefore, increased fetal sensitivity to cholinesterase-inhibiting pesticides would be expected. These issues of relative placental passage and potentially differing fetal and maternal sensitivities are important because the chief antidote atropine has potent agonistic properties. Therefore, there is the potential for a therapeutic maternal atropine dose being either subtherapeutic or toxic for the fetus.

Treatment. Most authors agree that the basic management of a pregnant woman with organophosphate poisoning should not differ from that for the nonpregnant patient, including appropriate supportive and respiratory care, gastrointestinal decontamination, and the administration of antidotes.[72] Data regarding the use of pralidoxime in pregnancy are scant, although reassuring. All reported live offspring postmaternal pralidoxime therapy during pregnancy had normal outcome.[12,66,67]

EPILOGUE

An overdose during pregnancy may be harmful for the fetus as well as the mother, but the timing is critical for many outcomes. Epidemiological studies on overdosed pregnant women reported a substantial increase in the risk of miscarriage, but no effect on the prevalence of congenital malformations, prematurity, or birth weight among fetuses surviving till birth.[4,22,73] However, the total number of cases examined is too low for drawing conclusions on individual drugs[4], and more data are needed to offer evidence-based counseling for the pregnant overdosed patient.

***PregTox* Network** at The Hospital for Sick Children, Toronto, Canada, is a unique clinical and research program, developed and launched on the twentieth anniversary of the Motherisk program. Its aim is to promote evidence-based practice on the risk, management, and outcome of poisoned pregnant women and their offspring.

The goals of ***PregTox*** are

- To provide authoritative, evidence-based information and to assist health-care professionals in treating poisoned pregnant women and their fetuses
- A commitment to collect and publish the data gathered regarding poisonings in pregnancy

There is an urgent need for prospective multi-center studies to investigate pregnancy outcome following acute poisoning in pregnancy. ***PregTox* Network** is a unique service in an attempt to fill this gap.

If you are interested in hearing more or have cases of poisoning in pregnancy that you would like to discuss or submit to this new collaboration, the ***PregTox*** team encourages you to contact us.

Please log on to *www.motherisk.org* and click on the ***PregTox*** icon or

Directly email to yfinkel@yahoo.com

Or call 1-800- 670-6126; Fax 1-416-813-7562

REFERENCES

1. Watson WA, Litovitz TL, Klein-Schwartz W, et al. 2003 annual report of the American Association of Poison Control Centers Toxic Exposure Surveillance System. *Am J Emerg Med.* 2004;22:335–404.
2. Riggs BS, Bronstein AC, Kulig K, et al. Acute acetaminophen overdose during pregnancy. *Obstet Gynecol.* 1989;74:247–253.
3. Czeizel A, Szentesi I, Szekeres I, et al. Pregnancy outcome and health conditions of offspring of self-poisoned pregnant women. *Acta Paediatr Hung.* 1984;25:209–236.
4. Flint C, Larsen H, Nielsen GL, et al. Pregnancy outcome after suicide attempt by drug use: a Danish population-based study. *Acta Obstet Gynecol Scand.* 2002;81:516–522.
5. Palatnick W, Tenenbein M. Aspirin poisoning during pregnancy: increased fetal sensitivity. *Am J Perinatol.* 1998;15:39–41.
6. Jones JS, Dickson K, Carlson S. Unrecognized pregnancy in the overdosed or poisoned patient. *Am J Emerg Med.* 1997;15: 538–541.

7. Cumpston KL, Erickson TB. Maternal-Fetal Toxicology. In: Erickson TB, Ahrens WR, Aks SE, Baum. C.R., Ling LJ, eds. *Pediatric Toxicology. Diagnosis and Management of the Poisoned Child.* New York: McGraw-Hill, Medical Pub. Division; 2005:15–25.
8. Kazancioglu R, Sahin S, Has R, et al. The outcome of pregnancy among patients receiving hemodialysis treatment. *Clin Nephrol.* 2003;59:379–382.
9. Eroglu D, Lembet A, Ozdemir FN, et al. Pregnancy during hemodialysis: perinatal outcome in our cases. *Transplant Proc.* 2004;36:53–55.
10. Weis OF, Muller FO, Lyell H, et al. Materno-fetal cholinesterase inhibitor poisoning. *Anesth Analg.* 1983;62:233–235.
11. Olenmark M, Biber B, Dottori O, et al. Fatal iron intoxication in late pregnancy. *J Toxicol Clin Toxicol.* 1987;25:347–359.
12. Sebe A, Satar S, Alpay R, et al. Organophosphate poisoning associated with fetal death: a case study. *Mt Sinai J Med.* 2005;72:354–356.
13. Weigand UW, Chou RC, Maulik D, et al. Assessment of biotransformation during transfer of propoxyphene and acetaminophen across the isolated perfused human placenta. *Pediatr Pharmacol (New York).* 1984;4:145–153.
14. Rayburn W, Aronow R, DeLancey B, et al. Drug overdose during pregnancy: an overview from a metropolitan poison control center. *Obstet Gynecol.* 1984;64:611–614.
15. Carpenter SP, Lasker JM, Raucy JL. Expression, induction, and catalytic activity of the ethanol-inducible cytochrome P450 (CYP2E1) in human fetal liver and hepatocytes. *Mol Pharmacol.* 1996;49:260–268.
16. Johnsrud EK, Koukouritaki SB, Divakaran K, et al. Human hepatic CYP2E1 expression during development. *J Pharmacol Exp Ther.* 2003;307:402–407.
17. Haibach H, Akhter JE, Muscato MS, et al. Acetaminophen overdose with fetal demise. *Am J Clin Pathol.* 1984;82:240–242.
18. Silverman JJ, Carithers RL, Jr. Acetaminophen overdose. *Am J Psychiatry.* 1978;135:114–115.
19. Wang PH, Yang MJ, Lee WL, et al. Acetaminophen poisoning in late pregnancy: a case report. *J Reprod Med.* 1997;42:367–371.
20. Roberts I, Robinson MJ, Mughal MZ, et al. Paracetamol metabolites in the neonate following maternal overdose. *Br J Clin Pharmacol.* 1984;18:201–206.
21. Li DK, Liu L, Odouli R. Exposure to non-steroidal anti-inflammatory drugs during pregnancy and risk of miscarriage: population based cohort study. *BMJ.* 2003;327:368.
22. McElhatton PR, Sullivan FM, Volans GN. Paracetamol overdose in pregnancy analysis of the outcomes of 300 cases referred to the Teratology Information Service. *Reprod Toxicol.* 1997;11:85–94.
23. Horowitz RS, Dart RC, Jarvie DR, et al. Placental transfer of N-acetylcysteine following human maternal acetaminophen toxicity. *J Toxicol Clin Toxicol.* 1997;35:447–451.
24. Selden BS, Curry SC, Clark RF, et al. Transplacental transport of N-acetylcysteine in an ovine model. *Ann Emerg Med.* 1991;20:1069–1072.
25. Richards R, Brooks SE. Ferrous sulphate poisoning in pregnancy (with afibrinogenaemia as a complication). *West Indian Med J.* 1966;15:134–140.
26. Strom RL, Schiller P, Seeds AE, et al. Fatal iron poisoning in a pregnant female. *Minn Med.* 1976;59:483–489.
27. Tran T, Wax JR, Philput C, et al. Intentional iron overdose in pregnancy—management and outcome. *J Emerg Med.* 2000;18:225–228.
28. Thomas RM, Skalicka AE. Successful pregnancy in transfusion-dependent thalassemia. *Arch Dis Child.* 1980;55:572–574.
29. Martin K. Successful pregnancy in beta-thalassemia major. *Aust Paediatr J.* 1983;19:182–183.
30. Singer ST, Vichinsky EP. Deferoxamine treatment during pregnancy: is it harmful? *Am J Hematol.* 1999;60:24–26.
31. Banner W, Jr, Tong TG. Iron poisoning. *Pediatr Clin North Am.* 1986;33:393–409.
32. Proudfoot AT, Simpson D, Dyson EH. Management of acute iron poisoning. *Med Toxicol.* 1986;1:83–100.
33. Manoguerra AS. Iron poisoning: report of a fatal case in an adult. *Am J Hosp Pharm.* 1976;33:1088–1090.
34. Rejent TA, Baik S. Fatal in utero salicylism. *J Forensic Sci.* 1985;30:942–944.
35. Corby DG. Aspirin in pregnancy: maternal and fetal effects. *Pediatrics.* 1978;62:930–937.
36. Earle R Jr. Congenital salicylate intoxication—report of a case. *Nord Hyg Tidskr.* 1961;265:1003–1004.
37. Lynd PA, Andreasen AC, Wyatt RJ. Intrauterine salicylate intoxication in a newborn: a case report. *Clin Pediatr (Phila).* 1976;15:912–913.
38. Bentur Y. Acute poisoning in pregnancy. *Harefuah.* 2001;140:770–775.
39. Netland KE, Martinez J. Abortifacients: toxidromes, ancient to modern—a case series and review of the literature. *Acad Emerg Med.* 2000;7:824–829.
40. Austin J, Ford MD, Rouse A, et al. Acute intravaginal misoprostol toxicity with fetal demise. *J Emerg Med.* 1997;15:61–64.
41. Bentov Y, Sheiner E, Katz M. Misoprostol overdose during the first trimester of pregnancy. *Eur J Obstet Gynecol Reprod Biol.* 2004;115:108–109.
42. Alfaro J, Von Muhlenbrock R, Burgos N, et al. Acute poisoning with methotrexate used as an abortifacient: description of 2 cases. *Rev Med Chil.* 2000;128:315–318.
43. Perrone J, Hoffman RS. Toxic ingestions in pregnancy: abortifacient use in a case series of pregnant overdose patients. *Acad Emerg Med.* 1997;4:206–209.
44. Committee on Environmental Health. Lead exposure in children: prevention, detection, and management. *Pediatrics.* 2005;116:1036–1046.
45. Bellinger DC. Lead. *Pediatrics.* 2004;113:1016–1022.
46. Lanphear BP, Dietrich K, Auinger P, et al. Cognitive deficits associated with blood lead concentrations <10 microg/dL in US children and adolescents. *Public Health Rep.* 2000;115:521–529.
47. Bellinger DC, Needleman HL. Intellectual impairment and blood lead levels. *N Engl J Med.* 2003;349:500–502.
48. Graziano JH, Popovac D, Factor-Litvak P, et al. Determinants of elevated blood lead during pregnancy in a population surrounding a lead smelter in Kosovo, Yugoslavia. *Environ Health Perspect.* 1990;89:95–100.
49. Shannon M. Severe lead poisoning in pregnancy. *Ambul Pediatr.* 2003;3:37–39.
50. Gulson BL, Mizon KJ, Korsch MJ, et al. Mobilization of lead from human bone tissue during pregnancy and lactation—a summary of long-term research. *Sci Total Environ.* 2003;303:79–104.
51. Gulson BL, Pounds JG, Mushak P, et al. Estimation of cumulative lead releases (lead flux) from the maternal skeleton during pregnancy and lactation. *J Lab Clin Med.* 1999;134:631–640.
52. Borja-Aburto VH, Hertz-Picciotto I, Rojas LM, et al. Blood lead levels measured prospectively and risk of spontaneous abortion. *Am J Epidemiol.* 1999;150:590–597.
53. Irgens A, Kruger K, Skorve AH, et al. Reproductive outcome in offspring of parents occupationally exposed to lead in Norway. *Am J Ind Med.* 1998;34:431–437.
54. Gonzalez-Cossio T, Peterson KE, Sanin LH, et al. Decrease in birth weight in relation to maternal bone-lead burden. *Pediatrics.* 1997;100:856–862.
55. Sowers M, Jannausch M, Scholl T, et al. Blood lead concentrations and pregnancy outcomes. *Arch Environ Health.* 2002;57:489–495.
56. Timpo AE, Amin JS, Casalino MB, et al. Congenital lead intoxication. *J Pediatr.* 1979;94:765–767.
57. Horowitz BZ, Mirkin DB. Lead poisoning and chelation in a mother-neonate pair. *J Toxicol Clin Toxicol.* 2001;39:727–731.
58. Tait PA, Vora A, James S, et al. Severe congenital lead poisoning in a preterm infant due to a herbal remedy. *Med J Aust.* 2002;19;177:193–195.
59. Tsoukali-Papadopoulou H, Njau S. Mother-fetus postmortem toxicologic analysis in a fatal overdose with mecarbam. *Forensic Sci Int.* 1987;35:249–252.
60. Gibson JE, Peterson RK, Shurdut BA. Human exposure and risk from indoor use of chlorpyrifos. *Environ Health Perspect.* 1998;106:303–306.
61. Deacon MM, Murray JS, Pilny MK, et al. Embryotoxicity and fetotoxicity of orally administered chlorpyrifos in mice. *Toxicol Appl Pharmacol.* 1980;54:31–40.

62. Wagner U, Schlebusch H, Diedrich K, et al. Accumulation of pollutants in the genital tract of sterility patients. *J Clin Chem Clin Biochem.* 1990;28:683–688.
63. Clavin T. Danger on your doorstep; the pesticide risks parents don't know about. *McCall's.* 1993;95–96.
64. Okumura T. Organophosphate poisoning in pregnancy. *Ann Emerg Med.* 1997;29:299–300.
65. Gadoth N, Fisher A. Late onset of neuromuscular block in organophosphorus poisoning. *Ann Intern Med.* 1978;88:654–655.
66. Karalliedde L, Senanayake N, Ariaratnam A. Acute organophosphorus insecticide poisoning during pregnancy. *Hum Toxicol.* 1988;7:363–364.
67. Kamha AA, Al Omary IY, Zalabany HA, et al. Organophosphate poisoning in pregnancy: a case report. *Basic Clin Pharmacol Toxicol.* 2005;96:397–398.
68. Benslama A, Moutaouakkil S, Charra B, et al. The intermediate syndrome during organophosphorus pesticide poisoning. *Ann Fr Anesth Reanim.* 2004;23:353–356.
69. Sudakin DL, Mullins ME, Horowitz BZ, et al. Intermediate syndrome after malathion ingestion despite continuous infusion of pralidoxime. *J Toxicol Clin Toxicol.* 2000;38:47–50.
70. Karlsen RL, Sterri S, Lyngaas S, et al. Reference values for erythrocyte acetylcholinesterase and plasma cholinesterase activities in children, implications for organophosphate intoxication. *Scand J Clin Lab Invest.* 1981;41:301–302.
71. Sanz P, Rodriguez-Vicente MC, Diaz D, et al. Red blood cell and total blood acetylcholinesterase and plasma pseudocholinesterase in humans: observed variances. *J Toxicol Clin Toxicol.* 1991;29:81–90.
72. Bailey B. Organophosphate poisoning in pregnancy. *Ann Emerg Med.* 1997;29:299.
73. Czeizel AE, Tomcsik M, Timar L. Teratologic evaluation of 178 infants born to mothers who attempted suicide by drugs during pregnancy. *Obstet Gynecol.* 1997;90:195–201.

CHAPTER 10

MATERNAL DISORDERS LEADING TO INCREASED REPRODUCTIVE RISKS

Shital Gandhi, Ruth R. Geist, and Alon Shrim

INTRODUCTION

When pregnancy and maternal medical disease coexist, there may be serious consequences for the mother, fetus, and future child. For example, maternal risks include preeclampsia in the hypertensive woman, increased vaso-occlusive crises in the presence of sickle cell disease, and functional deterioration or even death in patients with cardiac disease. The fetus or neonate is predisposed to congenital anomalies if the mother has uncontrolled diabetes, to hemorrhage if she suffers from autoimmune thrombocytopenia, and to congenital heart block in the presence of certain maternal antibodies. In later years, the child may exhibit manifestations of genetic transmission, as with thalassemia or Marfan syndrome, and in addition is subject to the potential repercussions from growing up in an environment rendered less secure by the mother's medical condition.

Aside from events that relate directly to the interaction between maternal health and pregnancy, there are risks arising from the drugs used to treat some underlying medical disorders. For example, warfarin (in a woman with a prosthetic heart valve) and valproic acid (in the treatment of seizure disorders) are known teratogens. Propylthiouracil, used in the management of hyperthyroidism, can result in fetal goiter and hypothyroidism. Other drugs, such as the chemotherapeutic agents and posttransplant immunosuppressants, are potentially dangerous and require further evaluations. In addition, drugs need to be evaluated not only for possible malformation risk, but also for their effect on neurocognitive outcomes.

Finally, certain maternal factors that relate primarily to lifestyle carry increased reproductive risks. Aside from the obvious disadvantages to maternal health brought on by alcohol, drug abuse, and dietary extremes, there are recognized corresponding fetal and neonatal hazards such as intrauterine growth restriction, placental abruption, stillbirth, and fetal alcohol syndrome.

MEDICAL DISEASES IN PREGNANCY

In this chapter, we summarize the interrelationship between a variety of maternal medical diseases and pregnancy outcome. Reproductive risks associated with maternal lifestyle and various specific medical therapies are dealt with in other chapters. Table 10-1 addresses the three essential questions one asks when a woman with a medical disease becomes pregnant:

1. What is the effect of the disease on pregnancy?
2. What is the effect of pregnancy on the disease?
3. What is the effect of the drugs used to manage this medical condition on the developing fetus?

The first question deals with pregnancy loss (abortion, stillbirth, neonatal death), congenital malformations, fetal and neonatal morbidities, and maternal complications peculiar to pregnancy, such as abruptio placentae and preeclampsia.

In the second question, we are asking whether pregnancy per se alters the course and prognosis of the disease, to what extent, and in what manner.

The third question incorporates the need to question whether the medical treatment should be altered because of possible adverse fetal effects.

For the purposes of this chapter, we have limited ourselves to medical disorders that are relatively common in pregnancy and to those that are not common but are associated with specific reproductive risks. Clearly, a complete list of medical conditions in pregnancy could not be incorporated into a single chapter, and the reader is directed to the references for further information.

The final column of Table 10-1 is headed "Practice points." Again, the details of management and the adjustments in medical care necessary during pregnancy are numerous. We have tried to highlight a few key points for each condition that may serve as valuable clinical tips.

DISCUSSION

During the past three decades, we have witnessed an explosion of activity directed toward the identification of the fetus at risk, the management of preterm labor, and the intensive care of the prematurely born neonate. These efforts have been accompanied by significant reductions in perinatal mortality and morbidity. More recently, the high-risk pregnancy arising from compromised maternal health has acquired a growing, if not novel importance, as evidenced by a proliferation of scientific articles as well as textbooks addressing this theme.[1–43]

There are several good reasons for intensified interest in the influence of maternal factors on reproductive risks.

First, advances in medical and surgical care have made pregnancy feasible in a variety of conditions in which previously the mother's life was seriously threatened. Examples include surgical correction of congenital heart disease, renal transplantation, and the medical management of systemic lupus erythematosus. These women are now healthy and thriving while still in their reproductive years, and are interested in considering starting a family.

Second, societal factors are altering the composition of the population at risk. With the advent of in vitro fertilization and the expansion of career options for women, many have delayed childbearing (comforted by the availability of prenatal diagnosis for advanced maternal age); thus, during pregnancy we are already increasingly seeing certain conditions that occur with aging, such as chronic hypertension and diabetes. Human immunodeficiency virus (HIV) remains a major public health risk (due to ongoing intravenous drug abuse plus high-risk sexual practices such as not using a condom, etc.) and vertical transmission to the neonate is possible, although now virtually preventable with the use of antiretroviral therapy.

Third, with the heightened awareness by members of the medical profession, as well as legislators and consumers, of the

Table 10-1
Maternal Disorders and Obstetric Outcome

CONDITION	EPIDEMIOLOGY/INCIDENCE	EFFECTS OF THE DISEASE ON PREGNANCY	EFFECTS OF PREGNANCY ON THE DISEASE	PRACTICE POINTS
AIDS[a] [1–4]	Current seroprevalence of AIDS in the United States: 3.8/100,000 in whites 59.2/100,000 in blacks 61.91100,000 in Hispanic HIV seroprevalence in all reproductive age women: 1.1–104/1000 In parts of Central Africa and Haiti, it may be 10–30% High-risk women: younger, prostitutes, IV drug abusers, women living outside major population centers 70% of women infection results from heterosexual transmission In the 1990s, the rate of increase of incidence was threefold in women compared to men	Vertical transmission averages 15–40% of nontreated infected mothers. Most occur peripartum (risk factors are preterm labor, coexisting STDs, and prolonged rupture of membranes) and less common can occur prenatally or postpartum via breast-feeding Vertical transmission may result in intrauterine growth retardation, increased risk of postpartum endometritis, neonatal AIDS Adverse fetal outcome correlates with low CD^{4+} cell proportion	No adverse impact of pregnancy on disease progression	Pregnant women who are HIV-positive should be counseled regarding the risks for the newborn Zidovudine and other antiretroviral treatment during pregnancy markedly reduce the rate of vertical transmission (the lower the viral load, the minimal the transmission rate) Efavirenz teratogenic. The efficacy of cesarean section for the prevention of vertical transmission has been suggested for women with viral loads more than 1000 copies per milliliter of plasma. Mouth-suction devices for clearing the newborn's airway should be avoided In the industrialized world, HIV-positive women are advised to refrain from breast-feeding (HIV is found in breast milk)
Anemia[1,2]	Most frequent maternal complication during pregnancy. WHO defines anemia in pregnancy/puerperium as hemoglobin (Hgb) <11 g/dL (110 g/L)	Maternal and perinatal outcomes differ markedly between different etiologies of anemia Please refer to specific type	Significant maternal complications with Hgb <6 g/dL (60 g/L)	Compete blood count in first trimester Consider screening for iron deficiency with serum ferritin (see iron deficiency anemia) Iron supplementation recommended even if Hgb not measured
Antiphospholipid antibodies: lupus anticoagulant and anticardiolipin antibodies.[1,5,6]	3–5% of general obstetrical population Only a fraction of these women will have a clinical syndrome related to these antibodies, such as recurrent miscarriages, maternal thrombosis (arterial and venous), and placental insufficiency	Increased rate of recurrent miscarriages, fetal wastage, stillbirth, growth restriction, and early-onset preeclampsia High incidence of venous and arterial thromboses, cerebral thrombosis, hemolytic anemia, thrombocytopenia, and pulmonary hypertension	Sometimes symptomatic disease occurs only during pregnancy	IgG anticardiolipin antibodies have clinical significance, not IgM. In women with high-titer antibodies and a history of recurrent early pregnancy loss or previous unexplained second- or third-trimester fetal death, therapy with aspirin 81 mg daily and prophylactic dose heparin should be initiated at diagnosis of pregnancy Women with a history of thrombosis due to antiphospholipid antibodies should be treated with therapeutic doses of heparin during pregnancy and for at least 6 weeks postpartum

				In absence of clinical manifestations, positive antiphospholipid antibodies do not require therapy Corticosteroids not beneficial
Asthma[1,7,8]	3.4–8.7% of pregnancies Incidence in pregnancy appears to be increasing	Significant relationship exists between level of chronic asthma control and infant gestational age, intrauterine growth retardation, and perinatal mortality Increased risk of preeclampsia with suboptimal control of disease	30% of women have worse airway obstruction in pregnancy Course unpredictable for first pregnancy, but severe asthma prior to pregnancy often associated with worsening during pregnancy; exacerbation usually between 28 and 36 weeks In 60% of women, the course of asthma is similar in subsequent pregnancies In 10%, asthma is exacerbated during labor and delivery; this is more frequent following cesarean section	Therapy should be guided by objective measures of airway obstruction, as subjective complaints are unreliable. Considered safe in pregnancy: inhaled β_2-selective agents, steroids, disodium chromoglycate, ipratropium. When needed, IV/PO steroids can be safely administered. Avoid Leukotriene modifiers because of lack of safety data in pregnancy Note: excessive use of inhaled β_2-agonists may suppress uterine contractions. For analgesia, prefer non-histamine-releasing narcotic (fentanyl) to meperidine or morphine. Epidural analgesia is ideal for labor. For postpartum hemorrhages, use $PGE_{2\alpha}$ and not $PGF_{2\alpha}$, as the latter can cause bronchospasm and oxygen desaturation.
Vitamin B_{12} deficiency[2,9]	Very rare. More likely encountered following partial or total gastric resection, Crohn's disease, ileal resection, bacterial overgrowth in the small bowel, or in strict vegans Normal level >200 pg/mL (150 pmol/L), but neurologic manifestations may occur with levels in the normal range. Serum methylmalonic acid and homocysteine levels are more sensitive tests	Pernicious anemia may be associated with infertility Except in transcobalamin II deficiency, the fetus is protected from deficiency because of efficient placental transfer Breast-fed neonates whose mothers have B_{12} deficiency may develop severe deficiency 4–12 months after birth	Maternal levels of vitamin B_{12} fall progressively during gestation to intermediate levels (80–120 pg/mL), because of decreased concentration of transcobalamins	Treatment is necessary for vitamin B_{12} <100 pg/mL (74 pmol/L) Levels 100–400 pg/mL (74–295 pmol/L) should have further testing with fasting serum methylmalonic acid and homocysteine levels Contrary to traditional wisdom, oral therapy is effective Breast-feeding is not recommended until deficiency corrected

(*Continued*)

Table 10-1
Maternal Disorders and Obstetric Outcome (*Continued*)

CONDITION	EPIDEMIOLOGY/INCIDENCE	EFFECTS OF THE DISEASE ON PREGNANCY	EFFECTS OF PREGNANCY ON THE DISEASE	PRACTICE POINTS
Cancer, acute leukemias[1,10]	0.9–1.2/100,000 pregnancies (two-thirds of cases are AM)	Increased risk for spontaneous abortion, premature deliveries, IUGR, stillbirths Increased risk of maternal bleeding and infection if peripheral blood counts are suppressed by chemotherapy Chemotherapy may increase risk of fetal abnormalities There are case reports of congenital leukemia in the newborns of women with leukemia	Pregnancy does not adversely affect course of disease. Overall, complete remission rate for standard induction chemotherapy is comparable to that in general population Suboptimal treatment and delay of therapy in attempt to protect the fetus may adversely affect chances of remission/cure	Once the diagnosis of acute leukemia has been made, treatment with multi-agent chemotherapy should not be delayed Fetal well-being should be followed up closely. Therapeutic abortion may be considered if disease is diagnosed in first trimester because of poor maternal prognosis and the effects of multidrug chemotherapy on the fetus If chemotherapy is administered close to time of delivery, neonatal hematological status should be assessed
Breast cancer[1,11]	The second most common malignancy during pregnancy. Complicating 1:1500–1:10,000 pregnancies About 3% of all breast cancer cases are diagnosed during pregnancy Early age at first full term pregnancy and increasing parity are associated with a reduced risk of breast cancer	Teratogenic risk when chemotherapy is used during first trimester (10%). Breast cancer is not transmitted vertically The effect of gestational exposure to chemotherapy on female fetuses is of concern because ova are formed during gestation Mutations/chromosomal aberrations produced in such gametes could result in embryopathology in the next generation; recessive mutations might not become manifest until subsequent generations	Patient and physician-related delays in diagnosis during pregnancy have been reported Stage-for-stage survival similar in pregnant and non-pregnant women, but diagnosis and treatment may be delayed by pregnancy, worsening prognosis Pregnancy may affect the course of breast cancer by altering the incidence, altering the ability to diagnose, or limiting therapeutic options	The risk of mammography is negligible for the fetus if appropriate shielding is used. Still ultrasound is more accurate in pregnancy Therapeutic abortion does not improve prognosis, therefore it should not be offered unless it is necessary to initiate chemotherapy in the first trimester. An additional pregnancy after completion of therapy most probably does not adversely affect the prognosis Radiotherapy is not recommended during pregnancy because fetal radiation exposure is substantial even with shielding Surgical and chemotherapeutic treatment as in nonpregnant women

Cervical cancer[1,11]	The most common malignant tumor encountered throughout pregnancy In situ: 0.13% Invasive: 0.005% About 2–5% are diagnosed during pregnancy	Unlike most pregnancy-related malignancies, in most cases—initiation of treatment cannot coexist with preservation of fetal life Conization can cause hemorrhage, abortion, rupture of membranes, and preterm delivery Rarely spread to either the fetus or placenta	Survival not influenced by pregnancy Mode of delivery does not alter prognosis; however, there is theoretical concern of implantation of cancer cells along the vaginal tract during vaginal delivery	Treatment of invasive cervical cancer in pregnancy depends on the stage of disease at diagnosis: with minimal disease, treatment may be deferred until fetal maturity is achieved Pregnancy termination may be advisable with more advanced stages when diagnosed before 24 weeks' gestation
Hodgkin's lymphoma[1,11]	1/1000–1/6000 pregnancies	Disease does not affect pregnancy outcome; however, during the first trimester, diagnostic and/or therapeutic radiological procedures may be hazardous to the fetus. Radiation doses >10 rads or full doses of chemotherapy during the first trimester can be deleterious to fetal health	Pregnancy does not affect course or prognosis Limitation in application of radiographic studies for staging	MRI should be considered instead of CT scan in the process of staging Therapeutic abortion may be advised if disease is diagnosed during the first trimester because of chemotherapy, irradiation, or aggressive/advanced disease (especially in advanced or infra diaphragmatic disease) If the disease is asymptomatic and diagnosed during second or third trimester, follow-up without treatment until early delivery might be considered
Melanoma[1,11]	One of the leading malignancies associated with pregnancy 0.14–2.8/1000 live births	Generally, no adverse effects Cases of metastases causing neonatal melanomas have been reported. They represent one-third to one-half of all tumors with fetal involvement	Influence of pregnancy on malignant melanoma still controversial Several studies suggest more advanced stage in pregnant patients Stage-for-stage survival rates similar	Primary lesion should be treated surgically as soon as diagnosis is made Prophylactic chemotherapy or immunotherapy should be avoided during pregnancy In case of active disease, chemotherapy should be given as indicated Placenta and fetus should be examined for signs of metastasis
Ovarian cancer[1,12]	1/10,000–1/50,000 deliveries 1/1000 pregnant patients undergoing surgery for adnexal mass About 5% of adnexal neoplasms in pregnancy are malignant	Fetus usually not affected. Increased rate of abortion and preterm deliveries due to torsion and rupture In advanced malignancy, fetal growth retardation may occur Possible virilization of a female fetus due to androgens produced by ovarian stromal tumors	Prognosis not altered by pregnancy Pregnancy does not promote/predispose to ovarian cancer but rather is considered protective to subsequent ovarian cancer	Exploratory laparotomy with staging procedure to evaluate an adnexal mass detected early in pregnancy should not be delayed 12% of ovarian masses may present as an acute surgical abdomen not allowing for planned surgery In advanced cases, hysterectomy with bilateral adnexectomy is indicated, but in certain circumstances, it is justified to remove the tumor and wait for lung maturity while giving chemotherapy

(*Continued*)

Table 10-1
Maternal Disorders and Obstetric Outcome (*Continued*)

CONDITION	EPIDEMIOLOGY/INCIDENCE	EFFECTS OF THE DISEASE ON PREGNANCY	EFFECTS OF PREGNANCY ON THE DISEASE	PRACTICE POINTS
				Postoperative therapy should be given in nearly all instances. Serum markers should be followed, as they indicate tumor progression (e.g., α-fetoprotein, hCG, LDH, CA-125)
Chlamydia trachomatis infection[1,2]	Prevalent in young women of lower economic status Cultured from up to 25% of women attending prenatal clinics, many of whom are asymptomatic	Vertical transmission intrapartum in at least 50% of infected women In infants of untreated mothers, ophthalmia neonatorum occurs in one-third and 10% develop pneumonia May increase risk of premature rupture of membranes, premature deliveries, and perinatal death, more so with recent infection Late postpartum endometritis is increased	Pregnancy does not alter the course of the disease	Infected pregnant women should be treated with erythromycin. The efficacy of eye prophylaxis with silver nitrate, erythromycin, or tetracycline in the prevention of Chlamydia conjunctivitis is not clear
Cystic fibrosis[1,13]	80% of females survive to adulthood; 4% become pregnant each year in the United States Fertility not affected in women who maintain normal weight and pulmonary function	Increased maternal and perinatal mortality related to degree of hypoxia and pulmonary infections For pregnancies that proceed beyond 20 weeks gestation, obstetric outcome is generally good. Increased rate of preterm deliveries (20%) Increased development of gestational diabetes mellitus.	Pulmonary hypertension and cor-pulmonale are absolute contraindications to pregnancy Cumulative maternal mortality of 7.9% at 6 months postpartum and 13.6% at 2 years Risk high if prepregnancy FVC <60%, FEV_1 <70%, and if rate of decline is rapid prior to pregnancy	Prepregnancy counseling is mandatory Follow-up with serial pulmonary function tests, also surveillance for respiratory infection, diabetes, and heart failure Treatment as in nonpregnant. Adequate nutrition is essential Mode of delivery is decided upon according to obstetrical guidelines Epidural analgesia is recommended during delivery or cesarean section
Cytomegalovirus (CMV) infection[1,14,15]	Primary infection in 1–4 % of pregnancies Seropositivity is more prevalent in lower socioeconomic class(85% vs. 55% in mid-upper class) Most common cause of perinatal infection, in the developed world	An infected fetus is more likely with maternal infection during first half of pregnancy >90% of primary infections and almost all recurrent infections are asymptomatic at birth. With primary infection later sequelae are common to develop	No change in incidence/severity of maternal disease.	Serologic screening is common in Europe but less so in America. Seronegative women should be warned to avoid contact with susceptible people or places

	Evidence for fetal infection in 0.5–2% of all neonates	Vertical transmission during pregnancy occurs in approximately 40% of infected gravidas with primary infection and in less than 1% after recurrent infection Congenital CMV includes small-for-gestational-age newborns, microcephaly, intracranial calcifications, chorioretinitis, sensorineural hearing loss hepatosplenomegaly, jaundice, petechiae or purpura, and thrombocytopenia There is also an increased rate of spontaneous abortion and later fetal loss		Primary infection is diagnosed by measuring IgM, IgG. IgG avidity is beneficial in dating infection Culture and PCR of amniotic fluid by amniocentesis allow diagnosis of >80% of infected fetuses (increased sensitivity when done after 21 weeks) Breast-feeding not contraindicated Recent study suggests treatment with CMV-specific hyperimmune globulin to be safe and effective for treatment and prevention of congenital CMV infection
Diabetes mellitus[1,2,16] Pregestational	Type I DM: 1% of pregnancies. Type II DM: prevalence in pregnancy increasing	*Maternal* Increased in frequency: chronic hypertension, probably pregnancy-induced hypertension, polyhydramnios, maternal mortality is low *Fetal/neonatal* Type I DM: rate of congenital malformations increased two to sixfold (7.5–12.9%). Data for Type II are unknown Preconceptional counseling recommended, as preconception hemoglobin A_{1C} (glycosylated hemoglobin) within 1% of upper limits of normal (6–7%) has decreased rate of malformations almost to levels seen in nondiabetic patients (2–3%) *Cardiac* and *neural tube* defects most common, followed by skeletal, GI, urinary tract abnormalities	Insulin requirements increase progressively during pregnancy Complications of diabetes: *Diabetic retinopathy:* nonproliferative usually does not progress; proliferative retinopathy may develop in pregnancy (<20%) or may progress. Should be assessed prepregnancy and during pregnancy by ophthalmology	Excellent preconceptional blood sugar control and in early pregnancy may reduce risk of fetal malformations Diabetic diet should be reviewed with a dietitian Multi-disciplinary approach involving obstetrician, endocrinologist, and dietician Intensive insulin therapy and monitoring is required; have basic ophthalmologic assessment, and 24-hour urine collection for protein and creatinine clearance (the latter to be repeated every month) Level II ultrasound and serum α-fetoprotein recommended in mid second trimester Cesarean delivery for obstetrical indications only

(*Continued*)

Table 10-1
Maternal Disorders and Obstetric Outcome (*Continued*)

CONDITION	EPIDEMIOLOGY/INCIDENCE	EFFECTS OF THE DISEASE ON PREGNANCY	EFFECTS OF PREGNANCY ON THE DISEASE	PRACTICE POINTS
		Increased perinatal mortality and morbidity (macrosomia, cesarean delivery, birth trauma, respiratory distress syndrome, hypoglycemia, hypocalcemia, hyperbilirubinemia, polycythemia) that *may* be decreased by good glycemic control	*Diabetic nephropathy:* proteinuria usually *increases* during pregnancy, whereas creatinine clearance may *decrease* in up to one-third of patients Associated with increased risk of fetal growth restriction, and can be very difficult to ascertain if superimposed preeclampsia is developing However, *most* values return to normal postpartum, following same rate of progression thereafter as in women who did not undertake a pregnancy	
Epilepsy[17,18]	0.3–0.5% of pregnancies	Higher rates of miscarriage Two- to threefold increase in malformations, especially facial clefts, cardiac malformations, and neural tube defects due to antiepileptic medications. Highest risk with polypharmacy and with the use of older antiepileptics Increase in seizures and neurodevelopment delay in the offspring has been noted, possibly due to medications (especially valproate)	Variable effect of pregnancy on seizure frequency; increased in 45%, unchanged in 50% and decreased in 5%	Prepregnancy counseling is crucial; consider switching to medications with less teratogenic effects, such as carbamazepine if seizure type allows Seizures must be controlled to avoid maternal and fetal injury; women should be encouraged to continue medications throughout pregnancy Adjust dose according to clinical status, rather than serum drug levels Vitamin K in the last month of pregnancy as prophylaxis for maternal and neonatal bleeding Folic acid 0.4–5 mg/day prepregnancy and in first trimester

Folic acid deficiency[1,19]	Frank megaloblastic anemia in 1170–1/250 pregnancies. WHO report I in 3 women worldwide suffer from folic acid deficiency 30–69% American women in low socioeconomic class have this deficiency	Prospective human studies show a cause-and-effect relationship between folate deficiency and increased risk for neural tube defects (both in normal population and high-risk families) The fetus and placenta extract folate from the maternal circulation so efficiently that the fetus is not anemic even when the mother is severely so	Pregnancy aggravates folic acid depletion	1 mg of supplemental folate is adequate for prophylaxis and overt folate deficiency Treatment should include iron as well Folate supplementation periconceptually and prenatally has been reported to reduce the risk for neural tube defects in the newborn
Gonorrhea[1,2]	Up to 7% of prenatal patients in North America have endocervical gonorrhea; 75–90% are asymptomatic In 40% there is concomitant chlamydia infection	Infection may have effect on pregnancy outcome in any trimester Untreated infection is associated with septic spontaneous abortions Vertical transmission occurs by ascending infection in the presence of ruptured membranes or by delivery through an infected birth canal Higher incidence of premature rupture of membranes, preterm labor and delivery, intrauterine growth retardation, and chorioamnionitis in untreated cases Newborn infection may involve eye, ear canal, oropharynx, stomach, anorectal mucosa, or hematogenous dissemination	Risk of noncervical infection and disseminated infection increase in pregnancy	Routine endocervical cultures are essential in early pregnancy and again at 28 weeks' gestation Treatment of an uncomplicated infection with ceftriaxone and topical application of 1% silver nitrate or erythromycin to the newborn's eyes dramatically decrease neonatal infection and ophthalmia neonatorum. If allergic to penicillin: spectinomycin and erythromycin Screening for syphilis and chlamydia should always precede treatment
Heart disease[1,20,21]	Heart disease complicates 1–4% of all pregnancies Congenital and rheumatic etiologies most common	Poor cardiovascular status associated with spontaneous abortions, intrauterine growth retardation, and premature labor Women with congenital heart disease (CHD) have a 3–10% risk of having a baby with CHD, especially in the presence of obstruction to left ventricular outflow	Cardiac output increases during pregnancy by 40%, peaking by the end of the second trimester. The vast majority of patients can be safely managed to term.	Management in high-risk obstetrical center recommended Rest and monthly examination are mainstays of therapy Warfarin should be changed to low molecular weight heparin either prior to conception or before 6 weeks' gestation. Close monitoring of level of anticoagulation with Anti-Xa levels is crucial to avoid thrombosis

(*Continued*)

Table 10-1
Maternal Disorders and Obstetric Outcome (*Continued*)

CONDITION	EPIDEMIOLOGY/INCIDENCE	EFFECTS OF THE DISEASE ON PREGNANCY	EFFECTS OF PREGNANCY ON THE DISEASE	PRACTICE POINTS
		Critical period of exposure for causing fetal warfarin syndrome is between 6–12 weeks' gestation, when 25% of babies are affected Fetal warfarin syndrome includes nasal hypoplasia and stippled epiphyses Intrauterine growth retardation, developmental retardation, eye defects, and hearing loss have also been described Exposure to warfarin after the first trimester may present a risk of CNS damage and stillbirth due to hemorrhage; however, degree of risk unclear and must be balanced against the benefit of warfarin to the mother (i.e., most effective drug in preventing valve thrombosis and embolic stroke)	Maternal mortality is 0.4% with New York Heart Association (NYHA) class I or II but increases to 4–7% with class III or IV. Pregnancy not recommended with high-risk cardiac lesions: any cardiac disease with class III or IV symptoms, unrepaired cyanotic CHD, critical aortic stenosis, primary pulmonary hypertension, Eisenmenger's syndrome, Marfan syndrome, or peripartum cardiomyopathy in previous pregnancy with persistent cardiac dysfunction Maternal complications include congestive heart failure and risk of aortic rupture in Marfan syndrome or coarctation of aorta (even if repaired)	Digoxin, β-adrenergic blockers, calcium channel blockers, and heparin are not teratogenic Angiotensin-converting enzyme inhibitors cannot be used during pregnancy Fetal echocardiography recommended at 18–20 weeks' gestation to rule out fetal CHD Delivery mode dictated mainly by obstetrical considerations Deterioration can occur in labor and especially postpartum American Heart Association does not consider delivery in either mode an indication for antibiotic prophylaxis
Hepatitis (viral)[1,22–24]	0.2% of pregnant women. However, 1–5% of adults may develop chronic infection and persistent viremia, depending on the pathological agent. Hepatitis C virus infection prevalence in pregnant women: 1.5–5.2%	Hepatitis A (HAV): no risk of vertical transmission.	The course of HAV, HBV, and HCV viral diseases is unaltered by pregnancy; thus risk of fulminant hepatitis is well below 2%.	Pregnant women in contact with HAV infective cases should receive immune globulin (0.02 mL/kg) as soon as possible Pregnant women exposed to HBV should receive HBIg (0.04–0.07 mL/kg) and the first of three 1-mL HBV vaccines as soon as possible, the second and third vaccines given 1 and 6 months later

		Hepatitis B (HBV): significant risk of vertical transmission from mother with acute or chronic hepatitis and from asymptomatic carriers. If maternal HBe antibody positive or HBe antigen negative, there is a 10–20% risk of perinatal infection. If maternal HBe antigen positive, the risk is 80–90% for either infantile hepatitis or carrier state. Hepatitis C (HCV): risk of vertical transmission of ~5%, but 22% if coinfected with HIV Transmission does not occur before third trimester Hepatitis E (HEV) virus disease increases fetal mortality In fulminant hepatitis, fetal wastage is >70%	Hepatitis E may be fulminant during pregnancy, with high mortality rates in third trimester (20%).	Prevention of HBV transmission currently dependent on identification of HB surface antigen (HbsAg) and HbeAg carriers among pregnant women and the recognition of acute HBV infection in the latter half of the pregnancy/postpartum period. Screening of all women in first trimester recommended Newborns of HbsAg-positive women should receive HBIg (0.5 mL within 1 hour and 0.5 mL HBV within a week of birth) Test infants for HbsAg and antiHBc at 1 year to determine treatment success. The presence of HbsAg ± IgM anti HBc indicates treatment failure, since the infant is actively infected Anti HBs alone suggests that vaccine-induced immunity can last approximately 5 years Boosters needed every 5 years for continued protection Immune globulins are ineffective for prevention or treatment of HCV There is no vaccine yet
Herpes simplex (HSV)[1,25–27]	About 22% of pregnant women are positive for HSV-2 and more than 2% acquire it during pregnancy Approximately 70% of newly acquired infections are not unrecognized Neonatal infection is acquired either intrauterine (5%), peripartum (85%) or post partum (10%) 20–50% of primary infections are due to herpes simplex virus type I (HSV-1), but >80% of recurrent infections are due to HSV-2 Women may shed virus in absence of clinical history of HSV infection Only 0.25–0.33% of women who deliver a neonate with HSV infection are symptomatic at the time of delivery	Neonatal HSV infection occurs in up to 1 in 3200 live births [mainly due to infection at the time of delivery]. Neonatal infections can 1. Be localized with skin, eye, and mouth manifestations 2. Have CNS involvement 3. Be disseminated Recurrent infections during pregnancy are a reservoir for neonatal infections. Perinatally acquired infections are still present in absence of maternal symptoms or lesions Recent case control study suggests twofold risk for CP when maternal HSB–B nucleic acids are detected. More research is needed!	Primary maternal infection during pregnancy associated with greater risk of recurrence and viral excretion during labor Recurrences tend to increase in frequency as pregnancy progresses. Overriding concern is transmission to baby, since maternal infection usually follows self-limited course	CDC recommends both virologic and type specific serologic tests for patients at risk for STD For symptomatic women, oral antiviral medications hasten lesion healing and reduce viral shedding For frequent recurrences of HSV, consideration might be given to oral acyclovir treatment starting at 36 weeks Pregnant women with history of HSV and no lesions or prodromal symptoms at the time of delivery can undergo vaginal delivery; however, they should also have cultures of previously affected areas and cervix done to document possible neonatal exposure Avoidance of invasive procedures is warranted Women with genital lesions or prodromal symptoms should be delivered by cesarean section as soon as possible after membrane rupture/onset of labor, ideally, within 4–6 hours

(*Continued*)

Table 10-1
Maternal Disorders and Obstetric Outcome (*Continued*)

CONDITION	EPIDEMIOLOGY/INCIDENCE	EFFECTS OF THE DISEASE ON PREGNANCY	EFFECTS OF PREGNANCY ON THE DISEASE	PRACTICE POINTS
Hypertensive disorders[1,28–30]	5–10% of all pregnancies. Chronic hypertension defined as elevated blood pressure prior to 20 weeks gestation. Risk of developing superimposed preeclampsia 20–25%. Gestational hypertension occurs after 20 weeks, with the majority occurring at term. No proteinuria present. Preeclampsia/eclampsia is a placental mediated disorder that occurs after 20 weeks, and is characterized by hypertension and proteinuria. Etiology unknown. Results in 20% of all maternal deaths. 70% have preeclampsia/eclampsia, 25% essential hypertension, 5% gestational hypertension.	In chronic hypertension, increased rate of intrauterine growth retardation (IUGR) abruptio placentae, and perinatal death with severe hypertension. 10–15% of gestational hypertension will develop preeclampsia. In preeclampsia, increased rate of the following proportional to degree of hypertension: spontaneous abortions, intra-uterine growth restriction and fetal death, abruptio placentae, prematurity, operative delivery, perinatal morbidity and mortality. Elevated uric acid independent predictor of fetal risk.	Incidence of chronic hypertensive complications unchanged. Acute hypertension (BP>170/110) associated with increase in maternal stroke.	Blood pressure usually decreases until 20 weeks gestation, then rises to reach previous levels by term Decreased maternal stroke is the only consequence of treating chronic hypertension in pregnancy other than possible decrease in fetal loss with treatment of essential hypertension in first trimester with methyldopa BP >160/100 mm Hg should be treated. Goal of treatment: diastolic BP ≤90 mm Hg. Methyldopa, labetalol safest drugs in pregnancy. Can add nifedipine and hydralazine for refractory hypertension Symptomatic severe hypertension (BP >170/110 mm Hg) should be treated with intravenous labetalol or hydralazine
Hyperthyroidism[31]	Rare 1:1000 pregnancies. Graves' disease most common etiology	In untreated women, there is increase in rate of stillbirths, low birth weight, neonatal death, premature birth, preeclampsia, and heart failure. Fetal/neonatal Graves' disease due to transplacental transfer of thyroid-stimulating IgG (TSAb) occurs in 1–2% of cases, especially with history of previously affected children. However, even presence of IgG TSAb confers a low risk of neonatal Graves' No adverse effects in subsequent growth or development	Tendency for increased activity of disease in first trimester and postpartum No change in natural history of disease TSAb activity in Graves' disease usually declines during pregnancy, with remission in almost all pregnancies with Graves' disease. Up to 30% of women can be titrated off medications in the third trimester; activity often increases postpartum	TSAb may be present even after thyroidectomy or radioactive iodine ablation; should be measured in all patients with history of Graves'. If present, increase fetal surveillance, looking for tachycardia, hydrops, goiter Treatment in pregnancy decreases risk of maternal thyroid storm. Propylthiouracil (in lowest possible dose) is the drug of choice in pregnancy; Methimazole is associated with aplasia cutis (localized absence of skin at the vertex or occipital area of the scalp) Thyroidectomy can be safely carried out in second trimester if needed

Hypothyroidism[32,33]	6/1000 women who carry pregnancy >20 weeks	Decreased fertility Possibly increased miscarriage, adverse fetal and perinatal outcomes When hypothyroidism is caused by iodine deficiency, cretinism may develop if no replacement therapy Severe maternal hypothyroidism is associated with decreased IQ	Thyroid requirements increase early in pregnancy (fifth week of gestation) by an average of 30%	Treatment improves fertility and probably pregnancy outcome TSH and free thyroid hormones should be repeated every trimester Subclinical hypothyroidism should be treated during pregnancy Screening *all* pregnant women is controversial, but recommended in women at increased risk (Type I diabetes, autoimmune conditions, and positive family history of thyroid dysfunction)
Immune thrombocytopenia purpura (ITP)[1,34,35]	Commonly occurs in women of child-bearing age and hence often seen in pregnancy Accounts for 4% of cases thrombocytopenia in pregnancy Etiology: autoimmune Often occurs in conjunction with other autoimmune conditions, such as systemic lupus erythematosus	*Maternal* If platelets <20,000/mm^3, blood loss may be increased during delivery. No increase in maternal mortality. *Fetal* Increased risk of stillbirth and fetal hemorrhage of <1% (most common causes are spontaneous abortion and hemorrhage) due to transplacental transfer of antiplatelet antibodies Incidence of neonatal thrombocytopenia (NATP) is 30–40% but severe NATP (i.e., platelets <50/mm^3) occur in 10–20% at delivery or in the first 3–5 days postpartum 1–4% of babies with NATP suffer from cerebral hemorrhage There is no correlation between maternal and fetal platelet count! Factors that indicate a high risk of NATP are controversial but include women with a previous history of ITP (especially if splenectomy), or a previous infant with NATP. These have a 20% risk of severe NATP	Thrombocytopenia tends to worsen Ideally, pregnancy should be postponed until remission	Treatment is as in nonpregnant state (i.e., steroids are first-line treatment, with intravenous γ-globulin as second line, and splenectomy as last resort) Maternal steroid treatment is of unproven benefit in increasing fetal platelet count Treatment should be initiated if maternal platelets are <10,000; if platelets are 10–30,000 in the second or third trimester or if there is maternal bleeding Goal of therapy: maternal platelets >50,000 or cessation of serious bleeding Note: regional anesthesia is usually not an option if platelets are <80,000 These pregnancies are best managed in a high-risk obstetric center Cordocentesis should be considered if indicators of high risk for NATP present (i.e., previous NATP, splenectomy) Cesarean section reserved for obstetrical indications unless the fetus is shown to be severely thrombocytopenic (i.e., by cordocentesis) In other circumstances, Cesarean section is of unproven benefit in decreasing rate of neonatal cerebral hemorrhage

(*Continued*)

Table 10-1
Maternal Disorders and Obstetric Outcome (*Continued*)

CONDITION	EPIDEMIOLOGY/INCIDENCE	EFFECTS OF THE DISEASE ON PREGNANCY	EFFECTS OF PREGNANCY ON THE DISEASE	PRACTICE POINTS
Inflammatory bowel disease, (IBD) Crohn's disease[36,37]	Not rare in pregnancy. Prevalence of inflammatory bowel disease in the United States ranges 1–2 million people: with peak incidence at 15–30 years	The effects on pregnancy outcome are unclear. There are controversial data Most report no effect of disease—no increase in adverse pregnancy outcome	Disease not adversely affected by pregnancy per se; disease remains quiescent in about 70% of pregnant women if in remission at time of conception 30% relapse during pregnancy if in remission at time of conception Highest risk of exacerbation in first trimester and puerperium Onset of Crohn's disease during pregnancy is associated with a poorer prognosis	Infertility is reversed with appropriate drug therapy resulting in remission Management of active disease should be similar to nonpregnant patients Safe: corticosteroids, sulfasalazine and its 5-aminosalicylic component (*5-ASA*), and antibiotics 6-Mercaptopurine and azathioprine should best be avoided Limited radiological investigations should not be postponed if results are likely to alter management
Iron deficiency anemia (IDA)[1,2]	75–80% of pregnant women with low hemoglobin have IDA	Severe IDA may be associated with increased risk of preterm birth, intrauterine growth retardation, stillbirths, and maternal deaths in the developing world	There is a 50% increase in plasma volume during pregnancy, leading to a dilutional anemia. Iron requirements increase If iron depletion present, without signs of deficiency, IDA may develop during/after gestation	IDA during pregnancy is primarily the consequence of plasma volume expansion without sufficient expansion of maternal red cell mass. Since demand for iron in pregnancy cannot be met by dietary iron alone, supplemental iron recommended (30–60 mg/day in nonanemic and 200–300 mg/day in IDA states)
Malaria[1,38]	Approx. 1000 cases of malaria in United States per year 13 cases of congenital malaria in United States/year, but 0.3% in immune mothers and 1–4% in nonimmune mothers—in endemic areas	Majority of malarial infections caused by *Plasmodium falciparum* Severe maternal disease causes—increased fetal wastage Increased rates of: miscarriages, preterm labor Placental malaria might lead to anemia	Pregnancy enhances the severity of *falciparum* malaria	Antimalarial prophylaxis advocated for mothers living in endemic areas May prescribe chloroquine or mefloquine as prophylaxis or for treatment

Multiple sclerosis (MS)[1,2]	10–75/100,000 pregnancies (same as general population)	Uncomplicated MS has no effect on pregnancy. Exacerbation episodes tend to occur in the first trimester and mainly in the puerperium (30–40%)	Relapse rate approximates that of nonpregnant state Women with severe debilitation may experience an increase in infections, fatigue, and pulmonary problems	Rest is an important component of optimal care in pregnancy. Urinary tract infections should be screened for and treated promptly. Avoid use of interferon in pregnancy for lack of adequate safety data.
Myasthenia gravis[1,2]	2–4/100,000 pregnancies (same as general population)	Neonatal myasthenia gravis occurs in 10–20% of newborns Newborn disease is more likely if the mother produces antibodies against embryonic acetylcholine receptors Newborn disease resolves in 2–6 weeks No adverse perinatal effects	One-third improves, one-third worsens, and one-third remains stable If diagnosed during pregnancy, mother is prone to more severe form of disease Exacerbations tend to occur in first trimester and puerperium, with improvement in second and third trimesters	Agents that potentiate neuromuscular blockade, such as curare, muscle relaxants, magnesium sulfate, or aminoglycosides should be avoided Regional anesthesia preferred. Narcotics must be used with care Mode of delivery is according to obstetrical considerations. Might consider forceps during second stage to overcome lack of maternal expulsive forces
Parvovirus B 19[39]	35–55% of women of childbearing age are seropositive (immune) Infection is estimated to occur in 1 in 400 pregnancies Estimated transmission across the placenta in 30% of infected women	Vertical transmission: in the first half of pregnancy (16%). Above 20 weeks' gestation (35%) Virus has affinity to erythroid precursor cells—causing anemia and hydrops Overall fetal loss rate of 10% Most common cause of fetal hydrops fetalis (this complication occurs however in only 1% of infected women) Fetal infection follows maternal infection in 25% of cases and resolves in most fetuses without sequelae Case reports of association with congenital birth defects, but no epidemiological studies May increase fetal loss	No effect on natural history of disease	Routine exclusion of pregnant women from work if a case of B 19 parvovirus is found is not recommended since low risk of adverse fetal outcome For women with positive serology—ultrasonographic fetal evaluation for hydrops is indicated Fetal transfusion for hydrops may improve outcome in some cases

(*Continued*)

Table 10-1
Maternal Disorders and Obstetric Outcome (*Continued*)

CONDITION	EPIDEMIOLOGY/INCIDENCE	EFFECTS OF THE DISEASE ON PREGNANCY	EFFECTS OF PREGNANCY ON THE DISEASE	PRACTICE POINTS
Renal disease[1,2,40,41]	Fertility decreased with severe chronic renal impairment. Uneventful pregnancy unusual when serum creatinine >3 mg/dL (265 μM), even in absence of maternal symptoms Outcome is usually successful when serum creatinine <1.5–2 mg/dL (133–177 μM), poly-arteritis is absent, and underlying renal disease is not scleroderma or poly-arteritis nodosa (PAN) Pregnancy outcome depends on the degree of associated hypertension and renal insufficiency Increased risk of preeclampsia and perinatal morbidity and mortality Acute glomerulonephritis: high rate of fetal loss, preterm deliveries, intrauterine growth restriction With nephrotic syndrome, significant peripheral edema may develop	Mild renal impairment (serum creatinine <1.4 mg/dL (124 μM), even with preserved renal function, pregnancy termination should be consid-ered in women with renal PAN or renal scleroderma Natural history of other renal diseases not affected, except possibly IGA nephropathy, focal glomerulosclerosis (FGS), membranoproliferative glomerulonephritis, and reflux nephropathy. Most show increase in glomeru-lar filtration rate, but 15% decrease near term is permissible Increased/appearance of protein-uria (may be nephrotic) common, up to 60% of patients Up to 50% develop hypertension High rates of preterm deliveries. Severe renal impairment (creatinine> 3 mg/dL = 265 μM): pregnancy should be dis-cour-aged because of risk of severe maternal complication hypertension, anemia, preeclampsia, high-grade proteinuria, and need for dialysis	Moderate renal impairment (creati-nine 1.5–2 mg/dL = 133–265μM) may suffer unpredictable, and at times irre-versible, loss of function during/after pregnancy In the absence of superimposed preeclampsia or severe placental abruption, long-term deterioration of mild renal dysfunction is not accelerated by pregnancy	Patient should be seen every 2–4 weeks for serial urine collections for protein and creatinine clearance and BP control to rule out asymptomatic bacteriuria Criteria of hypertension and proteinuria are unreliable for diagnosis of preeclampsia. Need to assess placental function with Doppler studies. Monitor for HELLP syndrome (Hemolysis, Elevated Liver enzymes, Low Platelets) Renal biopsy can definitively diagnose preeclampsia, but rarely recommended because of risks

Renal transplantation[1,42]	Prevalence increases as more successful outcome and the prompt return of ovulation in most women	High rate of spontaneous and therapeutic abortions 90% chance of successful outcome if pregnancy survives beyond first trimester Increased premature rupture of membranes and preterm labor	Glomerular filtration rate usually increases, as in healthy women However, there is no risk of glomerular sclerosis, since this rise is due to increased plasma flow, without changes in intraglomerular pressure	At least 2 years of good general health without hypertension required before conception Prednisone and azathioprine should be continued to avoid rejection The evidence concerning cyclosporine use during pregnancy is inconclusive, but there is no report to link its use to teratogenicity or mutagenicity. There is a paucity of data on tacrolimus, mycophenolate mofetil, and OKT3 There is still concern about the possibility of late effects of immunosuppression on the offspring (e.g., malignancy, germ-cell dysfunction, and malformations in the offspring's children)
Rheumatoid arthritis[1,2]	RA affects 1–2% of women of childbearing age and may present during pregnancy	Anti-Ro antibodies might be present in 5% of women with RA, (antibody has been associated with congenital heart block, but the risk is very low). Fetal echocardiogram at 20 weeks' gestation is recommended when maternal Anti-Ro is present Otherwise, no adverse effects on fetal outcome	75% of patients improve. Most do so in the first trimester, but may not improve until the third 25% worsen and may develop new joint lesions Relapse often occurs, usually within 2 months of delivery. Course during last pregnancy is predictive of course in current pregnancy	Many patients are able to stop non steroidal anti-inflammatory drugs and disease-remitting agents during pregnancy and are often managed with analgesics. NSAIDs decrease joint inflammation, although this may cause maternal complications (prolonged gestation and labor, ante- and postpartum hemorrhage) or neonatal pulmonary hypertension secondary to premature closure of ductus arteriosus (need to stop at 32 weeks) If needed, gold salts and chloroquine can be used. Azathioprine might be considered Corticosteroids are considered safe to use during pregnancy When cervical spine involvement exists, subluxation is common, more so during pregnancy Delivery mode is according to obstetrical considerations
Rubella infection[43,44]	Incidence declined from 0.45/100,000 in 1990 to 0.1/100,000 in 1999.	Congenital rubella might cause malformations, miscarriage or fetal death	Course of disease is unchanged by pregnancy Maternal disease is usually mild	Vaccination of seronegative women advised 48–72 hours postpartum Vaccine virus excreted in breast milk, but no contraindication to breast-feeding

(Continued)

Table 10-1
Maternal Disorders and Obstetric Outcome (*Continued*)

CONDITION	EPIDEMIOLOGY/INCIDENCE	EFFECTS OF THE DISEASE ON PREGNANCY	EFFECTS OF PREGNANCY ON THE DISEASE	PRACTICE POINTS
		Effects depends on gestational age at infection: infection during the first 16 weeks carries 90% for congenital rubella syndrome (CRS) As the duration of pregnancy increases, fetal infections are less likely to cause congenital malformations CRS includes one or more of the following: 1. Eye lesions 2. Heart disease 3. Sensorineural deafness 4. CNS defects 5. IUGR 6. Thrombocytopenia, anemia 7. Liver problems 8. Pneumonitis 9. Osseous changes Maternal infection confirmed by rubella-specific IgM or four-fold rise in rubella-specific IgG In utero infection diagnosed by rubella-specific antibody in cord blood		According to recent guidelines from the CDC, pregnancy should be deferred for only 1 month after vaccination
Sickle cell disease[45,46]	Incidence in black Americans: sickle cell trait: 1 in 12 HbS-S-1 in 576 HbS-C-1 in 2000 HbS-β-1 in 2000	>30% overall fetal wastage with increased risk of spontaneous abortions, infertility, prematurity, intrauterine growth retardation, and perinatal death, likely due to placental infarcts Prior to 1970, maternal mortality was as high as 10–12% and maternal morbidity up to 80–90%.	Vaso-occlusive crises increase, especially in the third trimester, labor, and puerperium Increased incidence of congestive heart failure (2–20%), pneumonia (3–15%), pyelonephritis (5–12%), pulmonary embolism (20–40%) and cholelithiasis (25% vs. 10% in nonpregnancy)	Sickle cell screen in early pregnancy is recommended for all black women Prepregnancy counseling and testing of partners is critical Prenatal diagnosis by amniocentesis, cordocentesis, or chorionic villus sampling is recommended Early and frequent prenatal assessment of pregnant women with this condition Supplemental folic acid Painful crises treated as in nonpregnant states (oxygen, fluids, transfusion, opiates)

		Fetal loss up to 50–60%. These figures have been markedly reduced as a result of improved obstetric and prenatal care; maternal mortality nowadays in the Western world is around 1%		Prophylactic transfusion reduces likelihood of occlusive crises, but no effect on fetal outcome Exchange transfusions by manual/ erythrocytapheresis techniques may be used for specific crises; not recommended prophylactically
Streptococcus group B (GBS)[47–49]	Between 10% and 30% of pregnant women are colonized in the vagina or rectum Invasive infection 0.23 per 1000 live births.	If causes urinary tract infection, increase rate of preterm premature rupture of membranes, preterm deliveries, postpartum endometritis, and chorioamnionitis Early-onset infection: peripartum infection during first week of life. Late-onset infection: after 1 week of age. Both might cause sepsis, pneumonia, or meningitis. High mortality and morbidity	Usually asymptomatic infection Might cause urinary tract infection: unlike asymptomatic carrier, demands treatment during pregnancy	Screen for vaginal and rectal GBS at 35–37 weeks' gestation Treatment during pregnancy: only in symptomatic cases (asymptomatic carriers—treat in labor) Intrapartum penicillin when: -Previous infant with GBS infection -GBS bacteriuria in current pregnancy -Premature labor -Positive screening at 35–37 weeks When screening not done: intrapartum fever >38°C membrane rupture >18 hours
Syphilis[1,50,51]	Approximately 100,000 cases of syphilis diagnosed annually in United States 350 cases of congenital syphilis per year Increase in prevalence in the late 1980s and 1990s	Vertical transmission can occur in any trimester; most severe fetal disease results from syphilis in early pregnancy In untreated early disease, 80% infantile mortality and morbidity 50% of infants born to women with untreated primary/ secondary syphilis will have congenital infection at birth	The course of syphilis is not altered by pregnancy	Pregnancy is commonly listed as an etiology for false-positive serology but recent studies do not show increased rate of such results in gravidas HIV-coinfected adults show extremely high titer or paradoxically negative titers with secondary syphilis Confirmatory tests as in nonpregnant state
Systemic lupus erythematosus (SLE)[1,52]	1:500 (In childbearing age)	Factors for pregnancy outcome: activity of disease, age, parity, coexisting medical conditions (e.g., renal failure), antiphospholipid antibodies (see separately) Usually SLE improves in a third of women, remains unchanged in a third, and worsens in a third	Conflicting data Most agree that pregnancy has no adverse effect on the course of disease No evidence for increased exacerbation postpartum	Should be followed in high-risk obstetrics unit Treatment is generally the same as in nonpregnant Prednisone is drug of choice for therapy, but no prophylactic treatment or increase in dosage recommended

(Continued)

Table 10-1
Maternal Disorders and Obstetric Outcome (*Continued*)

CONDITION	EPIDEMIOLOGY/INCIDENCE	EFFECTS OF THE DISEASE ON PREGNANCY	EFFECTS OF PREGNANCY ON THE DISEASE	PRACTICE POINTS
		Increased rate of stillbirths, IUGR, preterm deliveries, and perinatal mortality with active disease at conception and positive maternal antibodies (especially antiphospholipid). With lupus nephropathy, increased risk of preeclampsia (~63%) Positive anti-Ro antibody present in 20–80% of SLE patients and is associated with neonatallupus syndrome (NLS) Risk of NLS <5%. In presence of anti-Ro/anti-La—risk of congenital heart block <3%		If immunosuppression needed, azathioprine is preferred to cyclophosphamide Decreasing C3 or C4 levels useful for distinguishing SLE flare from preeclampsia
Toxoplasmosis[1,53]	25% of women of childbearing age susceptible Acute toxoplasmosis complicates 1–5/1000 pregnancies. Congenital infection in 1–2/1000 live births in United States 90% of acute toxoplasmosis infections are asymptomatic	The risk of fetal infection increases with duration of pregnancy. Overall, congenital infection in 40–60% of cases Most severe sequelae with transmission before 20 weeks' gestation Spontaneous abortion, stillbirth, and severe congenital infection occur exclusively with maternal infection in early pregnancy Congenital toxoplasmosis includes IUGR, hepatosplenomegaly, icterus, anemia, convulsions, intracranial calcifications, hydrocephalus or microcephalus, and mental retardation Asymptomatic/subclinical infection occurs in the majority of babies infected	Pregnancy does not alter course of disease	Preconception serology of high-risk women is key (i.e., women who have recently acquired cats, who handle kitty litter, eat raw/undercooked meat, or have had a recent mononucleosis-like illness) Seronegative individuals should avoid high-risk situations (as detailed above); serial serology should be performed throughout pregnancy Diagnosis made by serology: rising IgM is a good indicator of active, recent infection Treatment may decrease risk of congenital infection, but risk still remains substantial and there is no proof that the severity of congenital infection is modified Ultrasound is not sensitive enough to diagnose all cases of congenital infection Amniocentesis/cordocentesis/PCR assay are performed in some centers when acute infection occurs during pregnancy and therapeutic abortion is an option; treatment with spiramycin recommended while awaiting the procedure

Tuberculosis[1,54]	Prevalence increasing since 1985 as a result of HIV infection in population and considerable immigration from endemic areas	Congenital TB from intrauterine fetal infection is rare, and is usually seen only if the woman has tuberculous endometritis or military TB. However, can be fatal (fetal mortality close to 50%), mainly due to the failure to diagnose correctly	No increase in risk of progression to active disease; risk of such still greatest in the 1–2 years after infection Presentation and natural history of disease unchanged in pregnancy	Pregnant women generally react to purified protein derivative (PPD) testing in manner similar to general population Treatment depends on maternal disease status: 1) PPD positive, no active infection: controversial. Some advocate isoniazid (INH) only after delivery, others state is should be given in pregnancy at any gestational age. If the woman is HIV-positive, or has other risk factors for progression, she should be treated 2) Active pulmonary TB: treat with INH, rifampin, ethambutol, plus pyrazinamide if local resistance is high. Pyridoxine should also be given Drugs to avoid: ethionamide, streptomycin, amikacin, and kanamycin Higher risk of INH hepatitis in pregnancy Prophylactic treatment of the neonate with Vitamin K recommended because of possible complication of hemorrhagic disease of the newborn Neonatal management: 1) Prophylactic: Neonate born to a mother with active TB should be treated with isoniazid for the first 2–3 months of life or at least until the mother is known to be smear- and culture-negative. This treatment is necessary in order to avoid separation of mother and child 2) Therapeutic: Treat with four drugs if infant's PPD is positive or there is evidence of clinical disease
Urinary tract infection (UTI)[1,55]	Asymptomatic bacteriuria (ASB) occurs in 2–7% of women during pregnancy, most of whom have positive urine cultures at first antenatal visit 25% of untreated gravidas with ASB will develop acute UTI Pyelonephritis complicates 1–2% of pregnancies	Association of ASB with preeclampsia, anemia, prematurity, and fetal loss unproven Acute UTI can mimic/precipitate premature labor; role in etiology of intrauterine growth retardation, fetal death, or congenital abnormalities controversial	Pregnancy does not predispose women to ASB. However, higher risk of UTI in pregnancy than non-pregnant	All women should be screened for ASB at first antenatal visit Treatment of ASB prevents most of acute UTI cases Treatment can proceed with nitrofurantoin (for 10 days), ampicillin, or cephalexin. There are also single-dose and 3-day regimens

(*Continued*)

Table 10-1
Maternal Disorders and Obstetric Outcome (*Continued*)

CONDITION	EPIDEMIOLOGY/INCIDENCE	EFFECTS OF THE DISEASE ON PREGNANCY	EFFECTS OF PREGNANCY ON THE DISEASE	PRACTICE POINTS
			1–2% of gravidas with pyelonephritis develop respiratory complications, sometimes ARDS	One-third of women treated for ASB will have persistence/recurrence of infection; suppressive therapy should be considered in such women if close follow-up and treatment not possible Acute UTI usually caused by gram-negative bacteria Treatment of pyelonephritis in pregnancy requires hospitalization and intravenous ampicillin and gentamicin or cephalosporins
Urolithiasis[56]	Complicates 1:1500 pregnancies	Increase in symptomatic urinary tract infection; otherwise, course and outcome of pregnancy unchanged	Pregnancy has no effect on progression of nephrolithiasis Increased rate of spontaneous stone passage (70%) Pregnant women have fewer symptoms and pass stones more easily	Hydronephrosis (usually greater on right side) diagnosed by ultrasound is an unreliable sign for urethral obstruction Calcium oxalate stones are the most common in pregnancy The stones can usually be visualized by ultrasound, but if there is a diagnostic dilemma, radiography should be done Must be distinguished from acute pyelonephritis
Varicella[1,57,58]	90% of adults in nontropical areas are immune to varicella Incidence: 1–5/10,000 pregnancies	Congenital varicella syndrome (CVS) is characterized by intrauterine growth retardation, limb hypoplasia, brain atrophy, cutaneous and bony leg defects, mental retardation, and ocular lesions Risk for CVS only if encountered before 20 weeks' gestation 2% above baseline risk for birth defects Before 13 weeks reduced risk (~0.5%) Otherwise, no increase in pregnancy complications Varicella near term can cause disseminated varicella in newborn with high complication rate	It is not clear whether chickenpox during pregnancy has a higher complication rate than in adults in general However, maternal mortality rate of 41% has been reported due to chickenpox pneumonia	Exposed pregnant women should receive varicella zoster immune globulin (VZIG) within 96 hours of exposure. VZIG has been shown to reduce maternal complication rate Infants born to mothers who had chicken pox 5 days prior to delivery to 2 days' postpartum are at greatest risk of varicella of newborn; VZIG should, therefore, be given to these newborns

Venous thromboembolism[59,60]	Deep venous thrombosis (DVT) of lower extremities in 0.0004–0.007% of pregnancies antepartum, but up to 3% postpartum Pulmonary embolism (PE) occurs in 1:2700 to less than 1:7000 pregnancies Should test for underlying hypercoagulable states (e.g., antiphospholipid antibodies, deficiencies of antithrombin III, protein C, protein S, plasminogen or factor V Leiden gene mutation) once thrombosis occurs	Only a problem when maternal hemodynamic integrity is compromised No fetal effects unless oral anticoagulants are given If there is an associated thrombophilia (inherited or acquired), there is an increased risk of stillbirth, preeclampsia, growth restriction	Pregnancy is a hypercoagulable state Diagnosis of DVT best made by combined ultrasound Doppler technique Clinical suspicion of PE should be investigated objectively. Begin with chest X-ray, followed by either V/Q scan or CT scan (with PE protocol). V/Q preferable because of less radiation delivered to fetus	Warfarin teratogenic between 6 and 12 weeks' gestation (nasal hypoplasia, stippled epiphyses). Warfarin best avoided throughout pregnancy for the treatment of VTE as it may cause fetal CNS problems, and there are safe and effective alternatives (heparin). Low molecular weight heparin provides reliable anticoagulation. Monitor Anti-Xa levels. Heparin should be discontinued at onset of labor and restarted 6 hours postpartum, or once hemostasis achieved Anticoagulation should be continued for 6 weeks postpartum, or until 3 months of treatment achieved when DVT occurred in index pregnancy; warfarin and heparin are both safe for breast-feeding Prophylactic heparin (either unfractionated heparin 5000 units SC q 12 hours, or low molecular weight heparin, starting at 12 weeks' gestation) recommended for history of unexplained DVT in previous pregnancy, antiphospholipid antibodies, or other hypercoagulable states

importance of preventive medicine and quality of life, it is no longer sufficient merely to see a woman affected with a medical disorder safely through pregnancy and delivery. Rather, it is important to adopt a more global approach, which in an interdisciplinary fashion encompasses prepregnancy counseling and obstetrical care and, in addition, addresses the medical and social factors that might influence the well-being of the child, the mother, and the family.

REFERENCES

1. Cunningham FG, MacDonald PC, Gant NF, et al. *Williams Obstetrics.* Stamford, CT: Appleton & Lange; 2005.
2. De Swiet M. *Medical Disorders in Obstetric Practice.* Malden, MA: Blackwell Science; 2002.
3. Mofenson LM. Reducing the risk of perinatal HIV -1 transmission with zidovudine: results and implications of AIDS Clinical Trials Group protocol 076. *Acta Paediatr Suppl.* 1997;421:89–96.
4. Riley LE, Yawetz S. Case records of the Massachusetts General Hospital. Case 32-2005. A 34-year old HIV-positive woman who desired to become pregnant. *N Engl J Med.* 2005;353(16):1725–1732.
5. Carp HJ. Antiphospholipid syndrome in pregnancy. *Curr Opin Obstet Gynecol.* 2004;16(2):129–135.
6. Lassere M, Empson M. Treatment of antiphospholipid syndrome in pregnancy: a systematic review of randomized therapeutic trials. *Thromb Res.* 2004;114(5–6):419–426.
7. Gardner MO, Doyle NM. Asthma in pregnancy. *Obstet Gynecol Clin N Am.* 2004;31:385–413.
8. Wendel PJ, Ramin SM, Barnett-Hamm C, et al. Asthma treatment in pregnancy: a randomized controlled study. *Am J Obstet Gynecol.* 1996;175(1):150–154.
9. Snow CF. Laboratory diagnosis of vitamin B12 and folate deficiency. *Arch Intern Med.* 1999;159:1297.
10. Chelghoum Y, Vey N, Raffoux E, et al. Acute leukemia during pregnancy: a report on 37 patients and a review of the literature. *Cancer.* 2005;104(1):110–117.
11. Weisz B, Schiff E, Lishner M. Cancer in pregnancy: maternal and fetal implications. *Hum Reprod Update.* 2001;7(4):384–393.
12. Ferrandina G, Distefano M, Testa A, et al. Management of an advanced ovarian cancer at 15 weeks of gestation: case report and literature review. *Gynecol Oncol.* 2005;97(2):693–696.
13. Edenborough FP. Women with cystic fibrosis and their potential for reproduction. *Thorax.* 2001;56:649–655.
14. Nelson CT, Demmler GI. Cytomegalovirus infection in the pregnant mother, fetus and newborn infant. *Clin Perinatol.* 1997;4(1):151–160.
15. Nigro G, Adler SP, La TR, et al. Passive immunization during pregnancy for congenital cytomegalovirus infection. *N Engl J Med.* 2005;353(13):1350–1362.
16. Reece EA. Diabetes in pregnancy. *Obstet Gynecol Clin North Am.* 1996;23(1):29–45.
17. Zahn CA, Morrell MJ, Collins SD, et al. Management issues for women with epilepsy: a review of the literature. *Neurology.* 1998;51:949–956.
18. Kaaja E, Kaaja R, Hiilesmaa V. Major malformations in offspring of women with epilepsy. Neurology 2003;60(4):575–579
19. Holmes L, Harris I, Oakley GP, et al. Teratology society consensus on use of folic acid to reduce the risk of birth defects. *Teratology.* 1997;55(6):381.
20. Braunwald E, ed. *Braunwald's Heart Disease: A Textbook of Cardiovascular Medicine.* Philadelphia, PA: Saunders; 2004.
21. Siu S, Colman JM. Cardiovascular problems and pregnancy: an approach to management. *Cleve Clin J of Med.* 2004;71(12):977–985.
22. Centers for Disease Control, Immunization Practices Advisory Committee. Prevention of perinatal transmission of hepatitis B virus: prenatal screening of all pregnant women for hepatitis B surface antigens. *MMWR.* 1988;37:341.
23. Hadžić N. Hepatitis C in pregnancy. *Arch Dis Child Neonatal Ed.* 2001;84:F201–F204.
24. Kane MA. Hepatitis viruses and the neonate. *Clin Perinatol.* 1997;24:181–192.
25. Kohl S. Neonatal herpes simplex virus infection. *Clin Perinatol.* 1997;24(1):129–150.
26. ACOG practice bulletin. Management of herpes in pregnancy. Number 8 October 1999. Clinical management guidelines for obstetrician-gynecologists. *Int J Gynaecol Obstet.* 2000;68(2):165–173.
27. Gibson CS, MacLennan AH, Goldwater PN, et al. Neurotropic viruses and cerebral palsy: population based case-control study. *BMJ.* 2006;332(7533):76–80.
28. von Dadelszen P, et al. The complications of hypertension in pregnancy. *Minerva Med.* 2005;96:287–302.
29. Sibai BM. Treatment of hypertension in pregnant women. *N Engl J Med.* 1996;335(4):257–265.
30. Kaplan PW, Repke JT. Eclampsia. *Neurol Clin.* 1994;12(3):565–582.
31. Masiukiewicz US, Burrow GN. Hyperthyroidism in pregnancy: diagnosis and treatment. *Thyroid.* 1999;9(7):647–652.
32. Haddow JE, Palomaki GE, Allan WC, et al. Maternal thyroid deficiency during pregnancy and subsequent neuropsychological development of the child. *N Engl J Med.* 1999;341:549–555.
33. Alexander EK, Marqusee E, Lawrence J, et al. Timing and magnitude of increases in levothyroxine requirements during pregnancy in women with hypothyroidism. *N Engl J Med.* 2004;351(3):241–249.
34. George J, Woolf SH et al. Idiopathic thrombocytopenic purpura: a practice guideline developed by explicit methods for the American Society of Hematology. *Blood.* 1996;88(1):3–40.
35. Webert KE, Mittal R, Sigouin C, et al. A retrospective 11-year analysis of obstetric patients with idiopathic thrombocytopenia purpura. *Blood.* 2003;102:4306–4311.
36. Korelitz BI. Inflammatory bowel disease and pregnancy. *Gastrointest Endosc Clin N Am.* 1998;27:213–221.
37. Mottet C, Juillerat P, Gonvers JJ, et al. Pregnancy and Crohn's disease. *Digestion.* 2005;71(1):54–61.
38. Whitty CJ, Edmonds S, Mutabingwa TK. Malaria in pregnancy. *BJOG.* 2005;112(9):1189–1195.
39. Goff M. Parvovirus B19 in pregnancy. *J Midwifery Womens Health.* 2005;50(6):536–538.
40. Jones DC, Hayslett JP. Outcome of pregnancy in women with moderate or severe renal insufficiency. *N Engl J Med.* 1996;335(4):226–232.
41. Lindheimer MD, Katz AI. Gestation in women with kidney disease: prognosis and management. *Baillière's Clinical Obstetrics and Gynecology.* 1994;8:387–393.
42. Lessan-Pezeshki M. Pregnancy after renal transplantation: points to consider. *Nephrol Dial Transplant.* 2002;17:703–707.
43. Rubella vaccination during pregnancy-United States, 1971-1988. *MMWR.* 1989;38:289–293.
44. ACOG Committee Opinion: number 281, December 2002. Rubella vaccination. *Obstet Gynecol.* 2002;100(6):1417.
45. Charache S, Neibyl JR. Pregnancy in sickle cell disease. *Clin Haematol.* 1985;14:729.
46. Koshy M, Burd L, Wallace D, et al. Prophylactic red-cell transfusions in pregnant patients with sickle cell disease. *N Engl J Med.* 1989;319:1447–1452.
47. Schuchat A, Whitney C, Zanfwill K. Prevention of perinatal group B streptococcal disease: a public health perspective. *MMWR.* 1996;45:1.

48. Hannah ME, Ohlsson A, Wang EEL, et al. Maternal colonization with group B Streptococifus and prelabor rupture of membranes at term: the role of induction of labor. *Am J Obstet Gynecol.* 1997;177:780–785.
49. Baker CJ. Group B streptococcal infections. *Clin Perinatol.* 1997;24(1):59–70.
50. Centers for Disease Control. Recommendations for diagnosing and treating syphilis in HIV-infected patients. *MMWR.* 1988;37:600.
51. Genç M, Ledger WJ. Syphilis in pregnancy. *Sex Transm Inf.* 2000;76:73–79.
52. Ramsey-Goldman R. Pregnancy in systemic lupus erythematosus. *Rheum Dis Clin North Am.* 1988;14:169–185.
53. Kravetz JD, Federman DG. Toxoplasmosis in pregnancy. *Am J Med.* 2005;118(3):212–216.
54. Laibl VR, Sheffield JS. Tuberculosis in pregnancy. *Clin Perinatol.* 2005:32(3):739–747.
55. Le J, Briggs GG, McKeown A, et al. Urinary tract infections during pregnancy. *Ann Pharmacother.* 2004;38(10):1692–1701.
56. Maikranz P, Lindheimer M, Coe F. Nephrolithiasis in pregnancy. Renal Disease in Pregnancy. *Baillieres Clin Obstet Gynaecol.* 1994;8(2):375–386.
57. Pastuszak AL, Levy M, Schick B, et al. Outcome after maternal varicella infection in the first 20 weeks of pregnancy. *N Engl J Med.* 1994;330:901–905.
58. Enders G, Miller E, Cradock-Watson J, et al. Consequences of varicella and herpes zoster in pregnancy: prospective study of 1739 cases. *Lancet.* 1994;343:1543–1550.
59. Greer IA. Thrombosis series: Thrombosis in pregnancy: maternal and fetal issues. *Lancet.* 1999;353:1258–1265.
60. Ginsberg JS. Use of antithrombotic agents during pregnancy. *Chest.* 2001;119:22S–131S.

CHAPTER 11

DEPRESSION AND ANTIDEPRESSANT USE IN PREGNANCY

Sanjog Kalra and Adrienne Einarson

A substantial number of women of childbearing age suffer from depression. A recent American prevalence study screened 3472 pregnant women for depressive symptoms with the Centre for Epidemiologic Studies-Depression scale (CES-D). The authors found that, of the women surveyed, 20% scored above the cutoff for depressive symptoms with more than16 points.[1] A British study documented in 2001 that maternal depression during pregnancy has been relatively neglected in favor of postnatal depression, even though it is more prevalent and approximately 25% of post partum depressive episodes actually began during pregnancy.[2]

Recent evidence suggests that prevalence of depression during pregnancy varies throughout pregnancy, at 7.4% in the first trimester, 12.8% in the second trimester and 12.0% in the third trimester.[3] In this chapter, we provide a complete review of safety data regarding the use of antidepressants in pregnancy.

TRICYCLIC ANTIDEPRESSANTS (TCAs)

Although widely prescribed since their introduction, use of TCAs has decreased significantly. Their decline in popularity is most frequently attributed to the advent of newer medications with preferable side effect profiles. TCA exposure during the first trimester of pregnancy has been addressed in 3 prospective and over 10 retrospective studies examining an excess of 700 pregnancies and their outcomes. Although these studies have evaluated the risks associated with prenatal TCAs exposure as a group, both individual and pooled results of these studies suggest that TCA use in pregnancy is not associated with an increased risk of congenital malformations above the baseline.[4]

SELECTIVE SEROTONIN REUPTAKE INHIBITORS (SSRIs)

SSRI antidepressants, are amongst the most widely prescribed drugs in the world today. There are several hypotheses regarding the pharmacodynamic characteristics of these agents. The members of this class differ, however, in their respective affinities and selectivities for the 5-HT reuptake mechanism and their respective pharmacokinetics. SSRIs show remarkable selectivity towards the serotonergic system over the noradrenergic or cholinergic systems and as such, have much wider therapeutic windows and more favorable tolerability profiles compared to earlier antidepressant medications.[5]

Fluoxetine (Prozac)

Fluoxetine, a prototypical SSRI, is the most studied member of this group during pregnancy and is currently the only SSRI for which long-term neurodevelopmental studies have been completed. Fluoxetine has been shown to cross the placenta in both animal and human placental kinetics studies and crosses the placenta to a greater degree than all other SSRIs, with the exception of citalopram.[6]

To date, over 1700 pregnancies exposed to fluoxetine at varying stages of gestation have been examined. None of these 10 studies, of which 7 are prospective and 3 are retrospective have found any association with fluoxetine exposure and an increase in the risk of major malformations above the 1–3% baseline risk for malformations that exists in the general population.[7]

Paroxetine (Paxil)

To date, some data concerning the safety of prenatal paroxetine use is available. Published reports of 274 prospectively followed pregnancies exposed to paroxetine at varying stages of gestation are available. No evidence linking prenatal paroxetine use to an increase in the risk of major malformations above the baseline risk has been found.[7]

Citalopram (Celexa)

Citalopram is a relatively new SSRI antidepressant. Several studies evaluating the effects of gestational citalopram use are available. A human placental kinetics study showed that citalopram crosses the human placenta to a greater degree than all other SSRIs (with the exception of fluvoxamine, whose placental kinetics have yet to be examined.[6]

One study prospectively evaluated 364 women exposed to citalopram in early gestation. No statistically significant increase in the rate of major malformations above the baseline was observed in this study.[8] The most recent study evaluating the use of citalopram during pregnancy has been completed at The Motherisk Program. To date, this study has prospectively identified and assessed the outcome of 132 women exposed to citalopram 108 (81%) in the first trimester and 71 (54%) throughout the pregnancy. Results of this study did not find an increase above the baseline for major malformations.[9]

Sertraline (Zoloft)

Data on the safety of sertraline in pregnancy is available. In a study by Hendrick et al. sertraline was shown to cross the human placenta significantly less than all other SSRIs (with the exception of fluvoxamine, which was not evaluated).[6] To date, prospective data on 181 pregnancies from a data base[8] and a second multicenter, prospective, cohort controlled study followed 147 women exposed to sertraline in the first trimester and there was no increase in the rates of major malformations.[7]

Fluvoxamine (Luvox)

Very limited data is available regarding the use of fluvoxamine during pregnancy. To date, placental kinetics of this agent have not been established.

As part of a retrospective study by the European Network of Teratology Information Services (ENTIS), the outcomes of 66 women with early pregnancy exposure to fluvoxamine were examined. Of these women, 49 gave birth to live infants with 1 malformation amongst them. It should be noted that the rates of major malformations were no different than those observed in the general population.[10] As well 26 women exposed to fluvoxamine in the first trimester were included in the meta-analysis of newer antidepressants.[7]

OTHER ANTIDEPRESSANTS

Venlafaxine (Effexor)

Venlafaxine, a phenethylamine bicyclic derivative is a structurally novel agent indicated for the treatment of major depressive disorder, most often in SSRI refractory disease. Venlafaxine achieves its antidepressant effects via potentiation of central neurotransmission through selective noradrenaline and serotonin reuptake inhibition. It is associated with relatively mild adverse effects, likely owing to its low affinity for central cholinergic or histaminergic receptors.[11]

To date, one prospective study conducted by the Motherisk Program evaluating the safety of venlafaxine use in pregnancy is available. In this multicenter, prospective, comparison study, 150 women exposed in early gestation to venlafaxine (35 exposed throughout pregnancy) were examined. The rates of major malformations were not above baseline.[12]

Bupropion (Wellbutrin/Zyban)

Bupropion is marketed as both an antidepressant and an aid for smoking cessation. This aminoketone compound, which chemically unrelated to all tricyclic, tetracyclic and SSRI antidepressants achieves its antidepressant effects via a mechanism that is as yet not well understood but is thought to entail modifications of central dopaminergic and noradrenergic pathways.[13]

Manufacturer data is available on 226 pregnancies exposed to bupropion at various stages in pregnancy. The outcomes of these pregnancies suggest no increase in the rate of major malformations due to bupropion exposure.[14] A recent prospective study from The Motherisk program, was published that evaluated the safety of bupropion use in pregnancy, both as an antidepressant and as a smoking cessation aid. One hundred thirty-six women exposed to bupropion in early gestation or throughout pregnancy were prospectively identified and the outcomes of these pregnancies were compared to those of two comparison groups exposed to other antidepressants or nonteratogens. There were no reports of any malformations. This study examined the safety of bupropion in pregnancy, when used as an antidepressant and/or as a smoking cessation aid. As such, several comparisons were carried out both within and between groups. When compared to the nonteratogen comparison group, the number of spontaneous abortions seen in the group exposed to bupropion for either indication was significantly elevated (14.7% vs. 4.5%; $p < 0.009$). In contrast, when pregnancy outcomes in women using bupropion as an antidepressant only, (15.4%) were compared to those of women using other antidepressants (12.3%) or women exposed only to nonteratogens (6.7%), no significant differences in the rates of spontaneous abortions were found between groups ($p < 0.18$). As such, the above study did account for the effects of nicotine on pregnant outcome by matching the bupropion exposed group with comparators for smoking status and the number of cigarettes smoked per day. There were no differences in the rates of spontaneous abortions among the depressed and smoking women (15.4% vs. 16.2%).[15]

Trazodone and Nefazodone

Both trazodone and nefazodone are phenylpiperazine antidepressants whose antidepressant effects occur via central noradrenergic and serotonerigic reuptake inhibition. The sedative effects associated with trazodone are like due to its affinity for central cholinergic and α-adrenergic receptors.[16]

Currently, one study examining the safety of trazodone and nefazodone during pregnancy has been conducted, in which 147 women exposed to either drug in the first trimester (52 of whom continued either drug throughout gestation) were identified. Upon statistical analysis, no differences in the rates of major malformations were found between any of the groups. There were; however, more spontaneous abortions seen in both the nefazodone and trazodone exposed group (13.6%) and the antidepressant exposed group (11.5%) compared to the nonteratogen comparison group (8.1%), however, these differences did not reach statistical significance.[17]

Mirtazapine (Remeron)

Mirtazapine is a new antidepressant that potentiates central noradrenergic and serotonergic activity.[18] To date, there are no prospective, comparative studies that have been published regarding the safety of mirtazapine use in pregnancy. Currently, Motherisk is conducting a prospective, multicentre, comparative study on the safety of mirtazepine during pregnancy. Preliminary data (96 cases) shows no increase risk for major malformations.[19]

St. John's Wort (SJW)

The most common herbal therapy for depression in use today is *Hypericum perforatum*, more commonly known as St. John's Wort. This herbal agent is thought to mediate its antidepressant activities via hyperforin mediated inhibition of noradrenergic and serotonergic reuptake.[20] There are no prospective studies available on SJW use in pregnancy. Currently, Motherisk is conducting a study on the safety of St. John's Wort in pregnancy.

Monoamine Oxidase Inhibitors (MAOIs)

The use of MAOIs in pregnancy has not been well studied, mainly because they are used infrequently as drugs of *last resort.* Human data concerning MAOI safety during pregnancy is limited. A published case series associated MAOI use in pregnancy with an increased incidence of major malformations.[21] Specific details concerning the exposures or malformations, however, were unavailable.

Given the paucity of data available, its potential interactions with medications such as terbutaline (hypertensive crisis) and the availability of other more studied antidepressants, the use of MAOIs during pregnancy probably should be avoided.

Long-term Neurodevelopmental Effects of Antidepressants on the Offspring. Studies performed to date are limited (albeit reassuring), have not followed the exposed children further than 4 years old and have only been published on fluoxetine and TCAs, Nulman et al. from Motherisk, conducted a long-term assessment of temperament, mood arousability, activity level, distractibility and most importantly, global IQ and language development in children of

80 women exposed to TCAs and 55 women exposed to fluoxetine in the first trimester of pregnancy. Assessment of language development and IQ occurred between 16 and 86 months postnatal age. No significant differences between the groups were detected in any of the parameters examined.[22]

A second long-term neurodevelopmental follow-up conducted by the same author examined the offspring of 40 women exposed to TCAs and 46 women exposed to fluoxetine throughout gestation and compared them to those of 36 nonteratogen exposed women, in terms of language development, global IQ and temperament between 15 and 71 months postnatal age. In their analyses, this group also adjusted for the effects of duration and severity of maternal depression, duration of pharmacological treatment, number of depression episodes after delivery, maternal IQ, socioeconomic status, cigarette smoking, and alcohol use. No association between gestational use of TCAs or fluoxetine and language development, global IQ or temperament was observed. In contrast, global IQ was negatively associated with duration of depression and language development was negatively correlated with the number of postnatal depressive episodes, suggesting that the children of depressed mothers have decreased global IQ and language development in comparison to the children prenatally euthymic women.[23]

Abrupt Discontinuation Syndrome

Given that at least 50% of pregnancies are unplanned, many women may not become aware of their pregnancies well into the first trimester. These women may abruptly discontinue taking all medications, including antidepressants, in attempts to minimize drug exposure to their fetuses. Abrupt discontinuation of certain antidepressants may be associated with a *discontinuation syndrome*, characterized by any or all of the following: nausea and vomiting, diarrhea, diaphoresis, hot or cold flashes, tremors, excess lacrimation, syncope, anxiety, panic attacks, low energy, fatigue, and mood swings. Most critically, sudden discontinuation of antidepressants has been associated with relapse of the underlying psychiatric condition. Einarson and colleagues interviewed 36 pregnant women 1 month after they received counseling regarding the safety of antidepressant use in pregnancy. They found that 34 of these women discontinued their medication abruptly (28 on the advice of their health-care providers). Of these women, 26 (70.3%) reported deteriorating physical and psychological health. Eleven of these women reported suicidal ideation and 4 were admitted to hospital.[24]

Untreated Depression in Pregnancy

The issue of not treating depression during pregnancy is emerging as an important issue which requires addressing. A study found that untreated depression during pregnancy may have deleterious effects on peripartum and neonatal outcomes, such as more cesarean sections and a greater number of admissions to neonatal intensive care units.[25] A woman who is depressed may also make other poor decisions during her pregnancy, such as drinking alcohol and not attending her obstetrician's appointments, etc.[26] In addition, a woman who is depressed may also have difficulty bonding with her child after birth and may experience other adverse attachment behaviors.[27]

Increase Risk for Spontaneous Abortions

In several of the studies that have been published, a higher rate of spontaneous abortions in the antidepressant group compared to the nonteratogen group has been noted. However, because of the small sample sizes, there was no statistical significance in any of the results. Recently, at Motherisk we published a meta-analysis in which 15 potential articles, 6 cohort studies of 3567 women (1534 exposed, 2033 nonexposed) provided extractable data to assess the rates of spontaneous abortions. All were matched on important confounders. Tests found no heterogeneity [chi(2) 3.13; p = 0.98], and all quality scores were adequate (>50%). The baseline SA rate (95% CI) was 8.7% (7.5–9.9%; n = 2033). For antidepressants, the rate was 12.4% (10.8–14.1%; n = 1534), significantly increased by 3.9% (1.9–6.0%); RR was 1.45 (1.19–1.77; n = 3567). No differences were found among antidepressant classes.[28]

In summary, the body of evidence in the literature to date suggests that antidepressants as a group are relatively safe to take during pregnancy and women and their health care providers should not be unduly concerned if a woman requires treatment. Just as important, it must also be noted that evidence is emerging that untreated depression can exert its own risk, not only on maternal health but also on the health of the infant. It is logical that a woman who is in optimal mental health will be the best mother she can be to her baby. This evidence-based information will empower women and their healthcare providers to make an informed decision on whether or not to take an antidepressant during pregnancy.

REFERENCES

1. Evans J, Heron, J, Francomb H, et al. Cohort study of depressed mood during pregnancy and after childbirth. *BMJ.* 2001;323:257–260.
2. Marcus SM, Flynn HA, Blow FC, et al. Depressive symptoms among pregnant women screened in obstetric settings. Journal of Women's Health volume 12, number 4, 2003.
3. Bennett HA, Einarson A, Taddio A, et al. Prevalence of depression during pregnancy: systematic review. *Obstet Gynecol.* 2004;103(4): 698–709.
4. Wen SW, Walker M. Risk of fetal exposure to tricyclic antidepressants. *J Obstet Gynaecol Can.* 2004 Oct;26(10):887–892.
5. Preskorn SH, Fast GA. Therapeutic drug monitoring for antidepressants: efficacy, safety, and cost effectiveness. *J Clin Psychiatry.* 1991 Jun;52 Suppl:23–33.
6. Hendrick V, Stowe ZN, Altshuler LL, et al. Placental passage of antidepressant medications. *Am J Psychiatry.* 2003 May;160(5):993–996.
7. Einarson TR, Einarson A. Newer antidepressants in pregnancy and rates of major malformations: a meta-analysis of prospective comparative studies. *Pharmacoepidemiol Drug Saf.* 2005 Dec;14(12):823–827.
8. Ericson A, Kallen B, Wiholm B. Delivery outcome after the use of antidepressants in early pregnancy. *Eur J Clin Pharmacol.* 1999 Sep;55(7):503–508.
9. Sivojelezova A, Shubaiber SA, Einarson Koren G. Prospective comparative study of citalopram in pregnancy. In press: *Am J Obstet Gynecol.* 2005 Dec;193(6):2006–2009.
10. McElhatton PR, Garbis HM, Elefant E, et al. The outcome of pregnancy in 689 women exposed to therapeutic doses of antidepressants.

A collaborative study of the European Network of Teratology Information Services (ENTIS). *Reprod Toxicol.* 1996 Jul–Aug;10(4):285–294.
11. Ward HE. The newer antidepressants. *IM Inter Med.* 1997;18(7): 65–76.
12. Einarson A, Fatoye B, Sarkar M, et al. Pregnancy outcome following gestational exposure to venlafaxine: a multicenter prospective controlled study. *Am J Psychiatry.* 2001;158:1728–1730.
13. Ascher JA, Cole JO, Colin JN, et al. Bupropion: a review of its mechanism of antidepressant activity. *J Clin Psychiatry.* 1995 Sep;56(9):395–401.
14. Personal communication. Glaxo-Smith-Kline. Mississauga, Ontario, Canada 2004.
15. Chan B, Koren G, Fayez I, et al. Pregnancy outcome of women exposed to bupropion during pregnancy: A prospective comparative study. *Am J Obstet Gynecol.* 2005 Mar;192(3):932–936.
16. Product mongraph Bristol—Myersd Squibb. Monteal, Quebec, Canada 2001.
17. Einarson A, Bonari L, Voyer-Lavigne S, et al. A multicentre prospective controlled study to determine the safety of trazodone and nefazodone use during pregnancy. *Can J Psychiatry.* 2003 Mar;48(2):106–110.
18. Product Monograph, Organon Roseland New Jersey, USA, 2003.
19. Djulus J, Koren G, Wilton L, et al. Exposure to mirtazepine during pregnancy: a prospective comparative study of birth outcomes. (Abstract) 18th International OTIS meeting, St. Pete's Beach, Florida, USA, June 2005.
20. Goldman R, Koren G. Taking St. John's Wort during pregnancy. *Can Fam Physician.* 2003;49:29–30.
21. Cohen LS, Nonacs R. Assessment and treatment of depression during pregnancy: an update. *Psychiatr Clin North Am.* 2003 Sep;26(3): 547–562.
22. Nulman I, Rovet J, Stewart DE, et al. Neurodevelopment of children exposed in utero to antidepressant drugs. *N Engl J Med.* 1997; 336:258–262.
23. Nulman I, Rovet J, Stewart DE, et al. Child development following exposure to tricyclic antidepressants or fluoxetine throughout fetal life: a prospective, controlled study. *Am J Psychiatry.* 2002 Nov; 159(11):1889–1895.
24. Einarson A, Selby P, Koren G. Abrupt discontinuation of psychotropic drugs due to fears of teratogenic risk and the impact of counseling. *J Psychiatry Neurosci.* 2001;26(1):44-889–894.
25. Chung TK, Lau TK, Yip AS, et al. Antepartum depressive symptomatology is associated with adverse obstetric and neonatal outcomes. *Psychosom Med.* 2001;63:830–834.
26. Orr ST, Miller CA. Maternal depressive symptoms and the risk of poor pregnancy outcome. Review of the literature and preliminary findings. *Epidemiol Rev.* 1995;17:165–171.
27. Ashman SB, Dawson G, Panagiotides H, et al. Stress hormone levels of children of depressed mothers. *Dev Psychopathol.* 2002;14: 333–349.
28. Hemels ME, Einarson A, Koren G, et al. Antidepressant use during pregnancy and the rates of spontaneous abortions: a meta-analysis. *Ann Pharmacother.* 2005 May 22;39(5):803–809.

CHAPTER 12

NEONATAL POOR ADAPTATION SYNDROME FOLLOWING IN UTERO EXPOSURE TO ANTIDEPRESSANTS

Alaa Ali, Nobuko Taguchi, and Adrienne Einarson

BACKGROUND

Given that depression in pregnancy affects approximately 10–20% of women, there is a clinical demand for safe and effective treatment for these patients with an antidepressant medication.[1] Serotonin reuptake inhibitors (SSRI), serotonin and norepinephrine reuptake inhibitors (SNRI) are antidepressants being prescribed for depression, panic disorder, and obsessive-compulsive disorder during pregnancy. Due to the good documentation of efficacy, relatively few adverse effects, and safety in overdose, SSRIs/SNRIs are currently the drug of choice for pregnant women.[2]

A number of epidemiologic studies on hundreds of pregnant women exposed to SSRIs/SNRIs have been published. According to those studies, SSRIs/SNRIs prescribed for depression, panic disorder, and obsessive-compulsive disorder in pregnancy have not been found to increase the baseline rate of major malformations.[3]

Drugs that can cause dependence in adults have been reported to be associated with neonatal withdrawal syndrome.[4] Opiates (heroin, methadone, morphine, etc.), benzodiazepines and barbiturates are established as drugs that cause neonatal withdrawal symptoms.[5] There is no report in literature regarding adverse effects from bupropion, trazodone, nefazodone, mirtazapine. Affected infants have symptoms from different organs, most frequently from the central nervous system and the gastrointestinal system.

With the increasing number of the prescription of SSRIs/SNRIs, there were some reports describing complications in some babies whose mothers used a variety of SSRIs near term. Also, given that there were reports suggesting increased admission to the neonatal intensive care unit (NICU) in the neonates exposed to SSRIs during the last trimester, investigators assessed SSRI/SNRI use in late pregnancy and its relation to poor neonatal adaptation. This chapter focuses on the pharmacology of SSRIs/SNRIs, existing studies on neonatal poor adaptability, and the management of those neonates who developed adverse effects after the exposure to SSRIs/SNRIs in utero.

PHARMACOLOGY

The antidepressants in the SSRI group have different pharmacokinetic properties. Hence, they could possibly differ in their potential for causing poor neonatal adaptation effects. SSRI and SNRI act centrally by increasing levels of serotonin and/or norepinephrine. All members of these classes have been shown to cross the placenta and enter the fetal circulation in measurable quantities, but only the free fraction of any drug is available to cross the placenta. In a study by Hendrick et al, they examined the placental passage of various SSRIs in 38 women near term. They found that citalopram crossed the placenta to the greatest degree (as measured by ratios of umbilical cord to maternal serum drug concentrations), followed by fluoxetine, paroxetine, and sertraline.[6]

In adults receiving SSRIs, abrupt discontinuation of those medications has been associated with a withdrawal syndrome. Characterized by irritability, insomnia, nausea, vomiting, diarrhea, sweating, hot or cold flashes, tremors, dizziness, and vertigo. The syndrome has been shown in adults to be more prevalent with paroxetine than with fluoxetine and sertraline, possibly due to the shorter elimination half-life of the former.[7,8]

There are two main factors that contribute to the pharmacokinetic changes due to pregnancy: (1) maternal physiological changes, and (2) the effect of the placental fetal compartment.[9] Factors that affect drug absorption, distribution, metabolism, and elimination in pregnancy would include increased volume of distribution, decreased drug-binding capacity, decreased plasma albumin levels, increased hepatic metabolism due to liver enzyme induction, increased renal clearance, delayed gastric emptying, and decreased gastrointestinal motility.[10]

Theoretically, the longer the half-life, the lower the risk of these symptoms, because the drug is gradually excreted from the body of the newborn. This is the reason why the symptoms appear with different severity in different infants exposed to SSRIs in the last trimester. The reported rate of withdrawal reaction was 10 times higher with paroxetine (0.3/1000) than with sertraline and fluvoxamine (0.03), and 100 times higher than with fluoxetine (0.002).[11]

There are also pharmacokinetic differences in antidepressants, which could partially explain their different withdrawal effects. Sertraline and citalopram use cytochrome P450 3A3/4 and 2C19, and paroxetine and fluoxetine are mainly metabolized by 2D6. Paroxetine and fluoxetine inhibit the metabolism of 2D4, presenting a nonlinier kinetics, which produces a rise in the half-life with high doses or long-term treatment. Other enzymes such as 3A3/4, 2C19, and 2C9/10 are also induced in fluoxetine's metabolism, and its metabolites still have a pharmacological effect and a long half-life. In the case of paroxetine, due to the existence of another enzyme of high capacity and the fact that metabolites have no pharmacological effect, it has the shortest half-life among SSRIs, despite the potential increased half-life. In support of the kinetic explanation, venlafaxine, which has a rapid clearance, can also have a high level of withdrawal reaction.[12]

EXISTING DATA ON NEONATAL POOR ADAPTATION

SSRI withdrawal symptoms in adults include nonspecific symptoms such as dizziness, paresthesia, tremor, anxiety, nausea, and vomiting. The symptoms occur two days after the last dose and continue for an average of 10 days and these symptoms were explained as hyposerotonergic state.[8]

Along with reports describing complications in some babies whose mothers used a variety of antidepressants near term, there are some studies evaluating SSRIs in late pregnancy and its relation to neonatal poor adaptability syndrome (Table 12-1). Four of the existing studies, which we have identified, were prospective and two were retrospective studies. All those studies described a similar pattern of symptoms that are consistent with neonatal SSRI withdrawal (Table 12-1).

In Chamber's study regarding fluoxetine and neonatal poor adaptability, 31.5% of the infants exposed to fluoxetine in the last trimester had poor adaptation, including respiratory difficulty, cyanosis on feeding and shivering, which means that these symptoms are not rare. Chambers et al. identified a relative risk of 8.7 for this poor neonatal adaptation following exposure to SSRI near term.[13] Costi et al. found respiratory distress necessitating intensive care support in 9 cases out of 55 exposed to fluoxetine throughout pregnancy or near term. This had a relative risk of 9.3 for neonatal distress in the exposed group compared to the nonexposed group of infants in whom antidepressants were discontinued early in pregnancy.[14] Hendrick et al. detected respiratory difficulty, diagnosed as respiratory distress syndrome or transient tachypnea of the newborn, in 9 out of 85 babies exposed to fluoxetine, sertraline, paroxetine, citalopram and/or fluvoxamine throughout pregnancy, compared to 1 out of 53 infants experiencing respiratory symptom when antidepressant use was discontinued in early pregnancy.[15] Kallen examined 997 Swedish born infants exposed to antidepressants (558 of which were exposed to SSRIs) throughout pregnancy and they found significant risks for low Apgar score (OR 2.33), hypoglycemia (OR 1.62), neonatal convulsions (OR 1.9), and respiratory distress (OR 2.21) in these neonates.[16] Laine et al. compared 20 neonates exposed to fluoxetine or citalopram in utero with 20 matched controls. They noted significantly higher serotonin-related

Table 12-1
Epidemiological Studies on Neonatal Complications after Maternal SSRI Use in Late Pregnancy

STUDY	DESIGN	MEDICATIONS	OUTCOME
Chambers et al.	Prospective cohort study	Fluoxetine during 3rd trimester: n = 73 infants Fluoxetine during 1st and 2nd trimester only n = 101 infants	RR (95% CI) late versus early exposure Special care nursery 2.6 (1.1–6.9) Poor neonatal adaptation* 8.7 (2.9–26.6)
Costei et al.	Prospective cohort study	Paroxetine during 3rd trimester: n = 55 Control group: n = 54 (27 paroxetine during 1st and 2nd trimester and 27 nonteratogenic drugs)	12/55 infants exposed during 3rd trimester experienced complications (respiratory distress n = 9) OR for neonatal respiratory distress 9.53 (95% CI = 1.14–79.30)
Hendrick et al.	Large case series	Fluoxetine n = 73 Sertraline n = 36 Paroxetine n = 19 Citalopram n = 7 Fluvoxamine n = 3 Total n = 138 pregnant women, 131 at delivery	Investigators concluded that rate of neonatal complications after prenatal exposure to SSRIs (n = 28) within general population rates
Oberlander et al.	Prospective cohort study	SSRI (paroxetine, fluoxetine, or sertraline) ± clonazepam during 2nd and 3rd trimester n = 46 Nonexposed control group n = 23	Poor neonatal adaptation* (all with respiratory distress) in 14/46 (30%) of infants with SSRI exposure and 2/23 (9%) of control infants (likelihood ratio = 5.64, 95% CI = 1.1–25.3)
Kallen	Swedish Medical Registry data	Tricyclic antidepressants n = 395 SSRIs n = 558 (citalopram n = 285, paroxetine n = 106, fluoxetine n = 91 or sertraline n = 77) Other antidepressant n = 63 (venlafaxine n = 24)	OR (95% CI) SSRI-exposed infants compared with all infants in registry Respiratory distress 1.97 (1.38–2.83) Hypoglycemia 1.35 (0.90–2.03) apgar score 2.28 (1.27–4.10) Convulsions risk ratio 3.6 (1.0–9.3)
Sanz et al.	Analysis of WHO database of adverse drug reactions (Bayesian confidence propagation neural network)	Paroxetine n = 64 Fluoxetine n = 14 Sertraline n = 9 Citalopram n = 7 (1 patient receiving both paroxetine and paroxetine)	By November 2003, 93 suspected cases of SSRI-induced neonatal withdrawal reported and regarded as enough information to confirm a possible causal relation.

* Poor neonatal adaptation defined as reported jitteriness, tachypnea, hypoglycemia, hypothermia, poor tone, and respiratory distress, weak or absent cry or desaturation on feeding.

neurological symptoms in exposed versus nonexposed infants. The exposed infants had significantly lower umbilical cord blood concentrations of a serotonin metabolite, 5-hydroxyindolacetic acid (5-HIAA), compared to nonexposed infants. Interestingly, a significant, negative correlation was found between cord blood 5-HIAA concentrations and the presence of serotonin-related symptoms in the SSRI exposed neonates.[17] More recently in 2004, Oberlander et al. reported the appearance of symptoms reported in the previous studies was 30% of the SSRIs exposed in late pregnancy, when compared to 9% in controls (RR 3.3).[18] The increased risks for the appearance of a neonatal discontinuation syndrome following SSRI use near term suggest that neonates born to mothers using SSRI medication near term should be closely monitored.

Poor Neonatal Adaptation Syndrome. Clinical manifestation of poor neonatal adaptation includes symptoms, such as jitteriness, tachycardia, hypothermia, vomiting, hypoglycemia, irritability, constant crying, increased tonus, eating/sleeping difficulties, convulsions, respiratory distress which vary from transient and self-limiting, aspiration, pneumothorax, and infections. This syndrome occurs when infants who have been exposed in utero to certain drugs abruptly discontinue (due to the fact of being born) exposure to the drug at birth.[7]

Although the mechanism underlying these symptoms is not well understood, they may result from either a type of serotonin syndrome in the infant (a toxicity phenomenon) or from withdrawal. Serotonin syndrome is characterized by confusion, restlessness, myoclonus, hyperreflexia, diaphoresis, tremor, incoordination, and hyperthermia. It is typically encountered in adults taking more than one medication, which causes elevation in brain serotonin, although the mild serotoninergic symptoms may be encountered in patients receiving therapeutic doses of SSRIs.[14]

Withdrawal or Serotonergic Toxicity. Neonatal serum concentrations of SSRIs have been reported to be low after maternal use in late pregnancy, which is compatible with withdrawal syndrome rather than with serotonin syndrome. On the contrary, Knoppert et al. recently measured the infant serum paroxetine level for an infant who developed hypertonicity, arching and mouthing. They found paroxetine level was high while the infant was symptomatic, and the symptoms subsided with decreasing paroxetine concentration in the blood. Careful assessment of neonatal SSRI level will be necessary to distinguish between cases of withdrawal and those of serotonin toxicity.[19]

Management

Physicians should discuss the risks and benefits of taking untidepressants in pregnancy. If clinicians identify those cases with exposure to SSRIs/SNRIs in late pregnancy, it is important that the babies are observed for longer than the typical 1–2 days post partum, to be able to detect neonatal symptomatology. In most cases, infants with symptoms are treated conservatively with observation in a NICU. Respiratory support is seldom required. Investigation should be conducted to rule out exposure to other toxic agents (e.g., benzodiazepine, opioids, ethanol), infectious agents (e.g., bacterial and viral causes). Phenobarbital is most commonly used to mitigate the irritability, rigidity and seizures, due to its long-established safety record in neonates.[19]

If the symptoms are neonatal SSRI withdrawal syndrome, it would make sense to treat it with an SSRI with a long elimination half-life such as fluoxetine. Presently, fluoxetine is the only SSRI for which an oral solution is available. Although no prospective randomized control trials support its safety and efficacy of giving SSRI/SNRI to the baby, 1 case report describes an infant with signs of SNRI withdrawal and undetectable serum level of venlafaxine.[20]

Discontinuation of antidepressants during pregnancy can lead to serious maternal morbidity, including miscarriage, preterm birth, suicidal ideation, need for hospitalization and even replacing the drug with alcohol to combat withdrawal effects.[21] On the other hand, the neonatal syndrome appears to be a self limited and treatable transient condition. Based on the reports that showed in utero exposure to antidepressants can cause complications after birth, the FDA and Health Canada recently instructed manufacturers of antidepressants to issue warnings about perinatal complications associated with their products.[22,23] Given that the symptoms are usually self-limiting, this recommendation could bring mothers and their babies to an unreasonable health risk. Also, tapering the drug at the late pregnancy may increase the risk of postpartum depression. The overall health of the mother is an important determinant for the well-being of the infant. Thus, the transient neonatal symptoms may be less harmful, considering the potentially serious outcome to the mother's health.

In summary, the evidence suggests that discontinuation of clinically-needed antidepressants, for women near term, is unwarranted and may put the mother at an unjustified perinatal risk. Neonatal symptomatology occurs in a minority of cases, and is self-limited. A careful risk-benefit assessment should be done by a responsible health-care provider on a case by case basis, and the informed decision should be made by the patient.

REFERENCES

1. Bennett HA, Einarson A, Taddio A, et al. Prevalence of depression during pregnancy. Systemic review. *Obstet Gynecol.* 2004;103: 698–709.
2. American Academy of Pediatrics Committee on Drugs. Use of psychoactive medication during pregnancy and possible effects on the fetus and newborn. *Pediatrics.* 2000;105:880–887.
3. Einarson A, Einarson TR. Newer antidepressants in pregnancy and rates of major malformations: A meta-analysis of prospective comparative studies. *Pharmacoepidemiol Drug Saf.* 2005 Mar 1.
4. Webster PA. Withdrawal symptoms in neonates associated with maternal antidepressant therapy. *Lancet.* 1973;2:318–319.
5. American academy of Pediatrics. Committee on drugs. Neonatal drug withdrawal. *Pediatrics.* 1998;101:1079–1088.
6. Hendrick V, Stowe ZN, Altshuler LL, et al. Placental passage of antidepressant medications. *Am J Psychiatry.* 2003;160:993–996.
7. Rosenbaum JF, Fava M, Hoog SL, et al. Selective serotonin reuptake inhibitor discontinuation syndrome: a randomized clinical trial. *Biol Psychiatry.* 1998;44:77–87.
8. Newport JD, Hostetter A, Arnold A, et al. The treatment of postpartum depression: minimizing infant exposure. *J Clin Phyiachatry.* 2002;63 (suppl 7):31–44.
9. Koren G. Maternal-Fetal Toxicology: A Clinician's Guide. Dekker M (ed), New York 2001;2–8:767–789.
10. Stowe ZN, Nemeroff CB. Psychopharmacology during pregnancy and lactation. Textbook of Psychopharmacology. Schatzberg AF, Nemeroff CB (eds) American Psychiatric Press, Washington, DC 1998:823–837.

11. Price JS, Waller PC, Wood SM, et al. A comparison of the post-marketing safety of the four selective SSRIs including the investigation of symptoms occurring on withdrawal. *Br J Clin Pharmacol.* 1996; 42:757–763.
12. Sanz EJ, De-las-Cuevas C, Kiuru A, et al. Selective serotonin reuptake inhibitors in pregnant women and neonatal withdrawal syndrome: a database analysis. *Lancet.* 2005;365:482–487.
13. Chambers CD, Johnson KA, Dick LM, et al. Birth outcomes in pregnant women taking fluoxetine. *N Engl J Med.* 1996;335:1010–1015.
14. Costi AM, Kozer E, HO T, et al. Perinatal outcome following third trimester exposure to paroxetine. *Arch Pediatr Adolesc Med.* 2002; 156:1192–1132.
15. Hendrick V, Smith LM, Suri R, et al. Birth outcomes after prenatal exposure to antidepressant medication. *Am J Obstet Gynecol.* 2003; 188(3):812–815.
16. Kallen. Neonate characteristics after maternal use of antidepressants in late pregnancy. *Arch Pediatr Adolesc Med.* 2004;158:312–316.
17. Laine K, Heikkinen T, Ekblad U, et al. Effects of exposure to selective serotonin reuptake inhibitors during pregnancy on serotoenergic symptoms in newborns and cord blood monoamine and prolactin concentrations. *Arch Gen Psychiatry.* 2003;60:720–726.
18. Oberlander TF, Misri s, Fitzderald CE, et al. Pharmacologic factors associated with transient neonatal symptoms following prenatal psychotropic medication exposure. *J Clin Psychiatry.* 2004;65:230–237.
19. Koren G, Matsui D, Einarson A, et al. Is maternal use of selective serotonin reuptake inhibitors in the third trimester of pregnancy harmful to neonates? *CMAJ.* 2005;172:1457–1459.
20. deMoor RA, Mourad L, ter Haar J, et al. Withdrawal symptoms in a neonate following exposure to venlafaxine during pregnancy. *Ned Tijdschr Geneeskd.* 2003;147:1370–1372.
21. Einarson A, Selby P, Koren G. Abrupt discontinuation of psychotropic drugs during pregnancy: fear of teratogenic risk and impact of counseling. *J Psychiatry Neurosci.* 2001;26:44–48.
22. FDA Medwatch Drug Alert. http://www.fda/gov/medwatch/SAFETY/2004/may June 03, 2004.
23. Health Canada Online. Health Canada advisory of potential adverse effects of SSRIs and other antidepressants on newborns. August 9th 2004.

CHAPTER 13

CLINICAL MANAGEMENT OF SUBSTANCE USE DURING PREGNANCY

Lori E. Ross, Gideon Koren, and Meir Steiner

INTRODUCTION

Substance abuse and dependence are increasingly recognized as significant health concerns for women.[1–3] Epidemiological data from the National Comorbidity Survey (United States) indicate that among women aged 15–54, 22.6% meet criteria for lifetime dependence of tobacco, 8.2% for alcohol, and 5.9% for an illicit drug.[4]

Many women use substances during their childbearing years, and as a result, exposure to licit and/or illicit substances often occurs during pregnancy. Estimates of the prevalence of illicit substance use during pregnancy vary from centre to centre, with rates of 16% reported in the United Kingdom[5] and up to 44% reported in a high-risk urban population in the United States.[6] More recently, data from the National Household Survey on Drug Abuse in the United States found that between 1996–1998, 2.8% of pregnant women reported using illicit drugs.[7] This figure is likely an underestimate, due to the possibility of underreporting and the exclusion of individuals who were homeless, institutionalized, or living in drug treatment services. Marijuana was the illicit drug most commonly used during pregnancy, followed by cocaine[5,7] The majority of women who reported use of illicit drugs during pregnancy also reported use of cigarettes and/or alcohol.[7]

Substance use during pregnancy is of particular importance due to the potential health consequences not only for the mother, but also for the exposed fetus. Premature delivery, fetal distress and other ante- and neonatal complications have been associated with prenatal substance use.[6] It is very difficult to determine whether these complications result from direct effects of the drugs, or rather from behavioural factors often characteristic of women who use substances during pregnancy, including poor nutrition and inadequate prenatal care. Further, research is often confounded by high rates of alcohol and cigarette use, both of which have been independently associated with negative outcomes in babies exposed in utero.[8,9]

Substance-dependent pregnant women are a particularly difficult population to treat. Due to the disruptive effects of opiates and other drugs on the reproductive system,[10,11] substance dependent women often remain unaware of their pregnancies until well into the first trimester. Even upon acknowledgement of pregnancy, substance-dependent women may be reluctant to seek prenatal care or substance use services due to fear of experiencing stigma at the hands of health-care providers, or of having the baby or older children apprehended by child protection services.[12]

In this chapter, we review what is known about management of substance use during pregnancy. In particular, we focus on treatment for nicotine, alcohol, and opioid dependence, since pharmacotherapies for these substances are currently available and may be considered for use during pregnancy.

NICOTINE DEPENDENCE IN PREGNANCY

Smoking is the leading preventable cause of premature death and disability in Canadian women,[13] and cigarette smoking is the most common form of substance abuse during pregnancy.[14] Despite evidence that nearly half of smoking women quit during pregnancy,[15] recent studies suggest that at least 10% of North American women continue to smoke after their pregnancies are known.[15–17] Younger women and those with lower educational attainment may be particularly likely to smoke during their pregnancies, and in a recent Canadian study, nearly 80% of women who continued to smoke were daily smokers.[16]

Negative effects of cigarette smoking on the fetus have now been well established, and include risk of spontaneous abortion and a dose-dependent decrease in birth weight,[9] as well as increased risk for psychopathology in childhood and even adulthood.[18–20] However, if smoking is stopped or significantly reduced prior to 20-weeks gestation, birth weights are likely to be within the normal range.[21,22] Early and effective treatment of pregnant smokers is therefore a priority.

Counselling Interventions

Brief counselling interventions for smoking cessation have been recommended for pregnant smokers; however, they appear to be primarily effective for light to moderate smokers, and less effective for women who smoke more than one pack of cigarettes per day.[23] Effectiveness of counselling interventions may be enhanced through use of financial or other reward incentives, biochemical feedback on cotinine levels, and smoking cessation programs for the pregnant woman's partner.[17]

Nicotine Replacement Therapies

In nonpregnant populations, the addition of pharmacotherapy to behavioural counselling increases quit rates by 1.5-fold to 2-fold.[24] Nicotine replacement therapies (NRT), including the transdermal patch and chewing gum, aim to decrease cigarette smoking by providing a near-constant level of nicotine above the level which is associated with symptoms of nicotine withdrawal.[25] Although few studies have evaluated safety of NRT during pregnancy, it is thought to result in lower plasma nicotine levels than would heavy smoking,[26] and has the added benefit of eliminating exposure to other known toxins contained in cigarettes.[27,28] Available evidence suggests that short-term application of transdermal nicotine patch does not result in any adverse fetal effects.[29–31] While nicotine gum and patches have been associated with dose-related increases in maternal blood pressure and heart rate, these changes were less than those caused by smoking.[32]

Efficacy of NRT in pregnancy has been barely tested, and never in a study sufficiently powered to detect statistically significant differences in quit rates.[23] One randomized controlled trial of 30 women who smoked more than 15 cigarettes per day and were unable to quit during their first trimester found no statistically significant difference in quit rates between those receiving an 18-hour nicotine patch and those receiving a placebo patch.[33] A second randomized controlled trial of 250 women who smoked more than 10 cigarettes per day after the first trimester also found that nicotine patch (15 mg patches for 8 weeks, followed by 10 mg patches for 3 weeks) did not improve rates of smoking cessation in pregnancy, but was nonetheless associated with increased birth weights.[34] This suggests that NRT was associated with a decrease in total smoking. Another notable finding of this study is that salivary cotinine levels after 8 weeks of treatment were similar in patch users and in placebo-treated women,[34] suggesting that higher doses of NRT may have been required to achieve cessation in these women.

Based on these limited data, it has been proposed that NRT be considered for women who smoke more than 10 cigarettes daily, who are motivated to quit, and who have had at least one failed quit attempt with nonpharmacological therapies.[23,35] Pharmacotherapy, together with behavioral counselling, should be initiated as early as possible in pregnancy in order to minimize the negative effects of smoking on the fetus, and should be used for the shortest effective duration. The lowest effective dose of NRT is advised; however, pharmacokinetic research has demonstrated that clearance of nicotine and its principal metabolite, cotinine, is increased during pregnancy, meaning that higher than usual doses of NRT may be required to maintain efficacy.[36] Nicotine gum or spray may be a better choice than transdermal systems for some women, in that they result in smaller daily doses of nicotine and allow for better individual dose titration,[14] however, oral formulations may be poorly tolerated by women with nausea and vomiting during pregnancy.[23] When patches are used, measurement of cotinine levels prior to treatment can provide a marker for dose monitoring (aiming to achieve similar cotinine levels during use of patch as during *ad libitum* smoking). Sixteen or eighteen hour patches rather than twenty-four hour patches are preferred to minimize fetal exposure to nicotine.

Bupropion. Bupropion was first developed as the antidepressant Wellbutrin, but anecdotal observations of spontaneous smoking cessation in patients treated with the drug led to discovery of its use as an aid in smoking cessation. In non-pregnant populations, the sustained-release formulation of bupropion (Zyban) is typically used at a maximal dose of 300 mg/day.[23] No published studies have evaluated safety of bupropion administration during pregnancy for the purpose of smoking cessation. Immediate-release bupropion carries theoretical risk of seizure for some patients, which could have potentially serious effects on the fetus, and therefore it has been recommended that bupropion not be prescribed to women with history or symptoms of preeclampsia.[23] However, no reports of bupropion-related seizures during pregnancy appear in the literature, and results of a recent study suggest that bupropion use during pregnancy is not associated with an increase in risk for major malformations.[37] A recent controlled, prospective observational study found that of 22 pregnant smokers taking bupropion, 10 (45%) quit smoking, compared to only 3 women (14%) in the control group. This difference was statistically significant.[38] These data suggest that bupropion may prove to be a promising alternative to NRT in pregnant women.

Relapse Prevention. Relapse prevention should be considered a priority in recently nonsmoking postpartum women.[39] Estimates suggest that between half and two-thirds of women who successfully quit moking during pregnancy relapse within the first 6 months postpartum.[15,40] Relapse is predicted by concerns about weight gain[41], early weaning,[42] and a smoking partner.[43] Safety of NRT during lactation has not been evaluated; however, studies in smoking mothers have demonstrated that the amount of nicotine exposure via breastfeeding is comparable to that associated with passive smoking.[44]

ALCOHOL DEPENDENCE IN PREGNANCY

Compared to men, women become intoxicated after drinking smaller amounts of alcohol, develop alcohol-related health complications more quickly, and have a greater risk of dying from alcohol-related accidents.[3,45] Some of these differences may arise as a result of altered alcohol metabolism in women.[46,47] Women's lower total body water content results in less dilution of alcohol than in men, and ingestion of the same amount of alcohol, after correction for body weight, results in higher blood alcohol levels in women.[48] Women have also been reported to have less first-pass metabolism than men, as a result of a lower concentration of the enzyme alcohol dehydrogenase in the gastric mucosa.[49]

Alcohol is a known teratogen. Heavy drinking during pregnancy is strongly associated with fetal alcohol syndrome, and consumption of lesser quantities of alcohol is associated with fetal alcohol effects.[8,50] Data from the Canadian Community Health Survey suggest that while rates of alcohol use during pregnancy are decreasing, 14% of recent Canadian mothers reported drinking alcohol (any amount) during their last pregnancy.[51] A review of the literature revealed that studies of pharmacotherapies for alcohol dependence have largely not reported on treatment outcome in women[47], and data related to clinical management of alcohol dependent pregnant women are extremely scarce.

Alcohol Withdrawal

Women may require treatment for alcohol withdrawal during pregnancy or in particular, during labour; however, no research has examined the effectiveness of various available pharmacotherapies in pregnant women. Guidelines for treatment of alcohol withdrawal during pregnancy have been proposed by Miller & Raskin.[14] They suggest oral benzodiazepines (particularly lorazepam or diazepam) as the treatment of first choice, with other agents (e.g., carbamazepine, haloperidol, phenobarbital) used only for control of specific symptoms not adequately controlled by benzodiazepines. When carbamazepine or phenobarbital are used during pregnancy, supplementation with vitamins K and D is recommended to prevent neonatal hemorrhage.[14]

Disulfiram

Until recently, disulfiram was the most commonly used therapy to promote abstinence from alcohol. Disulfiram (Antabuse) is an aldehyde dehydrogenase inhibitor. By inhibiting the metabolism of alcohol, disulfiram causes an aversive physical reaction upon ingestion of alcohol, and so is used to prevent relapse.[52] In Canada and the United States, Antabuse is no longer commercially available; however, some pharmacies will prepare it, and so it continues to be prescribed.

The limited available data suggest that disulfiram is potentially teratogenic, particularly if taken with even a few drops of alcohol.[53,54] To date, 14 cases of in utero exposure to disulfiram have been reported; of these, eight neonates exhibited nonspecific abnormalities.[55] However, many of these cases were complicated by concomitant use of other substances, making it difficult to determine the relative contribution of disulfiram to the complications observed. There is also theoretical risk of fetal vulnerability to lead poisoning and decreased placental perfusion due to maternal shock when disulfiram is used during pregnancy.[14] Disulfiram therefore should be avoided during pregnancy.

Other Pharmacotherapies

Naltrexone (Revia) is another pharmacotherapy that may be prescribed for treatment of alcohol dependence. It is an opioid receptor antagonist, and acts to prevent relapse in alcohol and opioid addicts by blocking the positive effects of the drugs.[56] One report of 18 cases of opioid users treated with naltrexone in pregnancy revealed good outcomes,[57] but no research has investigated effectiveness or safety of naltrexone treatment for alcohol dependence in pregnancy.

In recent years, a number of other compounds have been studied as potential treatments for alcohol dependence. These include acamprosate[58] and the selective serotonin reuptake inhibitors (SSRIs), including fluoxetine,[59] citalopram,[60] fluvoxamine,[61] as well as dexfenfluramine.[62] No published studies have evaluated safety or efficacy of these agents during pregnancy, although the SSRIs are typically considered to be appropriate for use in treatment of depression during pregnancy.[63]

OPIOID DEPENDENCE DURING PREGNANCY

The number of women opioid users is growing.[64,65] However, negative effects on the fetus of heroin use seem to be less severe than those associated with heavy use of cigarettes or alcohol.[66] Possible risks such as low birth weight are difficult to separate from the effects of the impoverished and often chaotic lifestyles of heroin-dependent women. These lifestyle factors themselves pose serious risks to the fetus, including exposure to other teratogenic drugs (particularly alcohol), malnourishment, and HIV.[67]

Methadone Maintenance Therapy

Heroin dependence, and dependence on other opioids (e.g., Oxycodone-Oxycontin, Percocet) can be well-managed during pregnancy with methadone maintenance therapy (MMT).[67–69] MMT was discovered in the 1960s as the first effective pharmacotherapy for long-term heroin addicts, and is still first-line therapy today.[67] Methadone, like heroin, is an opioid, but unlike heroin, has a long half-life (at least 24-hours in humans) with slow onset of action, and can be taken orally.[56] Thus methadone can be administered once daily, preventing the cycles of intoxication and withdrawal associated with self-administering illicit opiates several times each day.[67]

MMT is reported to result in birth outcomes comparable to a general obstetrical population.[70] In particular, a meta-analysis of studies of the effects of maternal opiate use on infant birth weight found that while maternal heroin use was associated with a mean reduction of 489 g, use of methadone alone was associated with a reduction of only 279 g.[71] Similarly, maternal use of heroin has been associated with a 6.37-fold increase in neonatal mortality rates, compared to an increase of only 1.47-fold in women maintained on methadone.[72] Additional benefits of MMT over use of street heroin are clear: the longer half-life results in stable blood levels of opiates, allowing for the development of a regular schedule and routine in the mother-to-be, reducing the risk of spontaneous abortion, preterm labour and fetal distress that can result from opioid withdrawal,[73,74] and avoiding the health risks associated with intravenous drug use (e.g., HIV and Hepatitis C) and drug seeking activities.[67] Birth outcomes are best when women receive MMT in the context of comprehensive services (e.g., including prenatal care, services for substance-dependent partners, and child care services).[75]

Despite evidence of the benefits of MMT for opioid-dependent pregnant women, there is little research to guide clinical management in this population, and current recommendations are based upon clinical experience of service providers who work with this population. Pregnant opioid-dependent women are best managed at a specialized, multidisciplinary centre when possible.[76,77]

Cessation of methadone use is generally avoided during pregnancy because of the risk of preterm labour and fetal loss.[78] Further, rates of successful detoxification during pregnancy are relatively low: studies have reported recidivism rates as high as 50%.[79] In one study of 34 women who opted to undertake detoxification from heroin or methadone, 59% were successful and did not relapse, while 29% resumed opioid use and 12% opted for MMT.[80] These authors suggest that detoxification from methadone or other opioids may be possible for highly motivated pregnant patients under close medical supervision during the second trimester.[80] Attempts to taper doses or withdrawal from methadone or other opiods during pregnancy should therefore generally be avoided unless the patient insists, and detoxification should not be attempted prior to 14-weeks gestation or after 32 weeks gestation to avoid risk of spontaneous abortion or preterm labour.[81]

Methadone clearance increases significantly during pregnancy,[82] and changes in other pharmacokinetic parameters have also been observed.[67,83,84] As a result, outcomes may be improved with either split-dosing (twice daily)[85] or slightly increased doses in the third trimester.[86]

It is notable that MMT may alter the morphology of the non-stress test (NST), which measures the integrity of the fetal central nervous system in utero.[69] Specifically, higher incidences of non-reactive NSTs have been described in methadone maintained women, despite no increase in immediate neonatal outcomes.[87] In contrast, biophysical profiles do not seem to be altered by MMT.[88]

A notable potential effect of MMT exposure during pregnancy is the emergence of neonatal abstinence syndrome (NAS), which is thought to affect between 60–80% of babies exposed to methadone in utero.[89] Symptoms of NAS may include abnormal sleep patterns, weight loss, tremor, irritability, and hyperactivity.[89] For neonates requiring medical management of NAS, opioid treatment (e.g., with morphine sulphate, tincture of opium or paregoric) has been recommended over other treatments such as phenobarbital or diazepam.[90–92]

Some have suggested that methadone dose reduction should be attempted during the second trimester, in order to minimize fetal exposure and as such potentially reduce the risk for NAS.[70] However, the benefits of this approach should be carefully weighed against the potential risks of opioid withdrawal and relapse to use of street heroin. It is important that women be maintained on an adequate dose of methadone such that they do not use heroin or other opioids. This is particularly important in light of evidence that continued use of heroin during MMT may counteract its positive effects on neonatal birth weight and mortality: the worst neonatal outcomes were reported for infants of women using both methadone and heroin, relative to women using either methadone or heroin alone.[71,72] Further, it is not clear that maternal methadone dose during pregnancy is correlated with either the presence or severity of NAS.[93,94] In contrast, use of benzodiazepines[93] and heavy cigarette smoking[95] have both been associated with increased severity of NAS.

Buprenorphine

A newer potential alternative to MMT is the partial μ-receptor agonist buprenorphine.[96] Like methadone, buprenorphine is a synthetic opioid with a long duration of action (approximately 72 hours). In Europe and the UK, buprenorphine is widely available, unlike methadone which can only be accessed through specialized treatment centres, and therefore is commonly used. In North America, buprenorphine has been approved by both Health Canada and the U.S. Food and Drug Administration, but is not yet widely available.

Numerous case reports and uncontrolled studies now indicate that buprenorphine is well tolerated during pregnancy, and may be associated with relatively brief and mild NAS.[96,97] A milder NAS might be expected after in utero exposure to buprenorphine relative to methadone, due to its relatively limited transfer and metabolism across the placenta[98] and its partial (rather than full) opiod agonist properties.[90] Randomized controlled trials are currently underway to compare both maternal and infant outcomes in women treated with either buprenorphine or methadone.

Other Perinatal Considerations

Opioid dependence can have implications for anaesthetic administration during labour. Practitioners are often hesitant to administer opiates to methadone users, and this has frequently resulted in undertreatment of pain in a population with an already low pain threshold.[99] Narcotics with mixed agonist-antagonist properties (e.g., petazocine, butorphanol) are contraindicated due to risk of precipitating acute withdrawal.[100] Regional anaesthesia (i.e., epidural) is likely the best option.[78]

Studies of methadone use in lactating women suggest that breastfeed infants are exposed to less than 3% of the maternal methadone dose,[101] and the immunologic and attachment benefits of breastfeeding may be particularly valuable in this vulnerable population.[69] As such, so long as women are not using other substances and are free of viral infections, breastfeeding can be advocated for methadone-maintained women. Although breastfeeding has been suggested as a technique for gradually withdrawing the baby from methadone,[78] it is unlikely that the dose received in breast milk would be sufficient to prevent symptoms of NAS.[102] One study found that 58% of breastfed infants developed symptoms of NAS during ongoing MMT.[103] Symptoms of NAS have also been associated with abrupt cessation of breastfeeding at high maternal methadone doses.[104]

DETERMINANTS OF TREATMENT OUTCOME

Components of the Treatment Program

Substance use during pregnancy is a complex problem that is associated with many other risk variables, including poverty, poor nutrition, substance abuse by significant others, and domestic violence.[105] As such, multi-faceted treatment programs that address a variety of these risk factors have been advocated. However, few studies have evaluated the relative benefits of such comprehensive treatment programs.

Research in both pregnant and nonpregnant populations shows that retention in a treatment program is strongly associated with positive outcomes of that treatment (i.e., abstinence or reduction in use of substances).[75,106] A review of treatment programs for substance abusing pregnant women found that retention was improved in programs that provided support services such as child care, parenting education, and vocational training.[107] The Center for Substance Abuse Treatment in the United States has specifically addressed the proposed components of model treatment programs for pregnant substance using women.[108] According to these guidelines, treatment programs should be family-centered, staffed by an interdisciplinary team of professionals, address obstetrical and mental health needs, and facilitate access through provision of child care and transportation services. However, in a 1998 survey of treatment programs in the United States, only one in 16 provided on-site family planning services, and only 1 in 16 provided prenatal care.[109] Research and policy changes are needed to ensure provision of necessary services to pregnant substance users.

Comorbid Depression

Several studies have demonstrated that women with substance dependence are more likely than substance dependent men to present with comorbid depression,[110,111] though the magnitude of the sex difference is approximately equivalent to that in the general population. Few studies have examined mental health status among pregnant women accessing treatment for substance use, but similarly high rates of psychiatric comorbidity have been reported.[112,113]

When patients present with both symptoms of depression and substance abuse issues, thorough personal and family histories of both substance abuse and mood disorders should be taken to help differentiate whether the substance abuse is secondary to depression, or whether depressive symptomatology have developed in response the substances used (e.g., alcohol, which has dysphoric effects).[114] Untreated depression could increase risk for relapse upon discharge from substance abuse treatment,[115] and untreated depression during pregnancy may leave women vulnerable to developing postpartum depression.[116]

Current and Past Abuse

Adverse childhood experiences, and particularly childhood sexual abuse, are strongly associated with substance abuse in both women and men.[117] Since substantially more females than males are abused in childhood, this is particularly an issue for female substance dependent patients.[118] Violence during pregnancy is also a common problem in this population. In a recent Toronto-based study, 79% of women who used marijuana, crack, cocaine, or heroin during their pregnancies experienced one or more incidents of physical (including sexual) or emotional violence while pregnant.[119]

Childhood histories of experienced or witnessed abuse have been consistently associated with poorer outcomes in substance abuse treatment programs.[120–122] Screening for past abuse as well as current domestic violence should be incorporated in the history taking.[123] Treatment programs that acknowledge the impact of violence of women's health may be particularly helpful for substance dependent women.[119,124]

CONCLUSIONS

Women substance abusers present with a host of medical, psychiatric and psychosocial problems. They are more likely to be unemployed, receiving welfare, and to come from more dysfunctional families of origin than male substance abusers.[65,125] They are more likely to report lifetime histories of depression, anxiety, and suicide contemplation or attempt.[3,65] A frightening proportion of women substance abusers have been involved in current or past violent assault, including childhood sexual abuse.[119,126] Women who use substances during pregnancy may be particularly marginalized, and may face additional barriers in accessing treatment due to perceived stigma at the hands of health-care providers, and fear of having children removed from their care.[105] Treatment for substance dependent pregnant women should be nonjudgemental, should acknowledge that total abstinence may not always be a realistic treatment goal, and should work towards the best possible outcome for mother and baby as a unit.[78,127]

Considering the risk profile of pregnant, substance-using women, it may not be surprising that comprehensive treatment programs result in better outcomes than do standard programs for substance dependence. Holistic treatment programs that simultaneously address women's substance use, psychiatric, psychosocial, parenting, and obstetric/gynaecologic needs are likely to be proven the gold standard for clinical management of this population.[107,128]

ACKNOWLEDGEMENTS

The authors wish to acknowledge Pearl Isaac, Pharmacist, Centre for Addiction & Mental Health for her helpful review of an earlier draft of this manuscript, and Khatune Zannat for her help in the preparation of the manuscript.

REFERENCES

1. el Guebaly N. Alcohol and polysubstance abuse among women. *Can J Psychiatry.* 1995;40:73–79.
2. Blumenthal SJ. Women and substance abuse: A new national focus. In: Wetherington CL, Roman AB, eds. Drug addiction research and the health of women. Rockville: National Institutes of Health, 1998:13–32.
3. Greenfield SF. Women and alcohol use disorders. *Harv Rev Psychiatry.* 2002;10:76–85.
4. Anthony JC, Warner LA, Kessler RC. Comparative epidemiology of dependence on tobacco, alcohol, controlled substances, and inhalants: Basic findings from the National Comorbidity Survey. *Exp Clin Psychopharmacol.* 1994;2:244–268.
5. Sherwood RA, Keating J, Kavvadia V, et al. Substance misuse in early pregnancy and relationship to fetal outcome. *Eur J Pediatr.* 1999;158:488–492.
6. Ostrea EM Jr., Brady M, Gause S, et al. Drug screening of newborns by meconium analysis: a large-scale, prospective, epidemiologic study. *Pediatrics.* 1992;89:107–113.
7. Ebrahim SH, Gfroerer J. Pregnancy-related substance use in the United States during 1996–1998. *Obstet Gynecol.* 2003;101:374–379.
8. Jones KL, Smith DW. Recognition of the fetal alcohol syndrome in early pregnancy. *Lancet.* 1973;ii:989–992.
9. DiFranza JR, Lew RA. Effect of maternal cigarette smoking on pregnancy complications and sudden infant death syndrome. *J Fam Pract.* 1995;40:385–394.
10. Santen RJ, Sofsky J, Bilic N, Lippert R. Mechanism of action of narcotics in the production of menstrual dysfunction in women. *Fertil Steril.* 1975;26:539–548.
11. Kreek MJ. Medical complications in methadone patients. *Ann NY Acad Sci.* 1978;311:110–134.
12. Goldberg ME. Substance-abusing women: False stereotypes and real needs. *Soc Work.* 1995;40:789–798.
13. Pope M, Ashley MJ, Ferrence R. The carcinogenic and toxic effects of tobacco smoke: are women particularly susceptible? *J Gend Specif Med.* 1999;2:45–51.
14. Miller LJ, Raskin VD. Pharmacological therapies in pregnant women with drug and alcohol addictions. In: Miller NS, Gold MS, eds. Pharmacological therapies for drug & alcohol addictions. New York: Marcel Dekker, Inc., 1995:–1986.
15. Colman GJ, Joyce T. Trends in smoking before, during, and after pregnancy in ten states. *Am J Prev Med.* 2003;24:29–35.
16. Johnson IL, Ashley MJ, Reynolds D, et al. Prevalence of smoking associated with pregnancy in three Southern Ontario Health Units. *Can J Public Health.* 2004;95:209–213.
17. Melvin C, Gaffney C. Treating nicotine use and dependence of pregnant and parenting smokers: an update. *Nicotine Tob Res.* 2004;6 Suppl 2:S107–S124.
18. Brennan PA, Grekin ER, Mortensen EL, et al. Relationship of maternal smoking during pregnancy with criminal arrest and hospitalization for substance abuse in male and female adult offspring. *Am J Psychiatry.* 2002;159:48–54.
19. Silberg JL, Parr T, Neale MC, et al. Maternal smoking during pregnancy and risk to boys' conduct disturbance: An examination of the causal hypothesis. *Biological Psychiatry.* 2003;53:130–135.
20. Thapar A, Fowler T, Rice F, et al. Maternal smoking during pregnancy and attention deficit hyperactivity disorder symptoms in offspring. *Am J Psychiatry.* 2003;160:1985–1989.
21. Ahlsten G, Cnattingius S, Lindmark G. Cessation of smoking during pregnancy improves foetal growth and reduces infant morbidity in the neonatal period. A population-based prospective study. *Acta Paediatr.* 1993;82:177–181.
22. Klesges LM, Johnson KC, Ward KD, Barnard M. Smoking cessation in pregnant women. *Obstet Gynecol Clin North Am.* 2001;28: 269–282.
23. Benowitz N, Dempsey D. Pharmacotherapy for smoking cessation during pregnancy. *Nicotine Tob Res.* 2004;6 Suppl 2:S189–S202.
24. Coleman T, Britton J, Thornton J. Nicotine replacement therapy in pregnancy. *BMJ.* 2004;328:965–966.
25. Peters MJ, Morgan LC. The pharmacotherapy of smoking cessation. *Med J Aust.* 2002;176:486–490.
26. Hackman R, Kapur B, Koren G. Use of the nicotine patch by pregnant women. *N Engl J Med.* 1999;341:1700.
27. Scalera A, Koren G. Rationale for treating pregnant smokers with nicotine patches. *Can Fam Physician.* 1998;44:1601–1603.
28. West R, McNeill A, Raw M. Smoking cessation guidelines for health professionals: an update. Health Education Authority. *Thorax.* 2000;55:987–999.
29. Wright LN, Thorp JM Jr., Kuller JA, et al. Transdermal nicotine replacement in pregnancy: maternal pharmacokinetics and fetal effects. *Am J Obstet Gynecol.* 1997;176:1090–1094.
30. Ogburn PL Jr., Hurt RD, Croghan IT, et al. Nicotine patch use in pregnant smokers: nicotine and cotinine levels and fetal effects. *Am J Obstet Gynecol.* 1999;181:736–743.
31. Schroeder DR, Ogburn PL Jr., Hurt RD, et al. Nicotine patch use in pregnant smokers: smoking abstinence and delivery outcomes. *J Matern Fetal Neonatal Med.* 2002;11:100–107.
32. Dempsey DA, Benowitz NL. Risks and benefits of nicotine to aid smoking cessation in pregnancy. *Drug Saf.* 2001;24:277–322.
33. Kapur B, Hackman R, Selby P, et al. Randomized, double-blind, placebo-controlled trial of nicotine replacement therapy in pregnancy. *Curr Ther Resh.* 2001;62:274–278.
34. Wisborg K, Henriksen TB, Jespersen LB, et al. Nicotine patches for pregnant smokers: a randomized controlled study. *Obstet Gynecol.* 2000;96:967–971.

35. Walsh RA, Lowe JB, Hopkins PJ. Quitting smoking in pregnancy. *Med J Aust.* 2001;175:320–323.
36. Dempsey D, Jacob P III, Benowitz NL. Accelerated metabolism of nicotine and cotinine in pregnant smokers. *J Pharmacol Exp Ther.* 2002;301:594–598.
37. Chun-Fai-Chan B, Koren G, Fayez I, et al. Pregnancy outcome of women exposed to bupropion during pregnancy: a prospective comparative study. *Am J Obstet Gynecol.* 2005;192:932–936.
38. Chan B, Einarson A, Koren G. Effectiveness of bupropion for smoking cessation during pregnancy. *J Addict Dis.* 2005;24:19–23.
39. Levine MD, Marcus MD. Do changes in mood and concerns about weight relate to smoking relapse in the postpartum period? *Arch Women Ment Health.* 2004;7:155–166.
40. McBride CM, Pirie PL. Postpartum smoking relapse. *Addict Behav.* 1990;15:165–168.
41. Pomerleau CS, Brouwer RJ, Jones LT. Weight concerns in women smokers during pregnancy and postpartum. *Addict Behav.* 2000; 25:759–767.
42. Ratner PA, Johnson JL, Bottorff JL. Smoking relapse and early weaning among postpartum women: is there an association? *Birth.* 1999;26:76–82.
43. Mullen PD. How can more smoking suspension during pregnancy become lifelong abstinence? Lessons learned about predictors, interventions, and gaps in our accumulated knowledge. *Nicotine Tob Res.* 2004;6 Suppl 2:S217–S238.
44. Greenberg RA, Haley NJ, Etzel RA, et al. Measuring the exposure of infants to tobacco smoke. Nicotine and cotinine in urine and saliva. *N Engl J Med.* 1984;310:1075–1078.
45. Fuchs CS, Stampfer MJ, Colditz GA, et al. Alcohol consumption and mortality among women. *N Engl J Med.* 1995;332:1245–1250.
46. Thomasson HR. Gender differences in alcohol metabolism: Physiological responses to ethanol. New York: Plenum Press, 1995:163–179.
47. Romach MK, Sellers EM. Alcohol dependence: Women, biology, and pharmacotherapy. In: McCance-Katz EF, Kosten TR, eds. New treatments for chemical addictions. Washington: American Psychiatric Press, Inc., 1998:35–73.
48. Marshall AW, Kingstone D, Boss M, et al. Ethanol elimination in males and females: relationship to menstrual cycle and body composition. *Hepatology.* 1983;3:701–706.
49. Frezza M, di Padova C, Pozzato G, et al. High blood alcohol levels in women. The role of decreased gastric alcohol dehydrogenase activity and first-pass metabolism. *N Engl J Med.* 1990;322: 95–99.
50. Streissguth AP, Aase JM, Clarren SK, et al. Fetal alcohol syndrome in adolescents and adults. *JAMA.* 1991;265:1961–1967.
51. McCourt C, Paquette D, Pelletier L, et al. Make every mother and child count-Report on maternal and child health in Canada. 2005. Ottawa, Public Health Agency of Canada Publishers.
52. Chick J, Gough K, Falkowski W, et al. Disulfiram treatment of alcoholism. *Br J Psychiatry.* 1992;161:84–89.
53. Nora AH, Nora JI, Blue J. Limb reduction abnormalities in infants born to disulfiram-treated alcoholic mothers. *Lancet.* 1977;2:664.
54. Veghelyi PV, Osztovics M. Fetal-alcohol syndrome in child whose parents had stopped drinking. *Lancet.* 1979;2:35–36.
55. Reitnauer PJ, Callanan NP, Farber RA, et al. Prenatal exposure to disulfiram implicated in the cause of malformations in discordant monozygotic twins. *Teratology.* 1997;56:358–362.
56. Kreek MJ, LaForge KS, Butelman E. Pharmacotherapy of addictions. *Nat Rev Drug Discov.* 2002;1:710–726.
57. Hulse GK, O'Neill G, Pereira C, et al. Obstetric and neonatal outcomes associated with maternal naltrexone exposure. *Aust N Z J Obstet Gynaecol.* 2001;41:424–428.
58. Myrick H, Anton R. Recent advances in the pharmacotherapy of alcoholism. *Curr Psychiatry Rep.* 2004;6:332–338.
59. Gorelick DA, Paredes A. Effect of fluoxetine on alcohol consumption in male alcoholics. *Alcohol Clin Exp Res.* 1992;16:261–265.
60. Naranjo CA, Sellers EM, Sullivan JT, et al. The serotonin uptake inhibitor citalopram attenuates ethanol intake. *Clin Pharmacol Ther.* 1987;41:266–274.
61. Angelone SM, Bellini L, Di Bella D, et al. Effects of fluvoxamine and citalopram in maintaining abstinence in a sample of Italian detoxified alcoholics. *Alcohol.* 1998;33:151–256.
62. Romach MK, Sellers EM, Kaplan HL, et al. Efficacy of dexfenfluramine in the treatment of alcohol dependence. *Alcohol Clin Exp Res.* 2000;24:1534–1541.
63. Ross LE, Gunasekera S, Rowland M, et al. Pharmacotherapy for psychiatric disorders in pregnancy. Perinatal Stress, Mood and Anxiety Disorders. *Karger.* 2005:112–136.
64. Brands B, Blake J, Marsh D. Changing patient characteristics with increased methadone maintenance availability. *Drug Alcohol Depend.* 2002;66:11–20.
65. Chatham LR, Hiller ML, Rowan-Szal GA, et al. Gender differences at admission and follow-up in a sample of methadone maintenance clients. *Subst Use Misuse.* 1999;34:1137–1165.
66. Ostrea EM, Chavez CJ. Perinatal problems (excluding neonatal withdrawal) in maternal drug addiction: a study of 830 cases. *J Pediatr.* 1979;94:292–295.
67. Kreek MJ. Gender differences in the effects of opiates and cocaine. In: Frank E, ed. Gender and its effects on psychopathology. Washington: American Psychiatric Press, Inc., 2000:281–299.
68. Kandall SR, Doberczak TM, Jantunen M, et al. The methadone-maintained pregnancy. *Clin Perinatol.* 1999;26:173–183.
69. Wang E. Methadone treatment during pregnancy. *J Obstet Gynecol Neonat Nurs.* 1999;28:615–622.
70. Jha RR, Carrick P, Pairaudeau P, et al. Maternal opiate use: Pregnancy outcome in patients managed by a multidisciplinary approach. *J Obstet Gynecol.* 1997;17:331–334.
71. Hulse GK, Milne E, English DR, et al. The relationship between maternal use of heroin and methadone and infant birth weight. *Addiction.* 1997;92:1571–1579.
72. Hulse GK, Milne E, English DR, et al. Assessing the relationship between maternal opiate use and neonatal mortality. *Addiction.* 1998;93:1033–1042.
73. Zuspan FP, Gumpel JA, Mejia-Zelaya A, et al. Fetal stress from methadone withdrawal. *Am J Obstet Gynecol.* 1975;122:43–46.
74. Connaughton JF, Reeser D, Schut J, et al. Perinatal addiction: outcome and management. *Am J Obstet Gynecol.* 1977;129: 679–686.
75. Chang G, Carroll KM, Behr HM, et al. Improving treatment outcome in pregnant opiate-dependent women. *J Subst Abuse Treat.* 1992;9:327–330.
76. Kaltenbach K, Berghella V, Finnegan L. Opioid dependence during pregnancy. Effects and management. *Obstet Gynecol Clin North Am.* 1998;25:139–151.
77. Fischer G, Eder H, Jagsch R, et al. Maintenance therapy with synthetic opioids within a multidisciplinary program—A stabilizing necessity for pregnant opioid dependent women. *Arch Womens Ment Health.* 1998;1:109–116.
78. Wright A, Walker J. Drugs of abuse in pregnancy. *Best Pract Res Clin Obstet Gynaecol.* 2001;15:987–998.
79. Jarvis MA, Schnoll SH. Methadone treatment during pregnancy. *J Psychoactive Drugs.* 1994;26:155–161.
80. Dashe JS, Jackson GL, Olscher DA, et al. Opioid detoxification in pregnancy. *Obstet Gynecol.* 1998;92:854–858.
81. Kahan M, Brands B, Gourlay D. Methadone treatment for opioid dependence. In: Brands B, ed. Management of alcohol, tobacco and other drug problems. Toronto: Centre for Addiction and Mental Health, 2000:234–245.
82. Jarvis MA, Wu-Pong S, Kniseley JS, Schnoll SH. Alterations in methadone metabolism during late pregnancy. *J Addict Dis.* 1999; 18:51–61.
83. Kreek MJ. Methadone disposition during the the perinatal period in humans. *Pharmacol Biochem Behav.* 1979;11:1–7.

84. Pond SM, Kreek MJ, Tong TG, et al. Altered methadone pharmacokinetics in methadone-maintained pregnant women. *J Pharmacol Exp Ther.* 1985;233:1–6.
85. DePetrillo PB, Rice JM. Methadone dosing and pregnancy: impact on program compliance. *Int J Addict.* 1995;30:207–217.
86. Archie C. Methadone in the management of narcotic addiction in pregnancy. *Curr Opin Obstet Gynecol.* 1998;10:435–440.
87. Anyaegbunam A, Tran T, Jadali D, et al. Assessment of fetal well-being in methadone-maintained pregnancies: abnormal nonstress tests. *Gynecol Obstet Invest.* 1997;43:25–28.
88. Cejtin HE, Mills A, Swift EL. Effect of methadone on the biophysical profile. *J Reprod Med.* 1996;41:819–822.
89. Levy M, Spino M. Neonatal withdrawal syndrome: associated drugs and pharmacologic management. *Pharmacotherapy.* 1993;13:202–211.
90. Johnson K, Gerada C, Greenough A. Treatment of neonatal abstinence syndrome. *Arch Dis Child Fetal Neonatal Ed.* 2003;88:F2–F5.
91. Jackson L, Ting A, McKay S, et al. A randomised controlled trial of morphine versus phenobarbitone for neonatal abstinence syndrome. *Arch Dis Child Fetal Neonatal Ed.* 2004;89:F300–F304.
92. Langenfeld S, Birkenfeld L, Herkenrath P, et al. Therapy of the neonatal abstinence syndrome with tincture of opium or morphine drops. *Drug Alcohol Depend.* 2005;77:31–36.
93. Berghella V, Lim PJ, Hill MK, et al. Maternal methadone dose and neonatal withdrawal. *Am J Obstet Gynecol.* 2003;189:312–317.
94. Kuschel CA, Austerberry L, Cornwell M, et al. Can methadone concentrations predict the severity of withdrawal in infants at risk of neonatal abstinence syndrome? *Arch Dis Child Fetal Neonatal Ed.* 2004;89:F390–F393.
95. Choo RE, Huestis MA, Schroeder JR, et al. Neonatal abstinence syndrome in methadone-exposed infants is altered by level of prenatal tobacco exposure. *Drug Alcohol Depend.* 2004;75:253–260.
96. Johnson RE, Jones HE, Jasinski DR, et al. Buprenorphine treatment of pregnant opioid—dependent women: maternal and neonatal outcomes. *Drug Alcohol Depend.* 2001;63:97–103.
97. Kayemba-Kay's S, Laclyde JP. Buprenorphine withdrawal syndrome in newborns: a report of 13 cases. *Addiction.* 2003;98:1599–1604.
98. Nanovskaya T, Deshmukh S, Brooks M, et al. Transplacental transfer and metabolism of buprenorphine. *J Pharmacol Exp Ther.* 2002;300:26–33.
99. Scimeca MM, Savage SR, Portenoy R, et al. Treatment of pain in methadone-maintained patients. *Mt Sinai J Med.* 2000;67:412–422.
100. Hoegerman G, Schnoll S. Narcotic use in pregnancy. *Clin Perinatol.* 1991;18:51–76.
101. McCarthy JJ, Posey BL. Methadone levels in human milk. *J Hum Lact.* 2000;16:115–120.
102. Begg EJ, Malpas TJ, Hackett LP, et al. Distribution of R- and S-methadone into human milk during multiple, medium to high oral dosing. *Br J Clin Pharmacol.* 2001;52:681–685.
103. Wojnar-Horton RE, Kristensen JH, Yapp P, et al. Methadone distribution and excretion into breast milk of clients in a methadone maintenance programme. *Br J Clin Pharmacol.* 1997;44:543–547.
104. Malpas TJ, Darlow BA. Neonatal abstinence syndrome following abrupt cessation of breastfeeding. *N Z Med J.* 1999;112:12–13.
105. Siney C. Pregnancy and drug misuse. Chesire, England: Books for Midwives Press, 1999.
106. Stevens SJ, Arbiter N. A therapeutic community for substance-abusing pregnant women and women with children: process and outcome. *J Psychoactive Drugs.* 1995;27:49–56.
107. Howell EM, Heiser N, Harrington M. A review of recent findings on substance abuse treatment for pregnant women. *J Subst Abuse Treat.* 1999;16:195–219.
108. Center for Chemical Dependency Treatment. Treatment of the pregnant addict. 1994. Providence, RI, Behavioral Health Resource Press.
109. Chavkin W, Breitbart V, Elman D, et al. National survey of the states: policies and practices regarding drug-using pregnant women. *Am J Public Health.* 1998;88:117–119.
110. DiNitto DM, Webb DK, Rubin A. Gender differences in dually-diagnosed clients receiving chemical dependency treatment. *J Psychoactive Drugs.* 2002;34:105–117.
111. Sinha R, Rounsaville BJ. Sex differences in depressed substance abusers. *J Clin Psychiatry.* 2002;63:616–627.
112. Haller DL, Miles DR, Dawson KS. Factors influencing treatment enrollment by pregnant substance abusers. *Am J Drug Alcohol Abuse.* 2003;29:117–131.
113. Miles DR, Svikis DS, Haug NA, et al. Psychopathology in pregnant drug-dependent women with and without comorbid alcohol dependence. *Alcohol Clin Exp Res.* 2001;25:1012–1017.
114. De Bernardo GL, Newcomb M, Toth A, et al. Comorbid psychiatric and alcohol abuse/dependence disorders: psychosocial stress, abuse, and personal history factors of those in treatment. *J Addict Dis.* 2002;21:43–59.
115. Hill SY. Alcohol and drug abuse in women. In: Steiner M, Yonkers KA, Eriksson E, eds. Mood disorders in women. London: Martin Dunitz, 2000:449–468.
116. Robertson E, Grace S, Wallington T, et altewart DE. Antenatal risk factors for postpartum depression: a synthesis of recent literature. *Gen Hosp Psychiatry.* 2004;26:289–295.
117. Simpson TL, Miller WR. Concomitance between childhood sexual and physical abuse and substance use problems. A review. *Clin Psychol Rev.* 2002;22:27–77.
118. Jarvis TJ, Copeland J, Walton L. Exploring the nature of the relationship between child sexual abuse and substance use among women. *Addiction.* 1998;93:865–875.
119. Sales P, Murphy S. Surviving violence: Pregnancy and drug use. Journal of Drug Issues 2000;30:695–724.
120. Root MP. Treatment failures: the role of sexual victimization in women's addictive behavior. *Am J Orthopsychiatry.* 1989;59:542–549.
121. Hurley DL. Women, alcohol and incest: an analytical review. *J Stud Alcohol.* 1991;52:253–268.
122. Young AM, Boyd C. Sexual trauma, substance abuse, and treatment success in a sample of African American women who smoke crack cocaine. *Subst Abus.* 2000;21:9–19.
123. Greenfield SF. Women and substance use disorders. In: Jensvold MF, Halbreich U, Hamilton JA, eds. Psychopharmacology and women: Sex, gender, and hormones. Washington: American Psychiatric Press, Inc., 1996:299–321.
124. Stein JA, Leslie MB, Nyamathi A. Relative contributions of parent substance use and childhood maltreatment to chronic homelessness, depression, and substance abuse problems among homeless women: mediating roles of self-esteem and abuse in adulthood. *Child Abuse Negl.* 2002;26:1011–1027.
125. Collins L. Alcohol and drug addiction in women: Phenomenology and prevention. In: Ballou M, Brown LS, eds. Rethinking mental health and disorder: Feminist perspectives. New York: Guilford Press, 2002:351–375.
126. Winfield I, George LK, Swartz M, et al. Sexual assault and psychiatric disorders among a community sample of women. *Am J Psychiatry.* 1990;147:335–341.
127. Greaves L, Varcoe C, Poole N, et al. A Motherhood issue: Discourses on mothering under duress. 2002. Status of Women Canada.
128. Rowan-Szal GA, Chatham LR, Joe GW, et al. Services provided during methadone treatment. A gender comparison. *J Subst Abuse Treat.* 2000;19:7–14.

CHAPTER 14

FETAL ALCOHOL SPECTRUM DISORDER: THE CENTRAL NERVOUS SYSTEM TRAGEDY

Irena Nulman, Dafna Knittel-Keren, and Gideon Koren

INTRODUCTION

Alcohol is a legal, socially acceptable drug whose use is part of the lives of most American women. The spectrum of alcohol's teratogenic effects spans a wide continuum that includes craniofacial anomalies, growth deficiency, and central nervous system (CNS) dysfunction. Fetal alcohol spectrum disorder (FASD) is an expression of fetal alcohol-related abnormalities and may be seen in the offspring of women who drink throughout pregnancy or during critical times of fetal development. Presently, alcohol is the most common preventable cause of birth defects and the leading cause of mental retardation, ahead of Down's syndrome and cerebral palsy.

The previous decades have seen an accumulation of a large body of research into alcohol's teratogenicity. This chapter provides an overview of fetal alcohol toxicity, with a focus on the pharmacology of ethanol in women and fetus, epidemiology, diagnostic issues, and risk factors.

HISTORICAL PERSPECTIVE

While the role of alcohol in causing human teratogenicity was not proven until the 70s, the adverse effects of alcohol consumption during pregnancy have been noted throughout history. Several reviews of the history of alcohol & pregnancy are available.[1–3] *Judges 13:7* states "Behold, thou shalt conceive, and bear a son; and now drink no wine or strong drink." Plato is said to have proclaimed that children should not be made in bodies saturated with drunkenness. As well, Aristotle is reported to have stated that "Foolish, drunken and harebrained women most often bring forth children like unto themselves, morose and languid." During the gin epidemic of 1726, the College of Physicians Report to the British Parliament described parental drinking "a cause of weak, feeble and distempered children." In 1834, a report on drunkenness to the British House of Commons concluded that infants born to alcoholic mothers sometimes have a "starved, shriveled and imperfect look." The first scientific study on children of alcoholic mothers was reported in 1899 by Dr. William Sullivan, a Liverpool prison physician. He noted that maternal inebriety was unfavorable to normal development and that jailed and detoxified women had improved birth outcomes.

Little attention was paid to the plausibility of alcohol's teratogenicity until the last few decades. An article by Lemoine et al. published in 1968 in France, provided the first description in the medical literature of the effects of alcohol on the fetus.[4] It was not until 1973, however, with the independent observation of Jones and Smith, that a distinct dysmorphic syndrome associated with gestational alcoholism, the fetal alcohol syndrome (FAS), was described and recognized in the medical literature.[5,6] During the last 30 years, large number of articles have been published in the field of alcohol teratology.

Ethanol crosses the placenta, enters the fetal blood circulatory system, and can adversely affect the developing fetus in a number of ways. The critical features of FASD include intrauterine and postpartum growth restriction, specific facial changes and a complex and pervasive pattern of brain damage. FAS is the most severe presentation of the spectrum of fetal alcohol related abnormalities and the leading nongenetic cause of intellectual and developmental disabilities. Individuals with fetal alcohol abnormalities without full expression of FAS were said to have fetal alcohol effects (FAE) and partial FAE. These terms were originally developed for use in animal studies, a fact which caused considerable confusion. Various investigators believe therefore, that the term FAE should be used only in the research realm, not in the clinical domain.[7] Thus the term alcohol-related neurodevelopmental disorder (ARND) has replaced the term FAE in clinical settings.[8]

Due to the continuum of severity in growth impairments, neurobehavioral abnormalities, and unique facial traits that characterize individuals exposed to ethanol in utero, they are now commonly described by the term fetal alcohol spectrum disorder (FASD).[9]

ALCOHOL PHARMACOLOGY

Ethanol is a small molecule that is soluble in both water and lipids, enabling it to easily pass through cell membranes. It distributes throughout tissues and cells in proportion to their respective water contents. Therefore, highly vascular organs can equilibrate quickly with arterial blood and have an increased rate of alcohol distribution. During ethanol absorption, the brain, a highly vascular organ, achieves a higher ethanol concentrations more rapidly than most other organs.[10]

The metabolism of alcohol is almost entirely dependent on the liver[11], the only organ that contains the host of enzymes required to initiate the metabolic pathway.

The first step in the metabolism of ethanol is its conversion to acetaldehyde, a process catalyzed by alcohol dehydrogenase (ADH) (Fig. 14-1).

ADH is a general remover of hydrogen atoms from various compounds and is available in sufficient amounts to deal with ingested alcohol efficiently. ADH catalyzes the transfer of hydrogen atoms from ethanol to nicotinamide adenine dinucleotide (NAD), a cofactor for the reaction. Acetaldehyde is then oxidized to form acetate, which is later converted to carbon dioxide and water. For a given amount of ingested alcohol, women achieve higher blood alcohol levels due to their smaller body sizes and higher fat content, resulting in a smaller volume of distribution for alcohol and less gastric-ADH activity than in men, leading to less first—pass metabolism.[12,13]

Gender differences in ethanol metabolism are also influenced by the sex hormones. Testosterone, for example, depresses the activity of hepatic ADH,[14] resulting in a relative increase in ADH activity in the female liver before the age of 50–53.[15] There is also

$$\text{Ethanol} \xrightarrow[\text{ADH}]{\text{NAD+} \rightarrow \text{NADH}} \text{Acetaldehyde} \xrightarrow[\text{ALDH}]{\text{NAD+} \rightarrow \text{NADH}} \text{Acetate} \longrightarrow CO_2 + H_2O$$

Figure 14-1. Ethanol metabolism.

a delay in gastric emptying, which occurs during the luteal phase of a woman's menstrual cycle.

Among men and women with similar histories of alcohol abuse, more women incur liver injury than men[16], and such liver damage is typically more rapidly progressive in women than in men.[17] A similar pattern has been described for brain diminution, which occurs in women after significantly shorter ethanol exposure.[18]

The actual blood alcohol concentration is dependent on the amount of ethanol ingested, gastrointestinal motility, vascularity of the mucous membranes, and the concentration and distribution of water in each organ. Since pregnancy may influence these factors, one may expect that the disposition of alcohol in pregnancy will be altered. For obvious ethical reasons, there are no controlled studies on the pharmacokinetics of alcohol in pregnant women. However, one can examine information from observational human and experimental animal studies.

There is a delay in the emptying time of a pregnant woman's stomach, suggesting a lower peak alcohol concentration maintained for a longer duration.[19] In addition, pregnant women are in a state of water-volume expansion, including water volume from the fetus, placenta, uterus, and amniotic fluid. Since alcohol is distributed according to the water content of body compartments, and the pregnant women has a great volume of distribution of alcohol, this again should contribute to her lower peak blood alcohol concentrations.

Pregnancy-induced alteration in volume of distribution may have implications for the fetus because the effect of alcohol on the fetus varies with the change in water concentration throughout pregnancy. In early pregnancy, the fetal water concentration tends to be higher[20], increasing alcohol's volume of distribution within the fetus. This is meaningful, since ethanol crosses the placenta[21] and rapidly achieves equilibrium between maternal and fetal fluid.[22]

It has been suggested that the altered water content in the mother and fetus may favor the passage of ethanol across the placenta into the fetus. Rat studies reveal an increasing gradient of ethanol concentration in fetal blood, amniotic fluid, and intragastric fetal content when compared to maternal blood.[23–26]

Limited or no ethanol-related ADH activity has been found in the placenta[27] and the fetus itself has a low capacity to eliminate alcohol.[22] Ethanol concentration in the amniotic fluid at the end of pregnancy is associated with the contribution of fetal urine to the amniotic fluid.[28] Also at the end of pregnancy, the fetal sucking reflex develops which may contribute to the high ethanol concentration found in the fetal intragastric fluid.[23]

Pregnant rats have been found to have significantly lower levels of ADH activity compared to virgin female rats, irrespective of ADH isoenzyme distribution, tolerance, or malnutrition status.[23] The combination of low ADH activity in the fetal liver,[29] and marginal ethanol metabolism in the placenta means that maternal metabolism is responsible for the elimination of ethanol from both the mother and the fetus.

Ethanol freely passes into breast milk and achieves almost the same concentration as in the women's blood. Animal studies have shown that chronic ethanol administration results in a loss of mammary cell polarization, reduction in Golgi distyosomal elements, abnormalities in casein maturation and secretion, mammary gland, amino acid uptake, changes in pH and amount of lactose, lipoprotein lipase activity and a decrease in both absolute and relative mammary gland weight and protein content.[30,31] Alcohol interferes with prolactine secretion in lactating and nonlactating women.[32]

Subramanian (1996) points out that ethanol has a disruptive effect at the hypothalamic, pituitary, and mammary glands, which modulate mammary gland growth, initiation, and maintenance of lactation.[33]

EPIDEMIOLOGY OF ALCOHOL CONSUMPTION BY WOMEN

Over the years, the general tendency to drink is increasing. As well there has been an increase in the average weekly consumption of spirits from 0.8 units in 1992 to 1.9 units in 2000.[34] In a United States (U.S.) national survey, 61.5% of all women reported consuming alcohol in the previous year. Moreover, 75% of women aged 18–34 reported using alcohol in the preceding year, making alcohol the most widely used agent that can affect fetal development.[35] In England 46% of 15 year old girls were noted to have used alcohol in year 2000. According to Abel (1998), 49% of women drink some alcohol during pregnancy.[36] The 2004 CDC report addressed the overall prevalence of alcohol use during the last 3 months of pregnancy by women in eight states of the United States during 2000 and 2001. This prevalence ranged from 3.4% in Nebraska to 9.9% in Colorado. Women who were more than 35 years of age, non-Hispanic women, women with more than a high school education, and women with higher incomes reported the highest prevalence of alcohol use during pregnancy.[37]

One of the problems with alcohol consumption and the risk of FASD is that many women are not aware of their pregnancies for the first 4–6 weeks—in fact, a large number of pregnancies are unplanned. There is currently no evidence of a "risk-free" drinking level. Thus, women who are actively seeking to become pregnant should stop using alcohol (and other substances) as soon as they plan their pregnancies.

EPIDEMIOLOGY AND ECONOMIC BURDEN

FASD is generally believed to affect children of women who are considered to be "heavy" drinkers. However, heavy drinking is an ambiguous term that has been variously defined as consuming an average of two or more drinks per day[38], consuming five or more drinks during one two-hour period (binging) at least five times a month[39], or having a clinical diagnosis of alcohol abuse. Within this subpopulation of heavy drinkers, Abel's review of the literature found the incidence of FAS to be 4.3 per 100 live births in alcohol dependent women.[40] This figure represents only a small proportion of all the individuals who are affected physically, behaviorally and/or cognitively by alcohol toxicity.

The literature on FASD incidence and prevalence reflects variables known as "epidemiological inconsistencies." Discrepancies result from variation in study design, failure to estimate the amount and pattern of drinking, precise time of exposure during gestation, failure to include confounding factors, inclusion of different populations, and different reporting practices. Still, two seminal papers in FAS epidemiology have attempted to establish a universal FAS rate incorporating systematic analysis of various prospective studies. Abel (1998) reviewed the available epidemiological studies on FAS and calculated the prevalence of FAS based on geographical, ethnic and socio-economic variables.[36] He estimated, after an analysis of 29 prospective studies, a mean incidence of 0.97 cases per 1000 live births in the general obstetric population.

Prevalence appears to vary both among and within countries. The prevalence of FAS found in the United States ranges from 0.6 to 3 per 1000 in most populations, with some communities having higher rates. Subpopulation analysis within the United States showed that, in selected subpopulations in inner cities, the rates were 2.29 cases per 1000 compared to 0.26 cases per 1000 at sites were the population is middle class.[8] Since the annual birth rate in the United States is about 4 million, an estimated 2000–12,000 children with FAS are born each year.

Outside the United States, Harris and Bucens (2003) found the prevalence of FAS in the northern territory of Australia to be 0.68 per 1000.[41] In indigenous children, the prevalence was calculated to be between 1.87 and 4.7 per 1000 live births, which is comparable to the high rates in indigenous populations worldwide. The high-risk populations in Western Cape Province of South Africa were found to have a prevalence of FASD, 48.2 per 1000. In Moscow, Russia, 14.1% of assessed subjects were diagnosed with FASD.[42] Accurate estimates of incidence are hampered by differences in research methodology, even among populations and locations that are quite similar. On the other hand, in a study based in New Mexico, May (2000) found that rates were close to Abel's estimate of 0.97 per 1000.[43]

Combined rates of FAS and ARND are estimated to be at least 9.1 per 1,000. This higher figure underscores the importance of considering clinically the whole spectrum of severity. What is important to keep in mind is that nearly 1% of live births in North America are children born with problems related to prenatal alcohol use, clearly a preventable condition, representing a public health problem of appalling dimensions.[44]

The costs of FAS and related abnormalities are extremely high for the individual, family, education and health care system, and society at large. Just as it is difficult to assess the incidence or prevalence of FASD (FAS and ARND), it is also challenging to make a competent estimate of the costs associated with fetal alcohol abnormalities. Cost information usually falls into two categories: (1) total annual cost of FAS to the nation and (2) lifetime cost of each child born with FAS. Factors that affect such costs include: the incidence or prevalence rate that is used; health impacts and associated care/services that are considered, and the time period over which the estimate is based.[45]

The 10th Special Report to the U.S. Congress on Alcohol and Health estimated the annual cost of FAS in 1998 to be $2.8 billion (CDC website, 2005, frequently Asked Questions, para. 9). Other estimates for the annual economic impact have ranged as high as $9.7 billion.[46] Lupton et al. (2004) reported that the lifetime health cost in 2002 for one person with FAS was $2 million.[45] This is an average for all persons with FAS. Individuals with severe problems, such as profound mental retardation, have much higher costs. Klug and Burd (2003) estimated the mean annual cost of health care for children with FAS from birth through 21 years of age to be $2842 dollars (n = 45).[46] In contrast, the annual average cost of care for children who did not have FAS was $500. Prevention of one case of FAS per year in North Dakota would result in a cost savings of $128,810 in 10 years and $491,820 after 20 years.

CRITERIA FOR DEFINITION AND DIAGNOSTIC CHALLENGES

Jones and Smith (1973) coined the term Fetal Alcohol Syndrome (FAS) to describe children they observed born to mothers who were chronic alcoholics throughout gestation.[5] They noted that the affected children had a similar pattern of craniofacial, limb and cardiovascular defects associated with prenatal-onset growth and developmental delay. The criteria for diagnosis of FAS has been based on the presence of a triad of features: (1) prenatal and/or postnatal growth retardation (weight, length and/or height < 10th percentile), (2) CNS damage (signs of neurological abnormalities, developmental delay or intellectual impairment), and (3) characteristic facial dysmorphology (micropthalmia, short palpebral fissures (two standard deviations below the mean for age and gender), poorly developed philtrum, thin upper lip, and flattened maxillary area).[3]

Numerous problems have come to light that contribute to the difficulty in making the diagnosis of FASD. First, research has demonstrated that in prenatally alcohol-exposed individuals, the presence and/or degree of abnormalities can vary considerably. An affected individual may have an IQ ranging from the normal to the severely mentally retarded range, and may have physical features that range from normal to obvious anomalies. Correspondingly, a prenatally alcohol-exposed child may present with normal growth and physical features but with slight or substantial behavioral and cognitive abnormalities. Second, the phenotype of FAS varies with age and may alter or normalize as the child moves through childhood into adolescence and adulthood.[8] Third, many of the individual deficits seen in FASD are not pathognomonic for fetal alcohol exposure and similar deficits may be seen in isolation or in combination without any history of prenatal alcohol exposure. Consequently, when the phenotype is "incomplete" or "atypical" or the clinician is inexperienced in this diagnosis, FAS may be misdiagnosed.

Syndromes confused with FAS due to similar physical features may include: Aarskog syndorme, Williams syndrome, Noonan's syndrome, Dubowitz syndrome, Bloom syndrome, Fetal Hydantoin syndrome, maternal phenylketonuria (PKU) fetal effects, and Fetal Toluene syndrome. Other syndromes that may be confused for FAS due to similarities in the cognitive and behavioral profiles present include fragile X syndrome, velocardiofacial syndrome, Turner's syndrome, Opitz syndrome, and attention-deficit hyperactivity disorder.[47]

Presently it is not clear why there is so much overlap of physical phenotype between FAS, Fetal Toluene Syndrome and PKU. Hypotheses about how ethanol results in FAS/FASD includes the triggering of widespread neurodegeneration by apoptosis as the result of its N-methyl-D-aspartate antagonist and Gamma-aminobutyric acid mimetic properties[48], and disruption of cholesterol homoeostasis via its interaction with glial cells, particularly astrocytes.[49]

The neurobehavioural features of FASD, the ARND, can also be seen in other disorders, such as attention deficit disorder (ADHD), oppositional defiant disorder, specific learning disabilities, conduct disorder, and communication disorders, which are not pathogonomic to fetal alcohol exposure, and thus making the diagnosis difficult. The behavioral abnormalities may represent increased genetic susceptibility transmitted by affected parents who may be using alcohol as self-medication for anxiety, mood and personality disorders, or specific learning and attention problems.

A wide range of neurobehavioral abnormalities with low specificities have been found by a large number of investigators. These include: impairment in intellectual deficit with low average

I.Q., lower scores on arithmetic and memory tests[50]; a deficit in different components of attention and executive control functioning,[51] impaired information processing and visual spatial reasoning, impaired visual memory and verbal learning and memory function,[52–54] impaired motor functioning, speech and hearing performance, practical reasoning and eye and hand coordination,[55] behavioral and emotional deficits,[56] and behavioral regulation disorders as well as impaired judgment and poor adaptability.[57,58]

Evidence of a complex pattern of behavioral or cognitive impairment that is inconsistent with the developmental level and that cannot be explained by familial or genetic background, or environment alone may reflect ethanol toxicity in utero, clinically expressed as ARND.

A diagnosis of ARND represents a different, but not necessarily less severe spectrum, of alcohol abnormalities than a diagnosis of FAS. ARND was proposed for children who predominantly or in isolation exhibit neurodevelopment abnormalities. Specific morphologic, cognitive and/or behavioral markers indicative of ARND have not been defined. Moreover, abnormalities that result from other forms of brain insult (e.g., trauma, toxic, genetic, metabolic, etc.) may be similar to those that result from ARND, such that it is not possible to specify their cause.

Several attempts have been made to improve and clarify the criteria for diagnosis of affected individuals.[59–61] A comprehensive advancement was undertaken by the Institute of Medicine (IOM) of the National Academy of Sciences, Committee to Study Fetal Alcohol Syndrome.[62] The committee attempted to resolve the issues confusing the clinical and research communities by delineating five diagnostic categories for fetal alcohol related abnormalities (Table 14-1). The first category contains those individuals with a diagnosis of FAS (triad of symptoms as above) plus a confirmed history of maternal alcohol exposure (a pattern of excessive intake characterized by substantial, regular intake or heavy episodic drinking). The second group includes individuals with a diagnosis of FAS without a confirmed history of maternal alcohol exposure (accurate history not provided by birth mother, or inaccessible alcohol history for foster/adopted children). The third classification describes individuals as having partial FAS with confirmed maternal alcohol exposure. It includes those with confirmed alcohol exposure during gestation, some of the facial features of FAS, and evidence of growth, neurodevelopmental, behavioral and/or cognitive abnormalities. Two additional categories were devised in which to place individuals with a history of maternal alcohol exposure plus evidence of conditions that have been noted in clinical or animal alcohol teratology research. Category four, alcohol-related birth defects (ARBD), designates those with physical anomalies, while category five, ARND, describes those with neurodevelopmental abnormalities and/or behavioral or cognitive abnormalities.

Investigators have recognized that the birth defect known as FAS is only the "tip of the iceberg" of prenatal alcohol-related disabilities.[63] This viewpoint considers those with full expression of FAS as only a very small subsection of all the individuals affected physically, developmentally, behaviorally and/or cognitively by fetal alcohol exposure.

DYSMORPHOLOGY

As outlined above, FAS is characterized by a triad of features: pre- and/or postnatal growth deficiency, visceral defects, specific craniofacial anomalies, and CNS dysfunction. Abel (1996) reviewed neuropathological investigations utilizing ultrasound,[64,65] computed tomography (CT),[66] magnetic resonance imaging (MRI),[67–71] positron-emission tomography (PET),[72] and autopsy[73–77] clearly demonstrating the susceptibility of the brain to the teratogenic insults of alcohol. The affected brain typically is reduced in volume, and certain regions (e.g., basal ganglia, corpus callosum, anterior vermis of cerebellum) show a disproportionately large decrease in size. Other abnormalities seen including cerebral dysgenesis, enlarged ventricles, and abnormal neural/glial migration indicating that fetal-alcohol-related brain anomalies are structurally and functionally different than those seen in similarly developmentally disabled, functionally impaired, microcephalic children.[53,78,79] It is now apparent that a *unique* pattern of craniofacial anomalies is attributable to prenatal alcohol exposure. The unique configuration of the upper lip in humans is mainly determined by the existence of the philtrum. The philtrum consists of two structures, the lateral philtral ridges (two lateral ridges) and the midline philtral depression (the space between them). Research done on fetuses revealed that lateral philtral ridges start to develop at 14 weeks postconception. The orbicularis oris muscle (surrounding the mouth and controlling the lip movements) is detected at 11 weeks of pregnancy and, at 15–16 weeks, the muscle fibers from each lateral aspect of the lip cross towards the midline creating the two lateral philtral ridges and the midline philtral depression. Meanwhile, underneath the future philtral area, an area of loose connective tissue is found (11 weeks postconception) called the frenulum-associated connective tissue. This connective tissue seems to have a major role in the formation of the philtrum, perhaps by directing the orbicularis oris muscle fibers. Thus the formation of the philtrum is the result of an interaction between the connective tissues and the orbicularis oris muscle. Only the existence of both components will result in a normal philtrum-lip formation. A smooth upper lip is the result of the absence of philtral structures. Alcohol toxicity has been associated with the absence of frenulum-associated connective tissue, orbicularis oris muscle dysmorphology, and forebrain developmental abnormalities.[80] The forebrain plays a major role in the development of the midline portion of the upper lip, primarily through the neural crest cell mesoderm, which forms the midface region. Sulik et al. demonstrated that in mice, prenatal exposure to ethanol severely affects the development of the forebrain and the midface.[80] Deficiencies in neural plate development at early stages would lead, not only to abnormal brain morphogenesis, but also to deficient eye formation, since the eyes develop at later stages as evaginations from the neural epithelium. This shows that forebrain abnormalities caused by prenatal ethanol exposure may be the mechanism by which the philtrum fails to develop normally.

While growth deficiencies may normalize and craniofacial abnormalities may become less distinct with age, it is the brain injuries and their corresponding disabilities that are the hallmark of and the most unfortunate aspects of the prenatal alcohol effects. Normal sensory input is essential for the performance of higher cortical functions. Therefore, early impairment of sensory pathways may contribute to abnormal intellectual development.

Research into the developing visual system has shown that sensory impairment during critical period of postnatal maturation interferes with normal development of visual perception, neural synapses, myelination, and cell size, number, and organization.[81,82]

A wide range of ophthalmological abnormalities have been found to be associated with FAS, including microphthalmia, strabismus, visual impairment, short horizontal palpebral fissure, blepharoptosis, microcornia, corneal opacity, iris defects, cataracts,

Table 14-1
Diagnostic for Fetal Alcohol Syndrome (FAS) and Alcohol-Related Effects (10 M, 1996)

Fetal Alcohol Syndrome

1. FAS with confirmed maternal alcohol exposure
   A. Confirmed maternal alcohol exposure
   B. Evidence of a characteristic pattern of facial anomalies that includes features such as short palpebral fissures and abnormalities in the premaxillary zone (e.g., flat upper lip, flattened philtrum, and flat midface).
   C. Evidence of growth retardation, as in at least one of the following:
      - low birth weight for gestational age
      - decelerating weight over time not due to nutrition
      - disproportional low weight to height
   D. Evidence of CNS neurodevelopment abnormalities, as in at least one of the following:
      - decreased cranial size at birth
      - structural brain abnormalities (e.g., microcephaly, partial or complete agenesis of the corpus callosum, cerebellar hypoplasia)
      - neurological hard or soft signs (as age appropriate), such as impaired fine motor skills, neurosensory hearing loss, poor tandem gait, poor eye-hand coordination
2. FAS without confirmed maternal alcohol exposure
   B, C, and D as above
3. Partial FAS with confirmed maternal alcohol exposure
   A. Confirmed maternal alcohol exposure
   B. Evidence of some components of the pattern of characteristic facial anomalies

Either C or D or E

   E. Evidence of a complex pattern of behavior or cognitive abnormalities that are inconsistent with developmental level and cannot be explained by perception; deficits in higher level receptive and expressive language; poor capacity for abstraction or metacognition; specific deficits in mathematical skills; or problems in memory, attention, or judgment.

4. Alcohol-related birth defects (ARBD)
   List of congenital anomalies, including malformation and dysplasias
   Cardiac Atrial septal defects Aberrant great vessels
   Ventricular septal defects Tetralogy of Fallot
   Skeletal Hypoplastic nails Clinodactyly
   Shortened fifth digits Pectus excavatum and carinatum
   Radioulnar synostosis Klippel-Feil syndrome
   Flexion contractures Hemivertebrea
   Camptodactyly Scoliosis
   Renal Aplastic, dysplastic, hypoplastic kidneys Ureteral duplications
   Horseshoe kidneys Hydronephrosis
   Ocular Strabismus Refractive problems secondary to small globes
   Retinal vascular anomalies
   Auditory Conductive hearing loss Neurosensory hearing loss
   Other Virtually every malformation has been described in some patients with FAS.
   The etiologic specificity of most of these anomalies to alcohol teratogenesis remains uncertain
5. Alcohol-related neurodevelopment disorder (ARND)

Presence of:

   A. Evidence of CNS neurodevelopmental abnormalities, as in any one of the following:
      - decreased cranial size at birth
      - structural brain abnormalities (e.g., microcephaly, partial or complete agenesis of the corpus callosum, cerebellar hypoplasia)
      - neurological hard or soft signs (as age appropriate), such as impaired fine motor skills, neurosensory hearing loss, poor tandem gait, poor eye-hand coordination and/or:
   B. Evidence of a complex pattern of behavior or cognitive abnormalities that are inconsistent with developmental level and cannot be explained by familial background or environment alone, such as learning difficulties; deficits in school performance; poor impulse control; problems in social perception; deficits in higher level receptive and expressive language; poor capacity for abstraction or metacognition; specific deficits in mathematical skills; or problems in memory, attention, or judgment.

(Reprinted with permission from Fetal Alcohol Syndrome: Diagnosis, Epidemiology, Prevention, and Treatment. Copyright 1996 by the National Academy of Sciences. Courtesy of the National Academy Press, Washington, D.C.)

glaucoma, persistent hyaloid, and combinations of these abnormalities.[83–86]

Stromland and Hellstrom (1996) have suggested the eye to be a sensitive indicator of adverse effects of prenatal alcohol exposure.[87] Optic nerve hypoplasia (the most common anomaly in their studied cohort) and a large number of other ophthalmological signs were found to be persistent during 11 years of follow-up.

Similar observations have been made concerning sensory deprivation in the developing auditory system. FAS children were found to be at high risk for a variety of hearing disorders: delay in the maturation of the auditory system, congenital sensorineural hearing loss, conductive hearing loss secondary to recurrent otitis media, and central hearing disorders.[88] Hearing disorders are strongly associated with craniofacial anomalies, mental impairment, and ocular defects.[89]

Adequate hearing is necessary for proper speech, language and intellectual development. A child with hearing loss is more likely to exhibit hyperactivity, distractibility and learning disabilities.[89] FAS is one of the most common causes of childhood hearing, speech and language disorders.[90]

But by far, neurobehavioral sequelae of in utero alcohol toxicity is the most devastating in terms of the affected child's appropriate integration in society.

In a prospective, longitudinal study, focusing on the moderate amount of alcohol ingested by "social drinking," Streissguth et al.[58] looked at deficit in growth, morphology, and function—teratogenic outcomes found in children with FAS. The findings of the study were in accordance with the experimental animal literature.

At that relatively moderate level of alcohol exposure, it is neurobehavioral function which displays the most reliably enduring adverse effects of prenatal alcohol exposure.

To date, no method exists to quantify the brain damage caused by alcohol and its relation to dysfunctional behavior in an affected child. The behavior of children with fetal alcohol related abnormalities varies widely, and many other exposed offspring who do not exhibit full blown FAS show neurobehavioral deficits as severe as those of FAS.

SCREENING FOR MATERNAL ALCOHOL ABUSE AND NEONATAL EXPOSURE

Sensitive and specific biomarkers of alcohol drinking are needed to differentiate acute from chronic exposure to ethanol, alcohol abuse from social drinking, for screening, diagnosing, and monitoring alcohol consumption. Ethanol metabolites such as ethyl glucoronide (EtG), phosphatidyl ethanol (PEth), fatty acid ethyl esters (FAEEs), and sialic acid index of plasma apolipoprotein J (SIJ) have proven to be promising biomarkers.[91]

Screening Pregnant Women

Questionnaires. Alcohol use disorders may be formally diagnosed using DSM IV-TR and ICD-10 criteria. However, there is much interest in developing and using brief screening questionnaires and blood tests to aid with their diagnosis. Brief screening questionnaires for alcohol use disorders that have been validated include AUDIT, CAGE, CRAFFT, RAPS-QF, and RUFT-Cut,[92] TWEAK,[93] and others. There is considerable disparity regarding their sensitivities and specificities in different populations and different settings.

Blood Tests. Blood tests are often used as biological markers to screen for alcohol abuse. Measuring alcohol in the blood or in exhaled air reflects only recent drinking, so this test is of limited use. To detect significant chronic alcohol exposure in pregnant women, Stoler et al.[94] have suggested that the most sensitive combination of laboratory test results predicting maternal alcohol dependence are:

1. Elevated γ-glutamyl transpeptidase (GGT) level: > 0.50 μkat/L (45 U/L) (reflecting liver damage)
2. Lowered mean red cell volume (MCV): <98 fL
3. High carbohydrate-deficient transferrin (CDT) level: positive result is above 99th percentile (differs from lab to lab)
4. High whole blood-associated acetaldehyde (WBAA) level: >9.0μmol/L

These authors found that women who drink one or more ounces of absolute alcohol per day have at least one positive blood marker. They also found that the presence of two or more positive markers was predictive of smaller birth weight, length and head circumference.

Screening children for FASD

Early identification of children affected by prenatal alcohol use can help provide needed support, with the hope of decreasing or eliminating the costly and debilitating secondary disabilities.[58] Some studies have shown that screening can be useful to identify children at high risk of being affected by prenatal alcohol use before a formal diagnosis is made using the facial features, growth parameters, and impaired neurobehavioral function.[95,96] For example, Poitra and colleagues[97] reported results of effective screening using Burd's[98] rapid screening tool for FAS. These studies show that population screening may be efficient in identifying children for future formal testing of FASD.

Meconium. Determination of the amount and schedule of alcohol exposures in pregnancy is often unreliable. Even when the report on maternal dose is correct, it does not necessarily reflect the amount reaching the fetus. Ethanol cannot be measured in hair or meconium; however, its FAEE derivatives accumulate in meconium during the last 4 months of pregnancy.[99] Importantly, measurement of FAEEs in meconium has now emerged as a promising test for heavy maternal drinking in the second half of pregnancy.[100] To determine if pregnant woman is drinking during pregnancy, the Motherisk Clinic at the Hospital for Sick Children uses the TWEAK test to screen for problem drinking. Following birth, the infant's meconium is tested for FAEEs to determine if they were exposed in utero to excessive drinking.[93]

Usually the body's load of alcohol is eliminated from the body after conversion to acetaldehyde and water. Recent studies in adults have shown that circulating alcohol complexes with fatty acids to form FAEEs. FAEE have been found to be produced by the fetus due to continuous exposure to alcohol in utero. A study from Cleveland[101] has shown accumulation of FAEE in meconium (first neonatal stool). The presence of FAEE in meconium reflects alcohol exposure during the last 4 months of pregnancy. FAEE belong to a group of nonoxidative alcohol metabolites with emerging clinical significance in the diagnosis of alcoholism and alcohol related organ damage.[102,103]

The presence of FAEE in meconium has led to the development of the first noninvasive neonatal screening method[99] for identifying heavy maternal drinking in pregnancy and, hence for estimating the risk of FASD.

RISK FACTORS IN THE DEVELOPMENT OF FASD

Abel (1995) proposed two categories of maternal risk factors: permissive factors—predisposing behavioral, social, or environmental (e.g., alcohol consumption pattern, SES) factors, and provocative factors, or the biological condition (e.g., high blood alcohol concentration, decreased antioxidant status) that increase fetal vulnerability to alcohol at the cellular level.[40] The facts that not all children exposed to gestational alcohol consumption develop FASD and the reality that an increased incidence of FAS is associated with low socioeconomic status (SES) and African-American and Native American communities suggest that other risk factors may be interacting with the maternal alcohol exposure, thus further compounding the risk to the fetus. Such risk factors may include: *alcoholism in first degree relatives*. The most powerful predictor of alcohol abuse in any individual is the occurrence of alcoholism in first degree relatives. For those with a family history of alcohol abuse, the risk of developing an alcohol use disorder increases two- or threefold.[104] *Psychiatric disorders*. The presence of a psychiatric disorder is one of the most significant risk factors for alcohol misuse. The risk is particularly high in individuals affected by schizophrenia, major depression, bipolar disorders, anxiety disorders, and personality disorders.[105] The risk of alcohol use during pregnancy is also higher in women with psychiatric disorders. Thus, in addition to the potential damage by the alcohol alone, there may be other genetic and environmental adverse effects on the development of the fetus. As already discussed, the spectrum of severity of these abnormalities varies considerably. *Low socio-economic status (SES)*. Low SES is often related to poor maternal nutrition and health, decreased access to prenatal care and increased stress, each of which can theoretically adversely affect pregnancy outcome and could interact with the effects of alcohol on the developing fetus[64]. *Genetic factors*. Clinical reports on monozygotic and dizygotic twins have provided evidence for the involvement of genetic factors in risk vulnerability for FASD including FAS.[106] Theoretically, genetic factors in the mother and genetic factors in the fetus might affect the risk for FASD and other alcohol effects. Factors responsible for differences in alcohol metabolism, rates of transport of nutrients across the placenta and alteration in uterine blood flow, could influence the severity of fetal alcohol-induced damage. Ethanol is metabolized by enzymes in the liver: alcohol dehydrogenase (ADH) and cytochrome P4502E1 (CYP2E1) to acetaldehyde, which is then oxidized to acetate by aldehyde dehydrogenase (ALDH). Genetic variants of each of these enzymes occur. A high activity variant of ADH, (ADH2 $\times$ 2), and a low activity variant of mitochondrial ALDH, ALDH2 (ALDH2 $\times$ 2), have been conclusively associated with reduced risk of alcoholism.[107] Research to identify specific polymorphisms contributing to FASD is still at an early stage. To date, polymorphisms of only one of the genes for the alcohol dehydrogenase enzyme family, the ADH1B, have been demonstrated to contribute to FASD vulnerability. In comparison with ADH1B*1, both maternal and fetal ADH1B*2 have been shown to reduce risk for FAS in a mixed ancestry South African population. ADH1B*3 appears to afford protection for FASD outcomes in African-American populations.[106] *Use of illicit drugs*. Women who abuse alcohol also tend to abuse other illicit drugs.[108] Cocaine used in combination with alcohol produces cocethylene, an exceptionally toxic substance. The combination of maternal alcohol consumption and cigarette smoking increases the risk of low birth weight, microcephaly and hearing difficulties.[109] Poor maternal health, poor nutrition, poor prenatal care and other factors may influence the development and presentation of FASD.

Pattern of Drinking and Peak Blood Alcohol Concentration

Drinking patterns are typically characterized by average daily, weekly or monthly alcohol intake levels. However, the definitions of mild, moderate and heavy use vary considerably among studies, making generalizations and comparisons difficult. It is now evident that the pattern of drinking plays a crucial role in predicting the effects that alcohol has on the fetus. The amount of alcohol consumed has not been proven to be a meaningful predictor. Instead, the critical variable appears to be the woman's blood alcohol level. Research indicates that a single binge exposure with a high blood alcohol concentration (BAC) during a critical time in pregnancy is harmful to the embryo or fetus, and sufficient to produce a wide spectrum of physical and neurodevelopmental deficits.[110] This is particularly important for alcoholic women. Most such women decrease their consumption of alcohol during pregnancy, but when they do drink, they tend to binge.

Peak BACs are a function of both the dose and rate of alcohol consumption. Alcohol consumed in a binge pattern can rapidly produce higher BACs than daily amounts consumed in a slower or more spread out manner. A very different pattern of BACs might be achieved by two different types of women: those who spread 10 drinks throughout the day from morning to evening, and those who binge on 10 drinks in the evening.[111] This may explain some of the large variability in the prevalence of FASD in children of alcohol users.

As to specific effects on children, even two or three binges during the first trimester, or "social" binging by women who are not alcohol dependent are associated with a greater degree of disinhibited behavior in exposed children.[112] A prospective, longitudinal study by Streissguth et al. (1996) investigated children exposed in utero to a moderate amount of alcohol, characteristic of social drinking, and examined three types of teratogenic outcomes: deficits in growth, morphology, and function, all of which were evident in children with FAS.[110] They reported that neurobehavioral functioning, observed from the first day of life through 14 years, showed the most reliably persistent effects of prenatal alcohol exposure. These effects were dose-dependent and, in the school-age years, more salient in the children of mothers with binge-type drinking patterns. Learning problems were observed from 7 to 14 years of age, but problems with attention and speed of information processing were observable over the entire 14-year period. In the dose-response analysis, there was no evidence of a "risk-free" drinking level or any threshold level of prenatal alcohol exposure.

The high association between alcohol intoxication and unplanned or unprotected sexual activity is another area of concern. Unfortunately, women who engage in binge style alcohol consumption may increase their likelihood of engaging in unprotected sex and unplanned pregnancy and, consequently, may unknowingly expose their fetus to alcohol. This is particularly alarming in the teenage population, given their high rate of binge drinking, the rising rate of teenage pregnancy, and the tendency for adolescents to recognize their pregnancies later than adults.[113] Taken together, these variables make the offspring of teenagers significantly more susceptible to FASD.[111]

The Role of Timing During Gestation

The timing of alcohol exposure in pregnancy is critical in its effect on the developmental stages of the human fetus. Alcohol is a low molecular substance and is able to cross the placental barrier and enter the fetus. In the first 21 days of the fetal development the preliminary cellular organization of the embryo, begins to take place. If an excessive amount of alcohol is consumed before the blastocyst is embedded in the uterus, the impact can be so severe that the fetus is miscarried. In fact, both male and female alcohol intakes during the week of conception increase the risk of early pregnancy loss.[114] By the end of the 36th day, often long before the woman even realizes that she is pregnant, the neural tube is clearly present and open, and most of the rudimentary organs have already been formed, such as limbs, heart, brain, eyes, mouth, digestive tract, etc. It is therefore obvious that if alcohol is consumed during this critical period of rapid growth, malformations of the newborn such as heart defects, musculoskeletal abnormalities, mental handicap, etc., without any specific outward signs of FAS. Because there is a brain growth spurt towards the end of the last trimester then alcohol exposure at this later stage may affect brain development and function particularly. Of particular concern to the human situation is that about half of pregnancies are unplanned, and women often do not know they are pregnant for the first few weeks of this critical period.

Research with animal models has resulted in valuable insights into clarifying the importance of timing of prenatal alcohol exposure with respect to outcome, and the teratogenic mechanisms of prenatal alcohol toxicity of possible relevance to the human situation. For example, a mouse model of FAS strongly suggests that the facial dysmorphology (characteristic facial abnormalities) characteristic of FAS results from exposure during the first trimester and, or specifically, during the first 2 months of gestation.[80,115] However, the relationship becomes less clear in the examination of growth retardation. It appears that both early exposure (during the first 2 months of pregnancy) and exposure during the third trimester affect growth.[116,117] Effects on head circumference—and, by extension, brain growth—appear to be the most consistent and permanent outcomes exposure during these two periods. It is more difficult to examine behavioral effects than physical anomalies using a trimester approach, due to the nature of behavior development. Correlational studies suggest that early exposure may be more damaging to behavior than is later exposure, but some animal studies indicate that exposure in the third trimester may specifically affect the hippocampus and the cerebellum, leading to deficits in learning and motor skills.[118] In rats, a single exposure to high BACs can produce a severe loss of brain cells.[119] Microcephaly (small head size) is associated with alcohol consumption throughout pregnancy (all three trimesters). Animal studies have shown that while many areas of the brain are affected by maternal alcohol exposure, its effects seem to be particularly detrimental on the dorsal hippocampus,[120] possibly accounting for deficits in spatial memory of children born to mothers using alcohol during pregnancy.

POSSIBLE MECHANISMS CONTRIBUTING TO FASD

It is presently not possible to fully detail the mechanism with which ethanol exerts its effects during each stage of development. It has been postulated that fetal alcohol-induced CNS abnormalities are mediated through multiple mechanisms.[121] Prenatal alcohol exposure leads to disruption of most areas of brain development.[121]

A number of studies reported alterations in proliferation, neuronal migration, dendritic growth, conductivity among neurons and even neuronal death.[122–124]

Alcohol also has a number of detrimental effects on nonneuronal elements and may affect indirectly brain function by altering the development of microvasculature in cerebellum and hippocampus.[125]

As ethanol crosses the placenta and the blood brain barrier, it may affect the fetus directly, or indirectly through secondary effects on leading, for example, to constriction of umbilical vessels and resulting in insufficient oxygen supply.[126]

There is still a concern whether alcohol per se or acetaldehyde is the teratogen associated with fetal alcohol induced brain damage, since heavy alcohol consumption typically results in high levels of both alcohol and acetaldehyde. Jones et al. (1991) postulated that inhibition of aldehyde dehydrogenase, the enzyme that converts acetaldehyde to acetate, exacerbates the effects of alcohol on the fetus by raising the levels of acetaldehyde.[127]

Alcohol interferes with brain cell metabolism by decreasing protein synthesis and DNA methylation, mechanisms most commonly used to explain fetal growth retardation.

DNA methylation has been shown as one of the mechanisms involved in gene activity and function. The embryonic DNA is highly methylated and alcohol-induced inhibition of fetal DNA methylation may be associated with the teratogenic effects of alcohol described in FAS.[128]

Garro et al. also demonstrated that acetaldehyde is a 0^6-methylguanine transferase that has an important role in DNA repair activities. Espina et al. (1988) hypothesized that hypomethylation alters gene expression and may be responsible for the developmental abnormalities observed in FAS.[129]

Free Radical Damage

An alternate explanation for alcohol damage has been free-radical-induced mitochondrial damage. A study in fetal rat hepatocytes demonstrated that exposure to ethanol inhibits mitochondrial function and thus creates oxidative stress in the hepatocyte and a subsequent drop in ATP levels.[130] The excess amount of the intermediate of oxygen reduction, O_2, and other short-lived reactive oxygenated free radicals were found to be associated with anomalies observed in FAS.

Free radicals are molecules with one or more unpaired electrons which are known to be highly unstable, reactive and citotoxic.[131,132]

Radicals are normally scavenged by endogenous antioxidative enzymes; alterations of such balance by ethanol may increase oxidative stress,[132] which is highly damaging to cells. These disruptive mechanisms may affect proteins, lipids, chromosomes, and specific receptors.

Due to peroxidation, lipids may become free radicals themselves, and then may enhance chain reaction and membrane decomposition, manifested by changes in membrane fluidity and "leaking," levels of phospho-glyco-lipid compositions, and decrease in activity of calcium-ATPase, Na and K- ATPase, all of which have been shown in animal fetuses exposed prenatally to ethanol.[133–135]

Gangliosides, which are actively involved in cellular migration, cell-cell interaction, neurite outgrowth and other biological processes, were found to be decreased after alcohol administration ganglioside activities. Alcohol adversely interferes with interaction of water, membrane proteins, and gangliosides, leading to a new hydrogen bond and membrane fluidization. In animals prenatal gangliosides administration was found to antagonize some of the harmful fetal effects of prenatal alcohol.[136,137] Concentration of gangliosides and ganglioside-specific enzymes increase dramatically during brain development, therefore it has been suggested that prenatal alcohol exposure may affect the amount of gangliosides and their activity, thus contributing to the formation of FAS.

Alcohol induced cellular damage due to oxygen radicals may also occur independently at ischemia or hypoxia. Neural crest cells, which are devoid of superoxide dismutase, an enzyme that catalyzes the conversion of O_2 into H_2O_2 and O_2 and protects tissues against the deleterious effect of O_2, are extremely sensitive to alcohol exposure.[138] This sensitivity may account for facial and visceral malformations because those structures derive from neural crest cell.[138]

The CNS may be more vulnerable than other organs to alcohol exposure because of its high dependence on uninterrupted blood flow, high content of polyunsaturated fatty acids, and relatively low levels of free-radical scavenging enzymes and antioxidants.[40]

Micronutrients such as iron, zinc, selenium, manganese, riboflavin, niacin and tryptophan, β-carotene and vitamins E and C are needed for the free-radical scavenging enzymatic defense mechanisms. They stabilize free-radicals and inhibit their activities.

Alcohol abuse is associated with increase of cellular iron. The involvement of iron in free radical formation increases the potential for cellular damage especially in the brain where lipid peroxidation is very rapid.[132]

Zinc is known to be essential in the synthesis of protein, DNA, RNA, critical for cell duplication and is a cofactor in enzymes involved in free radical defense mechanisms, such as superoxide dismutase. Maternal alcohol intake can reduce fetal zinc levels and reduce the activity of superoxide dismutase. Zinc deficiency during development is teratogenic and in combination with prenatal alcohol exposure may interact synergistically to reduce fetal body and brain weight.[139]

Acetaldehyde production may also cause organic damage as it is an extremely reactive molecule and affects most tissues in the body. Although most of it is converted to acetate some will enter the bloodstream and reach a plateau when both the alcohol dehydrogenase and cytochrome P450 systems are saturated. Acetaldehyde forms stable adducts with amino acid residues in proteins. These adducts are antigenic, giving rise to antiadduct antibodies that can react with hepatocyte surface antigens causing the destruction of these liver cells. It is important to note that alcoholics achieve significantly higher acetaldehyde plateaus than nonalcoholics, even when the same blood alcohol level is attained. This is most likely due to the induction of the p450 system in alcoholics resulting in a faster conversion of ethanol to acetaldehyde.

Prostaglandins

Alcohol causes both a direct and indirect increase in prostaglandins in fetal tissues.[140] Increased prostaglandin levels lead to increased cyclic-AMP levels, which in turn may reduce the rate of cell division.[141] In the brain this process may interfere with stem cell division during neuronal proliferation. Following alcohol exposure in utero decreased brain weight has been observed in fetuses with increased prostaglandin E and cAMP levels. Inhibiting prostaglandin production (by injecting acetylsalicylic acid prior to ethanol introduction) halves the number of defective offspring in animal models.[142]

Amino Acid Transport

An additional proposed mechanism links ethanol-induced growth retardation to fetal malnourishment secondary to ethanol's interference with placental essential amino acid transport.[143] While this could explain the fetal growth retardation commonly seen in FAS, when ethanol is directly administered to rat fetuses, thereby circumventing the placenta, malformation and growth retardation can still be documented.[144]

Fetal Hypoxia

There is evidence that alcohol-related impairments of essential amino acids,[145] glucose[146] or vitamins and minerals[147] may be partly caused by impaired functioning of the oxygen-dependent Na-K ATPase membrane transport in the presence of hypoxia.[148] Ethanol metabolism increases the liver's demands for oxygen to metabolize alcohol resulting in oxygen deprivation.[149] This relative hypoxia may be further intensified by ethanol-induced contraction of umbilical arteries and veins, and impaired oxygen unloading from hemoglobin by acidification of the blood.[150]

It has been suggested that episodes of acidosis and hypoxia are operative in impairing neurological functioning of children with fetal alcohol syndrome. However, the theory of ethanol-induced hypoxia has recently been challenged, showing in pregnant ewes that maternal ethanol infusions actually produced a dose-dependent *increase* in uterine blood flow and fetal arterial oxygen pressure.[151]

Inhibition of Cell—Cell Adhesion

Another mechanism proposed for alcohol-induced damage is the sensitivity of L1-mediated neural cell adhesion molecules to ethanol. The L1 gene encodes for an essential cell membrane protein that helps the neuronal membranes stick to each other and to their extracellular matrix. Researchers have recently noted a startlingly similar picture of defects in people with FAS and in those with a rare genetic mutation in the cell adhesion molecule L1; mental retardation, hydrocephalus and agenesis of the corpus callosum have all been observed in children with L1 mutations and with fetal alcohol syndrome.[152]

Subsequent rat studies have demonstrated that ethanol nearly completely inhibited the stickiness of cell adhesion molecules at a blood alcohol level of 0.08%, a level defining legal intoxication in many U.S. states.[152]

The authors of this study concluded that "because L1 plays a role in both neural development and learning, ethanol inhibition of L1-mediated cell-cell interactions could contribute to FAS and ethanol-associated memory disorders."

Long Term Potentiation

Finally, alcohol has been observed to disrupt *long term potentiation* (LTP), a phenomenon that many neuroscientists believe is a prerequisite to memory and learning. LTP refers to long-lasting increases in the strength of synapses between neurons. In a study by Savage and Sutherland,[153] pregnant rats were treated with alcohol equivalents of maternal consumption of 2–3 drinks per day. The adult offspring of the ethanol-treated rats were later tested on a series of maze tests. Interestingly, they performed equally well as controls on standard water-maze learning tests but were strikingly worse when presented with a more difficult variation of the test. While controls learned the new maze after just one trial, the offspring of alcohol-ingesting mothers required seven or eight trials to learn the new maze. The brains of the ethanol-exposed offspring were later examined and it was found that their neurons showed markedly reduced LTP in the hippocampus, an area essential for memory formation. It was also discovered that these neurons failed to release an important neurotransmitter when faced with changing stimuli, which is a sign that the neurons had lost the plasticity required for learning.

This last theory may move very important in advancing our knowledge regarding the mechanism of FARA, because to date it proposes to explain how moderate drinking can induce teratogenesis. How much alcohol is considered damaging during pregnancy has never been definitively established because we lack a distinct model of teratogenesis for moderate doses of alcohol.

PRIMARY AND SECONDARY DISABILITIES

FASD has life-long physical, mental and behavioral consequences.[154] Streissguth has defined *primary disabilities* as those that are congenital and reflect a diagnosis of FAS or ARND.

They refer to the brain damage that results in impaired mental function of persons with FASD. They are measured by general intelligence, mastery of reading, spelling, math, and level of adaptive functioning, representing the CNS manifestations of FASD. Secondary disabilities are those with which an individual is not born with but develops as a consequence of the primary disability. *Secondary disabilities* are those not present at birth but occur as a result of the primary disabilities, and which can presumably be prevented or lessened by better understanding and appropriate interventions. They tend to occur as the result of relatively good cognition but poor social adaptability and judgment. Main categories include: mental health problems, disrupted school experience, trouble with the law, confinement (for mental health alcohol/drug problems, incarceration for crime), inappropriate sexual behavior, alcohol/drug problems, dependent living, and problems with employment. Secondary disabilities may possibly be at least partly ameliorated through better understanding and appropriate intervention. Secondary disabilities occur in adults as well as in children and adolescents.[154]

Streissguth carried out a study of 473 individuals to determine secondary disabilities associated with in utero alcohol exposure.[57] *Understanding the occurrence of secondary disabilities in clients with Fetal Alcohol Syndrome (FAS) and Fetal Alcohol Effects (FAE): Final Report to the Centers for Disease Control and Prevention (CDC).* Retrieved September 20, 2004, from http://www.cdc.gov/ncbddd/fas/secondary.htm.). The sample of 473 individuals included 178 with FAS and 295 with FAE. The range of I.Q. of individuals with FAS was from 29 to 120, with mean I.Q. of 79. Range of I.Q. of individuals with FAE was from 42 to 142, with mean I.Q. of 90. Only 16% of all the individuals with FASD in this study legally qualified as having mental retardation. This means that 86% of the individuals with FASD in this study have an I.Q. in the "normal" range and do not qualify for services for developmental disabilities. They nevertheless have impaired mental functioning caused by brain damage that is permanent and incurable. Adaptive behavior scores were low in both FAS and FAE subgroups (61 and 67 respectively). Ninety percent presented with one or more psychiatric conditions. Disrupted school experience and trouble with the law were reported in 60% of assessed individuals. Confinement and inappropriate sexual behavior were reported in 50%, alcohol or drug problems in 30%, and dependent living and problems with employment in 80% of the studied population. Rates of secondary disabilities were nearly equal for males and females.

Streissguth et al.[57,58,63] have pointed out that strong protective factors for secondary disabilities include receiving a diagnosis before age 6 (except mental health) and being diagnosed as FAS rather than ARND. These factors point to the importance of early diagnoses of ARND so that treatment and intervention can be started at the earliest possible age. They also suggest that patients with ARND have a greater chance of developing serious secondary disabilities.

MENTAL HEALTH PROBLEMS

In the Streissguth et al. study, mental health problems were the most prevalent secondary disability, experienced by 94% of the full sample.[57] Several others have shown an increased risk for cognitive disorders, psychiatric illness, or psychological dysfunction among children and adults with FAS/FASD. The most frequently diagnosed disorders have been attention problems, including ADHD; conduct disorder; alcohol or drug dependence; depression; or psychotic episodes. Other psychiatric problems, such as anxiety disorders, depression, eating disorders, and posttraumatic stress disorder, have also been reported for some patients.

Medical complications, developmental delays and psychiatric symptoms are often evident in children with FASD from birth. In the preschool period, eating disorders, bedwetting, speech delay, stereotypies, and ADHD have also been reported. Problems such as speech delay and stereotypies, and anxiety or sleep disorders, may occur during the early school age. Steinhausen, Nestler & Huth (1982) reported a prevalence rate of 63% for either a single or, more commonly, comorbid psychiatric disorders in children with FASD.[155] In the study of Streissguth et al.[57] during childhood, 60% of children with FASD had ADHD. In another study by O'Connor et al.[156] 87% of children evaluated because of heavy exposure to alcohol met the criteria for a psychiatric disorder. The majority (61%) were assigned a mood disorder diagnosis, 26% were diagnosed with major depressive disorder or adjustment disorder with depressed mood and 35% met criteria for bipolar disorder.

Factors such as increased severity of morphological (structural) damage, psychopathology and cognitive delay often cluster together in children who are severely affected by FASD. These children tend to come from extremely deprived backgrounds that include chronic maternal alcoholism and, often, paternal alcoholism. No study has yet disentangled the effects of alcohol from other environmental and genetic factors associated with poor neurocognitive achievement in children. Longitudinal studies have shown that even a stimulating environment with sensitive parents or a good institution only partially compensates for prenatally damaged intelligence.

Although cognitive deficits are over-represented among FASD children, mental functioning varies widely and some of these children may function at satisfactory academic levels at school, even though they may display behavior problems. Mattson, Riley, Gramling, Delis & Jones (1997) recruited alcohol-exposed children with or without the traditional diagnostic criteria for FAS and tested them with standard I.Q. tests.[157] Those without a diagnosis of FAS lacked both the pattern of facial features and prenatal or postnatal growth deficiency characteristic of the diagnosis. Both groups of alcohol-exposed children displayed significant deficits in overall I.Q. measures and deficits on most of the subtest scores compared to matched controls, with few significant differences between them.

The authors concluded that high levels of prenatal alcohol exposure are related to an increased risk for deficits in intellectual functioning regardless of the morphological characteristics and stressed the need for evaluating all children with intellectual deficiency for alcohol exposure in utero. Steinhausen, Willms, Metzke & Spohr (2004) studied the behavioral phenotype in children with FAS, FAE and in a group with intellectual disability of unknown cause.[158] They found significant differences in the behavioral profile between the two groups of children exposed to alcohol and the control group, but not between the FAS and FAE groups. Thus in utero exposure to alcohol may adversely affect behavior as well as I.Q. in the absence of full morphological characteristics of FAS.

Having FASD results in mental health problems in children, adolescents, and adults, most adolescents and young adults with FASD must learn to cope with persisting mental impairment and psychiatric disorders that can cause serious problems throughout life. In addition, a substantial proportion of these individuals remain dependent on support from others such as mental health and developmental disability professionals. There is evidence that adults with FAS or FAE are at substantial risk of developing, in particular, alcohol and substance abuse, depression, psychotic disorders and personality disorders.[159] In the study of Streissguth et al.[57] most adults with FASD had clinical depression. As well, 23% of the adults had attempted suicide and 43% had threatened to commit suicide.

ATTACHMENT DISORDER

Attachment disorders are the psychological result of negative experiences with caregivers, usually since infancy, that disrupt the exclusive and unique relationship between children and their primary caregiver(s). Though oppositional and defiant behaviors may be a manifestation of conduct disorder, they also may be the expression of disruptions in the mother-child relationship (i.e., attachment). There are several models describing the mother-child relationship. The interactive model, which suggests that child development results from a combination of factors, is one of the most salient for understanding the mother-child attachment.[160] The neonatal symptoms of CNS dysfunction in infants born to mothers who report drinking large quantities of alcohol during pregnancy include irritability, autonomic instability, decreased sucking response, motor immaturity, slow habituation, low levels of arousal and distorted sleep patterns. High-pitched crying, disturbed sleep and feeding difficulties often follow withdrawal symptoms and may persist for days or weeks.[160] Behavioral difficulties may continue into the preschool period and may be coupled with problems in cognitive functioning and sustained attention, emotional instability, increased activity level, rigidity, and irritability. These neurobehavioral effects may, in turn, affect attachment and mother-infant relationships.

O'Connor, Kogan & Findlay (2002) proposed that alcohol consumption following pregnancy was directly related to the mother's interaction with her child, resulting in a negative affective response in the child and an insecure attachment.[161] One of their models tested the hypothesis that independent and direct paths could be drawn between prenatal drinking and infant negative affect, maternal behavior, and attachment behavior. The model was based on the possibility that alcohol consumption affected the mother and infant independently. The results showed that prenatal alcohol exposure was highly related to attachment insecurity. Eighty percent of children who were exposed to alcohol during gestation were insecure, whereas 36% of unexposed children were insecure. Prenatal alcohol exposure also predicted child negative affect, which was related to lower levels of maternal emotional support of the child. However, when the mothers of the prenatally exposed children provided high levels of support, these children evidenced better coping skills and more secure attachment relations. Thus, the supportive presence of a mother may mediate the association between prenatal alcohol exposure and the child's security of attachment.

Streissguth et al. (2004) have shown that there are major problems with adaptive behavior for adolescents and adults with FAS and FAE.[162] In a study of 413 individuals, 80% of whom were not raised by their biological mother, the life span prevalence was 61% for disrupted school experiences, 60% for trouble with the law, 50% for confinement (in detention, jail, prison, or a psychiatric or alcohol/drug inpatient setting), 49% for inappropriate sexual behaviors on repeated occasions, and 35% for alcohol/drug problems. The authors report that the odds of escaping these adverse life outcomes are increased two- to fourfold by receiving the diagnosis of FAS or FAE at an earlier age and by being reared in good stable environments. These findings highlight the need to examine pathways for later maladaptation and therapy for the child at as early an age as possible. Future research might focus on studying the mechanisms of secure attachment and positive mother-child relationship, as a better understanding of this complex process would lead to early intervention before the primary attachment relationship becomes disturbed.

PREVENTION

Effective prevention of FASD is optimally approached from a multifaceted perspective. Publicity about the dangers of maternal drinking can intensify a woman's despair over the damage she may have done to the fetus and her inability to stop drinking. Campaigns must therefore be mounted that motivate at-risk women to reduce alcohol consumption, stress the potential for success in overcoming their addiction and encourage these women to seek prenatal care. The various specialties involved in treating pregnant, addicted women must be coordinated to deal with the complex medical and social issues.

It is clearly evident that alcohol exposure is associated with long-term physical, cognitive and behavioral disabilities as well as with verbal and visual deficits.[52] Strategies to alleviate FASD must include interventions targeting society at large, cultural and community groups, as well as medical and public health professionals. The pediatrician and family doctor's involvement in FASD should focus on prevention, early diagnosis and multidisciplinary treatment of this disorder once diagnosed. Providing physicians with tools to diagnose and manage FASD can have an impact on the most preventable form of neurodevelopmental deficit that affects children worldwide. Educating school nurses about FASD also is critical, because they are positioned within the community and have links to children, families, and healthcare systems.[163]

Approaches for prevention are typically classified as primary, secondary, and tertiary (see below).

Primary prevention. These efforts target the universal level, striving to ensure that society as a whole is aware of the hazards associated with using alcohol, particularly during pregnancy. The choice to refrain from alcohol use prior to and during pregnancy is the goal of primary prevention. Although prevention and treatment of maternal alcohol abuse are difficult and often unsuccessful, effective contraception is a more discernible focus for primary prevention efforts.

Secondary prevention. These efforts are initiated after the diagnosis of heavy alcohol consumption in early pregnancy is recognized. The physician should inform the woman about the risks posed to her fetus to date, potential risks if alcohol use is continued, and the possibility for termination of pregnancy. Realistic discussion about the life-long risks to the fetus should be conveyed to the mother. Cessation of alcohol use should be strongly encouraged if the woman chooses to continue the pregnancy and suitable follow-up for post delivery should be arranged.

Tertiary prevention. These efforts focus on early intervention and screening of children with FAS and ARND in an attempt to prevent the development of secondary disabilities. Maternal and fetal biological markers are effective screening methods for identifying maternal alcohol abuse and extent of fetal exposure.

A variety of programs have been developed to prevent drinking during pregnancy and the resulting health problems.[164] Some of these efforts include public service announcements and beverage warning labels to increase the public's knowledge about FAS. In selective prevention, women of reproductive age who drink alcohol are targeted by selective prevention or by indicated prevention. Approaches for selective prevention may involve screening pregnant women for alcohol consumption and counseling those women who do drink. In indicated prevention, high-risk women (e.g., women who have previously abused alcohol or have had a child with FAS or other alcohol-related effects) are targeted and typically offered repeated counseling over several years. Both selective and indicated prevention efforts can reduce maternal alcohol consumption and improve the outcome of the offspring. Furthermore, many excellent programs exist for treatment of alcohol abuse (see websites references).

SUMMARY

Alcohol is currently the most widely used substance resulting fetal malformation and intellectual disability. FASD in a child reflects maternal alcohol abuse. FASD and other disorders caused by alcohol use are permanent conditions for which there are no specific treatments. Prenatal exposure to alcohol can create a wide variety of abnormalities that are extensive and very problematic. Since alcohol is legal and socially acceptable, it is used on a much larger scale than any other known substances. In utero alcohol abuse is among the most common causes of congenital brain injury and neurobehavioral abnormalities in children and adults. The cognitive and neurobehavioral impairment in FASD has a wide range of clinical presentations that also can occur with quite a number of other disorders. FAS and ARND are permanent manifestations not found to be affected by time or environment. There is also no specific treatment for this disorder. FASD is not a childhood disorder. There is a long-term progression of the disorder into adulthood in which the maladaptive behaviours present a risk for a wide range of secondary disabilities. FASD also is closely associated with mental health disorders. Secondary disabilities that may develop include various social, behavior, and learning problems. Screening for maternal alcohol abuse and fetal exposure can lead to early diagnosis and early intervention.

There have been significant advances in understanding alcohol's harmful effects, but it is not yet fully clear how the timing of alcohol exposure, SES factors, prenatal care, maternal physical and mental health, genetic susceptibility, and other factors contribute to FASD. We do know that FASD is fully preventable and that the economic costs of alcohol-related abnormalities are extraordinarily high for society as a whole, the education and health care systems, the family, and those individuals affected.

WEBSITE REFERENCES

1. Alcoholics Anonymous: http://www.aa.org
2. Canadian Centre on Substance Abuse: Fetal Alcohol Spectrum Disorder (FASD) Information Service: http://www.ccsa.ca/CCSA/EN/Topics/Populations/FASDInformationService.htm
3. Centers for Disease Control and Prevention (CDC): http://www.cdc.gov/ncbddd/fas/
4. FAS Community Resource Centre: http://www.come-over.to/FASCRC
5. FASlink: Fetal Alcohol Disorders Society: http://www.acbr.com/fas/index.htm
6. FASworld: http://www.fasworld.com
7. Motherisk Alcohol and Substance Abuse Help Line: 1-877-FAS-INFO (1-877-327-4636); http://www.motherisk.org
8. National Institute on Alcohol Abuse and Alcoholism: http://www.niaaa.nih.gov
9. National Organization on Fetal Alcohol Syndrome: http://www.nofas.org
10. Office for National Statistics: http://www.statistics.gov.uk/pdfdir/health0304.pdf
11. Substance Abuse and Mental Health Services Administration (SAMHSA): Substance Abuse Treatment Facilit Locator: 1-877-FAS-INFO (1-877-327-4636); http://dasis3.samhsa.gov

REFERENCES

1. Warner RH, Rosett HL. The effects of drinking on offspring: an historical survey of the American and British literature. *J Stud Alcohol.* 1975;36:1395–1420.
2. Rosett HL, Weiner L. Alcohol and the fetus. New York: Oxford University Press, 1984.
3. Abel EL. Historical background. In: Abel EL, ed. Fetal alcohol syndrome. New Jersey: Medical Economics Books; 1990:1–11.
4. Lemoine P, Harousseau H, Borteyra JP, et al. Les enfants des parents alcooliques: anomalies observees a propos de 127-cas. *Ouest Med.* 1986;21:476–482.
5. Jones KL, Smith DW. Recognition of the fetal alcohol syndrome in early infancy. *Lancet.* 1973;2:999–1001.
6. Jones KL, Smith DW, Ulleland CH, et al. Pattern of malformation in offspring of chronic alcohol mothers. *Lancet.* 1973;1:1267–1271.

7. Aase JM, Jones KL, Clarren SK. Do we need the term "FAE"? *Pediatrics.* 1995;95:428–430.
8. Institute of Medicine of the National Academy of Sciences Committee to Study Fetal Alcohol Syndrome. Introduction. In K. Stratton, C. Howe & F. Battaglia (Eds.), *Fetal alcohol syndrome* (pp 17–32). Gainesville, FL: National Academy Press, 1996.
9. Streissguth AP, & O'Malley K. Neuropsychiatric implications and long-term consequences of Fetal Alcohol Spectrum Disorders. *Seminars in Clinical Neuropsychology,* 2000;5:177–190.
10. Goldstein DB. Pharmacology of Alcohol. New York: Oxford University Press, 1983:6.
11. Lundsgaard E. Alcohol oxidation as a function of the liver. *CR Lab Carlsberg Ser Chim.* 1938;22:333–337.
12. Frezza M, di Padova C, Pozzato G, et al. High blood alcohol levels in women: the role of decreased gastric alcohol dehydrogenase activity and first pass-metabolism. *New England Journal of Medicine.* 1990;322:95–99.
13. Seitz HK, Egerer G, Simanowski UA, et al. Human gastric alcohol dehydrogenase activity: effect of age, sex and alcoholism. *Gut.* 1993;34:1433–1437.
14. Teschke R, Wiese B. Sex-dependency of hepatic alcohol metabolizing enzymes. *J Endocrinol Invest.* 1982;5:243–250.
15. Maly IP, Sasse D. Intraacinar profiles of alcohol dehydrogenase and aldehyde dehydrogenase activities in human liver. *Gastroenterology.* 1991;101:1716–1723.
16. Morgan MY, Sherlock S. Sex-related differences among 100 patients with alcoholic liver disease. *Br Med J.* 1977;1:939–941.
17. Rankin JG. The natural history and management of the patient with alcoholic liver disease. In: Fisher MM, Rankin JG, eds. Alcohol and the liver. Vol. 3 of Hepatology: research and clinical issues. New York: Plenum Press, 1977,365–381.
18. Mann K, Batra A, Gunthner A, et al. Do women develop alcoholic brain damage more readily than men? *Alcohol Clin Exp Res.* 1992; 16:1052–1056.
19. Hinckers HJ. Characteristics of the physiology of alcohol during pregnancy: absorption of alcohol. In: The influences of alcohol on the fetus. *J Perinat Med.* 1978;6:3–19.
20. McCance RA, Widdowson EW. Water metabolism: *Cold Spring. Harbor. Symp. Quant. Biol.* 1954;19:155.
21. Dilts PV. Placental transfer of ethanol. *Am J Obstet Gynecol.* 1970; 107:1195–1198.
22. Guerri C, Sanchis R. Acetaldehyde and alcohol levels in pregnant rats and fetuses. *Alcohol.* 1985;2:267–270.
23. Traves C, Camps L, Lopez-Tejero D. Liver alcohol dehydrogenase activity and ethanol levels during chronic ethanol intake in pregnant rats and their offspring. *Pharmacol Biochem Behav.* 1995;52(1): 93–99.
24. Lopez-Tejero D, Ferrer I, Llobera M, et al. Effects of prenatal ethanol exposure on physical growth, sensory reflex maturation and brain development in the rat. *Neuropathological Applications to Neurobiology.* 1986;12:251–260.
25. Lopez-Tejero D, Arilla E, Colas B, et al. Low intestinal lactase activity in offspring from ethanol-treated mothers. *Biology of the Neonate* 1989;55:204–213.
26. Lopez-Tejero D, Llobera M, Herrera E. Permanent abnormal response to glucose load after prenatal ethanol exposure in rats. *Alcohol.* 1989;6:469–473.
27. Pares X, Farres J, Vallee BL. Organ specific alcohol metabolism: Placental X-ADH. *Biochem Biophys Res Commun.* 1984; 119:1047–1055.
28. Hayashi M, Shimazaki Y, Kamata S, et al. Disposition of ethanol and acetaldehyde in maternal blood, fetal blood and amniotic fluid in near-term pregnant rats. *Bull Environ Contam Toxicol.* 1991; 47:184–189.
29. Sanchis R, Guerri C. Alcohol-metabolizing enzymes in placenta and fetal liver: effect of chronic ethanol intake. *Alc Clin Exp Res.* 1986b; 10:39–44.
30. Sanchis R, Guerri C. Chronic ethanol intake in lactating rats: milk analysis. *Comp Biochem Physiol.* 1986a;85:107.
31. Vinas O, Vilarso S, Herrera E, et al. Effects of chronic ethanol treatment on amino acid uptake and enzyme activities in the lactating rat mammary gland. *Life Sci.* 1989;40:1745.
32. Volpi R, Chiodera P, Gramellini D, et al. Endogenous opiod medication of the inhibitory effect of ethanol on the prolactin response to breath stimulation in normal women. *Life Sci.* 1994;54:739.
33. Subramanian MG. Effects of ethanol on lactation. In: Fetal Alcohol Syndrome (Abel EL, ed.) Boca Raton, FL: CRC Press; 1996: 237–247.
34. *Office for National Statistics (U.K.).* Retrieved June 14, 2005, from http://www.statistics.gov.uk/pdfdir/health0304.pdf
35. Koren G, Nulman I. Teratogenic drugs and chemicals in humans. In: Koren G, editor. Maternal-fetal toxicology. New York: Marcel Dekker; 1994:33–48.
36. Abel EL. Why fetal alcohol abuse syndrome? In E. L. Abel (Ed.), *Fetal alcohol abuse syndrome* (pp. 7–8). New York: Plenum Press. 1998.
37. Phares TM, Morrow B, Lansky A, et al. Surveillance for disparities in maternal health-related behaviors—selected states, Pregnancy Risk Assessment Monitoring System(PRAMS), 2000–2001. Retrieved September 20, 2004, from http://www.cdc.gov/mmwr/preview/mmwrhtml/ss5304a1.htm
38. National Institute of Alcohol Abuse and Alcoholism. *Eighth special report to the U.S. Congress on alcohol and health.* Washington, DC: US Department of Health and Human Services, 1993.
39. Substance Abuse and Mental Health Service Administration. *National household survey on drug abuse.* Rockville, MD: US Department of Health and Human Services, 1996.
40. Abel EL. An update on incidence of FAS: FAS is not an equal opportunity birth defect. *Neurotoxicol Teratol.* 1995;Vol 17(4):437–443.
41. Harris KR, & Bucens IK. Prevalence of fetal alcohol syndrome in the top end of the northern territory. *Journal of Pediatrics and Child Health.* 2003;39:528–533.
42. Warren KR, Calhoun FJ, May PA, et al. Fetal Alcohol Syndrome: An international perspective. *Alcohol Clin Exp Res,* 2001; 25:202S–206S.
43. May PA. Epidemiological research on FAS in the United States. Abstract WS5:1. *Alcohol Clin Exp Res.* 2000;24(5):184A.
44. Sampson PD, Streissguth AP, Bookstein FL, et al. Incidence of fetal alcohol syndrome and prevalence of alcohol-related neurodevelopmental disorder. *Teratology.* 1997;56:317–326.
45. Lupton C, Burd L, & Harwood R. Cost of fetal alcohol spectrum disorders. *American Journal of Medical Genetics. Part C, Seminars in Medical Genetics,* 2004;127:42–50.
46. Klug MG, & Burd L. Fetal alcohol syndrome prevention: annual and cumulative cost savings. *Neurotoxicology and Teratology.* 2003; 25:763–765.
47. Institute of Medicine (I.O.M) of the National Academy of Sciences Committee to Study Fetal Alcohol Syndrome. Issues and research on fetal drug effects. In: Fetal Alcohol Syndrome. (Stratton D, Howe C, Battaglia F, eds.) Washington, D.C.: National Academy Press, 1996b:33–51.
48. Olney JW, Wozniak DF, Farber NB, et al. The enigma of fetal alcohol neurotoxicity. *Annals of Medicine.* 2002;34:109–119.
49. Guizzetti M, & Costa LG. Disruption of cholesterol homeostasis in the developing brain as a potential mechanism contributing to the developmental neurotoxicity of ethanol: An hypothesis. *Medical Hypotheses.* 2005;64:563–567.
50. Streissguth AP, & Little RE. Unit 5: Alcohol, pregnancy, and the Fetal Alcohol Syndrome: Second edition, Project Cork Institute Medical School Curriculum (Slide lecture series) on Biomedical education: Alcohol use and its medical consequences, produced by Dartmouth Medical School, 1994.
51. Noland JS, Singer LT, Arendt RE, et al. Executive functioning in preschool-age children prenatally exposed to alcohol, cocaine, and marijuana. *Alcohol Clin Exp Res.* 2003;27:647–656.

52. Kaemingk KL, Mulvaney S, Halverson PT. Learning following prenatal alcohol exposure: performance on verbal and visual multitrial tasks. *Archives of Clinical Neuropsychology.* 2003;18:33–47.
53. Mattson SN, Riley EP, Delis DC, et al. Verbal learning and memory in children with fetal alcohol syndrome. *Alcohol Clin Exp Res.* 1996;20:810–816.
54. Willford JA, Richardson GA, Leech SL, et al. Verbal and visuospatial learning and memory function in children with moderate prenatal alcohol exposure. *Alcohol Clin Exp Res.* 2004;28:497–507.
55. Adnams CM, Kodituwakku PW, Hay A, et al. Patterns of cognitive-motor development in children with Fetal Alcohol Syndrome from a community in South Africa. *Alcohol Clin Exp Res.* 2001;24:557–562.
56. Steinhausen HC, & Spohr HL. Long term outcome of children with fetal alcohol syndrome: Psychopathology, behavior, and intelligence. *Alcohol Clin Exp Res.* 1998;22:334–338.
57. Streissguth AP, Barr HM, Kogan J, et al. (1996, August). *Understanding the occurrence of secondary disabilities in clients with Fetal Alcohol Syndrome (FAS) and Fetal Alcohol Effects (FAE): Final Report to the Centers for Disease Control and Prevention (CDC).* Retrieved September 20, 2004, from http://www.cdc.gov/ncbddd/fas/secondary.htm
58. Streissguth AP, Bookstein FL, Sampson PD, et al. *The enduring effects of prenatal alcohol exposure on child development.* Ann Arbor, MI: University of Michigan Press, 1996b.
59. Clarren SK, Smith DW. The fetal alcohol syndrome. *N Eng J Med.* 1978;298:1063–1067.
60. Rosett HL. A clinical perspective of the fetal alcohol syndrome. *Alcohol Clin Exp Res.* 1980;4:119–122.
61. Sokol RJ, Clarren SK. Guidelines for use of terminology describing the impact of prenatal alcohol on the offspring. *Alcohol Clin Exp Res.* 1989;13:597–598.
62. Institute of Medicine (I.O.M) of the National Academy of Sciences Committee to Study Fetal Alcohol Syndrome. Diagnosis and clinical evaluation of fetal alcohol syndrome. In Fetal Alcohol Syndrome. (Stratton, K, Howe, C, Battaglia, F, eds.) Washington, D.C.: National Academy Press, 1996c:63–81.
63. Streissguth AP, Kopera-Fyre K, & Barr HM. (1996a). A preliminary report on primary and secondary disabilities in patients with fetal alcohol syndrome: why prevention is so needed. *Proceedings of the 1994 NIAAA FAS Prevension Conference.*
64. Abel EL & Hannigan JN. (1996) Risk factors pathogenesis.in Spohr HL & Steinhausen HC, Alcohol Pregnancy and Developing Child. Cambridge University Press, 1996; pp 63–75.
65. Ronen GM and Andrews WL, Holoprosencphaly as a possible embryonic alcohol effect. *J Am Med Assoc.* 1991;40:151.
66. Goldstein G and Arulanantham K. Neural tube defects and renal anomalies in a child with fetal alcohol syndrome. *J Pediatr.* 1978; 93:636.
67. Gabrielli O, Salvolini U, Coppa GV, et al. Magnetic resonance imaging in the malformative syndromes with mental retardation. *Pediatr Radiol.* 1990;21:16.
68. Schaefer GB, Shuman RM, Wilson DA, et al. Partial agenesis of the anterior corpus callosum: Correlation between appearances, imaging, and neuropathology. *Pediatr Neurol.* 1991;7:39.
69. Robin NH and Zackai EH. Unusual craniofacial dusmorphia due to prenatal alcohol and cocaine exposure. *Teratology.* 1994;50:160.
70. Mattson SN, Riley EP, Jernigan TL, et al. Fetal alcohol syndrome: A case report of neurophychological, MRI, and EEG assessment of two children. *Alc Clin Exp Res.* 1992;16:1001.
71. Coulter CL, Leech RW, Schaefer GB, et al. Midline cerebral dysgenesis, dysfunction of the hypothalamic-pituitary axis, and fetal alcohol effects. *Arch Neruol.* 1993;50:771.
72. Hannigan JH, Martier SS, Chugani HT, et al. Brain metabolilsm in children with fetal alcohol syndrome (FAS): A positron emission tomography study. *Alc Clin Exp Res.* 1995;19:53A.
73. Carren SK, Alvord EC, Sumi SM, et al. Brain malformations related to prenatal exposure to ethanol. *J Pediatr.* 1978;92:64.
74. Clarren SK. Neural tube defect and fetal alcohol syndrome. *J Pediatr.* 1979;95:328.
75. Clarren SK. Recognition of the fetal alcohol syndrome. *JAMA.* 1981;245(23):2436–2439.
76. Peiffer J, Majewski F, Fischbach H, et al. Alcohol embryo- and fetophathy; Neuropathology of 3 children and 3 fetuses. *J Neurol Sci.* 1979;41:125.
77. Wisniewski K, Dambska M, Sher JH, et al. A clinical neuropathology study of the fetal alcohol syndrome, *Neuropediatricss.* 1983; 14:197.
78. Mattson SN, Riley EP, Jernigan TL, et al. A decrease in the size of the basal ganglia following prenatal alcohol exposure: A preliminary report. *Nuerotoxicology.* 1994;16:283.
79. Riley EP, Mattson SN, Sowel ER, et al. Abnormalities of the corpus callosum in children prenatally exposed to alcohol. *Alcohol Clin Exp Res.* 1995;19(5):1198–1202.
80. Sulik KK, Johnston MC, Webb MA. Fetal alcohol syndrome: embryogenesis in a mouse model. *Science.* 1981;214:936–938.
81. Globus A and Scheibel AB. The effect of visual deprivationf on cortical neurons; A Goldy study. *Exp Neurol.* 1967;19:333–345.
82. Wiesel TN. Postnatal development of the visual cortex and the influence of environment. *Nature* 1982;299:583–592.
83. Stromland K.. Eye ground malformations in the fetal alcohol syndrome. *Neuropediatrics.* 1981;12:97–98.
84. Stromland K. Ocular abnormalities in the fetal alcohol syndrome. *Acta ophthalmol.* 1985;63:(Suppl 171)1–50.
85. Miller M, Epstein R, Sugar J, et al. Anterior segment anomalies associated with the fetal alcohol syndrome, 1984.
86. Chan T, Bowell R, O'Keefe M, et al.Ocular manifestation in fetal alcohol syndrome. *Br J Ophthalmol.* 1991;25:524–526.
87. Stromland R and Hellstrom A. Fetal alcohol syndrome—an opthalmological and socioeducational prospective study. *Pediatrics.*; 1996; 97:845–850.
88. Church MW, and Holloway JA. The effect of prenatal alcohol exposure on postnatal development of the brain stem auditory evoked potential in the rat. *Alcohol Clin Exp Res.* 1984;8:258–263.
89. Northern JL, and Down SM. Hearing in children, 3rd ed. Williams & Wilkins, Baltimore, 1984.
90. Church MW. The effects of prenatal alcohol exposure on hearing and vestibular function. In Spohr HL and Steinhausen HC (Eds.) Alcohol, Pregnancy and the Developing Child. Cambridge University Press, 1996.
91. Wurst FM, Alling C, Aradottir S, et al. Emerging biomarkers: new directions and clinical applications. *Alcohol Clin Exp Res.* 2005 Mar; 29(3):465–73.
92. Kelly TM, Donovan JE, Chung T, et al. Alcohol use disorders among emergency department-treated older adolescents: A new brief screen (RUFT-Cut) using the AUDIT, CAGE, CRAFFT, and RAPS-QF. *Alcohol Clin Exp Res.* 2004; 28:746–753.
93. Gareri J, Chan D, Klein J, et al. Motherisk Team. Screening for fetal alcohol spectrum disorder. *Canadian Family Physician.* 2005; 51:33–34.
94. Stoler JM, Huntington KS, Peterson CM, et al. The prenatal detection of significant alcohol exposure with maternal blood markers. *Journal of Pediatrics.* 1998;133:346–352.
95. Clarren, S. K., Randels, S. P., Sanderson, M., & Fineman, R. (2001). Screening for Fetal Alcohol Syndrome in primary schools: A feasibility study. *Teratology.* 63, 3–10.
96. Koren G, & Nulman I. *The Motherisk guide to diagnosing Fetal Alcohol Spectrum Disorder.* Toronto: The Hospital For Sick Children, 2002 (1).
97. Poitra BA, Marioin S, Dionne M, et al. A school-based screening program for fetal alcohol syndrome. *Neurotoxicol Teratol.* 2003; 25:725–729.
98. Burd L, Klug MG, Martsolf JT, et al. Fetal Alcohol Syndrome: Neuropsychiatric phenomics. *Neurotoxicol Teratol.* 2003; 25:697–705.

99. Koren G, Chan D, Klein J, et al. Estimation of fetal exposure to drugs of abuse, environmental tobacco smoke, and ethanol. *The Drug Monitor.* 2002;24:23–25.

100. Chan D, Klein J, Karaskov T, et al. Fetal exposure to alcohol as evidenced by fatty acid ethyl esters in meconium in the absence of maternal drinking history in pregnancy. *Ther Drug Monit.* 2004;26:474–481.

101. Bearer CF, Lee S, Salvator AE, et al. Ethyl linoleate in meconium: A biomarker for prenatal ethanol exposure. *Alcohol Clin Exp Res.* 1999;23:487–493.

102. Klein J, Karaskov T, & Koren G. Fatty acid ethyl esters—a novel biological marker for heavy in utero ethanol exposure: A case report. *The Drug Monitor.* 1999;21:644–646.

103. Moore CM, & Lewis D. Fatty acid ethyl esters in meconium: Biomarkers for the detection of alcohol exposure in neonates. *Clin Chim Acta.* 2001;312:235–237.

104. Bierut LJ, Dinwiddie SH, Begleiter H, et al. Familial transmission of substance dependence: Alcohol, marihuana, cocaine and habitual smoking. *Archives of General Psychology.* 1998;55:982–988.

105. Kessler RC, MacGonagle KA, Zhao S, et al. Lifetime and 12-month prevalence of DSM-II-R psychiatric disoders in the United States. *Archives of General Psychology.* 1994;51:8–19.

106. Warren KR, Li TK. Genetic polymorphisms: Impact on the risk of fetal alcohol spectrum disorders. *Birth Defects Res A Clin Mol Teratol.* 2005;73:195–203.

107. Higuchi S, Matsushita S, Masaki T, et al. Influence of genetic variations of ethanol-metabolizing enzymes on phenotypes of alcohol-related disorders. *Annals of the New York Academy of Sciences.* 2004;1025:472–480.

108. Gladstone J, Levy M, Nulman I, et al. Characteristics of pregnant women who engage in binge alcohol consumption. *Can Med Assoc J.* 1997;156(6):789–794.

109. Olsen J, Pereira A, Da, C, et al. Does maternal tobacco smoking modify the effect of alcohol on fetal growth? *Am J Public Health.* 1991;81:69–73.

110. Streissguth AP, Bookstein FL, & Barr HM. A dose—response study of the enduring effects of prenatal alcohol exposure: birth to 14 years. in Spohr HL & Steinhausen HC, Alcohol Pregnancy and Developing Child. Cambridge University Press.(pp 141–68); 1996.

111. Gladstone J, Nulman I, Koren G. Reproductive risks of binge drinking during pregnancy. Reprod Toxicol. 1996;10(1):3–13.

112. Nulman I, Rovet J, Kennedy D, et al. Binge alcohol consumption by non-alcohol-dependent women during pregnancy affects child behavior, but not general intellectual functioning: A prospective controlled study. *Archives of Women's Mental Health,* 2004;7:173–181.

113. Cornelius MD, Richardson GA, Day NL, et al. A comparison of prenatal drinking in two recent samples of adolescents and adults. *J Stud Alcohol.* 1994;55:412–419.

114. Henriksen TB, Hjollund NH, Jensen TK, et al. Alcohol consumption at the time of conception and spontaneous abortion. *American Journal of Epidemiology,* 2004;160:661–667.

115. Sulik KK, Johnston MC, Draft PA, et al. Fetal alcohol syndrome and DiGeorge anomaly: critical ethanol exposure periods for craniofacial malformations as illustrated in an animal model. *Am J Med Genet.* 1986;2:97–112.

116. Maier SE, Chen WJ, Miller JA, et al. Fetal alcohol exposure and temporal vulnerability regional differences in alcohol-induced microencephaly as a function of the timing of binge-like alcohol exposure during rat brain development. *Alcohol Clin Exp Res.* 1997; 21:1418–1428.

117. Middaugh LD, & Boggan WO. Postnatal growth deficits in prenatal ethanol-exposed mice: characteristics and critical periods. *Alcohol Clin Exp Res.* 1997;15:919–926.

118. Coles CD. Critical periods for prenatal alcohol exposure. Evidence from animal and human studies, 1991. http://www.fas-region3.com/files/critperiod.pdf

119. Goodlett CR, Marcussen BL, and West JR. A single day of alcohol exposure during the brain growth spurt induces brain weight restriction and cerebellar Purkinje cell loss. *Alcohol.* 1990;7:107–114.

120. Sakata-Haga H, Sawada K, Ohta K, et al. Adverse effects of maternal ethanol consumption on development of dorsal hippocampus in rat offspring. *Acta Neuropathologica (Berl).* 2003;105:30–36. Epub 2002 Sep 11.

121. West JR, Wei-Jung A Chen, Pantazis NJ. Fetal Alcohol Syndrome: The vulnerability of the developing brain and possible mechanisms of damage. *Metab Brain Dis.* 1994;9:291–322.

122. Miller MW. Effects of alcohol on the generation and migration of cerebral cortical neurons. *Science.* 1986;233:1308–1311.

123. Miller MW. Migration of cortical neurons altered by gestational expousre to alcohol. *Alcohol Clin Exp Res.* 1993;12:304–314.

124. Marcussen BL, Goodlett CR, Mahoney JC, et al. Alcohol-induced Purkinje cell loss during differentiation but not during neurogenesis. *Alcohol.* 1994;11:147–156.

125. Kelly SJ, Mahoney JC, West JR. Changes in brain microvasculature resulting from early postnatal alcohol exposure. *Alcohol.* 1990; 7:43–47.l

126. Mukherjee AB, Hodgen GD. Maternal ethanol exposure induced transient impairment of umbilical circulation and fetal hypoxia in monkeys. *Science.* 1982;218:700–701.

127. Jones KL, Chambers CC, Johnson KA. The effect of disulfiram on the unborn baby. *Teratology.* 1991;43:438.

128. Garro AJ, McBeth DL, Lima V, et al. Ethanol consumption inhibits fetal DNA methylation in mice. Implications for the fetal alcohol syndrome. *Alcohol Clin Exp Res.* 1991;15:395–398.

129. Espina N, Lima V, Lieber CS, et al. In vitro and in vivo inhibitory effects of ethanol and acetaldehyde on 06 methyl-guamine transferase. *Carcinogenesis.* 1988; 9:761–766.

130. Devi BG, Henderson GI, Frosto TA, et al. Effect of acute ethanol exposure on cultured fetal rat hepatocytes: relation to mitochondrial function. *Alcohol Clin Exp Res.* 1994; 18(6):1436–1442.

131. De Groot M, Littauer A. Hypoxia, reactive oxygen and cell injury. *Free Radic Biol Med.* 1989; 6:541–551.

132. Nordman R, Ribiere C, Ronach H. Implication of free radical mechanisms in ethanol-induced cellular injury. *Free Radic Biol Med.* 1992;12:219–239.

133. Arienti G, DiRenzo GC, Cosumi EV, et al. Rat brain microsome fluidity is modified by prenatal ethanol administration. *Neurochem Res.* 1993;18:335–338.

134. Burmistrov SO, Kotin AM, Borodkin YS. Changes in activity of antioxidative enzymes and lipid peroxidation levels in brain tissue of embryos exposed prenatally to ethanol. *Byull Eksper Biolog Medits.* 1991;112:606–607.

135. Murdoch RN, Edwards T. Alterations in the methylation of membrane phospholipids in the uterus and postimplantation embryo following exposure to teratogenic doses of alcohol. *Biochem Inter.* 1992;28:1029–1037.

136. Klemm WR. Dehydration: A new alcohol theory. *Alcohol.* 1990; 12:49–59.

137. Hungund BL, Mahadik SP. Role of gangliosides in behavioural and biochemical action of alcohol: cell membrane structure and function. *Alcohol Clin Exp Res.* 1993;12:329–339.

138. Davis WL, Crawford LA, Cooper OJ, et al. Ethanol induces the generation of reactive free radicals by neural crest cells in vitro. *J Cranifac Genet Devel Biol.* 1990;10:277–293.

139. Dreosti IE. Nutritional factors underlying the expression of the fetal alcohol syndrome. NY *Acad Sci.* 1993;628:193–204.

140. Collier HOJ, McDonald-Gibson WJ, Saeed SA. Letter: Stimulation of prostaglandin biosynthesis by capsaicin, ethanol, and tyramine. *Lancet.* 1975;1:702.

141. Pastan IH, Johnson GS, Anderson WB. Role of cyclic nucleotides in growth control. *Annual Review of Biochemistry.* 1975;44:491–522.

142. Pennington S. Ethanol—induced growth inhibition: the role of cAMP—dependentprotein kinase. *Alcohol Clin Exp Res.* 1988; 12:125–129.

143. Lin GWJ. Effect of ethanol feeding during pregnancy on placental transfer of alpha—aminoisobutyric acid in the rat. *Life Sci.* 1981; 28:595–601.

144. Brown NA, Goulding EH, Fabro S. Ethanol embryotoxicity: direct effects on mammalian embryos in vitro. *Science.* 1979;206:573.
145. Fisher SE, Inselman LS, Duffy L, et al. Ethanol and fetal nutrition: effects of chronic ethanol exposure on rat placental growth and membrane-associated folic acid receptor binding activity. *J Pediatr Gastroenterol Nutr.* 1985;4:645–649.
146. Snyder AK, Singh, SP, Pullen GL. Ethanol-induced intrauterine growth retardation: correlation with placental glucose transfer. *Alcohol Clin Exp Res.* 1986;10:167–170.
147. Schenker SJ, Johnson RF, Mahuren JD, et al. Human placental vitamin B6 (pyridoxal) transport: normal characteristics and effects of ethanol. Am J Physiol. 1992;262:R966–R974.
148. Fisher SE, Duffy L, Atkinson M. Selective fetal malnutrition: effect of acute and chronic ethanol exposure upon rat placental Na,K-ATPase activity. *Alcohol Clin Exp Res.* 1986;10:150–153.
149. Ugarte G, Valenzuela J. Mechanisms of liver and pancreas damage in man. In Biological Basis of Alcoholism, ed. Israel Y & Mardones J, pp 133–161. New York: Wiley, 1971.
150. Yang HY, Shum AYC, Ng HT, et al. Effect of ethanol on human umbilical artery and vein in vitro. *Gynecol Obstet Invest.* 1986; 21,131–135.
151. Reynolds JD, Penning DH, Dexter F, et al. Ethanol increases uterine blood flow and fetal arterial blood oxygen tension in the near term pregnant ewe. *Alcohol.* 1996;13(3):251–256.
152. Ramanathan R, Wilkemeyer MF, Mittal B, et al. Alcohol inhibits cell-cell adhesion mediated by human L1. *J Cell Biol.* 1996; 133:381–390.
153. Broun S. New experiments underscore warnings on maternal drinking. *Science.* 1996;273:738–739.
154. Streissguth AP, Aase IM, Clarren SK, et al. Fetal alcohol syndrome in adolescents and adults. *J Am Med Assoc.* 1991;265:1961–1967.
155. Steinhausen HC, Nestler V, & Huth H. Psychopathology and mental functions in the offspring of alcoholic and epileptic mothers. *J Am Acad Child Adolesc Psychiatry.* 1982;21:268–273.
156. O'Connor MJ, Shah B, Whaley S, et al. Psychiatric illness in a clinical sample of children with prenatal alcohol exposure. *Am J Drug Alcohol Abuse.* 2002b;28:743–754.
157. Mattson SN, Riley EP, Gramling L, et al. Heavy prenatal alcohol exposure with or without physical features of fetal alcohol syndrome leads to IQ deficits. *J Pediatr.* 1997;131:718–721.
158. Steinhausen HC, Willms J, Metzke CW, et al. Behavioural phenotype in foetal alcohol syndrome and foetal alcohol effects. *Developmental Medicine and Child Neurology,* 2004;45:179–182.
159. Famy C, Streissguth AP, & Unis AS. Mental illness in adults with fetal alcohol syndrome or fetal alcohol effects. *Am J Psychiatr.* 1998;155:522–554.
160. Coles CD & Platzman KA. Behavioral develpment in children prenatally exposed to drugs and alcohol. *Int J Addict.* 1993; 28:1393–1433.
161. O'Connor MJ, Kogan N, & Findlay R. Prenatal alcohol exposure and attachment behavior in children. *Alcohol Clin Exp Res.* 2002a; 26:1592–1602.
162. Streissguth AP, Bookstein FL, Barr HM, et al. Risk factors for adverse life outcomes in fetal alcohol syndrome and fetal alcohol effects. *J Dev Behav Pediatr.* 2004;25:228–238.
163. Caley LM, Kramer C, & Robinson LK. Fetal alcohol spectrum disorder. *The Journal of School Nursing,* 2005;21:139–146.
164. Hankin JR. Fetal alcohol syndrome prevention research. *Alcohol Research & Health.* 2002;26:58–65.

CHAPTER 15

DETERMINATION OF PRENATAL EXPOSURES

Joey N. Gareri, Julia Klein, and Gideon Koren

INTRODUCTION

Prenatal substance abuse is an ongoing concern, with significant impact on neonatal health and development.[1–11] Drug abuse in pregnancy exists across socioeconomic lines and has been consistently confirmed in numerous prevalence studies over the last decade.[12,13] Rates of prenatal drug use have been determined by maternal report, urine analysis, blood analysis, and meconium analysis ranging from 3.4 to 31% for cocaine, 1–12% for cannabis, 1.6–21% for opiates, and 0.1–4% for ethanol in general and high-risk populations.[13–17] Over the last two decades, the use of meconium as a matrix for assessing prenatal drug exposure has yielded a method exhibiting higher sensitivity, easier collection, and a larger window of detection than other traditional matrices.[18,19] In addition to its clinical utility in neonatal intervention and follow-up, the capability of meconium analysis to detect drugs of abuse and their multiple metabolites[20] provides a powerful research tool, assisting in the study of maternal-fetal drug disposition and metabolic capabilities specific to the fetus.[21–23]

While detecting neonatal withdrawal is one objective commonly listed in favor of neonatal drug screening, one study demonstrated that only 10% of screened infants with "withdrawal symptoms" tested positive for drugs of abuse, with 75% of infants with positive screens being asymptomatic.[24] In many cases, the benefit of screening lies mainly in the potential for intervention based on the developmentally detrimental lifestyle factors associated with prenatal drug abuse.[25] It is important to note that the use of unvalidated screening data to assess prenatal drug abuse can be unethical and at times dangerous.[26] The mass-spectrometer is the preferred detector for confirmational analysis due to its unequalled specificity.[24] Gas chromatography/mass spectrometry (GCMS) and liquid chromatography/mass spectrometry (LCMS) methods exhibit the ease of multi–sample processing in conjunction with reproducibility and high recovery rates for corresponding extraction procedures.[23,27]

The ability of meconium analysis to detect prenatal drug use across the latter two-thirds of pregnancy not only improves sensitivity over alternative screening matrices, but is customized to the detection of addicted behavior. Since meconium analysis cannot determine drug use in the first trimester, the method effectively protects against the labeling of mothers who ceased their drug or alcohol use upon the detection of pregnancy. In spite of increased sample preparation time relative to blood and urine, the long metabolic history, coupled with the ease and wide window of collection of meconium make it the ideal matrix for determining fetal drug exposure.

MECONIUM AS A MATRIX

Meconium comprises the neonate's first several bowel movements, identified most commonly by its dark green/black color and a lack of odor usually inherent to regular feces. It is a highly complex matrix consisting of water, desquamated epithelial cells from the gastrointestinal tract and skin, lanugo (fine neonatal hair), fatty material from the vernix caseosa, bile acids and salts, cholesterol and sterol precursors, blood group substances, enzymes, mucopolysaccharides, sugars, lipids, proteins, trace metals, various pancreatic and intestestinal secretions, as well as residue of swallowed amniotic fluid.[28–33]

The timing of formation of meconium has been variably reported from within the first trimester[34] to as late as five months of gestation.[35] The assertion that meconium begins to form at approximately 12 weeks of gestation is likely the most accurate. It is at this time that fetal swallowing of amniotic fluid begins,[31,33] and the formation of meconium has been evidenced at this time period by the presence of cocaine found in the meconium of early gestational fetuses.[30] Drugs of abuse are deposited into meconium by deposition from bile or urine via fetal swallowing.[31] Fetal swallowing is thought to be the mechanism by which drugs are concentrated in the meconium; as the fetus releases urine into the amniotic fluid, any excreted compounds and metabolites are then swallowed and ultimately deposited into the meconium.[30] Most drugs of abuse are capable of crossing the placenta at rates controlled by their molecular size, ionization state, lipophilicity, and degree of plasma protein or placental tissue binding.[32] Placental transfer of most drugs of abuse takes place primarily by passive diffusion due their small molecular size and high lipophilicity; because of this, placental blood flow may be the most critical limiting factor regarding drug transport to the fetus.[36] Ultimately, fetal exposure is a product of maternal consumption, metabolism and elimination, placental transfer and metabolism, and fetal metabolism.[32] These factors make meconium an optimal matrix for identifying in utero exposure as it is considered to be static once deposited in the fetal intestine,[27] a preserved record of the ultimate exposure by the fetus.

Urine contamination of meconium occurs when a neonate has been exposed to a compound near-term and evacuates drug-contained urine into a meconium soiled diaper. This phenomenon increases the sensitivity of meconium screening due to the augmentation of drug levels in the specimen. Urine contamination can however interfere with the development of dose-response relationships with regard to the level of drugs present in meconium. Urine-deposited drugs have not undergone the same degree of metabolism as meconium-deposited drugs, altering the expected relationships between drugs and metabolites in meconium.

The collection of meconium is noninvasive, making sample collection easy[12] and more successful than urine collection.[37] One major advantage of meconium is a relatively wide window for sample collection. Studies using zinc coproporphyrin (a meconium-specific bile pigment) as a marker have determined that meconium is fully evacuated by 125 hours postnatally.[28] Other markers of meconium excretion do not appear in the literature and are not used in the standard practice of meconium analysis. The texture and odor of the sample is used to qualitatively distinguish meconium from postnatally produced feces. The findings attributed to the study of zinc coproporphyrin have correlated well with the practice of meconium collection; while all meconium is evacuated by 125 hours postnatally, viable analysis appears to be optimal via collection within 72 hours, with the later stages of meconium excretion producing a transitional matrix of meconium and feces. Analysis of meconium for cocaine and opiates has demonstrated positive results upon third postnatal day sample collection.[38] While 99% of term infants pass their first formed stool by 48 hours, in extremely low birth weight infants, of particular interest in the drug-exposed neonatal population, median age of first stool is 3 days, with 90% of infants passing their first stool by day 12.[39] This window of opportunity for sample collection far beyond 48 hours postnatally is a remarkable advantage of this matrix.[24] In general, it can be assumed that in a general neonatal population, meconium can be reliably collected for drug analysis within the first three postnatal days.

Meconium is collected by scraping the contents (0.5 g minimum) of the soiled diaper into a specimen collection container. The thick, viscous nature of the substance makes collection quite easy. Meconium for drug analysis should be stored at −20°C or −80°C. For transport to external laboratories for analysis, it is advisable to store at −80°C until frozen and ship on dry ice.

PRENATAL COCAINE EXPOSURE AND DETECTION

Cocaine crosses the placenta via passive diffusion.[40] The metabolism of cocaine has been shown to be highly variable, with little consistency in the relative amounts of cocaine and its metabolites among specimens.[5–20] This fact, in combination with the potential augmentation of cocaine and metabolites in meconium by urine contamination in the diaper, has created difficulty in establishing a genuine dose-response relationship.[25–41] In spite of this, there is solid evidence correlating the frequency, timing, and amount of cocaine use by the mother with the amount of cocaine found in meconium by immunoassay.[30] The concentration of cocaine and metabolites in meconium diminishes rapidly 48 hours after birth, with the exception of benzoylecgonine, which remains detectable with relative frequency up to twice as long.[27]

Cocaine metabolites exhibit a diverse range of polarities[23] and are not uniformly distributed in meconium.[42] The metabolite of cocaine most commonly determined is the hydrolysis product benzoylecgonine. Low confirmation rates were reported for benzoylecgonine[26] prior to the discovery of several additional metabolites, which contributed significantly to immunoreactivity in screening methods.[20,23] Cocaine is almost never found alone in meconium, whereas certain metabolites can exist exclusively within a given sample. Benzoylecgonine and cocaethylene have both shared the distinction of being the sole immunoreactive cocaine metabolite present in meconium samples.[27] Different species of cocaine metabolites can also be associated with specific drug use patterns. Cocaethylene, norcocaethylene, and ecgonine ethyl ester are all associated with the concurrent abuse of cocaine and ethanol, while anhydroecgonine and anhydroecgonine methyl ester are pyrolytic products of cocaine indicative of "crack" cocaine use.[23]

Cocaine: Laboratory Analysis

Certain extraction procedures may exclude specific metabolites due to differences in pH that subsequently affect ionization state.[42] Extraction of cocaine and metabolites with methanol was found to result in the highest sensitivity and lowest limits of detection.[43] Inclusive extraction procedures have been developed for GCMS and LCMS, capable of extracting up to 15 metabolites of cocaine simultaneously.[20,23]

Table 15-1
Confounders in Assessing Poor Perinatal Outcome Associated with Illicit Drug Use[49,50]

Cigarette smoking
Concurrent alcohol use
Multiple drug use
Sexually transmitted disease
Poverty
Poor prenatal care
Poor nutrition (maternal)
Poor nutrition (post-natal)
Poor social environment (postnatal)

Various immunoassays [i.e., radioimmunoassay (RIA), enzyme-multiplied immunoassay technique (EMIT), enzyme-linked immunosorbent assay (ELISA)] are commonly used in initial toxicological screening for cocaine and cocaine metabolites. All methods are capable of achieving a high sensitivity of with cut-offs of 50 ng/g or lower for multiple cocaine-related compounds.[24,26,44] In order to increase specificity (i.e., limit the number of false positive results) the cut-off for positive samples is often set at 100 ng/g for cocaine or benzoylecgonine. The procedure used for extracting, isolating, and/or purifying cocaine and metabolites from meconium has a much more important effect on the sensitivity of a screening method than the immunoassay procedure itself.[26,29] GCMS and LCMS are capable of simultaneously identifying cross-reacting cocaine metabolites.[20,45] The cross-reactivity of specific cocaine metabolites due to structural similarity and affinity to the antibody complex will vary with the specific immunoassay screening method initially used. Information regarding cross-reactivity is generally provided within the respective immunoassay kit.

Cocaine: Clinical Implications

The clinical effects of prenatal exposure to cocaine are not conclusive. While some studies have claimed neuroteratogenicity as an adverse outcome related to prenatal exposure,[46] later systematic reviews could not detect long-term developmental consequences directly attributable to cocaine.[47] Associated effects such as dose-related decrease in fetal weight and head size,[2] prolonged hospitalization,[48] and increased early life problems[6] may not be due to cocaine itself, but rather due to a large number of confounders associated with prenatal drug abuse (Table 15-1).[49,50] Upon controlling for confounders, only placental abruption and premature rupture of membranes were found to be attributable to prenatal cocaine use.[1]

PRENATAL OPIATE EXPOSURE AND DETECTION

Animal studies have shown that opiates distribute readily across the placenta, resulting in peak fetal blood levels occurring relatively quickly post intravenous administration as studied with meperidine, methadone, and morphine.[36] Morphine distributes widely and variably into many fetal tissues, independent of administered dose.[19] Correlations have been demonstrated between higher dose, longer duration and later gestational timing of exposure and increased levels of morphine in meconium.[51] The extent of fetal exposure to different opiates, based on animal studies, is in the order of meperidine > methadone > morphine.[36] Heroin, based on its high degree of lipid solubility, would carry a high index of fetal exposure as it diffuses readily across the placenta as well as the blood-brain barrier. While this increased fetal exposure has not been specifically shown in animal studies, this mechanism of increased membrane permeability due to the addition of two acetyl groups to the morphine molecule is understood to be the mitigating factor in the pronounced central nervous system effects seen with heroin over the more peripheral activity of morphine.

Human studies have shown morphine detectable in meconium collected on the third postnatal day in 75% of subjects upon serial analysis.[52] Higher levels seen in second day-collected samples suggest that hydrolysis of glucuronidated morphine in meconium and subsequent reabsorption from the intestine occurs.[19] Morphine is extensively glucuronidated in the liver producing the major metabolites morphine-3-glucuronide (inactive), morphine-6-glucuronide (active), and normorphine.[36] Bound morphine is found in much higher concentrations in the bile than in other tissues and fluids[19], predicting ready deposition into meconium. Heroin is rapidly deacetylated in vivo to the active metabolite 6-monoacetylmorphine.[53] Fetal liver microsomes are also capable of N-dealkylating meperidine and methadone.[36] Fetal exposure is to opiates is mediated by placental clearance, maternal and fetal protein binding, and fetal microsome activity.[36]

Opiates: Laboratory Analysis

Acid and methanolic extractions can be used to extract opiates from meconium with varying degrees of success.[29,45,54] Levels of codeine, hydrocodone, and hydromorphone are known to increase markedly following acid hydrolysis of meconium, indicating a variable degree of glucuronidation in these compounds.[29] Simultaneous methanolic extraction of morphine, codeine, 6-monoacetylmorphine, hydrocodone, and hydromorphone is possible.[45]

Immunoassay analysis for opiates using FPIA and enzyme-based systems can exhibit significant cross-reactivity between illicit and prescribed opiates.[45,54] In spite of this, some radioimmunoassay systems for free morphine analysis have demonstrated negligible cross-reactivity with hydrocodone.[55] The immunoreactivity displayed by hydrocodone and its metabolite hydromorphone as well as meperidine and codeine warrants confirmational analysis in cases of opiate-positive screens in order to avoid unnecessary labeling or misdiagnosis. The sensitivities of the opiate immunoassays range from 25 ng/g to 100 ng/g,[54,56,57] however, the cutoff value for positive results is often set at 100 ng/g of meconium. GCMS confirmation of opiate-positive immunoassays is capable of determining multiple opiate metabolites, including morphine, codeine, 6-monoacetylmorphine, hydromorphone, and hydrocodone.[45,58] The cut-off of all these analytes is 50 ng/g.[45] Although the assay sensitivity was far below the cutoff levels, these levels were selected to minimize the number of unconfirmed positives. Naturally, the cut-off value is higher in the immunoassays than in the confirmatory methods because the immunoassays are specific for the entire group of opiates not for each individual opiate, while GC/MS exhibits very high specificity for each individual opiate.

Opiates: Clinical Implications

Withdrawal manifestations are the most significant concern regarding prenatal exposure to opiates.[7,8,25,59] It has been speculated that reabsorption of morphine from intestinal tissue and meconium may actually alleviate potential opiate withdrawal in addicted neonates, although this protective effect is rarely seen clinically.[11] The pronounced effects of withdrawal seen in neonates in the absence of large morphine concentrations in CNS tissues indicates a high neonatal sensitivity to morphine as determined by human case reports and studies in nonhuman primates.[19]

PRENATAL CANNABIS EXPOSURE AND DETECTION

The plant *Cannabis Sativa* produces over 50 unique compounds known as cannabinoids, with Δ^9-tetrahydrocannabinol (THC) being the most prevalent and psychoactive. Both human and animal studies have shown that cannabinoids cross the placenta, resulting in peak fetal levels after approximately 2 hours post inhalation.[36] Levels in the maternal circulation remain higher than those on the fetal side at all times after smoke inhalation, presumably due to extensive protein binding.[36,60] The higher frequency of episodic use of cannabis in pregnancy, compared to other drugs of abuse, limits the sensitivity of meconium analysis in detecting infrequent or isolated fetal cannabinoid exposure.[56] No dose-response relationship or correlations have been established regarding the level of use of marijuana in pregnancy and the levels of cannabinoids found in meconium. Upon serial analysis of meconium for cannabinoids, there is a 60% rate of subsequent detection if the initially collected sample was positive.[56]

THC is metabolized to the active compound 11-hydroxy-Δ^9-tetrahydrocannabinol (11-OH-THC), which is principally excreted in feces.[36] A subsequent metabolite, 11-nor-Δ^9-tetrahydrocannabinol-9-carboxylic acid (THC-COOH), is most often used in meconium analysis due to the fact that it is the major urinary metabolite of THC[56,61] and most immunoassays used for meconium are also used in urinalysis. 8β-hydroxy-Δ^9-tetrahydrocannabinol (8β-OH-THC) and 8β,11-dihydroxy-Δ^9-tetrahydrocannabinol (8β,11-diOH-THC) have also been identified as THC metabolites found in meconium.[62]

Cannabis: Laboratory Analysis

Extraction of cannabinoids for immunoassay can be carried out via normal saline, methanol, or acetic acid/diphenylamine in acetone, depending on the immunoassay in use.[61] Methanolic extraction of THC-COOH from meconium is capable of yielding a recovery as high as 79%.[45] For GCMS confirmation, an additional hexane/ethyl acetate extraction step is required.[45,61] Base hydrolysis improves the extraction of THC-COOH, indicating that it is significantly glucuronidated in meconium.[29,61] RIA, FPIA, EMIT, and ELISA are all used in screening for cannabinoids in meconium with variable limits of detection.[45] ELISA demonstrated a confirmation rate of 100% in one study confirmed by GCMS.[44] THC, 11-OH-THC, 8β-OH-THC, and 8β,11-diOH-THC are all considered major contributors to immunoreactivity when testing for THC-COOH using EMIT.[45] Immunoassay screening for cannabinoids demonstrates sensitivities ranging from 22.7 to 98%.[44,56] This range of sensitivity is likely due to differences in the relative study population as infrequent cannabis users are thought to increase the rate of false-negatives.[56]

The specificity of GCMS confirmational analysis in meconium testing for cannabinoids is dependant on the number of metabolites determined and the extraction procedure utilized. The use of THC-COOH as a primary analyte means that any extraction procedure that reduces the ration of THC-COOH/total cannabinoids will result in lower rates of confirmation.[45] This can be adjusted by optimizing THC-COOH extraction[44,61] or determining a greater number of potentially immunoreactive cannabinoids and THC metabolites via mass spectrometry.[29,45] GCMS confirmation of THC-COOH can produce a limit of detection as low as 2 ng/g.[61]

Cannabis: Clinical Implications

Infrequent use of cannabis in pregnancy may have little to no effect of the fetus;[3] however, it is not known if there is a threshold level use for adverse developmental effects that is any way related to the screening cut-off values.[4] Unlike other drugs of abuse, acute complications at birth are unlikely to occur via cannabis exposure alone.

AMPHETAMINES/PHENCYCLIDINE EXPOSURE AND DETECTION

Amphetamines and phencyclidine are used in pregnancy, although less extensively relative to other drugs of abuse.[15,57,63] Methamphetamine has been shown to cross the placenta within 30 seconds of intraperitoneal injections in animal studies. Peak concentrations are lower on the fetal side, but slower elimination results in prolonged fetal exposure relative to the mother.[64] While no dose-response relationship has been established for amphetamines in meconium, individual case reports show agreement between self-reported heavy prenatal use of methamphetamine and high concentrations (200–1000 ng/g) in meconium.[63] Animal studies of phencyclidine demonstrated somewhat slower placental transfer, reaching peak fetal levels 2 hours post parenteral administration. Phencyclidine appears to accumulate in fetal tissue, with fetal levels reaching 10-fold higher than maternal blood.[65]

Multiple derivatives and metabolites of amphetamine, including; 3,4-methylenedioxyamphetamine (MDA), 3,4-methylene-dioxy-methamphetamine (MDMA), 4-hydroxy-3-methoxy-methamphetamine (HMMA), 3,4-methylene-dioxyethyl-amphetamine (MDEA), *N*-methyl-1-(3,4-methylene-dioxyphenyl)-2-butanamine (MBDB) are extractable from meconium, but generally only the parent compounds (amphetamine/methamphetamine/MDMA) seem to be detected in routine practice.[63]

Amphetamines/Phencyclidine: Laboratory Analysis

For screening purposes, amphetamines and phencyclidine can be extracted using methanol. For confirmation by GCMS, amphetamines can be extracted from meconium by chloroform in basic conditions followed by derivatization.[45,57] Phencyclidine extraction has been reported using ethyl acetate.[45]

Screening for amphetamines and phencyclidine has been described via EMIT immunoassay. This method demonstrates a cutoff of 200 ng/g and 20 ng/g for amphetamines and phencyclidine, respectively.[45] It has been speculated, due to difficulties with confirmation, that unknown metabolites of phencyclidine contribute to immunoreactivity upon meconium screening.[29] Confirmation of amphetamines by LC-MS exhibits a limit of detection of 1 ng/g for all amphetamine derivatives listed above.[63] GCMS validation is also reported with limits of detection of 50 ng/g, and 3 ng/g for amphetamine/methamphetamine and phencyclidine, respectively.[45]

Amphetamines/Phencyclidine: Clinical Implications

Prenatal exposure to amphetamines has been linked to oral clefting, cardiac anomalies, and intrauterine growth retardation in both human and animal studies.[9] A comparison of phencyclidine-exposed neonates to matched cocaine-exposed neonates demonstrated a nearly twofold increase in incidence of intrauterine growth retardation, preterm labor, withdrawal/intoxication, and prolonged hospitalization.[10] While confounding factors (see Table 15-1) are thought to interfere with the definitive establishment of causality in cocaine-exposed neonates, the increased frequency with which these adverse effects are seen in phencyclidine-exposed neonates indicates that prenatal exposure is of significant clinical concern. While the adverse effects of these compounds are significant, the low incidence of prenatal use[15,57,63] dictates that screening is likely beneficial only upon suspicion of use. It is likely that designer drugs in this class (e.g., MDMA) are used mainly for recreational purposes and discontinued upon realization of pregnancy.[66]

CURRENT TRENDS IN ILLICIT DRUG DETECTION

ELISA is rapidly becoming the favored method for screening. While the assay sensitivity can be as low as 5 ng/g of meconium when 0.5 g of meconium is used for the analysis, the cutoff for the positive values is still kept rather high: 80–100 ng/g for cocaine, benzoylecgonine, opiates, and amphetamines, and 10 ng/g for PCP and cannabinoids.

For confirmation, LCMS is gaining in popularity, due to the fact that there is no need for derivatization and in most cases LCMS has a higher sensitivity than GCMS. These issues become extremely important when a small amount of meconium is available for testing. In many clinical cases there is not enough meconium for both: screening and confirmation and the analyst has to judge if it is more beneficial to perform a broad screening or a more specific test targeted to one specific family of drugs.

PRENATAL ETHANOL EXPOSURE AND DETECTION

Ethanol is a small molecule that distributes rapidly into total body water and passes readily across the placenta. Ethanol is cleared rapidly from the blood following pseudo-zero order kinetics[67] resulting in a limited window of detection in blood and urine. The use of multiple maternal markers for alcoholism was found to be ineffective in accurately detecting prenatal alcohol abuse,[68] warranting the need for a biomarker specific for pregnancy and directly related to fetal exposure.

Fatty acid ethyl esters (FAEE) are nonoxidative ethanol metabolites produced by the esterification of ethanol to free fatty acids, catalyzed primarily by FAEE synthases[69] (see Fig. 15-1). While the incorporation of fatty acids is tissue- and enzyme-dependent, human placenta, animal placenta, heart, and liver are all reported to have significant FAEE synthase activities.[70] Selected FAEE have been recovered from meconium at levels correlating well with maternal self-reported gestational alcohol consumption,[71,72] or tolerance for alcohol.[73] Several studies suggest the

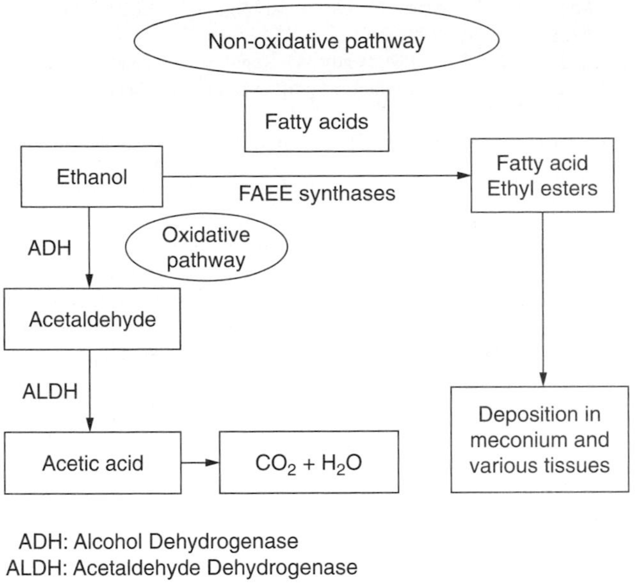

Figure 15-1. Ethanol Metabolism and the formation of Fatty Acid Ethyl Esters.

presence of individual FAEE species correlate well with maternal alcohol consumption;[71,74] however, it has been shown that the total level of multiple common FAEE (as opposed to one selected FAEE) quantified in meconium is a more reliable biomarker by providing a redundancy system for individual variability in fatty acid profiles.[72,75] One case report demonstrated cumulative FAEE levels in a confirmed drinker 34-fold higher than nondrinking controls.[72] The FAEE species of interest in meconium are ethyl laurate, ethyl myristate, ethyl palmitate, ethyl palmitoleate, ethyl stearate, ethyl oleate, ethyl linoleate, ethyl linolenate, and ethyl arachidonate.[76]

FAEE: Laboratory Analysis

FAEE are isolated from meconium via hexane/acetone and solid-phase extraction.[75,77] Since ethanol is also produced endogenously by gut flora,[78] the presence of low levels of FAEE in meconium are not necessarily indicative of exogenous ethanol. One study identified cumulative FAEE levels greater than 10,000 ng/g as being indicative of significant alcohol exposure.[77] A baseline study of the meconium of children born to 197 nondrinking women in two distinct populations yielded a positive cutoff of 2.0 nmol cumulative FAEE/g meconium with a sensitivity of 100% and specificity of 98.4%.[75] The longer-chain esters appear to be selectively expressed in alcohol-exposed populations, while the shorter-chain esters are more common in individuals who test below 2.0 nmol/g.[75] The baseline was established using gas chromatography with flame-ionization detection exhibiting a limit of detection of approximately 50 ng/g.[75] The use of molar concentrations when quantifying FAEE is a more accurate reflection of the amount of esterified ethanol due to the variability in molecular weights exhibited by the various FAEE species.

Confirmation of FAEE in meconium can be carried out using the above-mentioned method with a mass spectrometer instead of a flame ionization detector.[74,77] One study confirmed the presence of FAEE above 50 ng/g in 16.7% of a mixed general neonatal and neonatal intensive care unit population.[77]

Ethanol: Clinical Implications

Fetal alcohol spectrum disorder (FASD) is a detrimental outcome of maternal alcohol abuse during pregnancy. Clinical presentation of FASD consists of a complex pattern of behavioral or cognitive abnormalities that are inconsistent with the patient's level of development, familial and environmental background, and/or evidence of CNS neurodevelopmental abnormalities.[16] A delayed diagnosis may exacerbate the primary insult produced by prenatal alcohol exposure, warranting a neonatal screen in order to increase the capability of intervention. A spectrum of secondary disabilities such as trouble with law, mental health and behavioral problems, and low social adaptability may arise from the primary organic insult and are preventable with early intervention.[16,79] The use of molar concentrations as opposed to mass-based units when describing FAEE is necessitated by the variability in molecular weight between individual FAEE species.

REFERENCES

1. Addis A, Moretti ME, Ahmed SF, et al. Fetal effects of cocaine: an updated meta-analysis. *Reprod Toxicol.* 2001;15:341–369.
2. Church MW, Morbach CA, Subramanian MG. Comparative effects of prenatal cocaine, alcohol, and undernutrition on maternal/fetal toxicity and fetal body composition in the Sprague-Dawley rat with observations on strain-dependent differences. *Neurotoxicol Teratol.* 1995; 17:559–567.
3. Fried PA, Watkinson B. 36- and 48-month neurobehavioral follow-up of children prenatally exposed to marijuana, cigarettes, and alcohol. *J Dev Behav Pediatr.* 1990;11:49–58.
4. Goldschmidt L, Day NL, Richardson GA. Effects of prenatal marijuana exposure on child behavior problems at age 10. *Neurotoxicol Teratol.* 2000;22:325–336.
5. Konkol RJ, Murphey LJ, Ferriero DM, et al. Cocaine metabolites in the neonate: potential for toxicity. *J Child Neurol.* 1994;9:242–248.
6. Oro AS, Dixon SD. Perinatal cocaine and methamphetamine exposure: maternal and neonatal correlates. *J Pediatr.* 1987;111:571–578.
7. Ostrea EM, Chavez CJ, Strauss ME. A study of factors that influence the severity of neonatal narcotic withdrawal. *J Pediatr.* 1976; 88:642–645.
8. Ostrea EM, Chavez CJ. Perinatal problems (excluding neonatal withdrawal) in maternal drug addiction: a study of 830 cases. *J Pediatr.* 1979;94:292–295.
9. Plessinger MA. Prenatal exposure to amphetamines. Risks and adverse outcomes in pregnancy. *Obstet Gynecol Clin North Am.* 1998; 25:119–138.
10. Tabor BL, Smith-Wallace T, Yonekura ML. Perinatal outcome associated with PCP versus cocaine use. *Am J Drug Alcohol Abuse.* 1990; 16:337–348.
11. Zuspan FP, Gumpel JA, Mejia-Zelaya A, et al. Fetal stress from methadone withdrawal. *Am J Obstet Gynecol.* 1975;122:43–46.
12. Ryan RM, Wagner CL, Schultz JM, et al. Meconium analysis for improved identification of infants exposed to cocaine in utero. *J Pediatr.* 1994;125:435–440.

13. Ostrea EM Jr, Brady M, Gause S, et al. Drug screening of newborns by meconium analysis: a large-scale, prospective, epidemiologic study. *Pediatrics.* 1992;89:107–113.
14. Bibb KW, Stewart DL, Walker JR, et al. Drug screening in newborns and mothers using meconium samples, paired urine samples, and interviews. *J Perinatol.* 1995;15:199–202.
15. Lewis D, Moore C, Leikin JB, et al. Multiple birth concordance of street drug assays of meconium analysis. *Vet Hum Toxicol.* 1995; 37:318–319.
16. Institute of Medicine (IOM) of the National Academy of Sciences committee for Study Fetal Alcohol Syndrome. Fetal Alcohol Syndrome: Diagnosis, Epidemiology, Prevention and Treatment. In: Stratton K, Howe C, Battaglia F, editors. Fetal Alcohol Syndrome. National Academy Press, 1996.
17. Alcohol consumption among pregnant and childbearing-aged women—United States, 1991 and 1995. *MMWR Morb Mortal Wkly Rep.* 1997;46:346–350.
18. Samperiz S, Millet V, Arditti J, et al. [Value of toxicological research in newborn infants of addicted mothers by the study of several samples (urine, meconium, hair)]. *Arch Pediatr.* 1996;3:440–444.
19. Ostrea EM Jr, Lynn SM, Wayne RN, et al. Tissue distribution of morphine in the newborns of addicted monkeys and humans. Clinical implications. *Dev Pharmacol Ther.* 1980;1:163–170.
20. ElSohly MA, Kopycki W, Feng S, et al. Identification and analysis of the major metabolites of cocaine in meconium. *J Anal Toxicol.* 1999; 23:446–451.
21. Booze RM, Lehner AF, Wallace DR, et al. Dose-response cocaine pharmacokinetics and metabolite profile following intravenous administration and arterial sampling in unanesthetized, freely moving male rats. *Neurotoxicol Teratol.* 1997;19:7–15.
22. Bourget P, Roulot C, Fernandez H. Models for placental transfer studies of drugs. *Clin Pharmacokinet.* 1995;28:161–180.
23. Xia Y, Wang P, Bartlett MG, et al. An LC-MS-MS method for the comprehensive analysis of cocaine and cocaine metabolites in meconium. *Anal Chem.* 2000;72:764–771.
24. Ostrea EM Jr. Understanding drug testing in the neonate and the role of meconium analysis. *J Perinat Neonatal Nurs.* 2001;14:61–82.
25. Koren G, Chan D, Klein J, et al. Estimation of fetal exposure to drugs of abuse, environmental tobacco smoke, and ethanol. *Ther Drug Monit.* 2002;24:23–25.
26. Moore C, Lewis D, Leikin J. False-positive and false-negative rates in meconium drug testing. *Clin Chem.* 1995;41:1614–1616.
27. Abusada GM, Abukhalaf IK, Alford DD, et al. Solid-phase extraction and GC/MS quantitation of cocaine, ecgonine methyl ester, benzoylecgonine, and cocaethylene from meconium, whole blood, and plasma. *J Anal Toxicol.* 1993;17:353–358.
28. Gourley GR, Kreamer B, Arend R. Excremental studies in human neonates. Identification of zinc coproporphyrin as a marker for meconium. *Gastroenterology.* 1990;99:1705–1709.
29. Moore C, Negrusz A, Lewis D. Determination of drugs of abuse in meconium. *J Chromatogr B Biomed Sci Appl.* 1998;713:137–146.
30. Ostrea EM Jr, Romero A, Knapp DK, et al. Postmortem drug analysis of meconium in early-gestation human fetuses exposed to cocaine: clinical implications. *J Pediatr.* 1994;124:477–479.
31. Kwong TC, Ryan RM. Detection of intrauterine illicit drug exposure by newborn drug testing. National Academy of Clinical Biochemistry. *Clin Chem.* 1997;43:235–242.
32. Chan D, Klein J, Koren G. New Methods for Neonatal Drug Screening. *NeoReviews.* 2004;4:e1–e8.
33. Miller V, Holzel A. Growth and development of endodermal structures. In: Davis J, Dobbing J, editors. Scientific foundations in paediatrics. Philadelphia: WB Saunders, 1974:281–296.
34. Browne SP, Tebbett IR, Moore CM, et al. Analysis of meconium for cocaine in neonates. *J Chromatogr.* 1992;575:158–161.
35. Vaughan V, Litt I. Nelson Textbook of Pediatrics, 13th ed. Philadelphia: Saunders, 1987.
36. Szeto HH. Kinetics of drug transfer to the fetus. *Clin Obstet Gynecol.* 1993;36:246–254.
37. Maynard EC, Amoruso LP, Oh W. Meconium for drug testing. *Am J Dis Child.* 1991;145:650–652.
38. Ostrea EM Jr, Parks PM, Brady MJ. Rapid isolation and detection of drugs in meconium of infants of drug-dependent mothers. *Clin Chem.* 1988;34:2372–2373.
39. Verma A, Dhanireddy R. Time of first stool in extremely low birth weight (< or = 1000 grams) infants. *J Pediatr.* 1993;122:626–629.
40. Mofenson HC, Caraccio TR. Cocaine. *Pediatr Ann.* 1987;16:864–874.
41. Lombardero N, Casanova O, Behnke M, et al. Measurement of cocaine and metabolites in urine, meconium, and diapers by gas chromatography/mass spectrometry. *Ann Clin Lab Sci.* 1993;23:385–394.
42. Murphey LJ, Olsen GD, Konkol RJ. Quantitation of benzoylnorecgonine and other cocaine metabolites in meconium by high-performance liquid chromatography. *J Chromatogr.* 1993;613:330–335.
43. Clark GD, Rosenzweig IB, Raisys V, et al. The analysis of cocaine and benzoylecgonine in meconium. *J Anal Toxicol.* 1992;16:261–263.
44. Bar-Oz B, Klein J, Karaskov T, et al. Comparison of meconium and neonatal hair analysis for detection of gestational exposure to drugs of abuse. *Arch Dis Child Fetal Neonatal Ed.* 2003;88:F98–F100.
45. ElSohly MA, Stanford DF, Murphy TP, et al. Immunoassay and GC-MS procedures for the analysis of drugs of abuse in meconium. *J Anal Toxicol.* 1999;23:436–445.
46. Chen WJ, West JR. Cocaethylene exposure during the brain growth spurt period: brain growth restrictions and neurochemistry studies. *Brain Res Dev Brain Res.* 1997;100:220–229.
47. Frank DA, Augustyn M, Knight WG, et al. Growth, development, and behavior in early childhood following prenatal cocaine exposure: a systematic review. *JAMA.* 2001;285:1613–1625.
48. Joyce T, Racine AD, McCalla S, et al. The impact of prenatal exposure to cocaine on newborn costs and length of stay. *Health Serv Res.* 1995;30:341–358.
49. Graham K, Koren G. Characteristics of pregnant women exposed to cocaine in Toronto between 1985 and 1990. *CMAJ.* 1991; 144:563–8.
50. Volpe JJ. Effect of cocaine use on the fetus. *N Engl J Med.* 1992; 327:399–407.
51. Silvestre MA, Lucena JE, Roxas R Jr, et al. Effects of timing, dosage, and duration of morphine intake during pregnancy on the amount of morphine in meconium in a rat model. *Biol Neonate.* 1997;72:112–117.
52. Moriya F, Chan KM, Noguchi TT, et al. Detection of drugs-of-abuse in meconium of a stillborn baby and in stool of a deceased 41-day-old infant. *J Forensic Sci.* 1995;40:505–508.
53. Umans JG, Inturrisi CE. Pharmacodynamics of subcutaneously administered diacetylmorphine, 6-acetylmorphine and morphine in mice. *J Pharmacol Exp Ther.* 1981;218:409–415.
54. Moore CM, Deitermann D, Lewis D, et al. The detection of hydrocodone in meconium: two case studies. *J Anal Toxicol.* 1995; 19:514–518.
55. Smith ML, Hughes RO, Levine B, et al. Forensic drug testing for opiates. VI. Urine testing for hydromorphone, hydrocodone, oxymorphone, and oxycodone with commercial opiate immunoassays and gas chromatography-mass spectrometry. *J Anal Toxicol.* 1995;19:18–26.
56. Ostrea EM Jr, Knapp DK, Tannenbaum L, et al. Estimates of illicit drug use during pregnancy by maternal interview, hair analysis, and meconium analysis. *J Pediatr.* 2001;138:344–348.
57. Moriya F, Chan KM, Noguchi TT, et al. Testing for drugs of abuse in meconium of newborn infants. *J Anal Toxicol.* 1994;18:41–45.
58. Lester BM, ElSohly M, Wright LL, et al. The Maternal Lifestyle Study: drug use by meconium toxicology and maternal self-report. *Pediatrics.* 2001;107:309–317.
59. Reddy AM, Harper RG, Stern G. Observations on heroin and methadone withdrawal in the newborn. *Pediatrics.* 1971; 48:353–358.
60. Blackard C, Tennes K. Human placental transfer of cannabinoids. *N Engl J Med.* 1984;311:797.
61. Moore C, Lewis D, Becker J, et al. The determination of 11-nor-delta 9-tetrahydrocannabinol-9-carboxylic acid (THCCOOH) in meconium. *J Anal Toxicol.* 1996;20:50–51.
62. ElSohly MA, Feng S. delta 9-THC metabolites in meconium: identification of 11-OH-delta 9-THC, 8 beta,11-diOH-delta 9-THC, and

11-nor-delta 9-THC-9-COOH as major metabolites of delta 9-THC. *J Anal Toxicol.* 1998;22:329–335.

63. Pichini S, Pacifici R, Pellegrini M, et al. Development and validation of a high-performance liquid chromatography-mass spectrometry assay for determination of amphetamine, methamphetamine, and methylenedioxy derivatives in meconium. *Anal Chem.* 2004;76: 2124–2132.
64. Burchfield DJ, Lucas VW, Abrams RM, et al. Disposition and pharmacodynamics of methamphetamine in pregnant sheep. *JAMA.* 1991; 265:1968–1973.
65. Nicholas JM, Lipshitz J, Schreiber EC. Phencyclidine: its transfer across the placenta as well as into breast milk. Am *J Obstet Gynecol.* 1982;143:143–146.
66. Ho E, Karimi-Tabesh L, Koren G. Characteristics of pregnant women who use ecstasy (3, 4-methylenedioxymethamphetamine). *Neurotoxicol Teratol.* 2001;23:561–567.
67. Kalant H, Khanna J. The Alcohols. In: Kalant H, Roschlau W, editors. Principles of Medical Pharmacology, 6th ed. New York: Oxford University Press, 1998:303–316.
68. Stoler JM, Huntington KS, Peterson CM, et al. The prenatal detection of significant alcohol exposure with maternal blood markers. *J Pediatr.* 1998;133:346–352.
69. Laposata M. Fatty acid ethyl esters: ethanol metabolites which mediate ethanol-induced organ damage and serve as markers of ethanol intake. *Prog Lipid Res.* 1998;37:307–316.
70. Bearer CF, Gould S, Emerson R, et al. Fetal alcohol syndrome and fatty acid ethyl esters. *Pediatr Res.* 1992;31:492–495.
71. Bearer CF, Lee S, Salvator AE, et al. Ethyl linoleate in meconium: a biomarker for prenatal ethanol exposure. *Alcohol Clin Exp Res.* 1999; 23:487–493.
72. Klein J, Karaskov T, Korent G. Fatty acid ethyl esters: a novel biologic marker for heavy in utero ethanol exposure: a case report. *Ther Drug Monit.* 1999;21:644–646.
73. Yamashita T, Lee SC, Minnew S, et al. Meconium FAEE and maternal ethanol use. *Alcohol Clin Exp Res.* 1997.
Ref Type: Abstract
74. Bearer CF, Jacobson JL, Jacobson SW, et al. Validation of a new biomarker of fetal exposure to alcohol. *J Pediatr.* 2003;143:463–469.
75. Chan D, Bar-Oz B, Pellerin B, et al. Population baseline of meconium fatty acid ethyl esters among infants of nondrinking women in Jerusalem and Toronto. *Ther Drug Monit.* 2003;25:271–278.
76. Chan D, Caprara D, Blanchette P, et al. Recent developments in meconium and hair testing methods for the confirmation of gestational exposures to alcohol and tobacco smoke. *Clin Biochem.* 2004; 37:429–438.
77. Moore C, Jones J, Lewis D, et al. Prevalence of fatty acid ethyl esters in meconium specimens. *Clin Chem.* 2003;49:133–136.
78. Ostrovsky YM, Pronko PS, Shishkin SN, et al. An attempt to evaluate diagnostic and prognostic significance of blood endogenous ethanol in alcoholics and their relatives. *Alcohol.* 1989;6:97–102.
79. Streissguth AP, Barr HM, Kogan J, et al. Understanding the Occurrence of Secondary Disabilities in Clients with Fetal Alcohol Syndrome (FAS) and Fetal Alcohol Effects (FAE). 1.
Ref Type: Report

CHAPTER 16

OCCUPATIONAL EXPOSURES KNOWN TO BE HUMAN REPRODUCTIVE POISONS

Yedidia Bentur and Gideon Koren

INTRODUCTION

By the end of the twentieth century, there was a steady increase in the number of women joining the workforce. Moreover, women were taking jobs that were traditionally held by men only. With increased awareness of reproductive toxicity caused by chemicals, women in the reproductive age range and their families became troubled about potential hazards to unborn babies. Moreover, employers are often concerned about their liability in cases of women working with certain chemicals who experience adverse fetal outcome.

Several years ago, an American battery manufacturer tried to exclude all women of reproductive age from its production line, and a similar thrust has been tried by a Canadian nickel producer. In both cases the workers' unions rejected the manufacturers' attempts.

In comparison to therapeutic agents, our knowledge of reproductive toxicology of industrial chemicals in humans is in most cases sketchy or missing. Before marketing, the teratogenic potential of drugs must be tested in animals; no such data are required for industrial chemicals. In trying to identify adverse reproductive effects in humans of chemicals that have already been introduced into the workplace, one has to struggle with the plethora of methodological problems covered elsewhere in this book. Moreover, in most cases workers are exposed to more than one chemical, various routes of exposure may be involved, working conditions as well as circumstances of exposure can vary between or within working days, and the amount of absorbed chemicals is unclear. In addition, the potential presence of toxic industrial byproducts and metabolites further complicate the situation. Thus, it is often impossible to identify a chemical culprit causing reproductive toxicity.

Every chemical used in the workplace has safety exposure limits aimed at protecting the workers from toxicity. However, these standards were not meant to protect the fetus, and it is possible that airborne levels (e.g., of metallic mercury) that are safe for the mother may be hazardous for the developing organism.

It is beyond the scope of this chapter to discuss the toxic potential of every chemical that may be encountered during pregnancy. Because in the vast majority of cases reproductive toxicology has not been proven in women exposed in the workplace, we prefer to include only cases where such evidence is unequivocal. Every case in which a woman experiences clinical symptoms or signs that may be associated with chemical exposure should be investigated in depth. The nature and conditions of the work should be looked into, including ventilation and means of protection, and it should be determined whether a similar clinical picture exists in fellow workers.

If the clinical picture is consistent with the chemical(s) in question, exposure levels must be defined. We often find that women are reluctant to induce such an investigation or even to ask for the installation of safety measures because they are afraid of retaliation by the employer. While there is no simple solution for such a situation, the industrial counselor must explain to such women the seriousness of prolonged exposure. Many large plants have industrial hygienists, safety officers, or physicians on the staff, and these health professionals should assist pregnant workers.

Table 16-1 lists suggested steps in analyzing the reproductive hazard associated with chemicals to which women are occupationally exposed.

DEFINITIONS

The following definitions of workplace standards are commonly employed in discussing occupational standards:

PEL = permissible exposure limit set by the U.S. Occupational Safety and Health Administration (OSHA).
TLV = threshold limit value set by the American Conference of Governmental Industrial Hygienists (ACGIH).
REL = recommended exposure limit set by the U.S. National Institute for Occupational Safety and Health (NIOSH).
PEL, TLV, and REL refer to the airborne concentrations of a substance and represent conditions under which it is believed that nearly all workers may be repeatedly exposed, day after day, without adverse effects.
TWA = time-weighted average concentration for a normal 8-hour work day and a 40-hour work week to which nearly all workers may be repeatedly exposed, day after day, without adverse effects (NIOSH refers to a 10-hour work day). Usually the values above are expressed as TLV-TWA, PEL-TWA, or REL-TWA
STEL = short-term exposure limit, set by the ACGIH. It refers to the maximum concentration to which workers can be exposed for up to 15 minutes continuously provided that no more than four excursions per day are permitted, but with at least 60 minutes between exposure periods and provided the daily TLV-TWA is not exceeded.
IDLH = immediately dangerous to life or health, a concentration set by the standards completion program of the (U.S.) National Institute of Occupational Safety and Health (NIOSH), in conjunction with OSHA. Represents the maximum concentration from which (in the event of respirator failure), one could escape within 30 minutes without a respirator and without experiencing any escape-impairing symptoms or irreversible health effects.
Ceiling = the concentration that should not be exceeded during any part of the working exposure.

The exposure limits are given in parts per million (ppm) or parts per billion (ppb), or as milligrams per cubic meter (mg/m^3). The following formula converts these units:

$$\text{mg/m}^3 = \frac{\text{ppm} \times \text{molecular weight}}{24.5}$$

Table 16-1
A Clinical Approach to Reproductive Hazards of Chemicals

1. Obtain medical, obstetric, and genetic history from the patient.
2. Identify the chemicals in question by their safety sheets.
3. Obtain a detailed description of the work performed by the woman, length of exposure, and means of protection (ventilation system, respirator, mask, gown, gloves, hood, etc.).
4. Inquire about possible exposure from nearby workstations.
5. Identify symptoms and signs reported to be associated and their temporal relationship to the exposure.
6. Rule out underlying conditions that may cause a similar clinical picture (e.g., morning sickness in the first trimester).
7. Determine whether symptoms and signs are manifest in fellow workers.
8. Inquire about pregnancy outcome in other workers.
9. Find out whether periodic occupational monitoring, including risk assessment and biomonitoring is performed.
10. Obtain the most recent levels of the chemicals in question measured in the patient's particular area and their relationship to workplace standards such as TWA and BEI.
11. Obtain medical and occupational history of the spouse.
12. Try to understand the attitude of the woman and her supervisors toward her particular work and toward a possible change of job. Will a change of job affect her income or chances for promotion?
13. Before reporting to the woman on available information, read the data critically and be accurate in your description of what is known.
14. Advise the woman on possible safety measurements to reduce exposure (e.g., mask, gloves, ventilation, etc.), biologic and environmental monitoring, and targeted ultrasound. Discuss possible necessity of temporary change of job conditions, reassignment or even removal from work.

BEI = biologic exposure index set by the ACGIH. Biological monitoring of the chemical or its metabolite in blood or urine instituted to evaluate the total exposure from all sources, including dermal, ingestion or nonoccupational.

It should be noted that all these workplace standards are meant to protect the adult worker; it is unknown whether they also protect the fetus. Therefore, in counseling the occupationally exposed pregnant woman, the availability of occupational monitoring measurements may be useful mainly in three extreme situations:

1. Concentrations close to or below detectable level, in the absence of adverse effects, may suggest low fetal risk.
2. Concentrations higher than TLV (or PEL)-TWA or BEI may suggest that the fetus is at risk; the higher the concentration, the larger the possible risk.
3. Abnormal biochemical or hematological parameters (e.g., abnormal liver function tests after exposure to trichloroethylene). Even in the presence of normal occupational indices, this can represent target organ damage to the mother. In this circumstance, a similar damage to the fetus might be suspected.

This approach needs to be validated by controlled studies.

INTERPRETATION OF ANIMAL STUDIES WHEN NO INFORMATION ON PATIENTS EXISTS

For most of the chemicals in question, no epidemiological studies exist. In this case animal studies should not be ignored, rather, they should be continuously interpreted. Parameters that may be of help in this process include molecular similarity of the toxin to a known teratogen, dose, relationship between dose and workplace standards and the "no observable adverse effect level" (NOAEL), route of administration, duration of exposure, gestational age at exposure, species and number of species studied, type of birth defect induced and its incidence, and the greater sensitivity of humans to most developmental toxins.

SUMMARY OF HUMAN DATA

The following short statements summarize published human data on chemicals about which we have been consulted most frequently by pregnant women. Animal studies and chemicals infrequently cited are not included. The possible limitations of epidemiological studies on occupational exposures in pregnancy are discussed in Chap. 9.

ANESTHETIC GASES

There is no evidence to date that a single course of general anesthesia in early pregnancy is capable of inducing teratogenicity. A large prospective study has shown the safety of nitrous oxide.[1,2] Similarly, thiopental, enflurane, and halothane were not shown to cause untoward embryonic or fetal effects.[2] Reduced fertility was found among female dental assistants exposed to high levels of unscavenged nitrous oxide.[3] The same was found in a subgroup of Swedish midwives who assisted at more than 30 deliveries per month when nitrous oxide was used.[4] Increased rate of miscarriage among operating room personnel was observed in some studies.[5–7] However, methodological problems, mainly response bias, preclude any firm conclusions from their results.[8] No increased risk for spontaneous abortions was found among 352 pregnancies in dental assistants occupationally exposed to nitrous oxide.[9] However, another study demonstrated a relative risk of spontaneous abortion of 2.6 (95% CI, 1.3–5.0) associated with exposure of female-dental personnel to unscavenged nitrous oxide.[10] A lower birth weight was reported in term infants to midwives who used nitrous oxide; -77 g, 95% CI - 24–129 g.[11] Most epidemiological studies do not suggest that congenital anomalies occur more often than expected among children of women with occupational exposure to volatile anesthetics during pregnancy. No consistent difference has been observed in the types of patterns of congenital anomalies found in children born to these women when compared with controls.[12] No developmental differences were found in 40 children of female anesthesiologists and nurses exposed to waste gases in operating rooms. But, the mean score of gross motor ability was significantly lower in the exposed group compared to a matched control group.[13] The use of scavenging systems, including gas extraction devices, is recommended to minimize potential risks.

Workplace standards (nitrous oxide): TLV-TWA, 50 ppm; REL-TWA, 25 ppm. Every effort should be made to minimize chronic exposure to nitrous oxide.

Biomonitoring parameters (nitrous oxide) complete blood count, methemoglobin (BEI 1.5% of hemoglobin — nonspecific and semiquantitative, background interference), blood and urinary nitrous oxide (limited usefulness).

Cadmium

There is inconclusive evidence for the adverse effect of cadmium on male fertility.[14,15] Cadmium-metallothionein mobilized from the liver has been speculated to be the etiologic agent in pre-eclampsia, as the symptoms of cadmium toxicity resemble those of toxemia of pregnancy.[16] In smokers, placental levels were higher,[17] and this metal may accumulate in the fetus.[18] It may impair placental function by displacing zinc, thereby reducing birth weight.[19] However, an association between placental cadmium and birthweight was not found in another study.[20] In the presence of placental calcifications, birthweight decreased with increasing cadmium hair levels, especially if it was at least 0.3 ppm.[21] Teratogenic effects were not reported in exposed populations.[22] Adverse reproductive effects may include low birth weight,[23] fewer full-term deliveries, fewer multiple pregnancies, lower birth weight in preterm infants,[24] and poorer performance on intellectual and motor skills tests at 6 years of age.[25] No association was found between placental cadmium levels and birthweight in nonsmoking pregnant women exposed to low levels of smelter-derived cadmium. This was found in spite of higher mean placental cadmium levels compared to the control group.[26] Polish pregnant women exposed to high levels of cadmium in the soil had fewer full-term deliveries, fewer multiple (>3) pregnancies and preterm infants with lower birth weight than did a control group. Blood cadmium levels were higher in the exposed group (0.29 vs. 0.25 μg/dL) but blood lead levels were not significantly different (6.7 vs. 6.2 μg/dL).[27] An association was suggested between neonatal hair cadmium levels and lower birthweight.[28] Cadmium in combination with other heavy metals may have mutagenic effects, but evidence that cadmium alone has cytogenetic effects is as yet unconvincing.[29–32] Cadmium is classified by the International Agency for Research on Cancer (IARC) as human carcinogen and by the ACGIH as potential human carcinogen.

Workplace standards: TLV-TWA 0.01 mg/m^3; cadmium compounds as Cd 0.002 mg/m^3. *Biomonitoring parameters*: blood cadmium levels (normal levels differ between smokers and nonsmokers), urinary cadmium-spot or 24-hour collection (BEI 5 μg/g creatinine), urinary metallothionein, and *N*-acetylglucosaminidase.

Carbon Monoxide, Including Methylene Chloride

Carbon monoxide (CO) readily crosses the placenta and is eliminated from the fetal circulation more slowly than from the maternal circulation.[33] CO poisoning may result in fetal death, stillbirth, or severe neurological deficits.[34–36] However, toxicity of this sort has been seen most often in symptomatic maternal poisoning.[37] Mild chronic exposure from the second to the seventh month of gestation was associated with multiple fetal anomalies.[38] It seems that the fetus is more susceptible than the mother to CO, and some authors believe that there is no margin of safety for CO exposure to the fetus.[39] The risk to the fetus from chronic low level exposure is not well documented, and it was suggested that it may pose a risk to the fetus comparable to that from smoking in the mother.[40]

Methylene chloride is partially metabolized to CO (25–33%) and may induce CO toxicity. A possible increase in risk for spontaneous abortions was suggested but other solvents were also involved.[41,42] The U.S. Environmental Protection Agency (EPA) regards this substance as having "minimal teratogenic potential."[43] Concern was raised that occupational exposure to methylene chloride may reduce sperm concentrations.[44] For further discussion of methylene chloride, see "organic solvents" below. Methylene chloride is a suspected animal carcinogen.

Workplace standards: TLV-TWA, 25 ppm.

Biomonitoring parameters: carboxyhemoglobin (may differ between nonsmokers and smokers). Levels do not necessarily correlate with toxicity.

Cholinesterase Inhibitors

Organophosphates and carbamates are irreversible and reversible cholinesterase inhibitors, respectively. The potential of these pesticides to induce human developmental toxicity is unknown. Rodent studies are of concern, but they involve high doses that are unlikely to be encountered by pregnant women. Several case reports and poorly documented studies described malformations after high acute exposures to organophosphates[45–48] but not in others.[49–51] In one case report, a suicide attempt with carbofuran (a carbamate insecticide) resulted in fetal death.[52] An association between birth defects and prenatal exposure to chlorpyrifos was suggested in four anecdotal human reports.[53] A CDC review could not verify that these mothers were exposed to organophosphates and found no published literature supporting the hypothesis that chlorpyrifos causes serious birth defects in humans or animals.[54]

Workplace standards: TLV-TWA, 0.05 mg/m^3 for parathion, 0.1 mg/m^3 for chlorpyrifos, and 0.011 mg/m^3 for diazinon.

Biomonitoring parameters: erythrocyte (true) acetylcholinesterase (mainly), plasma (pseudo) butyrylcholinesterase (less important).

BEI of parathion is 0.5 mg/g creatinine as total *P*-aminopherol in urine; nonspecific.

Dibromochloropropane

Occupational exposure to the agricultural nematocide dibromochloropropane has been associated in men with elevated serum gonadotropins, oligospermia, azoospermia, and infertility.[55–57] The duration of the exposure may be related to the severity and reversibility of the injury.[58–60] A higher percentage of female infants were found after paternal exposure,[61–63] but not miscarriages and malformations.[64,65] No chromosomal abnormalities were found in offspring of exposed men.[66] Nondisjunction was found in exposed workmen.[67] Increased incidence of the frequency of Y chromosomes was not observed in women exposed to dibromochloropropane.[55] This agent may increase the risk of cancer.

Workplace standards: PEL-TWA, 0.001 ppm.

Biomonitoring parameters: sperm count, serum testosterone, follicle-stimulating hormone, luteinizing hormone as well as liver and kidney function tests.

Epichlorohydrin

Several studies showed epichlorohydrin to be mutagenic in workers; the exposure level in one of these studies was 0.13–1.3 ppm.[68,69] However, chromosomal aberrations in lymphocytes were not found in another study involving occupational exposure.[70] Epichlorohydrin is a testicular toxicant in animals[71] and is a metabolite of dibromochloropropane, which is also a known testicular toxicant in humans and animals.[55,56] An unpublished report of the Shell Oil Company claims no decrease in sperm count or hormonal activity among exposed workers, but no details are available.[72] Epichlorohydrin was classified by the IARC as a probable human carcinogen.

Workplace standards: TLV-TWA, 0.5 ppm.

Biomonitoring parameters: liver and kidney function tests.

Ethylene Dibromide (Dibromoethane)

Agricultural workers exposed to ethylene dibromide had reduced sperm concentrations and lower percentage of normal cells.[73,74] In one study, mean exposure levels were estimated at 88 ppb with peak levels of 262 ppb.[73] In the other study, marijuana use was more prevalent in the exposed group.[74] There was no effect of ethylene dibromide on fertility in wives of exposed workers in three chemical plants in southern United States; however, fertility was significantly reduced at the fourth plant.[75] Exposure levels in all plants was <5 ppm. The American Medical Association (AMA) concluded that as of 1980, there was no conclusive human evidence that this agent was a reproductive hazard.[76] Ethylene dibromide was classified by the NIOSH as a potential occupational carcinogen.

Workplace standards: TLV-TWA, not listed, PEL-TWA, 20 ppm; REL-TWA, 0.045 ppm.

Biomonitoring parameters: blood bromide levels, complete blood count, liver and kidney function tests.

Ethylene Oxide

Hospital workers exposed to 8-hour weighted mean ethylene oxide concentrations of 0.1–0.5 ppm had a higher incidence of spontaneous abortions; 16.7% versus 5.6% in controls. These workers were also exposed to glutaraldehyde and formaldehyde. However, the rate of miscarriages among controls was lower than expected.[77] Similar findings were found in other studies involving production of ethylene oxide, sterilizing operations (adjusted rate of spontaneous abortions of 16.1% compared to 7.8% in unexposed group), and dental hygienists who sterilized instruments.[78,79,80] Another study showed increased risk for spontaneous abortions (RR 2.5), preterm birth (RR 2.7), and postterm birth (RR 2.1) in dental assistants occupationally exposed to ethylene oxide together with mercury and nitrous oxide.[81] Some of these studies were criticized for their methodology. A case-control study did not confirm an association with spontaneous abortions and birth defects.[82] No increased risk for spontaneous abortions was found with self-reported exposure in female veterinarians.[83] Occupational exposure was demonstrated to increase frequency of sister chromatid exchange.[84–88] The reference dose for developmental toxicity from ethylene oxide was suggested to be 0.1–0.3 ppm; lower than occupational exposure standards.[89] Ethylene oxide is classified by the IARC as a human carcinogen and by the ACGIH as a suspected human carcinogen.

Workplace standards: TLV-TWA, 1 ppm, REL-TWA <0.1 ppm.

Biomonitoring parameters: chest x-ray, blood ethylene oxide (not clinically useful).

Formaldehyde

No increase in birth defects or spontaneous abortions was observed in women workers occupationally exposed to formaldehyde.[77,78] In contrast, an association of miscarriages was suggested in cosmetologists and laboratory workers.[90,91] The latter study did not show an increase in birth defects. A Soviet study reported excess menstrual disorders and low-birth-weight infants, but the women involved had done heavy lifting and the study had methodological problems.[92] Reduced fertility was found among female wood workers exposed to formaldehyde.[93] This study may have been subjected to recall and response bias. Formaldehyde is classified by the IARC as a human carcinogen and by the ACGIH as a suspected human carcinogen.

Workplace standards: TLV-TWA, not listed; TLV-ceiling, 0.3 ppm; REL-TWA, 0.016 ppm.

Biomonitoring parameters: urine formate; but the use of this substance for biological monitoring is questionable because of large normal variation.

Glutaraldehyde

Miscarriage rate adjusted for possible risk factors was not found to be increased in a questionnaire study of women undergoing surgical sterilization in hospitals.[77]

Workplace standards: TLV-ceiling, 0.05 ppm.

Biomonitoring parameters: liver and kidney function tests, chest x-ray, and pulmonary function tests, especially when respiratory tract irritation presents.

Halogenated Hydrocarbon Solvents

The reader is also referred to the discussion of organic solvents, below (see also Chap. 28).

Chloroprene

Soviet studies have suggested that chloroprene may induce menstrual disorders, decreased sperm motility, and changes in sperm morphology. It seems that high doses are more toxic to the testes, but the effect of near-TLV concentrations is unclear. A threefold increase in abortion rate was reported in wives of workers exposed to 0.3–1.9 ppm, but the significance of this finding is unclear.[94] A French study quoted in a NIOSH document observed impotence and reduced libido during overexposure to chloroprene which disappeared after removal from exposure.[95] There is limited evidence that this agent may be mutagenic in humans.[94] Functional disturbances in spermatogenesis and sperm morphological abnormalities were reported in workers exposed to chloroprene.[79] NIOSH considers this agent as a potential occupational carcinogen.

Workplace standards: TLV-TWA, 10 ppm.

Biomonitoring parameters: liver function tests; chest x-ray in overexposure.

Chloroform (See also Organic Solvents, Chap. 29)

Chloroform crosses the human placenta.[96] In 492 laboratory workers with first-trimester exposure to organic solvents, including chloroform, there was no increased frequency of congenital anomalies.[97]

A more recent study supports this finding.[91] Conflicting results were found on the association between chloroform and other trihalomethanes in drinking water and congenital anomalies.[98–100] An association was suggested between stillborn infants and chloroform concentration of 100 μg/L or more in drinking water; RR 1.56, 95% CI 1.04–2.34.[101] Conflicting results were also found in studies investigating the association between chloroform in drinking water and low birthweight.[102–104] Higher frequencies of acquired chromosomal aberrations were observed in women occupationally exposed to organic solvents, including chloroform, and in the children of these exposed women.[105] Chloroform was classified by the IARC as a possible human carcinogen.

Workplace standards: TLV-TWA, 10 ppm.

Biomonitoring parameters: liver and kidney function tests.

Hexachlorophene

Hexachlorophene was detectable in maternal and cord blood after vaginal use during labor of this bactericidal agent.[106] Occupational exposure of women medical personnel during hand washing was suggested to increase the frequency of a heterogeneous group of congenital malformations.[107] However, this study was criticized for its methodology, and a more comprehensive and careful epidemiological study could not confirm this association.[108] A similar conclusion was achieved in a case control study of children with various anomalies.[109] Maternal occupational exposure to hexachlorophene or phenylphenol during the sixth to ninth months of pregnancy was possibly associated with mental retardation, odds ratio 3.1, 90% CI 1.0–9.7[110] The AMA Council on Scientific Affairs concluded that pregnant women should not use hexachlorophene-containing products.[111]

Workplace standards: TLV-, PEL-, or REL-TWA, not listed.

Biomonitoring parameters: blood hexachlorophene levels; but correlation with clinical effects is not good.

Tetrachloroethylene (See also Organic Solvents, Chap. 29)

Women of reproductive age who work in dry-cleaning facilities may receive substantial exposure to tetrachloroethylene, since environmental air levels may range between 200 and 4000 mg/mL (30–540 ppm). Sperm from exposed dry-cleaning workers were found to be round, which is believed to be a mark of infertility.[112] Wives of dry-cleaning workers required longer periods of time to become pregnant, but they did not have fewer pregnancies or increased spontaneous abortions.[113] A case-control study of laundry and dry cleaning workers suggested high exposure to tetrachloroethylene be associated with increased risk of spontaneous abortions, odds ratio 3.4, 95% CI 1.0–11.2.[114] A later retrospective study supported this finding.[115] Other epidemiological studies could not find such an association.[116,117] The frequency of malformations was no greater than expected.[114,118] Maternal residence in a town in which drinking water contained twice the allowable concentration of tetrachloroethylene was associated with an increased risk for oral clefts; n = 83, OR 3.54, 95% CI 1.09–10.11.[119,120] Although limited epidemiological studies suggest that tetrachloroethylene may induce liver cancer, the data are not satisfactory to reach a definite conclusion on its carcinogenicity in humans.[121] It is classified by the IARC as a probable human carcinogen.

Workplace standards: TLV-TWA, 25 ppm.

Biomonitoring parameters: blood and expired air levels, liver and kidney function tests, urinalysis, urinary trichloroacetic acid and thioether.

BEI: 0.5 mg/L of tetrachloroethylene in blood prior to last shift or work week; 3.5 mg/L in urine at the end of shift at end of workweek—nonspecific and semiquantitative.

Trichloroethylene (See also Organic Solvents, Chap. 29)

Trichloroethylene has been reported to cross the placenta.[122] Controversy exists whether trichloroethylene can cause spontaneous abortions.[123,124] Methodological problems limit interpretation of the results. An increased incidence of congenital heart disease among offspring of mothers with first-trimester exposure to contaminated ground water was reported, but a direct cause-and-effect relationship has not been established.[125] Other studies could not confirm this association.[119,120,126] Contradicting results were also found regarding trichloroethylene contaminated drinking water and neural tube defects.[119,120,127] An insignificant increase was found for cleft palate and exposure to trichloroethylene based on occupation.[128] Although trichloroethylene may be carcinogenic in animals, this effect has not been clearly found in humans.[129] It is classified by the IARC as probable human carcinogen.

Workplace standards: TLV-TWA, 50 ppm.

Biomonitoring parameters: blood and breath levels, renal and liver. BEI: 2 mg/L of trichloroethanol in blood, 80 mg/L or 300 mg/g creatinine of trichloroacetic acid in urine; both should be sampled at the end of shift at end of workweek and are regarded as nonspecific.

Lead

For a detailed discussion the reader is referred to Chap. 29. Lead crosses the placenta[130] and accumulates in the fetus[131] It may induce abortions and prematurity[132,133] A dose-related association with minor malformations has been suggested.[134] Children with cord blood lead levels exceeding 10 μg/dL scored lower on developmental tests.[135] Lead was shown to cause infertility in exposed men[136] and possibly chromosomal aberrations[137] The latter association is still unclear.

Workplace standards: TLV-TWA, 0.05 mg/m^3, action level, 0.03 mg/m^3.

Biomonitoring parameters: blood lead levels (if employee's level ≥40 μg/dL or ≥30 μg/dL if he or she intends to have children, removal from exposure should be considered), erythrocyte protoporphyrin, and the lead mobilization test may be used to assess total body burden (especially if blood levels are borderline), complete blood count and a peripheral smear.

BEI is 30 μg/dL.

Mercury

Elemental (Metallic) Mercury. Occupational male exposure was reported to induce impotence and decreased libido,[138] but not infertility[139] Paternal exposure to mercury, confirmed by urinary levels, was suggested to be associated with spontaneous abortions.[140] Menstrual disorders were reported in several studies,[141,142] as well as infertility.[143] Mercury crosses the placenta, and fetal blood levels may be comparable or even higher than maternal level.[144–147] No increase in spontaneous abortions was found in female dental assistants and factory workers exposed to elemental mercury.[148,149,150] Increased rate of spontaneous abortions and stillbirth was found in female dentists and dental assistants.[151] Other authors also reported more spontaneous abortions (average exposure levels 0.08 mg/m^3), but it is difficult to separate the effects of other occupational exposures from those of mercury.[152,153] There are positive[151,154] and negative[149, 150, 155, 156] reports on the ability of metallic mercury to induce birth defects, especially neural tube defects. Maternal occupation in which low level exposure to mercury or mercury compounds may have occurred during pregnancy was found in a case control study to be associated with low birth weight; OR 1.8, 95% CI 1.1–2.8.[157] Higher cord blood mercury concentrations were associated with slightly decreased performance on neurobehavioral tests in a study of 917 7-year-old children.[158] Fetal and newborn toxic mercury level was estimated to be 3 μg/g.[159] Since daily uptake of mercury from dental amalgam is low (2–5 μg), it was suggested that restriction of amalgam therapy in pregnant women is unwarranted.[160] Amniotic fluid mercury concentrations were related to the occurrence of dental amalgam repairs but not to the number of amalgam fillings.[161] Dental restoration was associated with a significantly higher level of maternal and neonatal hair mercury.[162] In a study of sheep, mercury was shown to be released from maternal dental amalgam fillings and to be transferred to the fetus. Although no toxic effects were found, these authors recommended avoidance of the use of dental amalgams containing mercury.[163]

Workplace standards: TLV-TWA, 0.025 mg/m^3; suggested guideline in pregnancy, 0.01 mg/m^3.

Biomonitoring parameters: blood levels, preshift urine collection, kidney function tests, nerve conduction velocities.

Inorganic Mercury

This metal may cross the placenta[164] and affect central nervous system (CNS) development.[165] However, a specific embryopathy has not been reported. Indoor exposure to mercury-containing latex paint was shown to result in an increased urine mercury level.[166]

Workplace standards: TLV-TWA, 0.025 mg/m^3.

Biomonitoring parameters: as for elemental mercury.

BEI: 35 μg/g creatinine, preshift urine; 15 μg/L, blood, end of shift, end of workweek.

Organic Mercury. Pregnant women treated with mercurials had a higher incidence of spontaneous abortions.[167] Methyl mercury may accumulate in the fetus. This is suggested by higher blood mercury level found in infants born to mothers exposed to methyl mercury in contaminated bread.[168] Two epidemics of cerebral palsy, microcephaly, and psychomotor retardation were reported after *in utero* exposure to methyl mercury in Japan (contaminated fish) and Iraq (bread made of contaminated grain).[169–172]

Workplace standards: TLV-TWA, alkyl compounds, 0.01 mg/m^3, aryl compounds 0.1 mg/m^3.

Biomonitoring parameters: as for elemental mercury, hair analysis.

Organic Solvents

For more detailed discussion, the reader is referred to Chap. 16. Because of the complexity and diversity of exposure to organic solvents, adequate epidemiological studies are difficult to conduct and interpret. In spite of the many, sometimes serious, methodological limitations, most studies suggest that maternal occupational exposure to organic solvents is associated with adverse reproductive effects on fertility, spontaneous abortions, intrauterine growth and birth defects. However, these data cannot be used to incriminate organic solvents as a group as proven teratogens nor can this suspicion be quantitated. Using the precautionary approach is suggested when evaluating these exposures and in consulting the patients.

Workplace standards: TWA, according to the agents involved.

Biomonitoring parameters: according to the agents involved.

Organochlorine Insecticides

Endosulfan, Dieldrin, Chlordane. No occupational reproductive information is available.

Lindane

At least 10% can be absorbed through human skin.[173] Lindane crosses the human placenta,[174] and fetal levels are comparable to maternal level.[175,176] This insecticide may induce menstrual disorders, infertility,[177] excess blood loss after delivery, and lower birth weights.[178] Although anecdotal reports found higher placental, fetal and maternal blood lindane levels in cases of spontaneous abortions and premature deliveries,[178,179] other studies could not find a relationship between lindane levels and stillbirth[180] or other pathological conditions of pregnancy.[181] Lower levels of testosterone and other sex hormones[182] and reversible oligospermia and high ratio of dead sperm[183] were reported in males occupationally exposed to lindane.

Workplace standards: TLV-TWA, 0.5 mg/m^3.

Biomonitoring parameters: serum levels are not clinically useful.

DDT

DDT can cross the human placenta at term.[184,185] It is unclear whether the insecticide can induce pregnancy complications in human.[174,186–189] Although chlorinated hydrocarbons were found in seminal fluid and cervical mucus of infertility patients,[189] their role in reproductive problems is uncertain. Contradicting results were reported on the effects of organochlorine insecticides, including DDT, on birth weight.[190,191] The EPA banned the use of DDT because it is stored indefinitely in human tissue.

Workplace standards: TLV-TWA, 1 mg/m^3.

Biomonitoring parameters: serum levels may reflect cumulative exposure.

Heptachlor

No increase in the incidence of birth defects was observed in Hawaii in infants exposed *in utero* to milk contaminated with heptachlor.[192] The exposure could not be quantitated in either the study or the control group. After similar incidents in Arkansas, Missouri, and Oklahoma, one report on a neonate who developed gliosarcoma was noted, but heptachlor could not be established as the primary oncogen.[193] This agent may be mutagenic in human fibroblasts.[194]

Workplace standards: TLV-TWA, 0.05 mg/m^3.

Phenol

No clear association with birth defects was found in women occupationally exposed to phenol among other disinfectants.[109] Phenol may induce methemoglobinemia, especially in infants. Based on this possibility, it was suggested in one review that phenol may affect the human fetus.[195]

Workplace standards: TLV-TWA, 5 ppm.

Biomonitoring parameters: blood and urine free phenol or conjugated phenol, methemoglobin determination during or at end of shift, nonspecific.

BEI: 250 mg/g creatinine in urine, end of shift.

Polychlorinated Biphenyls and Polybrominated Biphenyls

In the Yusho epidemic in Japan (1968), pregnant women were exposed to rice oil contaminated with PCBs. The following adverse pregnancy outcomes were reported: stillbirth; gray-brown discoloration of skin, gingiva, and nails (cola-colored babies); parchment-like skin with desquamation; exophthalmos; teeth present at birth; conjunctivitis; and low birth weight.[196–201] Skin discoloration slowly disappeared after birth, and normal weight was gained afterward.[198–201] Persistent signs included recurrent acne and nail pigmentation.[202] In a similar epidemic in Taiwan (1979), children exposed *in utero* had developmental delay in addition to the foregoing abnormalities.[203] No association could be demonstrated between cord blood, placenta, and milk PCB levels and birth weight or head circumference.[204] Children exposed in these epidemics also scored lower than controls on developmental tests, especially those who had low birth weight and were more severely affected.[205] It seems that males were more susceptible to the teratogenic effects of PCBs.[196] Small head circumference and low birth weight were found in offspring of women exposed to PCB-contaminated fish in the Great Lakes.[206] The children exposed in the Great Lakes region of the United States also had small but significant impairment in short-term memory.[207] PCBs were suggested to adversely affect sperm quality.[208] Workplace exposure was also associated with low birth weight as well as shorter gestation.[209] PCBs are considered to be potential human carcinogens.[210]

Thirty-three farm children exposed *in utero* or in early pregnancy to PBBs were normal in growth and in results of physical examination and neurological assessment at the age of 37 months.[211]

Workplace standards: TLV-TWA: chlorodiphenyl (42% chlorine), 1 mg/m^3 (skin notation); chlorodiphenyl (54% chlorine), 0.5 mg/m^3 (skin notation).

Biomonitoring parameters: PCBs can be measured in blood, urine, milk, and adipose tissues. One should consider background levels.

Styrene

The reader is also referred to the discussion of organic solvents in Chap. 29. Two studies from the former Soviet Union showed low concentrations of styrene to be associated with menstrual disorders.[212, 213] However, a large American study on women exposed to styrene in reinforced plastics companies failed to show this association.[214] Styrene has been shown to cross the human placenta.[96] In a study on 2209 workers (511 females), again in the reinforced plastics industry, no increase in birth defects was found.[215] Chronic occupational exposures to styrene have sometimes been associated with chromosomal damage in germ cells and lymphocytes.[216–218]

Workplace standards: TLV-TWA, 20 ppm.

Biomonitoring parameters: urinary mandelic acid; other possible tests include phenylglyoxylic acid in urine and blood styrene level.

BEI: 400 mg/g creatinine in urine, end of shift.

2,3,7,8-Tetrachlorodibenzo-p-dioxin (TCDD, Dioxins)

There was no increase in malformations following the Seveso dioxin accident.[219] Another study suggesting that TCDD may have induced malformations and embryopathy in this accident[220] was shown to have methodological problems that invalidated its finding.[221] Males who were under 19 years of age when exposed to dioxin during the Seveso accident were found to have a large excess of female offspring.[222,223] No clear mechanism for such an effect has been proposed.[224] Offspring of Vietnam veterans exposed to Agent Orange (about 50% 2,4,5-trichlorophenoxyacetic acid contaminated by TCDD) were not found to have increased incidence of malformation.[225,226] The data of these studies could not address questions regarding association with defects of rare types or defects in offspring of selected groups of veterans. A large study could not uncover any convincing association between paternal exposure to dioxins among Vietnam veterans and adverse reproductive outcome. Four children had nervous system anomalies (anencephaly -1, spina bifida -3). The number was too small to be analyzed statistically, but there was an indication of an increasing rate with increasing paternal dioxin level.[227] A study involving 370 men occupationally exposed to TCDD and other dioxins in a Michigan plant did not reveal adverse reproductive outcome.[228] TCDD was classified by the IARC as a human carcinogen.

Workplace standards: TLV-TWA, not listed.

Biomonitoring parameters: liver and kidney function tests, complete blood count, serum lipids, prothrombin time, uroporphyrins, and fat biopsies.

Vinyl Chloride (Chloroethylene)

Impotence and loss of libido were reported by men occupationally exposed to vinyl chloride monomer.[229–231] Increased rate of miscarriages was found in wives of male vinyl chloride workers.[232] This study was criticized for its methodology of data collection and response bias.[233, 234] Later studies could not demonstrate such an association.[235–237] Although several studies suggested an association between congenital anomalies (especially CNS) and the presence in the community of vinyl chloride industries,[238–240] these reports should be considered to be inconclusive. The presence of other pollutants and personal factors were not controlled,[241] and there was no relation between parental occupation in a vinyl chloride plant and congenital anomalies in the offspring.[240,242] There have been anecdotal reports of increased fetal mortality in the offspring of male vinyl chloride monomer workers, and birth defects in communities near vinyl chloride monomer plants.[243–245] Mutagenicity studies on exposed workers are controversial, but it seems that chromosomal aberrations may be related to duration and extent of exposure, especially if greater than 20 ppm.[246] Vinyl chloride is a human carcinogen.

Workplace standards: TLV-TWA, 1 ppm.

Biomonitoring parameters: liver and kidney function tests; complete blood count; other tests may include urinary thiodiglycolic acid and uroporphyrins, as well as pulmonary function tests after exposure to dust.

RADIATION

For a detailed discussion on the effects of ionizing and non-ionizing radiation and video display terminals on pregnancy, the reader is referred to Chap. 18.

Eli Zalzstein, MD, Sovoka Medical Center, Beer Sheva, Isvael, contributed to previous editions of this chapter.

REFERENCES

1. Crawford JS, Lewis M. Nitrous oxide in early human pregnancy. *Anesthesia.* 1986;41:900–905.
2. Heinonen OP, Slone D, Shapiro S. Birth Defects and Drugs in Pregnancy. Littleton, MA: Publishing Sciences Group; 1977.
3. Rowland AS, Baird DD, Weinberg CR, et al. Reduced fertility among women employed as dental assistants exposed to high levels of nitrous oxide. *N Engl J Med.* 1992;327:993–997.
4. Ahlborg G Jr, Axelsson G, Bodin L. Shift work, nitrous oxide exposure and subfertility among Swedish midwives. *Int J Epidemiol.* 1996;25:783–790.
5. Ferstanding LL. Trace concentration of anesthetic gases. *Acta Anesth Scand.* 1982;75(suppl):38–43.
6. Tannenbaum TN, Goldberg RJ. Exposure to anesthetic gases and reproductive outcome: a review of the epidemiologic literature. *J Occup Med.* 1985;27:659–668.
7. Spence AA. Chronic exposure to trace concentration of anaesthetics. In: Gray TC, Nunn JS, Utting JE, eds. *General Anaesthetic.* 4th ed. London: Butterworth, 1980; pp. 189–201.
8. Axelsson G, Rylander R. Exposure to anaesthetic gases and spontaneous abortion: response bias in a postal questionnaire study. *Int J Epidemiol.* 1982;11:250–256.
9. Heidam LZ. Spontaneous abortions among dental assistants, factory workers, painters and gardening workers: a follow-up study. *J Epidemiol Community Health.* 1984;38:149–155.
10. Rowland AS, Baird DD, Shore DL, et al. Nitrous oxide and spontaneous abortion in female dental assistants. *Am J Epidemiol.* 1995;141:531–538.
11. Bodin L, Axelsson G, Ahlborg G Jr. The association of shift work and nitrous oxide exposure in pregnancy with birth weight and gestational age. *Epidemiology.* 1999;10:429–436.
12. Friedman JM. Teratogen update: anesthetic agents. *Teratology.* 1988;37:69–77.
13. Ratzon NA, Margolin PR, Hatch M, et al. Developmental evaluation of children born to mothers occupationally exposed to waste anesthetic gases. (Abstract). *Birth Defects Research.* 2003;67:316.
14. Schray SD, Dixon RL. Occupational exposures associated with male reproductive dysfunction. *Annu Review Pharmacol Toxicol.* 1985;25:567–592.
15. Keck C, Bramkamp G, Behre HM, et al. Lack of correlation between cadmium in seminal plasma and fertility status of nonexposed individuals and two cadmium-exposed patients. *Reprod Toxicol.* 1995;9:35–40.
16. Chisolm JG, Handorf CR. Further observations on the etiology of preeclampsia-mobilization of toxic cadmium metallothionein into the serum during pregnancy. *Med Hypoth.* 1996;47:123–128.
17. Cadmium and its compounds. In: Barlow SM, Sullivan FM, eds. *Reproductive Hazards of Industrial Chemicals.* London: Academic Press, 1982, pp. 136–177.
18. Sikorski R, Radomanski T, Paszkowski T, et al. Smoking during pregnancy and the perinatal cadmium burden. *J Perinat Med.* 1988;16:225–231.
19. Kuhnert PM, Kuhnert BR, Bottoms SF, et al. Cadmium levels in maternal blood, fetal cord blood and placental tissues of pregnant women who smoke. *Am J Obstet Gynecol.* 1982;142:1021–1025.
20. Frery N, Nessmann C, Girard F, et al. Environmental exposure to cadmium and human birthweight. *Toxicology.* 1993;79:109–118.
21. Loiacono NJ, Graziano JH, Kline JK, et al. Placental cadmium and birthweight in women living near a lead smelter. *Arch Environ Health.* 1992;47:250–255.
22. Tsvetkova RP. Materials on the study of the influence of cadmium compounds on the generative function. *Gig Tr Prof Zabol.* 1970;14:31–33.
23. American Medical Association, Council on Scientific Affairs. Effects of Toxic Chemicals on the Reproductive System. Chicago: AMA, 1985.
24. Laudanski T, Sipowiez M, Modzolewski P, et al. Influence of high lead and cadmium soil content on human reproductive outcome. *Int J Gynecol Obstet.* 1991;36:309–315.
25. Bonithon-Kopp C, Huel G, Moreau T, et al. Prenatal exposure to lead and cadmium and psychomotor development of the child at 6 years. *Neurobehav Toxicol Teratol.* 1986;8:307–310.
26. Loiacono NJ, Graziano JH, Kline JK, et al. Placental cadmium and birthweight in women living near a lead smelter. *Arch Environ Health.* 1992;47:250–255.
27. Laudanski T, Sipowicz M, Modzelewski P, et al. Influence of high lead and cadmium soil content on human reproductive outcome. *Int J Gynaecol Obstet.* 1991;36:309–315.
28. Frery N, Nessmann C, Girard F, et al. Environmental exposure to cadmium and human birthweight. *Toxicology.* 1993;79:109–118.
29. Shiraishi Y, Yoshida TH. Chromosomal abnormalities in cultured leukocyte cells from itai-itaie disease patients. *Proc Jpn Acad Sci.* 1972;48:248–251.
30. Shiraishi Y. Cytogenetic studies in 12 patients with itai-itai disease. *Hum Gene.* 1975;27:31–44.
31. Bui TH, Lindsten J, Nordberg GF. Chromosome analysis of lymphocytes from cadmium workers and itai-itai patients. *Environ Res.* 1975;9:187–195.
32. Leonard A, Deknude G, Gilliavod N. Genetic and cytogenetic hazards of heavy metals in mammals. *Mutat Res.* 1975;29:280–281.
33. Longo LD. The biological effects of carbon monoxide on the pregnant woman, fetus and newborn infant. *Am J Obstet Gynecol.* 1977;129:69–103.
34. Carbon monoxide. In: Barlow SM, Sullivan FM, eds. *Reproductive Hazards of Industrial Chemicals.* London: Academic Press, 1982, pp. 178–199.
35. Caravati EM, McElwee NE, Van Trigt M, et al. Carbon monoxide fetotoxicity (abstract). *Vet Hum Toxicol.* 1987;29:460.
36. Caravati EM, Adams CJ, Joyce SM, et al. Fetal toxicity associated with maternal carbon monoxide poisoning. *Ann Emerg Med.* 1988;17:714–717.
37. Koren G, Sharav T, Pastuszak A, et al. A multicenter, prospective study of fetal outcome following accidental carbon monoxide poisoning in pregnancy. *Reprod Toxicol.* 1991;5:397–M5.
38. Hennequin Y, Blum D, Vamos E, et al. *In utero* carbon monoxide poisoning and multiple fetal abnormalities. *Lancet.* 1993;341:240.
39. Waterman FK. *Occup Health Ont.* 1984;5:10–22. Quoted in Carbon Monoxide Monograph, Reprotext Information System. Denver, CO: Micromedex, 1992.
40. Carbon monoxide. In: *Reprotext Information System.* Denver, CO: Micromedex, 1992.
41. Taskinen H, Lindbohm ML, Hemminki K. Spontaneous abortions among women working in the pharmaceutical industry. *Br J Ind Med.* 1986;43:199–205.
42. Axelsson G, Lutz C, Rylander R. Exposure to solvents and outcome of pregnancy in university laboratory employees. *Br J Ind Med.* 1984;41:305–312.
43. Bayard S, et al. GRA & I (14), 1985. Quoted in Carbon Monoxide Monograph, Reprotext Information System. Denver, CO: Micromedex, 1992.
44. Kelly M. Case reports of individuals with oligospermia and methylene chloride exposures. *Reprod Toxicol.* 1988;2:13–17.
45. Ogi D, Hamada A. Reports on fetal deaths and malformations of extremities probably related to insecticide poisoning. *J Jpn Obstet Gynecol Soc.* 1965;17:569.
46. Romero P, Barnett PG, Nidling JE. Congenital anomalies associated with maternal exposure to oxydemeton-methyl. *Environ Res.* 1989;50:256–261.
47. Nora JJ, Nora AH, Sommerville RJ, et al. Maternal exposure to potential teratogens. *JAMA.* 1967;202:1065–1069.

48. Hall JG, Pailiser PD, Clarren SK, et al. Congenital hypothalamic hamartoblastoma, hypopituitarism, imperforate anus, and postaxial polydactyly—a new syndrome? Part 1: Clinical, causal and pathogenetic considerations. *Am J Med Genet.* 1980;7:47–74.
49. Gordon JE, Shy CM. Agricultural chemical use and congenital cleft lip and/or palate. *Arch Environ Health.* 1981;36:213–220.
50. Midtling JE, Barnett PG, Coye MJ, et al. Clinical management of field worker organophosphate poisoning. *West J Med.* 1985;142:514–518.
51. Karalliedde L, Senanayaka N, Ariaratnam A. Acute organophosphorous insecticide poisoning during pregnancy. *Hum Toxicol.* 1988;7:363–364.
52. Klys M, Kosun J, Pach J, et al. Carbofuran poisoning of pregnant woman and fetus per ingestion. *J Forensic Sci.* 1989;34:1413–1416.
53. Sherman JD. Chlorpyrifos (Dursban)-associated birth defects: report of four cases. *Arch Environ Health.* 1996;51:5–8.
54. Jackson RJ, Erickson JD, McGeehin M, et al. Possible teratogenic effects of intrauterine exposure to chlorpyrifos (Dursban). *Arch Environ Health.* 1999;54:141–143.
55. Whorton D, Krauss RM, Marshall S, et al. Infertility in male pesticide workers. *Lancet.* 1977;2:1259–1261.
56. Whorton D, Milby TH, Krauss RM, et al. Testicular function in DBCP exposed pesticide workers. *J Occup Med.* 1979;21:161–166.
57. Slutsky M, Levin JL, Levy BS. Azoospermia and oligospermia among a large cohort of DBCP applicators in 12 countries. *Int J Occup Environ Health.* 1999;5:116–122.
58. Lanham JM. Nine-year follow-up of workers exposed to 1,2-dibromo-3-chloropropane. *J Occup Med.* 1987;29:488.
59. Potashnik G, Yanai-Inbar I. Dibromochloropropane: an 8-year reevaluation of testicular function and reproductive performance. *Fertil Steril.* 1987;47:317–323.
60. Eaton M, Schenker M, Whorton MD, et al. Seven-year follow-up of workers exposed to1,2-dibromo-3-chloropropane. *J Occup Med.* 1986;28:1145–1150.
61. Goldsmith JR, Potashnik G, Israeli R. Reproductive outcomes in families of DBCP-exposed men. *Arch Environ Health.* 1984;39:85–89.
62. Potashnik G, Goldsmith J, Insler V. Dibromochloropropane-induced reduction of the sex ratio in man. *Andrologia.* 1984;16:213–218.
63. Goldsmith JR. Dibromochloropropane: epidemiological findings and current questions. *Ann N Y Acad Sci.* 1997;837:300–306.
64. Potashnik G, Phillip M. Lack of birth defects among offspring conceived during or after paternal exposure to dibromochloropropane. *Andrologia.* 1988;20:90–94.
65. Potashnik G, Porath A. Dibromochloropropane (DBCP): a 17-year reassessment of testicular function and reproductive performance. *J Occup Environ Med.* 1995;37:1287–1292.
66. Potashnik G, Abeliovich D. Chromosomal analysis and health status of children conceived to men during or following dibromochloropropane-induced spermatogenic suppression. *Andrologia.* 1985;17:291–296.
67. Kapp RW Jr, Picciano DJ, Jacobson CB. Y chromosomal nondisjunction in dibromochloropropane-exposed workmen. *Mutat Res.* 1979;64:47–51.
68. Kucerova M, Zhurkova VS, Polivkova Z, et al. Mutagenic effect of epichlorhydrin. *Mutat Res.* 1977;48:355–360.
69. Picciano D. Cytogenic investigation of occupational exposure to epichlorhydrin. *Mutat Res.* 1979;66:169–173.
70. Sram RJ, Landa I, Samkova I. Effect of occupational exposure to epichlorhydrin on the frequency of chromosome aberrations in peripheral lymphocytes. *Mutat Res.* 1983;122:59–64.
71. John JA, Quast JF, Murray FJ, et al. Inhalation toxicity of epichlorhydrin: effects on fertility in rats and rabbits. *Toxicol Appl Pharmacol.* 1983;68:415–423.
72. Epichlorhydrin. In: Barlow SM, Sullivan FM, eds. *Reproductive Hazards of Industrial Chemicals.* London: Academic Press, 1982, pp 287–295.
73. Ratcliffe JM, Elliott MJ, Wyse RK, et al. Semen quality in papaya workers with long-term exposure to ethylene dibromide. *Br J Ind Med.* 1987;44:317–326.
74. Takahashi W, Wong L, Rogers BJ, et al. Depression of sperm counts among agricultural workers exposed to dibromochloropropane and ethylene dibromide. *Bull Environ Contamin Toxicol.* 1981;27:551–558.
75. Wong O, Utidjian HMD, Karten VS. Retrospective evaluation of reproductive performance of workers exposed to ethylene dibromide. *J Occup Med.* 1979;21:98–102.
76. Ter Haar G. An investigation of possible sterility and health effects from exposure to ethylene dibromide. In: Ames B, Infante P, Reitz R, eds. *Ethylene Dichloride: A Potential Health Risk?* Cold Spring Harbor, NY: Cold Spring Harbor Laboratory, 1980, pp. 167–177.
77. Hemminki K, Mutanen P, Saloniemi I, et al. Spontaneous abortions in hospital staff engaged in sterilizing instruments with chemical agents. *Br Med J.* 1982;285:1461–1463.
78. Yabukova ZN, Shamova HA, Muftaknova FA, et al. Gynecological disorders in workers engaged in ethylene oxide production. *Kazan Med Zh.* 1976;57:558–560.
79. Hathaway GJ, Proctor NH, Hughes JP. Chemical Hazards of the Workplace, 4th ed. Van Nostrand Reinhold Company, New York, NY: 1996.
80. Bingham E, Cohrssen B, Powell CH. Patty's Toxicology, Vol 6, 5th ed. John Wiley & Sons, New York, NY: 2001.
81. Rowland AS, Baird DD, Shore DL, et al. Ethylene oxide exposure may increase the risk of spontaneous abortion, preterm birth, and post-term birth. *Epidemiology.* 1996;7:363–368.
82. Hemminki K, Kyyronen P, Lindbohm ML. Spontaneous abortions and malformations in the offspring of nurses exposed to anesthetic gases, cytostatic drugs and other potential hazards in hospitals, based on registered information of outcome. *J Epidemiol Community Health.* 1985;39:141–147.
83. Steele L, Wilkins J, Crawford J, et al. Occupational exposure to reproductive hazards among pregnant female veterinarians. *Am J Epidemiol.* 1989;130:834.
84. Laurent C, Frederic J, Leonard AY. Sister chromatid exchange frequency in workers exposed to high levels of ethylene oxide in a hospital sterilization service. *Int Arch Occup Environ Health.* 1984;54:33–43.
85. Stolley PD, Soper KA, Galloway SM, et al. Sister chromatid exchanges in association with occupational exposure to ethylene oxide. *Mutat Res.* 1984;129:89–102.
86. Yager JW, Hines CJ, Spear RC. Exposure to ethylene oxide at work increases sister chromatid exchanges in human peripheral lymphocytes. *Science.* 1983;219:1221–1223.
87. Schulle PA, Boeniger M, Walker JT, et al. Biologic markers in hospital workers exposed to low levels of ethylene oxide. *Mutat Res.* 1992;278:237–251.
88. Lerda D, Rizzi R. Cytogenetic study of persons occupationally exposed to ethylene oxide. *Mutat Res.* 1992;281:31–37.
89. Kimmel CA. Teratologic Evaluation of Ethylene Oxide. Govt Reports Announcements and Index (GRA&I), Issue 21, National Technical Information Services (NTIS), 1984.
90. John EM, Savitz DA, Shy CM. Spontaneous abortions among cosmetologists. *Epidemiology.* 1994;5:147–155.
91. Taskinen H, Kyyronen P, Hemminki K, et al. Laboratory work and pregnancy outcome. *J Occup Med.* 1994;36:311–319.
92. Shumillina AV. Menstrual and child-bearing functions of female workers occupationally exposed to the effects of formaldehyde. *Gig Tr Prof Zabol.* 1975;19:18–21.
93. Taskinen HK, Kyyronen P, Sallmen M, et al. Reduced fertility among female wood workers exposed to formaldehyde. *Am J Ind Med.* 1999;36:206–212.
94. Chloroprene. In: Barlow SM, Sullivan FM, eds. *Reproductive Hazards of Industrial Chemicals.* London: Academic Press, 1982; pp 239–252.

95. U.S. Department of Health, Education and Welfare. Criteria document for a recommended standard: Occupational exposure to chloroprene. DHFW (NIOSH) Publication No. 77-210. Washington, DC: USDHEW, 1977.
96. Dowty BJ, Laseter JL, Storer J. The transplacental migration and accumulation in blood of volatile organic constituents. *Pediatr Res.* 1976;10:696–701.
97. Axelsson G, Lutz C, Rylander R. Exposure to solvents and outcome of pregnancy in university laboratory employees. *Br J Ind Med.* 1984;41:305–312.
98. Aschengrau A, Zierler S, Cohen A. Quality of community drinking water and the occurrence of late adverse pregnancy outcomes. *Arch Environ Health.* 1993;48:105–113.
99. Dodds L, King WD. Relation between trihalomethane compounds and birth defects. *Occup Environ Med.* 2001;58:443–446.
100. Bove FJ, Fulcomer MC, Klotz JB, et al. Public drinking water contamination and birth outcomes. *Am J Epidemiol.* 1995;141:850–862.
101. King WD, Dodds L, Allen AC. Relation between stillbirth and specific chlorination by-products in public water supplies. *Environ Health Perspect.* 2000;108:883–886.
102. Gallagher MD, Nuckols JR, Stallones L, et al. Exposure to trihalomethanes and adverse pregnancy outcomes. *Epidemiology.* 1998;9:484–489.
103. Kramer MD, Lynch CF, Isacson P, et al. The association of waterborne chloroform with intrauterine growth retardation. *Epidemiology.* 1992;3:407–413.
104. Savitz DA, Andrews KW, Pastore LM. Drinking water and pregnancy outcome in central North Carolina: source, amount, and trihalomethane levels. *Environ Health Perspect.* 1995;103:592–596.
105. Funes-Cravioto F, Kalmodin-Hedman B, Lindsten J, et al. Chromosome aberrations in chemical laboratories and a rotoprinting factory and in children of women laboratory workers. *Lancet.* 1977;2:322–325.
106. Strickland DM, Leonard RG, Stavchansky S, et al. Vaginal absorption of hexachlorophene during labor. *Am J Obstet Gynecol.* 1983;147:769–772.
107. Halling H. Suspected link between exposure to hexachlorophene and malformed infants. *Ann NY Acad Sci.* 1979;320:326.
108. Baltzar B, Ericson A, Kallen B. Pregnancy outcome among women working in Swedish hospitals. *N Engl J Med.* 1979;300:627–628.
109. Hernberg S, Kurppa K, Ojajavri J, et al. Congenital malformations and occupational exposure to disinfectants: a case-referent study. *Scand J Work Environ Health.* 1983;9:55. Quoted in Hexachlorophene Monograph, Teris. Denver, CO: Micromedex, 1992.
110. Roeleveld N, Zielhuis GA, Gabreels F. Mental retardation and potential occupation. *Br J Ind Med.* 1993;50:945–954.
111. American Medical Association, Council on Scientific Affairs. Effects of Toxic Chemicals on the Reproductive System. Chicago: AMA, 1985.
112. Eskenazi B, Wyrobek AJ, Fenster L, et al. A study of the effect of perchloroethylene exposure on semen quality in dry cleaning workers. *Am J Ind Med.* 1991;20:575–591.
113. Eskenazi B, Fenster L, Hudes M, et al. A study of the effect of perchloroethylene exposure on the reproductive outcomes of wives of dry-cleaning workers. *Am J Ind Med.* 1991;20:593–600.
114. Kyyronen P, Taskinen H, Lindbohm ML, et al. Spontaneous abortions and congenital malformations among women exposed to tetrachloroethylene in dry cleaning. *J Epidemiol Community Health.* 1989;43:346–351.
115. Doyle P, Roman E, Beral V, et al. Spontaneous abortion in dry cleaning workers potentially exposed to perchloroethylene. *Occup Environ Med.* 1997;54:848–853.
116. Ahlborg G Jr. Pregnancy outcome among women working in laundries and dry-cleaning shops using tetrachloroethylene. *Am J Ind Med.* 1990;17:567–575.
117. Olsen I, Hemminki K, Ahlborg G, et al. Low birth weight, congenital malformations, and spontaneous abortions among dry-cleaning workers in Scandinavia. *Scan J Work Environ Health.* 1990;16:163–168.
118. Bosco MG, Figa-Talamanca L, Salerno S. Health and reproductive status of female workers in dry-cleaning shops. *Int Arch Occup Environ Health.* 1987;59:295–301.
119. Bove FJ, Fulcomer MC, Klotz JB, et al. Public drinking water contamination and birth outcomes. *Am J Epidemiol.* 1995;141:850–862.
120. Bove FJ. Public drinking water contamination and birthweight, prematurity, fetal deaths, and birth defects. *Toxicol Ind Health.* 1996;12:255–266.
121. Proctor NH, Hughes JP, Fischman ML, eds. *Chemical Hazards of the Workplace.* Philadelphia, PA: Lippincott, 1988; pp. 399–401.
122. Laham S. Studies on placental transfer of trichloroethylene. *Ind Med.* 1979;39:46–49.
123. Lindbohm ML, Taskinen H, Sallmen N, et al. Spontaneous abortions among women exposed to organic solvents. *Am J Ind Med.* 1990;17:449–463.
124. Windham GC, Shusterman D, Swan SH, et al. Exposure to organic solvents and adverse pregnancy outcome. *Am J Ind Med.* 1991;20:241–259.
125. Goldberg SJ, Lebowitz MD, Graver EJ, et al. An association of human congenital cardiac malformations and drinking water contaminants. *J Am Coll Cardiol.* 1990;16:155–164.
126. Susan SH, Shaw G, Harris JA, et al. Congenital cardiac anomalies in relation to water contamination, Santa Clara County, California 1981–1983. *Am J Epidemiol.* 1989;129:885–893.
127. Bove F, Shim Y, Zeitz P. Drinking water contaminants and adverse pregnancy outcomes: a review. *Environ Health Perspect.* 2002;110 (Suppl 1):61–74.
128. Lorente C, Cordier S, Bergeret A, et al. Maternal occupational risk factors for oral clefts. Occupational Exposure and Congenital Malformation Working Group. *Scand J Work Environ Health.* 2000;26:137–145.
129. Kimbrough RD, Michell FL, Houk VN. Trichloroethylene: an update. *J Toxicol Environ Health.* 1985;15:369–383.
130. Kostrial K, Moncilovic B. Transport of lead-203 and calcium-47 from mother to offspring. *Arch Environ Health.* 1974;29:28.
131. Rayegowda BK, Glass L, Evans HE. Lead concentration in newborn infants. *J Pediatr.* 1972;80:116.
132. Fahim MS, Fahim Z, Hall DG. Effects of subtoxic lead levels on pregnant women in the State of Missouri. In: *Proceedings of the International Conference on Heavy Metals in the Environmen.,* Toronto, Ont., Canada, October 27–31, 1975.
133. Nogaki K. On action of lead on body of lead refinery workers: Particularly conception, pregnancy and parturition in case of females and on vitality of their newborn. *Excerpta Med.* 1958;4:2176.
134. Needelman HL, Rabinowitz M, Leviton A, et al. The relationship between prenatal exposure to lead and congenital anomalies. *JAMA.* 1984;251:2956–2959.
135. Bellinger D, Leviton A, Watermaux C, et al. Longitudinal analysis of prenatal and postnatal lead exposure and early cognitive development. *N Engl J Med.* 1987;316:1037–1043.
136. Dekknudt GH, Leonard A, Ivanov B. Chromosome aberrations observed in male workers occupationally exposed to lead. *Environ Physiol Biochem.* 1973;3:132–138.
137. Rom WN. Effects of lead on the female reproduction: a review. *Mt. Sinai J Med.* 1976;43:542–551.
138. McFarland RB, Reigel H. Chronic mercury poisoning from a single brief exposure. *J Occup Med.* 1978;20:532–534.
139. Lauwerys R, Roels H, Geret P, et al. Fertility of male workers exposed to mercury vapor or to manganese dust: a questionnaire study. *Am J Ind Med.* 1985;7:171–176.
140. Cordier S, Deplan F, Mandereau L, et al. Paternal exposure to mercury and spontaneous abortions. *Obstet Gynecol Surv.* 1992;47:152–154.
141. Goncharak GA. Problems relating to occupational hygiene of women in production of mercury. *Gig Tr Prof Zabol.* 1977;5: 17–20.

142. Panaova Z, Dimitrov G. Ovarian function in women having professional contact with metallic mercury. *Akus Ginek.* 1974;13:29–34.
143. Rachootin P, Olsen J. The risk of infertility and delayed conception associated with exposures in the Danish workplace. *J Occup Med.* 1983;25:394–M2.
144. Lauwerys R, Buchet JP, Roels H, et al. Placental transfer of lead, mercury, cadmium and carbon monoxide in women: 1. Comparison of the frequency biological indices in maternal and umbilical cord. *Environ Res.* 1978;15:278–289.
145. Lien DC, Todoruk DN, Rajani HR, et al. Accidental inhalation of mercury vapour: respiratory and toxicologic consequences. *Can Med Assoc J.* 1983;129:591–595.
146. Baglan RJ, Brill AB, Schulert A, et al. Utility of placental tissue as an indicator of trace element exposure to adult and fetus. *Environ Res.* 1974;8:64–70.
147. Wannag A, Skajerasen J. Mercury accumulation in placenta and fetal membranes: a study of dental workers and their babies. *Environ Physiol Biochem.* 1975;5:348–352.
148. Heidam LZ. Spontaneous abortions among dental assistants, factory workers, painters and gardening workers: a follow-up study. *J Epidemiol Common Health.* 1984;38:149–155.
149. Brodsky JB, Cohen EN, Whitcher C, et al. Occupational exposure to mercury in dentistry and pregnancy outcome. *J Am Dent Assoc.* 1985;111:779–780.
150. Elghany NA, Stopford W, Bunn WB, et al. Occupational exposure to inorganic mercury vapour and reproductive outcomes. *Occup Med (Lond).* 1997;47:333–336.
151. Sikorski R, Juszkiewicz T, Paszkowski T, et al. Women in dental surgeries: reproductive hazards in occupational exposure to metallic mercury. *Int Arch Occup Environ Health.* 1987;59:551–557.
152. Goncharuk GA. Effect of chronic mercury poisoning on the immunological reactivity of offspring. *Gig Tr (Kiev).* 1971;7:73–75.
153. Panova Z, Ivanova S, Promeni V. Ovarialanta funktsiia: miakoi funktsionaini pokazateli na chernia drob pri profesionalen kontakt s metalen zhivak (purvo suobshtenie). *Akush Ginekol (Sofia).* 1976;15:133–137.
154. Kurppa K, Holmberg PC, Hemberg S, et al. Screening for occupational exposures and congenital anomalies. *Scand J Work Environ Health.* 1983;9:89–93.
155. Klinkova-Deutschor E. Teratogenoi vlivy zemiho prostredi. *Cesk Neurol Neurochir.* 1977;40:283–291.
156. Ericson A, Kallen B. Pregnancy outcome in women working as dentists, dental assistants or dental technicians. *Int Arch Occup Environ Health.* 1989;61:329–333.
157. Seidler A, Raum E, Arabin B, et al. Maternal occupational exposure to chemical substances and the risk of infants small-for-gestational-age. *Am J Ind Med.* 1999;36:213–222.
158. Dahl R, White RF, Weihe P, et al. Feasibility and validity of three computer-assisted neurobehavioral tests in 7-year-old children. *Neurotoxicol Teratol.* 1996;18:413–419.
159. Koos BJ, Longo LD. Mercury toxicity in the pregnant woman, fetus, and newborn infant. *Am J Obstet Gynecol.* 1976;126:390–409.
160. Larsson KS, Sagulin GB. Placental transfer of mercury from amalgam. *Lancet.* 1990;2:1251.
161. Luglie PF, Frulio A, Campus G, et al. Mercury determination in human amniotic fluid. *Minerva Stomatol.* 2000;49:155–161.
162. Razagui IB, Haswell SJ. Mercury and selenium concentrations in maternal and neonatal scalp hair: relationship to amalgam-based dental treatment received during pregnancy. *Biol Trace Elem Res.* 2001;81:1–19.
163. Vimy MJ, Takahashi Y, Lorscheider FL. Maternal-fetal distribution of mercury (203-Hg) released from dental amalgam fillings. *Am J Physiol.* 1990;258:R939–R945.
164. Mercury and its compounds. In: Barlow SM, Sullivan FM, eds. *Reproductive Industrial Chemicals.* London: Academic Press, 1982, pp. 386–406.
165. Choi BH. *Neurobiol Trace Elem.* 1983;2:197–235. Quoted in Mercury Monograph, Reprotext Information System. Denver, CO: Micromedex, 1992.
166. Agocs MM, Etzel RA, Parrish RG. Mercury exposure from interior latex paint. *N Engl J Med.* 1990;323:1096–1101.
167. Alfonso J, DeAlvarez R. Effects of mercury on human gestation. *Am J Obstet Gynecol.* 1960;80:145–154.
168. Amin-Zaki L, Ethassani SB, Majeed NU, et al. Intrauterine methylmercury poisoning in Iraq. *Pediatrics.* 1974;54:587–595.
169. Matsumoto H, Koya G, Takeuchi T. Fetal Minamata disease: a neuropathological study of two cases of intrauterine intoxication by a methyl mercury compound. *J Neuropathol Exp Neurol.* 1965;24:563–574.
170. Muramaki U. The effect of organic mercury on intrauterine life. *Acta Exp Med Biol.* 1972;27:301–306.
171. Marsh DO, Myers GJ, Clarkson TW, et al. Fetal methylmercury poisoning: Clinical and toxicological data on 29 cases. *Ann Neurol.* 1980;7:348–353.
172. Amin-Zaki L, Elhassani S, Majeed NR, et al. Perinatal methylmercury poisoning in Iraq. *Am J Dis Child.* 1976;130:1070–1076.
173. Feldman RJ, Maibach HI. Percutaneous penetration of some pesticide and herbicides in man. *Toxicol Appl Pharmacol.* 1974;28:126–132.
174. Saxena MC, Siddiqui MK, Bhargava AK, et al. Role of chlorinated hydrocarbon pesticides in abortions and premature labour. *Toxicology.* 1980;17:323–331.
175. Yoshimura M. *Kinki Daigaku Igaku Zasshi.* 1979;4:209–218. Quoted in Lindane Monograph, Reprotext Information System. Denver, CO: Micromedex, 1992.
176. Saxena MC. *Arch Toxicol.* 1984;48:127–134. Quoted in Lindane Monograph, Reprotext Information System. Denver, CO: Micromdex, 1992.
177. Ilina VI, Bleckherman NA. Deiaki dani pro stan sletsyfichnykh funksii zhinochoho orhanizmu v osib jaki pratsiuiut, z heksakhlortsykloheksanom. Pediatr Akush Ginekol 1974;1:46–49. Quoted in Lindane Monograph, Reprotext Information System. Denver: Micromedex, 1992.
178. Verzhanskii PS. Gumoral it regul rodovoi deyat lech EE. Narushenii 1976;88–91. Quoted in Lindane Monograph, Reprotext Information System. Denver: Micromedex, 1992.
179. Wassermann M, Ron N, Bercovici B, et al. Premature delivery and organochlorine compounds: polychlorinated biphenyls and some organochlorine insecticides. *Environ Res.* 1982;28:106–112.
180. Curley A, Copeland MF, Kimbrough RD. Chlorinated hydrocarbon insecticides in organs of stillborn and blood of newborn babies. *Arch Environ Health.* 1969;19:628–632.
181. Poradovsky K, Rosival L, Meszarosova A. Transplacentamy prienik pesticidov pocas fuziotogickej tehotnosti. *Cesk Gynekol.* 1977;42:405–410.
182. Tomczak S, Baumann K, Lehnert G. Occupational exposure to hexachlorocyclohexane: IV Sex hormone alterations in HCH-exposed workers. *Int Arch Occup Environ Health.* 1981;48:283–287.
183. Cranz C. *Contraception Fertil Sex.* 1981;9:421–423. Quoted in Lindane Monograph, Reprotext Information System. Denver, CO: Micromedex, 1992.
184. Cariati E, Acanfora L, Branconi F, et al. *p,p*-DDT in perinatal samples: report on maternal and neonatal measurements. *Biol Res Pregnancy Perinatol.* 1983;4:169–171.
185. Siddiqui MKJ, Saxena MC, Bhargava AK, et al. Chlorinated hydrocarbon pesticides in blood of newborn babies in India. *Pestic Monit J.* 1981;15:77–79.
186. Saxena MC, Siddiqui NW, Agarwal V, et al. A comparison of organochlorine insecticide contents in specimens of maternal blood, placenta and umbilical-cord blood from stillborn and live-born cases. *J Toxicol Environ Health.* 1983;11:71–79.
187. Leoni V, Fabiani L, Marinelli G, et al. PCB and other organochlorine compounds in blood of women with or without miscarriage: a hypothesis of correlation. *Ecotoxicol Environ Safety.* 1989;17:1–11.
188. Ron M, Cucos B, Rosenn B, et al. Maternal and fetal serum levels of organochlorine compounds in cases of premature rupture of membranes. *Acta Obstet Gynecol Scand.* 1988;67:695–697.

189. O'Leary JA, Davies JE, Feldman M. Spontaneous abortion and human pesticide residues of DDT and DDE. *Am J Obstet Gynecol.* 1970;108:1291–1292.
190. Torres-Arreola L, Berkowitz G, Torres-Sanchez L, et al. Preterm birth in relation to maternal organochlorine serum levels. *Ann Epidemiol.* 2003;13:158–162.
191. Gladen BC, Shkiryak-Nyzhnyk ZA, Chyslovska N, et al. Persistent organochlorine compounds and birth weight. *Ann Epidemiol.* 2003;13:151–157.
192. LeMarchand L, Kolonel LN, Siegel BZ, et al. Trends in birth defects for a Hawaiian population exposed to heptachlor and for the United States. *Arch Environ Health.* 1986;1:45–148.
193. Chadduck WM, Gollin SM, Gray BA, et al. Gliosarcoma with chromosome abnormalities in a neonate exposed to heptachlor. *Neurosurgery.* 1987;21:557–559.
194. Ahmed FE, Hart RW, Lewis NJ. Pesticide induced DNA damage and its repair in cultured human cells. *Mutat Res.* 1977;42:161–174.
195. Kuntz WD. The pregnant woman in industry. *Am J Ind Hyg Assoc.* 1976;37:423–426.
196. Kuratsure M, Yoshimura Y, Matsuzaka J, et al. Epidemiologic study on poisoning caused by ingestion of rice oil contaminated with a commercial brand of polychlorinated biphenyls. *Environ Health Perspect.* 1972;1:119–128.
197. Miller RW. Congenital PCB poisoning: a reevaluation. *Environ Health Perspect.* 1985;60:211–214.
198. Kodama H, Ota H. Studies on the transfer of PCB to infants from their mothers. *Jpn J Hyg.* 1977;32:567–573.
199. Funatsu I, Yamashita F, Ito Y, et al. Polychlorobiphenyls (PCB) induced fetopathy: 1. Clinical observation. *Kurume Med J.* 1972;19:43–51.
200. Taki I, Hisanaga S, Amagase Y. Report on Yusho (chlorobiphenyls poisoning) in women and their fetuses. *Fukuoko Acta Med.* 1969;60:471–474.
201. Yamashita F. Clinical features of polychlorobiphenyls (PCB)-induced fetopathy. *Paediatrician.* 1977;6:20–27.
202. Gladen BC, Taylor JS, Wu YC, et al. Dermatological findings in children exposed transplacentally to heat-degraded polychlorinated biphenyls in Taiwan. *Br J Dermatol.* 1990;22:799–808.
203. Rogan WJ, Gladen BC, Hung KL, et al. Congenital poisoning by polychlorinated biphenyls and their contaminants in Taiwan. *Science.* 1988;241:334–336.
204. Rogan WJ, Gladen BC, McKinaly JD, et al. Neonatal effects of transplacental exposure of PCBs and DDE. *J Pediatr.* 1986;109:335–341.
205. Yu M, Hsu C, Gladen BC, et al. *In utero* PCB/PCDF exposure: relation of developmental delay to dysmorphology and dose. *Neurotoxicol Teratol.* 1991;13:195–202.
206. Fein GG, Jacobson JL, Jacobson SW, et al. Prenatal exposure to chlorinated biphenyls effects on birth size and gestational age. *J Pediatr.* 1984;105:315–320.
207. Jacobson JL, Jacobson SW, Humphrey HEB. Effects of *in utero* exposure to polychlorinated biphenyls and related contaminants and cognitive functioning in young children. *J Pediatr.* 1990;116:38–45.
208. Rozati R, Reddy PP, Reddanna P, et al. Role of environmental estrogens in the deterioration of male factor fertility. *Fertil Steril.* 2002;78:1187–1194.
209. Taylor PR, Lawrence CE, Hwang HL, et al. Polychlorobiphenyls' influence on birthweight and gestation. *Am J Public Health.* 1984;74:1153–1154.
210. Letz G. The toxicology of PCBs: an overview for clinicians. *West J Med.* 1983;138:534–540.
211. Weil WB, Spencer M, Benjamin D, et al. The effect of polybrominated biphenyls in infants and young children. *J Pediatr.* 1981;98:47–51.
212. Pokrovskii VA. *Gig Prof Zabol.* 1967;11:17–20. Quoted in Styrene Monograph, Reprotext Information System. Denver, CO: Micromedex 1992.
213. Zlobina NS, Izyumora AS, Ragule NY. The effect of low styrene concentrations of specific functions of the female organism. *Gig Tr Prof Zabol.* 1975;12:21–25.
214. Lemasters GK, Hagen A, Samuels SJ. Reproductive outcomes in women exposed to solvents in 36 reinforced plastics companies: I. Menstrual dysfunction. *J Occup Med.* 1985:27:490–494.
215. Harkonen H, Tola S, Korkala ML, et al. Congenital malformations, mortality and styrene exposure. *Ann Acad Med Singapore.* 1984;13(suppl 2):40:404–407.
216. Meretoja T, Vainio H, Sorsa M, et al. Occupational styrene exposure and chromosomal aberrations. *Mutat Res.* 1977;56:193–197.
217. Meretoja T, Jarventaus H, Sorsa M, et al. Chromosome aberrations in lymphocytes of workers exposed to styrene. *Scand J Work Environ Health.* 1978;4(suppl 2):259–264.
218. Nordenson I, Beckmann L. Chromosomal aberrations in lymphocytes of workers exposed to low levels of styrene. *Hum Hered.* 1984;34:178–182.
219. Mastroiacovo P, Spagrolo A, Marni E, et al. Birth defects in the Seveso area after TCDD contamination. *JAMA.* 1988;259: 1668–1672.
220. Tognoi G, Bonaccarsi A. Epidemiological problems with TCDD (a critical review). *Drug Metab Rev.* 1982;13:447–M9.
221. Friedman JM. Does agent orange cause birth defects? *Teratology.* 1984;29:193–221.
222. Mocarelli P, Brambilla P, Gerthoux PM, et al. Change in sex ratio with exposure to dioxin. *Lancet.* 1996;348:409.
223. Mocarelli P, Gerthoux PM, Ferrari E, et al. Paternal concentrations of dioxin and sex ratio of offspring. *Lancet.* 2000;355:1858–1863.
224. Clapp R, Ozonoff D. Where the boys aren't: dioxin and the sex ratio. *Lancet.* 2000;355:1838–1839.
225. Donovan JW, MacLennan R, Adena M. Vietnam service and the risk of congenital anomalies: a case-control study. *Med J Aust.* 1984;140:394–397.
226. Erickson JD, Mulinare J, McClaim PW, et al. Vietnam veterans' risk for fathering babies with birth defects. *JAMA.* 1984;252:903–912.
227. Wolfe WH, Michalek JE, Miner JC, et al. Paternal serum dioxin and reproductive outcomes among veterans of Operation Ranch Hand. *Epidemiology.* 1995;6:17–22.
228. Townsend JD, Bodner KM, Van Peenen PFD, et al. Survey of reproductive events of wives of employees exposed to chlorinated dioxins. *Am J Epidemiol.* 1982;115:695–713.
229. Walker AE. A preliminary report of a vascular abnormality occurring in men engaged in the manufacture of polyvinyl chloride. *Br J Dermatol.* 1975;93:22–23.
230. Walker AE. Clinical aspects of vinyl chloride disease: skin. *Proc R Soc Med.* 1976;69:286–289.
231. Vinyl chloride. In: *Meditext, Healthcare Series.* Vol. 125, Thomson-Micromedex, Greenwood Village, CO, 2005.
232. Infante PF, McMichael AJ, Wagoner JK, et al. Genetic risks of vinyl chloride. *Lancet.* 1976;1:734–735.
233. Buffer PA. Some problems involved in recognizing teratognes used in industry. *Contrib Epidemiol Biostat.* 1979;1:118–137.
234. Paddle GM. Genetic risks of vinyl chloride. *Lancet.* 1976;1:1079.
235. Sanotsky IV, Davian RM, Glushchenko VI. Study of the reproductive function in men exposed to chemicals. *Gig Tr Prof Zabol.* 1980;5:28–32.
236. Lindbohm M, Hemminki K, Kyyronen P. Spontaneous abortions among women employed in the plastic industries. *Am J Ind Med.* 1985;8:579–586.
237. Mur JM, Manderean L, Deplan F, et al. Spontaneous abortion and exposure to vinyl chloride. *Lancet.* 1992;339:127–128.
238. Infante PF. Oncogenic and mutagenic risks in communities with polyvinyl chloride production facilities. *Ann NY Acad Sci.* 1976;271:49–57.
239. Edmonds LD, Falk H, Nissim JE. Congenital malformations and vinyl chloride. *Lancet.* 1975;2:1098.

240. Edmonds LD, Anderson CE, Flynt JW, et al. Congenital central nervous system malformations and vinyl chloride monomer exposure: a community study. *Teratology.* 1978;17:137–142.
241. Hemminki K, Vineis P. Extrapolation of the evidence on teratogenicity of chemicals between humans and experimental animals: chemicals other than drugs. *Teratogen Carcinog Mutagen.* 1985;5:251–318.
242. Theriault G, Iturra H, Gingras S. Evaluation of the association between birth defects and exposure to ambient vinyl chloride. *Teratology.* 1983;27:359–370.
243. Baxter PJ, Adams PH, Aw TC. Hunter's Diseases of Occupations, 9th ed. Oxford University Press, Inc., New York, NY, 2000.
244. Clemmesen J. International Commission for Protection against Environmental Mutagens and Carcinogens. ICPEMC working paper TG1/2/79. Mutagenicity and teratogenicity of vinyl chloride monomer (VCM): epidemiological evidence. *Mutat Res.* 1982;98:97–100.
245. Sever LE, Hessol NA. Toxic effects of occupational and environmental chemical on the testes. In: Thomas JA, Kovach KS, McLachlan JA eds. *Endocrine Toxicology*. Raven Press, New York, NY, 1985.
246. Vinyl chloride. In: Barlow SM, Sullivan FM, eds. *Reproductive Hazards of Industrial Chemicals.* London: Academic Press, 1982; pp 566–581.

CHAPTER 17

THE COMMON OCCUPATIONAL EXPOSURES ENCOUNTERED BY PREGNANT WOMEN

Yedidia Bentur and Gideon Koren

INTRODUCTION

It is clear from animal experiments and human epidemiological studies that industrial chemicals have the potential of being reproductive toxins. However, our knowledge of the reproductive toxicology of industrial chemicals in humans is sparse or absent. Before therapeutic agents are marketed, their teratogenic potential must be tested in animals; these data are not always required for chemicals. Other factors also may differ between medical and occupational exposures. In the workplace the exposure is usually to several chemicals, which may change between working days or even within a single day. In some cases one has to deal with possible unknown by-products. The amounts of the chemicals absorbed are often unclear, and the circumstances of exposure may vary from plant to plant or even within the same operation. Every chemical in the workplace has safety exposure limits aiming at protecting the worker. However, these standards were not designed to protect the fetus. Hence, even if exposure levels exists, one is never sure whether safe levels to the mother are also safe for her unborn child; lead is a good example of such a discrepancy.[1,2] An interesting attempt to approach this problem is illustrated by a study that suggested 20 ppm as a pregnancy guidance value for occupational exposure to toluene.[3] This value was based on "no observable adverse effect level" (NOAEL) of 500, 400, and 200 ppm in pregnant rabbits, rats, and mice and their offspring, respectively, and applying safety factors for interspecies and intraspecies variation.

In approaching the occupationally exposed woman, the following steps are suggested:

1. Obtain medical, obstetric, and genetic history from the patient and her spouse, including the use of cigarettes, alcohol, and drugs.
2. Identify the chemicals in question, if possible, by their material safety data sheets (MSDS).
3. Obtain a detailed description of the process the patients is operating, the work she performs, the length of exposure, and the means of protection used (ventilation system, hood, respirator, mask, gown, gloves, etc.).
4. Obtain information on possible exposure from nearby work stations.
5. Identify symptoms and signs reported to be associated with the chemicals and temporal relationship to the exposure.
6. Rule out underlying conditions that may cause a similar clinical picture (e.g., morning sickness).
7. Determine whether there are symptoms and signs manifest in fellow workers.
8. Ascertain the pregnancy outcome in other workers.
9. Obtain occupational history of the spouse.
10. Obtain the most recent levels of the chemicals in question or radiation measured in that particular area and their relation to the recommended threshold limit value-time-weighted average (TLV-TWA).
11. Find out whether employees are being regularly examined by an occupational physician and whether biological monitoring is done (e.g., blood lead levels, urinary phenol excretion, blood count for benzene, hepatic aminotransferase for carbon tetrachloride).
12. Try to understand the attitude of the woman and her supervisors toward her particular work and toward a possible change of job. Will a change of job affect her income or chances for promotion?
13. Search as many data sources as possible and evaluate the data critically to allow the patient to receive the most accurate information.
14. Convey the information to the patient, estimate the risk (if possible), and advise about ways to assess severity of exposure (i.e., environmental and biological measurements), on possible safety means to reduce exposure (ventilation, mask, gloves, etc.), the need for targeted ultrasound and possible removal from work.

The Motherisk Program in Toronto is an antenatal counseling service for health professionals, women, and their families dealing with exposures to drugs, chemicals, radiation, and infections in pregnancy and lactation. In 1990, between 40 and 50 telephone calls were processed daily. Women are referred to a clinic if they have been exposed to known or suspected teratogens, long-term drug therapy, new drugs on which there is sparse or no information, and drugs of abuse, or if they have experienced occupational exposure. After the expected day of confinement, follow-up of pregnancy outcome is performed, and all data are computerized for clinical and research use. In 1988, a total of 5040 telephone calls were received; 167 (3.3%) of them were due to occupational exposures to video display terminals (Table 17-1). This exposure is the one most frequently encountered in the workplace. Organic solvents were the concern of up to 150 of the callers, most of them entailing the use of oil-based paints, some of them at home. In 56 patients the exposure to organic solvents occurred in the workplace, and 24 of them were followed in the clinic (Table 17-2). In all, 29 patients were advised for exposure to lead (mostly in the form of paints); 6 were occupationally exposed, and 3 were seen in the clinic.

The Israel Poison Information Center, Haifa, Israel, provides teratological consultations 24 hours a day. It is mainly oriented to poisoning, radiation, chemical, and occupational exposures in pregnancy. In addition to textbooks, the Poison Center uses several computerized databases including Drugdex, Poisindex, Hazardous Substances Data Bank (HSDB), Registry of Toxic Effects of Chemical Substances RTECS), Reprotext, Reprotox, TERIS, Shepard's Catalog of Teratogenic Agents-online, Canadian Centre for Occupational Health and Safety-CCINFO, Toxline, and Medline.

The most common occupational exposures reported to the Poison Center in 2004 were hydrocarbons, including organic solvents (25.6%), gases (8.1%), ionizing radiation (5.8%), and metals (2.3%).

Table 17-1
Distribution of Telephone Consultations for Occupational Exposures in 1988

	EXPOSURES			
NUMBER OF CONSULTATIONS	VIDEO DISPLAY TERMINALS	ORGANIC SOLVENTS	LEAD	MISCELLANEOUS
5040	167	56	6	13

Most of the women occupationally exposed to organic solvents and all those exposed to ionizing radiation were laboratory technicians (academic or industrial). A small group of agricultural workers were exposed to insecticides, mainly organophosphates.

Different distribution of occupations among women and lack of awareness to reports on the use of video display terminals in pregnancy may explain the different pattern of calls between the programs in the two countries.

This chapter reviews the state of our knowledge on the reproductive hazards of these exposures and gives the clinician updated information with which to advise women.

EXPOSURES

Video Display Terminals

For discussion of this subject, the reader is referred to Chap. 32: "Ionizing and Nonionizing Radiation in Pregnancy."

Organic Solvents

In our clinics, we often counsel women who are occupationally exposed to numerous chemicals, most of which are organic solvents. A proper consultation in such cases is extremely difficult, because it is hard to estimate the predominant chemicals and their by-products. Even if one identifies the more toxic agents, it is still hard to assess the circumstances of exposure. For many chemicals one can measure neither airborne nor blood levels. Smelling the odor of organic solvents is not indicative of a significant exposure, because the olfactory nerve can detect levels as low as several parts per million, which are not necessarily associated with toxicity. For example, the odor threshold of toluene is 0.8 ppm, whereas TLV-TWA is 50 ppm. Finally, reproductive information on many solvents is at best sparse, either limited to animal studies or nonexistent.

Organic solvents are a structurally diverse group of low-molecular-weight chemicals that are liquids and are able to dissolve other organic substances.[4] They are ubiquitous in our industrialized society, both at work and at home, and they may be encountered as individual agents or in complex mixtures such as gasoline. Chemicals in the solvent class include aliphatic hydrocarbons (such as mineral spirits, varnish, and kerosene), aromatic hydrocarbons (benzene, toluene, xylene), halogenated hydrocarbons (carbon tetrachloride, trichloroethylene, methylcellosolve), aliphatic alcohols (methanol), ketones (methyl ethyl ketone, acetone), glycols (ethylene glycol), and glycol ethers (methoxyethanol).[5,6] Fuels are mixtures of various hydrocarbons.

The mechanisms by which many solvents exert their toxicity are unclear and may vary from one solvent to another. Halogenated hydrocarbons such as carbon tetrachloride may generate free radicals.[4] Simple aromatic compounds such as benzene may disrupt polyribosomes,[7] whereas some solvents are thought to affect lipid membranes and to penetrate tissues such as the brain, causing demyelination and degeneration (e.g., hexane). Other solvents may generate toxic metabolites (e.g., formic acid from methanol, glycolic acid from ethylene glycol). Organic solvents may also interfere with enzyme systems, affect membrane fluidity and cerebral blood flow.

Unintentional exposures may include vapors from gasoline, lighter fluid, spot removers, aerosol sprays, and paints.[8] The short-duration, low-level exposures may go undetected. More serious exposures occur mainly in industrial or laboratory settings during such manufacturing and processing operations such as dry cleaning, working with paint removers, thinners, floor and tile cleaners, and glues, and using laboratory reagents. Volatile substance inhalant abuse (e.g., gasoline or glue sniffing) is another source of exposure to organic solvents during pregnancy; although not occurring in the occupational setting.

Workers with short-term exposure to organic solvents experience fatigue, concentration disorder, feelings of drunkenness, dizziness, pneumonitis, and vomiting.[5] Long-term exposure (e.g., to benzene)

Table 17-2
Distribution of Occupational Exposures with Clinic Follow-Up in 1988

	NUMBER OF CASES	TOTAL CLINIC VISITS (%)[a]	OCCUPATIONAL EXPOSURES SEEN IN CLINIC (%)[b]
Organic solvents[c]	24	6.3	66.6
Video display terminals[d]	5	1.3	13.8
Lead[e]	3	0.8	8.3
Polychlorinated biphenyls	2	0.5	5.5
Miscellaneous[f]	5	1.3	13.8

[a] A total of 380 patients were seen in the clinic.
[b] Thirty-six patients with occupational exposures were monitored in the clinic.
[c] Two patients were exposed to organic solvents and lead.
[d] Four patients came to the clinic because of drug exposure.
[e] Two patients were exposed to lead and organic solvents.
[f] Each patient was exposed to multiple chemicals; no organic solvents.

may irreversibly affect the nervous system and liver and may cause blood disorders.

Most of the occupationally exposed women seen in our teratology counseling services were involved in manufacturing, processing, and application of paints and glues. Others were machinists, laboratory technicians, and dry cleaners.

It is beyond the scope of this chapter to review all the organic solvents, so we chose toluene as an illustrative example of exposure. This agent is used in a variety of mixtures and products. Also important, it is commonly involved in volatile substance inhalant abuse. Toluene is an aromatic hydrocarbon used as a solvent for paints, thinners, coatings, and glues.[5] It is a popular replacement for the more chronically toxic benzene solvents. Most exposures involve inhalation. About 50% of the inhaled dose is absorbed, whereas absorption is almost complete after oral administration.[5] Toluene inhalation by pregnant rats induced decreased fetal weight and retardation of skeletal growth.[9,10] No malformations were demonstrated in rats or mice after inhalation,[10,11] but oral administration to mice induced cleft palate.[12] Two other studies in rats showed exposure to 2000 ppm, but not to 600 ppm, to cause body weight suppression of dams and offspring, high fetal mortality, and embryonic growth retardation. No anomalies were observed. In one of these studies, exposure took place from 14 days before mating until day 7 of gestation.[13,14] The male reproductive system was also affected when inhalation of 2000 ppm began 60 days before pairing.[14] Fetal neuromotor abnormalities may be induced by inhalation of 800 mg/mL of toluene (more than twice the TLV-TWA) by pregnant rats.[15] However, subcutaneous injection of toluene (1.2 g/kg) to rats did not result in behavioral changes.[10] Exposure of pregnant rats to 1500 ppm toluene for 6 hours/day was associated with reduced birth weight, lower maternal weight gain and a depressant effect on maternal corticosterone.[16] A brief repeated exposure of pregnant rats to toluene (12,000 ppm for 15 minutes, twice daily from gestational day 8–20) caused growth restriction, malformations and impairment of biobehavioral development in the offspring.[17]

A retrospective cross sectional study of printing industry workers did not show a reduction of fecundity in males (n = 150) exposed to different concentrations of toluene. In female workers (n = 90) fecundability ratio (FR) was reduced; FR 0.48, 95% CI 0.29–0.77. An effect on hormonal regulation was proposed.[18] A study from 1977 compared pregnancy outcomes among 168 women occupationally exposed to varnishes containing toluene (55 ppm) with those of 201 control women.[19] While there were twice as many low-birth-weight infants in the toluene-exposed group, the two groups did not differ with regard to fertility, course of pregnancy, perinatal mortality, or adverse effects in the newborn. Unfortunately, congenital defects were not evaluated. It was suggested that occupational exposure to aromatic solvents, mainly to toluene, may be associated with various birth defects, predominantly renal-urinary or gastrointestinal.[20] Toluene-exposed shoe workers had a higher rate of spontaneous abortions: odds ratio 9.3, 95% confidence interval (CI) 1.0–84.7.[21] Chinese shoe workers exposed to toluene and benzene had a significantly higher rate of menstrual disorders and spontaneous abortions.[22] Significant association with spontaneous abortions was found among women laboratory workers (odds ratio 4.7, 95% CI 1.4–15.9). No association was found with congenital anomalies.[23]

Abuse of large quantities of pure toluene by inhalation throughout pregnancy was reported to result in microcephaly, central nervous system (CNS) dysfunction, minor craniofacial anomalies, and variable growth deficiencies in three patients.[24] These features resembled the pattern of malformations described in connection with exposure to alcohol or certain anticonvulsant medications and were name "fetal solvent syndrome." Pearson et al. proposed a common mechanism of craniofacial teratogenesis for toluene and alcohol—namely, a deficiency of craniofacial neuroepithelium and mesodermal component due to embryonic cell death.[25] More features of toluene embryopathy are discussed at the end of this section.

Due to confounding factors such as bias and exposure to multiple chemicals, the results of the occupational studies suggesting an adverse effect of toluene on pregnancy may be considered as "hypothesis generating."[26]

Many organic solvents are teratogenic and embryotoxic in laboratory animals, depending on specific solvent, dose, route of administration, and animal species.[4,7] Malformations described include hydrocephaly, exencephaly, skeletal defects, cardiovascular abnormalities, and blood changes. Other abnormalities include poor fetal development and neurodevelopmental deficits. In some of the studies exposure levels were high enough to induce maternal toxicity.

Adequate human epidemiological studies are difficult to conduct and most of them are retrospective. This is because of the complexity and diversity of organic solvents and because exposure usually involves more than one agent and different circumstances. In addition, studies are subjected to selection, recall and response bias and are not always controlled for other risk factors (age, smoking, etc.). Other confounders include small sample size, definition of exposure, assessment of exposure, measurement of airborne concentrations, biomonitoring, insensitive measures of effect, and inability to analyze dose-response relationship. Thus, epidemiological studies are often difficult to interpret.

Isolated case reports suggesting that solvent-related embryopathy may occur in humans have appeared for many years. In one report, five of nine women who gave birth to infants with caudal regression syndrome had been exposed to solvents, including xylene, trichloroethylene, methyl chloride, acetone, and gasoline.[27] These agents do not belong to the same subgroup of organic solvents, and it is impossible to identify the potential culprit.

Many epidemiological studies suggested association between adverse pregnancy outcome and exposure to organic solvents. However, most if not all of them, suffer from various methodological limitations. Among the common major drawbacks are the inability to identify the specific solvents involved, to quantitate the exposure, to separate the effects of the various solvents, inadequate control group and the retrospective design with its associated biases.

The following is a discussion of the various reproductive effects of organic solvents reported in epidemiological studies.

Fertility. Reduced fertility was found among female workers in various occupations: exposure to ethylene glycol ethers in the semiconductor industry, OR 4.6 in the high exposure group, 95% CI 1.6–3.3[28]; shoe factories, fecundability density ratio (FDR) 0.28, 95% CI 0.11–0.71[29]; dry cleaning shops, FDR 0.44, 95% CI 0.22–0.86[29]; metal industry, FDR 0.58, 95% CI 0.34–0.98[29]; printing industry with main exposure to toluene, fecundability ratio (FR) 0.47, 95% CI 0.29–0.77[18]; and biomedical research, FR 0.79, 95% CI 0.68–0.93.[30]

No reduced FDR was found in Finnish study of women occupationally exposed to various organic solvents.[31]

Several studies investigated the effect of paternal occupational exposure on semen quality and fertility; some of them have inconsistent results. FDR were reduced for high exposures and primigravida (FDR 0.35, 95% CI 0.19–0.66) but not for low or intermediate exposures and couples with at least one previous pregnancy.[32] A significant reduced implantation rate after IVF was found among couples with male partners (n = 21) exposed to presumably high levels of organic solvents in various occupations (e.g., printers, painters, floor layers), OR 0.29, 95% CI 0.06–0.91.[33] A Chinese study found decreased sperm motility and vitality in male workers (n = 24) exposed to benzene, toluene, and xylene. In addition, acrosin activity, γ-GT activity and LDH-C4 relative activity were lower and fructose concentration was higher compared to control. In some workers exposed to airborne concentrations exceeding the maximum allowable concentration, these three solvents were found in the blood and semen but not in control subjects.[34] A recent study reported a significant increase in FSH levels in male painters and millwrights compared to carpenters. LH, testosterone and time to pregnancy were not associated with solvent exposure.[35] A major limitation of this study is the reliability of exposure data, as some pregnancies occurred more then 20 years prior to the study. An insignificant increased risk of subfertility was found among spouses of male manufacturers exposed to mixtures containing ethylene glycol ethers.[28]

Spontaneous abortions. Spontaneous abortions were reported in 262 factory workers in Denmark; when controlled for gravidity, however, there was no longer a statistically increased risk.[36] No increased risk for miscarriages was found in university laboratory workers exposed to organic solvents. Conversely, shift work in these workers was related to a higher miscarriage rate (RR 3.2). This study did not demonstrate any differences in perinatal death rates or in the prevalence of malformations among women working with organic solvents when compared with controls.[37] Spontaneous abortions were found among women exposed to organic solvents during their work in a hospital laboratory,[38] in electronic plants,[39,40] in photolithography area in the semiconductor industry,[41] and in microelectronic equipment assembly plants.[42] In the latter study, the odds ratio of spontaneous abortions was 0.9 before the women began to assemble microelectronic components and increased to 5.6 after the commencement of this employment. A prospective observational controlled study reported miscarriage in 46.2% of occupationally exposed women compared to 19.2% in unexposed controls, p <0.01.[43] However, many of these studies are limited by recall bias, small sample size, wide confidence intervals, and variable exposures, which in many cases are not quantitated. In this respect, it is interesting to mention Lindbohm's study which examined the rate of medically diagnosed spontaneous abortions among women occupationally exposed to at least one of six organic solvents (styrene, trichloroethylene, xylene, tetrachloroethylene, toluene, and 1,1,1-trichloroethane) who were also biologically monitored. Reference values for hygiene standards were exceeded in 38% of styrene exposures and were reached in 15% of tetrachloroethylene exposures. The adjusted odds ratio of spontaneous abortions for solvent exposure was significantly increased (OR 2.2, 95% CI 1.2–4.1), especially for exposure to aliphatic hydrocarbons (OR 3.9, 95% CI 1.1–14.2), for graphite workers (OR 5.5, 95% CI 1.3–20.8), and for toluene-exposed shoe workers (OR 9.3, 95% CI 1.0–84.7).[44]

Confounding factors, again, are small sample size and multiple exposures in some cases.

Association of spontaneous abortions with exposure to aliphatic hydrocarbons, but not with the use of solvents as a group, was also suggested in a large case control study.[45] Among 561 pregnancies in female workers in two semiconductor plants in eastern United States, potential exposure to mixtures containing ethylene glycol ethers was associated with increased risks of spontaneous abortions (RR in the high exposure group 2.8, 95% CI 1.4–5.6). This risk exhibited a dose-response trend.[28] In a case-referent study, the odds ratio of spontaneous abortions was increased by paternal exposure to several organic solvents, maternal exposure to organic solvents, and maternal heavy lifting.[46] The cohort was too small to permit the evaluation of the effects of these parameters on congenital malformations. A prospective poison center study did not find an increased risk for miscarriage but the numbers were too small.[47]

The complexity of evaluating the effects of organic solvents may be illustrated in the following example. An Italian case-control study on female workers in shoe manufacturing exposed mainly to aliphatic hydrocarbons showed a RR of 3.85 (95% CI 1.24–11.9) for spontaneous abortions, if exposure was high. Air concentrations were below the TLVs.[48] However, when these authors repeated the study in another cohort about 10 years later, no such an association was found.[49]

A meta-analysis including five studies involving 2899 patients showed a tendency toward an increase in spontaneous abortions in occupational exposure to organic solvents; OR 1.25, 95% CI 0.99–1.58.[50]

Paternal exposure to ethylene glycol ethers was not associated with spontaneous abortions in one study.[28] But, a meta-analysis of 14 studies showed some tendency for it; OR 1.30, 95% CI 0.81–2.11, n = 1,2481.[51]

Intrauterine growth. A prospective cohort study of 3946 pregnant women whose occupational exposure to chemicals was assessed by a job matrix suggested that leather work might be associated with the birth of infants small for gestational age. This was suspected to be due to chlorophenols (p = 0.02) and aromatic amines (p = 0.05).[52] Maternal exposure to solvents in the petrochemical industry was significantly associated with reduced birth weight; −81.7g, 95% CI −106.3, −3.1.[53] Lower birth weight was also found in a prospective observational study; 3368 ± 795 g and 3536 ± 542 g in exposed and control subjects, respectively, p = 0.01.[43]

A study of birth outcomes was conducted at a U.S. Marine Corps Base at North Carolina, where drinking water was contaminated with volatile organic compounds, mainly tetrachloroethylene (PCE). Adjusted mean birth weight difference between PCE exposed and unexposed infants were −130 g (90% CI −236, −23) for mothers age 35 years or older and −104 g (90% CI −174, −34) for mothers with two or more previous fetal losses. Adjusted odds ratio for PCE exposure and small for gestational age were 2.1 (90% CI 0.9–4.9) for older mothers and 2.5 (90% CI 1.5–4.3) for mothers with two or more prior fetal losses.[54] Although not an occupational setting, this was a long-lasting exposure, thus making it relevant to the occupational setting.

A study from Wisconsin could not identify an increased risk for low birth weight and prematurity.[55]

Congenital anomalies. The association between occupational exposures to organic solvents was investigated in many studies; most of them were subjected to the various methodological limitations discussed above. These studies reported esophageal stenosis or atresia in babies of female laboratory workers,[56] omphalocele or gastroschisis in offspring of mothers in the printing industry,[57] and an association between increased risk of malformations and laboratory work in the pharmaceutical and paper industries.[58,59] A Mexican study suggested that children of ex-workers of the same factory who were in direct contact with methyl cellosolve and ethylene glycol without protection had peculiar facies, mental retardation, and musculoskeletal and sensorial abnormalities.[60] An experimental study supported this finding.[60] Case control studies of central nervous system defects in Finland showed an association with organic solvents.[61,62] However, when the study was extended for 3 more years, the authors could not prove this association.[63] A cumulative case referent study covering 3.5 years suggested an association of organic solvents with cleft palate.[64] A case-control study comparing maternal exposure to any organic solvent between 200 infants with oral clefts and 400 controls estimated the odds ratio to be 1.62 (95% CI 1.04–2.52). Comparison of nine subgroups of solvents showed only the odds ratio associated with halogenated aliphatic solvents to be significant (4.40, 95% CI 1.41–16.15).[65] The prevalence of exposure to organic solvents at work during the first trimester was 10.4% among 569 mothers of children with cardiovascular malformation, compared with 7.8% in the control group.[66] This retrospective study found an adjusted relative odds ratio of 1.3 for cardiovascular malformations and 1.5 for ventricular septal defects, both probably insignificant. In 1991 this group published assessments of risk factors for cardiovascular defects in general and ventricular septal defect (VSD) specifically in Finland and again found no significant association with exposure at work to organic solvents.[67,68] Maternal alcohol consumption during the first trimester was more common among mothers of VSD infants than among controls (47 vs. 38%, respectively $p < 0.05$).[68] Khattak et al. showed in a prospective observational study in 125 pregnant women exposed occupationally to organic solvents a significant increase in major malformations compared to controls; RR 13, 95% CI 1.8–99.5. Interestingly, 12 of the 13 malformations occurred among children of symptomatic exposed women while none in the asymptomatic exposed women; $p < 0.001$. In one patient this information was missing. Solvents involved included aliphatic and aromatic hydrocarbons, phenols, trichloroethylene, xylene, vinyl chloride, acetone and related compounds. Airborne levels of these chemicals were not provided.[43]

A small prospective study of poison center consultations and a study from an occupational reproductive health nurse consultation service did not find an increase in adverse reproductive outcome.[47,55]

In an interesting meta-analysis on pregnancy outcome following maternal exposure to organic solvents, only five studies fulfilled the inclusion criteria (case-control, cohort, first trimester) out of 559 studies found. The odds ratio for malformations (n = 7,036 patients) was 1.64, 95% CI 1.16–2.30.[50]

For paternal exposure to organic solvents, the following odds ratios were found in a meta-analysis: 1.47 (95% CI 1.18–1.83) for major malformations; 1.86 (95% CI 1.40–2.46) for any neural tube defect; 2.18 (95% CI 1.52–3.11) for anencephaly and 1.59 (95% CI 0.99–2.56) for spina bifida.[51] A study based on occupational titles in Denmark suggested that malformations of the CNS were related to fathers exposed to solvents and employed as painters; OR 2.8 and 4.9, respectively.[69]

Neurodevelopment. A study from California could not demonstrate any difference in neurobehavioral development and growth between children exposed in utero to organic solvents and a group of matched, unexposed children.[70] In a series of studies from Toronto involving about 30 patients each, children to mothers who worked with organic solvents scored lower on intellectual, language, motor and neurobehavioral functioning (e.g., receptive language, expressive language, graphomotor ability, visual-motor functioning, IQ). Visual-spatial ability and fine-motor ability were not different then controls.[71,72] The same group also reported increased risk of color vision, visual acuity and contrast sensitivity impairments.[73,74]

Miscellaneous effects. No correlation was found between laboratory work and sister chromatid exchanges and micronuclei in 59 Canadian laboratory workers. There was, however, an association between such exchanges and recent or past smoking.[75]

In a randomly selected group of 85 neonates, exposure to indoor volatile organic compounds was suggested to affect the immune status; OR 2.9 and 3.3 for elevated percentages of interleukin producing (IL-4) type 2 T cells and exposure to naphthalene and methylcyclopentane, respectively; OR 2.9 for reduced percentage of interferon type I T cells. Smoking during pregnancy, new carpets in the bedroom and home renovation were correlated with increased indoor air concentration of naphthalene, methylcyclopentane and trichloroethylene, respectively.[76]

A population-based case-control study including 790 incident cases of childhood acute lymphoblastic leukemia and matched healthy controls could not show that maternal occupational exposure to organic solvents before and during pregnancy played a major role in childhood leukemia. Adjusted OR for all solvents was 1.11 (95% CI 0.88–1.40); increased risks were found for 1,1,1-trichloroethane (OR 7.55, 95% CI 0.92–61.97), toluene (OR 1.88, 95% CI 1.01–3.47), mineral spirits (OR 1.82, 95% CI 1.05–3.14), alkanes (C5–C17); (OR 1.78, 95% CI 1.11–2.86) and mononuclear aromatic hydrocarbons (OR 1.64, 95% CI 1.12–2.41). Home exposure was not associated with increased risk.[77]

An association between exposure to organic solvents and pregnancy-induced hypertension (RR 2.4) and pre-eclampsia was suggested.[55,78] One of these studies also showed an increased risk for hydramnion (RR 5.2) and the offspring were more likely to have 5-minute Apgar scores less than 8 (RR 3.6).[55]

Fetal solvent syndrome. A discussion of organic solvents would be incomplete without mentioning the fetal solvent (or gasoline) syndrome. In 1979 a syndrome of anomalies (hypertonia, scaphocephaly, mental retardation, and other CNS effects) was suggested in two children in a small American Indian community where gasoline sniffing and alcohol abuse are common.[79] Four other children had similar abnormalities, but in their cases it was impossible to verify gasoline sniffing. The contribution of the lead in the gasoline or the alcohol abuse in producing these abnormalities is unclear. In another case, a child with nearly classic fetal alcohol syndrome was born to a mother with major addiction to solvents, mainly toluene.[80] Heavy alcohol consumption was also reported in that woman, and the authors questioned a possible interaction between solvents and alcohol. Toluene embryopathy was described in two additional children whose mothers probably did not abuse alcohol.[81] Paint sniffing, namely toluene, resulted in severe renal tubular acidosis in five pregnant women.[82] Fetal heart rate tracing and dynamic ultrasonographic examinations were normal in four of five. Fetal heart rate tracing and dynamic ultrasonographic examinations were normal in four of five. Three neonates exhibited growth retardation, and two had anomalies and hyperchloremic acidosis. Renal tubular acidosis was observed in more than half the women who abused toluene, especially in the long-duration abusers.[83] This study showed that among 21 newborns exposed to toluene in utero, preterm delivery, perinatal death, and growth retardation were significantly increased. Developmental delay was a common finding in these children. Two neonates were reported to have transient renal tubular dysfunction due to maternal toluene sniffing throughout the pregnancies. These infants were dysmature and had some dysmorphic features.[84] Another publication described a premature newborn with renal tubular acidosis probably due to maternal sniffing of paint containing toluene.[85] A study of 56 women from Manitoba who abused solvents in pregnancy reported renal tubular acidosis (5.6%) and adverse neurological sequelae in the mothers. Preterm delivery was reported in 21.4%; 16% of the infants had major anomalies, 12.5% fetal alcohol-like facial features and 10.7% had hearing loss.[86] Chronic maternal inhalation of carburetor fluid during pregnancy resulted in cerebral infarcts in the fetus leading to large areas of bilateral frontal cortical leukomalacia. The infant was born preterm and had acute fetal distress with significant metabolic acidosis at birth and initial hypotonia was followed by generalized hypertonicity.[87] It is important to remember that the mothers in many of these cases showed signs of solvent toxicity, indicating heavy exposure. In our experience this is not the case in most occupational exposures during pregnancy.

An animal study also demonstrated the adverse pregnancy outcome of "binge" exposure to toluene.[17]

In summary, adverse reproductive effects of organic solvents are a biologic plausibility. The complexity of exposure to organic solvents and the many confounders and limitations of the studies hinders the drawing of firm conclusions. The criteria required by evidence-based medicine are difficult to fulfill. Performing large, prospective, well-controlled, well-audited studies, with adequate quantitation of exposure to organic solvents, is problematic and cumbersome.

On one hand, the data presented cannot be used to incriminate organic solvents as proven reproductive poisons or teratogens nor can this suspicion be quantitated. One may even argue that such a ubiquitous exposure to solvents might be associated with adverse reproductive outcome by chance alone. On the other hand, the adverse effects of maternal exposure to organic solvents on fertility, spontaneous abortions, intrauterine growth, and congenital malformations suggested by most studies including a meta-analysis cannot be ignored.

Evidence on the effect of paternal exposure to organic solvents on pregnancy outcome is limited and variable.

We therefore suggest that exposures to organic solvents should be carefully identified, characterized and quantitated as much as possible. Possible risks should be indicated to the patient. Every effort should be made to minimize the exposure (e.g., reduced working hours and improved personal and environmental protection).[88] Removal from such work may be considered in selected workers and circumstances.

We believe that the precautionary principle in environmental medicine can be applied in the case of occupational exposure to organic solvents before or during pregnancy: (a) take preventive action in the face of uncertainty, (b) shift burden of proof to proponents of activity, (c) explore alternatives to possibly harmful actions, (d) increase public participation in decision making.[89]

In the meantime, high-quality epidemiological studies should be supported and performed.

Lead

The third most common occupational exposure in pregnancy encountered by the Canadian investigators was lead. It accounted for 29 (0.6%) of the telephone consultations provided by the Motherisk Program during 1988. Three of them were followed up in the Motherisk Clinic (Tables 17-1 and 17-2). The vast majority of lead exposures involved artists using glass staining techniques or workers in the paint manufacturing sector of the automotive and aircraft industries. Other occupational sources of lead exposure during pregnancy reported in the literature include printing, smeltering, and battery industries.[90] Not only is lead an occupational hazard, it also can enter the body from contaminated soil and drinking water,[91] by residence close to industrial areas, from a lead-exposed spouse,[92,93] and by consumption of moonshine whisky.[94] Other nonoccupational factors, which were shown to be associated with increased maternal or cord blood levels include the use of lead-glazed pottery and canned food, low socioeconomic status, and fall and winter seasons.[95,96] High milk intake and diets rich in calcium are associated with lower lead levels.[95,96,97]

Although it seems that blood lead levels in the United States are declining[98], including in cord blood,[99] much lower levels are now being considered toxic than in the past (<10 μg/dL in children[100] and <40 μg/dL in adults[101]). However, subtle toxicity was observed even in lower levels. The biologic exposure index (BEI) set by the American Conference of Governmental Industrial Hygienists (ACGIH) is 30 μg/dL. Lead poisoning is still a hazard in the industrialized countries, and pregnant women are at risk.

Lead crosses the placenta,[102,103] possibly by both passive diffusion and active transport,[103] and it is unclear whether placental permeability to lead is constant throughout gestation.[102,104–106] Transplacental transfer of lead has been shown in the human fetus as early as 12–14 weeks of gestation, along with increasing amounts of lead in fetal tissues with advancing gestational age.[107] Fetal bone and liver may have higher lead concentrations than maternal tissues.[108] Calciotropic factors determine the uptake and storage of lead in the bone compartment. Thus, pregnancy-induced changes in calcium-related regulatory factors may result in mobilization of lead from the bone to more bioavailable compartments in the mother and fetus.[90,109] Iron deficiency may further increase the susceptibility to lead toxicity.

During the late nineteenth and early twentieth centuries, women in the pottery and white lead industries used lead as an abortifacient[90]. European studies from that time found infertility, abortion, stillbirth, fetal death, and microcephaly to be associated with industrial lead exposure.[92,110–113] Even paternal lead exposure was found as early as 1860 to affect fertility and viability of the offspring.[114] Wives of lead workers were reported to have more abortions, stillbirths, and premature births than women in the general population.[92,115] Consequently, the employment of women in plants involving a lead hazard was forbidden.[116] Although these studies should be evaluated with consideration of the high fetal and neonatal loss for other working women at that time,[117] most of the studies from the nineteenth century and later, confirmed the early observations. For example, a study comparing the course and lead values in 249 pregnancies in Columbia, Missouri, with 253 occurring at the center of Americas' lead belt at Rolla, Missouri, showed that 96% versus only 70% were delivered at term.[118] In addition, 17% of the lead-exposed pregnancies had premature rupture of membranes, as compared with only 1% in the non-exposed group. Maternal and fetal blood lead levels in the cases of premature membrane rupture and preterm delivery were higher than in controls. Significantly higher lead concentrations were found in membranes of patients with stillbirths and preterm births, but there was a low correlation between membrane and antenatal blood lead concentrations.[119] A detailed Japanese study showed an increase in spontaneous abortions among female lead workers from a prelead rate of 45.6 per 1000 to 84.2 per 1000 (the rate in nonexposed employees was 59.1 per 1000).[120] A Danish study showed that when lead was used as an abortifacient, 60% of the pregnancies in the first trimester ended in abortion.[121] Moreover, women with a history of childhood lead poisoning were suggested to be at higher relative risk (RR) for having spontaneous abortions or stillbirths (RR 1.6, 95% CI, 0.6–4.0) and having children with learning disabilities (RR 3.0, 95% CI 0.9–10.2).[122] A dose-dependent decrease in hypothalamic gonadotropin-releasing hormone and somatostatin was found in lead-treated guinea pigs and their fetuses.[123] Although the relevance of these changes is unclear, they may partially explain decreased reproductive capacity.

A study from Boston (4354 cases) suggested that lead may be associated, in a dose-related fashion, with an increased risk for minor anomalies.[124] The relative risk increased from 1 at 0.7 μg/dL to 2.73 at the level of 24 μg/dL. The anomalies discovered did not have a specific pattern and were of little health consequence. They included hemangiomas (14 of 1000 births), hydrocele (27.6 of 1000 male infants), minor skin anomalies (12.2 of 1000 births), and undescended testicles (11 of 1000 male infants). A significant negative association was found between pre- and postnatal blood lead level and head circumference. Over the 1–35 μg/dL range of maternal blood lead level at 36 weeks of gestation, the estimated reduction in 6 months' head circumference was 1.9 cm, 95% CI 0.9–3.[125]

Lead also affects the male gonads; chromosomal alterations, as well as abnormalities in sperm count, vigor, and morphological features were demonstrated in workers and experimental animals.[126–128] Marital life records of lead-exposed men showed 24.7% of the marriages to be infertile compared with 14.8% in the nonlead control group. The rate of prematurity or stillbirth was 8.2%, whereas in the control group it was 0.2%.[128] In a case-referent study, a significant increase in spontaneous abortions was found in the wives of workers occupationally exposed to lead whose blood level was greater than 1.5 μmol/L (31 μg/dL) during or close to the time of spermatogenesis.[129] The adjusted odds ratio for low birth weight among infants whose fathers were potentially exposed to high levels of lead from 6 months before pregnancy to the end of it was 4.7, 95% CI 1.1–2. This effect was most prominent for low-birth-weight infants who were both preterm and small for gestational.[130]

Although increased numbers of chromosomal aberrations (gaps, breaks, fragments, chromatid aberrations) have been reported in lead workers, the contribution of lead itself is still unclear.[90]

Low level of exposure to lead (mean blood level 6.9 ± 3.3 μg/dL also seemed to have a small but demonstrable association with pregnancy-induced hypertension and elevated blood pressure at the time of delivery, but not with pre-eclampsia.[131,132] The association of lead with pregnancy-induced hypertension was also suggested in later studies.[133–136]

One of the main concerns regarding lead is its ability to cause neuropsychological impairment in children. In the late 1970s, half the children in the United States under 5 years of age had blood lead levels exceeding 20 μg/dL, and among urban African American children the figure approached 60%.[137] At this level a variety of enzymatic and neurophysiological processes are impaired. Until recently, it was not clear at what level deficits in children's learning and behavior become apparent, nor was the contribution of in utero exposure clearly identified. In a series of studies from Boston,[1,2] blood lead levels and development were monitored in a group of urban children from birth to the age of 2 years. No infant had a cord blood lead level exceeding 25 μg/dL, the level regarded at that time by the Centers for Disease Control as the upper normal limit for children. At all ages, children whose cord level was greater than 10 μg/dL scored lower in the Mental Development Index of the Bayley Scales (4.8-point difference between the low [<3 μg/dL] and high [>10 μg/dL] groups). At the age of 6 months, scores on the Psychomotor Development Index were not significantly related to cord blood lead level. Scores were not related to infants' postnatal blood lead levels. At the age of 57 months the performance of these children was tested on the McCarthy Scale of Children's Ability.[138] Surprisingly, at this age there was no association between prenatal lead exposure and children's cognitive function, except for children with high postnatal exposure (>10 μg/dL), particularly at 24 months of age. A study from Cincinnati obtained similar initial results.[139] Comparable to the Boston study, neuropsychological follow-up of the Cincinnati cohort, as assessed by the Kaufman Assessment Battery for Children at the age of 4 years, was inversely associated with higher neonatal blood lead level only in children from the poorest families.[140] The relationship between prenatal low level lead exposure and neurobehavioral development was not confirmed in another study.[141] However, the mean cord lead level was 8.1 μg/dL, which is lower than the cutoff point of 10 μg/dL suggested by the Boston study. A French study suggested that low level lead exposure in utero could affect the sociability of infants, possibly through a neurotoxic effect on the developing serotonergic system.[142] A more recent study using the Stanford-Binet Intelligence Scale at the age of 3 and 5 years showed that each 10 μg/dL increase in blood lead level was associated with 4.6 points decrease in IQ ($p = 0.004$). More importantly, an increase in lead levels from 1 to 10 μg/dL was associated with an IQ decline of 7.4 points.[143] This emphasizes the consequences of even very low exposure. A Mexican study suggested high maternal lead levels in the last two trimesters to be associated with altered baby cry and auditory function. The authors suggest this to contribute to developmental delays by affecting early communication between caretaker and baby.[144]

It is still unclear at what gestational age the fetus is most sensitive. Since the fetal brain develops throughout gestation, it is conceivable that lead deposition at any stage may be harmful. However, it seems that low-level prenatal lead-induced neurodevelopmental impairment may be reversible, provided the exposure is discontinued.

It has been suggested that cord blood levels above 15 μg/dL induce a modest decrease in fetal growth.[145] The on stature effect of lead exposure (in utero as well as during the first year of life) was transient 33 months of age, if subsequent exposure to lead was not excessive.[146] Another study could not confirm an association between prenatal lead exposure and neonatal size.[147]

These data suggest that low levels of lead delivered to the fetus may be toxic and may cause behavioral and developmental impairment. It led the Centers for Disease Control to reduce the acceptable level for young children from 2.5 μg/dL to 10 μg/dL.[100] Animal studies are consistent with these findings,[148–152] and it is possible that brain lead levels remain elevated longer than blood levels after short-term exposure.[153,154] It is also possible that the fetus is more sensitive to lead than the young child. Possible mechanisms for the brain damage include interference with embryonic nutrition and energy supply, competition with cations such as zinc, iron, or calcium,[155] interference with mitochondrial function[156] and synthesis of cytochromes, and effect on deoxyribonucleic acid synthesis.[157]

A study in Toronto found that about 90% of newborns had cord blood levels below 3 µg/dL and none above 10 µg/dL,[158] whereas in Boston, about one-third had such levels and one-third had levels exceeding 10 µg/dL. In Braunschweig, Germany, only 4.7% of the neonates had cord blood lead level above 10 µg/dL.[159] This range of results illustrates the difference between different urban environments.

The data above imply that it is important to detect, as early as possible, children potentially exposed in utero to excess lead. Several studies documented a high correlation between maternal and cord blood lead levels, usually being 80–98% of the maternal level.[93,102,105,160–163] In one of these studies, mean cord level was 10.1 µg/dL, compared with 10.3 µg/dL in the mother ($r = 0.6377$).[105] However, it is not advisable to assume lead exposure throughout pregnancy from a single blood measurement, because of the changes in maternal blood levels and placental permeability to lead.[2] An alternative method of assessing long-term lead exposure and estimating in utero exposure is head hair analysis, which reflects cumulative values.[164,165] A questionnaire was developed by the Centers for Disease Control that combined housing conditions, smoking status and high consumption of canned foods. This questionnaire is given to pregnant women for identification of children at risk for lead poisoning and has a sensitivity of 89.2% and a negative predictive value of 96.4%.[166] It cannot substitute biomonitoring of the pregnant woman in the workplace.

On the basis of the higher susceptibility of the fetal brain to lead, it may be argued that treatment should be instituted even when levels are low. From the chelating agents available, BAL (dimercaprol) is a very toxic compound that has been shown to induce skeletal abnormalities in fetal mice.[167] One woman who was treated for arsenic poisoning in the sixth month of pregnancy gave birth to a normal child.[168] Ethylenediaminetetraacetate (EDTA) is less toxic, but it can chelate calcium, zinc, and other trace elements and may adversely affect the fetus. In one case it was given at the eighth month of gestation (75 mg/kg/d for 7 days; maternal level of 240 µg/dL) without complication.[117] The infant was born normal with an undetected cord lead level. However, the sensitivity of the assay was very low (<60 µg/dL was undetectable). This infant had normal neurological and developmental assessments at the age of 4 years and 3 months. In another patient treated with calcium EDTA at the same gestational age, it appeared that the treatment did not adequately reduce the infant's lead burden[169]; this child had a blood lead level of 60 µg/dL at the time of delivery and radiological evidence of bony changes suggestive of prolonged exposure. A 17-year-old female in her 39th week of pregnancy who had a blood lead level of 79 µg/dL, with a corresponding amniotic fluid lead level of 90 µg/dL was treated with 3 g/day Ca-EDTA for 3 days. Eight days later, her blood lead level was 26 µg/dL. She delivered a normal-appearing girl, and the cord blood lead concentration was 79 µg/dL. Based on this result, the authors suggested a delay in the crossing of the placental barrier by Ca-EDTA.[170] D-Penicillamine is less effective than dimercaprol and Ca-EDTA, and in the doses used in lead poisoning it may cause connective tissue abnormalities (mainly cutis laxa) in human fetuses.[171] There is no experience with the use of the oral chelators 2,3-dimercaptosuccinic acid (DMSA) and dimercaptopropane-1-sulfonate (DMPS) in human pregnancy. At doses between 100 and 1000 mg/kg/day, DMSA induced increases in resorptions and in postimplantation loss, as well as reduced fetal weight, but there was no teratogenicity in rats.[172] Changes in mineral metabolism were suggested as one possible mechanism.[173] The therapeutic dose in adults is 30 mg/kg/day. Similar effects were observed with DMPS in mice.[174] Both chelators prevented arsenic teratogenicity and embryotoxicity in mice.[175,176]

However, three recently published studies have challenged the hypothesis that chelation therapy can improve neuropsychological outcome. The Treatment of Lead-Exposed Children Trial is a multicenter, randomized, double-blind, placebo-controlled study evaluating the effect of chelation therapy with dimercaptosuccininc acid-DMSA (up to three 26-days courses) on the neuropsychological and behavioral development of lead exposed children. Seven hundred and eighty children aged 12–33 months with blood lead levels between 20–44 µg/dL were enrolled; 647 of them remained at the study at the age of 7 years. DMSA caused an initial decrease in blood lead level but the decrease at 6 months and on was similar to the placebo group. DMSA therapy did not improve scores on tests of cognition, behavior, or neuropsychological function. At 36 months follow-up, cognition test scores had increased 4 points per 10 µg/dL fall in blood lead level from baseline to 36 months follow up and 5.1 points from 6 to 36 months only in the placebo group.[177–179]

These studies emphasize the need for environmental measures to prevent exposure to lead, for early detection and removal from the source of exposure. Quantitating lead burden by determining blood lead level is of utmost importance and will aid decision making.

In the case of a woman occupationally exposed to lead, it is important to measure her blood lead concentrations and compare them with the mean levels measured in the same city. Several women employed in stained glass workshops had lead levels well below or near the mean recently determined for women in Toronto,[158] indicating that their lead load was within the expected range. Should there be a substantially higher lead level in such patients, they would be advised to discontinue their occupational exposure.

At the present time chelation therapy of lead can be recommended in symptomatic or high-level exposures. Currently, the data are not sufficient enough to support institution of chelation in pregnant women with intermediate or low-level exposure.

More critical research is needed to assess the need for chelation treatment of lead in pregnancy, especially of low level exposures, to establish the criteria for instituting therapy, to evaluate the response and to identify the chelator of choice.

SUMMARY

Of the three most common occupational exposures in pregnancy, video display terminals do not represent a reproductive risk. Organic solvents are likely to exert various adverse effects but the evidence is not strong enough to incriminate them as a group as proven reproductive poisons. There is no clear evidence to state that maternal exposure to allowable levels causes fetal damage. Using the precautionary approach and minimizing exposure while monitoring the pregnancy is prudent. In the case of lead, a dose-response fetal risk appears to have been established, and lead levels should be monitored to avoid fetal risk. Chelation therapy is recommended in symptomatic or high-level exposures. Although useful in decreasing blood lead levels, it can not be recommended at this stage for low-level exposure during pregnancy.

REFERENCES

1. Bellinger DC, Needelman HL, Leviton A, et al. Early sensory-motor development and prenatal exposure to lead. *Neurobehav Toxicol.* 1984;6:387–402.
2. Bellinger DC, Leviton A, Waternaux C, et al. Longitudinal analysis of prenatal and postnatal lead exposure and early cognitive development. *N Engl J Med.* 1987;316:1037–1043.
3. Klimisch HJ, Helhnig J, Hoffmann A. Studies on the prenatal toxicity of toluene in rabbits following inhalation exposure and proposal of a pregnancy guidance value. *Arch Toxicol.* 1992;66:373–381.
4. Fabro S, Brown NA, Scialli AR. Is there a fetal solvent syndrome? *Reprod Toxicol Med Lett.* 1983;2:17–20.
5. Ellenhorn MJ, Barceloux DG. *Medical Toxicology: Diagnosis and Treatment of Human Poisoning.* New York: Elsevier, 1988; 940–1006.
6. Cornish HH. Solvents and vapors. In: Doull J, Klassen CD, Amdur MO, eds. *Casarett and Doull's Toxicology: The Basic Science of Poisons.* 2nd ed. New York: Macmillan, 1980;468–496.
7. Freedman ML. The molecular site of benzene toxicity. *J Toxicol Environ Health.* 1977;2(suppl):37–43.
8. Industrial solvents. In: Schardein JL, ed. *Chemically Induced Birth Defects.* New York: Marcel Dekker, 1985;645–658.
9. Hudak A, Rodics K, Stuber L, et al. The effects of toluene inhalation on pregnant cfy rats and their offspring. *Orsz Munka-Uzemegeszsegugui Intez Munkavedelm.* 1977;23(suppl):25–30.
10. da Silva VA, Malheiros LR, Paumgartten FJ, et al. Developmental toxicity of in utero exposure to toluene on malnourished and well nourished rats. *Toxicology.* 1990;64:155–158.
11. Hudak A, Ungvary G. Embryotoxic effects of benzene and methyl derivatives: toluene, xylene. *Toxicology.* 1978;11:55–63.
12. Nawrot PS, Staples RE. Embryofetal toxicity and teratogenicity of benzene and toluene in the mouse. *Teratology.* 1979;19:41A.
13. Ono A, Sekita K, Kaneko T, et al. Reproductive and developmental toxicity studies of toluene: I. Teratogenicity study of inhalation exposure to pregnant rats. *J Toxicol Sci.* 1995;20:109–134.
14. Ono A, Sekita K, Kaneko T, et al. Reproduction and developmental toxicity studies of toluene: II. Effects of inhalation exposure on fertility in rats. *J Environ Pathol Toxicol Oncol.* 1996;15:9–20.
15. da Silva VA, Malherios LR, Bueno FM. Effects of toluene exposure during gestation on neurobehavioral development of rats and hamsters. *Braz J Med Biol Res.* 1990;23:533–537.
16. Hougaard KS, Hansen AM, Hass U, et al. Toluene depresses plasma corticosterone in pregnant rats. *Pharmacol Toxicol.* 2003;92:148–152.
17. Bowen SE, Batis JC, Mohammadi MH, et al. Abuse pattern of gestational toluene exposure and early postnatal development in rats. *Neurotoxicol Teratol.* 2005;27:105–116.
18. Plenge-Bonig A, Karmaus W. Exposure to toluene in the printing industry is associated with subfecundity in women but not in men. *Occup Environ Med.* 1999;56:443–448.
19. Syrovadko ON. Working conditions and health status of women handling organosilicon varnishes containing toluene. *Gig Tr Prof Zabol.* 1977;21:15–19.
20. McDonald JC, Lavoie XX, Cote R, et al. Chemical exposures at work in early pregnancy and congenital defect: a case-referent study. *Br J Ind Med.* 1987;44:527–533.
21. Lindbohm ML, Taskinen H, Sallmen M, et al. Spontaneous abortions among women exposed to organic solvents. *Am J Ind Med.* 1990;17:449–M3.
22. Huang XY. Influence on benzene and toluene to reproductive function of female workers in leather shoe-making industry. *Chung Hua Yu Fang I Hsueh Tsa Chin.* 1991;25:89–91.
23. Taskinen H, Kyyronen P, Hemminki K, et al. Laboratory work and pregnancy outcome. *J Occup Med.* 1994;36:311–319.
24. Hersh JH, Podruch PE, Rogers G, et al. Toluene embryopathy. *J Pediatr.* 1985;106:922–927.
25. Pearson MA, Hoyme H. Toluene embryopathy: delineation of the phenotype and comparison with fetal alcohol syndrome. *Pediatrics.* 1994;93:211–215.
26. Bukowski JA. Review of the epidemiological evidence relating toluene to reproductive outcomes. *Regul Toxicol Pharmacol.* 2001;33:147–156.
27. Kucera J. Exposure to fat solvents: a possible cause of sacral agenesis in man. *J Pediatr.* 1968;72:857–859.
28. Correa A, Gray RH, Cohen R, et al. Ethylene glycol ethers and risks of spontaneous abortion and subfertility. *Am J Epidemiol.* 1996;143:707–717.
29. Sallmen M, Lindbohm ML, Kyyronen P, et al. Reduced fertility among women exposed to organic solvents. *Am J Ind Med.* 1995;27:699–713.
30. Wennborg H, Bodin L, Vainio H, et al. Solvent use and time to pregnancy among female personnel in biomedical laboratories in Sweden. *Occup Environ Med.* 2001;58:225–231.
31. Taskinen HK, Kyyronen P, Sallmen M, et al. Reduced fertility among female wood workers exposed to formaldehyde. *Am J Ind Med.* 1999;36:206–212.
32. Sallmen M, Lindbohm ML, Anttila A, et al. Time to pregnancy among the wives of men exposed to organic solvents. *Occup Environ Med.* 1998;55:24–30.
33. Tielemans E, van Kooij R, Looman C, et al. Paternal occupational exposures and embryo implantation rates after IVF. *Fertil Steril.* 2000;74:690–695.
34. Xiao G, Pan C, Cai Y, et al. Effect of benzene, toluene, xylene on the semen quality and the function of accessory gonad of exposed workers. *Ind Health.* 2001;39:206–210.
35. Luderer U, Bushley A, Stover BD, et al. Effects of occupational solvent exposure on reproductive hormone concentrations and fecundability in men. *Am J Ind Med.* 2004;46:614–626.
36. Heidan LZ. Spontaneous abortions among factory workers: the importance of gravidity control. *Scand J Soc Med.* 1983;11:81–85.
37. Axelson G, Liutz C, Rylander R. Exposure to solvents and outcome of pregnancy in university laboratory employees. *Br J Ind Med.* 1984;41:305–312.
38. Strandberg M, Sandback K, Axelson O, et al. Spontaneous abortions among women in hospital laboratory. *Lancet.* 1978;1:384–385.
39. Hemminki K, Franssilla E, Vainio H. Spontaneous abortions among female workers in Finland. *Int Arch Occup Environ Health.* 1980;45:123–126.
40. Lipscomb JA, Fenster L, Wrensch M, et al. Pregnancy outcomes in women potentially exposed to occupational solvents and women working in the electronics industry. *J Occup Med.* 1991;33:597–604.
41. Pastides H, Calabrese EJ, Hosmer DW Jr, et al. Spontaneous abortion and general illness symptoms among semiconductor manufacturers. *J Occup Med.* 1988;30:543–551.
42. Huel G, Mergler D, Bowler R. Evidence for adverse reproductive outcomes among women microelectronic assembly workers. *Br J Ind Med.* 1990;47:400–404.
43. Khattak S, K-Moghtader G, McMartin K, et al. Pregnancy outcome following gestational exposure to organic solvents: a prospective controlled study. *JAMA.* 1999;281:1106–1109.
44. Lindbohm ML, Taskinen H, Sallmen M, et al. Spontaneous abortions among women exposed to organic solvents. *Am J Ind Med.* 1990;17:449–463.
45. Windham GC, Shusterman D, Swan SH, et al. Exposure to organic solvents and adverse pregnancy outcome. *Am J Ind Med.* 1991;20:241–259.
46. Taskinen H, Anttila A, Lindbohm ML, et al. Spontaneous abortions and congenital malformations among the wives of men occupationally exposed to organic solvents. *Scand J Work Environ Health.* 1989;15:346–352.

47. Testud F, Lambert-Chhum R, Bellemin B, et al. Occupational toxic exposure and the pregnant woman. 2: results of a prospective study of 100 pregnancies. *J Gynecol Obstet Biol Reprod (Paris).* 2001;30:780–785.
48. Agnesi R, Valentini F, Mastrangelo G. Risk of spontaneous abortion and maternal exposure to organic solvents in the shoe industry. *Int Arch Occup Environ Health.* 1997;69:311–316.
49. Agnesi R, Valentini F, Meneghetti M, et al. Changes in risk factors for spontaneous abortion in an area with high concentrations of shoe manufacture after a preventive intervention. *G Ital Med Lav Ergon.* 2003;25Suppl(3):79–80.
50. McMartin KI, Chu M, Kopecky E, et al. Pregnancy outcome following maternal organic solvent exposure: a meta-analysis of epidemiologic studies. *Am J Ind Med.* 1998;34:288–292.
51. Logman JF, de Vries LE, Hemels ME, et al. Paternal organic solvent exposure and adverse pregnancy outcomes: a meta-analysis. *Am J Ind Med.* 2005;47:37–44.
52. Seidler A, Raum E, Arabin B, et al. Maternal occupational exposure to chemical substances and the risk of infants small-for-gestational-age. *Am J Ind Med.* 1999;36:213–222.
53. Ha E, Cho SI, Chen D, et al. Parental exposure to organic solvents and reduced birth weight. *Arch Environ Health.* 2002;57:207–214.
54. Sonnenfeld N, Hertz-Picciotto I, et al. Tetrachloroethylene in drinking water and birth outcomes at the US Marine Corps Base at Camp Lejeune, North Carolina. *Am J Epidemiol.* 2001;154:902–908.
55. Hewitt JB, Tellier L. Risk of adverse outcomes in pregnant women exposed to solvents. *J Obstet Gynecol Neonatal Nurs.* 1998;27: 521–531.
56. Meirik O, Kallen B, Gauffin U, et al. Major malformations in infants born of women who worked in laboratories while pregnant. *Lancet.* 1979;2:91.
57. Erickson DJ, Cochran WM, Anderson CE. Birth defects and printing. *Lancet.* 1978;1:385.
58. Hansson E, Jansa S, Wande H, et al. Pregnancy outcome for women working in laboratories in some of the pharmaceutical industries of Sweden. *Scan J Work Environ Health.* 1980;6:131–134.
59. Blomqvist U, Ericson A, Kallen B, et al. Delivery outcome for women working in the pulp and paper industry. *Scand J Work Environ Health.* 1981;7:114–118.
60. Saavedra-Ontiveros D, Reynoso-Arizmendi F, Prada-Garay N, et al. Industrial pollution due to organic solvents as a cause of teratogenesis. *Salud Publica Mex.* 1996;38:3–12.
61. Holmberg PC. Central nervous system defects in children born to mothers exposed to organic solvents during pregnancy. *Lancet.* 1979;2:177–179.
62. Holmberg PC, Nurminen M. Congenital defects of the central nervous system and occupational factors during pregnancy. *Am J Ind Med.* 1980;1:167–176.
63. Rantala K, Riala R, Nurniinen T. Screening for occupational exposures and congenital malformations. *Scand J Work Environ Health.* 1983;9:89–93.
64. Holmberg PC, Hernberg S, Kurppa K, et al. Oral clefts and organic solvent exposure during pregnancy. *Int Arch Occup Environ Health.* 1982;50:371–376.
65. Laumon B, Martin JL. Exposure to organic solvents during pregnancy and oral clefts: a case-control study. *Reprod Toxicol.* 1996;10:15–19.
66. Tikkanen J, Heinonen OP. Cardiovascular malformations and organic solvent exposure during pregnancy in Finland. *Am J Ind Med.* 1988;14:1–8.
67. Tikkanen J, Heinonen OP. Maternal exposure to chemical and physical factors during pregnancy and cardiovascular malformations in the offspring. *Teratology.* 1991;43:591–600.
68. Tikkanen J, Heinonen OP. Risk factors for ventricular septal defects in Finland. *Public Health.* 1991;105:99–112.
69. Olsen J. Risk of exposure to teratogens amongst laboratory staff and painters. *Dan Med Bull.* 1983;30:24–28.
70. Eskenazi B, Gaylord L, Bracken MB, et al. *In utero* exposure to organic solvents and human neurodevelopment. *Dev Med Child Neurol.* 1988;30:492–501.
71. Till C, Koren G, Rovet JF. Prenatal exposure to organic solvents and child neurobehavioral performance. *Neurotoxicol Teratol.* 2001;23: 235–245.
72. Laslo-Baker D, Barrera M, Knittel-Keren D, et al. Child neurodevelopmental outcome and maternal occupational exposure to solvents. *Arch Pediatr Adolesc Med.* 2004;158:956–961.
73. Till C, Westall CA, Rovet JF, et al. Effects of maternal occupational exposure to organic solvents on offspring visual functioning: a prospective controlled study. *Teratology.* 2001;64:134–141.
74. Till C, Westall CA, Koren G, et al. Vision abnormalities in young children exposed prenatally to organic solvents. *Neurotoxicol.* 2005;26:599–613.
75. Narod SA, Neri L, Risch HA, et al. Lymphocyte micronuclei and sister chromatid exchanges among Canadian federal laboratory employees. *Am J Ind Med.* 1988;14:449–456.
76. Lehmann I, Thoelke A, Rehwagen M, et al. The influence of maternal exposure to volatile organic compounds on the cytokine secretion profile of neonatal T cells. *Environ Toxicol.* 2002;17:203–210.
77. Infante-Rivard C, Siemiatycki J, Lakhani R, et al. Maternal exposure to occupational solvents and childhood leukemia. *Environ Health Perspect.* 2005;113:787–792.
78. Eskenazi B, Bracken MB, Holford TR, et al. Exposure to organic solvents and hypertensive disorders of pregnancy. *Am J Ind Med.* 1988;14:177–188.
79. Hunter AGW, Thompson D, Evans JA. Is there a fetal gasoline syndrome? *Teratology.* 1979;20:75–80.
80. Toutant C, Lippmann S. Fetal solvent syndrome. *Lancet.* 1979;1:1356.
81. Hersh JH. Toluene embryopathy: two new cases. *J Med Genet.* 1989;26:333–337.
82. Goodwin TM. Toluene abuse and renal tubular acidosis in pregnancy. *Obstet Gynecol.* 1988;71:715–718.
83. Wilkins HL, Gabow PA. Toluene abuse during pregnancy: obstetric complications and perinatal outcomes. *Obstet Gynecol.* 1991;77: 504–509.
84. Lindemann R. Congenital renal tubular dysfunction associated with maternal sniffing of organic solvents. *Acta Paediatr Scand.* 1991;80:882–884.
85. Erramouspe J, Galvez R, Fischel DR. Newborn renal tubular acidosis associated with prenatal maternal toluene sniffing. *J Psychoactive Drugs.* 1996;28:201–204.
86. Scheeres JJ, Chudley AE. Solvent abuse in pregnancy: a perinatal perspective. *J Obstet Gynaecol Can.* 2002;24:22–26.
87. Bharti D. Intrauterine cerebral infarcts and bilateral frontal cortical leukomalacia following chronic maternal inhalation of carburetor cleaning fluid during pregnancy. *J Perinatol.* 2003;23:693–696.
88. Saillenfait AM, Robert E. Occupational exposure to organic solvents and pregnancy. Review of current epidemiologic knowledge. *Rev Epidemiol Sante Publique.* 2000;48:374–388.
89. Kriebel D, Tickner J, Epstein P, et al. The precautionary principle in environmental science. *Environ Health Perspect.* 2001;109: 871–876.
90. Rom WN. Effects of lead on the female reproduction: a review. *Mt Sinai J Med.* 1976;43:542–551.
91. Baghurst PA, McMichael AJ, Vimpani GV, et al. Determinants of blood lead concentrations of pregnant women living in Port Pirie and surrounding areas. *Med J Aust.* 1987;146:69–73.
92. Hamilton A, Hardy HL. Hereditary lead poisoning. In: *Industrial Toxicology.* Acton, MA: Publishing Sciences, 1974, pp 119–121.
93. Lagerkvist BJ, Ekesrydth S, Englyst V, et al. Increased blood lead and decreased calcium levels during pregnancy: a prospective study of Swedish women living near a smelter. *Am J Public Health.* 1996;86:1247–1252.
94. Palmisano PA, Sneed RC, Cassady G. Untaxed whisky and fetal lead exposure. *J Pediatr.* 1969;75:869–872.

95. Farias P, Borja-Aburto VH, Rios C, et al. Blood lead levels in pregnant women of high and low socioeconomic status in Mexico City. *Environ Health Perspect.* 1996;104:1070–1074.
96. Rothenberg SJ, Karchmer S, Schnaas L, et al. Maternal influences on cord blood lead levels. *J Expo Anal Environ Epidemiol.* 1996;6:211–227.
97. Gulson BL, Mizon KJ, Palmer JM, et al. Blood lead changes during pregnancy and postpartum with calcium supplementation. *Environ Health Perspect.* 2004;112:1499–1507.
98. Annest JL, Pirkle JL, Makuc D, et al. Chronological trend in blood lead levels between 1976 and 1980. *N Engl J Med.* 1983; 308:1373–1377.
99. Hu H, Hashimoto D. Levels of lead in blood and bone of women giving birth in a Boston hospital. *Arch Environ Health.* 1996;51:52–58.
100. US Centers for Disease Control. Preventing lead poisoning in children: a statement by the Centers for Disease Control, Atlanta, October 1991. Quoted in Poisindex. Denver, CO: Micromedex, 1992.
101. OSHA.CFR. Code of Federal Regulations 29CFR 1910, 1025. Chap. XVII (7-188 ed), 1988, pp 832–870. Quoted in Poisindex. Denver: *Micromedex, 1992.*
102. Baltrop D. Transfer of lead to the human fetus. In: Baltrop D, Burland WL, eds. *Mineral Metabolism in Pediatrics.* Oxford: Blackwell Scientific, 1969; pp 135–151.
103. Kostial K, Momcilovic B. Transport of lead-203 and calcium-47 from mother to offspring. *Arch Environ Health.* 1974;29:28.
104. Alexander F, Delves H. Blood lead levels during pregnancy. *Arch Environ Health.* 1981;48:35–39.
105. Gershanick J, Brooks G, Little J. Blood lead values in pregnant women and their offspring. *Am J Obstet Gynecol.* 1974;119:508–511.
106. Lubin H, Caffo A, Reece R. A longitudinal study of interaction between environmental lead and blood lead concentrations during pregnancy, at delivery and in the first 6 months of life. *Pediatr Res.* 1978;12:425.
107. Rajegowda BK, Glass L, Evans HE. Lead concentration in newborn infants. *J Pediatr.* 1972;80:116.
108. Karlog O, Moller KO. Three cases of acute lead poisoning: analysis of organs for lead and observations on polarographic lead determinations. *Acta Pharm.* 1958;15:8–16.
109. Silbergeld EK. Lead in bone: implication for toxicology during pregnancy and lactation. *Environ Health Perspect.* 1991;91:63–77.
110. Oliver T. A lecture on lead poisoning and the race. *Br Med J.* 1911;1:1096–1098.
111. Rennert O. Uber eine hereditare Folge der chronischen Blievergiftung. *Arch Gynaecol.* 1881;16:109.
112. Chyzzer A. Des intoxications par le plomb se presentant dans le ceramique en Hongrie. *Natl Acad Sci (Budapest).* 1908;44:906–911.
113. Legge TM. Industrial lead poisoning. *J Hyg.* 1901;1:96.
114. Paul C. Etude sur l'intoxication lente par les preparations de plomb; de son influence pa le produit de la conception. *Arch Gen Med.* 1869;5:513–533.
115. Deneufbourg H. L'intoxication saturnine dans ses rapports avec la grossesse. *Thesis, Universite de Paris, 1905.*
116. Hamilton A. Industrial Poisons in United States. New York: Macmillan, 1929; pp 8–17, 110–115.
117. Angle CR, McIntire MS. Lead poisoning during pregnancy. *Am J Dis Child.* 1964;108:436–439.
118. Fahim MS, Fahim Z, Hall DG. Effects of subtoxic lead levels on pregnant women in the state of Missouri. In: *Proceedings of the International Conference on Heavy Metals in the Environment*, Toronto, Ocobert. 27–31, 1975.
119. Baghurst PA, Robertson EF, Oldfield RK, et al. Lead in the placenta, membranes, and umbilical cord in relation to pregnancy outcome in a lead-smelter community. *Environ Health Perspect.* 1991;90: 315–320.
120. Nogaki K. On action of lead on body of lead refinery workers: particularly conception, pregnancy and parturition in case of females and on vitality of their newborn. Excerpta Med. 1958;4:2176.
121. Pindborg S. On Solverglodforgifting i Denmark. *Ugeskr Lacg.* 1945;107:1–6.
122. Hu H. Knowledge of diagnosis and reproductive history among survivors of childhood plumbism. *Am J Public Health.* 1991;81:1070–1072.
123. Sierra EM, Tiffany-Castiglioni E. Effects of low-level lead exposure on hypothalamic hormones and serum progesterone levels in pregnant guinea pigs. *Toxicology.* 1992;72:89–97.
124. Needelman HL, Rabinowitz M, Leviton A, et al. The relationship between prenatal exposure to lead and congenital anomalies. *JAMA.* 1984;251:2956–2959.
125. Rothenberg SJ, Schnaas L, Perroni E, et al. Pre- and postnatal lead effect on head circumference: a case for critical periods. *Neurotoxicol Teratol.* 1999;21:1–11.
126. Deknudt GH, Leonard A, Ivanov B. Chromosome aberrations observed in male workers occupationally exposed to lead. *Environ Physiol Biochem.* 1973;3:132–138.
127. Lancranjan I, Popsecu H, Gavanescu O, et al. Reproductive ability of workmen occupationally exposed to lead. *Arch Environ Health.* 1975;30:396–401.
128. Stofen D. Less noted European papers on lead. In: *Proceedings of the International Symposium on Environmental Health Aspects of Lead.* Amsterdam 1972; pp 473–485.
129. Lindbohm ML, Sallmen M, Anttila A, et al. Paternal occupational lead exposure and spontaneous abortion. *Scand J Work Environ Health.* 1991;17:95–103.
130. Min YI, Correa-Villasener A, Stewart PA. Parental occupational lead exposure and low birth weight. *Am J Ind Med.* 1996;30:569–578.
131. Hardy HL. What is the status of knowledge of the toxic effects of lead on identifiable groups in the population? *Clin Pharmacol Ther.* 1966;7:713–722.
132. Rabinowitz M, Bellinger D, Leviton A, et al. Pregnancy hypertension, blood pressure during labor and blood lead levels. *Hypertension.* 1987;10:447–451.
133. Dawson EB, Evans DR, Kelly R, et al. Blood cell lead, calcium, and magnesium levels associated with pregnancy-induced hypertension and preeclampsia. *Biol Trace Elem Res.* 2000;74:107–116.
134. Vigeh M, Yokoyama K, Mazaheri M, et al. Relationship between increased blood lead and pregnancy hypertension in women without occupational lead exposure in Tehran, Iran. *Arch Environ Health.* 2004;59:70–75.
135. Rothenberg SJ, Kondrashov V, Manalo M, et al. Increases in hypertension and blood pressure during pregnancy with increased bone lead levels. *Am J Epidemiol.* 2002;156:1079–1087.
136. Sowers M, Jannausch M, Scholl T, et al. Blood lead concentrations and pregnancy outcomes. *Arch Environ Health.* 2002;57:489–495.
137. Mahaffey KR, Annest JL, Roberts J, et al. National estimates of blood lead levels: United States, 1976-1980: Association with selected demographic and socioeconomic factors. *N Engl J Med.* 1982;307:573–579.
138. Bellinger D, Solman J, Leviton A, et al. Low-level lead exposure and children's cognitive function in the preschool years. *Pediatrics.* 1991;87:219–227.
139. Dietrich KN, Kraft KM, Bornschein RL, et al. Low-level fetal lead exposure effect on neurobehavioral development in early infancy. *Pediatrics.* 1987;80:721–730.
140. Dietrich KN, Succop PA, Berger OG, et al. Lead exposure and the cognitive development of urban preschool children: The Cincinnati Lead Study cohort at age 4 years. *Neurotoxicol Teratol.* 1991; 13:203–211.
141. Cooney GH, Bell A, McBride W, et al. Neurobehavioral consequences of prenatal low level exposures to lead. *Neurotoxicol Teratol.* 1989;11:95–104.
142. Tang HW, Huel G, Campagna D, et al. Neurodevelopmental evaluation of 9-month-old infants exposed to low levels of lead in utero: involvement of monoamine neurotransmitters. *J Appl Toxicol.* 1999;19:167–172.

143. Canfield RL, Henderson CR Jr, Cory-Slechta DA, et al. Intellectual impairment in children with blood lead concentrations below 10 microg per deciliter. *N Engl J Med.* 2003;348:1517–1526.
144. Rothenberg SJ, Cansino S, Sepkoskic C, et al. Prenatal and perinatal lead exposure alter acoustic cry parameters of neonate. *Neurotoxicol Teratol.* 1995;17:151–160.
144. Belfinger D, Leviton A, Rabinowitz M, et al. Weight gain and maturing in fetuses exposed to low levels of lead. *Environ Res.* 1991;54: 151–158.
146. Shukla R, Dietrich KN, Bornschein RL, et al. Lead exposure and growth in the early preschool child: a follow-up report from the Cincinnati Lead Study. *Pediatrics.* 1991;88:886–892.
147. Greene T, Ernhart CB. Prenatal and preschool age lead exposure: relationship with size. *Neurotoxicol Teratol.* 1991;13:417–427.
148. Bushness PJ, Bowman RE. Persistence of impaired reversal learning in young monkeys exposed to low levels of dietary lead. *J Toxicol Environ Health.* 1979;5:1015–1023.
149. Levin ED, Bowman RE. The effect of pre or postnatal lead exposure on Hamilton Search Task in monkeys. *Neurobehav Toxicol Teratol.* 1983;5:391–394.
150. Mele PC, Bushnell PJ, Bowman RE. Prolonged behavioral effects of early postnatal lead exposure in rhesus monkeys: fixed-interval responding and interactions with scopolamine and pentobarbital. *Neurobehav Toxicol Teratol.* 1984;6:129–135.
151. Rice DC, Willes RF. Neonatal low-level lead exposure in monkeys (*Macaca fascicularis*): effect on two-choice non-spatial form discrimination. *J Environ Pathol Toxicol.* 1979;2:1195–1203.
152. Rie DC, Gilbert SG, Willes RF. Neonatal low-level lead exposure in monkeys: locomotor activity, schedule-controlled behavior, and the effects of amphetamine. *Toxicol Appl Pharmacol.* 1979;51:503–513.
153. Goldstein GW, Asbury AK, Diamond L. Pathogenesis of lead encephalopathy: uptake of lead and reaction of brain capillaries. *Arch Neurol.* 1974;31:382–389.
154. Hammond PB. The effects of chelating agents on the tissue distribution and excretion of lead. *Toxicol Appl Pharmacol.* 1971;18:296–310.
155. Mahaffey K, Michaelson A. Interactions between lead and nutrition. In: Needelman HL, ed. *Low level Lead Exposure: The Clinical Implications of Current Research.* New York: Raven Press, 1980; 159–200.
156. Holzman J, Hsu JS. Early effects of lead on immature rat brain mitochondrial respiration. *Pediatr Res.* 1976;10:70–75.
157. Choie DD, Richter GW. Stimulation of DNA synthesis in rat kidney by repeated administration of lead. *Proc Soc Exp Biol Med.* 1973;142:446–449.
158. Koren G, Cheung M, Klein J, et al. Lead exposure in mothers and infants in Toronto, 1989. *Can Med Assoc J.* 1990;142:1241–1244.
159. Meyer J, Genenich HH, Robra BP, et al. Determinants of lead concentration in the umbilical cord blood of 9189 newborns of a birth cohort in the government district of Braunschweig. *Zentralb Hugg Umweltmed.* 1992;192:522–533.
160. Angell NF, Lavery JP. The relationship of blood lead levels to obstetric outcome. *Am J Obstet Gynecol.* 1982;142:40–46.
161. Zetterlund B, Winberg J, Lundgren G, et al. Lead in umbilical cord blood correlated with the blood lead of the mother in areas with low, medium or high atmospheric pollution. *Acta Paediatr Scand.* 1977; 66:169–175.
162. Milman N, Christensen JM, Ibsen KK. Blood lead and erythrocyte zinc protoporphyrin in mothers and newborn infants. *Eur J Pediatr.* 1988;147:71–73.
163. Wan BJ, Zhang Y, Tian CY, et al. Blood lead dynamics of lead-exposed pregnant women and its effects on fetus development. *Biomed Environ Sci.* 1996;9:41–45.
164. Laker M. On determining trace element levels in man: the uses of blood and hair. *Lancet.* 1982;2:260–262.
165. Huel G, Everson RB, Manger I. Increased hair cadmium in newborns of women occupationally exposed to heavy metals. *Environ Res.* 1984;1:115–121.
166. Stefanak MA, Bourguet CC, Benzies-Styku T. Use of the Centers for Disease Control and Prevention childhood lead poisoning risk questionnaire to predict blood level elevations in pregnant women. *Obstet Gynecol.* 1996;87:209–212.
167. Schardein JL. Chemical antagonists. In: Schardein JL, ed. *Chemically Induced Birth Defects.* New York: Marcel Dekker, 1985; pp 534–545.
168. Kantor MI, Levin PM. Arsenical encephalopathy in pregnancy with recovery. *Am J Obstet Gynecol.* 1948;56:370–374.
169. Timpo AE, Amin JS, Casalino MB, et al. Congenital lead intoxication. *J Pediatr.* 1979;94:765–767.
170. Peral M, Boxt M. Radiographic findings in congenital lead poisoning. *Radiology.* 1980;136:83–84.
171. Briggs GG, Freeman RK, Yaffe SJ, eds. *Drugs in Pregnancy and Lactation.* 2nd ed. Baltimore, MD: Williams & Wilkins, 1986; p 331.
172. Domingo JL, Ortega A, Paternain JL, et al. Oral meso-2,3-dimercaptosuccinic acid in pregnant Sprague-Dawley rats-teratogenicity and alterations in mineral metabolism: I. Teratological evaluation. *J Toxicol Environ Health.* 1990;30:181–190.
173. Paternain JL, Ortega A, Domingo JL, et al. Oral *meso*-2,3-dimercaptosuccinic acid in pregnant Sprague-Dawley rats-Teratogenicity and alterations in mineral metabolism: II. Effect on mineral metabolism. *J Toxicol Environ Health.* 1990;30:191–197.
174. Bosque MA, Domingo JL, Pater JL, et al. Evaluation of the developmental toxicity of 2,3-dimercapto-l-propanesulfonate (DMPS) in mice: effect on mineral metabolism. *Toxicology.* 1990;62:311–320.
175. Domingo JL, Bosque MA, Piera V. Meso-2,3-dimercaptosuccinic acid and prevention of arsenite embryotoxicity and teratogenicity in the mouse. *Fundam Appl Toxicol.* 1993;17:314–320.
176. Domingo JL, Bosque MA, Llobelt JM, et al. Amelioration by BAL (2,3-dimercapto-l-propanol) and DMPS (sodium 2,3-dimercapto-1-propanesulfonic acid) of arsenite developmental toxicity in mice. *Ecotoxicol Environ Saf.* 1992;23:274–281.
177. Rogan WJ, Dietrich KN, Ware JH, et al, Treatment of Lead-Exposed Children Trial Group. The effect of chelation therapy with succimer on neuropsychological development in children exposed to lead. *N Engl J Med.* 2001;344:1421–1426.
178. Liu X, Dietrich KN, Radcliffe J, et al. Do children with falling blood lead levels have improved cognition? *Pediatrics.* 2002;110:787–791.
179. Dietrich KN, Ware JH, Salganik M, et al, Treatment of Lead-Exposed Children Clinical Trial Group. Effect of chelation therapy on the neuropsychological and behavioral development of lead-exposed children after school entry. *Pediatrics.* 2004;114:19–26.

CHAPTER 18

IONIZING AND NONIONIZING RADIATION IN PREGNANCY

Yedidia Bentur

INTRODUCTION

Radiation is an anxiety-provoking term. In the minds of many, it is impossible to separate the psychological and physical effects of the atomic bomb from the effects of low-dose ionizing radiation. This anxiety is only aggravated by our knowledge of the carcinogenic effects of high-level exposure to ionizing radiation in humans (e.g., radium-dial workers, uranium miners, patients who receive radiotherapy or isotope therapy, and the victims of high exposures following the bombings of Hiroshima and Nagasaki and the accident at Chernobyl). This anxiety and misunderstanding may explain in part the ignorance of the public and many scientists and physicians regarding the qualitative and quantitative effects of ionizing radiation in spite of the extensive studies that have been carried out. Another source of confusion is the fact that the term *radiation* is applied to various forms of ionizing and nonionizing radiation such as x-rays, ultrasound, and microwave. Therefore, it has even been suggested that *radiation* should be applied to high-energy ionizing radiation (x-rays, γ-rays, and radionuclides), whereas, radar, broadcast-range FM radio waves, diathermy, and microwaves should be termed *long-wavelength electromagnetic waves* or, in the case of ultrasound, *sound waves*.[1]

Despite the increase in concern regarding the effects of ionizing radiation on health and reproduction, the medical use of x-rays has continued to grow. In 1980, the number of x-ray procedures in the United States was 225 million (roughly equal to the total population.[2] Approximately 80 million fertile men and women were exposed to x-ray procedures in that year. About 30,000 fertile women may have been exposed to abdominal x-rays in early pregnancy.[3] In the United Kingdom, approximately 12% of the total radiation dose to the population is due to man-made irradiation; from that, about 94% is due to medical procedures.[4] About 21 million radiodiagnostic studies were carried out annually in 1977 in the United Kingdom, of which about 6% were fluoroscopic investigations.[5] Although fluoroscopies involve mainly the abdominal region and are associated with high-dose exposure, the use of gonadal shields is still low.[6]

It is in this context of anxiety, ignorance, and confusion and, on the other hand, increasing medical use of ionizing radiation, that the reproductive effects of diagnostic and therapeutic uses of ionizing radiation are reviewed here.

HISTORY

Until 1895, when Wilhelm Roentgen devised a method to generate x-rays, human beings were exposed only to natural sources of ionizing radiation. *Background radiation,* as this form of energy is also called, consists of electromagnetic and particulate forms of ionizing radiation coming from the sun and the stars; radionuclides in the soil; and γ- rays, x-rays, and α- and β-particles from rocks and air. Roentgen's invention introduced to science and medicine an enormous new source of ionizing radiation. The diagnostic uses of x-rays were developed rapidly following this discovery. In addition, this radiation was used for cancer therapy and also for tinea capitis,[7] enlarged tonsils and adenoids,[8] thymic enlargement,[9] and infertility.[10] In 1896 Antoine Becquerel discovered that certain elements emit radiation. It was not until 1906, after the French physicist accidentally burned himself while carrying a radioactive compound in his pocket, that the possible therapeutic uses of radioisotopes were conceived.

Only after the bombings of Hiroshima and Nagasaki in World War II had provided live evidence of the hazards posed by radiation, were serious studies conducted regarding its delayed genetic effects and somatic damage. The medical uses of x-rays were intensely scrutinized, with a particular focus on what harm might be done to developing humans, including the mutagenic and carcinogenic effects of ionizing radiation.

DEFINITIONS

Ionizing radiation can be expressed in units of exposure (roentgen), its absorbency into human tissue (rad, gray), and as the biological effectiveness of absorbed radiation (rem).[11]

The *roentgen* (R) is the international unit of x- or γ-radiation equal to the amount of radiation that produces, in 1 cm^3 of dry air at 0°C and standard atmospheric pressure, ionization of either sign equal to one electrostatic unit (esu) of charge.

The *rad* is a unit of absorbed dose of ionizing radiation equal to an energy of 100 ergs/s of irradiated material: 100 rad 1 Gy (gray) = 1 J/kg.

The *rem* (roentgen-equivalent man) is the dosage of an ionizing radiation that will cause the same biological effect as 1 R of x-ray or γ-ray dosage; 100 rem = 1 Sv (sievert).

The relationship between the absorbed energy (in rad or Gy) and the effectiveness of that energy in causing damage incorporates a factor called the *relative biological effectiveness* (RBE): 1 rem = 1 rad/RBE or 1 Sv = 1 Gy/RBE. Thus, RBE is a correction factor for predicting the biological effect of absorbed radiation. For radiation in soft tissue, RBE is about 1; hence rad and rem (or Gy and Sv) are often used interchangeably.

The density of the radiation-induced ionizations in any tissue is directly related to the energy transferred to the irradiated substance, which is expressed as the *linear energy transfer* (LET).

MECHANISM OF ACTION

X-rays and γ-rays are short wavelength electromagnetic rays. Ionizing radiation in the form of high-energy photons in γ-rays and lower energy x-ray photons can alter the normal structure of the biochemical components of a living cell through direct and indirect mechanisms.

The direct mechanism involves disrupting the atom's structure of biological molecules by adding sufficient energy to incite electron shells to free an electron from its atomic orbit and produce a charged or ionized compound and a free electron. The indirect mechanism involves the radiolysis of water (which makes up more than 60% of the content of living cells) to form radicals like OH, H^+, H_2, and H_2O_2. These reactive compounds can attack and disrupt neighboring molecules.

Particulate radiation is generated from the spontaneous disintegration of radioactive compounds, which results in the emission of alpha particles (helium nuclei), β-particles (electrons), and other forms of energy. Nuclear fission generates a variety of heavy charged particles, fission fragments, and unchanged neutrons. These subatomic particles can also disrupt the atomic structure of biological molecules by inducing ionizations.

Particulate radiation does not penetrate tissues deeply, but it does generate ions densely along a short path (high LET). X-rays and γ-rays penetrate tissues deeply but generate ions sparsely along their path (low LET).

The harm that follows from a single, random modification in a cell component (such as the genetic structure of stem cells) as a result of ionizing radiation (or any other toxin), termed a *stochastic effect*, may still allow the cells to proliferate. A nonstochastic effect is produced by numerous and/or repeated instances of damage. Stochastic effects can theoretically originate in a single deleterious effect, which can be associated with extremely low levels of radiation. Thus, an experimentally derived dose-response curve for effects such as carcinogenesis, mutagenesis, and maybe even abortions may not include a threshold dose below which no adverse effects occur. On the other hand, the dose-response curve for nonstochastic effects (i.e., cataract formation) would be expected to show a threshold dose, which defines the smallest dose of radiation that induces detectable harm.

Similarly, Smith[12] separates the harmful effects of ionizing radiation into two classes:

1. *Deterministic effects,* which result in loss of tissue function, usually at doses in excess of a few hundred millisieverts (tens of rems). Its dose-frequency relationship is sigmoid, and a tissue-specific dose threshold exists. This type of injury may also involve various compensatory and repair mechanisms. When the radiation dose is fractionated, there is greater repair and proliferation, hence increasing the tolerance of the tissue. This radiobiological observation of tolerance dose for most tissues guides the radiotherapist in judging the regimen to avoid unwanted side effects.
2. *Stochastic effects,* as discussed earlier. Since no dose threshold is assumed for these effects, there is great uncertainty as to how best to predict unavoidable injurious effects that may result, for instance, from exposure to an ionizing radiation dose equivalent to the natural background levels.

The expression of radiation-induced damage in humans depends not only on total dose, dose rate, LET, and fractionation and protraction of total doses, but also on repair mechanisms, bystander effects and exposure to chemical carcinogens, tumor promoters, other toxins and level of anticarcinogenic and antitumor promoting agents.[13]

BIOLOGICAL EFFECT

Before discussing the biological effect of ionizing radiation, it is important to refer to some of the findings of the review of the 30-year study of the survivors of the Hiroshima and Nagasaki bombings.[14] It was clearly shown in this study that radiation effects are dose-dependent. More than 90% of survivors received much less than 10 rad from the atomic bombs. The possibility that such survivors will develop any disease from atomic bomb exposure is no greater than those of unexposed individuals. Those who received higher doses have greater risks.

Testes

In various animal experimental studies, it was shown that prenatal doses of ionizing radiation between 50 and 500 rad can induce testicular hypoplasia and sterility.[11] This radiosensitivity differed among different animal species[15] and according to the gestational state[16]. Fertility data from radiotherapy patients[17] is often of limited value, because illness and simultaneous administration of cytotoxic agents can also alter sperm production.

In a study sponsored by the U.S. Atomic Energy Commission (AEC), normal men received large, defined doses of x-irradiation to the testes and were monitored for alterations in testicular cell populations, spermatogenesis, and fertility.[18,19] Testicular radiation doses of 15–100 rad caused a decline in the sperm count about 50 days after irradiation, probably through an effect on the spermatogonia. A 15-rad dose caused only oligospermia. Doses of 50–80 rad and higher produced aspermia within 2–6 months. A decline in the sperm count was produced in less than 50 days after a single dose of 400 rad. It seems that this higher dose affected the spermatids, which are produced in the later stages of spermatogenesis. This finding in humans of increased radiosensitivity at earlier stages of cell division is consistent with findings in experimental models.[20,21] The findings of the recovery phase in the AEC study suggested that repopulation of germinal cells becomes less and less efficient as radiation exposures increase.[19] Histological recovery (increasing number of spermatogonia) was observed about 7 months postirradiation doses of 100–600 rad. After 100 rad, the appearance of sperm in seminal fluid coincided with the earliest sign of histological recovery (7 months). But, sperm production was not detectable until 11 and 24 months after doses of 200 and 600 rad, respectively. Similar findings were observed in the mouse,[22] but its testicular tissue is significantly less radiosensitive than that of the human.[23] It was also suggested in the human study[19] that radiation interfered with normal gonadotropin production by Leydig cells, thereby causing an increase in their number as a compensatory mechanism. The complete recovery of normal sperm concentrations after doses of between 100 and 600 rad took between 9 months and 5 years.[19] Some men who had been accidentally exposed to large doses of radiation fathered children after even longer periods of time.[24] Mouse experiments suggest that fertility can return when the sperm count is only 10% of its normal density.[25]

Ovaries

In the prenatal period, radiation sensitivity is high in oogonia that are undergoing mitosis.[11] The mammalian primary oocyte arrested in meiosis has been found to have varying radiosensitivity, depending on the subject's age and the species studied.[26,27] In vitro studies indicate that the human oocyte may be among the most radioresistant structures,[28] whereas other studies show the mouse's oocyte to be among the most radiosensitive structures.[29,30] Irradiation was shown in animals to cause rapid changes in germ-cell structure characterized by a condensation of the chromosomes and damage to the nuclear envelope.[29,31] Damaged oocytes either undergo repair[32] or are eliminated from the ovary within days or weeks.[29,30] Doses of radiation sufficient to destroy most of the small primordial follicles have little effect on oocytes in Graafian follicles.[28] The radiation dose administered influences mainly the proportion of oocytes affected but not the time course of degenerative changes.[33]

It seems that exposure in utero to low-dose radiation has little effect on human fertility, although the data are very limited. A fertility study on 180 women showed that 1–5 rad of gonadal radiation during infancy did not significantly affect the number of children born or the age distribution of births when compared with control data.[34] Brent has estimated that acute doses below 25 rad absorbed by the fetus during gestation are unlikely to result in sterility in the human female or male.[15]

The observation in animals that moderate doses of radiation (50 rad) increased litter size, probably owing to superovulation,[29,35,36] may have provided the empirical basis for the treatment of infertile women with x-rays in the past.[10]

Other human data showed that radiotherapy involving 600 rad in women over 40 years of age induced permanent menopause[17]. Younger women exposed to this dose of radiation are likely to recover normal menstrual function and fertility. A fractionated dose of 2000 rad over 5–6 weeks is considered likely to produce complete sterility in 95% of girls and young women.[17] An extended period of amenorrhea is expected after radiation doses, which are inadequate to cause complete sterility.[11] Young women with postirradiation amenorrhea were reported to resume their menstrual cycle only after a successful pregnancy.[28,37,38]

Women with internal exposure to α-particle radiation while employed in the radium dial industry prior to 1930 had reduced fertility (i.e., reduced number of pregnancies and live births) if ovarian exposure exceeded 5Sv (500rem). Below this dose, no effect on fertility could be shown.[39]

Gestation

In a study looking at the outcome of pregnancy in survivors of Wilms' tumor, it was suggested that radiation induces somatic damage to abdominopelvic structures.[40] This type of radiotherapy involves gonadal exposure of about 900 rad (one exposure) or 1100–1600 rad in fractionated doses.[11] Among 114 pregnancies in women who had received abdominal radiotherapy for Wilms' tumor, an adverse outcome occurred in 34 (30%) in the form of perinatal deaths (17 pregnancies) and low-birth-weight infants (18 pregnancies).

In comparison, only in 2 (30%) out of 77 pregnancies in nonirradiated females with Wilms' tumor and in the wives of male patients with Wilms' tumor was there an adverse outcome. The absence of adverse outcomes in the pregnancies fathered by irradiated males suggests that radiation-induced germinal mutation is an unlikely explanation. This is supported by similar findings in other studies.[41,42] In addition, shortened trunk, scoliosis, fibrosis of the abdominal musculature, and functional impairment of visceral organs have been reported in women who received curative radiation for Wilms' tumor in childhood.[43–45] Possible mechanisms for this impaired gestation are reduced dispensability of the irradiated uterine musculature and the abdominal cavity as well as uterine vascular insufficiency.[11] This high risk of adverse pregnancy outcome should be considered in the counseling and prenatal care of women who have received abdominal radiotherapy for Wilms' tumor.

A British study showed that female survivors of childhood cancer who had been given abdominal or gonadal irradiation had excessive miscarriages (19%) compared with a control group of females with similar neoplasms who were not irradiated (9%).[46] Leukemic children who received prophylactic irradiation of the central nervous system had, in adulthood, lower fertility expressed as a lower first-birth rate (rate ratio 0.39) than those without radiation, indicating that doses of 18–24 Gy to the brain may possibly be a risk factor.[47] Hypothalamic or pituitary injury is a suggested mechanism. In both these studies,[46,47] there was no increased risk for congenital anomalies.

A Canadian study of women exposed to low-level ionizing radiation from diagnostic radiography for adolescent idiopathic scoliosis showed an insignificant increase in unsuccessful attempts at pregnancy and congenital malformations, a significant increase in spontaneous abortions (OR 1.35) and a significant decrease in stillbirth (OR 0.38). The adjusted OR for low birth weight was found to increase by quartiles of dose. The adjusted mean birth weight decreased with increasing dose by 37.6 g per cGy.[48] Dental radiography involving exposures higher than 0.4 mGy (40 mrad) was associated with an adjusted OR for a low birth weight infant of 2.27 (95% CI 1.11–4.66). This association was stronger in term low-birth-weigh infants (OR 3.61, 95% CI 1.46–8.92). Involvement of the hypothalamus-pituitary axis was postulated.[49] However, this study was criticized for confounders such as dental carries, radiation dose delivered to the thyroid, lead oxide powder on the radiographic films and lack of control for known risk factors.

Genetic Disorders

Demonstrating the genetic effects of ionizing radiation in humans is limited by the difficulty in establishing a causal link between chromosomal damage and radiation exposure in the presence of other environmental mutagens. Chromosomal abnormalities are believed to be associated with 50% of spontaneous abortions and 8–10% of stillbirths.[50] Radiation genetic damage cannot be distinguished from this high natural occurrence of human genetic disorders.

Animal studies have shown that radiation can induce subtle genetic abnormalities in small, short-lived organisms[51] and that repeated small doses of radiation caused fewer mutations than the equivalent amount of radiation administered as a single dose.[21,52] Animal data also suggest that radiation-induced point mutations could not account for even a small proportion of radiation-induced teratogenicity unless it simply involves cell death.[1] An increase in chromosomal breakage was observed in lymphocytes from pregnant women exposed in vitro to ionizing radiation. This increase in radiosensitivity was in strong correlation with the amount of pregnancy hormones, especially progesterone.[53] Upon looking at children born to radiation-exposed and unexposed survivors of the bombings of Hiroshima and Nagasaki, no significant difference was found regarding the incidence of stillbirths, congenital abnormalities, and neonatal fatalities.[54] An apparent increase in abnormal pregnancies that correlated with increasing radiation dose was not found to be statistically significant. The data also suggested an increase in congenital problems when either mother or father had been exposed to ionizing radiation, but no cumulative effect was present in the data collected for births in which both parents had been exposed to radiation.

A case-control study of 67 infants with trisomy 21 and their matched controls showed no association with medical radiography. The relative risk of trisomy for a radiographic examination involving direct irradiation of the ovaries prior to conception (mean ovarian dose 2.19 and 2.41 mGy for case and controls, respectively) was 0.8; the 95% confidence interval (CI) was 0.34–1.83.[55] There are no reports of excessive genetic disorders in geographical areas where the annual background radiation is known to be as high as 1.3 rem (10 times the average background exposure in the United States).[56,57] The Committee on the Biological Effects of Ionizing Radiation of the U.S. National Academy of Sciences has estimated that 50–250 rem would be the dose of radiation sufficient to double the natural human mutation rate.[51]

Preliminary results of an American and Danish study on survivors of childhood cancer who underwent radiotherapy (gonadal dose >100 mSv and >1000 mSv in 46% and 16% of the patients, respectively) did not show an increased risk for inherited genetic disease in the offspring.[58] Interestingly, a recent study examining atomic bomb survivors exposed *in utero* for translocation frequencies in blood lymphocytes at 40 years of age, found no increased frequency with dose, except for a small significant increase (<1%) at doses below 0.1 Sv. These findings suggest the existence of two subpopulations of fetal lymphoid precursor cells. One is small in number, sensitive to the induction of translocations and cell killing, but rapidly diminishing above 50 mSv. The other is larger and insensitive to registering damage expressed as chromosome aberrations.[59]

Table 18-1 shows the known spontaneous incidence of genetic disorders causing serious handicaps per million live-born, together with estimates of additional radiation-induced defects.

It seems that no correlation has been demonstrated between exposure to ionizing radiation and the incidence of genetic disorders in any human population at any dose level.[51,60] If medical and occupational exposures are kept within recommended limits, radiation is responsible for few if any of the genetic disorders occurring spontaneously.[61]

Teratogenesis

During the preimplantation period of gestation (0–2 weeks), the embryo is most sensitive to the lethal effect of radiation,[62,63] probably owing to genetic damage,[11,62] and is insensitive to its growth-retarding and teratogenic effects.[1] During early organogenesis, the embryo is very sensitive to the growth-retarding, teratogenic, and lethal effects of irradiation but can recover somewhat from the growth-retarding effects in the postpartum period.[1] It seems that the time period for radiation-induced multiple malformations other than of the central nervous system is the second to fourth week of gestation, representing 5% of the length of pregnancy, versus, for instance, 14% of the pregnancy in rat.[11] During the early fetal period, the fetus exhibits central nervous system sensitivity to radiation, and it can be growth retarded at term, from which it recovers poorly in the postpartum period; at the same period, however, the fetus has diminished sensitivity to multiple-organ teratogenesis.[64,65] During the later fetal stages, the fetus will not be grossly deformed by radiation. If the radiation exposure is high enough, it will sustain permanent cell depletion of various organs and tissues.[15,66] Cell death, mitotic delay, and disturbances of cell migration are among the mechanisms postulated for the irradiation effects, but it is difficult to determine which of them are most important in radiation-induced embryopathology. In addition, the same mechanism may not have the same importance in different stages of the pregnancy. For instance, cell death may be of minimal importance in the preimplantation period because of the embryo's capacity for repair and the pluripotent nature of each remaining viable cell at this early stage.[1,67,68] In later stages of the pregnancy, the fetus loses this ability and cell death then becomes a primary factor.

Tables 18-2 and 18-3 summarize the effects of different radiation doses at various stages of the pregnancy.

The classic effects of radiation on the developing mammal are gross congenital malformations, intrauterine growth retardation, and embryonic death. Central nervous system effects and growth retardation are the cardinal effects. Each of these effects has a dose-response relationship and a threshold exposure below which there is no difference between the irradiated population and the control population.[1]

Microcephaly and Mental Retardation. Many studies indicate that microcephaly is the most common malformation observed in human beings randomly exposed to high doses of radiation during pregnancy.[69–76] In Goldstein and Murphy's studies, where the radiation dose was greater than 100 rad, out of 75 pregnancies, there were 16 microcephalic children, and almost all were developmentally delayed.[70,71] A total of 28 children had severe disturbances of the central nervous system.

In another study, Dekaban reported that 22 of 26 infants exposed to hundreds of rad between the third and twentieth week of human gestation were microcephalic, developmentally delayed, or both.[69] Severe mental retardation following in utero exposure to the atomic bombs was not observed in any patient receiving in

Table 18-1
Estimated Genetic Effects of Radiation per Million Live-Born Offspring

GENETIC DISORDERS	INCIDENCE	ADDITIONAL EFFECTS OF EXPOSURE OF 1 rem/30-year GENERATION	
		FIRST GENERATION	AT EQUILIBRIUM*
Recessive	1000	Very few	Very slow increase
Autosomal dominant and X-linked	10,000	5–65	40–200
Irregularly inherited	90,000	Very few	20–900
Chromosomal aberrations	6000	10	Slight increase

* Refers to later generations when the rate of elimination of defective genes is balanced by the rate of additional mutations.
SOURCE: Adapted from Advisory Committee on the Biological Effects of Ionizing Radiation. The Effects on Populations of Exposure to Low Levels of Ionizing Radiation. Washington, DC: National Research Council, National Academy of Sciences, National Academy Press, 1980.

Table 18-2
A Compilation of the Effects of 10 Rad or Less Acute Radiation at Various Stages of Gestation in Rat and Mouse[a]

	STAGE OF GESTATION (days)				
FEATURE	PREIMPLANTATION	IMPLANTATION	EARLY ORGANOGENESIS	LATE ORGANOGENESIS	FETAL STAGES
Mouse	0–4.5	4.5–6.5	6.5–8.5	8.5–12.0	12–18
Rat	0–5.5	5.5–8	8–10	10–13	13–22
Corresponding human gestation period	0–9	9–14	15–28	28–50	50–280
Lethality	+[b]				
Growth retardation at term	–	–	–	–	–
Growth retardation as adult	–	–	–	–	–
Gross malformations (aplasia, hyperplasia, absence or overgrowth of organs or tissues)	±[c]	–	–	–	–
Cell depletions, minimal but measurable tissue hypoplasia	–	–	–	–	–
		–	–	–	–
Sterility	–	–	–	–	–
Significant increase in germ-cell mutations	±	±	±	±	±
Cytogenic abnormalities	–	–	–	–	–
Neuropathology	–[c]	–	–	–	–
Tumor induction[e,f]	–	–	±	±	±
Behavior disorders[g]	–	–	–	–	–
Reduction of life span[e]	–	–	–	–	–

[a] Dose fractionation or protraction effectively reduces the biological results of all the pathological effects reported to this table. (–) indicates no observed effect, (±) questionable but reported or suggested effect, (+) demonstrated effect.

[b] At this stage the murine embryo is most sensitive to the lethal effects of irradiation. With 10 rad in the mouse, Rugh reports a slight decrease in litter size in the mouse (64).

[c] Rugh reports exencephalia with 1 and 25 rad in a strain of mice with a 1% incidence of exencephalia. Others have not been able to repeat these results.[62]

[d] Recent reevaluation of the atomic bomb victims data suggests the possibility that mental retardation is a risk in the 10- to 20-rad range. This is not supported by most other data.

[e] The potential for mutation induction exists in the embryonic germ cells or their precursors. Several long-term studies indicate that considerably greater dose in mice and rats do not affect longevity, tumor incidence, incidence of congenital malformations, litter size, growth rate, or fertility.

[f] Stewart and others have reported that 2 rad increases the incidence of malignancy by 50% in the offspring. See text for discussion.

[g] Piontkovskii (cited in Reference 1) reports behavioral changes in the rat after 1 rad daily irradiation. This work has not been reproduced.

SOURCE: From Brent RL. The Effects of Embryonic and Fetal Exposure to X-ray, Microwaves and Ultrasound. In: Brent RL, Beckman DA, eds. Clinics in Perinatology, Teratology. Vol 13. Philadelphia, PA: Saunders, 1986, pp 615–648.

utero dose less than 50 rad.[77] It has also been documented that 10–20 rad of low-LET radiation will not increase the incidence of microcephaly in experimental animals.[15] A retrospective study showed that medical ionizing radiation of more than 300 mrad in the second and third trimesters is related to a significant yet minimal decrease in head circumference at birth.[78] Analysis of the data on survivors of atomic bombings in Japan using refined estimates of the absorbed dose in fetal tissues demonstrated that the highest risk for forebrain damage occurred at 8–15 weeks' gestational age.[79] These data were consistent with a linear dose response model, which did not indicate the existence of a threshold dose. The authors estimated the probability of increasing the incidence of mental retardation as 0.4%/rad of radiation (i.e., four additional cases of mental retardation for each 1000 births). In contrast, the data collected for in utero exposures after the fifteenth week of gestation were not linearly related to dose, suggesting that a nonlinear model with a threshold dose for radiation effects best fits the data for this period of gestation. During 8–15 weeks of gestation, the risk of impaired central nervous system development was five times greater than that estimated for 16–25 weeks. Radiation exposure before the eighth week of gestation and after the twenty-fifth week was not associated with an increased risk of mental retardation. Yoshimaru et al. assessed school performance of prenatally exposed survivors of the atomic bombings using the DS86 dosimetry system instituted in 1986. They found that damage to the fetus exposed at 16–25 weeks after fertilization appeared similar to that seen in the 8–15-week group.[80] Otake et al. reviewed 45 years' study on brain damage among prenatally exposed survivors of Hiroshima and Nagasaki.[81] Again, they noted an increased frequency of severe mental retardation, a diminution in IQ score and school performance, and increased occurrence of seizures among individuals exposed in the eighth through twenty-fifth week postconception, especially in the 8–15-week period. Sixty percent of those with severe mental retardation had small head size, and 10%

Table 18-3
A Compilation of the Effects of 10 Rad or Less Acute Radiation at Various Stages of Gestation in Rat and Mouse

	STAGE OF GESTATION (days)				
FEATURE	PREIMPLANTATION	IMPLANTATION	EARLY ORGANOGENESIS	LATE ORGANOGENESIS	FETAL STAGES
Mouse	0–4.5	4.5–6.5	6.5–8.5	8.5–12	12–18
Rat	0–5.5	5.5–8	8–10	10–13	13–22
Corresponding human gestation period	0–9	9–14	18–36	36–50	50–280
Lethality	+++[b,c]	+	++	±	–
Growth retardation at term	–	+	+++	++	+
Growth retardation as adult	–	+	++	+++	++
Gross malformations (aplasia, hyperplasia, absence or overgrowth of organs or tissues)	–	–	+++	±[d]	–[d]
Cell depletions, minimal but measurable tissue hypoplasia	–	–	±	++	+[k]
Sterility	–	–	±	–	++[e]
Significant increase in germ-cell mutations[f]	±	±	±	±	±
Cytogenic abnormalities[c,g]	±			+[a]	+[a]
Cataracts	–	–	+	+	+
Neuropathology	–	–	+++	+++	++
Tumor induction[h]	–	±	±	±	±
Behavior disorders[i]	–	–	±	±	±
Reduction of life span[j] (in nonmalformed embryos)	–	–	–	–	–

[a] Dose fractionation or protraction effectively reduced the biological result of all the pathological effects reported in this table.
[b] (–) no observed effect, (±) questionable but reported or suggested effect, (+) demonstrated effect, (++) readily apparent effect, (+++) occurs in high incidence.
[c] Russell (cited in Reference 1) reported that 200 rad increased the incidence of XO aneuploidy in 2–5% of offspring in mice with a spontaneous incidence of 1%. A dose of 100 rad kills substantial numbers of mouse and rat embryos at this stage, but the survivors appear and develop normally.
[d] One hundred rad produces changes in the irradiated fetus that are subtle and necessitate detailed examination and comparison with comparable controls.
[e] The male gonad in the rat can be made extremely hypoplastic by irradiation in the fetal stages with 15 rad. In the mouse the newborn female is most sensitive to the sterilized effects of radiation. Much of this research on other animals cannot be applied to the human.
[f] The potential for mutation induction exists in embryonic germ cells or their precursors. The relative sensitivity of the embryonic germ cells when compared to adult germ cells is not known. Several long-term studies in animals do not indicate any exceptional differences.
[g] Footnote refers to the aneuploidy produced in a strain of mice with a 1% incidence of spontaneous XO aneuploidy. Bloom (cited in Reference 1) has reported a much higher percentage of chromosome breaks in human embryos receiving 100–200 rad in utero than in adults receiving the same dose of irradiation. As yet there have been no diseases associated with this increase in frequency of chromosome breaks.
[h] Animal experiments and the data from Hiroshima and Nagasaki do not support the concept that in utero irradiation is much more tumorigenic than extrauterine irradiation. On the other hand, Stewart and colleagues[104,105,107] and many others report that irradiation from pelvimetry (2 rad) increases the incidence of leukemia and other tumors.
[i] A statistically significant increase in percentage of mental retardation occurs with this dose of radiation. On the other hand, normal intelligence has been found in children receiving much higher doses in utero.
[j] Animal experiments indicate that survivors of in utero irradiation have a life span that is longer than that of groups of animals given the same dose of radiation during their extrauterine life and the same life expectancy as nonirradiated controls.
[k] There is a consensus that the brain maintains a marked sensitivity to radiation throughout all of gestation. Mental retardation is a serious risk at this dose.
SOURCE: From Brent RL. The Effects of Embryonic and Fetal Exposure to X-ray, Microwaves and Ultrasound. In: Brent RL, Beckman DA, eds. Clinics in Perinatology, Teratology. Vol 13. Philadelphia, PA: Saunders, 1986, pp 615–648.

of survivors with small head size were mentally retarded. A linear dose-response model fitted the data. There was strong evidence of threshold at 0.12-0.23 Gy (12–23 rad) at 8–15 weeks' exposure (when two probably non-radiation-related cases of Down's syndrome were excluded) and a 0.21 Gy (21 rad) threshold at 16–25 weeks' exposure. Regression analysis of IQ scores and school performance showed greater linearity with the new dosimetry system (DS86) than with the old (T65DR). These two parameters were similar to those in a control group for those exposed in utero to doses under 0.1 Gy (10 rad). Reanalysis of these data using an exponential linear model suggested the 95% lower bound of the threshold for severe mental retardation to be 0.06–0.31 Gy (6–31 rad) and 0.25–0.28 Gy (25–28 rad) for exposures at 8–15 weeks and 16–25 weeks postovulation, respectively.[82]

Other studies of this population also suggest that in utero radiation may affect intelligence test scores, with the greatest sensitivity during the eighth to fifteenth weeks of gestation.[2,83] One estimate of the dose-response relationship was a 20-point loss on IQ tests for each additional Gy (100 rad) of exposure. The relationship between dose and intelligence test scores is not yet well established, and the findings have to be refined to a demonstrable level of statistical significance or clinical relevance.[2,83] Smith quotes two studies that demonstrated a downward shift in the Gaussian distribution of IQ with an estimated probability coefficient indicating a loss of 30 IQ points per sievert (100 rem) fetal dose at 8–15 weeks after conception.[12] A similar but smaller shift to lower intelligence was detectable following exposure through the period from 16 to 25 weeks but not at other periods of pregnancy.

The estimates above are associated with numerous uncertainties[11]: the number of subjects in each age-defined exposure group was small and estimates of fetal-absorbed dose and prenatal age at exposure cannot be confirmed.

During the 8th–15th weeks of human fetal development, there is a well-characterized period of neuronal proliferation and migration in which cells that begin in the ventricular regions of the growing brain migrate into the various layers of the emerging cerebral cortex.[84] The apparent absence of an effect prior to the eighth week suggests that neuronal proliferation is capable of adequately replacing lost cells, or the effects on cell migration during weeks 8–15 postconception may be the crucial component of cerebral damage caused by radiation.[11] In utero radiation doses as low as 15 cGy (15 rad) affected cell migration in developing rat cerebral cortex possibly through effect on the neural cell adhesion molecule N-CAM.[85] The finding of a small head size in the populations of affected neonates[86] is related to a reduction in cell number, which in turn could be due to impairment of neuronal proliferation and/or massive cell killing.[79] MRI imaging of the brain of some of the mentally retarded survivors of the atomic bomb revealed a large region of abnormally situated gray matter, suggesting an abnormality in neuronal migration. But, cell killing could also contribute importantly to the observed effects on cognitive function.[87]

The finding of mental retardation in infants with normal head size[70,71,83] could be explained by glial cell proliferation after irradiation, as shown in animal studies.[88]

Other Malformations

In two studies from 1929 on 75 pregnancies, quoted above, besides microcephaly and mental retardation (16 infants), two children were born with hypoplastic genitalia, one with cleft palate, and one with hypospadias, abnormality of the large toe, and abnormality of the ear.[70,71] There were various abnormalities of the eyes, including microphthalmia, cataracts, strabismus, retinal degeneration, and optic atrophy. In a study of 26 infants exposed to radiation between the 3rd and 20th weeks of gestation; 22 were seriously affected. The most frequent abnormalities reported were small size at birth and stunted growth, microcephaly, mental retardation, microphthalmia, pigmentary changes of the retina, genital and skeletal malformations, and cataracts.[69] All the malformed children exhibited growth retardation. The estimated protracted exposure was 250 rad. The patients were irradiated for dysmenorrhea, menorrhagia, myomata, arthritis or tuberculosis of the sacroiliac joint, and malignant tumors of the uterus or cervix. In 1930 a typical camptomelic dwarf was born to a woman who had received high-dose radiation from the second to the fifth months of gestation.[89] This rare syndrome had not been described prior to 1930, and the authors were not in a position to recognize its possible genetic cause.

Growth Retardation. Growth retardation, microcephaly, and mental retardation are predominant observable effects following acute exposures exceeding 50 rad (low-LET radiation).[1] Radiation-induced morphological malformations have never been reported in humans without the coexistence of growth retardation or a central nervous system abnormality (mainly microcephaly, mental retardation, and readily apparent eye malformations).[1] In a study mentioned above, growth retardation was reported in all children malformed in utero following large doses of maternal pelvic x-irradiation.[69] Impairment of growth was also detected among individuals who had been exposed in utero to gamma and neutron radiation in Hiroshima and Nagasaki.[90,91] The abnormal findings in this population included reduced height and weight[74,92] and reduced head and chest circumference.[86,93] Diagnostic irradiation involving less than 5 rad to the human fetus has not been observed to cause congenital malformations or growth retardation,[94-100] but not all such studies are negative.[101] Animal studies support the contention that gross congenital malformations will not be increased in a human pregnant population exposed to 5 rad or less.[1,102] In addition, most human exposures to extensive diagnostic radiation studies are fractionated and/or protracted. The likelihood of producing malformations with this type of radiation is lower than with an acute exposure to low-LET radiation.[103,104] One might suggest that functional or biochemical changes may be produced at low levels and with low incidence; so far this has not been proven, at least not regarding thyroid function, liver function, and fertility.[1]

Oncogenesis

Epidemiological studies involving adults and children have established the potential of ionizing radiation to induce leukemia and solid tumors.[51,105] It has also been shown that carcinoma of the thyroid was more prevalent in infants irradiated for thymic hyperplasia.[106] Einhorn has suggested that the period of organogenesis may be highly resistant to carcinogenesis, possibly because of the existence of highly active regulators influencing development that may control cancer.[107] However, a few studies have suggested that in utero radiation may be leukemogenic and may even induce other cancers.[108–111] The present estimate is that a 1- to 2-rad in utero radiation exposure increases the chance of leukemia developing in the offspring by a factor of 1.5-2.0 over the natural incidence.[1] In comparison, a 2-rad dose delivered to an adult population would not make a perceptible change in the incidence of leukemia even for very large population groups.[112,113] An investigation utilizing data on the incidence of neoplastic disease in twins exposed *in utero* to diagnostic obstetrical x-ray examinations suggested a 2.4-fold risk of childhood cancer.[114] Based on this finding and earlier estimates, the increase in neoplastic diseases associated with low-dose ionizing radiation is believed to range between 100 and 240 cases per million persons exposed per rad.[110,115,116] The British Oxford Survey of Childhood Cancer estimates the risk following human in utero irradiation for cancer induction, including leukemia, to be 0.022/Gy (0.00022/rad).[117] This risk, based on a survey of the doses (mean fetal dose 6 mGy or 0.6 rad) associated with United Kingdom routine obstetric radiology in late pregnancy in the period 1958–1961, was estimated to be 0.04–0.05/Gy or 0.004–0.005/rad (95% Cl, 0.008–0.095/Gy).[118]

Among the survivors of the atomic bombings exposed in utero, there were only 18 incident cases of cancer in the years 1950–1984, 5 of them in the zero-dose group.[119] Two of these patients had childhood cancer during the first 14 years of life; both were exposed to 0.30 Gy (30 rad) or more. All the others developed cancer in adulthood. The estimated relative risk for cancer at 1 Gy (100 rad) uterine dose was 3.77. The Life Span Study from Japan, based on the new DS86 dosimetry system, indicates an upper-bound of risk on 95% Cl of 0.028/Gy (0.00028/rad).[120] In a review of several studies dealing with this issue, it has been noted that when one considers the variety of control groups and the sampling variability, the results are remarkably consistent in showing an excessive frequency of leukemia among children whose mothers were exposed to radiation during pregnancy.[121]

A major criticism of these studies has focused on the possible confounding effects of selection factors leading to prenatal x-ray and the possibility that these selection factors may be independently related to increased risk of malignancy.[51] In some studies, the number of patients was small, whereas other studies could not demonstrate any increase in leukemia following higher in utero diagnostic radiological procedures[97,122] or exposure to doses, including the atomic bomb.[123,124] An identical increased risk of leukemia was reported whether the mother had received radiation from diagnostic procedures shortly before or after conception,[125] but this was not proven in another study.[126] It should be pointed out that siblings of leukemic children have an incidence of leukemia of 1:720 per 10 years, which is greater than the 1:2000 risk of leukemia following pelvimetric exposure and the 1:3000 probability of leukemia in the general population of children followed for 10 years (Table 18-4).[1] Cancer incidence and mortality were no higher for subjects with parents exposed to the atomic bomb (median doses 143 mSv; 14.3 rem and 133 mSv; 13.3 rem for exposed fathers and mothers, respectively) than for reference subjects (0–4 mSv; 0.4 rem). The incidence rates did not increase with increasing dose. When both parents were exposed, the adjusted risk ratio for all cancers was 0.97, 95% CI 0.70–1.36 and for cancer mortality 1.16, 95% CI 0.59–1.55.[127,128]

Occupational paternal periconceptional exposure to ionizing radiation was not associated with increased risk of childhood cancer in the offspring.[129] Other studies could not show an association between prenatal diagnostic X-ray examinations and pediatric leukemias.[130,131]

Two German studies concluded that under current conditions, exposure to ionizing radiation in Germany does not constitute risks of childhood malignancies that are relevant to public health.[132,133]

Doll et al. suggested that diagnostic radiography involving low-dose ionizing radiation of the order of 10 mGy (1 rad) received by the fetus may increase the risk of childhood cancer. The excess absolute risk coefficient at this level of exposure is approximately 6%/Gy.[134]

In addition, several animal studies could not demonstrate a significant increase in the incidence of cancer after in utero irradiation.[135–137]

At present, it is not clear whether radiation exposure during either preconception or postconception is a causative or associative factor in the increased incidence of leukemia.[1,138] Genetic or other environmental factors may be more important than prenatal diagnostic radiation in the production of leukemia. That Japanese bomb survivors exposed in utero to up to 500 rad apparently did not experience a significant increase in carcinogenesis proves the complexity of this issue. Smith, from the International Commission on Radiological Protection, concludes that in utero irradiation is not considered likely to significantly influence the lifetime risk of a person living to old age who is irradiated throughout life.[12]

Although it seems that a dose of less than 10 rad to the implanted embryo does not result in a significant increase in the incidence of congenital malformations, growth retardation, or fetal death, low-risk tumorigenic or genetic hazards cannot be ruled out.[1] It is one thing to avoid radiation because of a potential hazard, but it is another matter to recommend therapeutic abortion on this basis.

Table 18-4
Risk of Leukemia in Various Groups with Specific Epidemiological and Pathological Characteristics in Populations Followed Up for 10–30 Years

GROUP	APPROXIMATE RISK	INCREASED RISK OVER CONTROL POPULATION	OCCURRENCE
Identical twin of leukemic twin	1/3	1000	Weeks to months
Irradiation-treated polycythemia vera	1/6	500	10–15 years
Bloom's syndrome	1/8	375	<30 years old
Hiroshima survivors who were within 1000 m of the hypocenter	1/60	50	Average 12 years
Down's syndrome	1/95	30	<10 years old
Irradiation-treated patients with ankylosing spondylitis	1/270	10	15 years
Siblings of leukemic children	1/720	4	to 10 years
Children exposed to pelvimetry in utero (gestational exposure)	1/2000	1.5	<10 years
American white children <15 years old	1/2800	1	to 10 years

SOURCE: From Brent RL. The Effects of Embryonic and Fetal Exposure to X-ray, Microwaves and Ultrasound. In: Brent RL, Beckman DA, eds. Clinics in Perinatology, Teratology. Vol 13. Philadelphia, PA: Saunders, 1986, pp 615–648.

Rugh R, Duhamel L, Skaredoff L. Relation of the embryonic and fetal x-irradiation to life time average weights and tumor incidence in mice. Proc Soc Exp Biol Med. 1966;121:714–718.

RADIODIAGNOSIS IN PREGNANCY

Diagnostic radiology usually involves a radiation dose of 0.02–5.0 rad. Thus, from a clinical standpoint, estimating the risk of gestational effects from a dose of x-ray radiation smaller than 5 rad is of primary importance. The radiation risk, especially in diagnostic radiation, should always be evaluated with consideration of the normal risks of pregnancy. Spontaneous risks of pregnancy are two orders of magnitude greater than the theoretical risks of diagnostic radiation. Table 18-5 lists an estimation of the risks of radiation in the human embryo based on human epidemiological studies and mouse and rat radiation embryological studies. As can be seen from Tables 18-6 and 18-7, the maximum theoretical risk to the human embryo exposed to doses of 5 rad or less is extremely small.

Extrapolation of risk estimates after intrauterine exposures to the atomic bomb may not be applicable to low-level radiodiagnostic exposures. For instance, an analysis of data from Hiroshima and Nagasaki suggested that any dose of radiation between the eighth and fifteenth weeks of gestation could increase the risk of microcephaly and mental retardation by 0.4%/rad and possibly decrease intellectual development.[79] Not only was the cohort small, but also the doses of radiation at Hiroshima and Nagasaki that produced these effects came from uncontrolled radiation sources that differed significantly in the two cities.[139] For example, in Hiroshima, severe mental retardation was not found in individuals exposed in utero to less than 50 rad, whereas in Nagasaki the risk for central nervous system damage was not increased even at levels of 50–150 rad.[140] Consequently, exposure to the atomic bomb cannot be considered readily comparable to the low-LET, filtered radiation used in diagnostic radiology.[2]

It is estimated that the overall risk of malformations and cancer for fetuses exposed in utero during the first 4 months of the pregnancy ranges between 0 and 1 case per 1000 radiated by 1 rad.[141] This estimate is reinforced by the U.S. National Council on Radiation Protection, which stated that the risk of malformations at 5 rad or less was negligible when compared to the other risks of pregnancy.[142] For stochastic phenomena such as cancer and genetic anomalies, it is estimated that the current practice of radiology in the United States increases spontaneous frequency by less than 1 %.[143] Performing several radiodiagnostic procedures in a pregnant woman should be avoided, since the radiation dose may accumulate to a hazardous level, especially in the sensitive period of 8–15 weeks postconception.

There is general agreement that no woman should be denied a medically justified radiodiagnostic procedure because she is pregnant.[83,142] On the other hand, unnecessary use of x-ray procedures is not good medical practice either. The radiobiological concept that no radiation dose can be considered completely safe should be taken in account. Every effort should be made to reduce the radiation dose and biological damage but without sacrificing the benefits of radiation.[13] The immediate medical care of the mother should take priority over the risks of diagnostic radiation exposure to the embryo. Elective procedures such as employment examinations or follow-up examinations once a diagnosis has been made need not be performed on a pregnant woman even though the risk to the embryo is very small.[1] If other procedures can provide adequate information without exposing the embryo to ionizing radiation, they should be used. Examples of such alternative procedures are ultrasound and using a computed tomography (CT) scout view for pelvimetry and excretory urography; with these techniques, radiation doses are significantly lower than with conventional x-ray techniques.[144]

The International Commission on Radiological Protection recommended the 10-day rule with regard to the question of when during the menstrual cycle elective x-ray studies should be scheduled.[83] They pointed out that it is most improbable that a woman will be pregnant in the 10-day interval following onset of menstruation. This should be regarded as the time of choice to perform radiological examinations of the abdomen and pelvis in women of childbearing age.[83,142]

Table 18-5
Estimation of the Risks of Radiation in the Human Embryo Based on Human Epidemiological Studies and Mouse and Rat Radiation Embryologic Studies

EMBRYONIC AGE (days)	MINIMAL LETHAL DOSE (rad)	APPROXIMATE LD_{50} (rad)	MINIMUM DOSE (RAD) FOR PERMANENT GROWTH RETARDATION IN THE ADULT	INCREASED INCIDENCE OF MENTAL RETARDATION	MINIMUM DOSE FOR RECOGNIZED GROSS ANATOMIC MALFORMATION (rad)	MINIMUM DOSE FOR INDUCTION OF GENETIC CARCINOGENETIC AND MINIMAL CELL DEPLETION PHENOMENA
1–5	10	<100	No effect in survivors			Unknown
18–28	25–50	140	20–50	20–50[c]	20	Unknown
36–50	50	200	25–50	50[a]	50	Unknown
50–100	>50	>100	25–50	50[a]	–[b]	Unknown
To term	>100	Same as mother	>50	100		Unknown

[a] Information published by Otake and Shull[79] suggests an increased risk at lower exposures.
[b] Anatomical malformations of a severe type cannot be produced this late in gestation except in the genitourinary system and tissue hypoplasia in specific organ systems, such as the brain and testes.
[c] Severe CNS anatomic malformations more likely than mental retardation.
SOURCE: From Brent RL. The Effects of Embryonic and Fetal Exposure to X-ray, Microwaves and Ultrasound. In: Brent RL, Beckman DA, eds. Clinics in Perinatology, Teratology. Vol 13. Philadelphia, PA: Saunders, 1986, pp 615–648.

Table 18-6
Estimate of Risks of 1-Rad Exposure to the Developing Human Embryo

AGE (days)	MUTAGENIC EFFECT [a–c]	CHILDHOOD CARCINOGENIC EFFECT (STEWART)[d]	MAXIMUM CHILDHOOD CARCINOGENIC EFFECT (ABCC)[b,e]	GROSS CONGENITAL MALFORMATION, DEATH, GROWTH RETARDATION	PERMANENT CELL DEPLETION
1	No data	No data	No data	?[f]	No effect[b]
18–28	10^{-7} per locus	3.2×10^{-4}	5×10^{-6}	Same as controls	?
50		3.2×10^{-4}	5×10^{-6}		
Late fetus to term		3.2×10^{-4}	5×10^{-6}		

[a] Based on an estimated doubling dose for mutagenesis of 100 rad, assuming a linear dose-response curve and no threshold for mutagenic effects.
[b] The mutagenic effects have not been studied in the preimplantation period, or during the perimplantation period, the surviving embryos are not reduced in size even when the dose is very high, although at this stage the embryo is very sensitive to the lethal effects of radiation.
[c] The estimate is assumed to be adult risk because there was no increased carcinogenic effect in the population of exposed fetuses in Hiroshima and Nagasaki.
[d] Stewart's (cited in Reference 1) data would indicate that the embryo is more sensitive to the carcinogenic effect of radiation than the adult. This is a controversial matter, and others[65,124] feel that this association may be other than a radiation effect.
[e] Atomic Bomb Casualty Commission data on carcinogenesis do not indicate that the embryo and fetus are at increased risk. The risk presented is the same carcinogenic risk attributed to adults, assuming maximal effect at low doses—namely, a linear dose-response curve- and no threshold for carcinogenic effects.
[f] Radiation-induced embryonic death might possibly be a stochastic effect in the first few days of gestation, although the present data involving hundreds of embryos indicate no effect at 5–10 rad.

SOURCE: From Brent RL. The Effects of Embryonic and Fetal Exposure to X-ray, Microwaves and Ultrasound. In: Brent RL, Beckman DA, eds. Clinics in Perinatology, Teratology. Vol 13. Philadelphia, PA: Saunders, 1986, pp 615–648.

The pregnancy status of the patient can be determined in several ways:

1. Asking for the date of the last menstrual period and the previous menstrual period, and asking whether the patient could possibly be pregnant.
2. Performing a pregnancy test in cases of uncertainty regarding the pregnancy status.
3. Performing pregnancy tests on all women of reproductive age admitted to the hospital.

Using cost/benefit analysis and simple probability calculations, it was shown that as general public policy, pregnancy tests and elective scheduling procedures are of little value, especially when looking at the current estimates of the morbidity that is associated with low-dose radiodiagnostic procedures.[3] It is important to discuss with the patient why the diagnostic study is indicated even though she may be pregnant, as well as the possible risks to her offspring. Some authors recommend acquiring written consent before the procedure is initiated.[2]

When it has been decided to perform the radiodiagnostic examination, every effort should be made to minimize the expected fetal dose. This can be accomplished by modifying the examination by using only selected views (antero-posterior vs. postero anterior), by using efficient collimators, by the deliberate adjustment of maternal bladder volume, and by using lead apron protectors of the pelvic and abdominal areas.[3,16,145]

Guidelines for x-ray examinations of women in reproductive age and pregnant women issued by the Israeli Ministry of Health in the year 2000 include reducing the milliamp value as much as possible, narrowing the radiation beam to the examined area, shielding (i.e., lead apron) and recording fluoroscopy time and number of films taken. According to these guidelines, fetal exposure to <5 rem does not justify an abortion, fetal exposure to 5–10 rem between

Table 18-7
Risk of 0.5 rem (Maximum Permissible Exposure for Women Radiation Workers with Reproductive Potential)

RISK	0 rem	ADDITIONAL RISK OF 0.5 rem
Spontaneous abortion	150,000/10^6	0
Major congenital malformations	30,000/10^6	0
Severe mental retardation	5000/10^6	0
Childhood malignancy/10-year period	7000/10^6/10 years	166/10^6/10 years or 2.5/10^6/10 years (ABCC data)*
Early to late-onset genetic disease	100,000/10^6	Risk is in next generation
Total risk (using Stewart, cited in Reference 1)		166/10^6
Ratio of total risk to additional risk of radiation	1721:1	
Total risk (using ABCC data)[a] risk of radiation	285,700/10^6	2.5/10^6 (ABCC data)[a]
Ratio of total additional	114,280:1	

* Data from Atomic Bomb Casualty Commission

SOURCE: From Brent RL. The Effects of Embryonic and Fetal Exposure to X-ray, Microwaves and Ultrasound. In: Brent RL, Beckman DA, eds. Clinics in Perinatology, Teratology. Vol 13. Philadelphia, PA: Saunders, 1986, pp 615–648.

the third and the twelfth week from last menstrual period and gestational age of <12 weeks at consultation—abortion should be considered and if >10 rem fetal exposure, abortion is indicated.[146]

ESTIMATION OF RADIATION DOSE

Before reviewing the embryonic exposures from various radiodiagnostic procedures, it is important to review the unavoidable radiation the embryo receives (i.e., the background radiation), which includes cosmic rays from outer space; terrestrial radiation from ground and building materials, and naturally occurring radioisotopes ingested or inhaled[61,147] (Table 18-8). The total dose to the embryo is less than 100 mrad during the 9 months of pregnancy. This dose will vary in different parts of the world and at different elevations, owing to variation in the terrestrial and cosmic ray radiation. Actually, the embryonic/fetal dose during the pregnancy is less than the maternal because of the higher water content of the embryo.[147]

In evaluating the need for a radiodiagnostic procedure during pregnancy or in counseling a pregnant woman who has been inadvertently exposed to such a procedure, it is important to estimate the embryonic/fetal exposure. Whenever one is dealing with radiodiagnosis or radiotherapy, it is always recommended to obtain the estimated embryonic/fetal exposure dose from the radiologist involved in the procedure. This is essential because of the differences in radiation dose delivered by using different equipment and techniques, as discussed further on.

A few methods are available for estimating organ exposure dose in radiodiagnostic examinations:

1. Thermoluminescent dosimeters (TLD) enable direct measurement of entrance skin doses and doses to superficial organs of interest.[148]
2. The Monte Carlo technique is a mathematical method whereby entrance doses are converted to organ doses.[149] For some organs (thyroid, breast, testes, and lungs) the dose measured with TLD is often higher, probably as a result of the limitations of the Monte Carlo method in simulating actual irradiation.[148]
3. A computerized program is available to enable estimation of output parameters of an x-ray machine from a single test exposure and using the data for organ dose estimates.[150]
4. Experimentally determined normalized depth-dose curves can be used in conjunction with monographic localization of the embryo/fetus.[145]

Methods 1 and 2 are the most frequently used.

Table 18-9 summarizes the estimated fetal exposure for various radiodiagnostic procedures as found in several studies.[148-153] Fetal exposure is usually regarded as equivalent to uterine or ovarian exposure. The highest dose to the fetus is delivered by barium enema and urethrocystography, whereas the lowest doses are delivered by examinations of remote areas (i.e., skull, thorax). Table 18-10 shows the estimated fetal dose during CT.[153-156]

Fetal dose estimates vary among different studies, as can be readily seen in Table 18-9.

A few factors influence the fluoroscopic and radiographic radiation exposure[4]:

1. Type of x-ray equipment. Exposure may vary by a factor of 2 or more with the use of different intensifiers and cameras.
2. Differences in technique used by the radiologist may contribute to the variation of exposure by a factor of 1.7 for fluoroscopy and 25 for radiography. Differences in technique may involve variations in fluoroscopic exposure time, number of films taken, beam size, maintenance of image quality, and imaging area.
3. Automatic versus manual control of fluoroscopy.
4. Obesity index, which depends on height and weight of the patient.
5. Cooperation of the patient.
6. Method of estimation. For example, fetal radiation dose during fluoroscopy assisted surgical treatment of hip fractures normalized to entrance surface dose was 23% higher compared to dose normalized to dose area product. Dose normalized to dose area product showed a dependence on tube potential and tube filtration. Conceptus dose from such a procedure is usually less than 1 mGy (0.1 rad) during all trimesters.[157]

Conceptus radiation dose associated with fluoroscopic imaging during a cardiac catheter ablation procedure was estimated by anthropomorphic phantoms simulating pregnancy and thermoluminescent dosimeters. For a typical examination, the average radiation dose to the conceptus was <1 mGy (100 mrad) at all periods of gestation.[158]

Table 18-8
Exposures of a Pregnant Woman to Naturally Occurring Background Radiation During 9 Months of Pregnancy*

TYPE OF RADIATION	EXPOSURE (mrad/9 months) MOTHER SOFT TISSUE	EMBRYO SOFT TISSUE
Potassium 40 (^{40}K)	14–18	10–14[a]
Daughters of radium-226	–	–
Carbon 14 (^{14}C)	0.5–1.3	0.5–1.3
External terrestrial	36	36
Cosmic rays	37	37
Total exposure	90	<86

* The dosage to the embryo is less because the embryo has a higher water content and a higher extracellular volume than the adult. Ossification does not occur in the early stages of pregnancy; therefore, radium and strontium localization would occur only in the latter portion of gestation.

SOURCE: Adapted from Brent RL. Effects and risks of medically administered isotopes to the developing embryo. In: Fabro S, Scialli AR, eds. Drug and Chemical Action in Pregnancy. New York, NY: Marcel Dekker, 1986, pp 427–439.

MAGNETIC RESONANCE IMAGING

Magnetic resonance imaging (MRI) (interchangeably called nuclear magnetic resonance, NMR) may replace the CT scanner for some diagnostic imaging. With MRI, patients are subjected to very high magnetic fields (static, rapidly varying, and radiofrequency). The background magnetic field ranges from 36 to 70μT (Tesla), patients' exposure during MRI is up to about 2T and MRI operators may be exposed to 5-100mT.[159] Studies thus far have not indicated any potential hazard to the unborn child.[160,161] Mice exposed to MRI at the magnetic isocenter or at the entrance to the magnetic lumen had a significantly higher rate of eye malformations

Table 18-9
Average Fetal Exposure Dose in Various Radiodiagnostic Procedures (mrad)*

EXAMINATION	SWEDEN 1977 (151)	USA 1980 (152)	UK 1986 (149)	ITALY 1987 (148)	USA 1999 (153)
Head, sinus	<1	<0.01	<1	<1	4
Full spine		128		227	
Cervical spine	<1	<0.01		<1	2 (2 views)
Dorsal spine	<100	0.6	<1	<1	9
Lumbar spine	620	408	346		
Lumbosacral region	180	639		385	359
Shoulder, clavicle, sternum	<1	<0.01		<1	
Arm	<1				1
Pelvis	190	194	165	238	40
Hip and femur	370	128		51	213 (1 view)
Femur (lower two-thirds)	50				
Lower leg, knee	<1				1
Lungs, ribs	<3	0.5	<1		
Lung (photofluorography)	<10			<1	
Lungs and heart	<5	0.06	<1	<1	0.07
Abdomen	200	263	289	233	245 (multiple views)
Upper GI tract	56	48	360	151	56
Small intestine	180				6
Barium enema	700	822	1600	1534	3986
Cholecystography, Cholangiography	24	5	60		
Urography (IVP)	880	814	358	505	1398
Retrograde pyelography	800				
Urethrocystography	1500				
Pelvimetry	460				
Obstetrical abdomen	150				
Hysterosalpingography	590				
Cerebral angiography	<10				
Mammography		†			20
Dental (single exposure)	0.01				0.0001

* Fetal dose is considered as equivalent to uterine or ovarian dose.

† Not computed but treated as negligible relative to absorbed dose to the female breasts (212–766 mrad).

Table 18-10
Fetal Exposure During Computed Tomography

EXAMINATION	FETAL DOSE (mrad)[a]
Head	<50[b]
Chest	100[b]–450
Chest/abdomen	240
Abdomen	240–2600[b]
Abdomen/pelvis	640
Pelvis	730
Pelvimetry	250[c]
Lumbar spine	3500[d]

[a] Fetal dose is considered equivalent to ovary dose.

[b] 10 slices.

[c] 1 slice.

[d] 5 slices.

SOURCE: Adapted from Toppenberg KS, Hill DA, Miller DP. Safety of radiographic imaging during pregnancy. Am Fam Physician. 1999;59:1813–1818, 1820. Murphy F, Heaton B. Patient doses received during whole body scanning using an Elscint 905 CT scanner. Br J Radiol. 1985;58:1197–1201. Schonken P, Marchal G, Coenen Y, et al. Body and gonad doses in computer tomography of the trunk. J Belge Radiol. 1978;61:363–371. McCullough EC, Payne JT. Patient dosage in computed tomography. Radiology. 1978;129:457–463.

than controls.[162] However, the mouse strain used in this study was genetically prone to these malformations. MRI fields under clinically realistic conditions did not enhance the teratogenic effect of X-ray (30 rad) on the developing eye of the mouse strain C57B1/6J.[163] Prolonged midgestational exposure of mice to MRI conditions currently used for human clinical imaging did not cause overt embryotoxicity or teratogenicity. However, a slight significant reduction in fetal crown-rump length was observed after prolonged exposure.[164] Cultured lymphocytes exposed to MRI during growth and division did not exhibit an increase in chromatid or chromosome lesions.[165] The National Radiological Protection Board has indicated that although there is evidence to suggest that the developing embryo is not sensitive to the magnetic field encountered in NMR clinical imaging, more studies are needed to rule out adverse developmental effects. Until more conclusive evidence is available, it is therefore considered prudent to exclude pregnant women from this procedure during the first trimester, when organ development is taking place.[166]

More recent estimations suggest that MRI does not seem to be dangerous to the course of pregnancy.[167] Although MRI imaging is not recommended during the first trimester and use of contrast material is not recommended in pregnant patients, fast MRI is useful in various obstetric settings and acute conditions in pregnancy[168,169] and in the evaluation of the perinatal brain[170]. MRI is considered by some clinicians to be the method of choice for antenatal pelvimetry.[171,172] It was also suggested for evaluation of lumbar herniated disc in pregnancy.[173]

A questionnaire study of MRI workers suggested an adverse effect on fertility and birth weight. The relative risk for miscarriage was 1.27, 95% CI 0.92–1.77, p = 0.07.[174] The validity of this self-reported data was questioned.[159]

RADIOTHERAPY

Radiotherapy involves large doses of radiation that are likely to affect the fetus deleteriously, especially if given to the abdominal region. If the dose delivered to the embryo during the early organogenetic period is hundreds of rad, the embryo will probably be aborted. During the second and third trimesters there is high chance of irreversible damage to the central nervous system. If the fetus absorbs 50 rad or more at any time during gestation, there is a significant possibility that the fetus may be damaged.[1] As mentioned earlier, the fetal exposure dose should be estimated by the radiologist, and the parents should be informed about the real probability of malformations and damage to the central nervous system. In some instances the human fetus has survived and has even appeared normal after exposure to doses exceeding 50 rad,[69,175] but this of course should not be regarded as the rule.

OCCUPATIONAL EXPOSURE

A radiation worker is defined as one whose annual exposure exceeds 0.5 rem. The radiation dose that an occupational worker may receive in a year is 5 rem.

Women of childbearing age working regularly with radiation must be monitored by film or TLD badge.[176] Few workers, male and female, actually receive an annual dose approaching 5 rem.[61] If average annual exposure exceeds 3 rem or if there are peak periods of higher exposure, the worker of childbearing age may receive more than 0.5 rem in the first 2 months of the pregnancy.[61] Women radiologists can work without interruption during pregnancy if proper precautions are taken, even with a heavy daily workload.[177] The U.S. Nuclear Regulatory Commission suggests that women who are or expect to become pregnant and whose fetuses could receive 0.5 rem or more before birth seek ways to reduce their exposure within their present job or delay having children until they change job locations.[178]

Currently, the U.S. Nuclear Regulatory Commission requires that the radiation dose to the embryo/fetus during the entire pregnancy, due to occupational exposure of a declared pregnant woman, does not exceed 0.5 rem (5 mSv). The National Council on Radiation Protection and Measurement recommends a monthly equivalent dose limit of 0.05 rem (0.5 mSv) to the embryo/fetus once the pregnancy is known. Any monthly dose of less than 0.1 rem (1 mSv) may be considered as not a substantial variation. If the patient has already received a dose exceeding 0.5 rem in the period between conception and declaration of pregnancy, an additional dose of 0.05 rem is allowed during the remainder of the pregnancy. In addition, efforts to avoid substantial variation above a uniform monthly dose rate are required so that all the 0.5 rem allowed dose does not occur in a short period during the pregnancy.[179]

The Israel Ministry of Industry, Trade and Labor recommends that a woman in the reproductive age (up to 45 years) will not be exposed during her work or professional training to radiation dose equivalent (external and internal sources) exceeding 5 rem/year; average monthly exposure should not exceed 0.4 rem. A pregnant woman will not be exposed during her work or professional training to radiation dose equivalent (external and internal sources) of more than 1 rem during the entire pregnancy; average monthly exposure should not exceed 0.15 rem.[180]

PATERNAL IRRADIATION

The effects of radiation on the testes were discussed earlier in this chapter.

The Avon Longitudinal Study of Pregnancy and Childhood (ALSPAC) showed a downward but insignificant trend in birth weight and fetal growth in infants to fathers who received diagnostic x-ray examinations likely to deliver significant gonadal doses within 1 year prior to conception.[181]

A study looking at the proportion of malformations in children fathered by testicular cancer patients treated with radiotherapy did not reveal any difference compared to a control group or to the incidence of malformations in the general population.[182]

The effects of paternal irradiation have been studied in Hiroshima and Nagasaki survivors. No increases in malformations, fetal death rate, or birth weight were found.[183,184]

No association was found between occupational exposure to low-level ionizing radiation of male nuclear industry workers and infertility.[185] Occupational paternal periconceptional exposure to ionizing radiation was not associated with an increased risk for childhood cancer in the offspring.[133,186] No association was found between paternal occupational preconceptional irradiation and adverse pregnancy outcome.[187,188] Another study showed an association between childhood leukemia and paternal preconception occupational exposure involving radiation (odds ratio, 3.23; 95% CI, 1.36–7.22) as well as with other factors such as wood dust and benzene.[189] Ionizing radiation alone gave an odds ratio of 2.35 (95% CI, 0.95–6.22).

Preliminary results of the Oxford Survey of Childhood Cancers suggest preconception paternal exposure to radionuclides was associated with relative risk of 2.87 (95% CI, 1.15–7.13) for childhood cancer.[190] The association between paternal preconceptional radiation dose and childhood leukemia has not been confirmed by studies using objectively determined doses.[191]

The results of many of these studies are confounded by small numbers and multiple exposures of some parents.

COSMIC RAYS (AIR TRAVEL)

Exposure to cosmic rays varies with the change in altitude, latitude, and solar activity. The flux of cosmic rays increases by approximately 100% for every 1.5–2 km above sea level.[2] Assuming that a jet aircraft flies at an average altitude of 8 km, the mean dose rate is 0.84 μGy/h (84 μrad/h) compared to 0.04 μGy/h (4 μrad/h) at sea level. For example, the cosmic ray dose to a person flying from New York to Paris round trip is 31 μGy (3.1 mrem) for subsonic flight and 24 μGy (2.4 mrem) for supersonic flight (subsonic flight is usually at an altitude of approximately 11 km; supersonic flight is at about 19 km).[2] Although supersonic flights take place at higher altitudes, the overall absorbed dose is less, since the flight is faster by a factor of two to three.

The average annual effective dose equivalent from cosmic rays for airline crew members is 0.8 mSv (80 mrem). Astronauts on

Apollo space missions and lunar landings have been in the range of 2 mrem/h^2.

The European Directive on Radiation Protection requires that exposure of air crew to cosmic radiation should be assessed if it is likely to exceed 1 mSv/year (100 mrem/y).[192] Guidance for exposure of air crews was also issued by the U.S. Federal Aviation Administration.[193]

Estimation of the equivalent dose of galactic radiation was almost the same at all depths of the mother's abdomen.[194] But, in general, offspring of air pilots and cabin attendants did not seem to be at increased risk of adverse pregnancy outcome.[195]

COUNSELING THE PREGNANT WOMAN

In all instances of counseling parents concerning the hazards to the embryo/fetus exposed to radiation, biological knowledge is only one facet to be considered. As mentioned earlier, the hazards of exposure to diagnostic radiation (0.02–5 rad) present an extremely low risk to the embryo when compared with the "spontaneous" risks. More than 15% of human embryos abort spontaneously. About 3% may have major malformations, 4% have intrauterine growth retardation, and 8–10% have early- or late-onset genetic disease.[1]

A systematic approach of patient evaluation should be used to obtain the following information:

- Stage of pregnancy at time of exposure
- Menstrual history
- Previous pregnancy history
- History of congenital malformations and genetic diseases
- Other potentially harmful exposures and environmental factors during the pregnancy
- Maternal and paternal age
- Type of radiation study, dates, and numbers of studies performed
- Estimate of the fetal exposure by a radiologist or medical physicist
- Status of the pregnancy - wanted or unwanted
- Emotional maturity of the family
- Religion and ethical values of the family

The applicable abortion laws should also be taken into consideration.

This information should be evaluated with both patient and counselor to arrive at a decision. The information delivered to the patient should be clearly documented in the medical record, including the idea that every pregnancy has a risk of problems. It also should be conveyed that the notion of no increased risk does not mean that the counselor is guaranteeing the outcome of the pregnancy. The physician may consider performing an ultrasound examination to rule out radiation-induced microcephaly or growth retardation.

The maximal theoretical risk attributed to a 1-rad exposure, approximately 0.003%, is thousands of times smaller than the spontaneous risks of malformations, abortions, or genetic diseases.[1] Thus, the present maximal permissible occupational exposures of 0.5 rem for pregnant women and 5 rem for medical exposure are extremely conservative. There is no medical justification for terminating pregnancy because of radiation exposure in women exposed to 5 rad or less.[1] The specter of radiation hazards should not be invoked to circumvent a social or legal problem.

Although radiodiagnosis involves fetal doses of less than 5 rad, which are not considered to be teratogenic, many pregnant women exposed to it perceive their teratogenic risk as unrealistically high.[196] This may be due to the anxiety provoked by the term *radiation* and by misinformation. An effective counseling process in these cases was shown to reduce the perception of teratogenic risk from 25.5 ± 4.3% to 15.7 ± 3.0% ($p < 0.05$), thus preventing unnecessary termination of otherwise wanted pregnancies.[196]

The benefits of radiotherapy in cancers such as cervical and breast carcinomas and lymphomas should be weighed against the potential risk to the fetus. Information necessary for determining the potential reproductive effects of radiotherapy include gestational age, absorbed fetal dose-equivalent, dose-rate and risk periods (i.e., neuronal migration from proliferative zones). Appropriate abdominal shielding can reduce fetal dose by 50% or more.[197]

The ICRP advises that fetal dose below 10 rad (100mGy) should not be considered a reason for terminating a pregnancy.[198]

RADIONUCLIDES

Physics and Biology

An element has a fixed number of protons, which determines its atomic number, but it may have a variable number of neutrons. For instance, ^{12}C, ^{13}C, and ^{14}C, which have six, seven, and eight neutrons, respectively, are referred to as isotopes of carbon, and each of them is a nuclide. Many nuclides have an unstable nucleus, owing to too many or too few neutrons; they are called radionuclides (radioisotopes). They disintegrate spontaneously and emit various forms of energy, collectively called radiation. The rate of disintegration is measured in units such as becquerel (Bq) and curie (Ci); 1 Bq is 1 disintegration per second and 1 Ci is the rate of disintegration of 1 g of pure ^{226}Ra (1 Ci = 3.7×10^{10} Bq; 1 Bq = 27 pCi, 1 pCi/L = 37 Bq/m^3). The half-life is the time required for half of a sample of radionuclide to decay. Table 18-11 shows the half-life and type of radiation of various radionuclides.[199]

The heavy alpha particle (positively charged particles; helium nuclei) has a very high LET but penetrates tissue poorly (in contrast to x-rays and γ-rays). Therefore, radionuclides are relatively nonhazardous when used externally, but they can be toxic if ingested. The distribution of absorbed energy is rather uniform in embryos exposed to x-rays and γ-rays. Conversely, radionuclides have a predictable but variable energy distribution in the embryo, depending on placental permeability, fetal distribution or tissue affinity, and the nature of radiation emitted (alpha particle, beta particle—identical with electrons or positrons, but arising from the nucleus; γ-ray electromagnetic radiation with wavelength much shorter than that of light or any combination). For example, ^{131}I will be absorbed and incorporated readily into the fetus with the development of the thyroid, as will plutonium and strontium with the development of the skeletal system. Thus, estimating the absorbed dose and hazards of a radionuclide is more complex than estimating externally administered radiation.

The mechanism of action of this form of ionizing radiation as well as its potential to cause congenital malformations, central nervous system damage, growth retardation, or embryonic death was discussed earlier in this chapter.

Types of Radionuclide

The number of agents available in nuclear medicine has expanded rapidly, and 150 substances containing 74 different radionuclides from 36 elements have been in use.[200] Over the years, the use of particular radionuclides has changed, the frequency of various

Table 18-11
Physical[a] and Effective[b] Half-Life and Type of Radiation of Various Radioisotopes

RADIONUCLIDE	PHYSICAL $t_{1/2}$	EFFECTIVE $t_{1/2}$	RADIATION
^{137}Cs	30.1 years	70 days	β^-, e^-, γ
^{47}Ca	4.54 days	4.5 days	β^-, γ
^{14}C	5730 years	12 days	β^-
^{51}Cr	27.7 days	27 days	e^-, γ
^{57}Co	270 days	9 days	e^-, γ
^{58}Co	71 days	8 days	β^+, γ
^{60}Co	5.27 years	10 days	β^-, γ
^{67}Ga	78.26 h		γ
^{198}Au	65 h	62 h	β^-, e^-, γ
^{111}In	67 h		γ
^{113m}In	99.5 min		e^-, γ
^{123}I	13.2 h		γ
^{125}I	60 days	42 days	e^-, γ
^{131}I	8.06 days	8 days	β^-, e^- γ,
^{192}I	74 days		β^-, e^-, γ
^{59}Fe	44.6 days	42 days	β^-, γ
^{197}Hg	64.4h	55.2 h	e^-, γ
^{203}Hg	46.6 days	11 days	β^-, e^- γ,
^{32}P	14.3 days	14 days	β^-
^{40}K	1.28 × 10^9 years		e^-, β^-, γ
^{42}K	12.36 h	12 h	β^-, γ
^{75}Se	120 days		e^-, γ
^{22}Na	2.6 years	11 days	β^+, γ
^{24}Na	15.02 h	14 h	β^-, γ
^{85}Sr	64.8 days	64 days	e^-, γ
^{90}Sr	28.5 years	15 years	β^- (DR)[c]
^{35}S	87.4 days	44 days	β^-
^{99m}Tc	6.02 h		e^-, γ
^{201}Tl	73.5 h		Γ (DR)
^{204}Tl	3.8 years		B^-, γ
^{224}Ra	3.6 days	3.6 days	B, α (DR)
^{226}Ra	160 years	44 years	A, e^-, γ (DR)
^{3}H	12.35 years	12 days	B^-,
^{127}Xe	36.4 days		e^-, γ
^{133}Xe	5.25 days		B^-, e^- γ^-,
^{90}Y	64.1 days	64 h	B^-

[a] The time required for the activity to decrease by 50%.
[b] The time required for the amount of a particular specimen of a radionuclide in a system to be reduced to half its initial value as a consequence of both radioactive decay and other processes, such as biological elimination.
[c] Daughter radiation (daughter radionuc lide is the decay product of a radionuclide).
SOURCE: Adapted from Reynolds JEF, Prasad AB, eds. Martindale, The Extra Pharmacopeia. London, UK: Pharmaceutical Press, 1982, pp 1386–1400. Mettler FA, Moseley RD. Medical Effects of Ionizing Radiation. New York, NY: Grune & Stratton, 1985, pp 206–209.

procedures in nuclear medicine has increased, several procedures have been introduced, and others have been eliminated.[147] For example, placental localization with isotopes (even with ^{99m}Tc, which delivers a very low dose to the fetus) has been completely replaced by ultrasound.

Radioactive Iodine. The usual forms of iodine are ^{123}I, ^{125}I, and ^{131}I. Isotope ^{125}I is used to label minute doses of hormones for in vivo and in vitro assays; ^{123}1 is used for uptake studies; ^{131}I can be given bound to protein or as the inorganic ion. It is used for thyroid uptake scanning and treatment of thyrotoxicosis and thyroid carcinoma as well as for other medical purposes not related to the thyroid. Inorganic iodides readily cross the placenta, in contrast to protein-bound iodides. Over time, substantial amounts of iodide are released from the protein and then cross the placenta. The fetal thyroid has more affinity to iodides than does the maternal (Table 18-12), and it begins to absorb and incorporate the iodide by the tenth week of gestation.[141] Ablative doses of ^{131}I given to the mother may result in fetal thyroid destruction. So far, the lowest dose reported to destroy the fetal thyroid was 12.2 mCi in a fractionated manner; 9.2 mCi of ^{131}I was given after the 74th day of gestation.[201] There are no reports of immediate deleterious fetal effects from tracer doses of radioactive iodine (147), but there is a theoretical possibility of induction of thyroid carcinoma. The fetal whole-body dose consists mainly of gamma rays, whereas the fetal thyroid dose is a combination of gamma rays and beta particles. This makes the fetal whole-body dose significant compared with the thyroid dose.

Other Radionuclides. Many radionuclides are bound to macroaggregates and macromolecules; they cross the placenta in small amounts, and the radiation dose delivered to the fetus is very small. For example, ^{99m}Tc is used in many diagnostic procedures. Sodium ^{99m}Tc pertechnetate is used for thyroid imaging. The radiation dose delivered with this radionuclide is lower than that of iodide because of its short physical half-life and short duration in the thyroid (since little of it is organically bound).

Radioactive phosphorus or gold is used in the treatment of polycythemia or peritoneal malignancies. High-dose radioactive phosphorus may result in embryonic abnormality and death in animals; this is also the case for radioactive strontium.[202]

Inorganic radioactive potassium, sodium, phosphorus, cesium, thallium, selenium, chromium, iron, and strontium cross the placenta readily, but their use is very limited.

Dose Estimation

The dose to the embryo is dependent on the form of the radionuclide, the site of administration, and the nature of the disease. In any case of exposure to radionuclides during pregnancy, the

Table 18-12
Thyroidal Radioiodine Dose of the Fetus

GESTATION PERIOD	FETAL/MATERNAL RATIO (THYROID GLAND)	DOSE TO THYROID (FETUS) (rad/μCI)*
10–12 weeks	–	0.001 (precursors)
12–13 weeks	1.2	0.7
Second trimester	1.8	6
Third trimester	7.5	–
Birth imminent	–	8

* Rad/μCi of ^{131}I ingested by mother.
SOURCE: Adapted from Brent RL. Effects and risks of medically administered isotopes to the developing embryo. In: Fabro S, Scialli AR, eds. Drug and Chemical Action in Pregnancy. New York, NY: Marcel Dekker, 1986, pp 427–439. Fabro S, Brown NA, Scialli AR. Radionuclides in pregnancy. Reprod Toxicol (Med Lett). 1986;5:17–22.

embryonic dose should be calculated. Often this dose will be less than the maternal dose because the nature of the radionuclide limits its ability to cross the placenta. Methods to estimate the dose to the embryo from radionuclides have been devised.[203,204]

Adult administered activity in various clinical radiopharmaceutical procedures is presented in Table 18-13.[147,205–207] The estimated embryonic/fetal doses from several radionuclides and nuclear medicine procedures are shown in Tables 18-14 and 18-15.[208] Fetal exposure in most studies using ^{99m}Tc involve <500 mrad; in hepatobiliary Tc HIDA scan 150 mrad, in ventilation-perfusion scan 215 mrad (perfusion, Tc – 175 mrad; ventilation, ^{133}Xe –40 mrad) and ^{131}I at fetal thyroid tissue 590 rad.[153]

Table 18-13
Clinical Radiopharmaceutical Procedures

RADIOPHARMACEUTICAL	STUDY	ADULT ADMINISTERED ACTIVITY
^{32}*P*-Sodium phosphate	Therapy, polycythemia vera	2.3 mCi/m^2
^{51}Cr-albumin	GI protein loss	50 μCi IV
^{51}Cr-chromate	Red cell survival	160 μCi IV
^{51}Cr-chromate	Red cell mass	25 μCi IV
^{51}Cr-chromate	Red cell in vivo	160 μCi IV
^{51}Cr-chromate red blood cells	Spleen imaging	200 μCi IV
^{57}Co-vitamin B_{12}	Vitamin B_{12} absorption	0.5 μCi PO
^{60}Co-vitamin B_{12}	Vitamin B_{12} absorption	0.5 μCi PO
^{59}Fe-citrate	Iron absorption	5 μCi PO (700 μg ferrous ammonium sulphate, 300 mg ascorbic acid
^{59}Fe-citrate	In vivo counting for effective hematopoiesis	20 μCi IV
^{59}Fe-citrate	Iron plasma clearance and turnover	20 μCi IV
^{59}Fe-citrate	Iron red blood cell uptake	20 μCi IV
^{67}Ga-citrate	Tumor/abscess imaging	3–10 mCi IV
^{75}Se-selenomethionine	Pancreas imaging	250 μCi IV or 4 μCi/kg, whichever is less
^{99m}Tc-diphosphonate	Myocardial imaging	15 mCi IV
^{99m}Tc-diphosphonate or pyrophosphate	Bone imaging	15–25 mCi IV
^{99m}Tc-DTPA	Brain imaging	15–20 mCi IV (no perchlorate)
^{99m}Tc-DTPA	Kidney imaging	15 mCi IV
^{99m}Tc-DTPA iron ascorbate	Kidney imaging	15 mCi IV
^{99m}Tc-human serum albumin	Pericardial imaging	10 mCi IV
^{99m}Tc-human albumin microspheres	Lung perfusion study	3 mCi IV
^{99m}Tc-human serum albumin	Placenta imaging	1–2 mCi IV
^{99m}Tc-macroaggregated albumin	Lung perfusion study	3 mCi IV
^{99m}Tc-macroaggregates	Venous imaging for thrombosis	6 mCi IV
^{99m}Tc-pertechnetate	Vacular flow	20 mCi IV
^{99m}Tc-pertechnetate	Thyroid uptake when uptake is low, organification blocked	1–3 mCi IV
^{99m}Tc-pertechnetate	Thyroid scan	8–10 mCi IV
^{99m}Tc-pertechnetate	Ectopic gastric tissue (e.g., Meckel's diverticulum)	100 μCi/kg
^{99m}Tc-pertechnetate	Brain imaging	15–20 mCi IV (200 mg potassium perchlorate orally prior to exam)
^{99m}Tc-pertechnetate	Cartoid or cerebral hemisphere studies	20 mCi IV
^{99m}Tc-sulfur colloid	Bone marrow imaging	10 mCi IV
^{99m}Tc-sulfur colloid	Spleen imaging	3 mCi IV
^{99m}Tc-sulfur colloid	Liver imaging	3 mCi IV
^{111}In-DTPA	Cerebrospinal fluid rhinorrhea	0.5 mCi IT
^{123}I-iodide	Thyroid uptake	100 μCi PO
^{123}I-iodide	TSH thyroid uptake study	100 μCi PO (10 U Thytropar IM × 3 days prior to test)
^{123}I-iodide	T_3 suppression thyroid uptake	100 μCi PO (25 μg cytomel t.i.d. × 7 days prior to test)

Table 18-13
Clinical Radiopharmaceutical Procedures (*Continued*)

RADIOPHARMACEUTICAL	STUDY	ADULT ADMINISTERED ACTIVIT
^{123}I-iodide	Thyroid imaging	100 μCi PO
^{123}I-iodohipputate	Kidney function	1–2 mCi IV
^{123}I-iodohippurate	Kidney imaging	1–2 mCi IV
^{125}I-human serum albumin	Plasma volume	4 μCi IV
^{131}I-fibrinogen	Venous imaging for thrombosis	100 mCi
^{131}I-iodide	Thyroid uptake	10 μCi PO
^{131}I-iodide	TSH uptake study	10 μCi PO (10 U Thytropar IM × 3 days prior to test)
^{131}I-iodide	T3 suppression	10 μCi PO (25 μg cytomel tid × 7 days prior to test)
^{131}I-iodide	Thyroid imaging	100 μCi PO
^{131}I-iodide	Thyroid therapy	5–20 mCi PO for thyrotoxicosis; 75–100 mCi PO for thyroid cancer
^{131}I-iodohippurate	Kidney function	3.5 μCi/kg body weight IV, not to exceed 300 μCi
^{131}I-iodohippurate	Kidney imaging	200 μCi IV
^{131}I-oleic acid	Intestinal fat absorption studies	50 μCi PO
^{131}I-rose Bengal	Liver imaging	3 mCi IV
^{131}I-triolein	Intestinal fat absorption studies	50 μCi PO
^{127}Xe gas	Lung ventilation study	15 mCi by inhalation
^{133}Xe gas	Lung ventilation study	15 mCi by inhalation
^{129}Cs-chloride	Myocardial imaging	5–6 mCi IV
^{169}Yb-DTPA	Cerebrospinal fluid rhinorrhea	0.5 mCi IT
^{169}Yb-DTPA	Normal pressure hydrocephalus	1mCi IT
^{201}Tl-chloride	Myocardial imaging	1–3 mCi IV

SOURCE: Adapted from Brent RL. Effects and risks of medically administered isotopes to the developing embryo. In: Fabro S, Scialli AR, eds. Drug and Chemical Action in Pregnancy. New York, NY: Marcel Dekker, 1986, pp 427–439. Saenger EL. Protocol Book of Radioisotope Laboratory. Cincinnati, OH: University of Cincinnati Medical Center, 1976.
Kereiakes JG, Feller PA, Ascoi F, et al. Pediatric radiopharmaceutical dosimetry. In: Radiopharmaceutical Dosimetry Symposium. U.S. Department of Health, Education, and Welfare (Food and Drug Administration) Publication No 76-8044. Rockville, MD: US DHEW, Bureau of Radiological Health, 1976. Roedler HD, Kaul A, Hine GJ. Internal Radiation Dose in Diagnostic Nuclear Medicine. Berlin: Hoffman, 1978.

Table 18-14
Dose Estimated to Embryo from Radiopharmaceuticals

RADIOPHARMACEUTICAL	EMBRYO DOSE (rad/mCi ADMINISTERED)
^{99m}Tc-human serum albumin	0.018
^{99m}Tc-lung aggregate	0.035
^{99m}Tc-phospon0.02-0.022hate	
^{99m}Tc-polyphosphate	0.036
^{99m}Tc-sodium pertechnetate	0.029–0.037
^{99m}Tc-stannous glucoheptonate	0.040
^{99m}Tc-sulfur colloid	0.032
^{201}Tl-chloride	0.185
^{123}I-sodium iodide (15% uptake)-	0.032
^{131}I-sodium iodide (15% uptake)	0.100
^{131}I-sodium iodide (35% uptake)	0.185
^{123}I-rose bengal	0.130
^{131}I-rose bengal	0.680
^{67}Ga-citrate	0.292

SOURCE: Adapted from Kereiakes JG, Rosenstein M. Handbook of Radiation Doses in Nuclear Medicine and Diagnostic X-Ray. Boca Raton, FL: CRC Press, 1980, p 211. Smith EM, Warner GG. Estimates of radiation dose to the embryo from nuclear medicine procedures. J Nuclear Med. 1976;17:836–839. Kereiakes JG, Rosenstein M. Handbook of Radiation Doses in Nuclear Medicine and Diagnostic X-Ray. Boca Raton, FL: GRC Press, 1980, p 170.

Risk Estimation

Although it has been suggested that background and fallout radiation contribute to spontaneous mutation rate and congenital malformations, most studies have not found a correlation between levels of background radiation and any health hazard, including adverse pregnancy outcome.[200,209–211] It is important to remember these data when considering that many of the exposures from nuclear medicine procedures are within the order of magnitude of background radiation.

The reproductive effects of radionuclides have been less studied and less generalized than those of external radiation. This may be attributed to differences in placental permeability, nonrandom distribution of the radiation, existence of specific target organs, biological differences, or disease states that may affect the metabolism, and the exponential decrease in radiation dose rate over time. In addition, because the amount of energy absorbed over a given length of time (LET) is different for various radiations, 1-Gy aliquots from different radionuclides are not necessarily equally toxic.[200]

Teratogenic, embryonic/fetal, and growth-retarding effects in laboratory animals have been demonstrated for ^{137}Cs, ^{32}P, ^{89}Sr, ^{90}Sr, and [^{3}H]thymidine.[212] It is likely that similar effects could be demonstrated for any radionuclide if the exposure could be adjusted to deliver a cytotoxic dose of radiation to the embryo.

Table 18-15
Fetal Radiation Dose from Various Nuclear Medicine Procedures

STUDY	RADIOISOTOPE	FETAL DOSE (rad)
Pericardial imaging	^{99m}Tc-human serum albumin	0.18
Placenta imaging	^{99m}Tc-human serum albumin	0.018–0.036
Lung perfusion study	^{99m}Tc-lung aggregate	0.105
Brain imaging	^{99m}Tc-pertechnetate	0.555–0.74
Bone marrow imaging	^{99m}Tc-sulfur colloid	0.32
Bone scan	^{99m}Tc-phosphonate	0.4–0.55
Spleen imaging	^{99m}Tc-sulfur colloid	0.096
Liver imaging	^{99m}Tc-sulfur colloid	0.096
	^{131}I-rose bengal	2.04
Thyroid scan	^{99m}Tc-pertechnetate	0.232–0.290
Thyroid uptake (15% uptake)	^{123}I-iodide	0.0032
	^{131}I-iodide	0.001
Thyroid imaging (15% uptake)	^{131}I-iodide	0.01
Thyroid imaging (35% uptake)	^{131}I-iodide	0.0185
Thyroid therapy	^{131}I-iodide	0.05–2 (thyrotoxicosis) 7.5–15 (thyroid cancer)
Myocardial imaging	^{201}Tl-chloride	0.185–0.555
Tumor/abscess imaging	^{67}Ga-citrate	0.876–2.92

SOURCE: Adapted from Brent RL. Effects and risks of medically administered isotopes to the developing embryo. In: Fabro S, Scialli AR, eds. Drug and Chemical Action in Pregnancy. New York, NY: Marcel Dekker, 1986, pp 427–439. Kereiakes JG, Rosenstein M. Handbook of Radiation Doses in Nuclear Medicine and Diagnostic X-Ray. Boca Raton, FL: GRC Press, 1980, p 170.

Doses to the embryo from standard nuclear medicine procedures are low. This may not be the case for radioactive iodine used for the treatment of thyrotoxicosis and thyroid carcinoma. It is extremely important that a competent expert calculate the fetal dose in any case of fetal or embryonic exposure. If the calculated dose to the embryo is 10 rad or more (about 100 mSv), the offspring should be considered to have a significant risk of a radiation-induced abnormality.[200] The Collaborative Perinatal Project monitored 21 exposures to diagnostic radionuclides (^{131}I, mainly unbound) in the first trimester and found one malformation with standardized relative risk (SRR) of 0.72.[213] For exposures during the whole pregnancy, 3 out of 50 had malformations with SRR of 1.99. It is not mentioned what radionuclides were used in this group, and in addition the numbers were small. However, apart from the well-documented thyroid damage from radioactive iodine, there have been no controlled studies demonstrating an association between nuclear medicine procedures and adverse pregnancy outcome. Nevertheless, it is recommended that pregnant women not undergo radioisotope studies, unless mandated by the clinical condition (i.e., suspected pulmonary embolism). The use of radioactive iodine should be avoided during pregnancy unless essential for the medical care of the mother and there is no substitute. Even if administered during the first 5–6 weeks of human gestation, when the fetal thyroid has not yet developed, the total fetal dose should be estimated.

In any case of exposure to radionuclides when it is known that the patient is pregnant or in any case of inadvertent exposure, the guidelines outlined in the section on counseling the pregnant woman should be followed.

The Chernobyl Accident

Accidents in nuclear plants, such as that at Chernobyl in the former Soviet Union, may pose a threat to human reproduction. It seems obvious that lethal radiation levels were reached, and such an exposure can cause fetal damage. Air contamination and radionuclides deposited on the skin or the ground serve as an external source of irradiation, and the inhalation or ingestion of radionuclides in food (especially milk) is considered to be internal exposure. European cities reported doses of radiation of 0.1–1 mSv,[214] which is equivalent to an extra year of background radiation. There is no consistent proof that radiation level of exposure reached 0.1 Gy (10 rad).[215] Exposure to such levels is unlikely to increase the incidence of gross congenital malformations. An increase in adverse phenomena related to stochastic effects might be expected; for example, increased risk of thyroid carcinoma induced in young children by ^{131}I-contaminated milk[216] and a dramatic increase (over 100-fold in some areas) in childhood thyroid cancer in Belarus, Ukraine, and Bryansk.[217] In Greece, infants exposed in utero to ionizing radiation from the Chernobyl accident had two to six times (95% CI, 1.4–5.1) the incidence of leukemia compared to unexposed children. No significant difference in leukemia incidence was found among children aged 12–47 months and after preconception exposure.[218] In the heavily contaminated southern part of Germany, there was a higher rate of trisomy-21 among fetuses conceived during the period of greatest radioactive exposure.[219] In the geographical areas of Belarus that received at least 555 Bq/m^2 radioactive contamination, an apparent increase in congenital anomalies (i.e., multiple anomalies, polydactyly, and limb reduction defects) was reported. But, epidemiological studies are needed to establish this association.[220] In Finland there were no differences in the expected/observed rates of congenital malformations, preterm births, and stillbirths.[221] In Hungary no measurable germinal mutagenic effect was revealed[222] and in Norway no dose-response associations were observed with perinatal health problems.[223] In both countries the rate of live births[222] and the total number of pregnancies[223] somewhat decreased, although there was no increase in the rate of induced or legal abortions. Interestingly, on the other hand, there was an increased rate of termination of pregnancies in Greece and Denmark in the months after the Chernobyl accident, even though the radiation doses measured in these countries were not large enough to induce birth defects.[224,225] Thus, we see that high levels of anxiety can be invoked even by low amounts of radiation; in these two countries this anxiety caused more fetal deaths than the radiation itself. The importance of good and reliable counseling in such cases cannot be overemphasized.

RADON

Radon is an odorless, colorless, tasteless, and inert gas. It has several isotopes and radon daughters, all emitting mainly alpha radiation.

Radon in houses comes from building materials, the soil under the house, the water, and the domestic gas. Some building materials such as aerated concrete with alum shale and phosphogypsum from sedimentary ores have higher radium concentrations and cause enhanced radon concentrations indoors. Radon exhalation from walls, floors, and ceilings is dependent on radium concentration, emanation power, diffusion coefficient in the material, and quality and thickness of the applied sealant. Ventilation rate, as determined by meteorological conditions and human activities, has a strong influence on radon levels.

Radon and its daughters, after being attached to environmental airborne dust, stick to bronchial epithelial lining, releasing ionizing radiation (alpha particles) which may induce cancerous transformation.

Increased risk of lung cancer has been clearly documented in uranium miners and certain other miners exposed to radon and its daughters. The level of risk has not been so well quantitated in environmental exposure. There is an additive relationship between radon exposure and cigarette smoking for lung cancer risk.

No teratogenic effect was observed among the offspring of pregnant rats exposed to about 10,000 times the typical annual radon levels in houses.[226]

There are no human data on the effect of maternal exposure to radon during pregnancy. Since radon's main hazard is the ionizing radiation, a small risk cannot be excluded. The main emission consists of alpha particles, which do not penetrate tissues deeply but have high linear energy transfer. A study of 491 males employed at uranium mines revealed in their offspring low birth weight and a decreased male/female ratio.[227]

Indoor air concentration of radon should equal outdoor air concentration (0.2–0.7 pCi/L, or 7.4–26 Bq/m^3). Environmental standards for indoor residential air radon are 4–8 pCi/L (148–296 Bq/m^3), as guided by the Environmental Protection Agency and the National Council on Radiation Protection, respectively.

The action level set by the U.K. National Radiological Protection Board is 200 Bq/m^3 or 5.4 pCi/L.[228] On the year 2000, the U.S. Agency for Toxic Substances and Disease Registry (ATSDR) recommended remediation for homes with airborne radon concentrations of greater than 4 pCi/L (148 Bq/m^3).

VIDEO DISPLAY TERMINALS

Over the years, the microprocessor has brought video display terminals (VDTs) into offices and homes, and a massive increase in their use has been observed. It was estimated that in the United States 7 million people were occupationally exposed to VDTs in 1980.[229] The earliest complaints by operators of VDTs were concerned with visual problems and musculoskeletal discomfort.[166] Migraine, epilepsy (one case), and facial dermatitis were also reported.[166] The scale of expansion in the use of VDTs has prompted interest in the reproductive effects of radiation from these devices.

Physics

The VDT is a cathode ray tube that directs electrons at a screen coated with a fluorescent target, generally phosphor. The bombardment of the target with electrons causes the fluorescent material to emit light. Television sets operate in the same manner. The energy emitted by VDTs is in the form of electromagnetic radiation. It consists of ionizing radiation (x-ray), the biological effects of which have been discussed earlier in this chapter, and nonionizing radiation (ultraviolet, visible light, infrared, microwave, and electromagnetic fields), some of which can transmit energy to tissues as heat. It is important to remember that electromagnetic radiation decreases in proportion to the square of the distance between a point source and the observer. Therefore, one might expect a rapid decrease in radiation with increasing distance from the screen.

X-rays emitted by the cathode ray tube are entirely absorbed by the glass screen.[229] Several studies could not detect measurable ionizing radiation from VDTs (e.g., 0.01–0.05 mrad/h).[230–235]

Ultraviolet and visible light are emitted by the phosphor target of the VDT screen. The amount of ultraviolet radiation measured from VDTs is two to five orders of magnitude less than that of the environment.[231,233] The amount of heat produced from this type of radiation is estimated to be 1.75×10^{-6} cal.[236] In addition, the wavelength of ultraviolet radiation emitted from VDTs is not less than 336 nm;[233] the harmful range is considered to be higher than 300 nm.

No infrared radiation has been detected from VDTs tested.[231,233]

Nonionizing radiation in the form of microwave and extremely low frequency (ELF: 45–60 Hz) and very low frequency (VLF: 15 kHz) electromagnetic fields emitted from VDTs is in the same frequency range given off by most electrical appliances at home.[231,237] This amount of radiation is two orders of magnitude less than background.[233] Some VDTs are equipped with a flyback transformer, responsible for moving the arm of the cathode ray tube back and forth. People coming near the back casing of such a unit may be exposed to lower frequency electromagnetic radiation, with powers measured up to 800 mW/cm^2.[236] The casing can be modified to solve this problem.

Risk Estimation

Over the years, a few clusters of adverse pregnancy outcomes among women VDT operators were reported.[61,166,236] These clusters included spontaneous abortions, prematurity, neonatal respiratory disease, Down's syndrome, and birth defects. The malformations reported, which were different in each affected child, included clubfoot, underdeveloped eye, cleft palate, congenital heart defect, and neural tube defect. None of the reports of abnormal pregnancy presented a distinct or reproducible syndrome.

Current regulations require that x-ray emissions from any cathode ray tube be less than 0.5 mR/h at 5 cm.[61] Even at this maximum level, radiation exposure to the uterus (50 cm from the screen) would be minimal. A woman sitting at a VDT console for 30 hours a week would accumulate a maximum uterine dose of 0.006 rem during the first trimester, about one-quarter of the natural background radiation dose she would be receiving at the same time.[238] As the fetus grows, it may be physically closer to the terminal, but it would be shielded increasingly by the amniotic fluid.

The amount of nonionizing radiation emitted is very small and consists of frequencies that have not been shown to be harmful. Exposure to an improperly shielded flyback transformer would be associated with absorbing significant low frequency radio waves. Animal studies investigating magnetic field-induced abnormalities in chick embryos are inconclusive.[239–241]

Epidemiological studies dealing with these issues are fraught with pitfalls. A study reviewing occupations that might entail work with VDTs showed that in pregnancies in which a VDT had not been used, the rate of spontaneous abortions was 5.7%. The rate was 8.2 and 9.3% for women working with VDTs less and more than 15 hours weekly, respectively. In contrast, the rate of spontaneous abortions among women from groups not using VDTs was 7.8%.[242] These results were found later on by the authors themselves to be subjected to selection bias and recall bias.[243] In another study, response bias seemed to be a possible explanation for a suggested association with adverse reproductive effects.[244] Comparison of mothers of malformed children and their paired referents found no evidence that exposure to VDTs caused birth defects.[245] No mention was made in that report of miscarriages. Schnorr et al. compared a cohort of female telephone operators who used VDTs at work with a cohort of operators who did not use VDTs.[237] Operators who used VDTs had higher abdominal exposure to VLF electromagnetic fields (15 kHz), but not to ELF fields (45–60 Hz). VDT operators had no excess risk of spontaneous abortions, and there was no dose-response relation when the women's hours of VDT use per week were examined. In a case control study in Finland, no association was found between cardiovascular malformations and the use of VDTs at work or home among other parameters studied.[246] In another case control study the risk of congenital urinary tract anomalies was found not to be associated with VDTs.[247]

Based on the current data and the fact that a very large number of women are exposed occupationally to VDTs, it seems likely that the clusters reported were encountered by chance.[236] It appears that VDTs do not constitute a known radiation hazard.[61] In some countries, pregnant women may request a leave from working with VDTs, and they may be allowed to do so, based on the grounds of reducing worry.[248,249]

MICROWAVES, RADAR, RADIO WAVES, FM, AND DIATHERMY

Physics

Microwave, radar, radio wave, FM, and diathermy radiation sources all involve electromagnetic waves ranging in frequency from 27.5 MHz (diathermy) to 10^4–10^5 MHz (microwave communications).[1] The electromagnetic waves generated by diathermy are highly penetrating and can easily heat the human body. Microwaves of 2450 or 915 MHz produce hyperthermia but are less penetrating. Microwaves exceeding 10000 MHz produce significant hyperthermia at skin level but are minimally penetrating.[1] This type of radiation is incapable of producing ionizations within tissues.[15,250]

Biological Studies

Mice exposed during gestation days 0–19 to a 20-kHz magnetic field had a significant decrease in weight of whole brain, detectable on postnatal day 308. There was a decrease in DNA level and an increase in the activities of 2,3-cyclic nucleotide 3-phospodiesterase (marker for oligodendrocytes), nerve growth factor and acetylcholinesterase in the cortex.[251] Chick embryos exposed to 428-MHz radiofrequency radiation at a power density of 5.5 mW/cm^2 for more than 20 days had higher rates of embryo lethality and teratogenicity.[252] A few animal studies using a 27.12-MHz radiofrequency field showed an increased rate of resorption, incomplete cranial ossification, birth defects, reduced fetal weight, prenatal death, and reduced body weight in the exposed dams.[253–255] Those effects were related to increased maternal body temperature. In one study, 41.5°C was estimated to be a threshold temperature over which there is an increased incidence of adverse reproductive effects.[254] In another study, it appeared possible to ascribe some of the effects to a specific action of the radiofrequency radiation occurring independently of the rise in the temperature.[253] When 100-MHz radiofrequency was studied in rats, no increase in maternal colonic temperature or adverse pregnancy outcome was observed.[256] This exposure resulted in a specific absorption rate (SAR) of 0.4 W/kg, which corresponds to the maximum permissible level defined in 1982 by the American National Standards Institute. Since the unknowns and uncertainties are potentially significant, it was considered to apply a safety factor of 10, with a resultant SAR limit of 0.04 W/kg.[257] Individuals working near FM radio stations, radar, and microwave ovens are not exposed to the maximum permissible levels suggested for occupational and medical exposures.[1]

Human studies looking at adverse reproductive effects of radiofrequency radiation are controversial.[258] Investigations of human exposures to radiofrequency radiation are confounded by difficulties in determining the type and true extent of exposures, in selecting an appropriate control group for comparisons, in determining the existence and influence of many concomitant environmental factors, and in establishing the presence or measuring the frequency or severity of subjective complaints as well as objective findings in the studied populations.[258] In Danish physiotherapists exposed to high-frequency electromagnetic radiation, there was a lower rate of male children (23.5%), and these infants also had low birth weight[259] but no increase in congenital malformations.[260] In a case-control study, maternal exposure to microwave ovens was not found to be associated with cardiovascular malformations.[246]

A strong association between parental occupational exposures to electromagnetic fields could not be established; OR 2.8, 95% CI 0.9–8.7 for maternal exposure to radiofrequency radiation; OR 1.6, 95% CI 0.8–3.2 for paternal exposure to battery-powered forklifts.[261] The results of a recent study did not support the hypothesis that residential exposure to electromagnetic fields from power lines caused various congenital anomalies.[262]

Risk Estimation

There is no way to receive exposure from a microwave oven without bypassing several safety interlocks. In addition, it is easy to shield microwaves with a proper screen or metal foil.[1] If there was a door leak, it could theoretically result in a measurable exposure. But it should be remembered that electromagnetic radiation decreases in proportion to the square of the distance, so there should be no consequences several meters away from the microwave oven.

The eye and the embryo are most vulnerable to the thermal effects of microwave radiation because they cannot dissipate heat efficiently.[1] The nonthermal effects have not been clearly demonstrated, but they are still being investigated. There is no indication that this type of electromagnetic radiation can produce malignancy or mutations.[1] Microwave ovens properly handled should be regarded as safe.

Prenatal use of electric blankets and electrically heated water beds was not found to be associated with urinary tract anomalies unless subfertility existed.[247]

ULTRASOUND

Ultrasound is a widely used diagnostic modality in obstetrics and other fields. Its use in fetal monitoring and fetal diagnosis has expanded rapidly, and it has replaced obstetrical x-ray examinations. Deep tissue heating with ultrasound is a standard technique in physical therapy.

PHYSICS

Sound is a mechanical energy form in which small particles in a medium are made to oscillate. The oscillation of air molecules at frequencies of 20–20,000 Hz produces sound. Sound waves with a frequency above this range are called ultrasound. Medical ultrasound involves frequencies of 1–20 MHz, and the medium is water and tissues instead of air. The intensity of the sound energy, its alteration, and the exposure time determine the amount of energy reaching a given tissue.

In a diagnostic ultrasound examination, a significant proportion of the energy is absorbed and the rest is reflected. The reflection of the sound energy provides the basis for the imaging technique. The fraction of the energy absorbed produces heat within tissues. It is estimated that ultrasound intensities of 1 W/cm^2 will result in tissue temperature elevation of 0.8°C/min.[263] In Doppler fetal heart detectors, intensities are 0.75–75.0 mW/cm^2 (264). Intensities for diagnostic sector scanners may reach peak values of 2–200 mW/cm^2.[265] The theoretical temperature rise 2 cm from an external fetal monitor remains less than 1°C even after prolonged use.[263] In addition, further temperature loss occurs owing to removal of heat by circulating blood and by conduction of heat to other tissues.

The nonthermal effects include tissue disruption by the production of cavitation and streaming owing to the movement of particles in the sound field.[1] None of these effects occur with the energies utilized in diagnostic ultrasonography.[1]

Risk Estimation

In vitro studies have raised the possibility that commonly used ultrasound irradiation causes significant cellular damage.[266–270] Detectable biological effects from diagnostic ultrasound were not demonstrated in mammalian studies.[265,271,272] The American Institute of Ultrasound in Medicine concluded, in 1982, that there are no independently confirmed significant biological effects of ultrasound in mammals in the low megahertz frequency range and when intensities are below 100 mW/cm^2. Higher intensities with exposure time less than 500 seconds are not associated with biological effects as long as the product of intensity and exposure time is less than 50 J/cm^2.[265]

Epidemiological studies did not demonstrate that diagnostic ultrasound has any measurable or significant effects. The fetal anomaly rate was found to be 2.7%, which is comparable to the anomaly rate in the general population.[273] No difference was demonstrated in several measurements at birth, in neurological examination, or in developmental testing at 11–15 months of babies exposed antenatally to ultrasound done for amniocentesis.[274] Another study also did not find any difference in several birth parameters as well as neurological and cognitive testing at 7–12 years of age.[275] In addition, it was concluded that diagnostic ultrasound is safe with regard to the risk of childhood malignancy between birth and the sixth year.[135,276] After this period there appears to be a doubt, but the numbers are very small.

Therapeutic ultrasound involves higher intensity and may produce deep tissue heating. In a study where pregnant rats were exposed to shock-wave lithotriptor, fetuses located nearest the focal area of maximum shock-wave energy showed lower mean weight than controls but no recognizable gross or microscopic fetal damage.[277] Because of the potential of hyperthermia to induce birth defects, it is advisable to avoid this form of treatment during pregnancy.[265]

Another issue which drew attention is medical workers exposed to contact ultrasound waves, that is, no airspace between the energy source and the biological tissues. This is more hazardous than exposure to airborne ultrasound because air transmits less than 1% of this kind of energy. Although no definite conclusions could be drawn on its potential to cause adverse pregnancy outcome, avoiding unnecessary exposure of medical workers was suggested.[278]

Industrial ultrasound also involves very high intensities, and it is unlikely that there will be energy transfer to tissues.[265] The only exception is in the case of existence of a satisfactory coupling medium. In addition, standard safety precautions should provide adequate shielding of the ultrasound source.

LASER

Physics

The atomic nucleus is surrounded by electrons in orbits. When an electron is jumped, or excited, from an allowed orbit to a higher level, energy in the form of a photon is absorbed. When the electron returns to a lower energy state, a photon is omitted. This spontaneous emission can be accelerated if the excited state atom is struck by a photon of exactly the same energy as the spontaneously emitted photon. This accelerated process is called *stimulated emission,* and it yields two photons of the same energy level, which leaves the atom in exactly the same direction and phase.

Laser (light amplification by stimulated emission of radiation) is an active electron device that uses this process and converts input power into coherent electromagnetic radiation in the range of optic frequencies (ultraviolet, visible, or infrared). Unlike radiation emitted from the usual light sources, the laser produces a very narrow and intense beam of coherent light. The typical laser instrument consists of an energy input source, an active medium (atoms capable of undergoing stimulated emission), feedback mechanisms (totally and partially reflecting mirrors), and standard optical devices to focus the electromagnetic energy. The active medium may be solid (i.e., ruby crystal), liquid (i.e., tunable dyes), gas (i.e., helium-neon, carbon dioxide, argon ion), or a semiconductor. The choice of an active medium depends on the output power and wavelength required for a given application. Output may be delivered in a continuous wave, in a single pulse, or as a series of pulses. Carbon dioxide and excimer lasers produce extremely high output power, up to 10^9 W.

Lasers have various applications in the areas of materials processing, information handling, communication, research, arts and entertainment, and more. Examples of medical applications of lasers include surgery (carbon dioxide laser), various ophthalmological procedures (argon and excimer lasers), vaporization of lung tumors during bronchoscopy (neodymium:yttrium-aluminum-garnet laser), and coronary angioplasties (excimer laser).

The American National Standards Institute classified lasers into four classes (I–IV) in order of increasing risk of hazard.[279]

Biological Studies

The effects of laser in biological tissues can be divided into thermal and nonthermal; the latter may include driving chemical reactions, breaking atomic bonds, and creation of shock waves. Skin and eye damage is due mainly to denaturation of proteins resulting from hypothermia. Other hazards may include electrical shock, metal fumes released from processed material, and collateral radiation (e.g., intense light, arc lamps, ultraviolet radiation), which may induce delayed painful photokeratitis.[279] The magnitude of damage depends not only on the type of laser involved and its output power, but also on the duration of exposure.

Carbon dioxide laser surgery is used in obstetrics and gynecology via laparoscope for treatment of ectopic pregnancy[280] and intra-abdominally for reproductive pelvic surgical procedures (tubal anastomosis, adhesiolysis, etc.).[281]

Endoscopic fetal surgery by excimer laser (40 and 10 Hz) was studied in premature lambs.[282] Laser incisions were associated with smaller zones of devitalization compared to conventional cutting techniques using a scalpel. Albino rat embryos exposed to infrared laser beams (0.89 μm, 300 Hz for 256 and 128 seconds) had more preimplantation deaths and some disturbances in formation of the osseous skeleton.[283] Helium-neon lasers induced an increase in neuritic outgrowths of olfactory bipolar receptor cells in rat fetuses.[284]

Laser of chorionic plate vessels was found to improve significantly perinatal survival and reduce neurological morbidity in twin-twin transfusion syndrome compared with serial amnioreduction.[285] Successful obliteration of blood supply of a placental chorioangioma complicated by polyhydramnios using a diode laser at 25 weeks of gestation was reported. This was followed by an uneventful pregnancy and delivery and a healthy child at the age of 9 months.[286]

More studies are needed to evaluate the teratogenic potential of laser and its role in fetal therapy of malformations.

SUMMARY

It is well established that ionizing radiation may have adverse reproductive effects. At present, there is no indication that radiodiagnostic doses of ionizing radiation (<5 rad) during pregnancy increase the incidence of gross congenital malformations, intrauterine growth retardation, or abortion. The risks of acute exposures involving doses less than 5 rad are far below the spontaneous risks of the developing embryo. On the other hand, this does not mean that there are definitely no risks to the embryo exposed to low doses of ionizing radiation. It has not been determined whether there is a linear or exponential dose-response relationship or a threshold exposure for genetic, carcinogenic, cell-depleting, and life-shortening effects. Unnecessary x-ray or nuclear medicine procedures during pregnancy are not good medical practice, whereas medically indicated diagnostic roentgenograms are appropriate for pregnant women. A systematic approach of patient evaluation should be followed in any case of exposure during pregnancy and not only to consider the biological effects of ionizing radiation.

So far, it has not been proven that exposure to nonionizing radiation (VDT, microwave, ultrasound, etc.) below the maximal permissible level is associated with measurable adverse reproductive outcome. At present, ultrasound not only improves obstetrical care but also reduces the necessity of diagnostic x-ray examinations. Nevertheless, continued surveillance and more studies of potential risks are necessary.

REFERENCES

1. Brent RL. The Effects of Embryonic and Fetal Exposure to X-ray, Microwaves and Ultrasound. In: Brent RL, Beckman DA, eds. *Clinics in Perinatology, Teratology.* Vol 13. Philadelphia, PA: Saunders, 1986, pp 615–648.
2. Mettler FA, Moseley RD. *Medical Effects of Ionizing Radiation.* New York, NY: Grune & Stratton, 1985, pp 206–209.
3. Mossman KL. Medical radiodiagnosis and pregnancy: evaluation of options when pregnancy status is uncertain. *Health Phys.* 1985;48:297–301.
4. Rowley KA, Hill SJ, Watkins RA, et al. An investigation into the levels of radiation exposure in diagnostic examinations involving fluoroscopy. *Br J Radio.* 11987;60:167–173.
5. Kendall GM, Darby SC, Harries SV, et al. A frequency survey of radiological examinations carried out in National Health Service Hospitals in Great Britain in 1977 for diagnostic purposes, Report No NRPB-RI04. HMSO, National Radiological Protection Board, London, 1978.
6. Wall BF, Fisher ES, Shrimpton PC, et al. Current levels of gonadal irradiation from a selection of routine diagnostic x-ray examinations in Great Britain, Report No NRPB-RI05. HMSO. London: National Radiological Protection Board, 1980.
7. Albert RE, Omran AR, Brauer EW, et al. Follow-up study of patients treated by x-ray for tinea capitis. *Am J Public Health.* 1966;56:2114–2120.
8. Witherbee WD. Indications for roentgen therapy in chronic tonsillitis and pharyngitis. *Am J Roentgenol.* 1924;11:331–335.
9. Friedlander A. Status lymphaticus and enlargement of the thymus: with report of a case successfully treated by the x-ray. *Arch Pediatr.* 1907;24:490–501.
10. Kaplan II. The x-ray treatment of amenorrhea, with a report of 38 cases. *Am J Obstet Gynecol.* 1928;15:658–661.
11. Lione A. Ionizing radiation and human reproduction. *Reprod Toxicol.* 1987;1:3–16.
12. Smith H. The detrimental health effects of ionizing radiation. *Nuclear Med Commun.* 1992;13:4–10.
13. Prasad KN. Rationale for using multiple antioxidants in protecting humans against low doses of ionizing radiation. *Br J Radiol.* 2005;78:485–492.
14. Okada S, Hamilton HB, Egami N, et al. A review of thirty-year study of Hiroshima and Nagasaki atomic bomb survivors. *J Radiat Res (Tokyo).* 1975;16(suppl):1–164.
15. Brent RL. Radiation and other physical agents. In: Wilson JG, Fraser FC, eds. *Handbook of Teratology.* Vol. 1. New York, NY: Plenum, 1977, pp 153–223.
16. Brent RL. The effects of irradiation on the mammalian fetus. *Clin Obstet Gynecol.* 1960;3:928–950.
17. Lushbaugh CC, Casarett GW. The effects of gonadal irradiation in clinical radiation therapy: a review. *Cancer.* 1976;37:1111–1120.
18. Heller CG. Effects on germinal cell epithelium. In: Langham WH, ed. *Radiological Factors in Manned Space Flight.* National Radiation Council Publication No 1987. Washington, DC: National Academy of Sciences, NRC, 1967, pp 124–133.

19. Rowley MJ, Leach DR, Warner GA, et al. Effect of graded doses of ionizing radiation on the human testis. *Radiat Res.* 1974;59:665–678.
20. Lushbaugh CC, Ricks RC. Some cytokinetic and histopathologic considerations of irradiated male and female gonadal tissues. *Front Radiat Ther Oncol.* 1972;6:229–248.
21. Mandl AM. The radiosensitivity of germ cells. *Biol Rev Camb Phil Soc.* 1964;39:288–371.
22. Cattanach BM, Barlow JH. Evidence for the re-establishment of a heterogeneity in radiosensitivity among spermatogonial stem cells repopulating the mouse testis following depletion by x-rays. *Mutat Res.* 1984;127:81–89.
23. Withers HR, Hunter N, Barkley HT, et al. Radiation survival and regeneration characteristics of spermatogenic stem cells of mouse testis. *Radiat Res.* 1974;57:88–103.
24. Andrews GA, Hubner KF, Fry SA. Report of 21-year medical follow-up of survivors of the Oak Ridge Y-12 accident. In: *The Medical Basis of Radiation Accident Preparedness.* New York, NY: Elsevier/North Holland, 1980.
25. Searle AG, Beechey CV. Sperm-count, egg-fertilization and dominant lethality after x-irradiation of mice. *Mutat Res.* 1974;22:63–72.
26. Peters H, Levy E. Effect of irradiation in infancy on the fertility of female mice. *Radiat Res.* 1963;18:421–428.
27. Oakberg EF. Gamma ray sensitivity of oocytes of immature mice. *Proc Soc Exp Biol Med* 1962;109:763–767.
28. Baker TG. Radiosensitivity of mammalian oocytes with particular reference to the human female. *Am J Obstet Gynecol.* 1971; 110:746–761.
29. Mandl AM. Superovulation following ovarian x-irradiation. *J Reprod Fertil.* 1964;8:375–396.
30. Baker TG. The sensitivity in post-natal rhesus monkeys to x-irradiation. *J Reprod Fertil.* 1966;12:183–192.
31. Parsons DF. An electron microscope study of radiation damage in the mouse oocyte. *J Cell Biol.* 1962;14:31–48.
32. Sobels FH, ed. *Repair from Genetic Radiation Damage and Differential Radiosensitivity of Germ Cells.* Oxford, UK: Pergamon Press, 1963.
33. Mandl AM. A quantitative study of the sensitivity of oocytes to x-irradiation. *Proc R Soc [Biol].* 1959;150:53–71.
34. Mondorf L, Faber M. The influence of radiation on human fertility. *J Reprod Fertil.* 1968;15:165–169.
35. Lindop RJ, Sacher GA, eds. *Radiation and Aging.* London, UK: Taylor & Francis, 1966, p 307.
36. Hahn EW, Morales RL. Superpregnancy following pre-fertilization x-irradiation of the rat. *J Reprod Fertil.* 1964;7:73–78.
37. Jacox H. Recovery following human ovarian irradiation. *Radiology.* 1939;32:538–592.
38. Gans B, Bahary C, Levie B. Ovarian regeneration and pregnancy following massive radiotherapy for dysgerminoma. *Obstet Gynecol.* 1966;22:596–600.
39. Schieve LA, Davis F, Roeske J, et al. Evaluation of internal alpha-particle radiation exposure and subsequent fertility among a cohort of women formerly employed in the radium dial industry. *Radiat Res.* 1997;147:236–244.
40. Li FP, Gimbrere K, Gelber RD, et al. Outcome of pregnancy in survivors of Wilms' tumor. *JAMA.* 1987;257:216–219.
41. Lewis EB. Possible genetic consequences of irradiation of tumors in childhood. *Radiology.* 1975;114:147–153.
42. Schull WJ, Otake M, Neel JV. Genetic effects of the atomic bombs: a reappraisal. *Science.* 1981;213:1220–1227.
43. Bloomer WD, Heliman S. Normal tissue response to radiation therapy. *N Engl J Med.* 1975;293:80–83.
44. Riseborough EJ, Grabias SL, Burton RI, et al. Skeletal alterations following irradiation for Wilms' tumor. *J Bone Joint Surg [Am].* 1976;58-A:526–536.
45. Green DM, Jaffe N. Wilms' tumor: model of a curable pediatric malignant solid tumor. *Cancer Treat Res.* 1978;5:143–172.
46. Hawkins MM. Is there evidence of a therapy-related increase in germ cell mutation among childhood cancer survivors? *J Natl Cancer Inst.* 1991;83:1643–1650.
47. Nygaard R, Clausen N, Siimes MA, et al. Reproduction following treatment for childhood leukemia: a population-based prospective cohort study of fertility and offspring. *Med Pediatr Oncol.* 1991;19:459–466.
48. Goldberg MS, Mayo NE. Levy AR, et al. Adverse reproductive outcomes among women exposed to low levels of ionizing radiation from diagnostic radiography for adolescent idiopathic scoliosis. *Epidemiology.* 1998;9:271–278.
49. Hujoel PP, Bollen AM, Noonan CJ, et al. Antepartum dental radiography and infant low birth weight. JAMA. 2004;291:1987–1993.
50. Desforges JF. Current concepts in genetics. *N Engl J Med.* 1976;294:393.
51. Advisory Committee on the Biological Effects of Ionizing Radiation. *The Effects on Populations of Exposure to Low Levels of Ionizing Radiation.* Washington, DC: National Research Council, National Academy of Sciences, National Academy Press, 1980.
52. Russell WL, Russell LB, Kelly EM. Radiation dose rate and mutation frequency. *Science.* 1958;128:1546–1550.
53. Ricoul M, Sabatier L, Dutrillaux B. Increased chromosome radiosensitivity during pregnancy. *Mutat Res.* 1997;374:73–78.
54. Schull WJ, Otake M, Neel JV. Hiroshima and Nagasaki: a reassessment of the mutagenic effect of exposure to ionizing radiation. In: *Population and Biological Aspects of Human Mutation.* New York, NY: Academic Press, 1981, pp 277–303.
55. Francis J, Snee M. A case-control study of trisomy 21 and maternal preconceptional radiography. *Clin Radiol.* 1991;43:343–346.
56. Freire-Maia A, Krieger H. Human genetic studies in areas of high natural radiation. IX. Effects on mortality, morbidity and sex ratio. *Health Phys.* 1978;43:61–65.
57. George KP. Investigations on Human Populations Residing in High Background Radiation Areas of Kerala and Adjoining Regions. In: *Biological and Environmental Effects and Low-Level Radiation.* Vol 11. Vienna: International Atomic Energy Agency, 1976, pp 325–329.
58. Boice JD Jr, Tawn EJ, Winther JF, et al. Genetic effects of radiotherapy for childhood cancer. *Health Phys.* 2003;85:65–80.
59. Ohtaki K, Kodama Y, Nakano M, et al. Human fetuses do not register chromosome damage inflicted by radiation exposure in lymphoid precursor cells except for a small but significant effect at low doses. *Radiat Res.* 2004;161:373–379.
60. Ritenour RE. Health effects of low-level radiation: carcinogenesis, teratogenesis and mutagenesis. *Semin Nuclear Med.* 1986;16:106–117.
61. Jankowski CB. Radiation and pregnancy: putting the risks in proportion. *Am J Nurs.* 1986;86:260–265.
62. Brent RL, Bolden BT. The indirect effect of irradiation on embryonic development: III. The contribution of ovarian irradiation, oviduct irradiation and zygotic irradiation to fetal mortality and growth retardation in the rat. *Radiat Res.* 1967;30:759–773.
63. Russell LB, Russell WL. The effects of radiation on the preimplantation stages of the mouse embryo. *Anat Res.* 1950;108:521.
64. Rugh R. Major radiological concepts and ionizing radiation on the embryo and fetus. In: Haley TJ, Snider RS, eds. *Response of the Nervous System to Ionizing Radiation.* Vol 3. New York, NY: Academic Press, 1962.
65. Russell LB, Russell WL. An analysis of the changing radiation response of the developing mouse embryo. *J Cell Comp Physiol.* 1954;43:103–149.
66. Brent RL, Gorson RO. Radiation exposure in pregnancy. In: Moseley R, Baker DH, Gorson RO, eds. *Current Problems in Radiology.* Vol 2. Chicago: Year Book, 1972, pp 1–48.
67. Moore NW, Aflams CE, Rowson LEA. Development potential of single blastomeres of the rabbit egg. *J Reprod Fertil.* 1968;17:527–531.
68. Willadsen SM. A method for culture of micromanipulated sheep embryos and its use to produce monozygotic twins. *Nature.* 1979;217:298–300.

69. Dekaban AS. Abnormalities in children exposed to x-irradiation during various stages of gestation: tentative timetable of radiation injury to the human fetus. *J Nuclear Med.* 1968;9:471–477.
70. Goldstein L, Murphy DP. Microcephalic idiocy following radium therapy for uterine cancer during pregnancy. *Am J Obstet Gynecol.* 1929;18:189–195, 281–283.
71. Goldstein L, Murphy DP. Etiology of ill health in children born after maternal pelvic irradiation: 11. Defective children born after postconceptional maternal irradiation. *Am J Roentgenol.* 1929;22:322–331.
72. Miller RW. Delayed radiation defects in atomic bomb survivors. *Science.* 1969;166:569–574.
73. Plummer G. Anomalies occurring in children exposed in utero to the atomic bomb in Hiroshima. *Pediatrics.* 1952;10:687–692.
74. Wood JW, Johnson KG, Omori Y. In utero exposure to the Hiroshima atomic bomb. An evaluation of head size and mental retardation: twenty years later. *Pediatrics.* 1967;39:385–392.
75. Wood JW, Johnson KG, Omori Y, et al. Mental retardation in children exposed in utero to the atomic bombs in Hiroshima and Nagasaki. *Am J Public Health.* 1967;57:1381–1389.
76. Zappert J. Uber roentgenogene female microcephalie. *Monatsschr Kinderheildk.* 1926;34:490–493.
77. Blot WJ, Miller RW. Mental retardation following in utero exposure to the atomic bombs of Hiroshima and Nagasaki. *Radiology.* 1973; 106:617–619.
78. Bohnen NI, Ragozzino MW, Kurland LT. Brief communication: effects of diagnostic irradiation during pregnancy on head circumference at birth. *Int J Neurosci.* 1996;87:175–180.
79. Otake M, Schull WJ. In utero exposure to A-bomb radiation and mental retardation: a reassessment. *Br J Radiol.* 1984;57:409–414.
80. Yoshimaru H, Otake M, Fujikoshi Y, et al. Effect on school performance of prenatal exposure to the Hiroshima atomic bomb. *Nippon Eiseigaku Zasshi.* 1991;46:747–754.
81. Otake M, Schull WJ, Yoshimaru H. A review of forty-five years study of Hiroshima and Nagasaki atomic bomb survivors: brain damage among the prenatally exposed. *J Radiat Res (Tokyo).* 1991;32(suppl):249–264.
82. Otake M, Schull WJ, Lee S. Threshold for radiation-related severe mental retardation in prenatally exposed A-bomb survivors: a re-analysis. *Int J Radiat Biol.* 1996;70:755–763.
83. International Commission on Radiological Protection. Developmental Effects of Irradiation on the Brain of the Embryo and Fetus. Annals of the ICRP, Vol 16(4), Oxford, UK: Pergamon Press, 1986, p 43.
84. Dobbing J, Sands J. Quantitative growth and development of human brain. *Arch Dis Child.* 1973;48:757–767.
85. Fushiki S, Matsushita K, Yoshioka H, et al. In utero exposure to low-doses of ionizing radiation decelerates neuronal migration in the developing rat brain. *Int J Radiat Biol.* 1996;70:53–60.
86. Miller RW, Mulvihill JJ. Small head size after atomic irradiation. *Teratology.* 1976;14:355–358.
87. Schull WJ, Otake M. Cognitive function and prenatal exposure to ionizing radiation. *Teratology.* 1999;59:222–226.
88. D'Amato CJ, Hicks SP. Effects of low levels of ionizing radiation on the developing cerebral cortex of the rat. *Neurology.* 1965; 15:1104–1116.
89. Maroteaux P, Spranger J, Opitz JM, et al. Le syndrome camptomelique. *Presse Med.* 1971;79:1157–1162.
90. Mole RH. Consequences of pre-natal radiation exposure for postnatal development: a review. *Int J Radiat Biol.* 1982;42:1–12.
91. Lee S, Otake M, Schull WJ. Changes in the pattern of growth in stature related to prenatal exposure to ionizing radiation. *Int J Radiat Biol.* 1999;75:1449–1458.
92. Shohoji T, Pasternack B. Adolescent growth patterns in survivors exposed prenatally to the A-bombs in Hiroshima and Nagasaki. *Health Phys.* 1973;25:17–27.
93. Moriyama IW, Steer A, Hamilton HB. Radiation effects in atomic bomb survivors. Atomic Bomb Casualty Commission Technical Report, 1973, pp 6–73.
94. Kinlen LJ, Acheson FD. Diagnostic irradiation, congenital malformations and spontaneous abortion. *Br J Radiol.* 1968;41:648–654.
95. Nokkentred K. *Effects of Radiation upon the Human Fetus.* Munksgaard, Copenhagen, 1968, p 228.
96. Tabuchi A. Fetal disorders due to ionizing radiation. *Hiroshima J Med Sci.* 1964;13:125–173.
97. Tabuchi A, Nakagawa S, Hirai T, et al. Fetal hazards due to x-ray diagnosis during pregnancy. *Hiroshima J Med Sci.* 1967;16:49–66.
98. Vilumsen A. *Environmental Factors in Congenital Malformations.* Foreningen af Danske Laegestuderendes, Copenhagen, 1970.
99. Mossman K, Hill LT. Radiation risks in pregnancy. *Obstet Gynecol.* 1982;6:237–242.
100. Hammer-Jacobsen E. Therapeutic abortion on account of x-ray examination during pregnancy. *Dan Med Bull.* 1954;6:113–122.
101. Jacobsen L, Mellemgaard L. Anomalies of the eyes in descendants of women irradiated with small x-ray doses during age of fertility. *Acta Ophthalmol (Copenh).* 1968;46:352–354.
102. Brent RL. Irradiation in pregnancy. In: Sciarra JJ, ed. *Davis' Gynecology and Obstetrics.* Vol 2. New York, NY: Harper & Row, 1972, pp 1–32.
103. Brent RL. The response of the 9 and one-half-day-old-rat embryo to variations in dose rate of 150R X-irradiation. *Radiat Res.* 1971;45:127–136.
104. Brizzee KR, Brannon RB. Cell recovery in foetal brain after ionizing radiation. *Int J Radiat Biol.* 1972;21:375–378.
105. Bithell JF, Stewart AM. Prenatal irradiation and childhood malignancy: a review of British data from the Oxford Survey. *Br J Cancer.* 1975;31:271–287.
106. Favus MJ, Schneider AB, Stachura ME, et al. Thyroid cancer occurring as a late consequence of head-and-neck irradiation. *N Engl J Med.* 1976;294:1019–1025.
107. Einhorn L. Can prenatal irradiation protect the embryo from tumor development? *Acta Oncol.* 1991;30:291–299.
108. Stewart A, Webb J, Hewitt D. A survey of childhood malignancies. *Br Med J.* 1958;1:1495–1508.
109. Stewart A, Kneale GW. Changes in the cancer risk associated with obstetric radiography. *Lancet.* 1968;1:104–107.
110. Mole RH. Antenatal irradiation and childhood cancer: causation or coincidence? *Br J Cancer.* 1974;30:199–208.
111. Stewart A. The carcinogenic effects of low-level radiation: a reappraisal of epidemiologists' methods and observations. *Health Phys.* 1973;24:223–240.
112. Lewis EB. Leukemia and ionizing radiation. *Science.* 1957; 125:965–972.
113. Advisory Committee on the Biological Effects of Ionizing Radiations. *The Effects on Populations of Exposure to Low Levels of Ionizing Radiation.* Washington, DC: National Academy of Sciences, National Research Council, 1972.
114. Harvey EB, Boice JD, Honeyman M, et al. Prenatal x-ray exposure and childhood cancer in twins. *N Engl J Med.* 1985;312:541–545.
115. Jablon S, Kato H. Childhood cancer in relation to prenatal exposure to atomic-bomb radiation. *Lancet.* 1970;2:1000–1003.
116. United Nations Scientific Committee on the Effects of Atomic Radiation (UNSCEAR). Developmental effects of irradiation in utero. *Anex J.* 1977:655–725.
117. Bithell JF, Stiller CA. A new calculation of the carcinogenic risk of obstetric x-raying. *Stat Med.* 1988;7:857–864.
118. Mole RH. Fetal dosimetry by UNSCEAR and risk coefficients for childhood cancer following diagnostic radiology in pregnancy. *J Radiol Prot.* 1990;10:199–203.
119. Yoshimoto Y, Kato H, Schull WJ. A review of forty-five years study of Hiroshima and Nagasaki atomic bomb survivors: cancer risk among in utero-exposed survivors. *J Radiat Res (Tokyo).* 1991; 32(suppl):231–238.
120. Yoshimoto Y, Kato H, Schull WJ. Risk of cancer among children exposed in utero to A-bomb radiations, 1950-84. *Lancet.* 1988; 17:665–669.

121. Lilienfeld AM. Epidemiological studies of the leukemogenic effects of radiation. *Yale J Biol Med.* 1966;39:143–164.
122. Court Brown WM, Doll R, Hill RB. Incidence of leukaemia after exposure to diagnostic radiation in utero. *Br Med J.* 1960; 5212:1539–1545.
123. Burrow GN, Hamilton HB, Hrubec Z. Study of adolescents exposed in utero to the atomic bomb, Nagasaki, Japan. I. General aspects: clinical and laboratory data. *Yale J Biol Med.* 1964;36:430–444.
124. Kato H. Mortality in children exposed to the A-bombs while in utero. *Am J Epidemiol.* 1971;93:435–442.
125. Graham S, Levin MI, Lilienfeld AM. Preconception, intrauterine and postnatal irradiation as related to leukemia. *Natl Cancer Inst Monogr.* 1966;19:347–371.
126. Hoshino T, Itoga T, Kato H. Leukemia in the offspring of parents exposed to the atomic bomb at Hiroshima and Nagasaki. Presented to the Japanese Association of Hematology, March 28–30,1965.
127. Izumi S, Koyama K, Soda M, et al. Cancer incidence in children and young adults did not increase relative to parental exposure to atomic bombs. *Br J Cancer*. 2003;89:1709–1713.
128. Izumi S, Suyama A, Koyama K. Radiation-related mortality among offspring of atomic bomb survivors: a half-century of follow-up. *Int J Cancer.* 2003;107:292–297.
129. McKinny PA, Fear NT, Stockton D, UK Childhood Cancer Study Investigators. Parental occupation at periconception: findings from the United Kingdom Childhood Cancer Study. *Occup Environ Med.* 2003;60:901–909.
130. Naumburg E, Belloco R, Cnattingius S, et al. Intrauterine exposure to diagnostic X rays and risk of childhood leukemia subtypes. *Radiat Res.* 2001;156:718–723.
131. Shu XO, Potter JD, Linet MS, et al. Diagnostic X-rays and ultrasound exposure and risk of childhood acute lymphoblastic leukemia by immunophenotype. *Cancer Epidemiol Biomarkers Prev.* 2002;11:177–185.
132. Michaelis J. Recent epidemiological studies on ionizing radiation and childhood cancer in Germany. *Int J Radiat Biol.* 1998; 73:377–381.
133. Meinert R, Kaletsch U, Kaatsch P, et al. Associations between childhood cancer and ionizing radiation: results of a population-based case-control study in Germany. *Cancer Epidemiol Biomarkers Prev.* 1999;8:793 799.
134. Doll R, Wakeford R. Risk of childhood cancer from fetal irradiation. *Br J Radiol.* 1997;70:130–139.
135. Rugh R, Duhamel L, Skaredoff L. Relation of the embryonic and fetal x-irradiation to life time average weights and tumor incidence in mice. *Proc Soc Exp Biol Med.* 1966;121:714–718.
136. Brent RL, Bolden BT. The long-term effects of low-dosage embryonic irradiation. *Radiat Res.* 1961;14:453–454.
137. Brent RL, Bolden BT. Indirect effect of x-irradiation on embryonic development. V. Utilization of high doses of maternal irradiation on the first day of gestation. *Radiat Res.* 1968;36:563–570.
138. Miller RW. Epidemiological conclusions from radiation toxicity studies. In: Fry RJM, Grahn D, Griem ML, et al, eds. *Late Effects of Radiation.* London, UK: Taylor & Francis, 1970.
139. Loewe WE, Mendelson E. Revised dose estimates at Hiroshima and Nagasaki. *Health Phys.* 1981;41:663–666.
140. Blot WJ. Growth and development following prenatal and childhood exposure to atomic radiation. *J Radiat Res (Tokyo).* 1975;16:81–88.
141. Mole RH. Radiation effects on pre-natal development and their radiological significance. *Br J Radiol.* 1979;52:89–101.
142. National Council on Radiation Protection and Measurements. Medical Radiation Exposure of Pregnant and Potentially Pregnant Women, NCRP Report No 54. Washington, DC: Government Printing Office, 1979, p 320.
143. Hall EJ. Scientific view of low-level radiation risks. *Radiographics.* 1991;11:509–518.
144. Friedman WN, Rosenfield AT. Computed tomography in obstetrics and gynecology. *J Reprod Med.* 1992;37:3–18.
145. Ragozzino MW, Gray JE, Burke TM, et al. Estimation and minimization of fetal absorbed dose: data from common radiographic examinations. *AJR.* 1981;137:667–671.
146. Guidelines for the performance of Roentgen examinations to women in the reproductive age and pregnant women. Health Administartion, Report 33/2000, file 4/1/14, Ministry of Health, Israel, 2000.
147. Brent RL. Effects and risks of medically administered isotopes to the developing embryo. In: Fabro S, Scialli AR, eds. *Drug and Chemical Action in Pregnancy.* New York, NY: Marcel Dekker, 1986, pp 427–439.
148. Padovani R, Contento G, Fabretto M, et al. Patient doses and risks from diagnostic radiology in Northeast Italy. *Br J Radiol.* 1987; 60:155–165.
149. Shrimpton PC, Wall BF, Jones DG, et al. Doses to patients from routine diagnostic x-ray examinations in England. *Br J Radiol.* 1986;59:749–758.
150. McGuire EL, Dickson PA. Exposure and organ dose estimation in diagnostic radiology. *Med Phys.* 1986;13:913–916.
151. United Nations Scientific Committee on the Effects of Atomic Radiation (UNSCEAR). Sources and Effects of Ionizing Radiation. Report to the General Assembly, 1977, p 319.
152. Kereiakes JG, Rosenstein M. Handbook of Radiation Doses in Nuclear Medicine and Diagnostic X-Ray. Boca Raton, FL: CRC Press, 1980, p 211.
153. Toppenberg KS, Hill DA, Miller DP. Safety of radiographic imaging during pregnancy. *Am Fam Physician.* 1999;59:1813–1818, 1820.
154. Murphy F, Heaton B. Patient doses received during whole body scanning using an Elscint 905 CT scanner. *Br J Radiol.* 1985; 58:1197–1201.
155. Schonken P, Marchal G, Coenen Y, et al. Body and gonad doses in computer tomography of the trunk. *J Belge Radiol.* 1978; 61:363–371.
156. McCullough EC, Payne JT. Patient dosage in computed tomography. *Radiology.* 1978;129:457–463.
157. Damilakis J, Theocharopoulos N, Perisinakis K, et al. Conceptus radiation dose assessment from fluoroscopically assisted surgical treatment of hip fractures. *Med Phys.* 2003;30:2594–2601.
158. Damilakis J, Theocharopoulos N, Perisinakis K, et al. Conceptus radiation dose and risk from cardiac catheter ablation procedures. *Circulation.* 2001;104:893–897.
159. Robert E. Teratogen update: electromagnetic fields. *Teratology.* 1996;54:305–313.
160. Budinger TF. Nuclear magnetic resonance (NMR) in vivo studies: known thresholds for health effects. *J Cornput Assist Tomogr.* 1981;5:800–811.
161. Thomas A, Morris PG. The effects of NMR exposure in living organisms: a microbial assay. *Br J Radiol.* 1981;54:615–621.
162. Tyndall DA, Sulik KK. Effects of magnetic resonance imaging on eye development in the C57BL/6J mouse. *Teratology.* 1991; 43:263–275.
163. Tyndall DA. MRI effects on the teratogenicity of x-irradiation in the C57BL/6J mouse. *Magn Reson Imaging.* 1990;8:423–433.
164. Heinrichs WL, Fong P, Flannery M, et al. Midgestational exposure of pregnant BALB/c mice to magnetic resonance imaging conditions. *Magn Reson Imaging.* 1988;6:305–313.
165. Cooke P, Morris PG. The effects of NMR exposure on living organisms: II. a genetic study of human lymphocytes. *Br J Radiol.* 1981; 54:622–625.
166. Lee WR. Working with visual display units. *Am J Ophthalmol.* 1986;101:107–111.
167. Foulquier JN, LeBreton C. Radiodiagnosis and irradiated pregnancies *Ann Radiol (Paris).* 1997;40:225–236.
168. Nagayama M, Watanabe Y, Okumura A, et al. Fast MR imaging in obstetrics. *Radiographics.* 2002;22:563–580; discussion 580–582.
169. Levine D. Ultrasound versus magnetic resonance imaging in fetal evaluation. *Top Magn Reson Imaging* 2001;12:25–38.

170. Huppi PS, Inder TE. Magnetic resonance techniques in the evaluation of the perinatal brain: recent advances and future directions. *Semin Neonatol.* 2001;6:195–210.
171. Sigmund G, Bauer M, Henne K, et al. A technic of magnetic resonance tomographic pelvimetry in obstetrics. *ROFO Fortschr Geb Roentgenstr Nuklearmed.* 1991;154:370–374.
172. Tukeva TA, Aronen HJ, Karjalainen PT, et al. Low-field MRI pelvimetry. *Eur Radiol.* 1997;7:230–234.
173. LaBan MM, Viola S, Williams DA, et al. Magnetic resonance imaging of the lumbar herniated disc in pregnancy. *Am J Phys Med Rehabil.* 1995;74:59–61.
174. Evans JA, Savitz DA, Kanal E, et al. Infertility and pregnancy outcome among magnetic resonance imaging workers. *J Occup Med.* 1993;35:1191–1195.
175. Ronderos A. Fetal tolerance to radiation. *Radiology.* 1961; 76:454–456.
176. National Council on Radiation Protection and Measurements. Basic Radiation Protection Criteria, NCRP Publication No 39. Washington, DC: Government Printing Office, 1971.
177. Wagner LK, Hayman LA. Pregnancy and women radiologists. *Radiology.* 1982;145:559–562.
178. U.S. Nuclear Regulatory Commission. Instruction concerning prenatal radiation exposure. *Reg Guide.* 1975;8. 13 rev 1:3–4.
179. Instruction concerning prenatal radiation exposure. Regulatory Guide 8.13, US Nuclear Regulatory Commission, June 1999. *http://www.nrc.gov/reading-rm/doc-collections/reg-guides/occupational-health/active/8-13/*
180. Regulations of Women's work (work with ionizing radiation), Israel Ministry of Industry, Trade & Labor 1979. *http://www.moital.gov.il/NR/exeres/25BC96B3-753B-4A2F-8B64-AB1FBEB498D4.htm* (in Hebrew)
181. Shea KM, Little RE. Is there an association between preconception paternal x-ray exposure and birth outcome? The ALSPAC Study Team. Avon Longitudinal Study of Pregnancy and Childhood. *Am J Epidemiol.* 1997;145:546–551.
182. Senturia YD, Peckham CS, Peckham MJ. Children fathered by men treated for testicular cancer. *Lancet.* 1985;2:766–769.
183. Schull WJ, Neel JV. Atomic exposure and the pregnancies of biologically related parents. *Am J Public Health.* 1959;49:1621–1629.
184. Miller RW. Effects of ionizing radiation from the atomic bomb on Japanese children. *Pediatrics.* 1968;41:257–263.
185. Doyle P, Roman E, Maconochie N, et al. Primary infertility in nuclear industry employees: report from the nuclear industry family study. *Occup Environ Med.* 2001;58:535–539.
186. Draper GJ, Little MP, Sorahan T, et al. Cancer in the offspring of radiation workers: a record linkage study. Br Med J. 1997;315: 1181–1188.
187. Abrahamson S, Tawn EJ. Risk of stillbirth in offspring of men exposed to ionising radiation. *J Radiol Prot.* 2001;21:133–144.
188. Doyle P, Maconochie N, Roman E, et al. Fetal death and congenital malformation in babies born to nuclear industry employees: report from the nuclear industry family study. *Lancet.* 2000;356:1293–1299.
189. McKinney PA, Alexander FE, Cartwright RA, et al. Parental occupations of children with leukaemia in West Cumbria, North Humberside, and Gateshead. *Br Med J.* 1991;302:681–687.
190. Sorahan T, Roberts PJ. Childhood cancer and paternal exposure to ionizing radiation: preliminary findings from the Oxford Survey of Childhood Cancers. *Am J Ind Med.* 1993;23:343–354.
191. Wakeford R. The risk of childhood cancer from intrauterine and preconceptional exposure to ionizing radiation. *Environ Health Perspect.* 1995;103:1018–1025.
192. McAulay IR. Regulatory control of air crew exposure to cosmic radiation: the European approach. *Health Phys.* 2000;79:596–599.
193. Friedberg W, Copeland K, Duke FE, et al. Radiation exposure during air travel: guidance provided by the Federal Aviation Administration for air carrier crews. *Health Phys.* 2000;79:591–595.
194. Nicholas JS, Copeland KA, Duke FE, et al. Galactic cosmic radiation exposure of pregnant flight crewmembers. *Aviat Space Environ Med.* 2000;71:647–648.
195. Irgens A, Irgens LM, Reitan JB, et al. Pregnancy outcome among offspring of airline pilots and cabin attendants. *Scand J Work Environ Health.* 2003;29:94–99.
196. Bentur Y, Horlatsch N, Koren G. Exposure to ionizing radiation during pregnancy: perception of teratogenic risk and outcome. *Teratology.* 1991;43:109–112.
197. Greskovich JF Jr, Macklis RM. Radiation therapy in pregnancy: risk calculation and risk minimization. *Semin Oncol.* 2000;27:633–645.
198. International Commission on Radiological Protection. Pregnancy and medical radiation. *Ann ICRP.* 2000;30:iii–viii, 1–43.
199. Reynolds JEF, Prasad AB, eds. Martindale, *The Extra Pharmacopeia.* London, UK: Pharmaceutical Press, 1982, pp 1386–1400.
200. Fabro S, Brown NA, Scialli AR. Radionuclides in pregnancy. *Reprod Toxicol (Med Lett).* 1986;5:17–22.
201. Green GH, Gareis FJ, Shepard TH, et al. Cretinism associated with maternal sodium iodide[131] therapy during pregnancy. *Am J Dis Child.* 1971;122:247–249.
202. Sikov MR, Noonan TR. Anomalous development induced in embryonic rat by the maternal administration of radiophosphorus. *Am J Anat.* 1958;103:137–156.
203. Book SA, Goldman M. Thyroidal radioiodine exposure of the fetus. *Health Phys.* 1975;29:874–877.
204. Smith EM, Warner GG. Estimates of radiation dose to the embryo from nuclear medicine procedures. *J Nuclear Med.* 1976; 17:836–839.
205. Saenger EL. *Protocol Book of Radioisotope Laboratory.* Cincinnati, OH: University of Cincinnati Medical Center, 1976.
206. Kereiakes JG, Feller PA, Ascoi F, et al. Pediatric radiopharmaceutical dosimetry. In: *Radiopharmaceutical Dosimetry Symposium.* U.S. Department of Health, Education, and Welfare (Food and Drug Administration) Publication No 76-8044. Rockville, MD: US DHEW, Bureau of Radiological Health, 1976.
207. Roedler HD, Kaul A, Hine GJ. *Internal Radiation Dose in Diagnostic Nuclear Medicine.* Berlin: Hoffman, 1978.
208. Kereiakes JG, Rosenstein M. *Handbook of Radiation Doses in Nuclear Medicine and Diagnostic X-Ray.* Boca Raton, FL: GRC Press, 1980, p 170.
209. Brent RL. The prediction of human disease from laboratory and animal tests for teratology, carcinogenicity and mutagenicity. In: Lasagna L, ed. *Controversies in Therapeutics.* Philadelphia, PA: Saunders, 1980, pp 134–150.
210. Brent RL. Cancer risks following diagnostic radiation exposure. *Pediatrics.* 1983;71:288–289.
211. Brent RL. *The Effects of Ionizing Radiation, Microwaves and Ultrasound in the Developing Embryo: Clinical Interpretations and Applications of the Data.* Vol 14. Chicago: Year Book, 1984, pp 1–87.
212. Schardein JL, ed. *Chemically Induced Birth Defects.* New York, NY: Marcel Dekker, 1985, pp 659–668.
213. Heinonen OP, Sione D, Shapiro S. Diagnostic aids, technical aids and rare drugs. In: *Birth Defects and Drugs in Pregnancy.* Littleton, MA: PSG Publishing, 1977, pp 409–415, 444.
214. Webb GAM, Simmonds JR, Wilkins BT. Radiation levels in Eastern Europe. *Nature.* 1986;321:821–822.
215. Castronovo FP Jr. Teratogen update: radiation and Chernobyl. *Teratology.* 1999;60:100–106.
216. Baverstock KF. A preliminary assessment of the consequences for inhabitants of the UK of the Chernobyl accident. Int J Radiat Biol 1986; 50:III-XIII.
217. Rytomaa T. Ten years after Chernobyl. *Ann Med.* 1996;28:83–87.
218. Petridou E, Trichopoulos D, Dessypris N, et al. Infant leukaemia after in utero exposure to radiation from Chernobyl. *Nature.* 1996; 382:352–353.

219. Sperling K, Pelz J, Wegner RD, et al. Frequency of trisomy 21 in Germany before and after the Chernobyl accident. *Biomed Pharmacother.* 1991;45:255–262.
220. Lazjuk GI, Nikolaev DL, Novikova IV. Changes in registered congenital anomalies in the Republic of Belarus after the Chernobyl accident. *Stem Cells.* 1997;15 Suppl 2:255–260.
221. Harjulehto T, Rahola T, Suomola M, et al. Pregnancy outcome in Finland after the Chernobyl accident. *Biomed Pharmacother.* 1991;45:263–266.
222. Czeizel AE. Incidence of legal abortions and congenital abnormalities in Hungary. *Biomed Pharmacother.* 1991;45:249–254.
223. Irgens LM, Lie RT, Ulstein M, et al. Pregnancy outcome in Norway after Chernobyl. *Biomed Pharmacother.* 1991;45:233–241.
224. Trichopoulos D, Zavitsanos X, Koutis C, et al. The victims of Chernobyl in Greece: induced abortions after the accident. *Br Med J.* 1987;295:1100.
225. Knudsen LB. Legally induced abortions in Denmark after Chernobyl. *Biomed Pharmacother.* 1991;45:229–231.
226. Cross FT. A review of experimental animal radon health effects data. NTIS (National Information Service) Report/DE91-016710, 1991. Quoted in Shepard's Catalog of Teratogenic Agents, Healthcare Series Vol. 125, Thomson-Micromedex, Greenwood Village, CO, 2005.
227. Wiese WH, Skipper BJ. Survey of reproductive outcomes in uranium and potash mine workers: results of first analysis. *Ann Am Conf Govern Ind Hyg.* 1986;14:187–192.
228. Grainger P, Shalla SH, Preece AW, et al. Home radon levels and seasonal correction factors for the Isle of Man. *Phys Med Biol.* 2000;45:2247–2252.
229. Bergman T. Eye care health effects of video display terminals. *Occup Health Saf.* 1980;49:24,26–28,53–55.
230. Lazarus MG, Bourke JA. Problems associated with use of video display units by bank clerical staff. *Med J Aust.* 1982;2:186.
231. Letourneau EG. Are video display terminals safe? *Can Med Assoc J.* 1981;125:533.
232. Weiss MM, Peterson RC. Electromagnetic radiation emitted from video computer terminals. *Am Ind Hyg Assoc J.* 1979;40:300–309.
233. Weiss MM. The video display terminals: is there a radiation hazard? *J Occup Med.* 1983;25:98–100.
234. U.S. Radiological Health Bureau. An Evaluation of Radiation Emission from Video Display Terminals. U.S. Department of Health and Human Services (Food and Drug Administration) Publication No 81-8153. Washington, DC: Government Printing Office, 1981.
235. Hubar JS, Draus P. Determining the radiation exposure from visual display terminals used in dentistry. *J Can Dent Assoc.* 1991; 57:131–132.
236. Fabro S, Brown NA, Scialli AR. Video display terminals and human reproduction. *Reprod Toxicol (Med Lett).* 1984;3:1–4.
237. Schnorr TM, Grajewski BA, Hornung RW, et al. Video display terminals and the risk of spontaneous abortions. *N Engl J Med.* 1991;324:727–733.
238. Hirning CR, Aitken JH. Cathode-ray tube x-ray emission standard for video display terminals. *Health Phys.* 1982;43:727–731.
239. Delgado JMR, Leal J, Monteagudo JL, et al. Embryological changes induced by weak, extremely low frequency electromagnetic fields. *J Anat.* 1981;134:533–551.
240. Ubeda A, Leal J, Trillo MA, et al. Pulse shape of magnetic fields influences chick embryogenesis. *J Anat.* 1983;137:513–536.
241. Maffeo S, Miller MW, Carstensen EL. Lack of effect of weak low frequency electromagnetic fields on chick embryogenesis. *J Anat.* 1984;139:613–618.
242. McDonald AD, Cherry NM, Delorme C, et al. Work and pregnancy in Montreal-preliminary findings on work with visual display terminals. In: Pearce BG, ed. *Allegations of Reproductive Hazards from VDUs.* Loughborough: Humane Technology, 1984, pp 161–175.
243. McDonald AD, Chesy NM, Delorme C, et al. Visual display units and pregnancy: evidence from the Montreal survey. *J Occup Med.* 1986;28:1226–1231.
244. Goldhaber MK, Polen MR, Hiat RA. The risk of miscarriage and birth defects among women who use visual display terminals during pregnancy. *Am J Ind Med.* 1988;13:695–706.
245. Kurppa K, Holmberg PC, Rantala K, et al. Birth defects and video display terminals. *Lancet.* 1984;2:1339.
246. Tikkanen J, Heinonen OP. Maternal exposure to chemical and physical factors during pregnancy and cardiovascular malformations in the offspring. *Teratology.* 1991;43:591–600.
247. Li DK, Checkoway H, Mueller BA. Electric blanket use during pregnancy in relation to the risk of congenital urinary tract anomalies among women with a history of subfertility. *Epidemiology.* 1995;6:485–489.
248. Bergqvist U, Knave B. Video display work and pregnancy-research in the Nordic countries. In: Pearce BG, ed. *Allegations of Reproductive Hazards from VDUs.* Loughborough: Humane Technology, 1984, pp 49–53.
249. Bayne VJ. Paper outlining a trade union response to the allegations of reproductive hazards from VDUs. In: Pearce BG, ed. *Allegations of Reproductive Hazards from VDUs.* Loughborough: Human Technology, 1984, pp 111–126.
250. Brent RL. X-ray, microwave and ultrasound: the real and unreal hazards. *Pediatr Ann.* 1980;9:469–473.
251. Dimberg Y. Neurochemical effects of a 20 kHz magnetic field on the central nervous system in prenatally exposed mice. *Bioelectromagnetics.* 1995;16:263–267.
252. Saito K, Suzuki K, Motoyoshi S. Lethal and teratogenic effects of long-term low-intensity radio frequency radiation at 428 MHz on developing chick embryo. *Teratology.* 1991;43:609–614.
253. Tofani S, Agnesod G, Ossola P, et al. Effects of continuous low level exposure to radiofrequency radiation on intrauterine development in rats. *Health Phys.* 1986;51:489–499.
254. Lary JM, Conover DL, Johnson PH, et al. Dose-response relationship between body temperature and birth defects in radiofrequency-irradiated rats. *Bioelectromagnetics.* 1986;7:141–149.
255. Lary JM, Conover DL, Foley ED, et al. Teratogenic effects of 27.12 MHz radiofrequency radiation in rats. *Teratology.* 1982;26:299–309.
256. Lary JM, Conover DL, Johnson PH. Absence of embryotoxic effect from low-level (non-thermal) exposure of rats to 100 MHz radiofrequency radiation. *Scand J Work Environ Health.* 1983;9:120–127.
257. Cahill DF. A suggested limit for population exposure to radiofrequency radiation. *Health Phys.* 1983;45:109–126.
258. Roberts NJ Jr, Michaelson SM. Epidemiological studies of human exposure to radiofrequency radiation: a critical review. *Int Arch Occup Environ Health.* 1985;56:169–178.
259. Larsen AI, Olsen J, Svane O. Gender-specific reproductive outcome and exposure to high-frequency electromagnetic radiation among physiotherapists. *Scand J Work Environ Health.* 1991;17:324–329.
260. Larsen AI. Congenital malformations and exposure to high-frequency electromagnetic radiation among Danish physiotherapists. *Scand J Work Environ Health.* 1991;17:318–323.
261. De Roos AJ, Teschke K, Savitz DA, et al. Parental occupational exposures to electromagnetic fields and radiation and the incidence of neuroblastoma in offspring. *Epidemiology.* 2001;12:508–517.
262. Blaasaas KG, Tynes T, Lie RT. Risk of selected birth defects by maternal residence close to power lines during pregnancy. *Occup Environ Med.* 2004;61:174–176.
263. National Council on Radiation Protection Measurements. NCRP Report No 74, Bethesda, MD: NCRP, 1983, p 72.
264. World Health Organization, Environmental Health Criteria 22. WHO, Geneva, 1982.
265. Fabro S, Brown NA, Scialli AR. Ultrasound in industry and medicine. *Reprod Toxicol (Med Lett).* 1984;3:17–20.

266. Liebeskind D, Bases R, Mendez F, et al. Sister chromatid exchanges in human lymphocytes after exposure to diagnostic ultrasound. *Science.* 1975;205:1273–1275.
267. Haupt M, Martin AO, Simpson JL, et al. Ultrasonic induction of sister chromatid exchanges in human lymphocytes. *Hum Genet.* 1981;59:221–226.
268. Siegel E, Goddard J, James AE Jr, et al. Cellular attachment as a sensitive indicator of the effects of diagnostic ultrasound exposure on cultured human cells. *Radiology.* 1979;133:175–179.
269. Liebeskind D, Bases R, Elequin F, et al. Diagnostic ultrasound: effects on DNA and growth patterns of animal cells. *Radiology.* 1979;131:177–184.
270. Liebeskind D, Bases R, Koenigsberg M, et al. Morphological changes in the surface characteristics of cultured cells after exposure to diagnostic ultrasound. *Radiology.* 1981;138:419–423.
271. Au WW, Obergoenner N, Goldenthal KL, et al. Sister chromatid exchanges in mouse embryos after exposure to ultrasound in utero. *Mutat Res.* 1982;103:315–320.
272. Wegner RD, Obe G, Meyenburg M. Has diagnostic ultrasound mutagenic effects? *Hum Genet.* 1980;56:95–98.
273. Hellman LM, Duffus GM, Donald I, et al. Safety of diagnostic ultrasound in obstetrics. *Lancet.* 1970;11:1133–1135.
274. Scheidt PC, Stantey F, Bryla DA. One year follow-up of infants exposed to ultrasound in utero. *Am J Obstet Gynecol.* 1978; 131:743–748.
275. Stark CR, Orleans M, Haverkamp AD, et al. Short- and long-term risks after exposure to diagnostic ultrasound in utero. *Obstet Gynecol.* 1984;63:194–200.
276. Wilson MK. Obstetric ultrasound and childhood malignancies. *Radiography.* 1985;51:319–320.
277. Smith DP, Graham JB, Prystowsky JB, et al. The effects of ultrasound-guided shock waves during early pregnancy in Sprague Dawley rats. *J Urol.* 1992;147:231–234.
278. Magnavita N, Fileni A. Occupational risk caused by ultrasound in medicine. *Radiol Med (Torino).* 1994;88:107–111.
279. Krieger GR, Larson J. Lasers. In: Sullivan JB Jr, Krieger GR, eds. *Hazardous Materials Toxicology: Clinical Principles of Environmental Health.* Baltimore, MD: Williams & Wilkins, 1992, pp 1165–1174.
280. Koninckx PR, Witters K, Brosens J, et al. Conservative laparoscopic treatment of ectopic pregnancies using the CO_2 laser. *Br J Obstet Gynaecol.* 1991;98:1254–1259.
281. Kelly RW, Diamond MP. Intra-abdominal use of the carbon dioxide laser for microsurgery. *Obstet Gynecol Clin North Am.* 1991; 18:537–544.
282. Schmidt S, Decleer W, Gorissen-Bosselmann S, et al. Endoscopic fetal surgery by excimer laser: an experimental study in premature lambs. *J Perinat Med.* 1991;19:231–235.
283. Bandazhevskii IuI, Emel'ianchik IuM. Effect of infrared impulse laser irradiation on the development of albino rat embryos. *Arkh Anat Gistol Embriol.* 1991;100:15–18.
284. Mester AF, Snow JB Jr, Shaman P. Photochemical effects of laser irradiation on neuritic outgrowth of olfactory neuroepithelial explants. *Otolaryngol Head Neck Surg.* 1991;105:449–456.
285. Fox C, Kilby MD, Khan KS. Contemporary treatments for twin-twin transfusion syndrome. *Obstet Gynecol.* 2005;105:1469–1477.
286. Quarello E, Bernard JP, Leroy B, et al. Prenatal laser treatment of a placental chorioangioma. *Ultrasound Obstet Gynecol.* 2005;25:299–301.

CHAPTER 19

THE USE OF NATURAL HEALTH PRODUCTS IN PREGNANCY AND LACTATION: A CLINICIAN'S GUIDE

Anna G. Sivojelezova, Michael Gallo, Enkelejda Bollano, Heather Boon, and Gideon Koren

INTRODUCTION

Complementary and alternative medicine (CAM) is an umbrella term used to describe a number of health care therapies that are generally considered to fall outside the conventional medical model.[383] The use of CAM has increased dramatically, with the market in the United States estimated to be worth $27 billion.[384] In Canada a similar trend exists, with the market estimated to be $2.3 billion and almost three quarters of the population stating that they have used a form of CAM in their lifetime.[385]

Herbal medicine (also known as botanical medicine, phytotherapy, phytomedicine, herbalism, and herbology) is considered to be one of the primary complementary and alternative therapies.[383] In the United States, dietary supplement use increased from 14.2% in 1998–1999 to 18.8% in 2002.[462] In 2002, herbal supplement use in the Canadian adult population, excluding pregnant and breastfeeding women, was 13% in men and 16% in women.[463] In its most basic sense, herbal medicine can be simply defined as the use of plants and plant remedies in the treatment and prevention of disease.[387] Unfortunately the situation is more complex than this, with a number of different paradigms and philosophies present in clinical practice. This heterogeneous practice has led to a number of incongruities, most notably the wide variance in dosage that exists in erroneously referring to a homeopathic or nutritional supplement as a herbal medicine. Consequently it is often necessary for the clinician to confirm that the patient is actually taking a herbal medicine.[383]

A common misconception which exists among patients and practitioners alike is that the term safe and natural are interchangeable.[388,389] While this is not the case, it has led to added difficulties in assessing risk posed by herbal medicine. It is known that consumption of herbal medicine can result in direct adverse effects, such as allergic reactions, nausea, vomiting, and sedation.[388,390] In addition, the potential exists for herbal remedies to interact with conventional pharmacotherapy.[391] It is estimated that 15 million people annually (almost 20 of all prescription users) take either herbal or nutritional supplements concurrently with prescription drugs.[384] There seems to be reluctance on the part of consumers to report adverse drug reactions (ADR) resulting from herbal products when compared with conventional drugs.[392] When an ADR does occur there is a lack of systematic universal reporting. In addition, poor quality controls in manufacturing procedures have led to the erroneous reporting of serious adverse effects by herbal agents where adulterants are actually responsible.[63,390,393] Therefore, even when adverse effects and/or interactions with conventional drugs are reported in the literature, it is important to note whether the herbal product was authenticated. To complicate matters further, there is often a lack of disclosure on the part of the consumer to the health care provider when herbal remedies lead to ADR. It has been estimated that over 60 of users do not inform their primary physician that they are using CAM.[384] Canada has created the Natural Health Product Directorate (NHPD) to address some regulatory issues. Although the Natural Health Product Regulations came into force on January 1, 2004, a transition period will range from 2 years (for site licensing) to 6 years (for product licensing, for products already issued a drug identification number) until these regulations will come into full force.

Traditionally, women used herbal products in pregnancy for a variety of reasons, including pregnancy-related conditions (nausea and vomiting in pregnancy, constipation), to prepare for labor, to induce abortion, or for their overall well-being. In developing countries, plant products are still routinely administered to women during pregnancy and childbirth (470). Several surveys estimated that 12–59% of women used herbal products during pregnancy.[465,466–468] An Australian cross-sectional survey of vitamin, mineral and herbal supplementation during pregnancy determined that among 211 women the most prevalent herbal preparation used before conception was chamomile (5%); ginger was used by 20% of all women in the first trimester of pregnancy; chamomile displaced ginger in the second trimester of pregnancy (6%), and raspberry leaf as tea or capsules was the main herbal preparation during the third trimester (8%).[466] A Norwegian survey of pregnant women found that higher level of education and previous positive experience with herbal products were strong determinants of herbal therapy in pregnancy.[469] In this survey herbal product use increased from 20% in the first trimester of pregnancy to 26% in the third trimester.[469]

While the use of herbal medicine in pregnancy and lactation is prevalent due to a long history of use in pregnancy, during delivery, and lactation, it poses a number of concerns as clinically relevant sources of evidence-based information on the safety/risk of such products is lacking.[186] Health-care providers should be aware of several key factors during safety evaluation of a particular herbal product. Those herbal products that are considered generally toxic, such as some hepatotoxins (e.g., kava-kava), should be contraindicated not only in the general population, but also in pregnant women. Also, natural health products that have traditionally been used as abortifacients for the termination of pregnancy (e.g., black cohosh, golden seal, pennyroyal) should be intuitively contraindicated in pregnant women. Drug-herb interactions are also important to consider in pregnancy. Such interactions can affect the bioavailability, efficacy and adverse event profile of a herbal or a pharmaceutical agent.[470] For example, some herbs may enhance the effect of anticoagulant medications. Emmenagogues are agents that are used to stimulate and promote menstruation, and these agents may theoretically stimulate the uterus as well.[471] Other herbal medicines may exert hormonal effects (oestrogenic or adrogenic), thus should theoretically be avoided or used with caution during pregnancy.[471] In addition, certain plants may affect concurrent medical conditions in pregnancy (hypertensive or hyperglycaemic effects) or cause serious allergic responses (such as Roman or Russian chamomiles).[471]

The following chapter includes 40 of the most common herbal medicines discussed over the Motherisk counselling line. They are listed by species and family names. Each is identified by its primary constituents and pharmacological actions as reported in the literature. Many herbs exhibit lesser therapeutic actions that may not be covered in this chapter. Common uses are the main indications for each herb. Although variation in dose is possible for each herb, only standardized doses are listed. Adverse effects, cautions, contraindications, and drug interactions are based on reported clinical cases or possible theoretical concerns. This chapter is not intended to be an authorative text on herbal medicine. A number of excellent texts already exist, and readers are referred to them for more complete information.[1,2,53,288,394,464] Although the question of efficacy poses particular challenges for herbal medical practice, it is not addressed.

This chapter concentrates primarily on information relating to the use of these herbs in pregnancy and lactation and the safety/risk of such use. A review of the literature quickly shows that well controlled studies in this area are lacking. This chapter is intended to provide the clinician with a review of the available information on each herbal product and to list possible implications for pregnancy and lactation. It has been suggested that every health-care provider incorporates routine questioning of their patients regarding the use of herbal products (tinctures, teas, nutritional supplements, and medications from health food stores) in initial and subsequent obstetric visits.[472] Overall, it is best to limit the use of those herbal products with questionable safety and efficacy. However, health-care providers should remain informed of those CAM treatment modalities that are generally well studied and could be preferred to conventional pharmaceutical therapies.[472]

ALFALFA (MEDICAGO SATIVA L., FABACEAE)

Primary Constituents:
Saponins, isoflavone flavonoids (genistein, daidzein, formononetin), amino acids (canavanine), alkaloids, coumarins, carbohydrates, vitamins (A, B1, B6, B12, C, E, K) (1–6)
Primary Pharmacological Actions:
Nutritive;[1,7] hypercholesterolemic;[2,8,9] phytoestrogenic;[10,11] anticoagulant[10]
Common Uses:
Hypercholesterolemia; management of menopause and menstrual discomfort;[2] appetite stimulant;[478] dyspepsia; relief of pain from arthritis;[478] asthma; diuretic; diabetes[464]
Doses:[478]
Dried herb: 5–10 g, 3×/day
Fluidextract: 5–10 g dried equivalent, 3×/day (1:1; 25% alcohol)
Adverse Effects/Toxicology:
Gastrointestinal upset and diarrhea;[10] photosensitivity[12] and reactivation of systemic lupus erythematosus (SLE);[13–15,395] salmonella outbreaks from raw alfafa sprouts have been reported[397]
Cautions/Contraindications:
Discontinue use if allergic skin reaction occurs; patients with a history of SLE should avoid use,[13] women suffering coagulation disorders should be cautious[424]
Drug Interactions:
High vitamin K content may lead to interactions with anticoagulants;[1,2] phytoestrogenic properties of isoflavones suggests a possible interaction with hormone replacement therapy and oral contraceptives;[1] alfalfa contains saponins which interfere with the absorption or activity of vitamin E[396]
Implications for Pregnancy/Lactation:
Dietary use should not pose a risk; phytoestrogenic nature of herb would suggest caution in pregnancy, as well as women suffering from coagulation disorders should be cautious[424]

ALOE VERA (A. VERA [L.] BURM F., ALOEACEAE)

Primary Constituents:
Aloe vera gel: polysaccharides (acemannan), enzymes, vitamins, minerals[1,17–23]
Aloes: anthraquinone glycosides[24])
Primary Pharmacological Actions:
Aloe vera gel: immunostimulant;[25–32] antibacterial;[33,34] antimicrobial;[35] anti-inflammatory;[36–39] antiviral[40–42]
Aloes: laxative[2,18]
Common Uses:
Aloe vera gel: wound healing,[1,43] treatment of skin irritations (eczema, psoriasis)[2]
Aloes: constipation;[18] a bitter tonic;[478] emmenagogue[478]
Dose:
Aloe vera gel: strength varies between brands
Aloes: 50–200 mg 3×/day when used as a laxative; 28–907 g[478]
Adverse Effects/Toxicology:
Aloe vera gel: rare contact dermatitis[44–47]
Aloes: anthraquinone glycosides are colonic irritants;[7] chronic use may leadto severe cramping[1] and bloody diarrhea; kidney irritation and possible nephritis; electrolyte imbalances possible due to acute and chronic toxicity[18,24]
Cautions/Contraindications:
Aloe vera gel: discontinue use if skin reaction occurs
Aloes: chronic use for relief of constipation not recommended; not advised in patients with appendicitis, abdominal pain, or renal disease[1,2]
Drug Interactions:
None reported
Implications for Pregnancy/Lactation:
Conflicting reports of anti-implantation, abortifacient, and estrogenic effects in animal studies;[48,424] anthraquinone glycosides may lead to electrolyte imbalances and interfere with absorption of nutrients when used chronically; aloes should be considered contraindicated in pregnancy and lactation;[2] topical use of aloe vera gels is not expected to pose a risk in pregnancy[1]

BLACK COHOSH (CIMICIFUGA RACEMOSA [L.] NUTT, RANUNCULACEAE)

Primary Constituents:
Alkaloids, tannins, terpenoids, flavonoids (formononetin)[1,49,50]
Primary Pharmacological Actions:
Number of "endocrine active agents" have been identified with various pharmalogical properties including decreasing luteinizing hormone secretion and binding to estrogen receptors with no effect on follicle-stimulating levels[2,49,50]; debatable estrogenic effect in selected tissues (observed mainly in

the bones and fat tissues but not in ovaries or uterus);[398–400] hypotensive[51] and antibacterial actions[52] have been documented *in vitro* and *in vivo* for related species

Common Uses:

Management of premenstrual syndrome, dysmenorrhea, and menopause;[53,402] traditionally used to relax skeletal muscles and to ease nervous tension.[478]

Dose:[478]

Oral: Dried root or rhizome: 40–200 mg daily

Fluidextract: 40 mg dried equivalent (1:1, ethanol)

Tincture: 0.6–1.2 g dried equivalent (1:5, 60% ethanol)

Duration of use: May be used up to 6 months

Adverse Effects/Toxicology:

At higher doses headaches, nausea, vomiting, dizziness, nervous and cardiovascular depression may occur,[1,2] stomach/gastric pain,[53] acute hepatitis may occur[403,404]

Caution/Contraindications:

Limited toxicity at standard doses

Drug Interactions:

None reported

Implications for Pregnancy/lactation:

Contraindicated in pregnancy and lactation since known as an abortifacient,[429] estrogen effect is observed in selected body tissues.[1,54,398–401] Unconventional health care practitioners have been known to use this herb to aid delivery. One case report describes a newborn with severe neurologic impairments delivered by a woman, who was given a mixture of black and blue cohosh during labor (the causality has not been established).[405]

BLESSED THISTLE (CINICUS BENEDICTUS, ASTERACEAE OR COMPOSITAE)

Primary constituents:

Volatile oil, sesquiterpene lactone, tannins[464]

Primary Pharmacological Actions:

Antibacterial, antineoplastic[602]

Common uses:

Appetite stimulant,[603] antidiarrheal, expectorant, antibiotic,[439] antiseptic, antihemorrhagic, antiemetic;[478] promotion of lactation;[604] digestive bitter and digestive tonic;[478] topically, used as a vulnerary for wounds[439,478,602]

Dose:[478]

Oral: Dried herb: 4–6 g 1.5–3 g, 3×/day

Fluidextract: 1.5–2 g dried equivalent, 3×/day (1:1, 25% ethanol)

Tincture: 0.6–1.2 g dried equivalent, 3×/day (1:5, 25% ethanol)

Powder: 0.6–4 g

Infusion: 60 mL 1.5–2 g, 3×/day

Topical: Infusion: 60 mL

Adverse effects/Toxicology:

High dose greater than 5 g per cup of tea can cause stomach irritation and vomiting,[605] an allergic reaction can happen in individuals sensitive to the asteraceae/compositae family.

Cautions/Contraidications:

Not to be used in people allergic to the Asteraceae/Compositae family. Members of this family include ragweed, chrysanthemums, marigolds, daisies, etc. Contraindicated in individuals with infectious or inflammatory gastrointenstinal conditions.[606]

Drug Interactions:

Theoretically, due to claims that blessed thistle increases the production of stomach acid, it might interfere with antacids, sucralfate, H-2 antagonists, or proton-pump inhibitors (PPIs).[606]

Implications for Pregnancy/lactation:

Not commonly used in pregnancy, thus, the safety is not known. Traditionally, it is used to promote lactation, although no clinical data was found to support this application. Blessed thistle is virtually nontoxic, thus it should not be a concern during lactation at commonly used doses.[436]

BLUE COHOSH (CAULOPHYLLUM THALICTROIDES, BERBERIDACEAE)

Primary Constituents:

Alkaloids (anagyrine, N-methylcytosine, taspine), glycosides (caulosaponin)[600]

Primary Pharmacological actions:

Antispasmotic, laxative,[602] emmanogogue,[607] uterine stimulant,[440,607], anti-inflamatory.[439] Preliminary evidence suggests that blue cohosh might have estrogenic activity in animal models. It decreases luteninizing hormone (LH) and increases serum ceruloplasmin oxidase activity (a measure of estrogenic activity in the liver). It can enhance estradiol binding to estrogen receptors and increase the estradiol-induced transcription activity in estrogen-responsive cells[437]

Common Uses:

Colic, sore throat, cramps, hiccups, epilepsy, hysterics, to facilate childbirth[607,440]

Dose:[464]

Oral: dried rhizome or root: 0.3–1 g 3×/day

Liquid extract (1:1 in 70% alcohol): 0.5–1.0 mL 3×/day

Tea: 1 cup up to 3×/day, prepared by steeping the herb in 150 mL boiling water and then straining.

Adverse Effects/Toxicology:[464]

Gastrointestinal discomfort (diarrhea, cramps), chest pain (angina), hypertension, hyperglycemia.[439,608]

Cautions/Contraindications:

Should be avoided in patients with cardiovascular conditions such as angina and hypertension:[439,607,608] might worsen diabetes;[608] might worsen symptoms in patients with diarrhea;[439,607] due to estrogenic effects, women with hormone sensitive conditions should avoid blue cohosh (breast, uterine, or ovarian cancer; endometriosis and uterine fibroids)[609]

Drug Interactions:

Oral hypoglycemic drugs; might decrease the effectiveness of medcations used for diabetes and cardiovascular disorders;[439,607,608] can enhance the effects of nicotine[608]

Implications for Pregnancy:

Contraindicated in pregnancy. It was shown to be teratogenic;[438,440] uterine stimulant,[439] abortifacient,[441] possible antifertility effects.[439] In a national survey of registered midwifes 64% recommended the use of this herb to induce labor,[440] but based on available evidence should be avoided at any stage of pregnancy. Use of blue cohosh near term was reported to cause a life threatening toxicity in the infant.[442–444] Neonatal acute myocardial infarction (MI), congestive heart failure (CHF), and shock following maternal use of blue cohosh combination product used one month before delivery was reported.[442,444] One case report described a stroke in a

newborn, whose mother used blue and black cohosh during labor, however the causal relationship was not established.[443]
Implications for Lactation:
Not commonly used in breastfeeding, thus the safety is unknown.

BURDOCK (ARCTIUM LAPPA L., ASTERACEAE)

Primary Constituents:
Aldehydes, carbohydrates (inulin), polyacetylenes, volatileoils, sesquiterpene lactones (arctiopicrin)[1,55]
Primary Pharmacological Actions:
Folkloric evidence suggests diaphoretic;[55,56] diuretic;[55–58] laxative;[58] antipyretic properties;[55] hypoglycemic;[59] antibacterial;[52] antimicrobial;[1,59,60] antimutagenic;[1,55,61] fiber extracted from burdock root has been shown to protect against the potentially harmful effects of a number of artificial food additives in rats[7,62]
Common Uses:
Oral and topical use for skin conditions such as eczema and psoriasis;[1,55] orally, also used for rheumatic conditions and infection[2,55]
Dose:[478]
Oral: 2–6 g dried root, 3×/day
Infusion: 2–6 g dried root, 3×/day
Fluidextract: 2–8 g, 3×/day (1:1 in 25% alcohol)
Tincture: 0.8–1.2 g, 3×/day (1:10 in 45% alcohol)
Decoction: 25 g per 500 mL, 1×/day (1:20)
Topical: Tincture: 2.5–5 mL, 3×/day
Adverse Effects/Toxicology:
Temporary worsening of presenting symptoms is noted[2]
Caution/Contraindications:
Based on hypoglycemic action of root caution advised for diabetic patients;[1] potential for allergic reaction in individuals with a known allergy to the sunflower (Asteraceae) family, one case report of anaphylaxis[406]
Drug Interactions:
None reported; however, potential for interaction with oral hypoglycemic agents[1]
Implications for Pregnancy/Lactation:
Uterostimulant action has been noted *in vivo* suggesting caution in pregnancy;[1,55,63] use during lactation is not advised since sesquiterpene lactones are reported to be excreted in breast milk[64]

CALENDULA (CALENDULA OFFICLNALIS L., ASTERACEAE)

Primary Constituents:
Flavonoids, volatile oils, terpenoids, polysaccharides[1,65,66]
Primary Pharmacological Actions:
Anti-inflammatory action noted in vivo due possibly to inhibition of lipoxygenase activity;[7–69] immunostimulant;[70] antiviral;[71] antibacterial;[71,72] antineoplastic[71,73]
Common Uses:
Orally has been used for gastritis, ulcers, and minor digestive irritation;[1,2] applied topically for skin abrasions and minor burns[2,74]
Dose:[478]
Oral: Infusion: 1.0–2.0 g in 150 mL water
Fluidextract: 1–2 g dried equivalent (1:1, alcohol)
Tincture: 0.25–0.75 g dried equivalent, 3×/day (1:4, 25–35% ethanol)
Succus: 1–3 mL, 3×/day
Other dosage forms: equivalent to the above
Topical:
Ointment: 2.0–5.0 g of dried flowers in 100 g ointment
Infusion: 1.0–2.0 g in 150 mL water
Duration of use: may be used up to 7 days
Adverse Effects/Toxicology:
No reported toxicity
Cautions/Contraindications:
An allergic reaction can to occur in individuals sensitive to members of the sunflower (Asteraceae) family[2]
Drug Interactions:
Theoretically, concomitant use of calendula with barbiturates or other drugs with sedative properties can cause additive therapeutic and/or adverse effects[464]
Implications for Pregnancy/Lactation:
Oral use is not recommended in pregnancy since it has spermatocide, antiblastocist, and abortifacent effects;[439] traditionally used as an emmenagogue;[7] estrogenic activity would suggest avoidance in lactation as well;[75] extracts of this herb have been used externally to aid in postpartum wound healing[2]

CAPSICUM (CAPSICUM ANNUM L., SOLANACEAE)

Primary Constituents:
Capsaicinoids (capsaicin), volatile oils, carotenoids, vitamins A and C[1]
Primary Pharmacological Actions:
Capsaicin selectively inhibits the release of substance P, resulting in a number of clinical actions, most notably analgesia;[76] folkloric evidence suggests use as a digestive and cardiovascular stimulant[2]
Common Uses:
Topically, it is used for pain management,[77–81] such as in diabetic neuropathy;[82–86] HIV-neuropathy; pain in herpes zoster infections; for post-herpetic and trigeminal neuralgia,[88–92] as well as fibromyalgia. Capsicum is also used to aid digestion; as an antiflatulent; for colic; diarrea; cramps; toothaches; to improve peripheral circulation; to reduce blood clotting tendencies; motion sickness; alcoholism; malaria; yellow and other fever; for cholesterol reduction, and prevention of arteriosclerosis and heart disease.[464] It is also used as an inhalational provocation test to distinguish sensory hyperreactivity of the airways from asthma. It is also used to relieve muscle spasms, as a gargle for laryngitis, and as a deterrent to thumb-suckling or nail biting.
Dose:
Herb/fruit: 30–120 mg 3×/day
tincture: 0.3–1 mL daily (strength varies among topical products)
Adverse Effects/Toxicology:
If used internally, it can irritate mucosal membranes,[1] causing lacrimation and nasal secretions[76]; in excessive amounts can lead to gastroenteritis and hepatic or renal damage; can decrease blood coagulation. Topically used capsaicin can cause burning and uritcaria. Skin contact with fresh capsicum fruit can cause irritation or contact dermatitis. Inhalation of

capsicum can cause cough dyspnea, nasal congestion, eye irritation and allergic alveolitis[464]
Cautions/Contraindications:
Should be avoided by patients with a known skin allergy, gastric irritation, or hypertension[2]
Drug Interactions:
Caution is advised for patients on antihypertensive agents and monoamine oxidase inhibitors (MAOIs);[1] hepatic metabolism of drugs may be increased.[1,2,91] Possible interactions with ACE-inhibitors, aspirin, antiplatelet drugs, drugs with sedative properties, theophyline[464]
Implications for Pregnancy/Lactation:
Dietary amounts of capsicum should be considered safe in pregnancy and lactation. However, medicinal use should be avoided due to neurotoxicity observed in animal studies.[407,408] Hypertensive activity of this herb can be a concern among women with preeclampsia.[424] Extracts of leaves and stems are not used therapeutically, but in animal studies they have been shown to be uterine stimulants.[2,63] There are reports of dermatitis in breast-fed infants whose mothers' diet was heavily spiced with capsicum.[456]

CASTOR OIL (RICINUS COMMUNIS, RICINUS SANGUINES, EUPHORBIACEAE)

Primary Constituents:[464]
Glycerides; 89.5% of oil is composed of ricinoleic acid and 3% is composed of oleic acid.
Primary Pharmacological Actions:
Stimulant laxative;[610,612] promotes labor by producing hyperemia in the intestinal tract, which causes reflex stimulation of the uterus;[448] it may also increase the production of prostaglandins, which stimulate uterine activity.[449] Topically used as an emollient.[611]
Common Uses:
Constipation;[610] labor stimulation;[449,453,455] topically, used to dissolve cysts, growths or warts.[478]
Dose:[478]
Oral: 15 mL (for constipation)
For induction of labor: doses can vary from 5–120 mL. A single dose regimen of 60 mL dissolved in fruit juice is commonly used.
Adverse Effects/Toxicology:
Abdominal discomfort, cramps, nausea, faintness;[612,613] hypokalemia may occur due to fluid loss or malabsorption;[612,613] castor seeds contain a poisonous protein called ricin, however, pure oil seems to lack it
Cautions/Contraindications:
Contraidicated in intestinal/biliary obstruction, abdominal pain of unknown origin[450] and other biliary disorders[451]
Drug Interactions:
Theoretically, castor oil can increase the adverse effects of cardiac glycosides, corticosteroids, laxatives, potassium depleting diuretics.[614]
Implications for Pregnancy/Lactation:
Castor oil is commonly used to speed the onset of labor.[449] In a small prospective trial within 24 hours of administration of castor oil, 30 of 52 women (57.7%) began active labor compared to 2 of 48 (4.2%) women receiving no treatment.[449] This study was criticized for a small sample size and poor methodological quality.[452] There is a case report of amniotic fluid embolism at term attributed to maternal use of castor oil.[453] Another case report described uterine rupture which was thought to be associated with castor oil ingestion.[454] The use of castor oil near term has also been associated with a higher incidence of meconium passage in utero.[455] The safety of castor oil in breastfeeding has not been established.

CHAMOMILE, GERMAN (MATRICARIA RECUTITA L., ASTERACEAE)

Primary Constituents:
Coumarins, flavonoids (apigenin), volatile oils (chamazulene, (-) alpha-bisabolol, spiroethers)[1,92]
Primary Pharmacological Actions:
Anti-inflammatory;[92–94] spasmolytic;[92,93,95] antiulcerogenic;[92,93,96] hypnotic and anxyioltic actions;[97,98] anti-inflammatory properties (could be a result of the inhibition of leukotriene synthesis as well potential antioxidant properties)[99,100]
Common Uses:
Used orally as a digestive aid and for gastrointestinal discomfort (peptic ulcers, gastritis, colic, diarrhea);[2] insomnia, tension and anxiety;[1,92,93] applied topically for skin irritations;[93,101,102] hemorrhoids; mastitis; leg ulcers; skin; anogenital mucus membrane inflammation; bacterial skin diseases including those of the mouth and gums; for treatment and prevention chemotherapy or radiation induced oral mucositis.[514] When inhaled german chamomile is used to treat inflamation and irritation of the respiratory tract.[464]
Dose:[2,92]
Dried herb: 1–4 g 3×/day
Liquid extract: 1–4 mL 3×/day
Tincture: 3–10 mL 3×/day
Adverse Effects/Toxicology:
Allergic reactions following both oral and topical use have been reported[92,103,515] (including cases of anaphylactic reactions);[513,516,517,104,105] vomiting may occur following excessive doses[1,92]
Cautions/Contraindications:
Potential exists for cross-sensitivity in individuals known to be allergic to members of the sunflower (Asteraceae) family,[2,106] can exacerbate asthma, caution in people with coagulation disordes[424]
Drug Interactions:
The apigenin constituent is a central benzodiazepine receptorligand; therefore interaction with agents such as anxiolytics and hypnotics is possible,[98] anticoagulants, antiplatelet drugs and some medications that are metabolized by CYP450, such as lovastatin, ketoconazole, itraconazole, triazolam, etc.).[464]
Implications for Pregnancy/Lactation:
Traditional emmenagogue and abortifacient;[7,424] no teratogenicity reported, however, resorption of fetuses and reduction in birth weight has been observed in animal studies following administration of high doses;[2,107] caution advised with high dose, women suffering from coagulation disordes should be cautious;[424] no contraindications exist in pregnancy or lactation at this time. However, the concerns stated here for the therapeutic use of chamomile are generally not relevant to its common use as beverage tea.[473] An Australian cross-sectional survey of vitamin, mineral and herbal supplementation during pregnancy determined that among 211 women the most prevalent herbal preparation used before conception was

chamomile (5%); ginger was used by 20% of all women in the first trimester of pregnancy; chamomile displaced ginger in the second trimester of pregnancy (6%), and raspberry leaf as tea or capsules was the main herbal preparation during the third trimester (8%).[466]

CHASTE TREE (VITEX AGNUS-CASTUS L., VERBENACEAE)

Primary Constituents:
Iridoids (agnuside), alkaloids, flavonoids, volatile oils[1]
Primary Pharmacological Actions:
Low doses of approximately 120 mg/day are thought to diminish follicle stimulanting hormone (FSH) release and increase luteinizing hormone (LH) release, resulting in decreased estrogen levels and increased progesterone and prolatin levels. However, at higher doses of approximately 480 mg/day, chasteberry extract seems to result in decrease of prolactin release, but FSH and LH do not seem to be affected by higher doses of chasteberry.[457]
Common Uses:
Premenstrual syndrome, menstrual cycle irregularities, menopause;[108,109,411,412] mastodynia; acne resulting from a hormonal imbalance;[1,110] insufficient lactation; situations associated with hyperprolactinemia[111,112]
Dose:
Fruit: 0.5–1.0 g 3×/day[1]
Extract: 40 drops standardized to fruit content (9 g/100 mL) daily[2]
Adverse Effects/Toxicology:
Nausea, headache, diarrhea, dyspepsia, acne, pruritus, and menstrual irregularities have been reported to a limited degree;[2,108] some have alopecia, headaches, tiredness, agitation, tachycardia, and dry mouth while taking chasteberry. Allergic reactions can occur in some patients but typically resolve spontaneously when chasteberry is stopped.[464]
Cautions/Contraindications:
Patients on hormone therapy should avoid use[1]
Drug Interactions:
Patients on hormone therapy or oral contraceptives should avoid use;[1] possible interaction with dopamine antagonists such as haloperidol and metoclopramide[2]
Implications for Pregnancy/Lactation:
A case of multiple follicular development has been noted in patients undergoing unstimulated in vitro fertilization treatment with the use of herbal medicine containing chaste tree;[113] given the pharmacology of this herb, emmenagogue properties and uterine stimulant properties[424] use is not recommended during pregnancy. Although information is limited, stimulation of lactation has been noted without altering the composition of the breast milk.[1,2,457] Although still controversial, chaste tree may decrease breast milk production.[457]

CRANBERRY (VACCINIUM MACROCARPON AIT., ERICACEAE)

Primary Constituents:
Proanthocyanides, fructose, terpenoids, unidentified large molecular weight compound[2]
Primary Pharmacological Actions:
Have not been well established, however, cranberry is purported to inhibit bacterial adherence to the urinary tract[2,114–117]
Common Uses:
Prophylaxis use against urinary tract infections[18–120,421,422]
Dose:[2,118]
Capsules: 300–400 mg twice daily
Juice: 150–600 mL daily
Adverse Effects/Toxicology:
No evidence of toxicity
Cautions/Contraindications:
None reported
Drug Interactions:
A few described cases reports of interaction with warfarin.[418–420]
Implications for Pregnancy/Lactation:
Limited information on its safety in pregnancy or lactation

DANDELION (TARAXACUM OFFICINALE G.H. WEBER EX WIGGERS, ASTERACEAE)

Primary Constituents:
Terpenoids (triterpenoids), phytosterols, inulin, minerals (potassium), vitamin A[1,121]
Primary Pharmacological Actions:
Dandelion root used principally as a digestive aid and choleretic agent,[122] while the leaf exerts a diuretic action;[123] hepatoprotective;[124] antimicrobial;[125] hypoglycemic;[126] anti-inflammatory[127]
Common Uses:
Root suggested for hepatobiliary disorders, dyspepsia, and loss of appetite;[2] leaves used mainly for water retention[1]
Dose:[1]
Dried herb: 2–8 g of root or 4–10 g of leaves 3×/day
Liquid extract (leaves): 4–10 mL 3×/day
Tincture (root): 5–10 mL 3×/day
Adverse Effects/Toxicology:
Allergic reaction to herb can occur[1,128]
Cautions/Contraindications:
Allergic response possible in individuals with a known allergy to the sunflower (Asteraceae) family; caution suggested in cases of occlusion of the bile ducts, empyema, and paralytic ileus;[2] source of dandelion should be observed since reports of heavy metal contamination.[129] Consult a health care provider prior to use if you are on oral hypoglycaemic or psychoactive medications.[478] Discontinue use if hypersensitivity occurs such as contact dermatitis.[423]
Drug Interactions:
Possible interaction with dandelion leaves and diuretics[1]
Implications for Pregnancy/Lactation:
Folkloric evidence would suggest avoidance during pregnancy; however, generally not expected to be a concern if used in food amounts;[1] prudent to avoid high dose during pregnancy and lactation

DEVIL'S CLAW (HARPAGOPHYTUM PROCUMBENS DC., PEDALIACEAE)

Primary Constituents:
Carbohydrates, iridoids (harpaside, harpagoside), phenols[1,130–132]

Primary Pharmacological Actions:
Anti-inflammatory,[133,134] antirheumatic;[74,135,136] analgesic;[1] cardiovascular activity[137,138]
Common Uses:
Joint inflammation due to rheumatoid arthritis and gout;[1,427] indigestion and dyspepsia[2,56,139,140]
Dose:[478]
Oral (as a digestive aid):
Dried tuber: 0.5 g in decoction, 3×/day
Tincture: 0.2 g dried equivalent, 3×/day (1:5, 25% ethanol)
Fluid extract, tablet, capsule: equivalent to the above dose
Oral (inflammation of the joints):
Dried tuber: 1.5–2.5 g in decoction, 3×/day
Tincture, tablet, capsule: equivalent to the above dose.
Duration of use: Must be taken for a minimum of 2–3 months for beneficial effects to be demonstrated
Adverse Effects/Toxicology:
Headache, tinnitus, anorexia, diarrhea, loss of taste,[2,425] but serious adverse events have not been reported.[425]
Cautions/Contraindications:
Digestive bitter, therefore can theoretically increase stomach acid secretions and stimulate bile production; caution is advised in patients with active peptic ulcer and gall bladder disease;[1,2] should be used with caution in patients with hypertension or other cardiac conditions, since blood pressure and heart rate have been affected in animals; may cause hypoglycaemia, therefore diabetics should monitor their glucose levels closely when starting devil's claw.[464]
Drug Interactions:
One report of interaction with warfarin.[425,426]
Implications for Pregnancy/Lactation:
Safety in pregnancy and lactation has not been established; there is some doubt that devil's claw is a traditional abortifacient;[141] it may have some oxytocic effects[464]

DONG QUAI (ANGELICA SINENSIS [OLIV.] DIELS, APIACEAE)

Primary Constituents:
Furanocoumarins (bergapten), volatile oils[1,142,143]
Primary Pharmacological Actions:
Traditional use in gynecological disorders and obstetrics (see common uses); hypotensive;[144,145] antiarrhythmic;[144,145] antilipidemic;[1] analgesic.[146]
Common Uses:
Menopause;[147] dysmenorrhoea;[144,146] amenorrhea,[2,143,144] ulcers; anemia; constipation; in prevention and treatment of allergic attacks; treatment of skin depigmentation and psoriasis.[464]
Dose:
Dried herb: 1–2 g of root/rhizome or 2–5 g of leaves 3×/day
Liquid extract: 0.5–2.0 mL of root/rhizome or 2–5 mL of leaves 3×/day
Tincture: 0.5–2 mL of root/rhizome or 2–5 mL of leaves 3×/day
Adverse Effects/Toxicology:
Although not seen in angelica root specifically, concerns exist regarding the presence of furanocoumarins, which may result in possible photosensitization, resulting in a dermatitis-like skin reaction;[2,139,148] diarrhea possible since herb may exert a relaxant action on smooth muscle of digestive tract;[139] potentially carcinogenic and mutagenic.[464]
Cautions/Contraindications:
Folkloric evidence cautions against use in acute illnesses such as hypermenorrhea and hemorrhagic disease[144]
Drug Interactions:
Caution is recommended in patients receiving oral anticoagulants[1]
Implications for Pregnancy/Lactation:
Although widely used for gynecological disorders and obstetrics (including as a tonic aiding recovery postpartum and treatment of gestational hypertension),[2,149] considered a traditional emmenagogue and abortifacient;[7] first trimester use and patients with a history of spontaneous abortions cautioned since dong quai is known to influence uterine muscle in vitro (uterine stimulant and relaxant effects);[2,144,458,435] caution is prudent in pregnancy and lactation.

ECHINACEA (E. ANGUSTIFOLIA DC., E. PURPUREA [L.] MOENCH, E. PALLIDA [NUTT.] NUTT., ASTERACEAE)

Primary Constituents:
Carbohydrates (polysaccharides),[150,151] glycoproteins;[2] amides (alkamides),[152–154] caffeic acid derivatives (echinacoside, cichoric, cynarin)[155–158*]
Primary Pharmacological Actions:
Immunostimulatory action;[159–162] anti-inflammatory;[163,164] antibacterial;[2] antiviral;[165] antineoplastic[166]
Common Uses:
Upper respiratory tract (common cold and flu) and lower urinary tract infections[2,167]
Dose:[1]
Dried herb: 1 g 3×/day
Liquid extract: 0.25–1.0 mL 3×/day
Tincture: 1–2 mL 3×/day
Adverse Effects/Toxicology:
No reported toxicity
Cautions/Contraindications:
Should be avoided by individuals with a known allergy to the sunflower (Asteraceae) family;[53] caution in patients with progressive systemic diseases (tuberculosis, multiple sclerosis) and autoimmune conditions (diabetes mellitus, lupus, rheumatoid arthritis)[2,7]
Drug Interactions:
Immunostimulatory action suggests caution with immunosuppressant agents[2]
Implications for Pregnancy/Lactation:
In vitro studies of bacterial and mammalian cells and *in vivo* studies in mice have found no evidence of mutagenicity associated with Echinacea.[475] Some *in vitro* studies suggest possible impaired male fertility associated with Echinacea use.[476,477] This study found decrease in sperm movement at high concentration of Echinacea. It is not always possible to extrapolate results from *in vitro* or *in vivo* studies to humans. The first prospective controlled study completed at the Motherisk Program reported on pregnancy outcome of 206 women using Echinacea products. There were no statistical differences

* Although the three species are often considered interchangeable, their chemical constituents do differ.[2]

observed in the rates of major malformations as compared to the disease-matched group of women.[474] Safety during lactation has not been established.

EVENING PRIMROSE (OENOTHERA BIENNIS L., ONAGRACEAE)

Primary Constituents:
Fixed oils (linoleic acid and gamma linolenic acid)[1,168]
Primary Pharmacological Actions:
Essential fatty acid involved in prostaglandin bio synthetic pathways1,169
Common Uses:
Management of dermatological conditions (atopic eczema, psoriasis, acne);[170–174,464] gynecological disorders (premenstrual syndrome[175,176]; menopause[177]; mastalgia[178,179] and endometriosis[180]); psychiatric conditions;[1,181] diabetic neuropathy;[182] rheumatoid arthritis[183] multiple sclerosis;[184] Sjögren's syndrome;[180,185] used in pregnancy (prevention of preeclampsia, shortening the duration of labor, stimulating labor and preventing postdate deliveries).[464]
Dose:
Dose varies depending on the indication (standard adult dose is 2–8 g daily);[2] duration of use is up to 3 months[478]
Adverse Effects/Toxicology:
Gastrointestinal discomfort (indigestion, diarrhea, nausea) and headache have been reported to a limited degree;[1] one case report of noctural seizures associated with the use of evening primrose oil, black cohosh and chasteberry[478,588] and several case reports of seizures associated with the use of EPO in patients with or without known seizure disorders[430,431]
Cautions/Contraindications:
Caution advised for patients with a history of mania or epilepsy;[1,2] bleeding disorders[464]
Drug Interactions:
Possible concerns with phenothiazines, nonsteroidal anti-inflammatory drugs, corticosteroids, anticoagulants, and beta-adrenergic antagonists;[2] possibly with anesthesia, however other drugs were also involved[464]
Implications for Pregnancy/Lactation:
EPO has been used for prevention of preeclampsia, shortening the duration of labor, stimulating labor and preventing postdate deliveries. Data on the efficacy and the safety of EPO used to shorten labor or gestation is coflicting.[432,433] Use of EPO may increase the risk for pregnacy complications, including delayed rupture of membranes, oxytocin augmentation, arrest of descent and vacuum extraction.[432] In a randomized, double-blind, placebo-controlled study 43 women were given 450 mg of linoleic acid and 600 mg of calcium and 43 (placebo group) were given 450 mg of starch and 600 mg of lactose during the third trimester. This intervention seemed to reduce the incidence for preeclampsia.[334] In another placebo-controlled, partially double-blind, clinical trial in 150 women, a combination of evening primrose oil and fish oil was compared to magnesium oxide and to a placebo in preventing preeclampsia of pregnancy. Five women in the control group developed the triad of preeclampsia compared with two cases in each of the exposed groups.[335] The fatty acids found in evening prirose oil also occur naturally in breast milk so the administration of this oil to lactating mothers can increase the fatty acid content of their breast milk.[187]

FENUGREEK (TRIGONELLA FOENUM-GRAECUM L. FABACEAE)

Primary Constituents:
4-isoleucine, alkaloids (trigonelline, gentianin, carpaine), coumarin compounds, diosgenin[464,618]
Primary Pharmacological Actions:
Cardiotonic, hypoglycaemic;[615,616] diuretic, anti-inflamatory, antilypertensive, antiviral, hypoglycemic, anticholesteronic[439]
Common Uses:
Orally used as a tonic to promote appetite;[439,603] used for dyspepsia, gastritis;[439] lowering blood glucose in people with diabetes;[615,616] constipation; high cholesterol;[617] promotion of lactation;[618,446] bronchitis; tuberculosis; chronic cough; cancer; antipyretic;[620] topically, used for local inflammation,[603] myalgia, lymphadenitis, gout, wound, leg ulcer[604] and eczema.[605]
Dose:[478]
Oral: (dried) 1–6 g 3×/day
Daily dose: 6 g, 5–90 g seeds/day
Decoction: 31 g with 473 mL of water (for the stomach)
15 mL 3–5×/day; 0.5 g 3–5×/day (digestive tonic)
Topical: the powdered seeds are stirred with hot water to give a paste which is used for poultices, boils and carbuncles (50 g powdered seeds/250 mL water)
2–3 capsules 3×/day (for galactagoue effect)
Duration of use: For prolonged use, consult a health care provider
Adverse Effects/Toxicology:
Diarrhea and flatulence;[616] hypoglycemia with high doses;[610,619] occupational exposure to fenugreek can cause asthma;[610] inhalation of the seed powder or topical use of the paste applied to the scalp can cause an allergic reaction.[621]
Cautions/Contraindications:
Contraindicated in people allergic to fenugreek; caution in patients with diabetes blood glucose levels should be monitored closely.[439,610]
Drug Interactions:
Anticoagulants, corticosteroids, hypoglycemic drugs, insulin, MAOIs, hormone therapy[439]
Implications for Pregnancy/Lactation:
Contraindicated for oral use in amounts greater than those found in food due to its potential uterine stimulating activity.[439] Commonly used as a galactogogue. One study in a group of 10 women with infants born between 24 to 38 weeks gestation (nonplacebo-controlled), showed a significant increase in milk production, no adverse effects were reported.[446] One case of suspected GI bleeding in a premature infant has been reported (the causality not established).[447] Caution is advised in women with diabetes or on anticoagulants.[439]

FEVERFEW (TANACETUM PARTHENIUM [L.] SCHULTZ-BIP., ASTERACEAE)

Primary Constituents:
Sesquiterpene lactones (parthenolide), volatile oils, pyrethrins, flavonoids[1,188–190]
Primary Pharmacological Actions:
Analgesic;[189] anti-inflammatory;[191] antipsoriatic[189,190]
Common Uses:
Migraine prevention;[192–194,428] arthritis;[195] also used for menstrual irregularities, infertility, anemia, cancer, prevention of

miscarriage; toothaches; antiseptic and insecticide; stimulant and tonic; intestinal parasites[464]
Dose:[478]
Oral:
Dried leaf: 50–250 mg/day
Dried aerial parts: 50–200 mg/day
Tincture: 0.25–0.75 g/day (1:5, 25% ethanol), take with water
If standardized: equivalent to 0.2% dried weight of parthenolide daily, used as a marker of identity. Duration of use: consult a health care provider for use beyond 4 months
Adverse Effects/Toxicology:
Trials have reported mouth ulcers and gastrointestinal discomfort (abdominal pain, indigestion, diarrhea, flatulence);[139,193] "postfeverfew syndrome" has been described in the literature;[1,2,193] allergic contact dermatitis can occur with topical use of feverfew.[464]
Caution/Contraindications:
Individuals with known allergies to the sunflower (Asteraceae) family should avoid use[196,197]
Drug Interactions:
No reported cases; one review suggests possible interaction with anticoagulant therapy and NSAIDs[2,464]
Implications for Pregnancy/Lactation:
Traditional emmenagogue and abortifacient;[7,439] not recommended for use in pregnancy and lactation.

FISH OILS (OMEGA-3 FATTY ACIDS, LONG-CHAIN POLYUNSATURATED FATTY ACIDS [LCPUFA'S], DOCOSAHEXAENOIC ACID [DHA], EICOSAPENTAENOIC ACID [EPA], COD LIVER OIL, ETC.)

Primary Constituents:
There are two families of essential fatty acids (EFA's)—the n-3 family, which are primarily abundant in oil of marine animals or and the n-6 family, which are of vegetable origin.[479] The long-chain n-3 fatty acids include DHA and EPA. DHA and other polyunsaturated long-chain fatty acids are abundant in oily, dark-colored ocean fish, including salmon, tuna, mackerel, and sardines.[480]
Primary Pharmacological Actions:
The long-chain n-3 fatty acids may reduce the activity of eicosanoid promoters of the parturition process, particularly prostaglandins F and E, and increase the activity of eicosanoids with myometrial-relaxant properties, particularly prostacyclins.[479] EPA is an inhibitor of platelet aggregation because it is an effective substrate for cyclooxygenase and reduces TXA_2 concentration.[480]
Common Uses:[464]
Orally, fish oils are used for hyperlipidemia, coronary heart disease, hypertension, stoke, rheumatoid arthritis, psoriasis, attention deficit hyperactivity disorder, hypercholesterolemia, preeclampsia, recurrent miscarriages, preterm birth, intrauterine growth retardation, and others.
Dose:
In pregnant women: 2.7 g of fish oil per day (4 fish oil capsules providing 864 mg of EPA and 621 mg of DHA per day) was used in clinical trials,[480] although doses up to 6.1 g/day were also used in women with either threatening preeclampsia or intrauterine growth retardation[482] starting at 33 weeks gestation; For other indications, doses of 1–4 g of fish oils a day were used.[464]
Adverse Effects/Toxicology:
In studies of pregnant women receiving 2.7 g of fish oil per day (4 fish oil capsules providing 864 mg of EPA and 621 mg of DHA per day) no serious adverse effects were observed during pregnancy, labor and delivery.[480] Only mild side effects are reported, including belching and unpleasant taste (464). In one study conducted on pregnant women supplemented with fish oils there was a trend toward increased maternal blood loss during delivery (13% more than 500 mL).[481] At doses above 3 g/day, fish oils may cause bleeding.[464] Some fish oils (such as cod liver oil) could contain significant amounts of vitamins A and D.[464] Thus, if these supplements are used at high doses aver prolonged period of time there is a risk of toxicity. Some species of fish also contain environmental contaminants, such as methyl mercury and PCBs.[480]
Cautions/Contraindications:
Any treatment with fish oil supplementation should be stopped whenever pregnancy has gone beyond the preterm period;[482] women and infants should be monitored for any possible bleeding complications[479]
Drug Interactions:
None reported, but use with caution when combined with anticoagulant medications
Implications for Pregnancy/Lactation:
A number of randomised controlled trials, systematic reviews and a Cochrane Collaboration review addressed the role of long chain n-3 fatty acids on pregnancy duration and foetal outcome. The majority of clinical evidence supports the safety of fish oil supplementation in the latest stages of pregnancy or lactation. However, there is still limited evidence on the safety of fish oil supplementation in early stages or throughout pregnancy. FOTIP (fish oil trials in pregnancy) is the largest multicenter RCT, which was conducted in 19 European hospitals in seven countries during 1990 and 1996 recruiting 1619 pregnant women.[482] The results have shown a positive effect on length of pregnancy, but no benefit of fish oil supplementation for the primary prevention of preeclampsia or low birth weight. During pregnancy n-3 PUFA are incorporated into fetal brain and retinal lipids. Maternal supplementation of n-3 containing fish oils in pregnancy seems to carry some long-term beneficial effect on later cognitive and visual development of children.[483–486]
Recent study conducted in Ontario, Canada reported on inadequate dietary intake of n-3 fatty acids in a group of pregnant women in their second and third trimesters of pregnancy.[487] In 1990, Health and Welfare Canada recommended that pregnant women should be consuming a minimum of 1.36 g/day and 1.26 g/day of n-3 PUFA, respectively during the 2nd and 3rd trimesters.[487] The International Society for the Study of Fatty Acids and Lipids (ISSFAL) recommended a minimum of 300 mg/day of DHA for pregnant and lactating women.[487] In summary, supervised supplementation with long chain n-3 fatty acids in late (>18–20 weeks) pregnancy or breastfeeding does not appear to cause any major pregnancy or fetal risk at moderate doses. However, some experts believe that "giving fish is a gentler approach to tocolysis than providing pharmaceutical agents with potent physiological actions."[479] In addition, any treatment with fish oil supplementation should be stopped whenever pregnancy has gone beyond the preterm period.

Women and infants should be carefully monitored for any possible bleeding complications at high doses of n-3 fatty acids due to some theoretical and some clinically observed concerns.

FLAXSEED (LINUM USITATISSIMUM, LINACEAE)

Primary Constituents:
Alpha-linolinic acid, ligans, cyanogenic glycosides (linustatin, neolinustatin, linamarin), soluble fiber;[464] secoisolariciresinol diglucoside (SDG), 3-hydroxy-3methylglutaric acid (HMGA) and cinnamic acids[601]
Primary Pharmacological Actions:
Laxative,[614] antiatherogenic,[610,622,623] hypoglycaemic,[626] antioxidant,[625,627] antitumoral,[628] anti-inflammatory,[625] ligans have weak estrogenic effects and possible antiestrogenic effects.they seem to complete with endogenous steroids for various enzymes and receptors.this competition might reduce endogenous estrogen binding to estrogen receptors, resulting in an antiestrogenic effects.[461]
Common Uses:
Chronic constipation; colon damagedue to laxative abuse; diverticulitis; irritable bowel syndrome; irritable colon; gastritis; enteritis;[602] bladder inflammation;[614] hypercholesterolemia, atherosclerosis;[622,623] protection against cancer;[461,624] improvement of renal function in people with systemic lupus erythematosus (SLE) nephritis.[625] Topically, used as a poulitice for skin inflammation.[603] Ophtalmically, flaxseed is used for the removal of foreign bodies from the eye.[614]
Dose (478):
Source of fatty acids: up to 30 mL/day of flaxseed oil
Laxative: 5–10 g of whole or bruised seeds with 150 mL liquid, 3×/day (or 1:10 solid to liquid)
Flaxseed should be soaked in water before ingestion
Take at least 2 hours before or after any other medications
Duration of use: may be used up to 3 months
Adverse Effects/Toxicology:
Oral use may increase the number of bowel movements;[626] occasionally allergic and anaphylactic reactions have been reported after ingestion of flaxseed; workers processing flax products might be more likely to be hypersensitive.[610,629]
Cautions/Contraindications:
Use with caution in patients with bleeding disorders,[630] contraindicated in patients with gastrointestinal obstructions.[497]
Drug Interactions:[464,630]
Anticoagulant/antiplatelet agents (can increase bleeding time)
Implications for Pregnancy/Lactation:
In a study of 18 nonpregnant women supplementation with flaxseed powder (10 g/day for three menstrual cycles) lengthened luteal phases, but did not affect the levels of estradiol, estrone, progesterone, DHEA, prolactin, or SHBG concentrations as compared to control menstrual cycles in the same women.[409] Midfolicular phase testosterone levels were significantly higher during the flax cycles, and luteal phase progesterone/estradiol ratios were significantly higher.[462] In an animal study pregnant rats were given flaxseed (20 or 40% of the diet), or deffated flaxseed meal (13 or 26%). Although fertility and fetal development were not affected, the female rats experienced irregular estrous cycles, which appeared to be a dose-dependent effect.[459] Another study on flaxseed and its lignan precursor showed a negative effect on the birth weight and reproductive development of pups.[463] Due to lack of any human pregnancy studies and observed effects on sex hormones caution is advised in pregnancy or in planning stages. The only human study on lactation looked at seven women who took flaxseed oil supplementation (20 g/day for 4 weeks). This study observed increased breast milk levels of several omega-3 fatty acids (alpha-linolenic acid, eicosapentaenoic acid (EPA) and docosapentaenoic acid, but no increase in the levels of docoshexaenoic acid).[460]

GINGER (ZINGIBER OFFICINALE ROSCOE, ZINGIBERACEAE)

Primary Constituents:
Oleo-resin (gingerols, shogaols), carbohydrates, volatile oils[1,198]
Primary Pharmacological Actions:
Antiemetic/antinauseant;[2,199] antiulcerogenic;[200–203] anti-inflammatory;[204,205] hypoglycemic;[206] cardiotonic;[207] analgesic[208]
Common Uses:
Antinauseant;(motion sickness,[209,210] pregnancy,[211] drug-induced[212,213]) digestive aid (dyspepsia, gastrointestinal upset, flatulence, constipation);[214] management of inflammatory conditions (osteoarthritis, rheumatoid arthritis, myalgias);[2,215–217] helps to relieve pain associated with menstruation,[488] traditionally used as spasmolytic[489]
Dose (1):
Dried herb (rhizome): 0.25–1.0 g 3×/day
Tincture: 0.3–0.6 g dried equivalent, 3×/day (1:5, 90% ethanol) used with water[478]
Fluid extract: 0.125–0.25 g dried equivalent/day (1:2, 90% ethanol) taken with water[478]
Adverse Effects/Toxicology:
Low toxicity rating; it has Generally Recognized as Safe (GRAS) status in the States; heartburn and dyspepsia have been reported,[2] irritant effect in the mouth and throat[478]
Cautions/Contraindications:
None reported
Drug Interactions:
None reported, however, based on pharmacological actions caution advised when patients are using cardiac, diabetic, and anticoagulant therapy,[1,2] theoretically, may enhance barbiturate effect, and may interfere with acid-inhibiting drugs[464]
Implications for Pregnancy/Lactation:
Ginger is commonly used by pregnant women for the treatment of nausea and vomiting in pregnancy, for example, 20% of 211 pregnant women in their first trimester of pregnancy were taking ginger in one Australian study.[496] Several randomised-controlled clinical trials on the efficacy of ginger in the treatment of nausea and vomiting in pregnancy did not report any adverse outcomes or adverse effects.[211,491–495] No teratogenicity was seen in a study group of 27 patients taking 250 mg of powdered ginger 4×/day for the treatment of hyperemesis gravidarum.[211] A prospective cohort study of 187 pregnant women using ginger supplements in the first trimester of pregnancy did not reveal an increased risk of malformations or other pregnancy outcomes including the rates of miscarriages.[490] Although a traditional abortifacient at standard therapeutic doses, ginger appears safe during pregnancy at lower doses.[2,218]

GINKGO (GINKGO BILOBA L., GINKGOACEAE)

Primary Constituents:
Terpenoids (ginkolides), flavonoids (bilobides, flavone glycosides)[1,219,220]
Primary Pharmacological Actions:
Vasodilator;[219,221] spasmolytic;[222,223] antithrombotic;[224,225] antioxidant;[226–230] neuroprotective effect[231,232]
Common Uses:
Dementia,[233–235] memory impairment;[236–239] cerebral insufficiency;[219,240,241] intermittent claudication (242); Raynaud's syndrome (2); tinnitus;[243,244]; vertigo[245–247]
Dose (2):
Dried herb (leaves): 300 mg daily
Standardized extract: 40 mg 3×/day
Adverse Effects/Toxicology:
Rare, mild adverse reactions include gastrointestinal discomfort and headaches, dizziness, palpitations, restlessness, weakness, skin rash[1,497] spontaneous bleeding has also been reported[2,249]
Cautions/Contraindications:
None reported
Drug Interactions:
May potentiate the effect of anticoagulants, such as warfarin, aspirin[2]
Implications for Pregnancy/Lactation:
Safety in pregnancy and lactation has not been established

GLUCOSAMINE (2-ACETAMIDO-2-DEOXYGLUCOSE, GLUCOSAMINE SULPHATE, GLUCOSAMINE HYDROCHLORIDE, N-ACETYL-D-GLUCOSAMINE, ETC)

Primary Pharmacological Actions:
Glucosamine (GLS) becomes incorporated into proteoglycans, the building blocks of cartilage; available evidence from a number of randomized placebo-controlled trials (RCTs),[498,499] as well as from one meta-analysis[500] and a Cochrane review,[501] supports the use of GLS in the treatment of osteoarthritis (OA); it causes a disease-modifying effect (increases joint space width in OA),[502] and a pain-relieving and anti-inflammatory effect[508]
Common Uses:
Osteoarthritis; joint pain; used to maintain and slow down degradation of cartilage in chronic joint degenerative diseases
Dose (oral):
500 mg 3×/day, must be taken for at least 2 months to observe an effect[478]
Adverse Effects/Toxicology:
Low toxicity rating; well tolerated in multiple clinical trials with most common adverse effects involving reversible gastrointestinal symptoms;[501,510,511] based on animal *in vitro* and *in vivo* studies, GLS can interfere with glucose metabolism and result in insulin resistance, thus use with caution in patients with diabetes[505–508]
Cautions/Contraindications:
Use cautiously in patients with diabetes and asthma;[504] however, one RCT on patients with type 2 diabetes mellitus found no clinically significant alterations in glucose metabolism among 36 patients who used GLS orally;[503] since glucosamine is extracted from various shellfish use with caution in individuals with shellfish allergy
Drug Interactions:
Insufficient evidence
Implications for Pregnancy/Lactation:
Animal studies: GLS was not found to be teratogenic in mice following intra-placental and intra-amniotic injections;[514] it was found to decrease sperm-egg fusion in mice,[513] although it was not certain whether it will inhibit fertilization *in vivo*; one animal study suggested a possible *in vivo* teratogenic effect of high dose of GLS via activation of hexosamine pathway, leading to a state of hyperglycaemia, oxidative stress and inhibited expression of a gene responsible for neural tube closure[512]
Human studies: human data is scarce; a preliminary Motherisk cohort study prospectively followed-up 54 women with an early first trimester exposure to GLS supplements (data not published). There were no observed statistical differences in the rates of congenital malformations, spontaneous abortions, mean birth weights and other pregnancy outcomes, as compared to a nonexposed group of women (n = 54).
Due to limited human pregnancy and breastfeeding safety data, glucosamine use is not recommended.

GOLDENSEAL (HYDRASTIS CANADENSIS L., RANUNCULACEAE)

Primary Constituents:
Isoquinoline alkaloids (hydrastine, berberine, canadine)[1,250]
Primary Pharmacological Actions:
Antimicrobial;[58,251,252] astringent and antiseptic;[74,253] antipyretic;[253] antineoplastic[254,255]
Common Uses:
Orally, for infections of the upper respiratory[1] and genitourinary tract;[256–258] topically, as a mouthwash for sore gums and mouth, as well as for skin rashes, infections[464]
Dose (478):
Dried roots: 500–1000 mg, 3×/day
Tincture: 0.2–0.4 g dried equivalent, 3×/day (1:10, 60% ethanol) orally, take with water
Fluidextract: 0.3–1 g dried equivalent, 3×/day (1:1, 60% ethanol) orally, take with water
Adverse Effects/Toxicology:
Prolonged use is associated with digestive disorders and hallucinations;[464] toxicity at high dose can cause nausea, vomiting, diarrhea, hypotension, myocardiac depression, dyspnea, hyperreflexia, parasthesia, convulsions, and death through respiratory failure;[1,2,7] contact ulceration of mucosal membranes reported[1]
Cautions/Contraindications:
Contraindicated in hypertensive patients;[1,58] use with caution in patients with cardiovascular diseases and inflammatory gastrointestinal conditions[464]
Drug Interactions:
None reported, but there may be a few possible drug interactions
Implications for Pregnancy/Lactation:
Traditionally, contraindicated in pregnancy based on uterine stimulant actions of hydrastine, berberine, and canadine;[1,2,7,63] traditionally, it was used to regulate menstruation and as an abortifacient; in rats, orally administered berberine did not cause increased incidence of malformations, but caused a reduction in foetal body weight at high doses[515]

Human case reports: based on the fact that berberine affects bilirubin metabolism and has been reported to contribute to the risk of kernicterus in neonates, not recommended in pregnancy.[516] The safety during lactation has not been established; especially avoid using in infants with jaundice due to the above concerns[516]

GREEN TEA (CAMELLIA SINENSIS PLANT)

Primary Constituents:
Polyphenols (catechin, gallaogatechin, epicatechin, epigallocatechin, epicatechin gallate, and epigallocatechin gallate, [also known as EGCG]), caffeine, theobromine, and theophylline.
Primary Pharmacological Actions:
Contains polyphenols which are potent antioxidants, scavengers of free radicals; antitumor activity in animal models;[517,518,520,524] exerts antihyperglycemic effect in diabetic mice and promotes glucose metabolism in humans;[522,529] inhibits atherosclerosis by lipid, antioxidant and fibrinolytic mechanisms;[523,530] an inhibitor of dihydrofolate reductase (DHFR) activity *in vitro* at concentrations found in the serum of green tea drinkers (0.1–1.0 μmol/L)[532]
Common Uses:
Dietary beverage (commonly consumed in Asia, Japan); to prevent certain types of cancers;[517,518,520,521,527] used for gastrointestinal problems,[526] and to improve cognitive performance;[464] to protect skin from damaging effects of ultraviolet radiation,[525] cardiovascular disease[528]
Dose:
1–10 cups of brewed tea a day;[464] 500 mg capsules of 96% green extract containing polyphenols are available, equivalent to 2 cups of brewed green tea; in Phase I clinical trial a maximum tolerable dose was found to be 4.2 g/m^2 once daily or 1.0 g/m^2 three times daily of green tea capsules;[517] full clinical benefits of capsules are unknown
Caffeine content: in the first brew of 2.32 g of loose dry green tea leaves, 1 cup (6 oz) contains approximately 56 mg of caffeine,[519] but it can also range from 10–80 mg per cup[464]
Adverse Effects/Toxicology:
Well tolerated at moderate amounts; at a maximum tolerable dose some patients felt mild side effects such as insomnia, irritability, and nervousness, due to the caffeine content of green tea;[517] 50% of volunteers who ingested the equivalent of 10 Japanese cups of green tea a day for 3 months complained of mild abdominal bloating, heartburn, nausea, and insomnia (probably due to caffeine content).[518]
Cautions/Contraindications:[464]
Most concerns are highly theoretical and based on the fact that large amounts of caffeine may aggravate a number of medical conditions (such as hypertension, cardiac conditions, etc.)
Drug Interactions:[464]
Theoretically, green tea may promote anticoagulant activity of some medications (e.g., aspirin); caffeine found in green tea may also reduce the effectiveness of benzodiazepines or other psychotropic medications
Implications for Pregnancy/Lactation:
Due to caffeine content of green tea, pregnant or nursing mothers are advised to limit green tea intake to 2 cups a day.[521] The results of Motherisk study suggest a small but statistically significant increase in risk of spontaneous abortion and low birth weight babies in pregnant women consuming more than 150 mg of caffeine per day.[531] Pregnant women should be encouraged to be aware of dietary caffeine intake and to consume less than 150 mg of caffeine a day from all sources throughout pregnancy. Green tea extract in capsule formulations has not been adequately assessed in pregnancy or breastfeeding. Since EGCG (a component of green tea) was found to be a dihydrofolate reductase inhibitor in *in vitro* and *in vivo* studies at concentrations found in the blood of green tea drinkers, caution is recommended in the early stages of pregnancy. There is some evidence to suggest that green tea intake may reduce estrogen levels in the blood of postmenopausal women.[533]

HOPS (HUMULUS LUPULUS L., CANNABACEAE)

Primary Constituents:
Volatile oils, oleoresins, phenylflavonoids (nonsteroidal phytoestrogens), tannins[1,259]
Primary Pharmacological Actions:
Sedative;[74,253,259,260] spasmolytic[7,253]
Antimicrobial;[1,261,262] anti-inflammatory[263]
Common Uses:
Mood and sleep disturbances,[464] digestive aid, irritable bowel syndrome[57,253]
Dose:[478]
Dried inflorescence: 500–1000 mg, 3×/day
Tincture: 0.2–0.4 g dried equivalent, (1:5, 60% ethanol)
Fluidextract: 0.5–2 g dried equivalent, (1:1, 45% ethanol)
Adverse Effects/Toxicology:
Allergic response including anaphylactic reaction most frequently reported;[1,7,264,265] animal studies have shown hops can be fatal when administered parenterally[1]
Cautions/Contraindications:
Patients with a history of depression should avoid use,[1,2,253] not advised in patients with hormone-dependent cancers[535]
Drug Interactions:
Sedative action may potentiate the effects of hypnotics and alcohol[1,2]
Implications for Pregnancy/Lactation:
Contains 8-prenylnaringenin, a potent phytoestrogen,[536] a hormone substance with possible estrogenic activity;[7,58,266,534] antispasmodic activity in the uterus reported in vitro;[1] historical reports of female hops pickers and brewers with menstrual cycle irregularities and acne.[535] Based on the described estrogenic effects, hops should be avoided in pregnancy and lactation.

JUNIPER (JUNIPERUS COMMUNIS L., CUPRESSACEAE)

Primary Constituents:
Flavonoids, tannins, volatile etheric oils (monoterpenes, sesquiterpenes)[1,267]
Primary Pharmacological Actions:
Diuretic;[139] antiviral, antibacterial;[139,268,538] hypoglycaemic,[269,270] anti-inflammatory;[271] astringent[1]
Common Uses:
Genitourinary tract infections;[74,272] rheumatic conditions (arthritis);[56] cystitis;[2,272] digestive aid[56]

Dose[478]:
Oral (fruit):
Berries: 1–2 g, 3×/day, up to 10 g/day
Dried Berries Infusion: 2–3 g in 150 mL hot water, steep for 20 minutes, 3–4×/day
Fluidextract: 2–3 g dried equivalent, 3×/day (1:1, 45–64% ethanol)
Tincture: 0.2–0.4 g dried equivalent, 3×/day (1:5, 45% ethanol)
Oil: 20–100 mg
Adverse Effects/Toxicology:
Topical use documented to cause burning, erythema, inflammation, blistering, and possible contact dermatitis;[2] high oral dose associated with kidney and gastrointestinal irritation, nephrotoxicity, diuresis, albuminuria, hematuria, discolored urine, tachycardia, and hypertension;[1,7] one reported case of fever, severe hypotension, renal failure, hepatotoxicity, and severe cutaneous burns on the face following ingestion of home-made Juniperous oxycedrus extract[537]
Cautions/Contraindications:
Although refuted by a recent report,[273] herb generally considered contraindicated in kidney disease[2]
Drug Interactions:
Not advised in patients receiving hypoglycemic and diuretic agents[1]
Implications for Pregnancy/Lactation:
Traditionally, emmenagogue and abortifacient;[7,274–276] proposed uterostimulant, anti-implantation, and antifertility properties would suggest avoidance in pregnancy.[1,2,63,277]
Safety during lactation has not been established.

KAVA-KAVA [PIPER METHYSTICUM G. FORST, PIPERACEAE]

Primary Constituents:
Kavalactones (pyrones), alkaloids, flavonoids[278,279]
Primary Pharmacological Actions:
Anxiolytic;[280–282] spasmolytic;[279] analgesic;[283] neuroprotective;[284] anticonvulsant[285]
Common Uses:
Anxiety;[283,286,287] tension and restlessness;[2] headaches[74,283]
Dose:[2]
Dried herb: 1.5–3.0 g daily
Liquid extract: 3–6 mL daily (100 mg standardized kava extract two or three times daily)
Adverse Effects/Toxicology:
Allergic skin reactions resulting in a pruritic skin condition;[278,288] high dose associated with disturbances of vision (photophobia, diplopia, and oculomotor paralysis);[2] gastrointestinal discomfort;[2] equilibrium disturbances[283]
Health Canada issued a stop-sale order in August 2002 for all products containing kava. The department also requested the recall of these products from all levels of the market and issued an advisory to consumers, advising against the use of products containing kava. This advisory came in view of four cases of liver toxicity associated with the use of kava products reported in Canada. None of the Canadian cases resulted in death. Other foreign regulatory authorities have also received reports of liver toxicity associated with the use of kava, among which there were three fatalities. Individuals who have compromised liver function due to preexisting liver problems related to disease, age, or prior or current drug/alcohol abuse may be at particular risk of liver toxicity associated with kava use.[539]
Cautions/Contraindications:
Dopamine antagonism by kava suggests caution in Parkinson's disease;[289] contraindicated in depression[2]
Drug Interactions:
No reported interaction with centrally acting drugs, however, potential exists[2,290]
Implications for Pregnancy/Lactation:
Safety has not been established in pregnancy and lactation, avoid using

LACTOBACILLUS (PROBIOTICS, LACTOBACILLUS ACIDOPHILUS, L. PLANTARUM, L. CASEI, L. DELBRUECKII, L. RHAMNOSUS GG, L. GG, ETC)

Definition:
"Probiotics" are defined as live microorganisms, which when administered in adequate amounts confer a health benefit to the host[543]
Primary Pharmacological Actions:
Inhibit growth and adhesion of pathogens;[557,564] restore indigenous microflora; immune modulating response[564]
Common Uses:
For viral, antibiotic-induced, and traveler's diarrhoea (especially in infants and children);[544–547] urogenital infections (also during pregnancy);[548–550,564] investigated for lactose intolerance, necrotizing enterocolitis (in premature very low birth weight neonates),[551] alleviating symptoms of irritable bowel syndrome,[552] allergic diseases,[553–555] enhancement of immune response[556,557]
Dose:[464]
(Doses of Lactobacillus acidophilus preparations are based on the number of freeze-dried or liquid cultures of live bacteria.)
Adults (>18 years)
Capsules/tablets/liquid: a common dose is 1–10 billion live bacteria, in 3–4 divided doses, taken daily by mouth.
Vaginal suppository (for bacterial vaginosis): one to two suppositories, each containing 1–10 billion live bacteria, inserted into the vagina once or twice daily.
Children (<18 years)
For diarrhoea: 5–20 billion live Lactobacillus GG
Adverse Effects/Toxicology:
Low toxicity rating;[564] adverse-effects were not found in a large population receiving LGG in Finland or among preterm infants;[557] some cases of sepsis or endocarditis in adults, neonates and children were reported, primarily in immunosuppressed patients who had multiple risk factors[557–560]
Cautions/Contraindications:
Use with caution in immunosuppressed patients[557]
Drug Interactions:
Insufficient evidence
Implications for Pregnancy/Lactation:
In a retrospective collaborative drug surveillance program no congenital malformations were reported among 77 infants whose mothers took lactobacillus acidophilus in the first-trimester of pregnancy.[561] In a randomised placebo-controlled trial, the incidence of atopic eczema in infants exposed to Lactobacillus GG for 2–4 weeks prior to delivery and up to

6 months during breastfeeding was significantly lower at 2 years of age, as compared to a nonexposed group of children. No adverse effects were reported in this study, although probiotics were not administered to the women during organogenesis. Thirty six out of 64 infants in the treatment arm continued to receive probiotics orally during a postnatal period with no reported adverse effects.[554,562,563] In a number of other studies[550,565,566] probiotics were administered to pregnant women either starting at 14 weeks gestation or a few weeks prior to the expected date of delivery without any reported adverse pregnancy outcomes. In summary, there is insufficient number of studies on the safety of probiotics in the first trimester of pregnancy or on their long term use in pregnancy. However, due to their widespread use (especially in Europe) and lack of documented adverse pregnancy outcomes, the fetal risk is expected to be low. In view of several studies on the efficacy of probiotics for the treatment or prevention of diarrhea in infants and children, their use may be considered safe in breastfeeding.

LICORICE (GLYCYRRHIZA GLABRA L., FABACEAE)

Primary Constituents:
Coumarins, terpenoids (glycyrrhizin, glycyrrhetinic acid), flavonoids (isoflavones), volatile oils[1,291,292]
Primary Pharmacological Actions:
Gastroprotective and antiulcerogenic;[293,294] anti-inflammatory;[295,296] spasmolytic agent;[291] antibacterial;[297] antiviral;[298–300] antiparasitic;[301,302] hepatoprotective[303]
Common Uses:
Ulcers (gastric, duodenal, peptic);[291,304,305] canker sores and orofacial herpes;[306] coughs and bronchitis;[307,308] management of stress and fatigue;[2] premenstrual syndrome;[2] arthritis;[464] intravenously, used for viral hepatitis treatment[464]
Dose:[478]
Powdered root: 1–4 g, 3×/day or 1 cup of tea, TID
Fluidextract: 4–6 g dried equivalent, 3×/day, (1:1, 45–65% ethanol)
Licorice Extract: 600–2000 mg/day
Deglycyrrhizinated licorice: 760 mg, 3–6×/day
Adverse Effects/Toxicology:
Common adverse effects include headache, lethargy, and edema;[2] consumption of 50 g a day, or chronic use of longer than 6 weeks is documented to cause pseudohyperaldosteronism with hypertension and hypokalemia;[1,7,309] overconsumption has resulted in death;[308,310–312] since licorice can decrease serum testosterone and increase 17-hydroxyprogesterone it might cause decreased libido and sexual dysfunction in men;[464] can cause amenorrhea[464]
Cautions/Contraindications:
Not recommended in patients with cardiovascular, kidney, and liver disease[1,2]
Drug Interactions:
Possible interaction with hypoglycemic drugs (loop and potassium-sparing diuretics), cardiac glycosides, and hormonal therapy;[1,2] increases the half-life of hydrocortisone and prednisolone[2]
Implications for Pregnancy/Lactation:
Traditional emmenagogue and abortifacient;[7] although no clinical cases documented, one authoritative text suggests the action of licorice on estrogen may exacerbate gestational hypertension;[1] contains phytoestrogens and phytoprogestins;[540] heavy dietary licorice consumption (> 500 mg/week) among 95 Finnish women has been linked to increased risk of preterm delivery, possibly due to the effects on cortisol and prostaglandin metabolism in the placenta; however, information on licorice consumption during pregnancy was collected retrospectively.[541] Medicinal use during pregnancy and lactation would not be recommended.

MA HUANG (EPHEDRA SINICA STAPF., EPHEDRACEAE)

Primary Constituents:
Alkaloids (ephedrine, pseudoephedrine), tannins, volatile oils, flavonoid glycosides[2,313]
Primary Pharmacological Actions:
Cardiostimulant;[7,314] hypotensive/hypertensive;[7,313] bronchodilator;[314] decongestant[315]
Common Uses:
Weight loss;[316–320] bronchial asthma[58] and bronchitis[11,58]
Dose:
Food and Drug Administration (FDA) suggests a maximum dose of 8 mg of ephedrine every 6 hours up to 24 mg daily for no more than 7 days.[2,321]
Based on the Health Canada's advisory, the maximum allowable dosages for Ephedra/ephedrine in products is 8 mg ephedrine/single dose or 32 mg ephedrine/day. Products containing *Ephedra* which are marketed for traditional medicine, will continue to be available, provided they do not contain caffeine and that the ephedrine content does not exceed 8 mg/dose to a maximum of 32 mg/day.
Adverse Effects/Toxicology:
Reactions to ma huang or ephedrine include headache, restlessness, dizziness, insomnia, gastrointestinal discomfort, hypertension, palpitations, tachycardia, nausea, and vomiting;[7] high dose has been associated with hallucinations, paranoia, mania, and psychosis;[2,322,323] deaths have resulted from excessive use[324,325]
Cautions/Contraindications:
Due to the reported pharmacological actions, ma huang and ephedrine are not recommended in heart disease, hypertension, thyroid disease, diabetes, anxiety, glaucoma, impaired cerebral circulation, pheochromocytoma, and thyrotoxicosis[2]
In June, 2001 Advisory Health Canada is warning consumers not to use products containing the herb Ephedra, either alone or in combination with caffeine and other stimulants, for purposes of weight loss, body building or increased energy. Products containing Ephedra or ephedrine in combination with caffeine and other stimulants are of particular concern, since ephedrine may cause serious, possibly fatal, adverse effects in the body when combined with these ingredients.[542]
A review of a U.S. Food and Drug Administration database of adverse event reports collected between June 1, 1997, and March 31, 1999, identified 10 cases resulting in death and 13 cases resulting in permanent impairment that were considered to be possibly, probably, or definitely related to dietary supplements containing ephedra alkaloids. In Canada, a total of 60 adverse event reports have been received by Health Canada related to Ephedra or ephedrine, alone or in combination

with other products, previous to October 2000. This total includes two deaths, both suicides, which may or may not have been directly associated with the use of these products. Reported adverse events range from episodes that may indicate the potential for more serious effects, such as dizziness, tremors, headaches and irregularities in heart rate, to seizures, psychosis, heart attacks, and stroke.
Drug Interactions:
Actions may be potentiated by aspirin and stimulants such as caffeine;[321,326–328] avoid use with antidepressants and antihypertensives[2]
Implications for Pregnancy/Lactation:
No reported teratogenicity; ma huang not recommended in pregnancy and lactation due to uterostimulant properties of ephedrine[2]

PASSIONFLOWER (PASSIFLORA INCARNATA L., PASSIFLORACEAE, MORE THAN 500 SPECIES)

Primary Constituents:
Alkaloids, flavonoids (vitexin, orientin, swertisin, hyperoside, rutin, hesperidin, clorogenic acid),[1,329,330,596] other phytoconstituents[597]
Primary Pharmacological Actions:
Sedative/hypnotic;[56,331–334] anxiolytic;[335] spasmolytic;[253,331] analgesic[253,331]
Common Uses:
Indicated for symptoms of insomnia, tension, and restlessness[2,336]
Dose (1):
Dried herb: 0.25–1.0 g 3×/day
Liquid extract: 0.5–1.0 mL 3×/day
Tincture: 0.5–2.0 mL 3×/day
Adverse Effects/Toxicology:
A case of vasculitis has been reported with a herbal preparation containing passionflower;[337] due to cyanogenic constituents the toxicity of Passiflora species cannot be ruled out[597]
Cautions/Contraindications:
Excessive use may cause oversedation[1]
Drug Interactions:
No reported drug interactions in clinical practice; however, caution advised if patient is receiving centrally acting medications[2]
Implications for Pregnancy/Lactation:
Constituents have shown uterine stimulant activity in animal studies,[1] the plant constituent chrysin facilitates the body to produce more testosterone by inhibiting the aromatase enzyme responsible for the conversion of testosterone to estrogen;[597] passion flower extract was not found to be teratogenic in mice at maternal doses of 400 mg/kg/day;[410] caution is advised in pregnancy and lactation

PEPPERMINT (MENTHA X PIPERITA L., LAMINACEAE)

Primary Constituents:
Volatile oils (menthol), flavonoids, tannins[139,338]
Primary Pharmacological Actions:
Gastrointestinal;[139,253,339] spasmolytic;[53,340,341] antibacterial;[342,568] antifungal;[569] anti-inflammatory;[567] effective against type I allergic reactions[570,571]
Common Uses:
Gastrointestinal discomfort (nausea, vomiting, diarrhea, indigestion);[253,343] irritable bowel disease;[344,345] spastic colon;[346–348] colds and flu[253,343]
Dose:[478]
Oral (leaf): Dried leaf powder: 2–4 g, 3×/day
Tincture: 0.4–0.6 g dried equivalent, 3×/day, (1:5, 45% ethanol)
Tablet, capsule: 2–4 g of dried equivalent, 3×/day
Oral (oil): 0.05–0.2 mL, 3×/day
Adverse Effects/Toxicology:
The use of peppermint oil for irritable bowel disease has been reported to cause heartburn and esophageal reflux;[345] buccal products have been associated with contact irritation;[2] high dose can cause gastrointestinal upset and atrial fibrillation;[7,349] hemolysis and jaundice possible in cases of glucose-6-phosphate dehydrogenase deficiency[7]
Cautions/Contraindications:
Contraindicated in patients with achlorhydria and glucose-6-phosphate dehydrogenase deficiency,[2,345,350] not recommended in patients with chronic heartburn, severe liver damage, inflammation of the gallbladder, or obstruction of bile acids[572]
Drug Interactions:
None reported
Implications for Pregnancy/Lactation:
Traditional emmenagogue and abortifacient;[2,7] administration of large amounts of M. piperita and M. spicata teas to rats resulted in a decrease in spermatogenesis and plasma total testosterone levels.[573] However, the concerns stated here for the therapeutic use of peppermint are generally not relevant to its common use as beverage tea.[473]

RASPBERRY LEAF (RUBIS IDAEUS L.)

Primary Constituents:[464]
High tannin content, flavonoids, ellagic acid[580]
Primary Pharmacological Actions:
This herbal product has been reported to possess both uterine stimulating and relaxing effects in experiments conducted in animals, and in studies on isolated uterine strips;[576–578] these effects may be dose and tissue dependent; recent evidence suggests that there may be at least two components of this herb that are responsible for relaxant activity in an *in vitro* gastrointestinal preparation;[577] this herb may have some estrogenic effect[464]
Common Uses:
Tea prepared from red raspberry leaf is a popular traditional form of treatment during pregnancy for morning sickness, to prevent miscarriage, and to shorten and ease labor; also used for dysmenorrhea,[576] as well as it was traditionally used for diarrhoea, and as an astringent[577]
Dose:[464]
Can be used as tea, tinctures, tablets
Tea: 2 g of dried leafs steeped in 240 mL of boiling water for 5 minutes (for facilitation of labor); for other uses- 1 to 6 cups a day
Liquid extract: 1:1 in 25% alcohol, 4–8 mL 3×/day

Adverse Effects/Toxicology:
No serious side effects were reported among pregnant women taking raspberry leaf tablets, some developed constipation[575]
Cautions/Contraindications:
None reported
Drug Interactions:
None reported
Implications for Pregnancy/Lactation:
Red raspberry leaf tea is commonly used by midwifes and pregnant women primarily in the third trimester of pregnancy to prepare for labor. In an Australian study 8% of 211 surveyed pregnant women in their third trimester of pregnancy took red raspberry in capsules or teas.[574] However, to date there is only one randomized, placebo-controlled trial of 96 pregnant women who took 2.4 g/day of raspberry leaf tablets from 32 weeks of pregnancy until labor.[575] No major side effects were reported among women who took the herb. Women on red raspberry leaf tablets did not experience a shorter duration of labor; however they required fewer number of artificial rupture of membranes. There were no reported serious adverse effects in either the mothers or the infants in this study. Another retrospective observational study was conducted by the same authors to demonstrate the safety of raspberry leaf herb during pregnancy. Fifty-seven women consumed raspberry leaf in a variety of formulations, at various doses as early as 8 weeks' gestation. There were no reported complications.[579] Due to long-term traditional use and lack of documented adverse effects of red raspberry leaf, it seems relatively safe to use near the end of pregnancy under the supervision of a health care provider. Due to insufficient knowledge of its safety in early pregnancy avoid it, especially in larger amounts. No well documented studies exist on the safety of this product in breastfeeding. Probably safe as a beverage

SLIPPERY ELM (ULMUS RUBRA MUHL., ULMACEAE)

Primary Constituents:
Carbohydrates (mucilage), tannins[1]
Primary Pharmacological Actions:
Demulcent/emollient;[7,57,139,253] antitussive;[57,139,253] astringent[253]
Common Uses:
Orally used for gastrointestinal complaints (ulcers, gastritis, diarrhea),[1] and coughs;[139] traditionally has been used topically for wounds, sores, boils, and abscesses[2,253]
Dose:[1]
Powdered bark: 4–16 mL 3×/day
Liquid extract: 5 mL 3×/day
Adverse Effects/Toxicology:[464]
Contact dermatitis; pollen is an allergen
Cautions/Contraindications:
No reported contraindications
Drug Interactions:[464]
None reported; theoretically, may slow the absorption of orally administered drugs due to high mucilage content
Implications for Pregnancy/Lactation:
Traditionally, abortifacient actions reported with whole bark, however, powdered slippery elm unlikely to be a concern;[1] traditionally, sticks of slippery elm were inserted into the cervix, and when they swelled caused cervical dilation;[599] safety during lactation has not been established

ST. JOHN'S WORT (HYPERICUM PERFORATUM L., CLUSIACEAE)

Primary Constituents:
Anthraquinone (hypericin, isohypericin, protohypericin), flavonoids, phenols, tannins, volatile oils[1,351]
Primary Pharmacological Actions:
Antidepressant;[352–354] antiretroviral,[2,355–357] topical analgesic or anti-inflammatory,[581] traditionally has been used as an anticonvulsant, extracts of Hypericum perforatum aerial parts could contribute to the control of petit mal seizures in mice[582]
Common Uses:
Depression and mood disturbances,[358–362,584] topical analgesic and anti-inflammatory. Also used orally to treat cancer, HIV/AIDS, and as a diuretic.[464]
Dose:[1]
Dried herb: 2–4 g 3×/day
Liquid extract: 2–4 mL 3×/day
Tincture: 2–4 mL 3×/day
If standardized: 0.2–1.0 mg of total hypericin/day in 3 divided doses; or 900–1000 mg extract/day containing 0.3% hypericins or 5% hyperforin (or both) in 3 divided doses[478]
Adverse Effects/Toxicology:
Generally well tolerated in clinical trials, fewer drop out rates of patients in trials as compared to placebo or in comparison with standard antidepressants;[584] delayed hypersensitivity and photodermatitis have been reported in the literature;[1,363–365] phototoxicity in human lens epithelial cells;[583] other possible adverse effects include gastrointestinal discomfort (nausea), constipation, dizziness, dry mouth, sedation, and restlessness[2,364]
Cautions/Contraindications:
In cases of hypersensitivity or photodermatitis use should be discontinued; not recommended in patients with cardiovascular disease or pheochromocytoma,[2] not recommended in organ transplant patients on immunosupressants, patients on anti-HIV drugs; use with caution when coadministered with medications with a narrow therapeutic index; or agents used for photodiagnostic procedures.[586]
Drug Interactions:[586]
Based on antidepressant action of herb, should not be used in patients already receiving a conventional antidepressant agent (tricyclic antidepressants, selective serotonin reuptake inhibitors, monoamine oxidase inhibitors);[1,2] inducer of cytochrome P450 CYP3A4 liver enzyme and P-glycoprotein, thus may reduce efficacy of some coadministered medications, such as immmunosupressants (ciclosporine, tacrolimus); anti-HIV drugs, anticancer drugs, oral anticoagulants (digoxin), hormonal contraceptives; higher rates of intracyclic breakthrough bleeding were observed among patients coadministering St. John's Wort with low-dose oral contraceptives,[585] thus, there is a theoretical risk of poorer compliance and increased risk of unexpected pregnancies
Implications for Pregnancy:
In vitro/in vivo studies: slight *in vitro* uterotonic activity has been suggested;[366] animal studies: renal and hepatic damage was observed in the offspring of rats treated with 100–1000 mg/kg/day of hypericum extract prenatally and during breastfeeding, the lesions were more severe at higher doses;[587] no reproductive toxic effects were found in rats or dogs with oral

doses of 900 and 2700 mg/kg in another animal study;[588] female mice who were treated with this herb throughout gestation delivered pups which were not different in development and growth from the pups exposed to a placebo;[589] a similar study found lower birth weights among male offspring exposed to the herb *in utero*, but there were no long-term differences in later development[590]

Human case reports: a follow-up of a woman taking St. John's wort from 24 weeks gestation until delivery reported on a healthy neonate with normal physical and behavioral assessment during the first month of life[591]

Human clinical studies: none have been reported so far

Implications for Breastfeeding:

Animal studies: St. John's wort has been reported to adversely affect the quality and quantity of breast milk in cattle when consumed in large quantities, dose not specified[594]

Human studies: a decrease in plasma prolactin levels was found in healthy male volunteers after a single 2700 mg dose of St. John's wort;[592] hypericin and hyperforin were detected at minimal levels in breast milk of a woman who took 300 mg of St. John's wort three times a day, levels were not detected in infant's plasma.[593] One published case report describes an infant exposed to a maternal dose of 900 mg/day from 24 weeks gestation to 1 week prior to delivery, and then restarting on day 20 postpartum at a dose of 300 mg/day.[591] On days 4 and 33, behavioral assessment of the infant was normal. The only prospective cohort study followed up 33 breastfeeding women on St. John's wort therapy and compared the incidence of maternal and neonatal adverse outcomes to two comparison groups of women who either used conventional antidepressants or who were not exposed to any medications. Although no more women on this herbal product reported decreased milk production as compared to the unexposed women, there were five exposed infants who developed minor adverse effects (colic, drowsiness, lethargy), which did not necessitate any medical intervention.[594]

TEA TREE OIL (MELALEUCA ALTERNIFOLIA CHEEL, MYRTACEAE)

Primary Constituents:

Volatile oils (terpinen-4-ol and cineole)[367]

Primary Pharmacological Actions:

Antimicrobial and antiseptic[139]

Common Uses:

Fungal infections (including vaginal yeast infections)[368–370,371]

Dose:

Standard therapeutic levels do not exist; one report suggests oil should contain 30% or more of terpinen-4-ol and less than 15% of cineole[2,367]

Adverse Effects/Toxicology:

Topical use may result in skin irritation, or possible allergic contact dermatitis[372,595]

Cautions/Contraindications:

Oral use of tea tree oil would not be advised[2]

Drug Interactions:

None reported

Implications for Pregnancy/Lactation:

Safety in pregnancy and lactation has not been established; probably safe if used topically

UVA-URSI (ARCTOSTAPHYLOS UVA-URSI [L.] SPRENG., ERICACEAE)

Primary Constituents:

Flavonoids, iridoids, phenolic glycosides (arbutin, methylarbutin), tannins, terpenoids[2,373–376]

Primary Pharmacological Actions:

Antiseptic;[2] antimicrobial;[139,377] astringent[1,253]

Common Uses:

Urinary tract infections[139]

Dose[1]

Dried herb (leaves): 1.5–4.0 g 3×/day

Liquid extract: 1.5–4.0 g 3×/day

Adverse Effects/Toxicology:

High levels of hydroquinone were reported to cause tinnitus, nausea, vomiting, cyanosis, convulsions, collapse, and death[7]

Cautions/Contraindications:

Caution advised with chronic use and large doses; high tannin content suggests long-term use has the potential to lead to chronic liver impairment;[1] patients with a kidney disorder should avoid use[2]

Drug Interactions:

None reported

Implications for Pregnancy/Lactation:

Although no evidence of teratogenicity or harm, generally not recommended for use in pregnancy and lactation;[378] can have oxytocic effect;[464] arbutin did not affect reproduction or fetal development in rats at adult doses of 100 mg/kg/day[598]

WILD YAM (DIOSCOREA VILLOSA L., DIOSCOREACEAE)

Primary Constituents:

Steroidal saponins (dioscin, dioscorin) based on diosgenin[2]

Primary Pharmacological Actions:

Anti-inflammatory; antirheumatic; antispasmodic;[7,253,379] diosgenin is used as a precursor for commercial chemical synthesis of human steroidal hormones[464]

Common Uses:

Gastrointestinal discomfort (including irritable bowel disease);[2] rheumatism and arthritis;[7,253] "natural alternative" to hormone replacement therapy;[464] gynecological conditions (dysmenorrhea and ovarian pains)[2]

Dose[2]

Dried herb: 5–10 g 3×/day

Liquid extract: 1–2 mL 3×/day

Tincture: 2–4 mL 3×/day

Adverse Effects/Toxicology:

Ingestion of large amounts of wild yam tincture has caused emesis[464]

Cautions/Contraindications:

None reported; but avoid in hormone sensitive cancers/conditions[464]

Drug Interactions:

None reported

Implications for Pregnancy/Lactation:

Traditional contraceptive based on diosgenin content;[7,74] suggestions that diosgenin would be a substrate for steroidal substances such as progesterone and dehydroepiandrosterone (DHEA) have been refuted;[2,380–382] due to possible emmenagogue effect, use in pregnancy and lactation would not be advised[7]

REFERENCES

1. Newall CA, Anderson LA, Phillipson JD. *Herbal Medicines: A Guide for Health Care Professionals.* London, UK: The Pharmaceutical Press, 1996.
2. Boon H, Smith M. The Botanical Pharmacy. Toronto: Quarry Press, 1999.
3. Natelson S. Canavanine to arginine ratio in alfalfa (Medicago sativa), clover (Trifolium), and the jack bean (Canavalia ensiformis). *J Agric Food Chem.* 1985;33:413–419.
4. Natelson S. Canavanine in alfalfa (Medicago sativa). *Experentia.* 1985;41:257–259.
5. Polachek I, Zehavi V, Nairn M, et al. Activity of compound G2 isolated from alfalfa roots against medically important yeasts. *Antimicrob Agents Chemother.* 1986;30:290–294.
6. Berrang B, Davis KHJ, Wall ME, et al. Saponins of two alfalfa cultivars. *Phytochemistry.* 1974;13:2253–2260.
7. Koren G. *Maternal-Petal Toxicology: A Clinician's Guide.* 2nd ed. New York, NY: Marcel Dekker Inc., 1994.
8. Malinow MR, McLaughlin P, Stafford C. Alfalfa seeds: effects on cholesterol metabolism. *Experimentia.* 1980;36:562–563.
9. Molgaard J, Von Schenck H, Olsson AG. Alfalfa seeds lower low density lipoprotein cholesterol and apolipoprotein B concentrations in patients with type II hyperlipoproteinemia. *Atherosclerosis.* 1987;65:173–179.
10. Briggs C. Alfalfa. *Can Pharm J.* March 1994;(1):84–86.
11. Leung AY, Foster S. *Encyclopedia of Common Natural Ingredients Used in Food, Drugs and Cosmetics.* 2nd ed. Toronto/New York: John Wiley & Sons, 1996.
12. De Smet PA, et al. *Adverse Effects of Herbal Drugs.* 2nd ed. New York: Springer-Verlag, 1992.
13. Roberts JL, Hayashi JA. Exacerbation of SLE associated with alfalfa ingestion (letter). *N Engl J Med.* 1983;308(22):1361.
14. Malinow MR, Bardana EJ, Pirofsky B, et al. Systemic lupus erythematosus-like syndrome in monkeys fed alfalfa sprouts: role of a non-protein amino acid. *Science.* 1982;216:415–417.
15. Rosenthal GA. The biological effects and mode of action of L-canavanine, a structural analogue of L-arginine. *Q Rev of Biol.* 1977; 52:155–178.
16. Alcocer-Varela J, Iglesias A, Lorente L, et al. Effects of L-canavanine on T cells may explain the induction of systemic lupus erythematosus by alfalfa. *Arthritis Rheum.* 1985;28(1):52–57.
17. Shelton RW. Aloe vera, its chemical and therapeutic properties. *Int J Dermatol.* 1991;30(10):679–683.
18. Canigueral S, Vila R. Aloe. *Br J Phytother.* 1994;3(2):67–75.
19. Bruce WGG. Medicinal properties in the aloe. *Excelsa.* 1975;5:57–68.
20. Reynolds T. The compounds in aloe leaf exudates: a review. *Bot J Linnean Soc.* 1985;90:157–177.
21. Sabeh F, Wright T, Norton SJ. Purification and characterization of a glutathione peroxidase from the aloe vera plant. *Enzyme Protein.* 1993;47:92–98.
22. Yamaguchi I, Mega N, Sanada H. Components of the gel of Aloe vera (L.) *Burm. f. Biosci Biotechnol Biochem.* 1993;57(8): 1350–1352.
23. Afzal M, Ali M, Hassan RAH, et al. Identification of some prostanoids in aloe vera extracts. *Planta Med.* 1991;57:38–40.
24. The Lawrence Review of Natural Products. *Aloe. Monograph.* Levittown, PA: Pharmaceutical Information Associates, 1988.
25. Womble D, Helderman JH. Enhancement of allo-responsiveness of human lymphocytes by acemannan (Carrisyn). *Int J Immunopharmacol.* 1988;10(8):967–974.
26. Shida T, Yogi A, Nishimura H, et al. Effects of aloe extract on peripheral phagocytosis in adult bronchial asthma. *Planta Med.* 1985;51:273–275.
27. McDaniel HR, et al. An increase in circulating monocyte/macrophages is induced by oral acemannan in HIV-1 patients. *Am J Din Pathol.* 1990;94:516–517.
28. Egger SF, Brown GS, Kelsey LS, et al. Studies on optimal dose and administration schedule of a hematopoietic stimulatory b-(l,4)-linked mannan. *Int J Immunopharmacol.* 1996;18(2):113–126.
29. Marshall GD, Gibbons AS, Pamell LS. Human cytokines induces by acemannan. *J Allergy Immunol.* 1991;91:295.
30. Ramamoorthy L, Kemp MC, Tizard IR. Effects of acemnannan on the production of cytokine in a macrophage cell line RAW264.7. Joint Meeting of the European Tissue Repair Society and Wound Healing Society. Amsterdam: The Netherlands; 1993.
31. Zhang L, Tizard IR. Activation of a mouse macrophage cell line by acemannan: the major carbohydrate fraction from Aloe vera gel. *Immunopharmacology.* 1996;35:119–128.
32. Karaca K, Sharma JM, Nordgren R. Nitric oxide production by chicken macrophages activated by acemannan, a complex carbohydrate extracted from Aloe vera. *Int J Immunopharmacol.* 1995; 7(3):183–188.
33. Bruce WG. Investigations of antibacterial activity in the aloe. *S Afr Med J.* 1967;51:984.
34. Senzetti LJ, Salisbury R, Beal JL, et al. Bacteriostatic property of Aloe vera. *J Pharm Sci.* 1964;53:1287.
35. Heggers JP, Pineless GR, Robson MC. Dermaide/Aloe vera gel comparison of the antimicrobial effects. *J Am Med Technol.* 1979;41:293–294.
36. Hanley DC, Solomon WAB, Saffran B, et al. The evaluation of natural substances in the treatment of adjuvant arthritis. *J Am Podiatr Med Assoc.* 1982;72:275–284.
37. Davis RH, Leitner MG, Russo JM, et al. Anti-inflammatory activity of Aloe vera against a spectrum of irritants. *J Am Podiatr Med Assoc.* 1989;79:263–276.
38. Parish LC, Witkoski JA, Millikan LE. Aloe vera: its chemical and therapeutic properties. *Int J Dermatol.* 1991;30:679.
39. Davis RH, DiDonato JJ, Johnson RWS, et al. Aloe vera, hydrocortisone, and sterol influence on wound tensile strength and anti-inflammation. *J Am Podiatr Med Assoc.* 1994;84(12):614–621.
40. Kahlon JB, Kemp MC, Yawei N, et al. In vitro evaluation of the synergistic anti-viral effects of acemannan in combination with azidothymidine and acyclovir. *Mol Biother.* 1991;3:214–223.
41. McDaniel HR, et al. Extended survival and prognostic criteria for acemannan treated HIV-1 patients. *Antiviral Res.* 1990;13(1):117.
42. Kahlon JB, Kemp MC, Carpenter RH, et al. Inhibition of AIDS virus replication by acemannan in vitro. *Mol Biother.* 1991;13:127–135.
43. Davis RH, DiDonato JJ, Hartman GM, et al. Anti-inflammatory and wound healing activity of growth substance in aloe vera. *J Am Podiatr Med Assoc.* 1994;84(2):77–81.
44. Dominguez-Soto L. Photodermatitis to aloe vera. *Int J Dermatol.* 1992;31:372.
45. Hogan DJ. Widespread dermatitis after topical treatment of chronic leg ulcers and stasis dermatitis. *Can Med Assoc J.* 1988;138: 336–338.
46. Nakamura T, Kotajima S. Contact dermatitis from aloe arborescens. *Contact Dermtitis.* 1984;11(1):51.
47. Shoji A. Contact dermatitis to Aloe arborescens. *Contact Dermatitis.* 1982;8:164–167.
48. Tewari PV, Mapa HC, Chaturvedi RR. Experimental study on estrogemc activity of certain indigenous plants. *J Res Indian Med Yoga Homeopathy.* 1976;11:7–12.
49. Jarry H, Harnischfeger G. Untersuchugen zur endokrinen Wirksamkeit von Inhaltsstoffen aus Cimicifuga racemosa: Einfluss auf die Serumspiegel von Hypophysenhormonen ovariek- tomieter Ratten. *Planta Medica.* 1985;51:46–49.

50. Jarry H, Harnischfeger G, Duker E. Untersuchugen zur endokrinen Wirksamkeit von Inhaltss-toffen aus Cimicifuga racemosa: in vitro Bindung von Inhaltsstoffen an ostrogenrezeptoren. Ratten. *Planta Med.* 1985;51:316–319.
51. Genazzani E, Sorrentino L. Vascular action of acteina: active constituents of Actea racemosa. *Nature.* 1962;194:544–545.
52. Moskalenko S. Preliminary sreenmg of Far-Eastern ethnomedicinal plants for antibacterial activity. *J Ethnopharmacol.* 1986;15: 231–259.
53. Blumenmal M, Brusse WR, Goldberg A, et al. *The Complete Commission E Monographs.* Austin, TX: American Botanical Council, 1998.
54. Bradley P. *British Herbal Compendium.* Bournemouth, England: BHMA, 1992, p 239.
55. Chandler F, Osbome F. *Burdock. Can Phann J.* 1997;130(5):46–49.
56. Weiss R. *Herbal Medicine.* Beaconsfield, Quebec: Beaconsfield Publishers, 1988.
57. Wren R. *Potter's New Encyclopedia of Botanical Drugs and Preparations.* Saffron Walden: C.W. Daniel Company, 1988, p 362.
58. Mills S. *The Essential Book of Herbal Medicine.* 2nd ed. London: Penguin Publishers, 1991, p 677.
59. Bever B, Zahnd G. Plants with oral hypoglycemic action. *Q J Crude Drug Res.* 1979;17:139–196.
60. Cappalletti E, Trevisan R, Caniato R. External antirheumatic and antineuralgic herbal remedies in the traditional medicine of North-Eastern Italy. *J Ethnopharmacol.* 1982;6:161–190.
61. Morita K, Kada T, Namik M. Desmutagenic factor isolated from burdock (Arctium Lappa L.). *Mutat Res.* 1986;129:25–31.
62. Tsujita J, Takeda H, Ebihara K, et al. Comparison of protective activity of dietary fiber against the toxicities of various food colours in rats. *Nutr Rep Int.* 1979;20:635–642.
63. Farnsworth N, Bingel A, Cordell G, et al. Potential value of plants as sources of new antifertility agents. *J Pharm Sci.* 1975;64(4):535–598.
64. Panter KE, James LF. Natural plant toxicants in milk: a review. *J of Animal Sci.* 1990;68:982–994.
65. Willuhn G, Westhaus R. LolioUde (Calendin) from Calendula officianalis. *Planta Med.* 1987;53:304.
66. Vidal-Olivier E, Elias R, Faure F, et al. Flavonol glycosides from Calendula officianalis flowers. *Planta Med.* 1989;55:73–74.
67. Delia Loggia R, Tubaro A, Becker H, et al. The role of Triterpenoids in the topical anti-inflammatory activity of Calendula officianalis flowers. *Planta Med.* 1994;60:516–520.
68. Bezakova L, Masterova I, Paulikova I, et al. Inhibitory activity of isorhamnetin glycosides from Calendula officianalis L. on the activity of lipoxygenase. *Pharmazie.* 1996;51(2):126–127.
69. Akihisa T, Yasukawa K, Oinuma H, et al. Triterpene alcohols from the flowers of Compositae and their anti-inflammatory effects. *Phytochemistry.* 1996;43(6):1255–1260.
70. Wagner H. The immune stimulating polysaccharides and heteroglycans of higher plants: a preliminary communication. *Arzneimittelforschung.* 1984;34(6):659–661.
71. Boucaud-Maitre Y, Algernon 0, Raynaud J. Cytotoxic and antihumoral activity of Calendula officianalis extracts. *Pharmazie.* 1988;43:221–222.
72. Dumenil G, Chemli R, Balansard G, et al. Evaluation of antibacterial properties of marigold flowers and homeopathic mother tincture of Calendula off. *Ann Pharm Francoises.* 1980;36(6):493–499.
73. The Lawrence Review of Natural Products. *Calendula. Monograph.* Levittown, PA: Pharmaceutical Information Associates, 1987.
74. Chevallier A. *The Encyclopedia of Medicinal Plants.* London: Reader's Digest, 1996, p 336.
75. Banaszkiewicz W, Kowalska M, Mrozokiewizc A. Determination of the estrogenic activity of Calendula officinalis flowers in biological units. Poznan Towarz Pryjaciol Nauk, Wydzial Lekar, Prace Komisji Far 1963;14:53–63.
76. Locock RA. Capsicium. *Can Pharm J.* 1985;118:517–519.
77. Watson CP, Evans RJ. The postmastectomy pain syndrome and topical capsaicin: a randomized trial. *Pain.* 1992;51(3):375–379.
78. Deal CL, Schnitzer TJ, Lipstein E, et al. Treatment of arthritis with topical capsaicin: a double-blind trial. *Clin Ther.* 1991;13(3): 383–395.
79. McCarthy G, McCarty D. Effect of topical capsaicin on asteoarthritis of the hands. *J Rheumatol.* 1992;19:604–607.
80. Chesire WP, Snyder CR. Treatment of reflex sympathetic dystrophy with topical capsaicin. *Pain.* 1990;42:307–311.
81. Rayner HC, Atkins RC, Westerman RA. Relief of local stump pain by capsaicin cream (letter). *Lancet.* 1989;2(8674):1276–1277.
82. Donofrio PD, Walker F, Hunt V, et al. Treatment of painful diabetic neuropathy with topical capsaicin: a multicentre, double-blind, vehicle-controlled study. *Arch Intern Med.* 1991;151:2225–2229.
83. Dailey GE. Effect of treatment with capsaicin on daily activities of patients with diabetic neuropathy. *Diabetes Care.* 1992;15(2): 159–165.
84. Ross DR, Varipapa RJ. Treatment of painful diabetic neuropathy with topical capsaicin (letter). *N Engl J Med.* 1989;321(7):474–475.
85. Tandan R, Lewis GA, Krusinski PB, et al. Topical capsaicin in painful diabetic neuropathy: controlled study with long term follow-up. *Diabetes Care.* 1992;15(1):8–14.
86. Scheffler NM, et al. Treatment of painful diabetic neuropathy with capsaicin 0.075. *J Am Pediatr Med Assoc.* 1991;81(6):288–293.
87. Watson CP, Evans RJ, Wait VR, et al. Post-herpetic neuralgia: 208 cases. *Pain.* 1988;35:289–297.
88. Bernstein JE, Korman NJ, Bickers DR, et al. Topical capsaicin treatment of chronic postherpetic neuralgia. *J Am Acad Dermatol.* 1989;21:265–270.
89. Peikert A, Hentrich M, Ocas G. Topical 0.025 capsaicin in chronic post-herpetic neuralgia: efficacy, predictors of response and long-term course. *J Neural.* 1991;238(8):452–456.
90. Fusco BM, Alessandri M. Analgesic effect of capsaicin in idiopathic trigeminal neuraglia. *Anesth Analg.* 1992;74(3):375–377.
91. Kawada T, Hoziharak K, Iwai K. Effects of capsaicin on lipid metabolism in rats fed a high fat diet. *J Nutr.* 1986;116:1272–1278.
92. Mann C, Staba EJ. The Chemistry, pharmacology, and commercial formulations of chamomile. *Herbs Spices Med Plants.* 1984;1:235–280.
93. Berry M. The Chamomiles. *P/MTOZ J.* 1995;254:191–193.
94. Delia Loggia R, Carle R, Sosa S, et al. Evaluation of the anti-inflammatory activity of chamomile preparations. *Planta Med.* 1990;56:657–658.
95. Achterraath-Tuckennann U, Kunde R, et al. Pharmacological investigations with compounds of chamomile: V. Investigations on the spasmolytic effect of compounds of chamomile and kamillosan on the isolated guinea pig lleum. *Planta Med.* 1980;39:38–50.
96. Szelenyi I, Isaac O, Thiemer K. Pharmacological experiments with compounds of chamomile:III. Experimental studies of the ulceroprotective effect of chamomile. *Planta Med.* 1979;35:218–227.
97. The Lawrence Review of Natural Products. *Chamomile. Monograph.* St Louis, MO: Facts and Comparisons, 1991.
98. Viola H, Wasowski C, Levi de Stein M, et al. Apigenin, a component of Matricaria recutita flowers, is a central benzodiazepine receptors-ligand with anxiolyic effects. *Planta Med.* 1995;61:213–216.
99. Safayhi H, Sabieraj J, Sailer E, et al. Chamazulene: an antioxidant-type inhibitor of leukotriene B4 formation. *Planta Med.* 1994;60(5): 410–413.
100. Rekka E, Kourounakis A, Kourounakis P. Investigation of the effect of chamazulene on lipid peroxidation and free radical processes. *Res Commun Mol Pathol Pharmacol.* 1996;92(3):361–364.
101. Tubaro A, Zilli C, Redaelli C, et al. Evaluation of anti-inflammatory activity of a chamomile extract topical application. *Planta Medica.* 1986;50(4):359.
102. Korting H, Schafer-Korting M, Hart H, et al. Anti-inflammatory activity of hamamelis distillate applied topically to the skin. *Eur J Din Pharmacol.* 1993;44:315–318.

103. Van Ketel W. Allergy to Matricaria chamomila. *Contact Dermatitis.* 1987;16:50–51.
104. Benner M, Lee H. Anaphylactic reaction to chamomile tea. *J Allergy Clin Immunol.* 1973;52:307–308.
105. Casterline C. Allergy to Chamomile Tea. *JAMA.* 1980;4:330–331.
106. Hausen B. The sensitizing capacity of Compositae plants:!!!. Test results and cross reactions in Compositae-sensitive patients. *Dermatologica.* 1979;159:1–11.
107. Habersing S, Leuschner F, Isaac O, Theimer K. Pharmacological studies with compounds of chamomile:IV. Studies on toxicity of (—) alpha bisabolol. *Planta Med.* 1979;37:115–123.
108. Houghton P. Agnus castus. *Pharm J.* 1994;253:720–721.
109. Loch E, Bohnert K, Peeters M. The treatment of menstrual disorders with Vitex Agnus castus tincture. *Frauenarzt.* 1991;32:867–870.
110. Amann W. Akne vulgaris und Angus castus (Agnolyt). *Z Allg Med.* 1975;51:1645–1648.
111. Milewicz A, Gejdel E, Sworen H, et al. Vitex agnus-castus extract in the treatment of luteal phase defects due to latent hyperprolactinemia: results of a randomised placebo-controlled double-blind study. *Arzneim Forsch Drug Res.* 1993;43:752–756.
112. Bohnert K. The Use of Vitex agnus castus for Hyperprolactinemia. *Q Rev Nat Med.* 1997;5:19–21.
113. Cahill D, Fox R, Wardle P, et al. Multiple follicular development associated with herbal medicine. *Hum Reprod.* 1994;9(8):1469–1470.
114. Ofek I, Goldhar J, Zafriri D, et al. Anti-Escherichia coli adhesion activity of cranberry and blueberry juices (letter). *N Engl J Med.* 1991;324:1599.
115. Zafriri D, Ofek I, Adar R, et al. Inhibitory activity of cranberry juice on adherence of type I and type P fimbriated Escherichia coli to eucaryotic cells. *Antimicrob Agents Chemother.* 1989;33(1):92–98.
116. Schmidt D, Sobota A. An examination of the anti-adherence activity of cranberry juice on urinary and nonurinary bacterial isolates. *Microbios.* 1988;55:173–181.
117. Sobota AE. Inhibition of bacterial adherence by cranberry juice: potential use for the treatment of urinary tract infection. *J Urol.* 1984;131:1013–1016.
118. Gibson L, Pike L, Kilboum JP. Effectiveness of cranberry juice in preventing urinary tract infections in long-term care facility patients. *J Naturopath Med.* 1991;2(1):45–47.
119. Avorn J, Manone M, Gurwitz JH, et al. Reduction of bacteriuria and pyuria after ingestion of cranberry juice. *JAMA.* 1994;271:751–754.
120. Haverkom MJ, Mandigers J. Reduction of bacteriura and pyuria using cranberry juice. *JAMA.* 1994;272(8):590.
121. Williams C, Goldstone F, Greenham J. Flavonoids, Cinnamic acids and coumarins from the different tissues and medicina preparations of Taraxacum officinale. *Phytochemistry.* 1996;42(1):121–127.
122. Blanchert K. Dandelion leaves are rich source of vitamins and minerals. *Alt Comp Ther.* 1995;1(2):115–117.
123. Racz-Kotilla E, Racz G, Solomon A. The action of Taraxacum officinale extracts on the body weight and diuresis of laboratory animals. *Planta Med.* 1974;26:212–217.
124. Stelling K, Salama S, Salib M. Phytotherapy as an adjunct in Cancer Treatment. *Can J Herb.* 1995(winter):34–36.
125. CordatosE. Taraxacum Officinale: Textbook of Natural Medicine. Seattle: Bastyr University; 1992.
126. Akhtar MS, et al. Effects of Portulaca oleracae (kulfa) and Taraxacum officinale (dhudhal) in normoglycaemic and alloxan-treated hyperglycaemic rabbits. *J Pakistan Med Assoc.* 1985;35:207–210.
127. Mascolo N et al. Biological screening of Italian medicinal plants for anti-inflammatory activity. *Phytother Res.* 1987;1:28–29.
128. Lovell C, Rowan M. Dandelion Dermatitis. *Contact Dermatitis.* 1991;25:185–188.
129. Cook C, Sgardelis S, Pantis J, et al. Concentrations of Pb, Zn and Cu in Taraxacum spp. In relation to urban pollution. *Bull Environ Contam Toxicol.* 1994;53:204–210.
130. Burger J, Vincent Brant E, Ferreira D. Iridoid and phenolic glycoside from Harpogophytum. *Phytochemistry.* 1987;26:1453–1457.
131. Czygan F, Krueger A. Pharmaceutical biological studies of the genus harpagophytum: Part 3. Distribution of the iridoid glycoside harpagoside in the different organs of Harpagophytum procumbens and Harpagophytum zeyheri. *Planta Med.* 1977;31:305–307.
132. Ziller K, Franz G. Analysis of the water-soluble fraction from the roots of Harpogophytum-procumbens. *Planta Med.* 1979;37:340–348.
133. Lanhers M, Fleurentin J, Mortier F, et al. Anti-inflammatory and analgesic effects of an aqueous extract of Harpagophytum procwnbens. *Planta Med.* 1992;58:117–123.
134. Soulimani R, Younos C, Mortier F, et al. The role of stomachal digestion on the pharmacological activity of plant extracts, using as an example of Harpagophytum procumens. *Can J Physiol Pharmacol.* 1994;72(12):1532–1536.
135. Pinget M, Lecomte A. The effects of harpagophytum capsules (Arkocaps) in degenerative rheumatology. *Med Actuelle.* 1985;12: 65–67.
136. Grahame R, Robinson B. Devil's Claw (Harpagophytum procumbens): pharmacological and clinical studies. *Ann Rheum Dis.* 1981;40:632.
137. Circosta C, Occhiuta F, Ragusa S, et al. A drug used in traditional medicine: Harpagophytum procumbens DCIL Cardiovascular activity. *J Ethnopharmacol.* 1984;11:259–274.
138. Costa De Pasquale R, Busa G, et al. A drug used in traditional medicine: Harpagophytum procumbens DC: III. Effects on hyperkinetic ventricular arrythmias by reperfusion. *J Ethnopharmacol.* 1985;13:193–199.
139. Tyier V. *Herbs of Choice. The Therapeutic Use of Phytomedicinals.* Binghamton, NY: Pharmaceutical Products Press, 1994, p 209.
140. Occhiuto F, Circosta C, Ragusa S, et al. A drug used in traditional medicine: Harpagophytum procumbens DC: Cardiovascular activity. *J Ethnopharmacol.* 1984;11:259–274.
141. Foster S, Chongxi Y. *Herbal Emissaries: Bringing Chinese Herbs to the West.* Rochester,VT: Healing Arts Press; 1992, p 356.
142. Duke JA. *Handbook of Medicinal Herbs.* Boca Raton, FL: CRC, 1985.
143. Noe J. Angelica Sinensis: a monograph. *J Naturopath Med.* 1997;7(1):66–72.
144. Zhu D. Dong Quai. *Am J Chinese Med.* 1987;15:117–125.
145. Mei QB, Yi TJ, Cui B. Advances in the pharmacological studies of radix Angelica Sinensis (Oliv) Dils (Chinese Danggui). *Chinese Med J.* 1991;104(9):776–781.
146. Belford-Courtney R. Comparison of Chinese and Western uses of Angelica sinesis. *Aust J Med Herb.* 1993;5(4):87–91.
147. Hudson T, Standish L, Breed C, et al. Clinical and endocrinological effects of a menopausal botanical formula. *J Naturopath Med.* 1997;7(1):73–82.
148. Opdyke DLJ. Angelica root oil. *Food Cosmet Toxicol.* 1975; 13(Suppl):713.
149. Guo TL, Zhuo XW. Clinical observations on the treatment of the gestational hypertension syndrome with Angelica and Paeonia powder. *Chinese J Mod Dev Tradit Med.* 1986;6(12):714–716.
150. Luettig B, Steinmuller C, Gifford GE, et al. Macrophage activation by the polysacchande arabinogalactan isolated from plant cell cultures of Echinacea purpurea. *J Nati Cancer Inst.* 1989;81(9): 669–675.
151. Steinmuller C, Roesler J, Grottrup E, et al. Polysaccharides isolated from plant cell cultures of Echinacea purpurea enhance the resistance of immunosuppressed mice against systemic infections with Candida albicans and Listeria monocytgenes. *Int J Immunopharmacol.* 1993;15(5):605–614.
152. Muller-Jakic B, Breu W, Probstle A, et al. In vitro inhibition of cyclooxygenase and 5-lipoxygenase by alkamides from Echinacea and Achillea species. *Planta Med.* 1994;60:37–40.
153. Bauer R, et al. Alkamides from the roots of Echinacea angustifolia. *Phytochemistry.* 1989;28:505–508.
154. Bohlman F, Hoffmann M. Further amides from Echinacea purpurea. *Phytochemistry.* 1983;22:1173–1175.

155. Hobbs C. The chemistry and pharmacology of Echinacea species. *Herbal Gram (Suppl).* 1994;30:1–7.
156. Bauer R, Khan AI, Wagner H. TLC and HPLC Analysis of Echinacea pallida and E. angustifolia rots. *Plant Med.* 1988;54:426–430.
157. Hobbs C. Echinacea-a literature review. *Herbalgram.* 1994;30:33–47.
158. Houghton PJ. Echinacea. *Pharm J.* 1994;253:342–343.
159. Melchart D, Linde K, Worku F, et al. Immunomodulation with echinacea—a systemic review of controlled clinical trials. *Phytomedicine.* 1994;1:245–254.
160. Wagner H, et al. Immunologically active polysaccharides of Echinacea purpurea cell cultures. *Phytochemistry.* 1988;27: 119–126.
161. Dorn M, Knick E, Lewith G. Placebo-controlled, double-blind study of Echinacea pallidae radix in upper respiratory tract infections. *Compl Ther Med.* 1997;5:40–42.
162. Schoneberger D. The influence of immune-stimulating effects of pressed juice from Echinacea purpuraea on the course and severity of colds: results of a recent double-blind study (in German). *Forum Immunol.* 1992;8:2–12.
163. Tubaro A, Tragni E, Del Negro P, et al. Anti-inflammatory activity of a polysacchande fraction of Echinacea angustifolia. *J Pharm Pharmacol.* 1987;39:567–569.
164. Tragni E, Tubaro A, Melis S, et al. Evidence from two classical irritation tests for an anti-inflammatory action of a natural extract, echinacea B. *Food Chemical Toxicol.* 1985;23:317–319.
165. Wacker A, Hilbig W. Virus inhibition by Echinacea purpurea. *Plant Med.* 1978;33:89.
166. Lersch C, Zeuner M, Bauer A, et al. Nonspecific immunostimulation with low doses ofcyclophosphamide (LDCY), thymostimulin, and Echinacea purpurea extracts (echinacin) in patients with far advanced colorectal cancers: preliminary results. *Cancer Invest.* 1992;10(5):343–348.
167. The Lawrence Review of Natural Products. Echinacea. Levittown, PA: Pharmaceutical Information Associates, 1990.
168. Brigg CJ. Evening primrose. *Rev of Pharm Can.* 1986;119(5): 249–254.
169. Li Wan Po A. Evening primrose oil. *Pharm J.* 1991;246:670–676.
170. Morse PF, Horrobin DF, Manku MS, et al. Meta-analysis of placebo-controlled studies of the efficacy of Epogam in the treatment of atopic eczema: relationship between plasma essential fatty acid changes and clinical response. *Br J Dermatol.* 1989;121:75–90.
171. Schalin-Karrila M, Manila L, Jansen CT, et al. Evening primrose oil in the treatment of atopic eczema: effect on clinical status, plasma phospholipid fatty acids and circulating blood prostaglandins. *Br J Dermatol.* 1987;117:11–19.
172. Stewart JCM, et al. Treatment of severe and moderately severe atopic dermatitis with evening primrose oil (Epogam); a multicentre study. *J Nutr Med.* 1991;2:9–15.
173. Wright S, Burton JL. Oral evening primrose seed oil improves atopic eczema. *Lancet.* 1982;2:1120–1122.
174. Lovell CR, Burton JL, Horrobin DF, et al. Treatment of atopic eczema with evening primrose oil. *Lancet.* 1981;1:278.
175. Collins A, Cerin A, et al. Essential fatty acids in the treatment of premenstrual syndrome. *Obstet Gynecol.* 1993;81:93–98.
176. Lurie S, Borenstein R. The premenstrual syndrome. *Obstet Gynecol Survey.* 1990;45(4):220–228.
177. Chenoy R, Hussain S, Tayob Y, et al. Effect of oral gamolemc acid from evening primrose oil on menopausal flushing. *BMJ.* 1994;308(6927):501–503.
178. Wetzig NR. Mastalgia: a 3 year Australian study. *Aust NZ J Surg.* 1994;64(5):329–331.
179. Pye JK, Mansel RE, Hughes LE. Clinical experience of drug treatments for mastalgia. *Lancet.* 1985;2:373–377.
180. Horrobin DF. Gammalinolenic acid: an intermediate in essential fatty acid metabolism with potential as an ethical pharmaceutical and as a food. *Rev Contemp Pharmacother.* 1990;1:1–45.
181. Holman C, Bell A. A trial of evening primrose oil in the treatment of chronic schizophrenia. *J Orthomolec Psychiatry.* 1983;12:302–304.
182. Keen H, Payan J, Allawi J, et al. Treatment of diabetic neuropathy with gamma-linolenic acid. *Diabetes Care.* 199;16:8–15.
183. Horrobin DF. Nutritional and medical importance of gamma-linolenic acid. *Prog Lipid Res.* 1992;31:163–194.
184. Dwokin R, et al. Linoleic acid and multiple sclerosis: a reanalysis of three double-blind trials. *Neurology.* 1984;34:1441–1445.
185. Oxholm P, Manthorpe R, Prause J, et al. Patients with primary Sjogren's syndrome treated for two months with evening primrose oil. *Scand J Rheumatol.* 1986;15(2):103–108.
186. Lepik K. Safety of herbal medications in pregnancy. *Can Pharm J.* 1997;130(3):29–33.
187. Cant A, Shay J, Horrobin DF. The effect of maternal supplementation with hnolemc and gamma-linolenic acids on the fat composition and content of human milk. *J Nutr Sci Vitaminol.* 1991;37:573–579.
188. Groenewegen W, Knight D, Heptinstall S. Progress in the medicinal chemistry of the herb feverfew. *Prog Med Chem.* 1992;29:217–238.
189. Awang D. Herbal medicine: feverfew. *Can Pharm J.* 1989;122:266–270.
190. Berry M. Feverfew. *Pharm J.* 1994;253:806–808.
191. Sumner H, Salan U, Knight D, et al. Inhibition of 5-lipoxygenase and cyclo-oxygenase in leukocytes by feverfew. *Biochem Pharmacol.* 1992;43:2313–2320.
192. Murphy JJ, Hepinstall S, Mitchell JRA. Randomized double-blind placebo-controlled trial of feverfew in migraine prevention. *Lancet.* 1988;2:189–192.
193. Johnson ES, Kadam NP, Hylands DM, et al. Efficacy of feverfew as prophylactic treatment of migraine. *BMJ.* 1985;291:569–573.
194. Diamond S. Herbal therapy for migraine: an unconventional approach. *Postgrad Med.* 1987;197–198.
195. Pattrick M, Hepinstall S, Doherty M. Feverfew in rheumatoid arthritis: a double-blind, placebo controlled study. *Ann Rheum Dis.* 1989;48:547–549.
196. Rodriguez E, Epstein W, Mitchell J. The role of sesquiterpene lactones in contact hypersensitivity to some North and South American species of feverfew (Parthenium compositae). *Contact Dermatitis.* 1977;3:155–162.
197. Hausen B, Osmundsen P. Contact allergy to parthenolide in Tanacetum paithenium schulz-Bip (feverfew, Asteraceae) and cross-reactions to related sesquiterpene lactone containing compositae species. *Acta Derm Venereal.* 1983;63(4):308–314.
198. Awang DVC. Ginger. *Can Pharm J.* 192;125:309–311.
199. Holtmann S, Clarke AH, Scherer H, et al. The anti-motion sickness mechanism of ginger: a comparative study with placebo and dimenhydrinate. *Acta Otolaryngol (Stockh).* 1989;198(3–4):168–174.
200. Pengelly A. Ginger extracts prevent ulcers. *Aust J Med Herb.* 1993;59(2):73.
201. Yamahara J, Mochizuki M, Rong HQ, et al. The anti-ulcer effect in rats of ginger constituents. *J Ethnopharmacol.* 1988;23:299–304.
202. Al-Yahya MA, Rafatullah S, Mossa JS, et al. Gastroprotective activity of ginger Zingiber officinale Rose. in albino rats. *Am J Chinese Med.* 1989;17(1–2):51–56.
203. Sertie J, Basile A, Oshiro T, et al. Preventative anti-ulcer activity of the rhizome extract of Zingiber officinale. *Fitoterapia.* 1992;63:55–59.
204. Brown D. Anti-Inflammatory potential of ginger. *Q Rev Nat Med.* 1993;Spring:17.
205. McCaleb R. Ginger and atractylodes as an anti-inflammatory. *Herbalgram.* 1993;29:19.
206. Tanabe M, Chen YD, Saito KI, et al. Cholesterol biosynthesis inhibitory component from Zingiber officinale Roscoe. *Chem Pharm Bull.* 1993;41(4):710–713.
207. Shoji N, Iwasa A, Takemoto T, et al. Cardiotonic principles of ginger (Zingiber officinale Roscoe). *J Pharm Sci.* 1982;71(10): 1174–1175.
208. Mustafa T, Srivasava KC. Ginger (Zingiber officinale) in migraine headaches. *J Ethnopharmacol.* 1990;29(3):267–273.

209. Brown D. Antimotion sickness action of ginger questioned. *Q Rev Nat Med.* 1993;Spring:15–16.
210. Mowrey DB, Clayson DE. Motion sickness, ginger, and psychophysics. *Lancet.* 1982;1:655–657.
211. Fischer-Rasmussen W, Kjaer Dahl C, et al. Ginger treatment of hyperemesis gravidarum. *Eur J Obstet Gynecol Reprod Biol.* 1990;38:19–24.
212. Bon ME, Wilkinson DJ, Young JR, et al. Ginger root: a new antiemetic. The effect of ginger root on postoperative nausea and vomiting after major gynaecological surgery. *Anaesthesia.* 1990;45(8):669–671.
213. Phillips S, Ruggier R, Hutchinson S. Zingiber officinale (ginger)-an antiemetic for day case surgery. *Anaesthesia.* 1993;48(8):715–717.
214. Platel K, Srinivasan K. Influence of dietary spices or their active principles on digestive enzymes of small intestinal mucosa in rats. *Int J Food Sci Nutr.* 1996;47(1):55–59.
215. Srivastava KC, Mustafa T. Ginger (Zingiber officinale) and rheumatic disorders. *Med Hypoth.* 1989;29:25–28.
216. Srivastava KC, Mustafa T. Ginger (Zingiber officinale) in rheumatism and musculoskeletal disorders. *Med Hypoth.* 1992;39:342–348.
217. Sharma JN, Srivastava KC, Gan EK. Suppressive effects of eugenol and gingeroil on arthritic rats. *Pharmacology.* 1994;49(5):314–318.
218. Fulder S, Tenne M. Ginger as anti-nausea remedy in pregnancy: the issue of safety. *Herbalgram.* 1996;3:47–50.
219. Kleijnen J, Knipschild P. Ginkgo biloba. *Lancet.* 1992;340:1136–1139.
220. Sticher 0. Quality of Ginkgo preparatons (review). *Planta Med.* 1993;59(1):2–11.
221. Jung F, Mrowietz C, Kiesewetter H, et al. Effect of Ginkgo biloba on fluidity of blood and peripheral microcirculation in volunteers. *Arzneimittelforscung.* 1990;40(5):589–593.
222. Stucker O, Pons C, Duverger JP, et al. Effects of Ginkgo biloba extract (Egb 761) on arteriolar spasm in a rat creaser muscle preparation. *Int J Microcirculation Clin Exp.* 1996.
223. Puglisi L, Salvadori S, Gabrielli G, et al. Pharmacology of natural compounds: I. Smooth muscle relaxant activity induced by a Ginkgo biloba L. extract on guinea-pig trachea. *Pharmacol Res Commun.* 1988;20(7):573–589.
224. Bourgain RH, Andries R, Braquet P. Effect of ginkgolide PAF-acether antagonists on arterial thrombosis. *Adv Prostaglandin Thromboxane Leukotriene.* 1987.
225. Bourgain RH, Macs L, Andries R, et al. Thrombus induction by endogenic paf-acether and its inhibition by Ginkgo biloba extracts in the guinea pig. *Prostaglandins.* 1986;32(1):142–144.
226. Kose K, Dogan P. Lipoperoxidation induced by hydrogen peroxide in human erythrocyte membranes. 2. Comparison of the antioxidant effect of Ginkgo biloba extract (EGb 761) with those of water-solubl anipid-soluble antioxidants. *J Int Med Res.* 1995;23(1):9–18.
227. Kose K, Dogan P. Lipoperoxidation induced by hydrogen peroxide in human erythrocyte membranes. 1. Protective effect of Ginkgo biloba extract (EGb 761). *J Int Med Res.* 1995;23(1):1–8.
228. Oyama Y, Chikahia L, Ueha T, et al. Ginkgo biloba extract protects brain neurons against oxidative stress induces by hydrogen peroxide. *Brain Res.* 1996;712(2):349–352.
229. Rong Y, Geng Z, Lau BH. Ginkgo biloba attenuates oxidative stress in macrophages and endothelial cells. *Free Radio Biol Med.* 1996;20(1):121–127.
230. Shen JG, Zhou DY. Efficiency of Ginkgo biloba extract (EGb 761) in antioxidant protection against myocardial ischemia and reperfusion injury. *Biochem Mol Biol Int.* 1995;35(1):15–34.
231. Ramassamy C, Clostre F, Christen Y, et al. Prevention by a Ginkgo biloba extract (GBE 761) of the dopaminergic neurotoxicity of MPTP. *J Pharmacol.* 1990;42(11):785–789.
232. Brailowsky S, Montiel T, Medina-Ceja L. Acceleration of functional recovery from motor cotex ablation by two Ginkgo biloba extracts in rats. *Rest Neural Neurosa.* 1995;8:163–167.
233. Le Bars PL, Katz MM, Berman N. et al. A placebo-controlled, double-blind, randomized trial of an extract of Ginkgo biloba for dementia. *JAMA.* 1997;278:1327–1332.
234. Kanowski S, Herrman WM, Stephan K, et al. Proof of efficacy of the Ginkgo biloba special extract EGb 761 in outpatients suffering from mild to moderate primary degenerative dementia of the Alzheimer type or multi-infarct dementia. *Pharmacopsychatry.* 1996;29:47–56.
235. Hofferberth B. The efficacy of EGb 761 in patients with senile dementia of the Alzheimer type-a double-blind, placebo-controlled study on different levels of investigation. *Hum Psychopharmacol.* 1994;9:215–222.
236. Semlitsch HV, Anderer P, Saletu B, et al. Cognitive psychophysiology in nootropic drug research effects of Ginkgo biloba on event-related potentials (P300) in age-associated memory impairment. *Pharmacopsychiatry.* 1995;28(4):134–142.
237. Petkov VD, Kehayov R, Belcheva S, et al. Memory effects of standardized exttracts of Panax ginseng (G115), Ginkgo biloba (GK 501) and their combination Gincosan (PHL 00701). *Planta Med.* 1993;59(2):106–114.
238. Stoll S, Sceuer K, Pohl O, et al. Ginkgo biloba extract (EGb 761) independently improves changes in passive avoidance learning and brain membrane fluidity in the aging mouse. *Pharmacopsychiatry.* 1996;2(4):144–149.
239. Winter E. Effects of an extract of Ginkgo biloba on learning and memory in mice. *Pharmacology, Biochem Behav.* 1991;38(1):109–114.
240. Vesper J, Hansge KD. Efficacy of Ginkgo biloba in 90 outpatients with cerebral insufficiency caused by old age. *Phytomedicine.* 1994;1:9–16.
241. Vorberg G. Ginkgo biloba extract (GBE): a long term study of cerebral insufficiency in geriatric patients. *Clin Trials J.* 1985;22:149–157.
242. Mouren X, Calliard PH, Schwarz F. Study of the anti-ischemic action of EGb 761 in Ac treannent of periphera arterial occlusive disease by TcP02 determination. *Angiology.* 1994;45:413–417.
243. Holgers KM, Axelsson A, Pringle I. Ginkgo biloba extract for the treatment of tinnitus. *Audiology.* 1994;33(2):85–92.
244. Coles R. Trial of an extract of Ginkgo biloba (EGB) for tinnitus and hearing loss [letter] *Clin Otolaryngol.* 1988;13(6):501–502.
245. Haguenauer JP, Cantenot F, Koskas H, et al. Treatment of equilibrium disorders with Ginkgo biloba extract: a multicenter double-blind drug vs. placebo study (French). *Presse Med.* 1986;15(31):1569–1572.
246. Lacour M, Ez-Zaher L, Raymond J. Plasticity mechanisms in vestibular compensation in the cat are improved by an extract of Ginkgo biloba (EGb 761). *Pharmacol Biochem Behav.* 1991;40(2):367–379.
247. Yabe T, Chat M, Malherbe E, et al. Effects of Ginkgo biloba extract (EGb 761) on the guinea pig vestibular system. *Pharmacology, Biochem Behav.* 1992;42(4):595–604.
248. Gaby AR. Ginkgo biloba extract: a review. *Alt Med Rev.* 1996;1(4):236–242.
249. Rowin J, Lewis SL. Spontaneous bilateral subdural hematomas associated with chronic Ginkgo biloba ingestion. *Neurology.* 1996;46(6):1775–1776.
250. El-Masry S, Korany MA, Aboudonia AH. Colorimetric and spectrophotometric determinations of hydrastis alkaloids in pharmaceutical preparations. *J Pharm Sci.* 1980;69:597–598.
251. Bergner P. Goldenseal and the common cold: the antibiotic myth. *Med Herb.* 1997;97;8(4):1–10.
252. Amin A, Subbaiah T, Abbasi K. Berberine sulphate: antimicrobial activity, bioassay, and mode of action. *Can J Microbiol.* 1969;15(9):1067–1076.
253. Hoffmann D. *Holistic Herbal.* Rockport, ME: Element Books, 1996, p 256.
254. Nishino H, Kitagawa K, Fujiki H, et al. Berberine sulphate inhibits tumour-promoting activity of telecidin in two stage carcinogenesis on mouse skin. *Oncology.* 1986;43:131–134.
255. Zhang R, Dougherty D, Rosenblum M. Laboratory studies of berberine used alone and in combination with 1,3-Bis (2-chloroethyl-l-nitrosurea) to treat malignant brain tumours. *Chinese Med J.* 1990;103(8):658–665.

256. Marie Snow J. Hydrastis canadensis. *Protocol J Bot Med.* 1997; 2(2):25–28.
257. Rabbani GH, Butler T, Knight J, et al. Randomised controlled trial of berberine sulphate therapy for diarrhea due to enterotoxigenic Escherichia coli and Vibrio cholerae. *J Infect Dis.* 1987;155: 979–984.
258. Khin-Maung U, Myo-Kin, Nyunt-Nyaunt-Wai, et al. Clinical trial of beberine in acute watery diarrhea. *BMJ.* 1985;291:1601–1605.
259. Hansel R, et al. The sedative-hypnotic principle of hops. 3. Communication: Contents of 2-methyl-3-butene-2-ol in hops and hop preparations. *Planta Med.* 1982;45:224–228.
260. Wohlfart R, Wurm R, Hansel R, et al. Detection of sedative-hypnotic active ingredients in hops: 5. Degradation of bitter acids to 2-methyl-3-buten-2-ol, a hop constituent with sedative hypnotic activity. *Arch Pharm.* 1983;316(2):132–137.
261. Langezaal CR, Chandra A, Scheffer JJ. Antimicrobial screening of essential oils and extracts of some Humulus lupulus L. cultivars. *Pharm Week.* 1992;14(6):353–356.
262. Schmalrec AF, Teuber M. Structural features determining the antibiotic potencies of natural and synthetic hop bitter resins, their precursors and derivatives. Can J Microbiol 1975; 21:205–212.
263. Yasukawa K, Yamaguchi A, Arita J, et al. Inhibitory effect of edible plant extracts on 12-O-tetradecanoylphorbol-13-acetate-induced ear oedema in mice. *Phytother Res.* 1993;7:185–189.
264. O'Donovan W. Hops dematitis. *Lancet.* 1924;2:597.
265. Newmark FM. Hops allergy and terepene sensitivity: an occupational disease. *Ann Allergy.* 1978;41:311–312.
266. Kumai A, Okamoto R. Extraction of hormonal substance from hops. *Toxicol Lett.* 1984;21(2):203–207.
267. Friedrich H, Engelshowe R. Tannin producing monomeric substances in Juniperus communis. *Planta Med.* 1978;33:251–257.
268. Markanen T. Antiherpetic agent(s) from juniper tree (Juniperus communis): preliminary communication. *Drugs Exp Clin Res.* 1981; 7:69–73.
269. Sanchez de Medina F, Gamez M, Jimenez I, et al. Hypoglycemic activity of juniper "berries." *Planta Med.* 1994;60(3):197–200.
270. Swanson-Flatt S, Day C, Bailey C, et al. Traditional plant treatments for diabetes: studies in normal and streptozotocin mice. *Diabetologia.* 1990;33(8):462–464.
271. Mascolo N, et al. Biological screening Italian medicinal plants for anti-inflammatory activity. *Phytother Res.* 1987;1;28–31.
272. Bergner P. Juniper berries. *Med Herb.* 1994;6(2):13.
273. Schilcer H, Heil BM. Nephrotoxicity of juniper berry preparations: a critical review of the literature from 1844 to 1993. *Zeitschr Phytother.* 1994;15:203–213.
274. Prochnow L. Experimental contribution to the knowledge of the activity offolkloric abortifacients. *Arch Int Pharmacol Ther.* 1911;21:313–319.
275. Gunn JWC. The action of the emmenagogue oils on the human uterus. *Pharmacol Exp Ther.* 1921;16:485.
276. Datnow MW. An experimental investigation concerning toxic abortion produced by chemical agents. J Obstet Gynecol Br Emp 1928; 35:693.
277. Prakash A. Biological evaluation of some medicinal plant extracts for contraceptive efficacy. *Contracept Del Sys.* 1984;5(3):9–10.
278. Singh Y, Blumenthal M. Kava: an overview. *Herbalgram.* 1997;39:3–54.
279. Hansel R (trans Clay A, Reichert R). Kava-kava in modem drug research: portrait of a medicinal plant. *Q Rev Naf Med.* 1996;4(4):259–274.
280. Jussogie A, Scmiz A, Heimke C. Kavapyrone extract enriched from Piper methysticum as modulator of the GABA binding site in different regions of the rat brain. *Psychopharmacology (Berlin).* 1994;116:469–474.
281. Davies L, Drew C, Duffield P, et al. Kava pyrones and resin: studies on GABA(A), GABA(B), and benzodiazepine binding sites in the rodent brain. *Pharmacol Toxicol.* 1992;71(2):120–126.
282. Gebner B, Cnota P. Extract of Kava-kava rhizome in comparison with diazepam and placebo. *Zeitschr Phytother.* 1994;15:30–37.
283. Bone K. Kava-A safe herbal treatment for anxiety. *Br J Phythother.* 1993/94;3(4):147–153.
284. Backhauss C, Krieglstein J. Extract of kava and its methysticin constituents protect brain tissues against ischemic damage in rodents. *Eur J Pharmacol.* 1992;215:265–269.
285. Kretzschmar R, Meyer H. Comparative experiments on the anticonvulsant efficacy of Piper methysticum pyrone bonds (German). *Arch Int Pharmacodyn.* 1969;177:261–277.
286. Lehmann E, Kinzler E, Friedemann J. Efficacy of a special kava extract (Piper methysticum) in a patients with states of anxiety, tension and excitedness of non-mental origin-a double-blind placebo-controlled study of four weeks treatment. *Phytomedicine.* 1996;3(2):113–119.
287. Schuiz V, Hubner W, Ploch M. Clinical trials with phyto-psychopharmacological agents. *Phytomedicine.* 1997;4(4):379–387.
288. Schuiz V, Hansel R, Tyier V. *Rational Phytotherapy: A Physicians' Guide to Herbal Medicine.* Berlin: Springer-Verlag, 1998, p 306.
289. Schelosky L, et al. Kava and dopamine antagonism. *J Neurol Neurosurg Psychiatry.* 1995;58:639–640.
290. Almeida J, Grimsley E. Coma from the health food store: interaction between kava and alprazolam. *Ann Intern Med.* 1996;125:940–941.
291. Chandler RF. Licorice more than just a flavour. *Can Pharm J.* 1985;September:421–424.
292. Kitagawa I, Chen WZ, Hori K, et al. Chemical studies of Chinese licorice-roots: I. Elucidation of five new flavonoid constituents from the roots of Glycyrrhiw glabra L. collected in Xinjiang. *Chem Pharm Bull (Tokyo).* 1994;42(5):1056–1062.
293. Baker ME. Licorice and enzymes other than 11 beta-hydroxysteroid dehydrogenase: an evolutionary perspective. *Steroids.* 1994;59(2): 136–141.
294. Murray MT. *The Healing Power of Herbs.* Rocklin, CA: Prima Publishing, 1992; p 246.
295. Kroes BH, Beukelman CJ, van den Berg AJ, et al. Inhibition of human complement by beta-glycyrrhetinic acid. *Immunology.* 1997;90(1):115–120.
296. Mauricio I, Francischetti B, Monteiro RQ, et al. Identification of glycyrrhizin as a thrombin inhibitor. *Biochem Biophys Res Commun.* 1997;225:259–263.
297. Mitscher L, Park Y, Dark D. Antimicrobial agents from higher plants. Antimicrobial isoflavonoids from glycyrrhiza glabra L. var. typica. *J Nat Prod.* 1980;43:259–260.
298. Utsunomiya T, Kobayash M, Pollard RB, et al. Glycyrrhizin, an active component of licorice roots, reduces morbidity and mortality of mice infected with lethal doses of influenza virus. *Antimicrob Agents Chemother.* 1997;41(3):551–556.
299. Hirabayashi K, Iwata S, Matsumoto H, et al. Antiviral activities of glycyrrhizin and its modified compounds against human immunodeficiency virus type 1 (HIV-1) and Herpes simplex virus type 1 (HSV-1) in vitro. *Chem Pharm Bull.* 1991;39:112–115.
300. Baba M, Shigeta S. Antiviral activity of glycyrrhizin against varicella zoster virus in vitro. *Antivir Res.* 1987;7:999–1007.
301. Chen M, Theander TG, Christensen SB, et al. Licochalcone A, a new antimalarial agent, inhibits in vitro growth of the human malaria parasite Plasmodium falciparum and protects mice from P. yoelii infection. *Antimicrob Agents Chemother.* 1994;38(7): 1470–1475.
302. Chen M, Christensen SB, Blom J, et al. Licochalcone A, a novel antiparasitic agent with potent activity against human pathogenic protozoan species of Leishmania. *Antimicrob Agents Chemother.* 1993;37(12):2550–2556.
303. Sato H, Goto W, Yamamura J, et al. Therapeutic basis of glycynhizin on chronic hepatitis B. *Antivir Res.* 1996;30(2–3):171–177.
304. Glick L. Deglycyrrinated liquorice for peptic ulcer. *Lancet.* 1982;2:817.
305. Tewari SN, Wilson AK. Deglycyrrhizinated liquorice in duodenal ulcer. *Practitioner.* 1972;210:820–825.
306. Poswillo DE, Roberts GL. Topical carbenoxolone for orofacial herpes simplex infections. *Lancet.* 1981;2:142–144.

307. Anderson DM, Smith WG. The antitussive activity of glycyrrhetinic acid and its derivatives. *J Phar Pharmacol.* 1961;13:396–404.
308. De Smet PAGM, Keller K, Hansel R, et al. *Adverse Effects of Herbal Drugs.* 3rd ed. New York, NY: Springer-Veriag, 1997, pp 67–87.
309. Walker BR, Edwards CR. Licorice-induced hypertension and syndromes of apparent mineralocorticoid excess. *Endocrinol Metab Din North Am.* 1994;23(2):359–377.
310. Basso A, Dalla Paola L, Erie G, et al. Licorice ameliorates postural hypotension caused by diabetic autonomic neuropathy. *Diabetes Care.* 1994;17(11):1356.
311. Nielsen I, Pedersen RS. Life-threatening hypokalemia caused by liquorice ingestion. *Lancet.* 1984;1:1305.
312. Chamberlain TJ. Licorice poisoning, pseudoaldosteronism, heart failure. *JAMA.* 1970;213:1343.
313. Olin B. *The Review of Natural Products; The Ephedras.* St. Louis, MO: Facts and Comparisons, a Walters Kluwer Company, 1995.
314. Lee T, Stitze R. Adrenomimetic drugs. In: Craig C, Stitzel R, eds. *Modem Pharmacology.* 4th ed. New York, NY: Little, Brown, 1994, p 907.
315. Bowman W, Rand M. *Textbook of Pharmacology.* London: Blackwell Scientific Publications, 1980.
316. Murray M. *The Healing Power of Herbs.* 2nd ed. Rocklin, ME: Prima Publishing; 1995, p. 410.
317. Norregaard J, Jorgesen S, Mikkelsen KL, et al. The effect of ephedrine plus caffeine on smoking cessation and postcessation weight gain. *Clin Pharmacol Ther.* 1996;60(6):679–686.
318. Breum L, Pedersen JK, Ahlstrom F, et al. Comparison of an ephendrine/caffeine combination and dexfenfluramine in the treatment of obesity: a double-blind multi-centre trial in general practice. *Int J Obesity Pel Metab Disord.* 1994;18(2):99–103.
319. Astrup A, Lundsgaard C, Madsen J, et al. Enhanced thermogenic responsiveness during chronic ephedrine treatment in man. *Am J Clin Nutr.* 1985;42(1):83–94.
320. Pasquali R, Baraldi G, Cesari MP, et al. A controlled trial using ephedrine in the treatment of obesity. *Int J Obesity.* 1985;9(2): 93–98.
321. Nightingale SL. From the Food and Drug Administration. *JAMA.* 1997;278(1):15.
322. Doyle H, Kargin M. Herbal stimulant containing ephedrine has also caused psychosis (letter; comment). *BMJ.* 1996;313:756.
323. Capwell R. Ephedrine induced mania from a herbal diet supplement. *Am J Psychiatry.* 1995;152:647.
324. Josefson D. Herbal stimulant causes US deaths (news). *BMJ.* 1996;312(7043):1378–1379.
325. Maron B, Shirani J, Poliac L, et al. Sudden death in young competitive athletes. *JAMA.* 1996;276:199–204.
326. Dulloo A. Ephedrine, xanthines and prostaglandin-inhibitors: action and interactions in the stimulation of thermogenesis. *Int J Obesity.* 1993;17(suppl. 1):S35–S40.
327. Hoton TJ, Geissler CA. Aspirin potentiates the effect of ephedrine on the thennogenic response to a meal in obese but not lean women. *Int J Obesity.* 1991;15(5):359–366.
328. Dulloo AG, Miller DS. Aspirin as a promoter of ephedrine-induced thermogenesis: potential use in the treatment of obesity. *Am J din Niitr.* 1987;45(3):564–569.
329. Proliac A, Raynaud J. The presence of C-B-D-6-glucopyranosyl-C-a-L-arabinopyranosyl-8-apigenin in leafy stems of Passiflora incarnata. *Pharmaw.* 1986;41:673–674.
330. Pietta P, Manera E, Ceva P. Isocratic liquid chromatographic method for the simultaneous determination of Passiflora incamata L. and Crataegus monogyna flavonoids in drugs. *J Chromatogr.* 1986;357:233–238.
331. Bergner P. Passion flower. *Med Herb.* 1995;7(1–2):13–14, 26.
332. Meier B. Passiflora incamata L.—passion flower: portrait of a medicinal plant. *Q Rev Nut Med.* 1995;3(3 fall):191–202. (Translated from the German. Zeitschr Phytother 1995;16:15–26
333. Soulimani R, Younos C, Jarmouni S, et al. Behavioural effects of Passiflora incamata L. and its indole alkaloid and flavonoid derivatives and maltol in the mouse. *J Ethnopharmacol.* 1997;57(1): 11–20.
334. Speroni E, Minghetti A. Neuropharmacological activity of extracts from Passiflora incamata. *Planta Med.* 1988;54:488–491.
335. Wolfman C, Viola H, Paladini A, et al. Possible anxiolytic effects of chrysin, a central benzodiazepine receptor ligand isolated from Passiflora coerulea. *Pharmacol Biochem Behav.* 1994;47(1):1–4.
336. Bourin M, Bougerol T, Guitton B, et al. A combination of plant extracts in the treatment of outpatients with adjustment disorder with anxious mood: controlled study versus placebo. *Fundam Din Pharmacol.* 1997;11(2):127–132.
337. Smith GW, Chalmers TM, Nuki G. Vasculitis associated with herbal preparation containing Passiflora extract (letter). *Br J Rheumatol.* 1993;32(1):87–88.
338. The Lawrence Review of Natural Products. *Peppermint. Monograph.* St. Louis, MO: Facts and Comparisons, Lippincott Company, 1990.
339. Murray M. The clinical uses of peppermint. *Am J Nat Med.* 1995;2(2):10–13.
340. Hills JM. Aaronson PI. Mechanism of action of peppermint oil on GI smooth muscle. *Gastroenterology.* 1991;101:55–65.
341. Taylor BA, Luscombe DD, Duthie HL. Inhibitory effects of peppermint oil and menthol on isolated human coli. *Gut.* 1984;25: A1168–1169.
342. Pattnaik S, Subramanyam VR, Kole C. Antibacterial and antifungal activity of ten essential oils in vitro. *Microbios.* 1996;86(349): 237–246.
343. Foster S. *Peppermint: Metha x Piperita.* Austin, Texas: American Botanical Council; 1991.
344. Dew MJ, Evans BK, Rhodes J. Peppermint oil for the irritable bowel syndrome: a multicentre trial. *Br J Din Pract.* 1984;38:394–398.
345. Rees WDW, Evans BK, Rhodes J. Treating irritable bowel syndrome with peppermint oil. *BMJ.* 1979;October 6:835–836.
346. Sparks MJ, O'Sullivan P, Herrington AA, et al. Does peppermint oil relieve spasm during barium enema? *Br J Radiol.* 1995,68(812):841–843.
347. Jarvis LJ, Hogg JIC, Houghton CD. Topical peppermint oil for the relief of spasm at barium enema. *Din Radial.* 199;46:A435.
348. Leicester RJ, Hunt RH. Peppermint oil to reduce colonic spasm during endscopy. *Lancet.* 1982;2:989.
349. Thomas J. Peppermint fibrillation. *Lancet.* 1962;1:222.
350. Olowe SA, Ransome-Kuti O. The risk of jaundice in glucose-6-phosphate de-hydrogenase deficient babies exposed to menthol. *Arch Toxicol.* 1984;7(suppl):408.
351. Wagner H, Bladt S. Pharmaceutical quality of hypericum extracts. *J Geriatr Psychiatry Neurol.* 1994;7(suppl 1):S65–S68.
352. Ozturk Y. Testing the antidepressant effects of Hypericum species on animal models. *Pharmacopsychiatry.* 1997;30(suppl 2):125–128.
353. Butterweck V, Wall A, Lieflander-Wulf U, et al. Effects of the total extract and fractions of Hypericum perforation in animal assays for antidepressant activity. *Pharmacopsychiatry.* 1997;30:117–124.
354. De Smet PA, Nolen WA. St John's wort as an antidepressant (editorial; comment) (see comments). *BMJ.* 1996;313(7052):241–242.
355. Diwu Z. Novel therapeutic and diagnostic applications of hypocrellins and hypericins. *Photochem Photobiol.* 1995;61(6):529–539.
356. Lopez-Bazzocchi I, Hudson JB, Towers GNH. Antiviral activity of the photoactive plant pigment hypericin. *Photochem Photobiol.* 199;54(1):95–98.
357. Hudson JB, Lopez-Bazzocchi I, Towers GNH. Antiviral activities of hypericin. *Antivir Res.* 1991;15:101–112.
358. Volz HP. Controlled clinical trials of hypericum extracts in depressed patients—an overview. *Pharmacopsychiatry.* 1997; 30(suppl 2):72–76.
359. Linde K, Ramirez G, Mulrow C, et al. St John's wort for depression—an overview and meta-analysis of randomised clinical trials. *BMJ.* 1996;313:253–258.
360. Sommer H, Harrer G. Placebo-controlled double-blind study examining the effectiveness of an hypericum preparation in 105 mildly

depressed patients. *J Geriatr Psychiatry Neural.* 1994;7(Suppl 1): S9–S11.

361. Hasgen KD, Vesper J, Ploch M. Multicenter double-blind study examining the antidepressant effectiveness of the hypericum extract LI 160. *J Geriatr Psychiatry Neurol.* 1994;7(suppl 1):S15–S18;
362. Awang DVC. St John's wort: herbal medicine. *CJ RFC.* 1991;124:33–35.
363. Brockmoller J, Reum T, Bauer S, et al. Roots I. Hypericin and pseudohypericin: pharmacokinetics and effects on photosensitivity in humans. *Pharmacopsychiatry.* 1997;30(suppl 2):94–101.
364. Vorbach EU, Amoldt KH, Hubner WD. Efficacy and tolerability of St. John's wort extract LI 160 versus imipramine in patients with severe depressive episodes according to ICD-10. *Pharmacopsychiatry.* 1997;30 (suppl 2):81–85.
365. Woelk H, Burkard G, Grunwald J. Benefits and risks of the hypericum extract LI 160: drug monitoring study with 3250 patients. *J Geriatr Psychiatry Neurol.* 1994;7(suppl 1):S34–S38.
366. Kerb R, Brockmoller J, Staffeldt B, et al. Single-dose and steady-state pharmacokinetics of hypericin and pseudohypericin. *Antimicrob Agents Chemother.* 1996;40(9):2087–2093.
367. Altaian P. Australian tea tree oil. *Aust J Pharmacy.* 1988; 69:276–278.
368. Williams L, Home V. A comparative study of some essential oils for potential use in topical applications for the treatment of the yeast Candida albicans. *Aust J Med Herb.* 1995;7(3):57–62.
369. Buck D, Midorf D, Addino J. Comparison of two topical preparations for the treatment of onychomycosis: Melaleuca atemifolia (tea tree) oil and clotrimazole. *J Fam Pract.* 1994;38:601–605.
370. Tong MM, Altmann PM, Barnetson RS. Tea tree oil in the treatment of tinea pedis. *Aust J Dermatol.* 1992;33:145–149.
371. Bassett IB, Pannowitz DL, Barnetson RS. A comparative study of tea-tree oil versus benzoyl peroxide in the treatment of acne. *Med J Aust.* 1990;153:455–458.
372. Tisserand R, Balacs T. *Essential Oil Safety: A Guide for Health Care Professionals.* London: Churchill Livingstone, 1995, p 279.
373. Kerikas GA, et al. Isolation of piceoside from Arctostaphylos uva-ursi. *Planta Med.* 1987;53:307–308.
374. Jahodar L, et al. Unedoside in Arctostaphylos uva-ursi roots. *Pharmazie.* 1981;36:294–296.
375. Jahodar L, Leifertova I, Lisa M, et al. Investigation of iridoid substances in Arctostaphylos uva-ursi. *Pharmazie.* 1978;33:536–537.
376. The Lawrence Review of Natural Products. *Uva ursi. Monograph Systems.* Levittown, PA: Pharmaceutical Information Associates, 1987.
377. Moskalnko SA. Preliminary screening of far-Eastern ethnomedicinal plants for antibacterial activity. *J Ethnopharmacol.* 1986;15:231–259.
378. Houghton P. Bearberry, dandelion and celery. *Pharm J.* 1995;255: 272–273.
379. Briggs CJ. Herbal medicine: Dioscorea: the yams—a traditional source of food and drugs. *CPJ.* RPC 1990;413–415.
380. Hudson T. Wild Yam, Natural progesterone: unraveling the confusion. *Townsend Lett Doctors Patients.* 1996;July:125–127.
381. Araghiniknam M, Chung S, Nelson-White T, et al. Antioxidant activity of dioscorea and dehydrepiandrosterone (DHEA) in older humans. *Life Sci.* 1996;59(11):147–157.
382. Dollbaum C. Lab analysis of salivary DHEA and progesterone following ingestion of yam-containing products. *Townsend Newsl Doctors.* 1996;159:104.
383. Smith M, Boon H, Burman D. Alternative medicine: a survival guide for pharmacists. *Can Pharm J.* 1996;129:36–42.
384. Eisenberg D, Davis R, Ettner S, et al. Trends in alternative medicine use in the United States, 1990-1997. *JAMA.* 1998;280:1569–1575.
385. Frazer Institute. Alternative medicines in Canada: use and public attitudes. Vancouver; Canada: *http://www.fraserinstitute.ca/pps/21/* 1999.
386. Johnston B. One-third of nation's adult use herbal remedies. *Herbalgram.* 1997;40:49.
387. Barnes J. Herbal Medicine. *Pharm J.* 1998;260:344–348.
388. Ernst E, De Smet P. Risks associated with complementary therapies. In: Dukes M, ed. *Meyler's Side Effects of Drugs.* Berlin: Elsevier, 1996;1427–1454.
389. Boon H, Brown J, Gavin A, et al. Breast cancer survivors' perception of complementary snd alternative medicine (CAM): making the decision to use or not to use. *Qual Health Res.* 1999;9(5): 639–653.
390. Shaw D, Leon C, Kolev S, et al. Traditional remedies and food supplements: a 5-year toxico-logical study (1991-5). *Drug Safety.* 1997;17:342–356.
391. Miller L. Herbal Medicinals: Selected clinical considerations focusing on known or potential drug-herb interactions. *Arch Intern Med.* 1999;158:2200–2211.
392. Barnes J, Mills S, Abbot N, et al. Different standards for reporting ADRs to herbal remedies and conventional OTC medicines: face to face interviews with 515 users of herbal remedies. *Br J Din Pharmacol.* 1998;45:496–500.
393. Raman A, Jamal J. 'Herbal' hayfever remedy found to contain conventional drugs. *Pharm J.* 1997;258:105–106.
394. Phytotherapy ESCo. In: ESCOP, ed. *ESCOP Monographs.* Exeter, UK: 1996–1997.
395. Fugh-Berman A. 5-Minute Herb and Dietary Supplement Consult. Philadelphia, PA: Lippincott Williams and Wilkins; 2003.
396. Leung AY, Foster S. Encyclopedia of Common natural Ingredients Used in food, drugs and Cosmetics. 2nd ed. NewYork, NY: John Wiley & Sons; 1996.
397. Proctor ME, Hamacher M, Tortorello ML, et al. Multistate outbreak of Salmonella serovar Muenchen infections associated with alfalfa sprouts grown from seeds pretreated with calcium hypochlorite. *J Clin Microbiol.* 2001;39(10):3461–3465.
398. Seidlova-Wuttke D, Hesse O, Jarry H, et al. Evidence for selective estrogen receptor modulator activity in a black cohosh (Cimicifuga racemosa) extract: comparison with estradiol-17beta. *European Journal of Endocrinology.* 2003;149(4):351–362.
399. Mahady GB. Is black cohosh estrogenic? *Nutrition Reviews.* 2003;61(5 Pt 1):183–186.
400. Seidlova-Wuttke D, Jarry H, Becker T, et al. Pharmacology of Cimicifuga racemosa extract BNO 1055 in rats: bone, fat and uterus. *Maturitas.* 2003;44(1):S39–S50.
401. Liske E, Haggi W, Henneicke-Von Zepelen HH, et al. Physiological investigation of a unique extract of black cohosh (cimicifugae racemosae rhizoma): a 6-month clinical study demonstrates no significant estrogenic effect. *J Women' health Gender-Based Med.* 2002; 11(2):163–174.
402. Pockaj BA, Loprinzi CL, Sloan JA, et al. Pilot evaluation of black cohosh for the treatment of hot flashes in women. *Cancer Investigation.* 2004;22(4):515–521.
403. Whiting PW, Clouston A, Kerlin P. Black cohosh and other herbal remedies associated with acute hepatitis. *Medical Journal of Australia.* 2002;177(8):440–443.
404. De Smet PAGM. Health risks of herbal remedies: an update. *Clinical Pharmacology & Therapeutics.* 2004;76(1):1–17.
405. Gunn TR, Wright IM. The use of black and blue cohosh in labour [letter]. *N Z Med J.* 1996;109:410–411.
406. Sasaki Y, Kimura Y, Tsunoda T, et al. Anaphylaxis due to burdock. *International Journal of Dermatology.* 2003;42(6):472–473.
407. Pellicer F, Picazo O, Leon-Olea M. Effect of red peppers (Capsicum frutescens) intake during gestation on thermonociceptive response of rat offspring. *Behavioural Brain Research.* 2001;19(2):179–183.
408. Kirby ML, et al. Effects of prenatal capsacicin treatment on fetal activity, opiate receptor binding and acid phosphatases in the spinal cord. *Exp Neurol.* 1982;76:298–308.
409. Phipps WR, Martini MC, Lampe JW, et al. Effect of Flax Seed Ingestion on the Menstrual Cycle. *Journal of Clinical Endocrinology and Metabolism.* 1993;77(5):1215–1219.
410. Hirawaka T, et al. Reproductive studies of Passiflora incarnate extract. Teratological study. Kiso to Rinsho 15:3431–51, 1981. cited by Shepard TH: Catalog of teratogenic agents, Seventh edition, Baltimore, Johns Hopkins University Press, 1992, p 305.
411. Huddleston M, Jackson EA. Is an extract of the fruit of agnus castus (chaste tree or chasteberry) effective for prevention of symptoms of

premenstrual syndrome (PMS)? *Journal of Family Practice.* 2001;50(4):298.

412. Costemale T, Potherat JJ. The chaste tree (Vitex agnus castus (L.) - gattilier (Fr.)) and premenstrual syndrome. *Actualites Pharmaceutiques.* 2004;432:56–57.
413. Reider N, Sepp N, Fritsch P, et al. Anaphylaxis to camomile: clinical features and allergen cross-reactivity. *Clinical & Experimental Allergy.* 2000;30(10):1436–1443.
414. Mazokopakis EE, Vrentzos GE, Papadakis JA, et al. Wild chamomile (Matricaria recutita L.) mouthwashes in methotrexate-induced oral mucositis. *Phytomedicine.* 2005;12(1–2):25–27.
415. Rudzki E, Rapiejko P, Rebandel P. Occupational contact dermatitis, with asthma and rhinitis, from camomile in a cosmetician also with contact urticaria from both camomile and lime flowers. *Contact Dermatitis.* 2003;49(3):162.
416. Thien FC. Chamomile tea enema anaphylaxis. *Medical Journal of Australia.* 2002;175(1):54.
417. Jenesen JE, Reider N, Fritsch R, et al. Fatal outcome of anaphylaxis to chamomile-containing enema during labour: a case study. *J Allergy Clin Immunol.* 1998;102:1041–1042.
418. Suvarna R, Pirmohamed M, Henderson L. Possible interaction between warfarin and cranberry juice. *BMJ.* 2003;327(7429):1454.
419. Isele H. Fatal bleeding under warfarin plus cranberry juice. Is it due to salicylic acid? *MMW Fortschritte der Medizin.* 2004;146(11):13 (Letter, German).
420. Grant P. Warfarin and cranberry juice: an interaction? *Journal of Heart Valve Disease.* 2004;13(1):25–26.
421. Raz R, Chazan B, Dan M. Cranberry juice and urinary tract infection. *Harefuah.* 2004;143(12):891–894, 909 (Hebrew).
422. Jepson RG, Mihaljevic L, Craig J. Cranberries for preventing urinary tract infections. *Cochrane Database of Systematic Reviews.* 2004;(2):CD001321.
423. Lovell CR, Rowan M. Dandelion dermatitis. *Contact Dermatitis.* 1991;25(3):185–188.
424. Johns T. Sibeko L. *Pregnancy Outcomes in Women Using Herbal Therapies. Birth Defects Research. Part B, Developmental and Reproductive Toxicology.* 2003;68(6):501–504.
425. Bedard M. Devil's claw. *Canadian Pharmaceutical Journal.* 2001;134(10):20–32.
426. Izzo AA, Di Carlo G, Borrelli F, et al. Cardiovascular pharmacotherapy and herbal medicines: The risk of drug interaction. *International Journal of Cardiology.* 2005;98(1):1–14.
427. Wegener T, Lupke NP. Treatment of Patients with Arthrosis of Hip or Knee with an Aqueous Extract of Devil's Claw (Harpagophytum procumbens DC.). *Phytotherapy Research.* 2003;17(10):1165–1172.
428. Pittler MH, Ernst E. Feverfew for preventing migraine. *Cochrane Database of Systematic Reviews.* 2004;(1):CD002286.
429. Bruce A, Buehler K. Interactions of herbal products with conventional medicines and potential impact on pregnancy review. *Birth defects research (partB).* 2003;68:494–495.
430. Holman CP, Bell AF. A trial of evening primrose oil in the treatment of chronic schizophrenia. *J Orhtomolecular Psych.* 1983;12:302–304.
431. Vaddadi KS. The use of gamma-linolenic acid and linoleic acid to differentiate between temporal lobe epilepsy and schizophrenia. *Prostaglandins Med.* 1981;6(4):375–379.
432. Dove D, Johnson P. Oral evening primrose oil: its effect on length of pregnancy and selected intrapartum outcomes in low-risk nulliparous women. *Journal of Nurse-Midwifery.* 1999;44(3):320–324.
433. Gallagher S. Omega 3 oils and pregnancy. *Midwifery Today with International Midwife.* 2004;(69):26–31.
434. Herrera JA, Arevalo-Herrera M, Herrera S. Prevetion of preeclampsia by linoleic acid and calcium supplementation: a randomized controlled trial. *Obstet Gynecol.* 1998;91:585–590.
435. D'Almeida A, Carte JP, Anatol A, et al. Effects of a combination of evening prirose oil (gamma linoleic acid) and fish oil (eicosapentaenoic+ docahexaenoic acid) versus magnesum, and versus placebo in preventing pre-eclampsia.*Women Health.* 1992;19(2–3):117–131.
435. Upton R (ed). *American Herbal Pharmacopoeia and Therapeutic Compendium.* Dang gui root. Santa Cruz, CA: American Herbal Pharmacopoeia; 2003.
436. Hale T. Medications and Mothers' Milk. 11th ed. Amarillo, TX: Pharmasoft Publishing; 1992-2004.
437. Eagon PK, Elm MS, Hunter DS, et al. *Medicinal herbs: modulation of estrogen action.* Era of Hope Mtg, Dept Defence; breast Cancer Res Porg, Atlanta, CA; 2000.
438. American health consultants. Blue Cohosh: a word of caution. *www.ahcpud.com/ahc_root_html/hot/archive/atwh 1099.html* (accessed January 31, 2005).
439. Newall CA, Anderson LA, Philson JD. *Herbal Medicine: A Guide for Healthcare Professionals.* London, UK: The Pharmaceutical Press; 1996.
440. McFarlin BL,Gibson MH,O'Rear J, et al. A national survey of herbal preparation use by nurse-midwives for labor stimulation. Review of the literature and recommendations for practice. *J Nurse Midwifery.* 1999;44:205–216.
441. Mcguffin M, et al (ed). American herbal products Association's Botanical Safety Handbook. CRC Press LLC: New York, NY; 1997.
442. Jones TK, et al. Profound neonatal congestive heart failure caused by maternal consuption of blue cohosh herbal medication. *J Pediatr.* 1998;132:550–552.
443. Finkel RS, Zarlengo KM. Blue cohosh and perinatal stroke. *N Eng J Med.* 2004;351:302–303.
444. Wright IM. Neonatal effects of maternal consumption of blue cohosh. *J Pediatr.* 1999;134:384–385.
445. Flynn TJ, Kennelly EJ, Mazzola EP, et al. Screening of the dietary supplement blue cohosh for potentially teratogenic alkaloids using rat embryo culture. *Teratology.* 1998;57:219.
446. Swafford S, Berens P. Effect of fenugreek on breastmilk porduction. *ABM News and Views.* 2000;6(3) (Abstract).
447. DH. Personal communication. 2001.
448. Gennaro A. Reminton. *The Science and Practice of Pharmacy.* 19th ed. Lippincott: Williams&Wilkins, 1996.
449. Garry D, Figueroa R, Guillaume J, et al. Use of castor oil in pregnancy at term. *Altern Ther Health Med.* 2000;6:77–79.
450. Gruenwald J, et al. PDR for herbal Medicines. 1st ed. Montvale, NJ: Medical Economics Company, Inc., 1998.
451. Schulz V, Hansel R, Tyler VE. *Rational Phytotherapy: A Physicians Guide to Herbal Medicine.* Terry C.Telger, tranl. 3rd ed. Berlin, GER: Springer, 1998.
452. Kelly AJ, Kavanagh J, Thomas J. Castor oil, bath and/or enema for cervical priming and induction of labour. *Cochrane Database of Systematic Reviews.* 2001;(2):CD003099.
453. Steingrub JS, Lopez T, Teres D, et al. Amniotic fluid embolism associated with castor oil ingestion. *Critical Care Medicine.* 1988;16(6):642–643.
454. Sicuranza GB, Figueroa R. Uterine rupture associated with castor oil ingestion. *Journal of Maternal-Fetal & Neonatal Medicine.* 2003;13(2):133–134.
455. Mitri F, Hofmeyr GJ, Van Gelderen CJ. Meconium during labour—self-medication and other associations. South African Medical Journal. Suid-Afrikaanse Tydskrif Vir Geneeskunde. 1987;71(7):431–433.
456. Cooper RL, Cooper MM. Red pepper-induced dermatits in breast-fed infants. *Dematol.* 1996;93(1):61–62.
457. Mills S, Bone K. Principles and Practice of Phytotherapy. London, UK: Churchill Livingstone, 2000.
458. Foster S. Tyler's Honest Herbal. 4th ed., Binghamton, NY: Haworth Herbal Press, 1999.
459. Collins TF, Sprando RL, Black TN, et al. Effects of flaxseed on reproduction and development of rats. *Teratology.* 2002;61:331.
460. Francois CA, Connor SL, Bolewicz LC, et al. Supplementing lactating women with flaxseed oil does not increase docosahexaenoic acid in their milk. *American Journal of Clinical Nutrition.* 2003;77(1): 226–233.

461. Lampe JW, Martini MC, Kurzer MS, et al. Urinary ligan and isoflavonoid extretion in premenopausal women consuming flaxseed powder. *Am J Clin Nutr.* 1994;60:122–128.

462. Kelly JP, Kaufman DW, Kelley K, et al. Recent trends in use of herbal and other natural products. *Arch Intern Med,* 2005;165(3):281–286.

463. Troppmann L, Johns T, Gray-Donald K. Natural health product use in Canada. *Can J Public Health.* 2002;93(6):426–430.

464. Jellin JM, Gregory PJ, Batz F, et al. Pharmacist's Letter/Prescriber's Letter Natural Medicines Comprehensive Database. 4th ed. Stockton, CA: Therapeutic Research Faculty; 2002.

465. Pinn G, Pallett L. Herbal medicine in pregnancy. *Complement Ther Nurs Midwifery.* 2002;8(2):77–80.

466. Maats FH, Crowther CA. Patterns of vitamin, mineral and herbal supplement use prior to and during pregnancy. *Aust N Z J Obstet Gynaecol.* 2002;42(5):494–496.

467. Glover DD, Rybeck BF, Tracy TS. Medication use in a rural gynecologic population: prescription, over-the-counter, and herbal medicines. *Am J Obstet Gynecol.* 2004;190(2):351–357.

468. Nordeng H, Havnen GC. Use of herbal drugs in pregnancy: a survey among 400 Norwegian women. *Pharmacoepidemiol Drug Saf.* 2004;13(6):371–380.

469. Nordeng H, Havnen GC. Impact of socio-demographic factors, knowledge and attitude on the use of herbal drugs in pregnancy. *Acta Obstet Gynecol Scand.* 2005;84(1):26–33.

470. Buttar HS, Jones KL. What do we know about the reproductive and developmental risks of herbal and alternate remedies? *Birth Defects Res B Dev Reprod Toxicol.* 2003;68(6):492–493.

471. Johns T, Sibeko L. Pregnancy outcomes in women using herbal therapies. *Birth Defects Res B Dev Reprod Toxicol.* 2003;68(6):501–504.

472. Conover EA. Herbal agents and over-the-counter medications in pregnancy. *Best Pract Res Clin Endocrinol Metab.* 2003;17(2):237–251.

473. McGauffin M, Hobbs C, Upton R, et al. *Americam Herbal Products Association's: Botanical Safety Handbook.* New York, NY: CRC Press LLC; 1997.

474. Gallo M, Sarkar M, Au W, et al. Pregnancy outcome following gestational exposure to Echinacea: a prospective controlled study. *Arch Intern Med.* 2000;160(20):3141–3143.

475. Mengs U, Claire CB, Poiley JA. Toxicity of *Echinacea purpurea*: acute, subacute and genotoxicity studies. *Arzneimittelforschung.* 1991;41:1076–1081.

476. Ondrizek RR, Chan PJ, Patton WC, et al. An alternative medicine study of herbal effects on penetration of zona-free hamster oocytes and the integrity of sperm deoxyribonucleic acid. *Fertility Sterility.* 1999;71:517–522.

477. Ondrizek RR, Chan PJ, Patton WC, et al. Inhibition of human sperm motility by specific herbs used in alternative medicine. *J Assisted Reprod Genet.* 1999;16:87–91.

478. Natural Health Products Directorate's Compendium of Monographs, *http://www.hc-sc.gc.ca/hpfb-dgpsa/nhpd-dpsn/monograph_compendium_list_e.html* (accessed March-May, 2005).

479. Olsen SF, Secher NJ, Bjornsson S, et al. The potential benefits of using fish oil in relation to preterm labor: the case for a randomized controlled trial? *Acta Obstet Gynecol Scand.* 2003;82(11):978–982.

480. McGregor JA, Allen KG, Harris MA, et al. The omega-3 story: nutritional prevention of preterm birth and other adverse pregnancy outcomes. *Obstet Gynecol Surv.* 2001;56(5 Suppl 1):S1–S13.

481. Olsen SF, Sorensen JD, Secher NJ, et al. Randomised controlled trial of effect of fish-oil supplementation on pregnancy duration. *Lancet.* 1992;339(8800):1003–1007.

482. Olsen SF, Secher NJ, Tabor A, et al. Randomised clinical trials of fish oil supplementation in high risk pregnancies. Fish Oil Trials In Pregnancy (FOTIP) Team. *BJOG.* 2000;107(3):382–395.

483. Decsi T, Koletzko B. N-3 fatty acids and pregnancy outcomes. *Curr Opin Clin Nutr Metab Care.* 2005;8(2):161–166.

484. Helland IB, Smith L, Saarem K, et al. Maternal supplementation with very-long-chain n-3 fatty acids during pregnancy and lactation augments children's IQ at 4 years of age. *Pediatrics.* 2003;111(1):e39–e44.

485. Malcolm CA, McCulloch DL, Montgomery C, et al. Maternal docosahexaenoic acid supplementation during pregnancy and visual evoked potential development in term infants: a double blind, prospective, randomised trial. *Arch Dis Child Fetal Neonatal Ed.* 2003;88(5):F383–F390.

486. Dunstan JA, Prescott SL. Does fish oil supplementation in pregnancy reduce the risk of allergic disease in infants? *Curr Opin Allergy Clin Immunol.* 2005;5(3):215–221.

487. Denomme J, Stark KD, Holub BJ. Directly quantitated dietary (n-3) fatty acid intakes of pregnant Canadian women are lower than current dietary recommendations. *J Nutr.* 2005;135(2):206–211.

488. Felter HW, Lloyd JU. *King's American Dispensatory.* 18th edition. Sandy, OR: Eclectic Medical Publications;1983.

489. Bradley PR, editor. *British Herbal Compendium Vol. 1.* Bournemouth, UK: British Herbal Medicine Association;1992.

490. Portnoi G, Lu-Ann Chng, Karimi-Tabesh L, et al. Prospective comparative study of the safety and effectiveness of ginger for the treatment of nausea and vomiting in pregnancy. *Am J Obstet Gynecol.* 2003;189:1374–1377.

491. Vutyavanich T, Kraisarin T, Ruangsri R. Ginger for nausea and vomiting in pregnancy: Randomized, double-masked, placebo-controlled trial. *Obstet Gynecol.* 2001;97:577–582.

492. Keating A, Chez RA. Ginger syrup as an antiemetic in early pregnancy. *Altern Ther.* 2002;8:89–91.

493. Smith C, Crowther C, Willson K, et al. A randomized controlled trial of ginger to treat nausea and vomiting in pregnancy. *Obstet Gynecol.* 2004;104:639–645.

494. Sripramote M, Lekhyananda N. A randomized comparison of ginger and vitamin B6 in the treatment of nausea and vomiting of pregnancy. *J Med Assoc Thai.* 2003;86(9):846–853.

495. Willetts K, Ekangaki A, Eden J. Effect of a ginger extract on pregnancy-induced nausea: a randomised controlled trial. *Australian and New Zealand Journal of Obstetrics and Gynaecology.* 2003;43:139–144.

496. Maats FH, Crowther CA. Patterns of vitamin, mineral and herbal supplement use prior to and during pregnancy. *Aust N Z J Obstet Gynaecol.* 2002;42(5):494–496.

497. Sierpina VS, Wollschlaeger B, Blumenthal M. Ginkgo biloba. *Am Fam Physician.* 2003;68(5):923–926.

498. Bruyere O, Pavelka K, Rovati LC, et al. Glucosamine sulfate reduces osteoarthritis progression in postmenopausal women with knee osteoarthritis: evidence from two 3-year studies. *Menopause.* 2004;11(2):138–143.

499. Reginster JY, Deroisy R, Rovati LC, et al. Long-term effects of glucosamine sulphate on osteoarthritis progression: a randomised, placebo-controlled clinical trial. *Lancet.* 2001;357(9252):251–256.

500. McAlindon TE, LaValley MP, Gulin JP, et al. Glucosamine and chondroitin for treatment of osteoarthritis: a systematic quality assessment and meta-analysis. *JAMA.* 2000;283(11):1469–1475.

501. Towheed TE, Anastassiades TP, Shea B, et al. Glucosamine therapy for treating osteoarthritis. *Cochrane Database Syst Rev.* 2001;(1):CD002946.

502. Bruyere O, Honore A, Ethgen O, et al. Correlation between radiographic severity of knee osteoarthritis and future disease progression. Results from a 3-year prospective, placebo-controlled study evaluating the effect of glucosamine sulfate. *Osteoarthritis Cartilage.* 2003;11(1):1–5.

503. Scroggie DA, Albright A, Harris MD. The effect of glucosamine-chondroitin supplementation on glycosylated hemoglobin levels in patients with type 2 diabetes mellitus: a placebo-controlled, double-blinded, randomized clinical trial. *Arch Intern Med.* 2003;163(13):1587–1590.

504. Tallia AF, Cardone DA. Asthma exacerbation associated with glucosamine-chondroitin supplement. *J Am Board Fam Pract.* 2002;15(6):481–484.

505. Kaneto H, Xu G, Song KH, et al. Activation of the hexosamine pathway leads to deterioration of pancreatic beta-cell function

through the induction of oxidative stress. *J Biol Chem.* 2001;276(33):31099–31104.
506. Monauni T, Zenti MG, Cretti A, et al. Effects of glucosamine infusion on insulin secretion and insulin action in humans. *Diabetes.* 2000;49(6):926–935.
507. Yoshikawa H, Tajiri Y, Sako Y, et al. Glucosamine-induced beta-cell dysfunction: a possible involvement of glucokinase or glucose-transporter type 2. *Pancreas.* 2002;24(3):228–234.
508. Muller-Fassbender H, Bach GL, Haase W, et al. Glucosamine sulfate compared to ibuprofen in osteoarthritis of the knee. *Osteoarthritis Cartilage.* 1994;2(1):61–69.
509. Virkamaki A, Daniels MC, Hamalainen S, et al. Activation of the hexosamine pathway by glucosamine in vivo induces insulin resistance in multiple insulin sensitive tissues. *Endocrinology.* 1997;138(6):2501–2507.
510. Russell AL. Glucosamine in osteoarthritis and gastrointestinal disorders: an exemplar of the need for a paradigm shift. *Med Hypotheses.* 1998;51(4):347–349.
511. Anderson GD. Glucosamine part III: dosing, safety and side-effects. *Dynamic Chiropract.* 1998;16:28–30.
512. Horal M, Zhang Z, Stanton R, et al. Activation of the hexosamine pathway causes oxidative stress and abnormal embryo gene expression: involvement in diabetic teratogenesis. *Birth Defects Res A Clin Mol Teratol.* 2004;70(8):519–527.
513. Okabe M, Yagasaki M, Matzno S, et al. Glucosamine enhanced sperm-egg binding but inhibited sperm-egg fusion in mouse. *Experientia.* 1989;45(2):193–194.
514. Didock KA, Jackson D, Robson JM. The action of some nucleotoxic substances in pregnancy. *Br J Pharmacol.* 1956;11:437–441.
515. Price CJ, George JD, Marr MC, et al. Developmental toxicity evaluation of berberine chloride dehydrate (BCD) in Sprague-Dawley (CDN) rats. *Teratology.* 2001;63:279.
516. Chan E. Displacement of bilirubin from albumin by berberine. *Biol Neonate.* 1993;63:201–208.
517. Fujiki H, Suganuma M, Imai K, et al. Green tea: cancer preventive beverage and/or drug. *Cancer Lett.* 2002;188(1–2):9–13.
518. Fujiki H, Suganuma M, Okabe S, et al. Cancer prevention with green tea and monitoring by a new biomarker, hnRNP B1. *Mutat Res.* 2001;480–481:299–304.
519. Hicks MB, Hsieh YH, Bell LN. Tea preparation and its influence on methylxanthine concentration. *Food Research International.* 1996;29(3–4):325–330.
520. Kaszkin M, Beck KF, Eberhardt W, et al. Unravelling green tea's mechanisms of action: more than meets the eye. *Mol Pharmacol.* 2004;65(1):15–17.
521. Kaegi E. Unconventional therapies for cancer: 2. Green tea. The Task Force on Alternative Therapies of the Canadian Breast Cancer Research Initiative. *CMAJ.* 1998;158(8):1033–1035.
522. Tsuneki H, Ishizuka M, Terasawa M, et al. Effect of green tea on blood glucose levels and serum proteomic patterns in diabetic (db/db) mice and on glucose metabolism in healthy humans. *BMC Pharmacol.* 2004;4(1):18.
523. Vinson JA, Teufel K, Wu N. Green and black teas inhibit atherosclerosis by lipid, antioxidant, and fibrinolytic mechanisms. *J Agric Food Chem.* 2004;52(11):3661–3665.
524. Nakazato T, Ito K, Miyakawa Y, et al. Catechin, a green tea component, rapidly induces apoptosis of myeloid leukemic cells via modulation of reactive oxygen species production in vitro and inhibits tumor growth in vivo. *Haematologica.* 2005;90(3):317–325.
525. Morley N, Clifford T, Salter L, et al. The green tea polyphenol (-)-epigallocatechin gallate and green tea can protect human cellular DNA from ultraviolet and visible radiation-induced damage. *Photodermatol Photoimmunol Photomed.* 2005;21(1):15–22.
526. Koo MW, Cho CH. Pharmacological effects of green tea on the gastrointestinal system. *Eur J Pharmacol.* 2004;500(1–3):177–185.
527. Laurie SA, Miller VA, Grant SC, et al. Phase I study of green tea extract in patients with advanced lung cancer. *Cancer Chemother Pharmacol.* 2005;55(1):33–38.
528. Sano J, Inami S, Seimiya K, et al. Effects of green tea intake on the development of coronary artery disease. *Circ J.* 2004;68(7):665–670.
529. Kobayashi Y, Suzuki M, Satsu H, et al. Green tea polyphenols inhibit the sodium-dependent glucose transporter of intestinal epithelial cells by a competitive mechanism. *J Agric Food Chem.* 2000;48(11):5618–5623.
530. Son DJ, Cho MR, Jin YR, et al. Antiplatelet effect of green tea catechins: a possible mechanism through arachidonic acid pathway. *Prostaglandins Leukot Essent Fatty Acids.* 2004;71(1):25–31.
531. Koren G. Caffeine during pregnancy: in moderation. *Can Fam Physician.* 2000;46:801–803.
532. Navarro-Peran E, Cabezas-Herrera J, Garcia-Canovas F, et al. The antifolate activity of tea catechins. *Cancer Res.* 2005;65(6):2059–2064.
533. Wu AH, Arakawa K, Stanczyk FZ, et al. Tea and circulating estrogen levels in postmenopausal Chinese women in Singapore. *Carcinogenesis.* 2005;26(5):976–980.
534. Chadwick LR, Nikolic D, Burdette JE. et al. Estrogens and congeners from spent hops (Humulus lupulus). *Journal of Natural Products.* 2004;67(12):2024–2032.
535. Piersen CE. Phytoestrogens in botanical dietary supplements: implications for cancer. *Integr Cancer Ther.* 2003;2(2):120–138.
536. Milligan S, Kalita J, Pocock V, et al. Oestrogenic activity of the hop phyto-oestrogen, 8-prenylnaringenin. *Reproduction.* 2002;123(2): 235–242.
537. Koruk ST, Ozyilkan E, Kaya P, et al. Juniper tar poisoning. *Clin Toxicol (Phila).* 2005;43(1):47–49.
538. Barrero AF, Quilez del Moral JF, Lara A, et al. Antimicrobial activity of sesquiterpenes from the essential oil of Juniperus thurifera. *Planta Med.* 2005;71(1):67–71.
539. Health Canada: *http://www.hcsc.gc.ca/english/protection/ warnings/ 2002/2002_56e.htm* (accessed May 17, 2005).
540. Piersen CE. Phytoestrogens in botanical dietary supplements: implications for cancer. *Integr Cancer Ther.* 2003;2(2):120–138.
541. Strandberg TE, Andersson S, Jarvenpaa AL, et al. Preterm birth and licorice consumption during pregnancy. *Am J Epidemiol.* 2002;156(9):803–805.
542. Health Canada Warnings/Advisory for June 14, 2001: *http://www.hc-sc.gc.ca/english/protection/warnings/ 2001/2001_ 67e.htm* (accessed May 17, 2005).
543. FAO/WHO. Evaluation of Health and Nutritional Properties of Powder Milk and Live Lactic Acid Bacteria. Food and Agriculture Organization of the United Nations and World Health Organization Expert Consultation Report. Available at: *ftp://ftp.fao.org/ docrep/fao/meeting/009/y6398e.pdf*
544. de Roos NM, Katan MB. Effects of probiotic bacteria on diarrhea, lipid metabolism, and carcinogenesis: a review of papers published between 1988 and 1998. *Am J Clin Nutr.* 2000;71(2):405–411.
545. Van Niel CW, Feudtner C, Garrison MM, Christakis DA. Lactobacillus therapy for acute infectious diarrhea in children: a meta-analysis. *Pediatrics.* 2002;109(4):678–684.
546. Pochapin M. The effect of probiotics on Clostridium difficile diarrhea. *Am J Gastroenterol.* 2000;95(1):S11–S13.
547. Gorbach SL. Probiotics and gastrointestinal health. *Am J Gastroenterol.* 2000 Jan;95(1):S2–S4.
548. Reid G, Bocking A. The potential for probiotics to prevent bacterial vaginosis and preterm labor. *Am J Obstet Gynecol.* 2003;189(4): 1202–1208.
549. Shalev E. Ingestion of probiotics: optional treatment of bacterial vaginosis in pregnancy. *Isr Med Assoc J.* 2002;4(5):357–360.
550. Hoyme UB, Saling E. Efficient prematurity prevention is possible by pH-self measurement and immediate therapy of threatening ascending infection. *Eur J Obstet Gynecol Reprod Biol.* 2004;115(2): 148–153.
551. Lin HC, Su BH, Chen AC, et al. Oral probiotics reduce the incidence and severity of necrotizing enterocolitis in very low birth weight infants. *Pediatrics.* 2005;115(1):1–4.
552. Schultz M, Balfour Sartor R. Probiotics and inflammatory Bowel diseases. *Am J Gastroenterol.* 2000;95(1):S19–S21.

553. Ishida Y, Nakamura F, Kanzato H, et al. Clinical effects of Lactobacillus acidophilus strain L-92 on perennial allergic rhinitis: a double-blind, placebo-controlled study. *J Dairy Sci.* 2005;88(2):527–533.
554. Rautava S, Kalliomaki M, Isolauri E. Probiotics during pregnancy and breast-feeding might confer immunomodulatory protection against atopic disease in the infant. *J Allergy Clin Immunol.* 2002;109(1):119–121.
555. Rautava S, Isolauri E. The development of gut immune responses and gut microbiota: effects of probiotics in prevention and treatment of allergic disease. *Curr Issues Intest Microbiol.* 2002;3(1):15–22.
556. Cunningham-Rundles S, Ahrne S, Bengmark S, et al. Probiotics and immune response. *Am J Gastroenterol.* 2000;95(1):S22–S25.
557. Alvarez-Olmos MI, Oberhelman RA. Probiotic agents and infectious diseases: a modern perspective on a traditional therapy. *Clin Infect Dis.* 2001;32(11):1567–1576.
558. Thompson C, McCarter YS, Krause PJ, et al. Lactobacillus acidophilus sepsis in a neonate. *J Perinatol.* 2001;21(4):258–260.
559. De Groote MA, Frank DN, Dowell E, et al. Lactobacillus rhamnosus GG bacteremia associated with probiotic use in a child with short gut syndrome. *Pediatr Infect Dis J.* 2005;24(3):278–280.
560. Land MH, Rouster-Stevens K, Woods CR, et al. Lactobacillus sepsis associated with probiotic therapy. *Pediatrics.* 2005;115(1):178–181.
561. Aselton P, Jick H, Milunsky A, et al. First-trimester drug use and congenital disorders. *Obstet Gynecol.* 1985;65(4):451–455.
562. Kalliomaki M, Salminen S, Arvilommi H, et al. Probiotics in primary prevention of atopic disease: a randomised placebo-controlled trial. *Lancet.* 2001;357(9262):1076–1079.
563. Kalliomaki M, Salminen S, Poussa T, et al. Probiotics and prevention of atopic disease: 4-year follow-up of a randomised placebo-controlled trial. *Lancet.* 2003;361(9372):1869–1871.
564. Reid G, Devillard E. Probiotics for mother and child. *J Clin Gastroenterol.* 2004;38(6):S94–S101.
565. Schultz M, Gottl C, Young RJ, et al. Administration of oral probiotic bacteria to pregnant women causes temporary infantile colonization. *J Pediatr Gastroenterol Nutr.* 2004;38(3):293–297.
566. Dennemark N, Meyer-Wilmes M, Schluter R. Screening and treatment of bacterial vaginosis in the early second trimester of pregnancy: a sufficient measure for prevention of preterm deliveries? *International Journal of STD & AIDS.* 1997;8(1):38–39.
567. Juergens UR, Stober M, Schmidt-Schilling L, et al: Antiinflammatory effects of eucalyptol (1.8-cineole) in bronchial asthma: inhibition of arachidonic acid metabolism in human blood monocytes ex vivo. *Eur J Med Res.* 3:407–412, 1998.
568. Tassou CC, Drosinos EH, Nychas GJ. Effects of essential oil from mint (Mentha piperita) on Salmonella enteritis and Listeria monocytogenes in model food systems at 4 degrees and 10 degrees. *C J Appl Bacteriol.* 78:1995;593–600.
569. Sarbhoy AK, Varshney JL, Maheshwari ML, et al: Efficacy of some essential oils and their constituents on few ubiquitous molds. *Zentralbl Bacteriol Naturwiss.* 133:1978:723–725.
570. Arakawa T, Ishikawa Y, Ushida K. Volatile sulfur production by pig cecal bacteria in batch culture and screening inhibitors of sulfate reducing bacteria. *J Nutr Sci Vitaminol.* 46:193–198,2000.
571. Inoue T, Sugimoto Y, Masuda H, et al: Effect of pepper-mint (Mentha piperita L.) extracts on experimental allergic rhinitis in rats. *Biol Pharm Bull.* 24:92–95,2001.
572. Sigmund DJ, McNally EF. The action of a carminative on the lower esophageal sphincter. *Gastroenterology.* 56:13–18,1969.
573. Akdogan M, Ozguner M, Kocak A, et al. Effects of peppermint teas on plasma testosterone, follicle-stimulation hormone, and leutenizing hormone levels and testicular tissue in rats. *Urology.* 2004;64:394–398.
574. Maats FH, Crowther CA. Patterns of vitamin, mineral and herbal supplement use prior to and during pregnancy. *Aust N Z J Obstet Gynaecol.* 2002;42(5):494–496.
575. Simpson M, Parsons M, Greenwood J, et al. Raspberry leaf in pregnancy: its safety and efficacy in labor. *J Midwifery Womens Health.* 2001;46(2):51–59.
576. McFarlin BL, Gibson MH, O'Rear J, et al. A national survey of herbal preparation use by nurse-midwives for labor stimulation. Review of the literature and recommendations for practice. *J Nurse Midwifery.* 1999;44(3):205–216.
577. Rojas-Vera J, Patel AV, Dacke CG. Relaxant activity of raspberry (Rubus idaeus) leaf extract in guinea-pig ileum in vitro. *Phytother Res.* 2002;16(7):665–668.
578. Bamford DS, Percival RC, Tothill AU. Raspberry leaf tea: a new aspect to an old problem. *Br J Pharmacol.* 1970;40(1):161.
579. Parsons M, Simpson M, Ponton T. Raspberry leaf and its effect on labour: safety and efficacy. *J Aust Coll Midwives.* 1999 Sep;12(3):20–25.
580. Gudej J, Tomczyk M. Determination of flavonoids, tannins and ellagic acid in leaves from Rubus L. species. *Arch Pharm Res.* 2004;27(11):1114–1149.
581. Rabanal RM, Bonkanka CX, Hernandez-Perez M, et al. Analgesic and topical anti-inflammatory activity of Hypericum canariense L. and Hypericum glandulosum Ait. *J Ethnopharmacol.* 2005;96(3):591–596.
582. Hosseinzadeh H, Karimi GR, Rakhshanizadeh M. Anticonvulsant effect of Hypericum perforatum: role of nitric oxide. *J Ethnopharmacol.* 2005;98(1–2):207–208.
583. He YY, Chignell CF, Miller DS, et al. Phototoxicity in human lens epithelial cells promoted by St. John's Wort. *Photochem Photobiol.* 2004;80(3):583–586.
584. Linde K, Berner M, Egger M, et al. St John's wort for depression: meta-analysis of randomised controlled trials. *Br J Psychiatry.* 2005;186:99–107.
585. Pfrunder A, Schiesser M, Gerber S, et al. Interaction of St John's Wort with low-dose oral contraceptive therapy: a randomized controlled trial. *Br J Clin Pharmacol.* 2003;56(6):683–690.
586. Mannel M. Drug interactions with St John's wort: mechanisms and clinical implications. *Drug Safety.* 2004;27(11):773–797.
587. Gregoretti B, Stebel M, Candussio L, et al. Toxicity of Hypericum perforatum (St. John's wort) administered during pregnancy and lactation in rats. *Toxicol Appl Pharmacol.* 2004;200(3):201–205.
588. Upton R, Graffa WE, Buneing D, et al. St John's wort monograph. *Am Herbal Pharmacopoeia.* 1997;1:32.
589. Rayburn WF, Gonzalez CL, Christensen HD, et al. Effect of prenatally administered Hypericum (St John's wort) on growth and physical maturation of mouse offspring. *Am J Obstet Gynecol.* 2001;184:191–195.
590. Rayburn WF, Christensen HD, Gonzalez CL. Effect of antenatal exposure to Saint John's wort (Hypericum) on neurobehavior of developing mice. *Am J Obstet Gynecol.* 2000;183:1225–1231.
591. Grush LR, Nierenberg A, Keefe B, et al. St John's wort during pregnancy. *JAMA.* 1998;280:1566.
592. Franklin M, Chi J, McGavin C, et al. Neuroendocrine evidence for dopaminergic actions of hypericum extract (LI 160) in healthy human volunteers. *Biol Psychiatry.* 1999;46:581–584.
593. Clier CM, Schafer MR, Schmid-Siegel B, et al. St. John's wort (Hypericum perforatum): is it safe during breastfeeding? *Pharmacopsychiatry.* 2002;35:29–30.
594. Lee A, Minhas R, Matsuda N, et al. The safety of St. John's wort (Hypericum perforatum) during breastfeeding. *J Clin Psychiatry.* 2003;64(8):966–968.
595. Veien NK, Rosner K, Skovgaard GL. Is tea tree oil an important contact allergen? *Contact Dermatitis.* 2004;50(6):378–379.
596. Muller SD, Vasconcelos SB, Coelho M, et al. LC and UV determination of flavonoids from Passiflora alata medicinal extracts and leaves. *J Pharm Biomed Anal.* 2005;37(2):399–403.
597. Dhawan K, Dhawan S, Sharma A. Passiflora: a review update. *J Ethnopharmacol.* 2004;94(1):1–23.
598. Itabashi M, et al. Reproductive studies with arbutin in rats by subcutaneous administration. *Iyakuhin Kenkyu.* 1998;19:282–297. English abstract.
599. Castleman M. *The Healing Herbs: The Ultimate Guide.* Emmaus, PA, Rodale Press 1991:342–344.

600. Ganzera M, Dharmaratne HR, Nanayakkara NP, et al. Determination of saponins and alkaloids in Caulophyllum thalictroides (blue cohosh) by high-performance liquid chromatography and evaporative light scattering detection. *Phytochem Anal.* 2003;14(1):1–7.
601. Prasad K. Hypocholesterolemic and antiatherosclerotic effect of flax lignan complex isolated from flaxseed. *Atherosclerosis.* 2005;179(2):269–275.
602. Leung AY, Foster S. *Encyclopedia of common Natural Ingredients Used in Food, Drugs and Cosmetics.* 2nd ed. New York, NY: John Wiley & Sons, 1996.
603. Blumenthal M, et al. *The Comlete german Commission E Monographs: Therapeutic Guide to Herbal Medicines.* Trans. S. Klein. Boston, MA: American Botanical Council, 1998.
604. Herbs for Milk Production Breastfeeding/Nursing/Parenting, *www.gentlebirth.org/archives.*
605. McGuffin M, et al. *American Herbal Products Association's Botanical Safety Handbook.* Boca Raton, FL: CRC Press, 1997.
606. Brinker F. Herb *Contraindications and Drug Interactions.* 2nd ed. Sandy, OR; Eclectic Medical Publications, 1998.
607. Foster S, Tyler VE. *Tyler's Honest Herbal: A Sensible Guide to the use of Herbs and Related Remedies.* 3rd ed, Binghamton, NY: Haworth Herbal Press, 1993.
608. Fetrow CW, Avila JR. *Professional's Handbook of Complementary & Alternative Medicines.* Springhouse, PA: Springhouse Corporation, 1999.
609. Hegarty VM, May HM, Khaw K. Tea drinking and bone mineral density in older women. *Am J Clin Nutr.* 2000;71:1003–1007.
610. *The Review of Natural Products by Facts and Comparisons.* St.Louis, MO: Wolters Kluwer Co, 1999.
611. Fetrow CW, Avala JR. *Professional's Handbook of Complementary and Alternative Medicines.* Springhouse Corporation, 1999.
612. Covington TR, et al. *Handbook of Nonprescription Drugs.* Washington, DC: Am Pharmaceutical Assn, 1996.
613. Mc Kevoy GK, ed. *AHFS Drug Information.* Bethesda, MD: American Society of Health-System Pharmacists, 1998.
614. Gruenwald J, et al. *PDR for Herbal Medicines.* 1st ed. Montvale, NJ: Medical Economics Company, Inc., 1998.
615. Hertog MGL, Sweetnam PM, Fehily AM, et al. Antioxidant Flavonols and ischemic heart disease in Welsh population of men: the Caerphilly Study. *Am J Clin Nutr.* 1997;65:1489–1494.
616. Sharma RD, et al. Effect of fenugreek seeds on blood glucose and serum lipids in type I diabetes. *Eur J Clin Nutr.* 1990;44;301–306.
617. Lininger SW. *The Natural Pharmacy.* 1st ed Rocklin, CA: Prima Publishing; 1998.
618. Betzold CM. Galactagogues. *Journal of Midwifery & Women's Health.* 2004;49(2):151–154.
619. Madar Z, Thorne R. Dietary fiber. *Prog Food Nutr Sci.* 1987;11:153–174.
620. Basch E, Ulbricht C, Kuo G, et al. Therapeutic applications of fenugreek. *Alternative Medicine Review.* 2003;8(1):20–27.
621. Patil SP, Niphadkar PV, Bapat MM. Allergy to fenugreek (trigonella foenum graecum). *Ann Allergy Astma Immunol.* 1997;78(3): 297–300.
622. Bierenbaum ML, Reichstein R, Watkins TR. Reducing atherogenic risk in hyperlipemic humans with flaxseed supplementation: a preliminary report. *J Am Coll Nutr.* 1993;12(50):501–504.
623. Jenkins DJ, Kendall CW, Vidgen E, et al. Health aspects of partially defatted flaxseed, including effects on serum lipids, oxidative meaures, and ex vivo androgen and progestin activity: a controlled, crossover trial. *Am J Clin Nutr.* 1999;69:395–402.
624. Haggans CJ, Hutchins AM, Olson BA, et al. Effect of flaxseed consumption on urinary estrogen metabolites in postmenopausal women. *Nutr Cancer.* 1999;33(2):188–195.
625. Clark WF, Parbatani A, Huff MW, et al. Flaxseed : a potential treatment for lupus nephritis. *Kidney Int.* 1995;48:475–480.
626. Cunnane SC, Ganguli S, Menard C, et al. High alpha-linolenic acid flaxseed (linum usitatissmum) some nutritional properties in humans. *Br J Nutr.* 1993;69;443–453.
627. Prasad K. Dietary flax seed in prevention of hypercholesterolemic atherosclerosis. *Atherosclerosis.* 1997;132:69–76.
628. Thompson LU, Rickard SE, Orcheson LJ, et al. Flaxseed and its ligaanan and oil components reduce mammary tumor grouth at a late stage of carcinogenesis. *Carcinogenesis.* 1996;17(6):1373–1376.
629. Alonso L, Marcos ML, Blanco JD, et al. Anaphylaxis caused by linseed (flaxseed) intake. *J Allergy Clin Immunol.* 1996;98(2): 469–470.
630. Nordstrom DC, Honkanen VE, Nasu Y, et al. Alpha-linolenic acid in the treatment of rheumatoid arthritis. A double-blind, placebo-controlled and randomized study: flaxseed vs. safflower seed. *Rheumatol Int.* 1995;14(6):231–234.

CHAPTER 20

FOLIC ACID AND CONGENITAL BIRTH DEFECTS: A REVIEW

Y. Ingrid Goh and Gideon Koren

HISTORY

Folic acid (folate, vitamin B9, pteroylglutamic acid, pteroylglutamate) is a water-soluble vitamin. Its name is derived from folium, the Latin translation for leaf.[1] The history of folic acid dates back to the early 1930s when Lucy Wills discovered a factor in yeast that was able to correct macrocytic anemia in pregnant women.[1–3] To corroborate these findings, Wills conducted a study investingating the effect of diet modification in albino rats with macrocytic anemia caused by Bartonella infection.[1] The results from this study prompted the recommendation of yeast or Marmite (a yeast extract) supplementation to pregnant women suffering from macrocytic anemia in Bombay.[3]

Folic acid was first isolated from spinach in 1941,[4] following which, it was synthesized by Bob Stokstad in 1943.[1] Folic acid was found to be effective in treating megaloblastic anemia of all types: megaloblastic anemia of sprue, celiac disease, pregnancy, and malnutrition, as well as Addisonian pernicious anemia.[1,5,6] The association of folate deficiency and anemia was illustrated in a famous experiment conducted Victor Herbert.[7] Herbert monitored the sequence of hematological events as he voluntarily ate a folate-deficient diet for 4 months.[7]

Not only was folic acid found to be useful in treating anemia during pregnancy, Jack Metz et al. showed a decreased risk of premature births in undernourished populations that were prophylactically given folic acid.[8] The enzymes involved in mammalian folate metabolism were later isolated and purified in the 1970s.[9]

PHARMACOKINETICS

The term folic acid generally refers to the fully oxidized form of the chemical compound, which is not naturally available in foods. On the other hand, the term folate refers to a group of compounds that have the same vitamin activity but encompasses both folic acid and naturally occurring folates. Folates are composed of a pteridine ring, p-aminobenzoic acid, and may contain one to six glutamate molecules that are joined by peptide linkages (Fig. 20-1).[1,10] Natural folates are found in the form of polyglutamates. These are relatively heat labile molecules that may be destroyed by storage, processing, and cooking[11] and are not readily absorbed by the body in this form. As such, the absorption of dietary folate must occur in a two-step process.[12] Natural folates have to be metabolized by conjugases in the upper small intestine into monoglutamates,[11,13,14] which are then absorbed into the body by specific carriers located on the cell membrane of the proximal small intestine.[12,15,16] In contrast, synthetic folates are relatively stable as monoglutamates,[10] and have a better bioavailability compared to natural folates since they are rapidly absorbed in the unmodified or in the reduced or methylated form.[12,17–19]

Absorption across the enterocyte brush border membrane can occur by two means: high-capacity transporter that is pH dependent or low-capacity facilitated diffusion that is pH independent.[12] Of the two, the pH-dependent transporter is the prominent route through which folate is absorbed.[12,20] This anion exchange mechanism, however, is a saturable process.[14] After entering the cell, the transported folate monoglutamates are reconstructed into a polyglutamate chain by folylpolyglutamate synthetase.[14] The majority of folate is stored in the liver[12,19,20] and folate metabolism occurs in the cytoplasm and mitochondria.[14] Polyglutamyl folates are then hydrolyzed to folylmonoglutamates by pteroyl-g-glutamylhydrolase.[14] Those in turn are metabolized into 5-methyl-H4PteGlu1 within the enterocyte and transported to peripheral tissues, where it is converted to monoglutamyl tetrahydrofolate by methionine synthase.[14,21] Its one-carbon unit metabolism synthesizes three products in the cytoplasm: 10-formyltetrahydrofolate, methylene tetrahydrofolate, and 5-methyltetrahydrofolate.[22] The primary form of folate found in serum is 5 methyl-tetrahydrofolate[23] the chemically active form of folic acid, which is a cofactor for a variety of biosynthetic pathways.[24] These three products are required for the synthesis of purine rings; conversion of deoxyuridine monophosphate to deoxythymidine monophosphate; and the remethylation of homocysteine to methionine, respectively.[22] Methionine is converted to s-adenosylmethionine, which acts as a cofactor for many methylation reactions including the methylation of DNA, RNA proteins, and neurotransmitters.[10,11,25,26]

Folic acid is required for the synthesis of methionine from homocysteine.[14] Its ability to transfer methyl groups results in the recycling of homocysteine back to methionine.[10] The single carbon units from this final product are used for nucleotide biosynthesis including pyrimidines, thymidine, and purines, and the synthesis of DNA.[10,15,26–29] As such, all new cell formation is dependent on the adequate supply of folate. Folate also plays a role in protein metabolism by meditating the interconversion of serine and glycine and playing a role in hisitidine catabolism.[30] Therefore, folate deficiency in rapidly dividing cells may lead to alterations in DNA synthesis and chromosomal aberrations.[31,32] When the hypomethylation of DNA occurs, DNA strand breakage and abnormal gene expression may result.[33–38] Folate is degraded through the process of irreversible oxidative cleavage for the C9-N10 bond. This results in the formation of pteridine and p-aminobenzoylglutamate as degradation products.[14]

Folic acid is essential for growth and differentiation, repair, and host defense[11] and hence it is essential for fetal development. In order to be transported to the fetus, folate monoglutamates are transported by folate receptor, Folbp1, that are highly expressed in the embryo and fetus. In fact, it is also prominently expressed in the neural folds prior to the closure of the neural tube.[39] During embryogenesis and fetal growth, nucleic acid, and protein synthesis are reliant on the supply of folate and as such the requirement for maternal folate increases during this period of cell formation.[10] A deficient folate supply or problem in its metabolism may result in impaired cell formation and tissue growth.[30] As such, nucleic

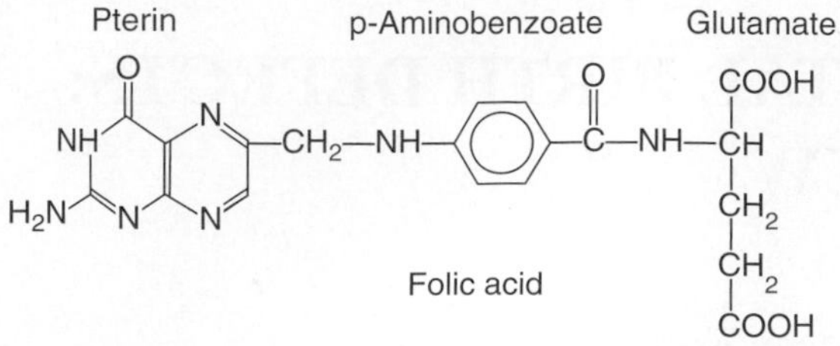

Figure 20-1. Folic acid.

acids will not be synthesized and cells will be unable to manufacture enough DNA for mitosis therefore resulting in abnormal cell division.[10] Proteins, lipids and myelin will also not be methylated due to the inhibition of the methylation cycle. Since cells are rapidly dividing during the fetal period, they are most susceptible to irregularities in DNA production. Folate deficiency or impairments in genetic folate metabolism are proposed mechanisms that cause congenital birth defects.[10]

Congenital Birth Defects

Congenital birth defects can range in their severity—they can be life-threatening or may result in disability that interferes with growth or function. Congenital birth defects are the most common cause of perinatal and infant mortality in the United States and Canada.[40,41] It is estimated that congenital birth defects affect 5% of individuals[42]; however, only 2–3% are recognized at birth.[43] It has been proposed that folic acid supplementation may correct folate levels in deficient mothers or compensate for innate folate metabolism abnormalities to decrease the risk of congenital birth defects.[44] The following review will highlight studies in which folic acid has been suggested to decrease the risk of birth defects.

Neural Tube Defects

Neural tube defects (NTDs) comprise of malformations of the cranium, spine, and nervous system that range from benign to serious in nature. NTDs can be classified as open such as anencephaly, myeloschisis, meningomyelocele, and spina bifida. Closed neural tube defects include encephalocele, and meningocele. Affecting 0.5–8/1000 live births, NTDs are among the most prevalent forms of congenital birth defects.[45] The CDC estimates that 3000 infants are born with NTDs in the United States each year.[46] In Canada NTDs are estimated to occur in 0.58/1000 births or 195 cases.[47] In addition, it is estimated that NTDs affect 300,000 infants worldwide.[48] Spina bifida and anencephaly alone are estimated to occur in 1/1000 pregnancies in the United States.[49]

NTDs are a major cause of mortality in newborns secondary to congenital heart defects.[45] The prevalence of NTDs varies by geographic region and ethnicity. The prevalence is highest in Celtic and the western part of the British Isle,[50] Newfoundland,[51] Eastern U.S.,[52,53] and Sikhs.[54] Conversely, there is a low prevalence of NTDs in the African population.[55] NTDs are present at moderate incidence in the Hispanic population.[55,56]

The exact mechanism by which folate supplementation prevents NTDs and its recurrence is not known.[45] Studies suggesting the effectiveness of folate supplementation in decreasing NTDs date back to the 1960s.[57] Smithells et al. were the first to suggest the possibility of this relationship in a case-control study from 1960 to 1966 where they noted that prenatal multivitamin supplementation resulted in a 7/1000 incidence of NTDs, whereas unsupplemented mothers had a 22/1000 incidence of delivering a child with NTDs.[57] As a follow-up to this study, Smithells et al. conducted a case-control study evaluating prenatal multivitamin supplementation in English and Irish women who had previously delivered a child with NTDs.[58] Prenatal multivitamin supplementation in 137 women resulted in a 0.6% recurrence rate of having a child with NTD.[58] In contrast, 187 control women had a 5.0% recurrence rate of NTDs.[58] Two other nonrandomized prospective studies by Smithells and colleagues in the early 1980s also supported the protective effect of folic acid.[59,60] In one study, NTDs occurred in 1/204 children (0.5%) born to folate-supplemented women versus 13/205 children (4.0%) born to unsupplemented women.[59] The second study had similar findings where 3/429 children (0.7%) born to folate-supplemented women had NTDs versus 24/510 children (4.7%) born to unsupplemented women.[60] The results from these observational studies endorsed the need to conduct a randomized control trial; however, they were not permitted to conduct a randomized control trial based on ethical consideration. They therefore conducted a cohort study of women who had a previous child with a NTD. Of the women receiving folic acid supplementation 2/234 (0.9%) delivered a child with NTD, compared to 11/215 (5.1%) children to unsupplemented women.[61]

At the same time, an observational study by Laurence et al. examining the diets of women who delivered a child with NTD found a possible relationship with poor prenatal nutrition.[62] Their results prompted them to conduct a small double-blinded randomized-controlled trial where half of the women who previously delivered a child with a NTD received 4 mg folic acid during pregnancy.[63] Supplementation resulted in 0/44 children born with a NTD whereas 6/61 children were born with NTDs to women in the unsupplemented group.[63] Despite these results, the study was limited by the small participant size.

An observational study by Sheppard et al. investigated the effect of folate supplementation in women who had a child with prior NTD.[64] They identified 227 women who were fully supplemented during pregnancy and observed no recurrence of NTD.[64] Of the 213 women who were partially supplemented, two women delivered a second child with NTDs.[64] An Atlanta case-control study by Mulinare et al. compared 347 babies affected with NTDs with 2829 healthy controls.[65] A protective effect of NTDs was observed in mothers who supplemented with multivitamins during pregnancy (RR = 0.40, 95% CI = 0.25–0.63).[65] Another case-control study conducted in Australia found that prenatal supplementation with folic acid consumption in early pregnancy also resulted in a decrease risk of NTD (OR = 0.7, 95% CI = 0.27–1.82).[66]

A large cohort study conducted by Milunsky et al. investigated the importance of the time of initiation and duration of use of folic acid-fortified multivitamin supplementation and its role of decreasing the risk of NTDs.[67] Of the 22,776 women they examined during pregnancy, nine children with NTDs were born to 7261 women who supplemented with multivitamin before and after conception.[67] On the other hand, 29 NTDs occurred among 12,297 women who reported taking multivitamins only in their first trimester of pregnancy.[67] Eleven NTDs occurred in women who did not supplement during their pregnancy.[67] All things considered, they found that the prevalence of NTDs were 1.1/1000 and 3.5/1000 for women with and without multivitamin supplementation in the first

6 months of their pregnancy, respectively.[67] When the data were separately analyzed by multivitamin fortification with folic acid, the prevalence for NTDs was 0.9/1000 and 3.2/1000 for supplementation in the first 6 weeks of pregnancy and after 7 weeks of pregnancy, respectively.[67] On the other hand, women who took multivitamins that were not supplemented with folic acid in the first 6 weeks of pregnancy had a prevalence of 3.2/1000 for NTDs.[65] Another cohort study conducted by Vergel et al. found no recurrence of NTDs among offspring of women who were supplementing with 5 mg of folic acid.[68] On the other hand there was a 3% recurrence rate in unsupplemented women.[68] Contrary to these studies, a case-control study from the Atlanta Birth Defects Registry could not find a statistically significant difference in NTDs in 573 multivitamin supplemented women and 546 controls.[69] This study might have been limited by recall bias. In addition, the investigators were not able to identify all of the infants; they only identified recurrent cases.

Perhaps of the most definitive research addressing the benefits of folic acid supplementation in decreasing the risks of NTDs was the multicentre randomized double-blind trial instigated by the United Kingdom Medical Research Council.[70] The aim of this trial was to evaluate the efficacy of 4 mg folic acid to prevent recurrent NTD in women who had previously delivered a child affect with NTD.[70] The trial took place in seven countries and recruited 1817 women who were randomized to one of four groups: folic acid (4 mg), folic acid (4 mg) and a multivitamin, multivitamin without folic acid, or no supplementation at all. Participants were asked to commence supplementation 1 month prior to conception and through the first 12 weeks of their pregnancy. In this trial Wald and colleagues showed that women randomized to the folic acid group had a 1.0% chance of having a child with a NTD (RR = 0.28, 95% CI = 0.12–0.71).[70] On the other hand, women in the unsupplemented arm did not have a statistically significant chance of decrease in NTD (RR = 0.8, 95% CI = 0.37–1.72).[70] Overall, supplementation with folic acid resulted in decreasing the recurrence of NTD by 72% (6/593 folate supplemented versus 21/602 in control).[70]

Another prominent trial evaluating folic acid fortified multivitamin supplementation during pregnancy was a double-blinded randomized control trial where 2104 women who did not have a previous child with NTD were randomized to a 0.8 mg folic acid fortified multivitamin, while 2052 women were randomized to a multivitamin containing trace supplementation.[17] Fortification commenced at least 1 month prior to pregnancy and continued to at minimum the second missed menstrual period.[17] Twenty-eight malformations were noted in the folic acid fortified group, whereas 47 malformations were noted in the trace supplement group.[17] There were 0/2104 NTDs in the folic acid fortified group, whereas there were 6/2052 NTDs in the trace element group.[17]

In 1992, Holmes-Siedle et al. emulated Smithell's original protocol of a cohort study investigating the effect of multivitamin supplementation in women who previously delivered a child with NTD.[71] They also found that supplementation reduced the risk for recurrence.[71] A case-control study by Werler et al. of 436 cases of children with NTDs and matched with 2615 healthy controls inquired women regarding their use of folic acid during pregnancy.[72] Their results indicated that 57% and 48% of women did not supplement with folic acid in both the NTDs and control group, respectively.[72] This infers that folic acid does have a significant effect of decreasing the risk of NTD by 60% (RR = 0.4, 95% CI = 0.2–0.6).[72] Another large case-control study by Czeizel also showed that folate supplemented women had 0/2471 NTDs whereas 6/2391 with NTD in the unsupplemented group.[73]

Ulrich et al. conducted and case-control observational study from January 1983 to March 1986.[74] During this period they identified 10,629 women with folic acid supplementation, 2742 women without folic acid supplementation.[74] They found seven children with NTDs born to 8293 women who used supplementation during in their pregnancy.[74] Conversely there were no NTDs in 2742 women who did not supplement with folic acid. This result may be attributed to the fact that the majority of women participating in this study started folic acid after finding out they were pregnant. A case-control study by Berry et al. investigated folic acid supplementation between 1993 to 1995.[75] 102 children with NTDs were born to 130, 142 women supplementing with folic acid. On the other hand, 173 children with NTDs were born to 117,689 women who were not supplementing with folic acid.[75]

An Indian randomized controlled trial found that supplementation with multivitamins decreased the recurrence of NTDs by 60%.[76] The recurrence rate was 2.92% in the multivitamin group as opposed to 7.04% in the placebo group.[76] Similarly, Thompson et al. showed a 65% risk reduction in NTDs (OR = 0.35, 95% CI = 0.17–0.72) in their case-control study conducted between 1992 to 1997.[77] More recently, a cohort-controlled study Czeizel et al. found that multivitamin supplementation decreased risk of NTDs.[78] Confirming the findings from their initial cohort study, this study showed that NTDs occurred in one supplemented pregnancy, whereas it occurred in nine unsupplemented pregnancies (OR = 0.11, 95% CI = 0.01–0.91).[78]

To investigate whether the dosage of folic acid affects the rate of reduction, a case-control study conducted by the California Birth Defects Monitoring Program from June 1989 to May 1991 investigated 538 children with NTDs compared with 540 controls. Women who reported any use of folic acid had an overall lower risk of having a child with NTDs (OR = 0.60, 95% CI 0.46–0.79).[79] Women taking folic acid 0.4–0.9 mg had a further reduced risk. Women who supplemented with less than 0.4 mg did not have important reductions in risk (OR = 0.99, OR = 0.92, respectively).[79] The only available study investigating serum folate concentrations found an inverse relation between maternal cell folate and the risk of NTD.[80] In a follow-up to this study, Daly et al. showed in a case-control study that women receiving <150 μg, >400 μg of folic acid had a 6.6/1000 and 0.8/1000 chance of NTD, respectively.[81] Supplementation at different doses of 100 μg, 200 μg, and 400 μg resulted in a 22%, 41%, and 47% decreased risk in NTD, respectively.[81] Another study investigating dosing variations of folic acid corroborated this result as they noted that 100 μg, 200 μg, and 400 μg folic acid decreased NTD by 18%, 35%, and 53%, respectively.[82]

Oral Clefts

The risk of a child being born with cleft lip with or without cleft palate is 1/1000.[83,84] The chance of occurrence of cleft palate alone is 1/2500.[83,84] In fact the first studies to investigate the possibility of multivitamin's effectiveness in preventing birth defects were specifically aimed at preventing the recurrent of oral clefts with or without cleft palate.[85–87] These studies found that multivitamin supplementation resulted in a 48% decrease in oral clefts (OR = 0.52, 95% CI = 0.34–0.80).[85–88] These results were supported in an animal study by Peer et al. where they pretreated Swiss albino mice receiving cortisone treatment with vitamin B6 and folic acid or folic acid alone.[89] They noted a protective effect in supplemented mice compared to unsupplemented mice.[89] The rate of mice with oral clefts due to cortisone treatment were vitamin B6 and folic acid 3/21, folic acid 21/98 and no treatment 38/49.[89]

A retrospective study of women who gave birth to children with oral clefts found that the incidence of oral clefts in multivitamin supplementation was 3.1% whereas the incidence without supplementation was 4.8%, accounting for a 30% reduction.[90] This was also supported by a case-control study by Tolarova et al. where they reported three oral clefts in 184 multivitamin supplemented women whereas there were 77 oral clefts among 1901 unsupplemented women.[91] These results were challenged by the randomized-controlled study of Czeizel et al. where they noted that supplementation of a folate fortified multivitamin resulted in no statistically significant reduction of oral clefts.[17]

In 1995 Shaw et al. conducted a case-control study from 1987 to 1989 comparing 731 folic acid fortified multivitamin supplemented mothers to 734 controls.[79] They showed that multivitamin supplementation decreased the risk of oral cleft by 25–50%.[79] A 50% decrease in rates of cleft palate with cleft lip was observed (OR = 0.5, 95% CI = 0.36–0.68), while cleft palate without cleft lip decreased by 27% (OR = 0.73, 95% CI = 0.46–1.2).[79] Tolarova et al. conducted a prospective intervention study where they asked 221 women who had a history of a child with cleft lip with or without cleft palate to supplement with 10 mg of folic acid at least 2–3 months prior to conception and continued at least 3 months post conception.[92] This regimen resulted in decreased the recurrence of oral cleft in high-risk families by 65.4% (OR = 0.35).[92] An 82.6% decrease was noted in families who had a history of females affected by oral clefts or a history of unilateral clefts.[92]

In contrast a case-control study by Hayes et al. of the Slone Epidemiology Unit Birth Defects Study in 1996 found no significant association between folic acid supplementation and oral clefts (OR = 1.2, 95% CI = 0.7–2.0) with or without cleft palate (OR = 0.9, 95% CI = 0.5–1.7).[93] In a case-control study by Czeizel et al. observing women using 4 mg of folic acid during the periconceptional period, a significant decrease in cleft lip with or without cleft palate was detected.[94] In addition, a case-control study by Werler et al. found a 60% decrease in cleft palate (OR = 0.4, 95% CI = 0.2–0.9) and a 30% decrease in cleft palate with cleft lip (OR = 0.7, 95% CI = 0.4–1.1).[7] Moreover, a case-control study in Brazil from September 1991 to August 1992 found a statistically significant inverse association between cleft palate and intake of vitamins in the first 4 months of pregnancy (RR = 0.58).[95]

Another challenge to the proposed protective effects of folic acid for oral clefts was a cohort study by Czeizel et al. who observed no protective effect in 5488 supplemented as compared to 5821 unsupplemented women in their randomized control trial.[96] They postulated that higher doses of folic acid was required compared to the quantities found in prenatal vitamins in order to decrease the incidence of orofacial clefts.[73] Similarly, a case-control study in Maryland from 1992 to 1998) found no protective effect against cleft palate (OR = 0.70, 95% CI = 0.31–1.56) or cleft palate with or without cleft lip (OR = 0.59 CI = 0.33–1.09).[97] This may be attributable to the fact that there were a low proportion of women who supplemented prior to 3 months pregnancy.[97]

Congenital Heart Defects

Congenital heart defects (CHD) are the most prevalent major birth defects. Congenital heart defects are estimated to affect CHD 1/120 live births[98–100], and conotruncal heart defects specifically have a prevalence of 0.8/1000.[101] The randomized controlled study conducted by Czeizel et al. showed that women randomized to 0.8 mg folic acid fortified multivitamin had 50% less children with congenital heart defects compared to women in the trace group (10 vs. 20 children).[17] These differences were especially prominent as conotruncal defects and septal defects.[17] Another intervention study by Czeizel et al. shows that folic acid fortified multivitamin supplementation decreased the occurrence of CHDs by 52%.[73] This result, however, was not statistically significant (RR = 0.48, 95% CI = 0.23–1.03).[73] They later conducted a cohort study that indicated that folic-fortified multivitamin supplementation decreased CHDs (OR = 0.60, 95% CI = 0.38–0.96).[78]

The CDC conducted a population control-based study by examining births from 1968 to 1980 and found that periconceptional multivitamin supplementation was associated with a 40% decrease in risk of conotruncal cardiovascular defects.[102] A 52% decreased risk was observed for isolated conotruncal defects (RR = 0.48, 95% CI = 0.20–0.89).[102] In addition, a population-based case-control study of the California Birth Defects Monitoring Program from 1987 to 1988 found that women taking folic acid 1 month prior conception to 2 months post conception had a 35% decreased risk for conotruncal defects compared to unsupplemented mothers (OR = 0.65, 95% CI = 0.44–0.96).[103] Moreover, a case-control study by Botto in 1996 found that multivitamin supplementation decreased conotruncal heart defects by 43% (OR = 0.57, 95% CI = 0.33–1) versus unsupplemented mothers.[101] In addition, decreases in transposition of great arteries by 64% (OR = 0.36, 95% CI = 0.15–0.89); isolated conotruncal effects by 66% (OR = 0.41, 95% CI = 0.2–0.84); isolated transposition of great arteries by 66% (OR = 0.34, 95% CI = 0.13–0.93) were observed.[101] Differences were also observed in teratology of fallot; truncus arteriosus; double outlet right ventricle.[101]

More studies have supported the effectiveness of folic acid to decrease the risk of CHDs. A case-control study of the Baltimore Washington Infant Study from April 1987 to December 1989 found that women with high intakes of folate had a decreased risk for cardiac outflow tract defects.[104] An Atlanta case-control study from 1968 to 1990 noted that prenatal multivitamin supplementation decreased occurrence of heart defect (OR = 1.8, 95% CI = 1.4–2.4); tricuspid atresia (OR = 5.2); obstructive defects (OR = 2.7); transposition of great arteries (OR = 1.9); ventral septal defect (OR = 1.8) compared to unsupplemented mothers.[98] In a recent cohort-controlled study conducted by Czeizel et al. observed that women taking multivitamin supplementation had a protective effect against congenital heart defect (OR = 0.6, 95% CI = 0.38–0.96).[78] There was a prominent difference in the rate of ventricular septal defects: 5 cases were observed in the multivitamin supplemented group versus 19 in the unsupplemented group (OR = 0.26, 95% CI = 0.09–0.72).[78]

Urinary Tract Anomalies

The prevalence of genital and urinary tract anomalies is estimated to be approximately 1/135 births in the general population.[105] In their randomized control study, Czeizel et al. noted that there was a decrease in the rate of congenital urinary tract anomalies (CUTA) in women who took folic acid fortified multivitamins (two cases) as opposed to the trace multivitamin group (nine cases).[73] Supplementation with folic-fortified multivitamin resulted in a 78% reduced risk in CUTA compared to the unsupplemented (RR = 0.22, 95% CI = 0.05–0.99).[73] To further investigate the possibility of an association of supplementation and the onset of urinary tract abnormalities Li et al. conducted a retrospective case-control trial.[106] Using the Washington State Birth Defect Registry and matched 118 cases of children born with CUTA to 369 controls from January 1990 to December 1991.[106] Supplementation with folic acid-fortified multivitamin in the first trimester was associated with an 85% reduction in risk of having a child with CUTA (OR = 0.15, 95% CI = 0.05–0.43).[106] In addition, with continued supplementation through the second and third trimester, a greater decrease was observed (OR = 0.31, 95% CI = 0.09–1.02).[106] Supplementation prior to pregnancy was not associated with the reduction of CUTA.[106] The most prominent decrease was noted in hydronephrosis (OR = 0.12, 95% CI = 0.04–0.38) compared to other UTAs (OR = 0.31, 95% CI = 0.06–1.56).[106] In addition, a cohort-controlled trial conducted by Czeizel et al. in 2004, observed a reduction in stensosis/atresia of the pelvicuretic junction in women with multivitamin supplementation compared to women who were not supplemented (OR = 0.19, 95% CI = 0.04–0.86).[78] There was, however, no significant difference in UTA.[78]

Limb Defects

The prevalence rate for all types of limb deficiency in the general population is 0.69/1000.[107] In their randomized control study, Czeizel et al. noted that there was one case of limb defect in the multivitamin supplemented group whereas there were five cases in the control group.[17] The most significant study with respect to prenatal multivitamin supplementation and limb defects was a case-control study by Shaw et al. who showed that the supplementation of folic acid fortified multivitamin 1 month prior to conception to 2 months post conception was associated with a 35% decrease in limb defects (OR = 0.65, 95% CI = 0.43–0.99).[101] Daily supplementation of <0.4 mg had a slightly small risk of decrease (OR = 0.63, 95% CI = 0.40–1.0) than >0.4 mg (OR = 0.71, 95% CI = 0.44–1.2).[101]

Omphalocele

Omphalocele occurs in 1/4000–1/6000 pregnancies in the general population.[108–111] A case-control study by Botto et al. of women in Atlanta examined the incidence of omphalocele in women with and without multivitamin supplementation from 1968 to 1980.[112] They found that 73 and 3029 children with omphalocele were born to supplemented and unsupplemented women, respectively.[112] Overall, periconceptional use of multivitamin was associated with a 60% reduction in nonsyndromic omphalocele (OR = 0.4, 95% CI = 0.2–1.0).[112]

Pyloric Stenosis

In the randomized-control study conducted by Czeizel et al. two cases of hyperpyloric stenosis were observed in the folic acid-fortified multivitamin group compared to eight cases in the trace multivitamin group.[17] In contrast, a study by Correa et al. did not corroborate this protective effect.[105]

Imperforate anus

The prevalence of imperforate anus is 0.2–0.67/1000.[84,113] Myers et al. conducted a cohort study from October 1993 to September 1995.[114] They noted that folic acid supplementation resulted in a 0.16/1000 rate of imperforation, whereas unsupplemented women had a rate of 0.31/1000.[114] This implies a decrease of 50% associated with folic acid supplementation.[114]

Pediatric Brain Tumours

The incidence of childhood primary nonmalignant and malignant brain and central nervous system tumors is 0.04/1000.[115] Specifically, neuroblastomas and medulloblastoma are the most common pediatric solid tumours.[115,116] Neuroblastoma is the most common cancer in infants and the third most common form of cancer in children.[117] Medulloblastoma is a benign or malignant form of cancer that is usually located in the cerebellum.[116] Also known as a primitive neuroectodermal tumour (PNET), medulloblastomas occur in 1 of 5 brain tumours.[116]

Despite being the leading cause of childhood cancer deaths in developed countries, little is known about the etiology of these tumours.[118] A case-control study by Preston-Martin found that prenatal supplementation with multivitamins may decrease brain tumours (OR = 0.6, p = 0.12).[119] A case-control study of maternal multivitamin supplementation and the risk of primitive neuroectodermal tumors (PNET) of the brain in children was conducted from 1986 to 1989 showing protective trends with folate intake (OR = 0.38; p = 0.005).[120] In addition, multivitamin use during the first 6 weeks of pregnancy was associated with decreased risk of brain tumours (OR = 0.56; P = 0.02).[120] Another case-control study by this group also suggested a decreased risk of astrocytoma.[118] All the above findings were reaffirmed by Preston-Martin et al. where they observed that prenatal multivitamin supplementation decreased brain tumors including PNET and astrocytoma.[121]

An international case-control study of primary pediatric brain tumors from 1976 to 1994 of 1051 cases and 1919 controls found that supplementation in the first 2 trimesters of pregnancy decreased brain tumors by (OR = 0.7, 95% CI = 0.5–0.9).[122] This reduction was furthered by supplementation in all three trimesters (OR = 0.5, 95% CI = 0.3–0.8).[122] Multivitamin supplementation one month prior to conception or while breastfeeding had no effect on the overall outcome.[122] In addition, Thorne et al. conducted a retrospective population-based study of children diagnosed with brain tumors from 1976 to 1991 in Avon, England.[123] From 1976 to 1984 there were 16 tumors identified whereas from 1985 to 1991 there were two tumors identified.[123] This corresponds to an initial of 9.6 per million to a 1.7 per million decreased incidence.[123] As periconceptional multivitamin supplementation was introduced in the 1980s there may be an association with the decline of medulloblastoma.[123] Moreover, an interventional time series analysis observed a 0.157/1000 to 0.062/1000 decrease after the introduction of folic acid fortification of flour with an adjusted incidence (RR = 0.38, 95% CI = 0.23–0.62).[124]

Genetics and Maternal Disease

Genetic polymorphisms may be responsible for variability in folate available to the fetus.[125] The absorption of folate can be hindered by the mutation of 677 C $\rightarrow$ T substitution in the 5,10-methylenetetrahydrofolate reductase (MTHFR) gene. This mutation results in a thermolabile variant C677T with decreased enzyme specific activity and elevated homocysteine concentrations.[126–129] The frequency of homozygous polymorphism varies in different ethnic groups from 5 to 25%.[128,130–134] In Caucasian and Asian populations TT homozygotes are present at approximately 12%.[135] African Americans have a very low prevalence,[135] whereas Hispanics of Mexican heritage have a high prevalence.[135,136] The homozygousity of the C677T allele variant for MTHFR doubles the risk associated with having an infant with spina bifida.[137] In addition, the MTHFR polymorphism involving a A → C substitution at base pair 1298 results in a benign allele unless it is present in combination with C677T.[138] With both polymorphisms present, the specific activity of MTHFR is lower by two-thirds.[138] MTHFR polymorphisms may also contribute to an increased incidence of Down syndrome.[139–142] Other genetic alternations may result in the alteration of folate absorption. Lammier et al. conducted a case-control study of comparing 421 cases of children with oral clefts and 299 controls. They found that despite taking vitamins, variations of acetyl-N-transferase 1(NAT-1) NAT1095 resulted in a twofold increased risk of oral clefts.[143]

Celiac disease results in the malabsorption of folic acid.[144] This disease causes an immune inflammatory response when the gastrointestinal tract is exposed to gluten. Since gluten is commonly found in bread, women may abstain from eating it to prevent triggering this response. Hence, they do not benefit from folic acid fortified flour, which was introduced to decrease the risk of having a newborn with a congenital malformation.

Folate Antagonists

There are two types of folic acid antagonists: dihydrofolate reductase inhibitors and folate antagonists that affect the absorption metabolism or degradation or folate. Dihydrofolate reductase inhibitors include agents such as methotrexate (amethopterin), aminopterin, sulfasalazine, pyrimethamine, triamterene, trimethoprim, and 5-flurouracil. Folate antagonists inhibit dihydrofolate reductase, an essential step in reducing folic acid to tetrahydrofolic acid, therefore preventing the synthesis of DNA and cell reproduction.[145] The second group of folate antagonists includes carbamazepine, phenytoin, primidone, phenobarbital, and valproic acid. Robert et al. first described the association of NTDs with valproic acid.[146] Myelomeningocele and anencephaly are the most common NTD associated with antiepileptic drug exposure.[145] A case-control study of women using folic acid antagonists in early pregnancy suggested an increased risk in NTDs, cardiovascular defects, oral clefts, and urinary tract defects.[147]

Recommendations

The above evidence suggests the benefit of folic acid supplementation in reducing the risk of NTD, oral clefts, congenital heart defects, and other congenital malformations. Since folic acid is not endogenously synthesized, it must be obtained from external sources such as dark-green leafy vegetables; other vegetables including asparagus, brussel sprouts, and cauliflower; fruits including citrus fruits, banana, and strawberries; beans; some forms of meat; diary; whole grains and breakfast cereals.

With respect to potential adverse events arising to folic acid supplementation, there has been one report of hypersensitivity.[150] Folic acid may interfere with zinc homeostasis or interact with other drugs rendering them less effective.[148,149] In addition, folic acid may mask colbalmin vitamin B12 deficiency.[151] By masking this deficiency it may increase the neurological complications associated with this deficiency.[15]

Given the prevailing evidence suggesting the importance of folate in the prevention of birth defects, the U.S. Public Health Service and Institute of Medicine placed separate recommendations that women of childbearing potential should fortify their diet with 400 μg of folic acid.[152,153] This recommendation is identical to that of Health Canada and the European Union.[154,155] In addition the FDA mandated the fortification of folic acid in staple foods in January 1998.[156] This has resulted in the addition of 100 μg of folic acid to grains.[156]

Since as many as 50% pregnancy are unplanned[157] and the neural tube closes around 23–28 days post conception, many women will have missed the opportunity for supplementation because they are unaware that they are pregnant. Therefore, unless they are actively planning pregnancy, this crucial period for supplementation may be missed. As such the recommended dietary allowance of folic acid is 400 μg. Women who consume folate antagonists, have folate deficiencies, or have had a previous child with a NTD are recommended to ingest higher doses of folic acid (5 mg).[158]

REFERENCES

1. Hoffbrand AV, Weir DG. The history of folic acid. *Br J Haematol.* 2001;113(3):579–589.
2. Wills L, Mehta MM. Studies in "pernicious anaemia" of pregnancy. I. Preliminary report. *Indian J Med Res.* 1930;17:777–792.
3. Wills L. Treatment of "pernicious anaemia of pregnancy" and "tropical anaemia" with special reference to yeast extract as curative agent. *BMJ.* 1931;1:1059–1064.
4. Mitchell HK, Snell EE, Williams RJ. The concentration of "folic acid." *J Am Chem Soc.* 1941;63:2284.
5. Moore CV, Bierbaum OS, Welch AD, et al. The activity of synthetic Lactobacillus carei factor (folic acid) as an antipernicious anemia substance. I. Observations on four patients, two with Addisonian perivirus anemias, one with nontropical sprue and one with pernicious anemia of pregnancy. *J Lab Clin Med.* 1945;30: 1056–1069.
6. Vilter RW, Spies TD, Koch MV. Further studies on folic acid in the treatment of macrocytic anemia. *5th Medical Journal (Nashville).* 1945;38:781–785.
7. Herbert V, Zalusky R. Interrelation of vitamin B12 and folic acid metabolism: folic acid clearance studies. *J Clin Invest.* 1962; 41:1263–1276.
8. Metz J, Stevens K, Krawitz S, et al. The plasma clearance of injected doses of folic acid as an index of folic acid deficiency. *J Clin Pathol.* 1961;14:622–625.
9. Stokstad EL. Early work with folic acid. *Fed Proc.* 1979; 38(13):2696–2698.
10. Locksmith GJ, Duff P. Preventing neural tube defects: the importance of periconceptional folic acid supplements. *Obstet Gynecol.* 1998;91(6):1027–1034.
11. Hall J, Solehdin F. Folic acid for the prevention of congenital anomalies. *Eur J Pediatr.* 1998;157(6):445–450.
12. Van Dyke DC, Stumbo PJ, Mary JB, et al. Folic acid and prevention of birth defects. *Dev Med Child Neurol.* 2002;44(6):426–9.
13. Czeizel AE. Reduction of urinary tract and cardiovascular defects by periconceptional multivitamin supplementation. *Am J Med Genet.* 1996;62:179–183.
14. Stover PJ. Physiology of folate and vitamin B12 in health and disease. *Nutr Rev.* 2004;62(6 Pt 2):S3–12.
15. Bailey LB. Folate and vitamin B12 recommended intakes and status in the United States. *Nutr Rev.* 2004;62(6 Pt 2):S14–20.
16. Suh JR, Herbig AK, Stover PJ. New perspectives on folate catabolism. *Annu Rev Nutr.* 2001;21:255–282.

17. Czeizel AE, Dudas I. Prevention of the first occurrence of neural-tube defects by periconceptional vitamin supplementation. *N Engl J Med.* 1992;327:1832–1835.
18. Gregory JF III. The bioavailability of folate. In: Bailey LB, editor. Folate in Health and Disease. New York: Marcel Dekker Inc, 1995: 195–236.
19. Rivey MP, Schottelius DD, Berg MJ. Phenytoin—folic acid: a review. *Drug Intell Clin Pharm.* 1984;18:292–301.
20. Malatack JJ, Moran MM, Moughan B. Isolated congenital malabsorption of folic acid in a male infant: insights into treatment and mechanisms of defects. *Pediatrics.* 1999;104:1133–1137.
21. Gregory JF III. Case study: folate bioavailability. *J Nutr.* 2001; 131:1376s–1382s.
22. Wagner C. Biochemical role of folate in cellular metabolism. In: Bailey LB, editor. Folate in Health and Disease. New York: Marcel Dekker Inc, 1995:23–42.
23. Butterworth CE Jr, Bendich A. Folic acid and the prevention of birth defects. *Annu Rev Nutr.* 1996;16:73–97.
24. Kruschwitz HL, McDonald D, Cossins EA, et al. 5-formyltetrahydropteroylpolyglutamates are the major folate derivatives in Neurospora crassa conidiospores. *J Biol Chem.* 1994;269: 28757–28763.
25. Clarke S, Banfield K. S-adenosylmethionine-dependent methyltransferases. In: Carmel R, Jacobson DW, editors. Homocysteine in Health and Disease. Cambridge: Cambridge Press, 2001:63–78.
26. Rosenblatt DS. Inherited disorders of folate transport and metabolism. In: Scriver CR, Beaudet AL, Sly WS, Valle D, editors. The Metabolic and Molecular Basis of Inherited Disease, seventh ed. New York: McGraw-Hill, 1995:3111–3149.
27. Ramakrishnan U. Micronutrients and pregnancy outcome: a review of the literature. *Nutr Res.* 1999;19(1):103–59.
28. Mudd SH. Vascular disease and homocysteine metabolism. In: Smith U, Eriksson S, Lindgarde F, editors. Genetic susceptibility to environmental factors: a challenge for public intervention. Stockholm: Almqvist & Wiksell, 1988:11–24.
29. Zhao R, Russell RG, Wang Y, et al. Rescue of embryonic lethality in reduced folate carrier-deficient mice by maternal folic acid supplementation reveals early neonatal failure of hematopoietic organs. *J Biol Chem.* 2001;30:276(13):10224–10228.
30. Hibbard BM. Folates and the fetus. *S Afr Med J.* 1975; 49(30):1223–1226.
31. Heath CW. Cytogenic observations in vitamin B12 and folate deficiency. *Blood.* 1966;27:800–15.
32. Sutherland GR, Ledbetter DH. Report of the committee on cytogenic markers. *Cytogenet Cell Genet.* 1989;51:452–8.
33. Wainfan E, Poirier LA. Methyl groups in carcinogenesis: effects on DNA methylation and gene expression. *Cancer Res.* 1992; 52(7S):2071–7.
34. Christman JK, Sheikhnejad G, Dizik M, et al. Reversibility of changes in nucleic acid methylation and gene expression induced in rat liver by severe dietary methyl deficiency. *Carcinogenesis.* 1993; 14:551–7.
35. Pogribny IP, Basnakian AG, Miller BJ, et al. Breaks in genomic DNA and within the p53 gene are associated with hypomethylation in livers of folate/methyl-deficient rats. *Cancer Res.* 1995;55:1894–1901.
36. Pogribny IP, Miller BJ, James SJ. Alternations in hepatic p53 gene methylation patterns during tumor progression with folate/methyl deficiency in the rat. *Cancer Lett.* 1997;115:31–38.
37. Pogribny IP, Muskhelishvili L, Miller BJ, et al. Presence and consequence of uracil in preneoplastic DNA from folate/methyl-deficient rats. *Carcinogenesis.* 1997;18:2071–6.
38. James SJ, Pogribna M, Pogribny IP, et al. Abnormal folate metabolism and mutation in the methylenetetrahydrofolate reductase gene may be maternal risk factors for Down syndrome. *J Clin Nutr.* 1999; 70:495–501.
39. De Franchis R, Sebastio G, Mandato C, et al. Spina bifida, 677CÆT mutation, and role of folate. *Lancet.* 1995;346:1703.
40. Center for Disease Prevention, Infant mortality-United States. *JAMA.* 1996;275:980.
41. Canadian Perinatal Surveillance System, Infant Mortality 2002; http://www.phac-aspc.gc.ca/rhs-ssg/factshts/mort_e.html. Accessed May 1, 2005.
42. Christianson RE, Berg BJ van den, Milkovich L, et al. Incidence of congenital anomalies among white and black lives births with long-term follow-up. *Am J Public Health.* 1981;71:1333–1341.
43. Marden PM, Smith DW, McDonald MJ. Congenital anomalies in the newborn infant, including minor variations. A study of 4,412 babies by surface examination for anomalies and buccal smear for sex chromatin. *J Pediatr.* 1964;64:357–371.
44. Scott JM, Weir DG, Molloy WA, et al. Folic acid metabolism and mechanisms of neural tube defects. In Bock, G. and Marsh, J. editors, Neural Tube Defects. Ciba Foundation Symposium, Vol. 181. John Wiley & Sons, Chichester, 1994:180–191.
45. Fleming A. The role of folate in the prevention of neural tube defects: human and animal studies. Nutr Rev 2001;59(8 Pt 2):S13–20.
46. Center for Disease Prevention, Spina bifida and anencephaly before and after folic acid mandate—United States, 1995–1996 and 1999–2000. MMWR 2004;53:362–365.
47. Health Canada, Congenital anomalies in Canada—A Perinatal Health Report, 2002. Ottawa: Minister of Public Works and Government Services Canada, 2002, page 8.
48. Shibuya K, Murray CJL. Congenital anomalies. In: Murray CJL, Lopez AD, editors. Boston: Harvard University Press, 1998: 455–512.
49. Cragan JD, Roberts HE, Edmonds LD, et al. Surveillance for anencephaly and spina bifida and the impact of prenatal diagnosis—United States, 1985–1994. *Morb Mortal Wkly Rep.* 1995;44(SS-4):1–13.
50. Elwood JH. Major central nervous system malformations notified in Northern Ireland, 1969–1973. *Dev Med Child Neurol.* 1976; 18(4):512–520.
51. Frecker M, Fraser FC. Epidemiological studies of neural tube defects in Newfoundland. *Teratology.* 1987;36:355–361.
52. Center for Disease Prevention, Congenital malformations surveillance report January–December 1979–1980.
53. Greenberg F, James LM, Oakley GP Jr. Estimates of birth prevalence rates of spina bifida in the United States from computer-generated maps. *Am J Obst Gynecol.* 1983;145:570–573.
54. Baird PA. Neural tube defects in the Sikhs. *Am J Med Genet.* 1983; 16(1):49–56.
55. Lary JM, Edmonds LD. Prevalence of spina bifida at birth—United States, 1983–1990: a comparison of two surveillance systems. *MMWR CDC Surveill Summ.* 1996;45(2):15–26.
56. Shaw GM, Jensvold NG, Wasserman CR, et al. Epidemiologic characteristics of phenotypically distinct neural tube defects among 0.7 million California births, 1983–1987. *Teratology.* 1994;49(2):143–149.
57. Smithells RW. Incidence of congenital abnormalities in Liverpool, 1960–64. *Br J Prev Soc Med.* 1968;22(1):36–37.
58. Smithells RW, Sheppard S, Schorah CJ. Vitamin deficiencies and neural tube defects. *Arch Dis Child.* 1976;51(12):944–950.
59. Smithells RW, Sheppard S, Schorah CJ, et al. Possible prevention of neural-tube defects by periconceptional vitamin supplementation. *Lancet.* 1980;1(8164):339–340.
60. Smithells RW, Sheppard S, Schorah CJ, et al. Vitamin supplementation and neural tube defects. *Lancet.* 1981;2(8260–61):1425.
61. Smithells RW, Nevin NC, Seller MJ, et al. Further experience of vitamin supplementation for prevention of neural tube defect recurrences. *Lancet.* 1983;1(8332):1027–1031.
62. Laurence KM, James N, Miller M, et al. Increased risk of recurrence of neural tube defects to mothers on a poor diet and possible benefits of dietary counseling. *BMJ.* 1980;281:1542.
63. Laurence KM, James N, Miller MH, et al. Double-blind randomised controlled trial of folate treatment before conception to prevent recurrence of neural-tube defects. *Br Med J.* (Clin Res Ed) 1981; 282(6275):1509–1511.

64. Sheppard S, Nevin NC, Seller MJ, et al. Neural tube defect recurrence after "partial" vitamin supplementation. *J Med Genet.* 1989; 26(5):326–329.
65. Mulinare J, Cordero JF, Erickson JD, et al. Periconceptional use of multivitamins and the occurrence of neural tube defects. *JAMA.* 1988;260:3141–3145.
66. Bower C, Stanley FJ. Dietary folate as a risk factor for neural-tube defects: evidence from a case-control study in Western Australia. *Med J Aust.* 1989;150(11):613–619.
67. Milunsky A, Jick H, Jick SS, et al. Multivitamin/folic acid supplementation in early pregnancy reduces the prevalence of neural tube defects. *JAMA.* 1989;262(20):2847–2852.
68. Vergel RG, Sanchez LR, Heredero BL, et al. Primary prevention of neural tube defects with folic acid supplementation: Cuban experience. *Prenat Diagn.* 1990;10(3):149–152.
69. Mills JL, Rhoads GG, Simpson JL, et al. The absence of a relation between the periconceptional use of vitamins and neural-tube defects. National Institute of Child Health and Human Development Neural Tube Defects Study Group. *N Engl J Med.* 1989;321(7):430–435.
70. Prevention of neural tube defects: results of the Medical Research Council Vitamin Study. MRC Vitamin Study Research Group. *Lancet.* 1991;338(8760):131–137.
71. Holmes-Siedle M, Dennis J, Lindenbaum RH, et al. Long term effects of periconceptional multivitamin supplements for prevention of neural tube defects: a seven to 10 year follow up. *Arch Dis Child.* 1992;67(12):1436–1441.
72. Werler MM, Hayes C, Louik C, et al. Multivitamin supplementation and risk of birth defects. *Am J Epidemiol.* 1999;150(7):675–682.
73. Czeizel AE, Dudas I, Metneki J. Pregnancy outcomes in a randomised controlled trial of periconceptional multivitamin supplementation. Final report. *Arch Gynecol Obstet.* 1994;255(3):131–139.
74. Ulrich M, Kristoffersen K, Rolschau J, et al. The influence of folic acid supplement on the outcome of pregnancies in the county of Funen in Denmark. Part III. Congenital anomalies. An observational study. *Eur J Obstet Gynecol Reprod Biol.* 1999;87(2):115–118.
75. Berry RJ, Li Z, Erickson JD, et al. Prevention of neural-tube defects with folic acid in China. China-U.S. Collaborative Project for Neural Tube Defect Prevention. *N Engl J Med.* 1999;341(20):1485–1490.
76. Central Technical Co-ordinating Unit, ICMRCentral Technical Co-ordinating Unit, ICMR. Multicentric study of efficacy of periconceptional folic acid containing vitamin supplementation in prevention of open neural tube defects from India. *Indian J Med Res.* 2000; 112:206–211.
77. Thompson SJ, Torres ME, Stevenson RE, et al. Periconceptional multivitamin folic acid use, dietary folate, total folate and risk of neural tube defects in South Carolina. *Ann Epidemiol.* 2003; 13(6):412–418.
78. Czeizel AE, Dobo M, Vargha P. Hungarian cohort-controlled trial of periconceptional multivitamin supplementation shows a reduction in certain congenital abnormalities. *Birth Defects Res A Clin Mol Teratol.* 2004;70(11):853–861.
79. Shaw GM, Lammer EJ, Wasserman CR, et al. Risks of orofacial clefts in children born to women using multivitamins containing folic acid periconceptionally. *Lancet.* 1995;346(8972):393–396.
80. Daly LE, Kirke PM, Molloy A, et al. Folate levels and neural tube defects, implications for prevention. *JAMA.* 1995;274:1696–1702.
81. Daly S, Mills JL, Molloy AM, et al. Minimum effective dose of folic acid for food fortification to prevent neural-tube defects. *Lancet.* 1997;350:1666–1669.
82. Wald NJ, Law M, Jordan R. Folic acid food fortification to prevent neural tube defects. *Lancet.* 1998;351(9105):834.
83. Itikala PR, Watkins ML, Mulinare J, et al. Maternal multivitamin use and orofacial clefts in offspring. *Teratology.* 2001;63(2):79–86.
84. Moore KL, Persaud TV. The developing human: clinically oriented embryology. Philadelphia, PA: WB Saunders Company, 1998.
85. Conway H. Effect of supplemental vitamin therapy on the limitation of incidence of cleft lip and cleft palate in humans. *Plast Reconstr Surg.* 1958;22(5):450–453.
86. Douglas B. The role of environmental factors in the etiology of so-called congenital malformations. I. Deductions from the presence of cleft lip and palate in one of identical twins, from embryology and from animal experiments. *Plast Reconstr Surg.* 1958;22(2):94–108.
87. Peer LA, Gordon HW, Bernhard WG. Effect of vitamins on human teratology. *Plast Reconstr Surg.* 1964;34:358–362.
88. Douglas B. The role of environmental factors in the etiology of so-called congenital malformations. II. Approaches in humans; study of various extragenital factors; theory of compensatory nutrients, development of regime for first trimester. *Plast Reconstr Surg.* 1958; 22(3):214–229.
89. Peer LA, Bryan WH, Strean LP, et al. Induction of cleft palate in mice by cortisone and its reduction by vitamins. *J Int Coll Surg.* 1958;30(2):249–254.
90. Briggs RM. Vitamin supplementation as a possible factor in the incidence of cleft lip/palate deformities in humans. *Clin Plast Surg.* 1976;3(4):647–652.
91. Tolarova M. Orofacial clefts in Czechoslovakia. Incidence, genetics and prevention of cleft lip and palate over a 19-year period. *Scand J Plast Reconstr Surg Hand Surg.* 1987;21(1):19–25.
92. Tolarova M, Harris J. Reduced recurrence of orofacial clefts after periconceptional supplementation with high-dose folic acid and multivitamins. *Teratology.* 1995;51(2):71–78.
93. Hayes C, Werler MM, Willett WC, et al. Case-control study of periconceptional folic acid supplementation and oral clefts. *Am J Epidemiol.* 1996;143(12):1229–1234.
94. Czeizel AE. Folic acid and prevention of birth defects. *JAMA.* 1996; 275(21):1635–1636.
95. Loffredo CA. Epidemiology of cardiovascular malformations: prevalence and risk factors. *Am J Med Genet.* 2000;97(4):319–325.
96. Czeizel AE, Timar L, Sarkozi A. Dose-dependent effect of folic acid on the prevention of orofacial clefts. *Pediatrics.* 1999;104(6):e66.
97. Beaty TH, Wang H, Hetmanski JB, et al. A case-control study of nonsyndromic oral clefts in Maryland. *Ann Epidemiol.* 2001; 11(6):434–442.
98. Botto LD, Mulinare J, Erickson JD. Occurrence of congenital heart defects in relation to maternal mulitivitamin use. *Am J Epidemiol.* 2000;151:878–884.
99. Lin AE, Herring AH, Amstutz KS, et al. Cardiovascular malformations: changes in prevalence and birth status, 1972–1990. *Am J Med Genet.* 1999;84(2):102–110.
100. Johnson KC, Rouleau J. Temporal trends in Canadian birth defects birth prevalences, 1979–1993. *Can J Public Health.* 1997;88: 169–176.
101. Botto LD, Khoury MJ, Mulinare J, Erickson JD. Periconceptional multivitamin use and the occurrence of conotruncal heart defects: results from a population-based, case-control study. *Pediatrics.* 1996;98(5):911–917.
102. Botto LD, Khoury MJ, Mulinare J. Periconceptional use of vitamins and the prevention of conotruncal heart defects: evidence from a population-based case-control study. *4th Ann Epidemic Intell Serv Conf.* 1995;56.
103. Shaw GM, O'Malley CD, Wasserman CR, et al. Maternal periconceptional use of multivitamins and reduced risk for conotruncal heart defects and limb deficiencies among offspring. *Am J Med Genet.* 1995;59(4):536–545.
104. Scanlon KS, Ferencz C, Loffredo CA, et al. Preconceptional folate intake and malformations of the cardiac outflow tract. Baltimore-Washington Infant Study Group. *Epidemiology.* 1998;9:95–98.
105. Correa-Villasenor A, Cragan J, Kucik J, et al. The Metropolitan Atlanta Congenital Defects Program: 35 years of birth defects surveillance at the Centers for Disease Control and Prevention. *Birth Defects Res A Clin Mol Teratol.* 2003;67(9):617–624.
106. Li DK, Daling JR, Mueller BA, et al. Periconceptional multivitamin use in relation to the risk of congenital urinary tract anomalies. *Epidemiology.* 1995;6(3):212–218.
107. McGuirk CK, Westgate MN, Holmes LB. Limb Deficiencies in Newborn Infants. *Pediatrics.* 2001;108(4):e64.

108. Calzolari E, Volpato S, Bianchi F, et al. Omphalocele and gastroschisis: a collaborative study of five Italian congenital malformation registries. *Teratology.* 1993;47(1):47–55.
109. Calzolari E, Bianchi F, Dolk H, et al. Omphalocele and gastroschisis in Europe: a survey of 3 million births 1980–1990. EUROCAT Working Group. *Am J Med Genet.* 1995;58(2):187–194.
110. Calzolari E, Bianchi F, Dolk H, et al. Are omphalocele and neural tube defects related congenital anomalies?: Data from 21 registries in Europe (EUROCAT). *Am J Med Genet.* 1997;72(1):79–84.
111. Forrester MB, Merz RD. Epidemiology of abdominal wall defects, Hawaii, 1986–1997. *Teratology.* 1999;60(3):117–123.
112. Botto LD, Mulinare J, Erickson JD. Occurrence of omphalocele in relation to maternal multivitamin use: a population-based study. *Pediatrics.* 2002;109(5):904–908.
113. Spouge D, Baird PA. Imperforate anus in 700,000 consecutive liveborn infants. *Am J Med Genet.* 1986;2S:151–161.
114. Myers MF, Li S, Correa-Villasenor A, et al. China-US Collaborative Project for Neural Tube Defect Prevention. Folic acid supplementation and risk for imperforate anus in China. *Am J Epidemiol.* 2001; 154(11):1051–1056.
115. Central Brain Tumor Registry of the United States, Primary brain tumours in the United States Statistical Report, 1997–2001. http://www.cbtrus.org/reports//2004–2005/2005report.pdf. Accessed May 1, 2005.
116. National Cancer Institute, General information about childhood medulloblastoma. http://www.cancer.gov/cancerinfo/pdq/treatment/childmedulloblastoma/Keypoint1. Accessed May 1, 2005.
117. American Cancer Society, What are key statistics about neuroblastoma?http://www.cancer.org/docroot/cri/content/cri_2_4_1x_what_are_the_ key_statistics_for_neuroblastoma_31.asp. Accessed May 1, 2005.
118. Bunin GR, Kuijten RR, Boesel CP, et al. Maternal diet and risk of astrocytic glioma in children: a report from the Childrens Cancer Group (United States and Canada). *Cancer Causes Control.* 1994; 5(2):177–187.
119. Preston-Martin S, Yu MC, Benton B, et al. N-Nitroso compounds and childhood brain tumors: a case-control study. *Cancer Res.* 1982; 42(12):5240–5245.
120. Bunin GR, Kuijten RR, Buckley JD, et al. Relation between maternal diet and subsequent primitive neuroectodermal brain tumors in young children. *N Engl J Med.* 1993;329(8):536–541.
121. Preston-Martin S, Pogoda JM, Mueller BA, et al. Maternal consumption of cured meats and vitamins in relation to pediatric brain tumors. *Cancer Epidemiol Biomarkers Prev.* 1996;5(8):599–605.
122. Preston-Martin S, Pogoda JM, Mueller BA, et al. Prenatal vitamin supplementation and risk of childhood brain tumors. *Int J Cancer.* 1998;11S:17–22.
123. Thorne RN, Pearson AD, Nicoll JA, et al. Decline in incidence of medulloblastoma in children. *Cancer.* 1994;74(12):3240–3244.
124. French AE, Grant R, Weitzman S, et al. Folic acid food fortification is associated with a decline in neuroblastoma. *Clin Pharmacol Ther.* 2003;74(3):288–294.
125. Molloy AM, Daly S, Mills JL, et al. Thermolabile varient of 5,10-methylenetetrahydrofolate reductase associated with low red cell folates: implications for folate intake recommendations. *Lancet.* 1997;1591–1593.
126. Motulsky AG. Nutritional ecogenetics: homocysteine-related arteriosclerotic vascular disease, neural tube defects, and folic acid. *Am J Hum Genet.* 1996;58(1):17–20.
127. Jacques PF, Bostom AG, Williams RR, et al. Relation between folate status, a common mutation in methylenetetrahydrofolate reductase, and plasma homocysteine concentrations. *Circulation.* 1996;93:7–9.
128. van der Put NM, Steegers-Theunissen RP, Frosst P, et al. Mutated methylenetetrahydrofolate reductase as a risk factor for spina bifida. *Lancet.* 1995;346(8982):1070–1071.
129. Engbersen AM, Franken DG, Boers GH, et al. Thermolabile 5,10-methylenetetrahydrofolate reductase as a cause of mild hyperhomocysteinemia. *Am J Hum Genet.* 1995;56(1):142–150.
130. Whitehead AS, Gallagher P, Mills JL, et al. A genetic defect in 5,10 methylenetetrahydrofolate reductase in neural tube defects. *QJM.* 1995;88(11):763–766.
131. Ou CY, Stevenson RE, Brown VK, et al. 5,10 Methylenetetrahydrofolate reductase genetic polymorphism as a risk factor for neural tube defects. *Am J Med Genet.* 1996;63(4):610–614.
132. Frosst P, Blom HJ, Milos R, et al. A candidate genetic risk factor for vascular disease: a common mutation in methylenetetrahydrofolate reductase. *Nat Genet.* 1995;10(1):111–113.
133. van der Put NM, Eskes TK, Blom HJ. Is the common 677C → T mutation in the methylenetetrahydrofolate reductase gene a risk factor for neural tube defects? A meta-analysis. *QJM.* 1997; 90(2):111–115.
134. van der Put NM, van den Heuvel LP, Steegers-Theunissen RP, et al. Decreased methylene tetrahydrofolate reductase activity due to the 677C → T mutation in families with spina bifida offspring. *J Mol Med.* 1996;74(11):691–694.
135. Botto LD, Yang Q. 5,10-Methylenetetrahydrofolate reductase gene variants and congenital anomalies: a HuGE review. *Am J Epidemiol.* 2000;151(9):862–877.
136. Barber R, Shalat S, Hendricks K, et al. Investigation of folate pathway gene polymorphisms and the incidence of neural tube defects in a Texas hispanic population. *Mol Genet Metab.* 2000;70(1):45–52.
137. Botto LD, Moore CA, Khoury MJ, et al. Neural-tube defects. *N Engl J Med.* 1999;341:1509–1519.
138. Chango A, Boisson F, Barbe F, et al. The effect of 677C → T and 1298A → C mutations on plasma homocysteine and 5,10-methylenetetrahydrofolate reductase activity in healthy subjects. *Br J Nutr.* 2000;83(6):593–596.
139. Barkai G, Arbuzova S, Berkenstadt M, et al. Frequency of Down's syndrome and neural-tube defects in the same family. *Lancet.* 2003; 361(9366):1331–1335.
140. Al-Gazali LI, Padmanabhan R, Melnyk S, et al. Abnormal folate metabolism and genetic polymorphism of the folate pathway in a child with Down syndrome and neural tube defect. *Am J Med Genet.* 2001;103(2):128–132.
141. Hobbs CA, Sherman SL, Yi P, et al. Polymorphisms in genes involved in folate metabolism as maternal risk factors for Down syndrome. *Am J Hum Genet.* 2000;67(3):623–630.
142. James SJ, Pogribna M, Pogribny IP, et al. Abnormal folate metabolism and mutation in the methylenetetrahydrofolate reductase gene may be maternal risk factors for Down syndrome. *Am J Clin Nutr.* 1999;70(4):495–501.
143. Lammer EJ, Shaw GM, Iovannisci DM, et al. Periconceptional multivitamin intake during early pregnancy, genetic variation of acetyl-N-transferase 1 (NAT1), and risk for orofacial clefts. *Birth Defects Res A Clin Mol Teratol.* 2004;70(11):846–852.
144. Ciacci C, Cirillo M, Auriemma G, et al. Celiac disease and pregnancy outcome. *Am J Gastroenterol.* 1996;91(4):718–722.
145. Lloyd ME, Carr M, McElhatton P, et al. The effects of methotrexate on pregnancy, fertility and lactation. *QJM.* 1999;Oct;92(10):551–563.
146. Robert E, Guibaud P. Maternal valproic acid and congenital neural tube defects. *Lancet.* 1982;2(8304):937.
147. Hernandez-Diaz S, Werler MM, Walker AM, et al. Folic acid antagonists during pregnancy and the risk of birth defects. *N Engl J Med.* 2000;343(22):1608–1614.
148. Hardman JG, Limbird LE, Molinoff PB, et al. Goodman & Gilman's The Pharmacological Basis of Therapeutics, 10th Edition, New York: McGraw-Hill, 2001:1519–1538.
149. Alhadeff L, Gualtiers T, Lipton M. The toxic effects of water soluble vitamins. *Nutr Rev.* 1984;42:33–40.
150. Mitchell DC, Vilter RW, Vilter CF. Hypersensivity to folic acid. *Ann Intern Med.* 1949;31:1102–1105.
151. Campbell NR. How safe are folic acid supplements? *Arch Intern Med.* 1996;156:1638–1644.
152. Centers for Disease Control and Prevention. Recommendations for the use of folic acid to reduce the number of cases of spina bifida and other neural tube defects. *MMWR Recomm Rep.* 1992;41(RR-14):1–7.

153. Institute of Medicine. Food and Nutrition Board. Dietary Reference Intakes: Thiamin, riboflavin, niacin, vitamin B6, folate, vitamin B12, pantothenic acid, biotin, and choline. National Academy Press. Washington, DC, 1998.
154. Government of Canada, Folic acid accessed http://www.hc-sc.gc.ca/hp-gs/know-savoir/folic-folique_e.html. Accessed May 1, 2005.
155. European Union, Country-Specific Chapters http://europa.eu.int/comm/health/ph_projects/2001/rare_diseases/fp_raredis_2001_a2_01_en.pdf Accssed May 1, 2005.
156. Food and Drug Administration. Food Additives Permitted for Direct Addition to Food for Human Consumption; Folic Acid (Folacin). *Federal Register.* 1996;61(44):8781–8797. http://www.cfsan.fda.gov/~lrd/fr96305c.html.
157. Forrest JD. Epidemiology of unintended pregnancy and contraceptive use. *Am J Obstet Gynecol.* 1994;170(5 Pt 2):1485–1489.
158. Crawford P, Appleton R, Betts T, et al. Best practice guidelines for the management of women with epilepsy. The Women with Epilepsy Guidelines Development Group. *Seizure.* 1999;8(4):201–217.

CHAPTER 21

TERATOGEN INFORMATION SERVICES AROUND THE WORLD

Antonio Addis, Myla E. Moretti, and Lavínia Schüler-Faccini

INTRODUCTION

The worldwide publicity of the thalidomide disaster revolutionized the way pharmacotherapy is utilized during pregnancy. Although many drugs and chemicals and a multitude of environmental factors were accused of being human teratogens, to date only a very limited group of agents have been conclusively associated with an increased of risk of congenital malformations.[1] Nevertheless, in the subsequent decades increasing numbers of pregnant women and their health-care providers have sought out advice and information on the fetal safety or risk of drugs, chemicals, and radiation.

Several factors can account for the requests for information on exposures during pregnancy, namely:

- It is estimated that about half the pregnancies in North America are unplanned[2,3] and so, numerous pregnant women expose their fetuses to substances taken for a variety of indications before they actually know about their pregnancy status.
- The use of drugs during pregnancy is not a rare event. International surveys have shown that up to 85% of pregnant women are exposed to an average of 2.5 medications during the gestational period.[4,5]
- For both ethical and methodological reasons, pregnant women are usually not included in pre-marketing drug investigations. Consequently, most drugs cannot be labeled for use during pregnancy and as a result, it is not unusual to find statements such as, "Safe use in pregnancy has not been established. Therefore, it should not be administered to women of child-bearing potential unless the expected benefits to the patients markedly outweigh the possible hazards to the fetus" within the product inserts or sources such as the Physicians Desk Reference and the Canadian Compendium of Pharmaceuticals and Specialties.[6]
- Because pharmacotherapy in pregnancy has become an orphan of research, human data in this area are scarce. Much of the information is based on animal, anecdotal or retrospective reports.
- The movement towards an "information age" has led patients to seek out more health information, and although their health care providers may encourage them to do so, the internet and mass media in general is fraught with inaccuracies and a lack of evidence based information.

In light of these issues, many drug information services over the past few decades found the need to become more oriented towards the evaluation of drugs as it relates to teratogenic risk. This has evolved into the creation or development of what is today known as the Teratology Information Service (TIS).

TIS have been implemented in various states, provinces and countries around the world. As of 2005, several dozen TIS were operational in North America, Europe, and elsewhere.[7] By describing their function and role, this chapter reviews the structure and activities of the TIS around the world and their unique potential to advance our knowledge on human teratogenesis.

STRUCTURE AND FUNCTION OF TERATOGEN INFORMATION SERVICES

Most TIS operate as a question/answer service, that is, they respond directly to questions posed by individual patients or health care providers. The services primary functions are usually conducted over the phone. Generally, each TIS has designed specific and detailed data forms to document these interactions. This begins with documenting the patient history and nature of the question, and concludes with documentation of advice or information given. While the various TIS will differ slightly in this documentation and data collection process, all services aim to review the relevant information needed to address the safety/risk for a particular case.

The TIS are operated by health professionals drawn from varied medical backgrounds, including genetic counselors, nurses, toxicologists, and pharmacists. Virtually all services are directed by physicians, most commonly geneticists, but also clinical pharmacologists-toxicologists, epidemiologists, and obstetricians. Frequently they are comprised of a multidisciplinary team, providing a broader scope of knowledge. At present there is no standardized process of training health professionals for their task as teratogen information specialists and as such training varies substantially among the TIS. The Organization of Teratology Information Specialists (OTIS) has created a comprehensive training and educational package that may be used by individual centers when new team members join a program and is distributed to new services that join the organization.

The scheme in Fig. 21-1 depicts the process by which most TIS work. While some TIS postpone the reply to the caller several days, most tend to answer as soon as possible. In the best case, replies occur within the initial call. Many TIS record all contacts and queries to the service in a specialized database and a selected number will perform follow up activity after pregnancy to obtain information on the health of the mother and newborn and other details pertaining to the pregnancy and its outcome. In some programs the information given to women or health professionals over the telephone is followed by a letter, while in other programs no such letters are sent. Furthermore, selected patients may need to be referred to geneticists, obstetricians, or to other medical specialists as the situation demands.

Networking of TIS

Through the years a number of formal and informal relationships between the TIS have been forged. These relationships have created an extraordinary opportunity for information exchange and

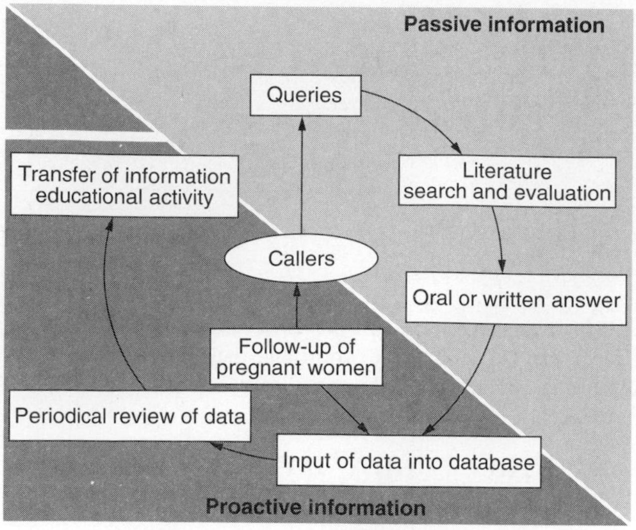

Figure 21-1. Working method of teratogen information services.

research collaborations and have resulted in two larger formal organizations. The OTIS is a nonprofit umbrella coalition of TIS in the United States and Canada, and has been in existence some 15 years. There are currently close to 20 services represented in this organization that meets annually in June and more recently has hosted a smaller, educational and research meeting, in January. Through their web site (www.otispregnancy.org) members can exchange information and update their directory listing, while the public can benefit from a number of information sheets, summaries of research endeavors and locate a service in their area. A similar organization, the European Network of Teratology Information Services (ENTIS) is actually a network with representatives from Europe, South America and the Middle East (www.entis-org.com). This group also meets annually and has a membership, which has been steadily increasing in recent years. TIS also exist in Australia and Asia, and although they have not created a formal network to date, their members are often very active in one of the established TIS networks, namely OTIS and ENTIS.

The TIS organizations have long recognized and embraced the need to network. The organization, meetings, and regular communications presents a number of advantages such as the increased ability to exchange data and establishes a tool for the enhanced transfer of information as it relates to exposures during pregnancy. Geographic, economic, political, and medical practice characteristics create different realities across countries and frequently the dilemmas surrounding risks and safety during pregnancy also differ significantly. Together TIS networks have worked to diminish these barriers. Moreover, teratogenic cases are rare events, requiring a large number of exposures before a single event is identified, and associations established. The communication and collaboration across these centers has made it possible to deal with questions single sites can not answer individually. For example, it was the collaboration between different centers in Brazil and around the world that made it possible to share information regarding the teratogenicity associated with the use of misoprostol during the first trimester of pregnancy.[8,9]

There is an urgent need to disseminate accurate and evidence based information on the use of drugs during pregnancy, particularly when data is limited. The mission of the new generation of TIS is to contribute not only to the optimal dissemination of information but also to the production of original data on the risks and safety of therapies in pregnancy.

Sources of Information

Typically there are three types of sources from which the TIS retrieve information necessary to answer queries from patients and health care providers.

Primary source of information: All TIS have access to one or many medical literature indexing databases such as Medline or Embase. Using appropriate search strategies one is able to identify the most recent literature published on a particular topic and have the citations readily available. The use of these databases, simplifies the task of answering a query with the most up-to-date data at their fingertips.

Secondary source of information: Most TIS use one or more specialized database programs specifically focused on reproductive toxicology, such as ReproTox[10], Teris[11], or ReproText[12] All programs contain summarized texts in the area of clinical teratology and frequently cover related fields such as diseases in pregnancy, drug abuse toxicology, infectious agents in pregnancy and chemical exposures.

Tertiary source of information: With regular attendance at academic meetings and participation in research projects TIS frequently have access to unpublished reports of studies or reviews as it relates to exposures in pregnancy. Meeting abstracts may reveal details of studies years before they appear in the peer reviewed literature. The development of TIS networks has facilitated and encouraged regular contact with colleagues in the area who may currently be conducting studies and for which preliminary results may be available. Tertiary sources may also include registries, maintained by the manufacturer[13]or other third parties, as well as reports to several regulatory bodies including the FDA.

Generating New Information Proactively. Problem oriented drug information centres, such as the TIS, are the obvious place where doubts and misperceptions converge. It follows logically that the TIS may be the ideal observatory for the informational needs in the area of maternal and fetal toxicology. These needs have been tended to in recent years with varied epidemiological methods. Tools such as the meta-analysis or prospective observational studies have been increasingly applied to better investigate the risks of exposure to xenobiotics in pregnancy.

Typically, when a TIS must reach an informed opinion concerning the possibility of teratogenic effects of a given therapeutic modality, it often faces contradicting and sometimes controversial results generated by different study methodologies or even different investigators. For a TIS it is vital to deliver the most updated and objective summary of the literature. In this context the meta-analytical approach[14,15] offers an important opportunity for a better understanding of risk or safety after exposure to drugs or other agents during pregnancy. On the other hand, the increasing numbers of women who contact TIS around the world each day are becoming an important cohort.[16] If observed prospectively, and when compared to adequate controls, they may serve as the obvious research subject and will assist investigators in providing optimal knowledge on the safety of the exposures.

The TIS truly is a unique and exemplary model of a "bench-to-bedside" establishment. Starting from the summary of literature to answer queries, to the ability to perform pharmacoepidemiologic studies with data collected at their very centers and then translating that information back into new evidence for the consumer, the TIS completes the full circle (Fig. 21-1).

The Meta-analysis

Each answer that the TIS produce requires a summary of the literature. However, the problem of how to analyze the literature in order to arrive at an overall conclusion concerning the relationship of a drug and a given outcome is not a new one. Meta-analysis is a well established strategy useful in clarifying the status of therapeutic modalities because it objectively combines and quantifies the data regarding risk or efficacy of drug (or other) exposures from a number of epidemiological studies. Because most studies investigating teratogenic risk are limited in size the meta-analysis of studies of similar design is becoming increasingly employed to clarify potential risks. The TIS, most notably the Motherisk program, has conducted a number of meta-analyses in this area. While individually, some observational cohorts or case-control studies have had limited power to clarify teratogenic risk, meta-analysis has been crucial in establishing and defining the correct risk levels for some common drugs (e.g., spermicides, Bendectin) initially fraught with conflicting study results.

The Collaborative Multicentre Study

In the past, most of the data regarding the use of drugs or any other agents during pregnancy came from animal models or retrospective analysis. With the exception of isotretinoin, animal studies have frequently been unable to accurately predict agents which were identified as teratogenic in humans, including thalidomide initially. Moreover, post marketing studies based on retrospective analysis suffer greatly from the human recall bias. That is, women treated with drugs for chronic illness or mothers who give birth to malformed children, may recall their treatments differently as compared to women who took an over-the-counter drug or those who had a healthy baby. Finally, premarketing studies can rarely provide information regarding a drug's teratogenic. Such trials generally exclude pregnant women due to obvious ethical considerations and so data would generally be limited by very small number of patients who may have become pregnant in the trial.

With the international development of TIS, an extraordinary source of data for prospective observational research has emerged. Pregnant women taking prescription or over-the-counter drugs voluntarily call the TIS for risk-assessment counseling, usually during the first trimester. Since the exposure data are recorded prospectively, the probability of recall bias is reduced, and follow-up of exposed pregnancies can extend well beyond parturition. Furthermore, contact with relevant physicians and direct examination of the child by specially trained investigators provides accurate and highly detailed information on the outcome of a particular case.

Some of the most well established TIS, which by now have accumulated impressive cohorts of patients, have been conducting follow-up analyses on a number of different exposures during pregnancy. Table 21-1 highlights some of the studies conducted as a collaboration of various TIS around the world. Few investigative groups have had the ability to consistently accrue cases and report on reproductive toxicology outcomes in the manner that the TIS have.

Table 21-1
Examples of Recent Multicentre Studies Conducted by TIS Collaborations

DRUGS	NUMBER OF TIS INVOLVED	LOCATIONS	TOTAL EXPOSED SUBJECTS	TOTAL CONTROLS	REFERENCE
Asthma medications	15	Canada, USA	654	303	Bakhireva et al.[17]
Dipyrone	4	Israel, Italy	108	108	Bar-Oz et al.[18]
Bupropion	2	Canada, USA	136	133	Chan et al.[19]
Haloperidol/Penfluridol	4	Germany, Israel, Italy, Netherlands	215	631	Diav-Citrin et al.[20]
Proton Pump Inhibitors	8	Finland, France, Germany, Greede, Israel, Italy, Netherlands	295	868	Diav-Citrin et al.[21]
H2-Blockers	18	Brazil, Finland, France, Germany, Greece, Israel, Italy, Netherlands, Spain, Switzerland, UK	553	1390	Garbis et al.[22]
Permethrins	2	Australia, Canada	113	113	Kennedy et al.[23]
Amoxicillin/ Clavulinic Acid	2	Israel	191	191	Berkovitch et al.[24]
Loratadine	4	Brazil, Canada, Israel, Italy	161	161	Moretti et al.[25]
Metoclopramide	6	Brazil, Canada, Israel, Italy	175	175	Berkovitch et al.[26]
Methimazole	10	Germany, Israel Italy, France, Netherlands	241	1089	DiGianantonio et al.[27]
Venlafaxine	7	Brazil, Canada, Italy, USA	150	300	Einarson et al.[28]

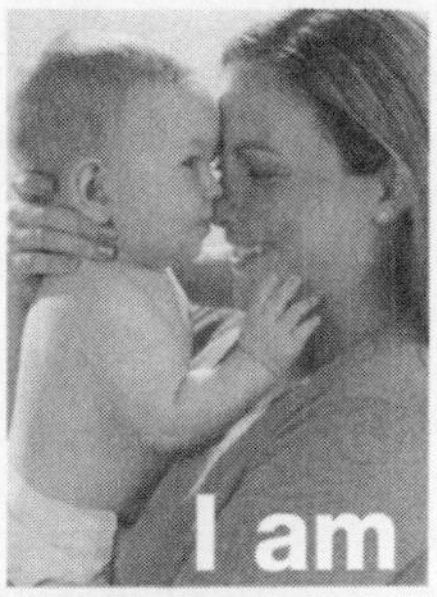

PREGNANT

Pregnancy Wallet Guide
to the safety of products
and medication when pregnant

MOTHERISK
TREATING THE MOTHER – PROTECTING THE UNBORN

There are some risks with every pregnancy. For every 100 pregnancies, 2 or 3 babies will be born with a birth defect, by chance alone.

The brands named in this brochure are not being endorsed but are given as examples to help you identify and recognize medications.

This information is presented as an educational service. It is not intended as a substitute for the medical care and advice of your physician.

Medications

How does it affect me and my baby?

Although most medicines are generally safe to take during pregnancy, you should always consult your practitioner or Wal-Mart pharmacist first.

Non-medicinal alternatives should always be your first step in managing your condition. One example is resting, drinking lots of fluid and using a vaporizer to control cold symptoms. Another example would be increasing dietary fibre and fluid intake and exercising for constipation.

Allergy & Cold Medications

- Antihistamines that make you sleepy are generally safe, i.e. chlorpheniramine (ChlorTripolon®), diphenhydramine (Benadryl®)
- For nasal congestion, try using nasal sprays for a few days, i.e. saline solution (Salinex®), xylometazoline (Otrivin®), or oral decongestants, i.e. pseudoephedrine (Sudafed®)
- Expectorants to reduce phlegm, i.e. guaifenesin (Robitussin plain®) and cough suppressants, i.e. dextromethorphan (Benylin DM®) are generally safe products that can be used for a short time

Anti-nausea Medications

- Check with your doctor before using
- Diclectin,® a prescription drug has been approved by Health Canada.
- Dimenhydrinate (Gravol®) can be used for "breakthrough vomiting"

Asthma Medications

- Most asthma medications are safe and should be used as directed by your physician

Heartburn Medications

- Use products that say "No Sodium" or "Sodium-Free"
- Calcium carbonate (Tums®, Rolaids®), aluminum hydroxide & magnesium hydroxide (Maalox®), and alginic compound (Gaviscon®) are safe products

Laxatives

- For constipation, it is best to eat high fibre (bran cereal) or use bulk forming agents, i.e. psyllium (Metamucil®)
- Do not use stimulant laxatives
- Stool softeners are safe, i.e. docusate calcium (Surfak®) or docusate sodium (Colace®)

Lice Medication

- For lice, products that contain permethrins (Nix®) or pyrethrins (R+C®) are preferred. Use as directed on the package

Prescription Medication

- Sometimes a prescription medication is necessary for the safety of both the mother and the baby.
- Your doctor will choose the safest and most effective medicine for you depending on your individual circumstances.
  For example:
  - If you are diabetic continue to monitor your blood sugar levels and use medicine prescribed by your doctor.
  - If you have epilepsy, your doctor will prescribe medicine to control seizures.
  - If you get an infection, your doctor may prescribe safe antibiotics such as penicillin, cephalosporins and erythromycin.

Pain Killers

- Acetaminophen (Tylenol®) is safe
- ASA and non-steroidal anti-inflammatory drugs, i.e. ibuprofen (Advil®), naproxen (Naprosyn®) are also safe in the first 6 months but should be avoided in late pregnancy (last 3 months)
- Codeine is safe for occasional use

Vaginal Creams & Ovules

- Most vaginal creams and suppositories (Canesten®, Micatin®) are safe
- Apply or insert gently as directed by your doctor
- Do not use iodine-containing products

Products

What commonly used products should I be careful around?

Alcohol

- It is best not to drink any alcohol when you are pregnant.
- There is no known safe amount or safe time to drink during pregnancy.
- Alcohol can affect a baby's development

Caffeine

- Small amounts (1½ cups of coffee per day) are generally safe
- Large amounts (more than 1½ cups of coffee per day) may increase the chances of miscarriage, premature delivery and low birth weight

Cigarette Smoking

- No smoking is best when you are pregnant, but if you cannot quit, cut down as much as possible
- Smoking increases the risk of low birth weight, miscarriage and premature delivery
- These risks may be reduced if you quit smoking as soon as you can
- Second hand smoke should also be avoided

Hair Colours and Perms

- Occasional use of these products, as directed, is safe
- Use products in well-ventilated areas

Household Cleaners

- Most products are safe for use as directed
- Use products in well-ventilated areas with appropriate safeguards (i.e. gloves)
- Do not use industrial-strength products in the home
- If you feel sick while cleaning, stop and check with your doctor

Household Paints

- If you are painting, use latex (water soluble) paints in well-ventilated areas
- Do not use oil-based paints
- If you feel sick while painting, stop and check with your doctor

Insecticides

- Try using a mineral oil based product such as Skin-so-Soft®
- Read labels of products and use ones that contain less than 30% DEET, sparingly

Pesticides

- It is best to avoid pesticides if possible
- For home interiors (after spraying), stay out of the home 2 – 3 times longer than recommended by the manufacturer
- Ventilate the area well by opening windows after spraying
- If applying to lawn, do not walk on the grass for the recommended amount of time

Sugar Substitutes or Sweeteners

- Moderate amounts of artificial sweetening agents, i.e. aspartame (NutraSweet®), saccharin (Sweet N Low®), sodium cyclamate (Sugar Twin®), sucralose (Splenda®) are safe

Video Display Terminals or Computer Terminals

- Using a computer is safe, at home or office
- They do not emit harmful radiation and are not an increased risk to you or the baby

Vitamins

- Compounds containing high amounts of Vitamin A (more than 8000 IU) should be avoided
- The use of folic acid (at least 0.4 mg per day) is recommended while planning for and in early pregnancy to protect newborns from neural tube defects (spina bifida)
- All other prenatal multi-vitamins are safe

X-rays

- Make sure your practitioner and x-ray technician know that you are pregnant
- The amount of radiation from x-ray is generally very small and is not a problem
- Wear a lead apron over the belly

Pregnancy Helplines

Safety/risk of drugs and chemicals
416-813-6780

Nausea and Vomiting of Pregnancy
1-800-436-8477

HIV and HIV Treatment
1-888-246-5840

Alcohol and Substance Use
1-877-FAS-INFO

For Further Information Call:

SickKids
MOTHERISK
TREATING THE MOTHER – PROTECTING THE UNBORN
www.motherisk.org

Developed by the Motherisk Program in co-operation with Algoma Best Start and

WAL★MART®

Figure 21-2. Pregnancy wallet card on the risks and safety of common exposures during pregnancy developed by the Motherisk program (a Canadian TIS).

Disseminating Information

As part of their proactive service, several TIS are involved in the production of information material for widespread dissemination of information on risk and safety after environmental or therapeutic exposures during pregnancy. The internet and creation of individual and organizational web sites has tremendously expanded the TIS ability to disseminate such materials. Individual TIS frequently produce their own brochures, pamphlets or information sheets for local distribution. For example the Motherisk program (a Canadian TIS) has developed a *pregnancy wallet card* on the risks and safety of common exposures during pregnancy (Fig. 21-2). This is a handy, wallet-size pamphlet, with answers to the most frequent questions asked by pregnant women about over-the-counter and household exposures. Some TIS produce their own newsletters or create regular *updates* and columns in a number of medical journals or therapeutic bulletins (e.g., Motherisk Update in Canadian Family Physician or the Drugs in Pregnancy and Lactation column in Ob/Gyn News). OTIS members have put significant efforts into creating a comprehensive collection of *fact sheets*, which are available on their website (http://otispregnancy.org/otis_fact_sheets.asp) as PDF files. Many of the fact sheets have also been translated into Spanish and French and individual OTIS members frequently distribute them to patients or while at educational meetings and conferences. The production of these materials is important to the progress of the TIS as an establishment that is proactive in its endeavors to communicate accurate information to the patient and public at large.

As an establishment that is proactive in its endeavors to communicate accurate information to the patient and public, the production of these materials is important to the progress and development of TIS.

TIS in Developing Countries

In South America, starting in 1990, nine TIS were created. These services were linked to the ECLAMC (Latin American Collaborative Study of Congenital Malformations), a hospital-based birth defects registry operating since 1967 in this continent. The social, political and economical characteristics as well as the health needs in developing countries presents unique challenges for the establishment of TIS in these countries. These characteristics include; large segments of the population with low education and economic means, high incidence of infectious and deficiency diseases, low financial support for health and research, poor drug control measures, governmental instability which may affect health policy, and few or no legalized means for voluntary termination of pregnancy. These challenges are most clearly illustrated by the continued frequent reports of congenital rubella syndrome[29,30] or to the ongoing occurrence of thalidomide embryopathy in regions where its use for leprosy is still a necessity and maternal misuse is common.[31] The case of misoprostol and its widespread use as attempts to induce abortion in countries where women do not have legal access to such medical procedures is another unfortunate example of the challenges in the developing world.[8,9,32]

In this context, the TIS have played essential role in both disseminating information and producing important data to further medical knowledge in these areas.

PERSPECTIVES ON THE FUTURE

It is difficult to determine whether the absolute number of TIS is increasing around the world, despite the clear need for such services. The reality is that this is somewhat of a moving target. While many clinicians and researchers have shown an interest and initiative by starting new services, particularly in Eastern Europe and Asia, the status of those as well as more established services is tenuous. Sadly, government and other funding agencies have not always led the way in providing support. For example, in the most recent years OTIS has seen significant decreases in the number of TIS within the organization, usually a result of cuts in federal or state funding. Even many remaining services operate on a year to year basis; not knowing if they will secure renewed funding. There is no doubt that many in the medical community share the knowledge, ability and desire to establish and maintain a TIS, but the challenges of funding sustainability are more predominant than ever before.

The TIS is the most simple, accessible and direct way for patients and health care providers to obtain personalized information on maternal and fetal toxicology. The effectiveness of these services is evidenced by the prevention of unnecessary pregnancy termination[33] and in their ability to allay fears by promoting good clinical choices in the appropriate treatment of maternal disease in pregnancy. Each time annual meetings bring new faces, the vision for the future of TIS is brighter. A continued existence and growth of the TIS and its networks will provide immediate benefit to patients today, and more importantly, by creating new knowledge about maternal-fetal toxicology, generations of future patients will also reap the rewards.

CONCLUSIONS

The past decade has brought tremendous changes to many TIS; they now play a principal role in the production of new data about maternal-fetal toxicology. More often, the TIS is looked to as a model for both the service it provides, and the research methods it utilizes. TIS team members are recognized world wide as knowledge leaders in their field. Their approach to generate hypotheses and research ideas in the very service where doubts and queries arise is an ideal illustration of the junction between research and clinical care.

REFERENCES

1. Koren G, Pastuszak A, Ito S. Drugs in pregnancy. *N Engl J Med.* 1998 April 16;338(16):1128–1137.
2. Henshaw SK. Unintended pregnancy in the United States. *Fam Plann Perspect.* 1998 January;30(1):24–29, 46.
3. Brown SS, Eisenberg L, Committee on Unintended Pregnancy IoM. *The best intentions: unintended pregnancy and the well-being of children and families.* Washington, D.C: National Academy Press; 1995.
4. Medication during pregnancy: an intercontinental cooperative study. Collaborative Group on Drug Use in Pregnancy (CGDUP). *Int J Gynaecol Obstet.* 1992 November;39(3):185–196.
5. Irl C, Hasford J. The PEGASUS project—a prospective cohort study for the investigation of drug use in pregnancy. PEGASUS Study Group. *Int J Clin Pharmacol Ther.* 1997 December; 35(12):572–576.

6. Canadian Pharmaceutical Association i. *Compendium of pharmaceuticals and specialties (Canada)*. 2005.
7. Leen-Mitchell M, Martinez L, Gallegos S, et al. Mini-review: history of organized teratology information services in North America. *Teratology.* 2000 April;61(4):314–317.
8. Schuler L, Pastuszak A, Sanseverino TV, et al. Pregnancy outcome after exposure to misoprostol in Brazil: a prospective, controlled study. *Reprod Toxicol.* 1999 March;13(2):147–151.
9. Pastuszak AL, Schuler L, Speck-Martins CE et al. Use of misoprostol during pregnancy and Mobius' syndrome in infants. *N Engl J Med.* 1998 June 25;338(26):1881–1885.
10. REPROTOX®. 2005. Bethesda, MD., The Reproductive Toxicology Center.
11. TERIS (The Teratogen Information System). 2005. Bethesda, MD., The Reproductive Toxicology Center.
12. REPROTEXT® Database. Dabney BJe, editor. 2005. Englewood, Colorado, MICROMEDEX, Inc.
13. Shields KE, Wiholm BE, Hostelley LS, et al. Monitoring outcomes of pregnancy following drug exposure: a company-based pregnancy registry program. *Drug Saf.* 2004;27(6):353–367.
14. Egger M, Schneider M, Smith GD. Spurious precision? Meta-analysis of observational studies. *BMJ.* 1998 January 10;316(7125):140–144.
15. Stroup DF, Berlin JA, Morton SC, et al. Meta-analysis of observational studies in epidemiology: a proposal for reporting. Meta-analysis Of Observational Studies in Epidemiology (MOOSE) group. *JAMA.* 2000 April 19;283(15):2008–2012.
16. Chambers CD, Braddock SR, Briggs GG, et al. Postmarketing surveillance for human teratogenicity: a model approach. *Teratology.* 2001 November;64(5):252–261.
17. Bakhireva LN, Jones KL, Schatz M, et al. Asthma medication use in pregnancy and fetal growth. *J Allergy Clin Immunol.* 2005 September; 116(3):503–509.
18. Bar-Oz B, Clementi M, Di Giantonio E, et al. Metamizol (dipyrone, optalgin) in pregnancy, is it safe? A prospective comparative study. *Eur J Obstet Gynecol Reprod Biol.* 2005 April 1; 119(2):176–179.
19. Chan BCF, Koren G, Fayez I, et al. Pregnancy outcome of women exposed to bupropion during pregnancy: a prospective comparative study. *Am J Obstet Gynecol.* 2005 March;192(3):932–936.
20. Diav-Citrin O, Shechtman S, Ornoy S et al. Safety of haloperidol and penfluridol in pregnancy: a multicenter, prospective, controlled study. *J Clin Psychiatry.* 2005 March;66(3):317–322.
21. Diav-Citrin O, Arnon J, Shechtman S, et al. The safety of proton pump inhibitors in pregnancy: a multicentre prospective controlled study. *Aliment Pharmacol Ther.* 2005 February 1;21(3):269–275.
22. Garbis H, Elefant E, Diav-Citrin O, et al. Pregnancy outcome after exposure to ranitidine and other H2-blockers. A collaborative study of the European Network of Teratology Information Services. *Reprod Toxicol.* 2005 March;19(4):453–458.
23. Kennedy D, Hurst V, Konradsdottir E, et al. Pregnancy outcome following exposure to permethrin and use of teratogen information. *Am J Perinatol.* 2005 February;22(2):87–90.
24. Berkovitch M, Diav-Citrin O, Greenberg R, et al. First-trimester exposure to amoxycillin/clavulanic acid: a prospective, controlled study. *Br J Clin Pharmacol.* 2004 September;58(3):298–302.
25. Moretti ME, Caprara D, Coutinho CJ, et al. Fetal safety of loratadine use in the first trimester of pregnancy: a multicenter study. *J Allergy Clin Immunol.* 2003 March;111(3):479–483.
26. Berkovitch M, Mazzota P, Greenberg R, et al. Metoclopramide for nausea and vomiting of pregnancy: a prospective multicenter international study. *Am J Perinatol.* 2002 August;19(6):311–316.
27. Di Gianantonio E, Schaefer C, Mastroiacovo PP, et al. Adverse effects of prenatal methimazole exposure. *Teratology* 2001 November; 64(5):262–266.
28. Einarson A, Fatoye B, Sarkar M, et al. Pregnancy outcome following gestational exposure to venlafaxine: a multicenter prospective controlled study. *Am J Psychiatry.* 2001 October;158(10):1728–1730.
29. Lanzieri TM, Parise MS, Siqueira MM, et al. Incidence, clinical features and estimated costs of congenital rubella syndrome after a large rubella outbreak in Recife, Brazil, 1999–2000. *Pediatr Infect Dis J.* 2004 December;23(12):1116–1122.
30. Robertson SE, Featherstone DA, Gacic-Dobo M, et al. Rubella and congenital rubella syndrome: global update. *Rev Panam Salud Publica.* 2003 November;14(5):306–315.
31. Castilla EE, Ashton-Prolla P, Barreda-Mejia E, et al. Thalidomide, a current teratogen in South America. *Teratology.* 1996 December; 54(6):273–277.
32. Pollack AE, Pine RN. Opening a door to safe abortion: international perspectives on medical abortifacient use. *J Am Med Womens Assoc.* 2000;55(3 Suppl):186–188.
33. Koren G, Pastuszak A. Prevention of unnecessary pregnancy terminations by counselling women on drug, chemical, and radiation exposure during the first trimester. *Teratology.* 1990 June;41(6):657–661.

CHAPTER 22

MOTHERISK: THE TORONTO MODEL FOR COUNSELLING IN REPRODUCTIVE TOXICOLOGY

Myla E. Moretti

INTRODUCTION

No doubt by this point in the text you are well aware of the lessons that the thalidomide tragedy has taught us. The potential dangers of drugs, chemicals and radiation and their abilities to disrupt normal fetal development have since been well documented.[1] For close to 50 years and nearly two generations later, women and their health care providers have approached the issue of exposures in pregnancy with both hesitation and extreme caution. For women, the media (such as newspapers, books, and television), word of mouth and physicians may all provide information and advice about such exposures. Frequently this advice, although well meaning, may be unsolicited and is frequently given by those who are not fully informed. Since the media has clearly shown its ability to skew the information it presents[2] and since physicians may not have the relevant literature available in their office, the need for a service to provide accurate information about the effects of exposures in pregnancy and lactation is crucial. This highly specialized information service, known as the Teratology Information Service (TIS) has appeared primarily across Europe and North America, although services now exist in parts of Asia, Australia, and South America.

The TIS functions mainly, to provide information to health care providers and the public about the effects of drugs, chemicals, radiation and infections in pregnancy on both the mother and her unborn child. Due to the fact that patients may continue to have exposures while breastfeeding and since infant development continues into this postpartum period many TISs will also provide information about these exposures in lactating patients. Services can be solely open to health care providers, to patients, or they may provide information to the public at large. Depending on the nature or mandate of the service there may be a consultation involved, specific to each patient, rather than the simple dissemination of information in a generic fashion. The purpose of this chapter is to describe the Motherisk Program, located at the Hospital for Sick Children in Toronto, Ontario, Canada. Special emphasis will be placed on the day-to-day operations of the services which have evolved over the last 20 years.

INCEPTION

The Motherisk Program, originally a clinical consultation service began its operation in September of 1985.[3] Some 2–3 years later it expanded to include a telephone consultation service, which remains its largest component to date, averaging greater than 150 calls per day from across the country. The most common calls to the program have not changed significantly over the years, namely calls regarding antibiotics, analgesics and antipyretics, cough, cold and allergy remedies, and cosmetic products continue to constitute a large proportion of the inquiries to the service as do calls about antidepressants. Increasingly women with multiple chronic diseases and/or exposures to drugs of abuse are the subject of the information service. Perhaps patient awareness of the potential for xenobiotics to affect fetal development has increased and more importantly patients who may not have even considered pregnancy 10 or even 5 years ago are today living with their disease and having children.

MANDATE

The goal of Motherisk is threefold:

1. To provide authoritative information and guidance to pregnant or breast-feeding patients and their health care providers regarding the fetal risks associated with drug, chemical, infection, disease and/or radiation exposure during pregnancy or lactation.
2. To research unanswered question on the safety of drugs, chemicals, infection, disease, and radiation during pregnancy and lactation.
3. To maintain a vital training and educational program in the area of reproductive and developmental toxicology at the undergraduate, graduate, and postgraduate levels.

Over the last 20 years of its existence the Motherisk program has grown into a service, which today is able to provide this authoritative information based on much of its own research in the area of maternal-fetal medicine.

THE TEAM MEMBERS

The Motherisk team consists of numerous individuals from various areas of the health care sciences. Although some team members affiliated with the program are based at other hospitals, most of team members are based within the Division of Clinical Pharmacology and Toxicology at the Hospital for Sick Children. Table 22-1, highlights the various team members and their specialties. The postdoctoral MD fellows training within the Division of Pharmacology and Toxicology are on call for Motherisk for at least 1 week every 2 months. During their on-call rotation they consult patients or health care providers over the telephone for consults, which require more expertise than is initially available at the first intake call with the information specialist. The fellows also participate weekly in clinic consultations and perform and supervise much of the research conducted within the program. The information specialists spend most of their time with the telephone consultations and also participate in the various research endeavors. Other team members are used as consultants for specific cases where unique expertise is required and they may also participate in research projects. While the coordinator overseas the day-to-day operations and activities of the information specialists, the assistant director and director oversee the operations of the program as a whole.

Table 22-1
Motherisk Team Members

Full-time
- Director—pediatrician/clinical pharmacologist and toxicologists
- Senior scientists—pediatricians, neurologist, pharmacologist/toxicologist
- Assistant director—MSc clinical pharmacology
- Clinical fellows—MD subspecializing in clinical pharmacology/toxicology
- Medical secretary
- Information specialists—BSc

Part-time/occasional
- Addiction specialists—physician, PhD
- Clinical pharmacologist—physicians
- Geneticists—physicians
- Genetics Counsellors—MSc
- Medical information specialist—clinical pharmacists
- Medical toxicologist—physicians
- Pediatrician—Physician
- Psychologist—PhD
- Psychometrist—MSc
- Statisticians—PhD

Students
- Graduate—pharmacology and toxicology, pharmacy, genetics
- Undergraduate—pharmacology, toxicology, medicine, pharmacy, midwifery

THE TELEPHONE CONSULTATION

The telephone consultation is available to both health professionals and the public at large. While calls from patients form the bulk of the consultations, health care providers, mainly physicians, comprise 20% of the calls to the service daily. The telephone service operates between 9:00 AM and 5:00 PM Monday to Friday (EST) and closes only for Canadian statutory holidays. During these hours of operation, calls are received immediately by an information specialist. Due to a high volume of calls, at some times in the day, calls are kept in sequence by a queuing system until an information specialist (counselor) is available. Initially, calls are documented and screened by the information specialist to obtain relevant details of the patient's medical history and to determine if the call can be satisfactorily answered over the telephone. While this is the case for greater than 95% of the calls to the service some are referred for a clinic appointment, or when a patient is not able to travel to the clinic in Toronto, to the physician on call. Each week approximately 7–10 patients are seen in the clinic additional 15–20 patients are referred to the on-call staff for consultation. Furthermore, physician callers who wish to discuss the risks with multiple or alternative drug protocols are generally referred to the team member on-call. While the decision to refer a call to clinic is at the discretion of the information specialist, the following are criteria or guidelines the information specialists use to determine which patients should be referred to clinic:

1. Patient has a chronic illness (e.g., epilepsy, lupus, inflammatory bowel disease)
2. Patient reports substance abuse (e.g., alcohol, cocaine, heroin, hallucinogens, tranquilizers)
3. Patient has or may have exposure to known or suspected teratogen during pregnancy (e.g., anticonvulsants, antineoplastics, misoprostol, organic solvents, isotretinoin, benzodiazepines, systemic steroids)
4. Pregnancy is complicated by psychosocial problems
5. Patient's physician has made referral to clinic
6. Patient has complicated multiple exposures
7. Patient expresses desire to be seen in clinic despite not meeting any of the criteria above (e.g., high maternal anxiety, previous pregnancy with adverse outcome)

Regardless of the exposure or magnitude of risk all calls to the program are documented firstly on the Telephone Intake form displayed in Fig. 22-1 (a, b). This telephone report form has undergone significant changes since the inception of the telephone service, a reflection of the changes in volume of calls, type of calls and the needs of the research protocols. It has become clear that quality of the form is essential for proper identification of potential risk factors in a particular patient. Patients are asked details of their obstetrical and medical histories and vitamin intake. The interview also includes ascertaining any exposure to drugs, which may include prescription, non-prescription or illicit drugs. If the primary concern is regarding an infectious disease, radiation or chemical exposure these parameters are also recorded (Fig. 22-1b). Beyond the identification of the particular exposure, determining the amount (or dose or level), timing and duration of exposure are all particularly important. The timing, relative to gestational age may alter the information presented to the patient. For example, lithium is known to be associated with cardiac anomalies. A patient may contact the service in her 16th week of pregnancy concerned that she may need to be started on lithium, due to her difficulties in coping with day-to-day activities. Since cardiac formation is known to be complete by this point the patient can be assured that commencing therapy will pose no harm to her fetus. At the same time, the patient will be informed that continuation of treatment throughout the duration of pregnancy remaining may be associated with neonatal lithium toxicity. As the infant clears the drug from his systemic circulation, these effects will disappear, something both mother and her physician should be aware of. Likewise, doses or levels of exposure are critical for risk assessment. Certain exposures (such as radiation or vitamin A) may present different outcomes depending on the amount of maternal exposures.

The obstetrical and medical histories are also critical in defining risk for a patient. Often, when ascertaining medical history, it becomes apparent that a patient may have some underlying disease for which she takes medication, but which may not have been the primary reason for contacting the service. Obtaining obstetrical history may highlight risks that the patient may not have been aware of or even questioned. For example, a previous terminated pregnancy with a known neural tube defect warrants discussion as the patient should be advised to take higher doses of folic acid when planning another pregnancy, again not likely the primary reason for contacting the service. As with medication, determining exact gestational ages becomes critical with maternal infectious diseases. Varicella, rubella and other infectious disease may pose different risks depending on the gestational age at the time of acute maternal infection, which many patients are unaware of before the call.

HSC The Hospital for Sick Children **MOTHERISK IntakeForm**

DEMOGRAPHICS

Patient Name ____________________

Home Phone ____________ Work Phone ____________

Date of Birth ____________

CVS Yes ❑ No ❑

Amnio Yes ❑ No ❑ Advised ❑

Results ____________

Referred By ____________

CurrentMD Type ____________ MD Phone ____________

CALLER ____________________

Contact Number ____________________

Identity ____________________

INCOMING:

date: ____________ time: ____________

counsellor: ____________

completed ❑ Passed to Fellow: ❑

OUTGOING:

date: ____________ time: ____________

completed by: ____________

PREGNANCY

NOT PREGNANT:
general info ❑ planning ❑ retrospective ❑ breast-feeding ❑

LMP (d/m/y) ____________ every ______ days

Currently: weight ______ kg lb gestation ______ wk mos

EDC (d/m/y) ____________ by dates ❑ by ultrasound ❑

G____ **P**____ **SA**____ **TA**____ **ectopic**____ **molar**____

Stillbith______ Other pregnacies____________

Defects in previous pregnancies no ❑ yes ____________

Most recent ultrasound in current pregnancy: not yet ❑

at: ______ weeks reason: ____________ results: ____________

MEDICAL HISTORY

Kidney No ❑ Yes ____________
Heart No ❑ Yes ____________
Hypertension No ❑ Yes ____________
Diabetes No ❑ Yes ____________
Respiratory No ❑ Yes ____________
Thyroid No ❑ Yes ____________
Psychiatric No ❑ Yes ____________
Epilepsy No ❑ Yes ____________
GI tract No ❑ Yes ____________
Other ____________

Vit/Min? No ❑ Yes ____________
NVP No ❑ Yes ____________

Alcohol No ❑ Yes ____________
Smoking No ❑ Yes ____________
Cocaine No ❑ Yes ____________
Marijuana No ❑ Yes ____________
Other ____________

EXPOSURE

DRUG Infections & Chemicals - reverse	**Start**	**Stop**	**Dose/ Route**	**Indication**	Advice as per MRS
	❑ not yet	❑ ongoing			
	❑ not yet	❑ ongoing			
	❑ not yet	❑ ongoing			
	❑ not yet	❑ ongoing			
	❑ not yet	❑ ongoing			
	❑ not yet	❑ ongoing			
	❑ not yet	❑ ongoing			

ADVICE

Baseline risk explained **yes** ❑ **no** ❑ **Risk no >1-3%** ❑

Clinic date/ time: ____________

bring translator ❑ language spoken ____________

DISCUSSED folic acid ❑ amount advised: ____________

ultrasound ❑ MSDS requested ❑

Referred to: NVP line ❑ FAS line ❑ HIV line ❑

Referred back to MD for suggestions of medications ❑

MO-RISK intake form DC.01

Figure 22-1a. The Telephone Intake Form
Front (page 3) of intake form used to document maternal characteristics, drug exposures, and advice given.
Back (page 4) of intake form used to document exposure to chemicals, infectious disease, and infant details in the case of calls regarding breastfeeding.

INFECTIOUS DISEASES

❑ Chlamydia ❑ Chicken pox ❑ CMV
❑ Genital herpes ❑ Red Measles ❑ Group B strep
❑ Coxsackie ❑ Hepatitis B ❑ Hepatitis C
❑ Shingles ❑ Syphilis ❑ Toxoplasmosis
❑ Roseola ❑ Rubella ❑ Parvovirus B19
other: ______

Exposed only ❑ Infected ❑
date of diagnosis: ______

Disease clinically diagnosed (patient): ❑ yes ❑ no

Patient had disease in the past: ❑ yes ❑ no ❑ unsure

SYMPTOMS (patient): ______

Date of contact with infected person: ______

Date of lesions on infected person: ______

TYPE OF CONTACT:
❑ blood ❑ oral ❑ household
❑ lesions ❑ mucosal ❑ daycare
❑ sexual ❑ fecal ❑ hospital
❑ other ______

OCCUPATIONAL EXPOSURES

Chemical: ______

Radiation/ Accidental: ______
Occupation: ______

Period of time in practice: ______

EXPOSURE
dose (if applicable): ______

type: direct secondary

where: factory office home school other ______

route: skin oral inhalation other ______

duration: minutes hours days other: ______ ❑ none

barrier: gloves mask respirator fumehood
other ______ ❑ none

side effects (patient): nausea vomiting diarrhea rash
headache tremors blurred vision
other ______

side effects (colleagues): ______

______ ❑ none

BREASTFEEDING

Infant Data	Breast-feeding info	Advice				
		#	BF chapter	Hale	Briggs	Safe
Date of birth ______	# times breastfed in 24 hr period ______					
Gestational age at birth ____wks	Formula? Yes No Solids? Yes No					
Birth weight ____lb ____oz	age started ______ age started ______					
(______ g)	# times/day ______ # times/day ______					

Reference Advice/Additional Information:

Figure 22-1b.

Although precise risks of chemical exposures in pregnancy remain to be elucidated, counselors obtain as many details of the type and duration of exposure, type of protection used and presence of adverse events which may be indicative of excessive exposure.

Ruling out all other risks the callers are subsequently counseled on the effects of the substance constituting the primary reason for the call. All calls are completed with the explanation of the baseline risks for major malformations in the general population. It is critical that patients understand and are aware of this baseline risk and for most callers, that their particular risk is not elevated above this. There is often also a brief discussion of the availability of amniocentesis, for patients who may have risks of chromosomal anomalies, and of the benefits of folic acid supplementation for all patients planning a pregnancy.

Each day, some 30% of the calls received by the program pertain to drug use in a lactating patient. As with exposures in pregnancy a telephone intake form is filled out (Fig. 22-1a and b) documenting medical history. Along with maternal data and demographics the back (Fig. 22-1b) of the form contains an area to document brief details pertaining to the infant. Namely, date of birth, gestational age, birth weight, and feeding habits. All of these parameters are critical in formulating a risk assessment. Counselors use the information in conjunction with milk excretion data in several reference materials to determine if the infant is likely to experience adverse events. Infant age, for example is critical because neonates and premature infants exhibit varied drug clearance rates such that they may be more susceptible to drugs through breast milk. On the other hand, older infants who receive most of their nutrition from solid foods and receive smaller volumes of breast milk throughout the day are less likely to experience adverse effects from drugs in breast milk since they will be exposed to less drug.

While documentation is quite rigorous for each phone call, it has become apparent that this process is essential for both adequate counselling and accurate information collection, which is used in follow-up and for research purposes. Although some calls each day are prolonged, with experience, counsellors reach a level of proficiency and thoroughness that allows them to complete between 30 and 40 calls each day. Patients can expect to spend 6–7 minutes, on average, with the counselor. Counselors subsequently spend an additional 2–3 minutes after each call to complete documentation.

Currently the Motherisk program receives and responds to nearly 3000 calls per month, a total of some 35,000 calls annually. This exhibits quite a contrast to the 300 calls we were receiving annually in the first year of the telephone service. Since all calls to the program will be answered, we can receive calls from across North America and very occasionally Europe; usually Canadians calling from abroad. Virtually all of the calls, however, originate from Canada and the bulk of these from the greater Toronto area (area codes 416, 905, and 647). However, about 35% of callers are contacting us long distance. Twenty percent of the calls are from health care practitioners, two-thirds of these being physicians; the remaining are from the patient herself or her partner.

As discussed earlier, calls vary significantly in the type of question as well as the number of exposures. The average number of exposures questioned is 2.7 per call. When divided by exposure type, prescription medications are the most common query (45%) followed by over-the-counter products (31%), illicit or recreational substances (5%), infectious diseases (5%), cosmetic agents (5%), and finally, chemicals (4%).

SPECIALIZED SERVICES

While the general Motherisk service just described constitutes the bulk of our activities and continues to grow in volume each year the program offers several other specialized services to patients and health care providers. Many of these services were initiated with a strong mandate for a particular research project, however the clinical activities have far exceeded the anticipated response and they now operate well beyond completion of the primary study. Moreover, the services present unique opportunities to reach the nation as a whole, by offering toll-free lines and bilingual services (English and French).

Nausea and Vomiting in Pregnancy (NVP) Program

The first of our specialized services created is that which we refer to as the NVP line. Instituted in early 1996 the NVP service was initiated to conduct a study on the behavior and attitudes of women suffering from NVP in Canada and the United States with special focus on terminations of otherwise wanted pregnancies.[4] The study documented current advice, NVP management practices[5], maternal morbidity, risk perceptions[6] and the effects of NVP on quality of life.[7] After studying nearly 7000 patients who called the line, the service evolved to provide counseling to pregnant women and health care providers about nausea and vomiting during pregnancy and related sequelae.[8] This counseling includes information about potential treatments for NVP, including both pharmacologic[9] and nonpharmacologic[10] therapies and provides support to patients who frequently have had no where else to turn. The NVP program continues to study the effects of NVP and its treatment on the outcome of pregnancy and the health of the mother and fetus. The result is over 20 original research and reviews published in the medical literature.[4–7,11–26] This bilingual service operates from Monday to Friday, 9:00 AM to 5:00 PM EST. Patients calling during these hours will generally have immediate contact with an information specialist who will provide specific counselling about the management and treatment of NVP. Depending on suitability and patient consent the caller may also be asked to participate in a particular research study.

HIV Healthline and Network

Initial team meeting for the Motherisk HIV Healthline and Network began in the fall of 1997, which was officially launched at a press conference on World AIDS Day, December 1, 1997.[27] The objectives of the program are as follows:

- To provide information and counseling on all issues involved in HIV and its care during pregnancy and lactation
- To establish a national network of healthcare providers interested in this area of maternal-fetal medicine
- To study the short- and long-term fetal risk/safety of antiretroviral therapy in pregnancy be creating a national registry of HIV infected pregnancies

There is an urgent need to provide information to pregnancy women about these issues. In addition, this population of women with HIV represents a different group of patients with unique concerns, very different from those using the general Motherisk service. This service is an extension of Motherisk's primary service and is also a significant collaboration with the pediatric HIV/AIDS program and The Hospital for Sick Children.[28,29] This collaboration allows patients to receive care from Motherisk information specialists, pediatric infectious disease physicians, nurses, social workers, and others in the community. Women, their families, and their healthcare providers can call this confidential toll-free service and obtain evidence-based information about HIV and its treatment in pregnancy from a counsellor trained specifically in the medical and social issues of these patients.

Along with counseling about fetal risks patients are given referrals to healthcare providers in their own community who care for pregnant women with HIV/AIDS. Patients can remain anonymous although those interested in participating in the national registry provide contact details so that network members can obtain detailed medical information and conduct follow-up. Since physicians from across the country are already network members. Patients continue to receive care through their own healthcare provider and still participate in the national registry. All children in the Toronto area born to mothers with HIV/AIDS in pregnancy are followed by the pediatric HIV program and The Hospital for Sick Children. Children are monitored for HIV status and with this new Motherisk service, all will have long term follow-up as well. Data collected from intake to follow-up is standardized and is similar to other Motherisk services, with modifications specific for maternal illness. Data collection forms are provided to all network members so data can be documented at a site near the patient and consistently across the network. All data is then maintained by a centralized secure database in Toronto.

As informed HIV testing of all pregnant women has become a reality in Canada,[30] the need for continued research in this area is obvious. Still today, some women will learn of their HIV status for the first time in pregnancy.

Alcohol and Substance Use Helpline

The newest of our specialized services is the Motherisk Alcohol and Substance Use Helpline.[31] Established in late 1998, this toll-free service operates 8:00 AM to 8:00 PM EST and is sponsored by the Brewers Association of Canada. Dedicated counselors provide information and counseling to pregnant women, healthcare providers, and adoptive parents about the risks of alcohol, smoking, and other substance use in pregnancy. The number of calls to the Alcohol and Substance Use Helpline has increased rapidly, with over 10,000 calls since its inception. The efforts of this service will help us to continue researching the effects of these agents on the child exposed in utero and to develop practice guidelines to deal with such patients.[32–35] Once again because of the highly sensitive nature of their exposures, counselors are committed to providing information and resources even when the caller wishes to remain anonymous. One of the key features of the service is an extensive database of patient resources available across Canada. If a need is identified by either the caller or the counselor, patients can be given information and referrals to agencies in their home community. This means that patient will have access to a variety of services such as treatment, housing, addiction counseling, and other support agencies.

THE CLINIC CONSULTATION

Each week between seven and ten patients are referred to the clinic, which is held at the Hospital for Sick Children. Some patients self refer while others are referred by their physician. All patients are seen by one of the team physicians, who provide verbal consultation regarding the exposures in pregnancy as well as obtain a more detailed patient history in order to determine the presence of other potential risk factors. The current form used to document this consultation is seen in Fig. 22-2. As is visible from the form, we obtain much more detailed contact information from the patient as well as any physicians that she may be under the care of. All of these parameters become much more relevant in the event that we need to recontact or follow-up on this patient as described later in this chapter. There is a thorough interview with the patient and often her partner also and detailed medical, obstetrical, and family history information is all used in the risk assessment and counseling process. As with telephone counseling the detailed history is particularly useful for the consulting physician who may become aware of other risk factors necessary to providing accurate and complete information and her physician.

THE FOLLOW-UP INTERVIEW

Pregnancy follow-up is an integral part of the program. Regular follow-ups are conducted daily, with the data being used to enrich the current status of knowledge on the safety of exposures in pregnancy. Follow-up usually occurs in the child's first or second year of life although depending on the primary objective of the follow-up, may occur earlier or later in the child's life. Most follow-ups are conducted directly with the mother, over the telephone. Since the number of daily consultations prohibits follow-up on all patients contacting the service most follow-ups are conducted as part of a particular research protocol.

During the telephone follow-up details of the course and outcome of pregnancy are documented on standardized forms (Fig. 22-3). Subsequent to this telephone interview a letter is sent to the child's physician who confirms and technically defines the child's medical conditions, health status and/or malformations. In addition to our standard follow-up, selected cohorts of patients undergo a more detailed follow-up in person. This more comprehensive interview may include examination by a pediatrician or geneticist or psychological testing, depending on the specific objectives or research questions.

INFORMATION RESOURCES

Both the telephone and clinical consultation service use a variety of resources to provide information to patients and health care providers. In order to assist the process of providing a standardized, cohesive, response to patients and health practitioners, team members use our internally created individual drug statements as their primary resource. This collection of reproductive risk monographs updated with the help of all team members, and maintained by the assistant director, forms the basis for patient consultation. They are also included in the consult summary letters sent to physicians after their patient is seen in clinic. A number of other resources are used when formulating a risk assessment for a particular patient. These include standard reference texts in the area,[36–38] peer reviewed literature searches from Medline EMBASE, Current Contents and Science Citation Index, and specialized databases such as ReproTox, TERIS, Shepard's catalog and ReproRisk. In addition, team members regularly participate in meta-analyses and systematic reviews of exposures in pregnancy. In particular, when the existing literature for a particular agent is

MOTHERISK PROGRAM

CLINIC FOR PREGNANCY EXPOSURE RISK COUNSELLING
DIVISION OF CLINICAL PHARMACOLOGY,
THE HOSPITAL FOR SICK CHILDREN, TORONTO, ONTARIO

ID NUMBER: ____________

CONSULTATION DATE (d/m/y) ____________

CONSULTATION BY: ____________

MATERNAL DATA

FULL NAME: ____________ Biological father's name: ____________

Address: ____________ Address: same as mother ☐ ____________

Date of birth (dd/mmm/yy) ____________ Date of birth (dd/mmm/yy) ____________

Home Telephone: (____) ____________ Home Telephone: same ☐ (____) ____________

Work Telephone: (____) ____________ Work Telephone: (____) ____________

Maternal Race: ☐ White ☐ Black ☐ Indo-Asian ☐ Hispanic ☐ Oriental Asian ☐ Other: ____________ **Marital Status:** ☐ married/common law ☐ single ☐ divorced ☐ widowed

Send MR letter to Dr. ____________ Dr. ____________

Street Address: ____________

City/Postal Code: ____________

Geographically stable relative: Name: ____________ Home telephone: (____) ____________

Relationship to patient: ☐ mother ☐ father ☐ aunt ☐ uncle ☐ cousin ☐ grandparent ☐ sister ☐ brother

OBSTETRICAL HISTORY

*gravidity*____ *parity*____ *spontaneous abortion <20wks*____ *fetal death ≥ 20weeks*____ *therapeutic abortion*____

Details on previous pregnancies: ____________

Contraception

Method	Start Date	Stop Date	Duration of Use	Pregnancy due to failure?
☐ none			____d☐ wk☐ mo☐ yr ☐	yes☐ no☐
☐ abstinence			____d☐ wk☐ mo☐ yr ☐	yes☐ no☐
☐ rhythm			____d☐ wk☐ mo☐ yr ☐	yes☐ no☐
☐ condom			____d☐ wk☐ mo☐ yr ☐	yes☐ no☐
☐ diaphragm			____d☐ wk☐ mo☐ yr ☐	yes☐ no☐
☐ IUD			____d☐ wk☐ mo☐ yr ☐	yes☐ no☐
☐ oral pill			____d☐ wk☐ mo☐ yr ☐	yes☐ no☐
☐ spermicide			____d☐ wk☐ mo☐ yr ☐	yes☐ no☐

Name of Pill ____________

Ovulatory Drugs ☐ no ☐ yes Name: ____________ Start: ____________ Stop: ____________

PREGNANCY INFORMATION

LMP (dd/mmm/yy) ____________ Certain? ☐Yes ☐No Cycle every ____ days x ____ days bleeding

EDC (dd/mmm/yy) ____________ Planned Pregnancy? ☐Yes ☐No

Current Gestational Age ________ ☐ weeks ☐ months by: ☐ dates ☐ ultrasound

Weight pre-pregnancy ________ ☐ kg ☐ lb current ________ ☐ kg ☐ lb

Pregnancy diagnosed at ________ wks ☐ months ☐ By which method? ☐ blood test ☐ urine test ☐ ultrasound

Ultrasounds? ☐ No ☐ Yes at ____ ☐ wks ☐ months Results: ☐ Normal ☐ Other ____________

at ____ ☐ wks ☐ months Results: ☐ Normal ☐ Other ____________

Amniocentesis ? ☐ Yes at ____ ☐ wks ☐ months Reason: ____________

Results: ____________

☐ No - Patient has discussed topic with physician already? ☐ Yes ☐ No

PRIMARY EXPOSURE INFORMATION

A. Over-the-counter and Prescription Medications and/or Radiation

Drug Name or Radiation Type	Start Date	Stop Date	Dose/Route/ Frequency	Indication
1.		☐ ongoing exposure		
2.		☐ ongoing exposure		
3.		☐ ongoing exposure		
4.		☐ ongoing exposure		
5.		☐ ongoing exposure		
6.		☐ ongoing exposure		

	Prescribing physician	*Side Effects*	*Comments*
1.			
2.			
3.			
4.			
5.			
6.			

Figure 22-2. The Clinic Consult Form.

B. Chemical Exposures

Occupation Title: ________________ ☐ maternal ☐ paternal

CHEMICAL NAME →	1.	2.	3.
Where is patient exposed?	Home [ ] factory [ ] office [ ] school [ ] studio [ ]	home [ ] factory [ ] office [ ] school [ ] studio [ ]	Home [ ] factory [ ] Office [ ] school [ ] Studio [ ]
Type of exposure *direct use* *In same area when chemical used*	[ ] [ ]	[ ] [ ]	[ ] [ ]
Purpose of chemical?			
START DATE of exposure			
STOP DATE of exposure			
For how long?	____ min [ ] hr [ ] days [ ]	____ min [ ] hr [ ] days [ ]	____ min [ ] hr [ ] days [ ]
Per day? week?	day [ ] week [ ]	day [ ] week [ ]	day [ ] week [ ]
Ventilation during exposure? *hood with power exhaust* *general - wall & roof fan, ceiling vent* *natural - open windows & doors*	None [ ] [ ] [ ] [ ]	None [ ] [ ] [ ] [ ]	None [ ] [ ] [ ] [ ]
Barriers during exposure? *gloves* *mask* *respirator* *apron, helmet, goggles*	[ ] cartridges yes [ ] no [ ] [ ] [ ] ____	[ ] cartridges yes [ ] no [ ] [ ] [ ] ____	[ ] cartridges yes [ ] no [ ] [ ] [ ] ____
Can patient smell or taste fumes or vapors during work?	yes [ ] no [ ]	yes [ ] no [ ]	yes [ ] no [ ]
Can other employees smell or taste fumes or vapors?	yes [ ] no [ ]	yes [ ] no [ ]	yes [ ] no [ ]
Side effects during exposure?	Patient Others NONE [ ] [ ] diarrhea [ ] [ ] dizziness [ ] [ ] headache [ ] [ ] nausea /vomit [ ] [ ] rash [ ] [ ] visual [ ] [ ] other ____	Patient Others NONE [ ] [ ] diarrhea [ ] [ ] dizziness [ ] [ ] headache [ ] [ ] nausea /vomit [ ] [ ] rash [ ] [ ] visual [ ] [ ] other ____	Patient Others NONE [ ] [ ] diarrhea [ ] [ ] dizziness [ ] [ ] headache [ ] [ ] nausea /vomit [ ] [ ] rash [ ] [ ] visual [ ] [ ] other ____

C. Herbal Exposure

INGREDIENT →	1.	2.
Indication?		
Amount	____ mg [ ] mL [ ] g [ ] % [ ]	____ mg [ ] mL [ ] g [ ] % [ ]
Exposure route	inhale [ ] skin [ ] oral [ ] inject [ ] other [ ]	inhale [ ] skin [ ] oral [ ] inject [ ] other [ ]
Start date		
Stop date		
Side effects during exposure?	NONE [ ] diarrhea [ ] headache [ ] nausea [ ] rash [ ] visual changes [ ] vomiting [ ] OTHER ____	NONE [ ] diarrhea [ ] headache [ ] nausea [ ] rash [ ] visual changes [ ] vomiting [ ] OTHER ____

D. Infectious Disease

AGENT	1.
Date of contact	
Contact type	direct with lesions [ ] oral [ ] school [ ] resp. secretions [ ] day-care [ ] household [ ] other ____
Date lesions seen on contact person	____
Patient had disease	N [ ] Y [ ] when ____
Method of diagnosis or contact	
Disease diagnosed in patient? *•by whom?*	N [ ] Y [ ] ____
Patient had relevant vaccinations? *date & type*	N [ ] Y [ ] ____

E. :Social Drug Use

Ethanol ☐N ☐Y wine during pregnancy: ____ glass ☐ bottle ☐ per day ☐ week ☐ weekend ☐ month ☐
beer during pregnancy: ____ glass ☐ bottle ☐ per day ☐ week ☐ weekend ☐ month ☐
liquor during pregnancy: ____ glass ☐ bottle ☐ per day ☐ week ☐ weekend ☐ month ☐
Date ethanol ingestion stopped ____ when pregnancy diagnosed ☐
additional information: ____

Tobacco ☐N ☐Y during pregnancy: ____ cigarettes per day ☐ week ☐ weekend ☐ month ☐
Date tobacco exposure stopped ____ when pregnancy diagnosed ☐
additional information ____

Cocaine ☐N ☐Y during pregnancy ____ per day ☐ week ☐ weekend ☐ month ☐
Marijuana ☐N ☐Y during pregnancy ____ per day ☐ week ☐ weekend ☐ month ☐
Heroin ☐N ☐Y during pregnancy ____ per day ☐ week ☐ weekend ☐ month ☐
LSD ☐N ☐Y during pregnancy ____ per day ☐ week ☐ weekend ☐ month ☐
Date above exposure stopped ____ when pregnancy diagnosed ☐
additional information ____

F. Miscellaneous Exposures

Radiation during pregnancy? ☐N ☐Y Describe (include type and dates): ____

Heat/Hyperthermia? ☐N ☐Y Describe (include type and dates): ____
(Jacuzzi, Saunas, Electric Blanket)

PAST MATERNAL MEDICAL HISTORY

Cancer ☐N ☐Y ____
Cardiovascular ☐N ☐Y ____
Central nervous system ☐N ☐Y ____
Diabetes ☐N ☐Y ____
Epilepsy ☐N ☐Y ____
Hematology ☐N ☐Y ____
Hypertension ☐N ☐Y ____
Renal disease ☐N ☐Y ____
Thyroid disease ☐N ☐Y ____
Other ____

GENETIC DISEASE/FAMILY HISTORY OF MALFORMATIONS ☐ no ☐ yes

Relative	Biological Family of Fetus	Condition
____________	☐ maternal ☐ paternal	____________
____________	☐ maternal ☐ paternal	____________
____________	☐ maternal ☐ paternal	____________
____________	☐ maternal ☐ paternal	____________
____________	☐ maternal ☐ paternal	____________

BIOLOGICAL FATHER DATA

Drug Name or Radiation Type	Start Date	Stop Date	Dose/Route/ Frequency	Indication
1.		☐ ongoing exposure		
2.		☐ ongoing exposure		

More details about medical condition: ____

Ethanol ☐N ☐Y wine _____ glass ☐ bottle ☐ per day ☐ week ☐ weekend ☐ month ☐
beer _____ glass ☐ bottle ☐ per day ☐ week ☐ weekend ☐ month ☐
liquor _____ glass ☐ bottle ☐ per day ☐ week ☐ weekend ☐ month ☐

Tobacco ☐N ☐Y _____ cigarettes per day ☐ week ☐ weekend ☐ month ☐

Cocaine ☐N ☐Y __________ per day ☐ week ☐ weekend ☐ month ☐
Marijuana ☐N ☐Y __________ per day ☐ week ☐ weekend ☐ month ☐
Heroin ☐N ☐Y __________ per day ☐ week ☐ weekend ☐ month ☐
LSD ☐N ☐Y __________ per day ☐ week ☐ weekend ☐ month ☐

SES

Mother

Occupation: ______________________

☐ unemployed ☐ homemaker

Highest Level of Education completed (circle one only)

Elementary: grade 5 6 7 8
High School: grade 9 10 11 12 13
College: 1 2 3 years
University: 1 2 3 years Bachelor
Graduate: Masters PhD PostDoctoral

Father

Occupation: ______________________

☐ unemployed

Highest Level of Education completed (circle one only)

Elementary: grade 5 6 7 8
High School: grade 9 10 11 12 13
College: 1 2 3 years
University: 1 2 3 years Bachelor
Graduate: Masters PhD PostDoctoral

Figure 22-2. (Continued)

VISUAL ANALOG

☐ currently pregnant
☐ planning a pregnancy
☐ retrospective

A. Tendency to continue / terminate pregnancy

would not terminate pregnancy ———————————— *will terminate pregnancy*

B. Patient's perception of risk of major birth defects in the fetus

NONE ***no chance*** *that baby will be born with birth defect* ———————————— ***100%*** *baby will definitely be born with a birth defect*

C. Patient's perception of baseline risk for birth defects in the general population

____

Pregnancy Follow Up
MOTHERISK PROGRAM

ID NUMBER ________________

Date of Interview: ________________

Interviewer: ________________

A. GENERAL

Mother's FIRST NAME ________________ Street Address ________________

Mother's LAST NAME ________________ City/Province ________________

Telephone (H) ____________ (W) ____________ Postal Code ________________

B. PREGNANCY OUTCOME

How did your pregnancy end? ☐ Live birth ☐ Miscarriage (<20 wks) ☐ Fetal Death (≥20wks) ☐ Elective abortion

If miscarriage, fetal death or elective abortion:

At how many weeks? ________

Were defects detected? ☐ No ☐ Yes

If Yes, describe ________________

How? By ☐ ultrasound ☐ amniocentesis

done at ________ weeks

If live birth: ☐ boy ☐ girl

Child's FIRST NAME ________________

Child's LAST NAME ________________

Child's DATE OF BIRTH ________________

Child's doctor ________________

street address ________________

city/province ________________

telephone ________________

C. DISEASES COMPLICATING PREGNANCY

Details: *diagnosis onset medication/doses hospitalization?*

Amniotic fluid alterations	☐ No ☐ Yes	
Cancer	☐ No ☐ Yes	
Cardiovascular	☐ No ☐ Yes	
Central nervous system	☐ No ☐ Yes	
Dermatology	☐ No ☐ Yes	
Ears, eyes, nose, throat	☐ No ☐ Yes	
Endocrine	☐ No ☐ Yes	
Gastrointestinal	☐ No ☐ Yes	
Genito-urinary	☐ No ☐ Yes	
Hematology	☐ No ☐ Yes	
Infectious Disease	☐ No ☐ Yes	
IUGR/growth problems	☐ No ☐ Yes	
Musculo-skeletal	☐ No ☐ Yes	
Psychiatric	☐ No ☐ Yes	
Respiratory	☐ No ☐ Yes	
OTHER		

TELEPHONE LOG

DATE/TIME	NUMBER DIALED	RESULT <VM>Verbal Message <MM>Machine Message <Busy> <OS>Out of Service <W>wrong number<NA>No Answer

D. EXPOSURES DURING PREGNANCY

- Did you use any **herbal** preparations?
- Did you use any **vitamins** (prenatal or other supplements)?
- Did you use anything for **allergies, anxiety, colds, constipation, depression, diarrhea, headache, heartburn, pain, weightloss**?

Over-the-Counter/Prescription medications and Radiation

	Drug Name or Radiation Type	Start Date	Stop Date	Dose (mg,g,mL)	Frequency (od,qhs,bid,tid)
1			ongoing ☐		
2			ongoing ☐		
3			ongoing ☐		
4			ongoing ☐		

	Indication for Medication	*Prescribing Physician*	*Details about medical condition*
1.			
2.			
3.			
4.			

Social Drugs/Others		Dose	Frequency	Started	Stopped
Ethanol	wine [] ☐ no	______ ounce [ ]	per day [] week [] weekend [] month []		
	liquor [] ☐ no	______ glass [ ]			
	beer [] ☐ no	______ bottle [ ]			
Tobacco	☐ no	______ cigarettes	per day [] week [] weekend [] month []		
Cocaine	☐ no		per day [] week [] weekend [] month []		
Heroin	☐ no		per day [] week [] weekend [] month []		
Marijuana	☐ no		per day [] week [] weekend [] month []		
Heat	jaccuzi [] ☐ no		per day [] week [] weekend [] month []		
	electric blanket [] ☐ no		per day [] week [] weekend [] month []		
Radiation	☐ no		per day [] week [] weekend [] month []		
Exercise	☐ no		per day [] week [] weekend [] month []		

Occupation during pregnancy (what does she do?) ________________

Started ____________ Stopped ____________ Reason for Stopping ____________

EXPOSURES? chemical ☐ no ☐ yes: ________________

computer ☐ no ☐ yes: ________________

radiation ☐ no ☐ yes: ________________

noise/vibration ☐ no ☐ yes: ________________

E. TESTS DURING PREGNANCY

1. Triple screening	☐ no ☐ yes:	at ____ weeks	Reason ____________
2. Amniocentesis	☐ no ☐ yes:	at ____ weeks	Reason ____________
3. Glucose Tolerance Test	☐ no ☐ yes:	at ____ weeks	Reason ____________
4. Ultrasound	☐ no ☐ yes:	at ____ weeks	Reason ____________
		at ____ weeks	Reason ____________
		at ____ weeks	Reason ____________
5. Chorionic villus sampling	☐ no ☐ yes:	at ____ weeks	Reason ____________
6. Other ____________	☐ no ☐ yes:	at ____ weeks	Reason ____________

RESULTS: # ___: ____________
___: ____________
___: ____________
___: ____________
___: ____________

F. DELIVERY INFORMATION

Maternal

Weight pre-pregnancy ______ lb ______ kg
gain ______ lb ______ kg
Total length of labour ________ hours
PROM? ☐ no ☐ yes: ______ hours before onset of labour
(Premature Rupture of Membranes)

Method ☐ vaginal, vertex ☐ C/S emergency
☐ vaginal, breech ☐ C/S repeat
☐ C/S scheduled
reason: ____________

Assistance: ☐ vacuum
☐ forceps

Hemorrhage? ☐ no ☐ yes
Transfusion? ☐ no ☐ yes
Pain relief? Anaesthetics ☐ no ☐ yes
epidural ☐ no ☐ yes
analgesic ☐ no ☐ yes
specify: ____________

Neonatal

Hospital/City ____________
Gestational age at birth ______ weeks ______ days
Birth weight ______ lb ______ oz (________ grams)
1 oz=28.4 g

Head Circumference ________ cm
Length ________ cm
Apgar scores 1 minute ______ 5 minute ______

A ppearance
P ulse
G rimace
A muscle activity
R espiration

Fetal Monitoring ☐ no ☐ yes external [ ] internal [ ]
explain ____________
Fetal distress ☐ no ☐ yes
explain ____________
Meconium ☐ no ☐ yes

For our own documentation, which will help other women exposed to the same drug that you were exposed to, would you share with us whether your child was born with any birth defects?

DEFECTS ☐ no ☐ yes Refused to answer ☐

____
____
____
____

Figure 22-3. The Follow-Up Form.

G. NEONATAL HEALTH

Health in hospital intensive care? ☐ no ☐ yes Home at: ________ days
____
____
____

Breast feeding ☐ no ☐ yes stopped ______ months
Medication during lactation ? ☐ no ☐ yes (specify details in section D)
Name: ____________
Infant side effects? ☐ no ☐ yes: ____________
Formula feeding ☐ no ☐ yes started ______ months stopped ______ months
Solids ☐ not yet ☐ yes started ______ months type: ____________
Problems with feeding? ☐ no ☐ yes explain: ____________

Infant health problems since discharge from hospital?

			Details: *diagnosis onset medication dose hospitalization?*
Cancer	☐ No	☐ Yes	____________
Cardiovascular	☐ No	☐ Yes	____________
Central nervous system	☐ No	☐ Yes	____________
Dermatology	☐ No	☐ Yes	____________
Ears, eyes, nose, throat	☐ No	☐ Yes	____________
Endocrine	☐ No	☐ Yes	____________
Gastrointestinal	☐ No	☐ Yes	____________
Genito-urinary	☐ No	☐ Yes	____________
Hematology	☐ No	☐ Yes	____________
Infectious Disease	☐ No	☐ Yes	____________
Musculo-skeletal	☐ No	☐ Yes	____________
Respiratory	☐ No	☐ Yes	____________
OTHER ____________			

H. MILESTONES

At what age did the infant first:		*Normal range*
Smile (recognition)	________	[2 months]
Lift head on own	________	[3 months]
Sit unaided	________	[6-8 months]
Crawl	________	[8-10 months]
Stand on own	________	[8-10 months]
Speak first word	________	[8-12 months]
Walk unaided	________	[12-15 months]

Infant's age at followup ________ months
Infant's weight ________ kg (______ lb ______ oz)
as of: ☐ follow up ☐ last MD visit
Infant's height/length ______ cm (______ inches)
as of: ☐ follow up ☐ last MD visit
Last MD visit : ____________ (date or baby's age)

I. CONSENT

We would like to send a letter to your child's doctor to confirm medical details of this follow-up. May we have your verbal permission to send this?

OBTAINED CONSENT? ☐ No ☐ Yes

Date letter sent: ____________ Date letter received: ____________

inconsistent or controversial the systematic reviews are an effective way to summarize the data and reach an overall consensus about the risks or safety in human pregnancy. Additionally, as new reports or studies concerning exposures in pregnancy or lactation are published they are brought to weekly rounds attended by all team members where they are critically appraised and reviewed. For new agents, and periodically for older agents, the manufacturer is consulted regarding any unpublished reports concerning the drug. This includes both animal reproductive/teratology studies as well as postmarketing surveillance reports in humans. These may be in the form of a registry collated and updated by the manufacturer periodically or voluntary reports of inadvertent pregnancy exposure. Information collected throughout this process is then summarized and incorporated into the reproductive risk monographs for further use by all team members.

TECHNICAL SUPPORT

Operation within the Hospital for Sick Children allows the program, and all staff members, to be connected to a hospital-wide information network, which provides access to the library and various literature retrieval sources. In addition, as a teaching centre the hospital is affiliated with the University of Toronto. The university also provides further access by faculty, graduate students and postgraduate trainees to numerous other catalogues databases and electronic journals directly via the internet. The ability to search and retrieve literature from an individual workspace has dramatically changed the way researchers and clinicians access information and update their knowledge base. For Motherisk it has increased efficiency by allowing for more rapid identification and retrieval of relevant reference material. As an example, the program subscribes to the computerized and on-line ReproTox Database.[39] This comprehensive resource provides details reproductive summaries on an extensive list of agents. The subscription provides quarterly updates for the desktop version and more frequent updates at its web site summaries.

EDUCATION

Throughout the academic year, including the summer session, undergraduate, graduate, and postgraduate trainees (research fellows) all participate in daily activities and research activities within the Motherisk program. Undergraduate students from the University of Toronto, usually members of the departments of pharmacology, toxicology, or pharmacy, conduct their own research projects, alone or within a group, under the supervision of other team members. Prior to commencing research activities, however, new students undergo intensive training, which includes a series of formal lectures, reading assignments, and observation. Medical students also conduct research projects or may briefly attend the program as an observer. Graduate students and postgraduate trainees often conduct several research projects of their own along with supervising undergraduate activities. Various annual meetings, such as the OTIS meeting provide a forum for trainees to present their research results to peers and colleagues outside of the program. The educational activities of the program have proven to be an invaluable learning experience for students and faculty alike and have provided ongoing opportunities for expanding our research endeavors.

FINANCIAL SUPPORT

Each year the hospital allocates a portion of its funds from the Ontario Ministry of Health to the Motherisk program. This funding supports the positions of three counselors and minimal administrative costs. Furthermore, some positions are filled as part of the educational curriculum of trainees. Since counseling and follow-up may ultimately contribute to research activities, funding for some counseling, administrative support and computer costs is often supplemented with external research or service grants. In addition to the director, several team members also participate as principal investigators and are able to secure their own funding for projects and trainees frequently obtain educational funds to conduct their research.

SUMMARY

Ensuring the well being of all unborn children is impossible without appropriate resources and informed patients. Antiquated attitudes have propagated misinformation among medical professionals and lay persons alike. Our own experience has shown that this has often resulted in disastrous outcomes, such as termination of an otherwise wanted pregnancy[40,41] or irrational fears and inadequate maternal treatment. Settings such as are own, are ideal in promoting evidence based risk assessments to large numbers of patients and health care providers, while maintaining educational and research portfolios.

The Motherisk program has initiated and sustained an effective approach to counseling in the field of reproductive toxicology. Time and experience have proven invaluable as we have striven to accomplish our goals of providing authoritative information on infant or fetal risk after maternal exposure to drugs, chemicals, or infectious diseases. Moreover, our prospective method of data collection minimizes recall bias and enables us to accurately accumulate patient details and pregnancy outcome data routinely. These activities allow us to provide information in areas for which there are shortcomings in the current medical literature. We look forward to the changes and challenges the next decade brings.

REFERENCES

1. Koren G, Pastuszak A, Ito S. Drugs in pregnancy. *N Engl J Med.* 1998;338:1128–1137.
2. Koren G, Klein N. Bias against negative studies in newspaper reports of medical research. *JAMA.* 1991;266:1824–1826.
3. Koren G, Feldman Y, Shear N. Motherisk—A new approach to drug/chemical teratogenicity. *Vet Hum Toxicol.* 1986;28:563–565.
4. Mazzotta P, Stewart DE, Koren G, et al. Factors associated with elective termination of pregnancy among Canadian and American women with nausea and vomiting of pregnancy. *J Psychosom Obstet Gynaecol.* 2001;22:7–12.
5. Mazzotta P, Maltepe C, Navioz Y, et al. Attitudes, management and consequences of nausea and vomiting of pregnancy in the United States and Canada. *Int J Gynaecol Obstet.* 2000;70:359–365.
6. Mazzotta P, Magee LA, Maltepe C, et al. The perception of teratogenic risk by women with nausea and vomiting of pregnancy. *Reprod Toxicol.* 1999;13:313–319.

7. Magee LA, Chandra K, Mazzotta P, et al. Development of a health-related quality of life instrument for nausea and vomiting of pregnancy. *Am J Obstet Gynecol.* 2002;186:S232–S238.
8. Anonymous. Motherisk Helpline for women suffering from nausea and vomiting during pregnancy (NVP). *The Motherisk Newsletter.* 1998;Spring:5.
9. Mazzotta P, Gupta A, Maltepe C, et al. Pharmacologic treatment of nausea and vomiting during pregnancy. *Can Fam Physician.* 1998; 44:1455–1457.
10. Leduc C. Treating morning sickness by non-pharmacological means. *The Motherisk Newsletter.* 1998;Spring:6–7.
11. Mazzota P, Magee L, Koren G. Therapeutic abortions due to severe morning sickness. Unacceptable combination. *Can Fam Physician.* 1997;43:1055–1057.
12. Magee LA, Mazzotta P, Koren G. Evidence-based view of safety and effectiveness of pharmacologic therapy for nausea and vomiting of pregnancy (NVP). *Am J Obstet Gynecol.* 2002;186:S256–S261.
13. Mazzotta P, Stewart D, Atanackovic G, et al. Psychosocial morbidity among women with nausea and vomiting of pregnancy: prevalence and association with anti-emetic therapy. *J Psychosom Obstet Gynaecol.* 2000;21:129–136.
14. Bishai R, Mazzotta P, Atanackovic G, et al. Critical appraisal of drug therapy for nausea and vomiting of pregnancy: II. Efficacy and safety of diclectin (doxylamine-B6). *Can J Clin Pharmacol.* 2000;7:138–143.
15. Emelianova S, Mazzotta P, Einarson A, et al. Prevalence and severity of nausea and vomiting of pregnancy and effect of vitamin supplementation. *Clin Invest Med.* 1999;22:106–110.
16. Mazzotta P, Loebstein R, Koren G. Treating allergic rhinitis in pregnancy. Safety considerations. *Drug Saf.* 1999;20:361–375.
17. Koren G, Magee L, Attard C, et al. A novel method for the evaluation of the severity of nausea and vomiting of pregnancy. *Eur J Obstet Gynecol Reprod Biol.* 2001;94:31–36.
18. Koren G, Boskovic R, Hard M, et al. Motherisk-PUQE (pregnancy-unique quantification of emesis and nausea) scoring system for nausea and vomiting of pregnancy. *Am J Obstet Gynecol.* 2002;186: S228–S231.
19. Levichek Z, Atanackovic G, Oepkes D, et al. Nausea and vomiting of pregnancy. Evidence-based treatment algorithm. *Can Fam Physician.* 2002;48:267–268, 277.
20. Boskovic R, Einarson A, Maltepe C, et al. Diclectin therapy for nausea and vomiting of pregnancy: effects of optimal dosing. *J Obstet Gynaecol Can.* 2003;25:830–833.
21. Baggley A, Navioz Y, Maltepe C, et al. Determinants of women's decision making on whether to treat nausea and vomiting of pregnancy pharmacologically. *J Midwifery Womens Health.* 2004;49:350–354.
22. Einarson A, Maltepe C, Navioz Y, et al. The safety of ondansetron for nausea and vomiting of pregnancy: a prospective comparative study. *BJOG.* 2004;111:940–943.
23. Koren G, Maltepe C. Pre-emptive therapy for severe nausea and vomiting of pregnancy and hyperemesis gravidarum. *J Obstet Gynaecol.* 2004;24:530–533.
24. Koren G, Maltepe C, Navioz Y, et al. Recall bias of the symptoms of nausea and vomiting of pregnancy. *Am J Obstet Gynecol.* 2004; 190:485–488.
25. Koren G, Piwko C, Ahn E, et al. Validation studies of the Pregnancy Unique-Quantification of Emesis (PUQE) scores. *J Obstet Gynaecol.* 2005;25:241–244.
26. Atanackovic G, Navioz Y, Moretti ME, et al. The safety of higher than standard dose of doxylamine-pyridoxine (Diclectin) for nausea and vomiting of pregnancy. *J Clin Pharmacol.* 2001;41:842–845.
27. King S. A Motherisk HIV Healthline update. *The Motherisk Newsletter.* 1998;Fall:3,8.
28. Ratnaplan S, King S, Koren G. Testing women for HIV. *Can Fam Physician.* 1997;43:1349–1351.
29. Anonymous. The Motherisk HIV Healthline and Network. *The Motherisk Newsletter.* 1998;Spring:5.
30. Jayaraman GC, Preiksaitis JK, Larke B. Mandatory reporting of HIV infection and opt-out prenatal screening for HIV infection: effect on testing rates. *CMAJ.* 2003;168:679–682.
31. Anonymous. New toll-free helpline—Alcohol and substance usein pregnancy. *The Motherisk Newsletter.* 1998;Fall:2.
32. Djulus J, Moretti M, Koren G. Marijuana use and breastfeeding. *Can Fam Physician.* 2005;51:349–350.
33. Sarkar M, Djulus J, Koren G. When a cocaine-using mother wishes to breastfeed: proposed guidelines. *Ther Drug Monit.* 2005;27:1–2.
34. Ho E, Karimi-Tabesh L, Koren G. Characteristics of pregnant women who use ecstasy (3, 4-methylenedioxymethamphetamine). *Neurotoxicol Teratol.* 2001;23:561–567.
35. Ho E, Collantes A, Kapur BM, et al. Alcohol and breast feeding: calculation of time to zero level in milk. *Biol Neonate.* 2001;80:219–222.
36. Koren G. *Maternal-fetal toxicology: a clinician's guide.* 3rd ed., rev. and expanded ed. New York: Marcel Dekker;2001.
37. Briggs GG, Freeman RK, Yaffe SJ. *Drugs in pregnancy and lactation—A reference guide to fetal and neonatal risk.* 7th ed ed. Philadelphia, Pa: Lippincott Williams & Wilkins;2005.
38. *Drugs and Human Lactation.* 2 ed. Amsterdam: Elsevier;1996.
39. *Reproductive Toxicology.* Bethesda, MD.:2005.
40. Koren G, Pastuszak A. Prevention of unnecessary pregnancy terminations by counselling women on drug, chemical, and radiation exposure during the first trimester. *Teratology.* 1990;41:657–661.
41. Koren G, Bologa M, Long D, et al. Perception of teratogenic risk by pregnant women exposed to drugs and chemicals during the first trimester. *Am J Obstet Gynecol.* 1989;160:1190–1194.

CHAPTER 23

THE WAY WOMEN PERCEIVE TERATOGENIC RISK: HOW IT CAN INFLUENCE DECISION MAKING DURING PREGNANCY REGARDING DRUG USE OR ABORTION OF A WANTED PREGNANCY

Adrienne Einarson

The practice of medicine is an evolving process, which changes as time goes by. What was an effective treatment last year may well be harmful this year. In fact, the pendulum can swing very widely from one extreme to the other at any given time and in the field of teratology, this has been especially true. Prior to the 1950s it was thought that there was a "placental barrier" through which nothing could cross, so it did not matter to what a woman was exposed during her pregnancy. However, since the thalidomide tragedy, it is widely believed that women should not be exposed to anything as it could potentially harm the fetus. Each exposure should be individually evaluated, and evidence-based information given to the woman and her healthcare provider, to allow them to make an informed decision on whether or not to take a particular drug and the like during pregnancy. At Motherisk and at other groups, some studies have been carried to assess how women and their health care providers perceive teratogenic risk. Below are some examples of studies that have been carried out in this area.

EFFECTS OF FRAMING ON TERATOGENIC RISK PERCEPTION IN PREGNANT WOMEN AND THEIR HEALTH CARE PROVIDERS

We examined the effects of information presentation (framing) on women's perception of fetal risk, and their intention to use a safe drug during pregnancy. Participants were successive female Motherisk callers (already, or planning to be, pregnant) seeking information about use of allergy-related drugs during pregnancy. Drugs included oral formulations, nasal sprays, and injections; none had been shown to increase teratogenic risk above baseline, 125 participants were included: 64 in the positive frame and 61 in the negative frame. However, only 105 participants were successfully contacted in follow-up. All women successfully contacted in follow-up agreed to participate.

After completing a standard intake form, callers were invited to participate in a study assessing "different ways of presenting information to callers." After giving verbal consent, callers were randomly assigned to baseline teratogenic-risk information in the positive (55 women) or negative (50) frame. Callers who received negatively-framed baseline information (the standard form of counseling at Motherisk) were told: "In every pregnancy, there is a 1–3% chance that a woman will give birth to a child who has a major birth defect. This/these drug(s) [insert applicable drug name] has/have not been shown to change that." Callers receiving positively framed baseline information were told: "In every pregnancy, there is a 97–99% chance that a woman will give birth to a child who does not have a major birth defect. This/these drug(s) [insert applicable drug name] has/have not been shown to change that."

Follow-up calls to participants were made 1–4 days after the first call. During follow-up, women were asked to (1) rate their likelihood of having a child with a birth defect as a result of using allergy-related drugs on a 5-point scale ranging from 1, "very low", to 5, "very high", with 3 being "moderate"; (2) rate their likelihood of having a child with a birth defect as a result of using allergy-related medications on a 100-point scale ranging from zero, "0% or absolutely no chance", to 100, "100% or definite chance"; and (3) indicate whether or not they were going to take the drug(s) in question. Data were compared between the framing groups with the Mann-Whitney U test (question 1), unpaired t test (2), and (3). In terms of risk perception, the two scales gave almost the same information. Binomial tests and one-sample t tests against the values of 3, 4, and 5 together (five-point scale) and 50 (100-point scale), respectively, showed that both groups estimated their risk of having a child with a birth defect as a result of allergy-related drug use as being low (all p values <0.05). Participants who had received positively-framed information, however, gave lower estimates of risk than those who received negatively-framed information.

This difference, though, was significant only for the 100-point risk estimation scale ($p = 0.0484$). Previous research, with a validated in-clinic visual analogue scale, has shown that mean estimates are 25% before Motherisk counseling.

Results showed no significant difference in the proportion of callers who said that they would take the medication in question. (A "no" decision included those who said "no" and those who said "no, probably not." Under positive framing, 10 women responded "no" and 23 women responded "no, probably not." Under negative framing, seven women said "no", and 29 said "no, probably not"). However, there was a tendency for callers receiving information in the positive frame to respond with "yes" more so than callers in the negative frame ($p = 0.126$). Almost twice as many women responded "yes" under positive, compared with negative, framing, 34% versus 20%, respectively. However, this difference was not significant and even with positive framing more than 65% of women chose not to take their medication. An additional É‘2 analysis was done with three categories instead of two: "yes," "no," and "no, probably not." The result (É‘2 = 3.43, $p = 0.180$), though nonsignificant, suggested that the increased proportion of "yes" responses under positive framing (by comparison with negative framing) came from callers switching from "no, probably not" to "yes," rather than from "no" to "yes."

Our results accord with those of previous work showing that framing manipulations can alter risk perceptions as well as decision-making. We showed that presentation of teratogenic risk information to women in terms of the probability of giving birth to a normal child lowers their perception of risk, and increases the likelihood that they will take their medication, more than does presentation of the same information in terms of the probability of giving birth to a malformed child. Subtle changes in framing do make a substantial difference to people's responses.[1]

HOW MISPERCEPTION OF TERATOGENIC RISK, IMPACTS ON WHETHER A WOMAN USES A NEEDED DRUG IN PREGNANCY

Nausea and vomiting of pregnancy (NVP) affects up to 80% of all women to some degree during their pregnancies. Diclectin (doxylamine and pyridoxine [vitamin B6]) has been on the Canadian market for many years and is indicated as the drug of choice for the treatment of NVP. However, some women choose not to treat NVP with pharmacologic measures, perhaps due to a persistent fear of teratogenic risk. The objective of this study was to determine the factors that influence a woman's decision not to treat NVP with pharmacologic measures. Fifty-nine women recruited from the Motherisk Nausea and Vomiting Helpline completed a questionnaire. All were informed that Diclectin was considered safe for use during pregnancy. At a follow-up telephone call, 34% were not using any pharmacologic treatment, and of those who were taking the drug, 26% were using less than the recommended dose. Reasons cited for not using the medication were insufficient safety data, preference for nonpharmacologic methods, and being made to feel uncomfortable by the physician. Of the women who did use Diclectin, the most convincing reassuring information that it was safe to use came from friends and family.[2]

The World Health Organization predicts that by 2012, depression will be the number one disease in the world. Thus, many women who become pregnant will require treatment with antidepressants. We are aware that women and their health care providers remain hesitant to prescribe and take these drugs during pregnancy, despite evidence of the relative safety. The objectives of our study were: (1) To determine perception of risk of antidepressant drugs by pregnant women with depression, (2) to determine the efficacy of evidence-based counseling, and (3) to identify determinants that influence women in their decision-making regarding the continuation/discontinuation of antidepressants during pregnancy. Women who called the Motherisk program requesting information about the safety of an antidepressant during pregnancy were compared with two other groups: (1) Women who called about antibiotic use (i.e., nonteratogenic drugs used short-term) and (2) women who called about gastric medications (i.e., nonteratogenic drugs used long-term). Their perception of risk was measured before and after evidenced-based information was given and determinants of decision-making were also evaluated.

We recruited 100 women taking antidepressants during pregnancy and 100 in each comparison group. Despite receiving evidence-based reassuring information, 15% of antidepressant users, compared to 4% using gastric drugs and 1% using antibiotics, chose to discontinue their medication. The main determinants of decision-making were based on: information received prior to calling Motherisk, family and friends advice, the internet, sequence of advice given, and if a women was undecided at the time of call.

Women continue to fear taking antidepressants during pregnancy, more so than non psychiatric drugs, however, evidence based counseling can lower this fear, although not totally. Deciding whether to continue to take a medication or not during pregnancy, is a complex decision for women and their healthcare providers to make (see Table 23-1).

In both these studies, we demonstrated that despite the fact that women are given reassuring information regarding the safety of exposures during pregnancy, their increased perception of risk cannot be completely eradicated.[3]

HOW THE LABELING OF DRUGS USED IN PREGNANCY AFFECT PERCEPTION OF TERATOGENIC RISK

The objectives of this study were the following: (1) to characterize the perception of teratogenic risk by pregnant women and their partners and by health professionals and (2) to examine the most reassuring way to present data on a drug for nausea and vomiting of pregnancy that has been proven to be safe to the fetus. A convenience sample of pregnant Canadian women and their partners, pharmacists, nurses, physicians, and hospital workers were asked to choose the *safest* among four drugs by statements describing their safety. Although the text of all four was similar, the title and narrative were modified to be more or less *reassuring* by the use of more or less terms such as malformations and abnormalities. Health professionals rated the teratogenic risk significantly lower than the parents, but even they rated the drugs as not safe, despite a scientifically reassuring text. Sixty percent of the 240 participants, regardless of their perception of teratogenic risk, believed the four drugs were of similar risks. However, in the other 40%, the

Table 23-1
Effectiveness of Counseling

PERCEPTION OF RISK (PRECOUNSELING)*	PERCEPTION OF RISK (POSTCOUNSELING)	P VALUE
87% of depressed women rated risk of antidepressants as greater than 1–3%	12% of depressed women rated risk of antidepressants as greater than 1–3%	<0.001
56% of women with gastric problems rated risk of medications as greater than 1–3%	4% of women with gastric problems rated risk of medications as greater than 1–3%	<0.001
22% of women with infections rated the risk of medications greater than 1–3%	2% of women with infections rated the risk of medications greater than 1–3%	<0.001

* Actual baseline rate for major malformations in the general population is 1–3%.

less reassuring text led to higher teratogenic perception, and the more reassuring options tended to decrease the false perception of teratogenic risk. It was concluded that in general, four different versions of reassuring text describing a scientifically proven safe drug in pregnancy did not lead expecting parents to believe they were safe. Among those who did not rank the four drugs as having equal safety/risk, the less reassuring text led to a higher perception of teratogenic risk. Even health professionals reading the labels describing safe drugs rated them as unsafe. Presently, the perception of teratogenic risk is strong even for safe drugs and is difficult to change even with evidence-based facts.[4]

UNREALISTIC FEARS OF RADIATION EXPOSURE

There is great concern about exposure to radiation during pregnancy, so much so, that some women will go through with an elective abortion of a wanted pregnancy, because of the perceived teratogenic risk. We conducted two studies to quantify this misperception. In our first study, we interviewed women attending the clinic at the Motherisk Program for counseling about diagnostic radiation in pregnancy (n = 50) and compared them with a control group of women exposed to nonteratogenic drugs and chemicals (n = 48). Before receiving known information about the specific exposure, women exposed to radiation assigned themselves a significantly higher teratogenic risk compared with the control group (25.5 +/− 4.3% vs. 15.7 +/− 3.0% for major malformations, $P < 0.01$). The post-consultation perception of teratogenic risk did not differ between the two groups. Special consideration and attention should be given when counseling pregnant women exposed to low-dose ionizing radiation, as their misperception of teratogenic risk may lead them to unnecessary termination of their pregnancy.[5]

The objective of our second study was to determine family physicians' and obstetricians' perceptions of the risk of major fetal malformations associated with exposure to radiation from radiography and CT during early pregnancy. Structured questionnaires were sent to 400 family physicians and 100 obstetricians selected randomly across Ontario, Canada. The physicians were informed about the 1–3% baseline risk for major malformations and were asked about their perceptions of the risk to the fetus associated with an abdominal radiograph and an abdominal CT scan during early pregnancy and whether they would recommend a therapeutic abortion after such exposure.

Fifty-five percent (218/400) of the family physicians and 69% (69/100) of the obstetricians responded to our questionnaire. Forty-four percent of family physicians estimated the risk associated with an abdominal radiograph to be 5% or greater, and 61% estimated the risk associated with an abdominal CT scan to be 5% or greater. Eleven percent of obstetricians estimated the risk associated with radiographs to be 5% or greater ($p < 0.001$), and 34% estimated the risk associated with CT scans to be 5% or greater ($p < 0.001$). Among family physicians, 1% recommended an abortion if the fetus was exposed to radiation from radiography and 6% after exposure to radiation from CT. None of the obstetricians recommended an abortion after exposure to radiation from an abdominal radiograph, but 5% recommended an abortion after exposure to radiation from an abdominal CT scan in early pregnancy. Our survey showed that physicians who care for pregnant women perceive the teratogenic risk associated with an abdominal radiograph and an abdominal CT scan to be unrealistically high during early pregnancy.[6]

HIGH PERCEPTION OF TERATOGENIC RISK OF DRUGS COMMONLY USED BY PREGNANT WOMEN

Another group assessed the perception teratogenic risk of common medication by professionals and lay people. A visual-analogue scale was used to measure the perceived percentage of mothers who will deliver a child with a malformation, including those exposed to a list of drugs. Fifteen general practitioners, 10 gynecologists, 106 preclinical students, 150 students in their clinical training, 81 pregnant women, and 63 nonpregnant women were interviewed.

The perception of the teratogenic risk related to medication used in pregnancy was higher than the recognised risk in all groups, and for all drugs. The risk associated with safe medications was perceived to be higher by nonpregnant women as compared with the pregnant women. Pregnant women perceived the medication associated risk to be higher than physicians did for all drugs included in the questionnaire.[7]

TERMINATION OF PREGNANCY BECAUSE OF UNREALISTIC FEARS OF TERATOGENIC RISK

The main goal of counseling women on their teratogenic risk is to present to them an accurate, up-to-date estimate of their specific risks. However, the same data may be received and interpreted very differently by different patients, leading them to individual conclusions and finally to the decision to continue or terminate pregnancy. While pregnancies are terminated for a variety of reasons, incorrect perception of a teratogenic risk may be an important factor. As documented by the Greek experience after the Chernobyl disaster, even an unbiased suggestion of adverse fetal outcome may prompt women to terminate pregnancy "to be on the safe side."[8]

As part of our approach to counseling pregnant women at Motherisk concerned about exposure to drugs, chemicals, or radiation, we measured their tendency to terminate their pregnancy by using a visual analogue scale (VAS). Analysis of 78 cases where women had less than 50% tendency to continue pregnancy before they were advised by us reveals that 61 decided to continue their pregnancy after the consultation (57 normal, healthy infants, four miscarriages) and 17 terminated. Women who continued their pregnancy significantly changed their tendency after we discussed relevant information with them (from 34.3 +/− 2.5% to 84.5 +/− 3.3%, $P < 0.00001$), whereas most of those who eventually terminated pregnancy did not change their tendency to continue pregnancy beyond the 50% mark (from 24.8 +/− 5.4% to 45.1 +/− 9.8%) ($P > 0.1$). Only two of the women who terminated their pregnancy were exposed to teratogenic drugs; however, in most other cases, other obvious reasons, unrelated to the exposure in question, were identified by the women as leading reasons for termination. An appropriate intervention in early pregnancy can prevent unnecessary pregnancy terminations by correcting misinformation and thereby decreasing the unrealistically high perception of risk by women exposed to nonteratogens.[9]

After confirming the clinical relevance of the VAS, we now use the information collected, not only for epidemiological endpoints, but also for individual cases. For example, if after the interview the woman has a tendency of termination higher than 50%, it is probably that she will not continue her pregnancy. If we are impressed that the teratogenic risk is the main reason for her tendency, and not other social, psychological, or personal reasons, we extend the interview to explain again the lack of risk associated with her exposure.

In summary, the aim at the Motherisk program is to give accurate up-to-date evidence-based information of exposures during pregnancy. Over the years we have realized, that this is not always enough to allay a woman's fears regarding teratogenicity of certain drugs and other exposures. We found that high initial risk perception was associated with less chance of continuing the medication or continuing the pregnancy. Despite receiving reassuring information, many women still decide to discontinue the medication or sometimes the pregnancy. Discontinuers of medication often reported that the first source that they discussed the safety of the medication use in pregnancy was negative and advised discontinuation. Consequently, it appears that the sequence of advice received is also important to those women in their decision-making.

However, most women who are given reassuring information by the Motherisk team, do continue on in their pregnancy without concern about their particular exposure.

REFERENCES

1. Jasper JD, Goel R, Einarson A, et al. Effects of framing on teratogenic risk perception in pregnant women. *Lancet.* 2002 May 11; 359(9318):1702.
2. Baggley A, Navioz Y, Maltepe C, et al. Determinants of women's decision making on whether to treat nausea and vomiting of pregnancy pharmacologically. *J Midwifery Womens Health.* 2004 Jul–Aug; 49(4):350–354.
3. Bonari L, Koren G, Einarson TR, et al. Use of antidepressants by pregnant women: Evaluation of perception of risk, efficacy of evidence based counseling and determinants of decision making. (In press) Archives of Women's Mental Health 2005.
4. Pole M, Einarson A, Pairaudeau N, et al. Drug labeling and risk perceptions of teratogenicity: a survey of pregnant Canadian women and their health professionals. *J Clin Pharmacol.* 2000 Jun;40(6):573–577.
5. Bentur Y, Horlatsch N, Koren G. Exposure to ionizing radiation during pregnancy: perception of teratogenic risk and outcome. *Teratology.* 1991 Feb; 43(2):109–112.
6. Ratnapalan S, Bona N, Chandra K, et al. Physicians' perceptions of teratogenic risk associated with radiography and CT during early pregnancy. *AJR Am J Roentgenol.* 2004 May;182(5):1107–1109.
7. Sanz E, Gomez-Lopez T, Martinez-Quintas MJ. Perception of teratogenic risk of common medicines. *Eur J Obstet Gynecol Reprod Biol.* 2001 Mar;95(1):127–131.
8. Trichopoulos D, Zavitsanos X, Koutis C, et al. The victims of Chemobyl in Greece: Induced abortions after the accident. *Br Med J.* 1987;295:1100.
9. Koren G, Pastuszak A. Prevention of unnecessary pregnancy terminations by counseling women on drug, chemical, and radiation exposure during the first trimester. *Teratology.* 1990 Jun;41(6):657–661.

PART II

MASTER; MOTHERISK ARCHIVES OF SYSTEMATIC AND EVALUATIVE REVIEWS

The field of reproductive toxicology struggles with wide gaps of knowledge regarding human exposure. Even when epidemiological human studies are published, they often contradict each other and the practicing clinician cannot put them into clinical context.

In 1988, we conducted the first systematic review, dedicated to the most commonly used drug for morning sickness, Bendectin, which was removed from the American market in 1983. The method used for this study was developed and has been refined since then by Tom Einarson of the University of Toronto and Motherisk team. This method (Chap. 24), was directly operative in the Health Canada review of diclectin (the generic form of Bendectin), leading the Canadian government to label the drug for morning sickness and hence support its use by millions of Canadian women. This meta-analysis, of the largest number of studies ever conducted in pregnancy for one drug, has ever since served as a benchmark of what could be done to ensure safe use of medications.

Since then the Motherisk program has conducted and published over 40 systematic reviews and meta-analyses involving fetal exposure to drugs, chemicals, and infectious agents.

This volume is the first attempt to put this knowledge under one roof. MASTER (Motherisk Archives of Systematic and Evaluative Reviews) will be also updated online as more systematic reviews are updated and published.

Alejandro A. Nava-Ocampo, MD and
Gideon Koren, MD

SECTION 1

METHODOLOGICAL ASPECTS

CHAPTER 24

A METHOD FOR META-ANALYSIS OF EPIDEMIOLOGICAL STUDIES

Thomas R. Einarson, J. Steven Leeder, and Gideon Koren

THOMAS R. EINARSON, Ph.D., is a Pharmacist with the MotheRisk Program, Division of Clinical Pharmacology, Department of Pediatrics, Hospital for Sick Children, and a member of the Faculty of Pharmacy, University of Toronto; J. STEVEN LEEDER, Pharm. D., is a Pharmacist with the MotheRisk Program, and a Fellow of the Medical Research Council of Canada; and GIDEON KOREN, M.D., is the Director of the MotheRisk Program, and a career scientist of the Ontario Ministry of Health, Toronto, Ontario. Reprints: Thomas R. Einarson, Ph.D., Faculty of Pharmacy, University of Toronto, 19 Russell St., Toronto, ON M5S IA1.

Abstract

This article presents a stepwise approach for conducting a meta-analysis of epidemiological studies based on proposed guidelines. This systematic method is recommended for practitioners evaluating epidemiological studies in the literature to arrive at an overall quantitative estimate of the impact of a treatment. Bendectin is used as an illustrative example. Meta-analysts should establish a priori the purpose of the analysis and a complete protocol. This protocol should be adhered to, and all steps performed should be recorded in detail. To aid in developing such a protocol, we present methods the researcher can use to perform each of 22 steps in six major areas. The illustrative meta-analysis confirmed previous traditional narrative literature reviews that Bendectin is not related to teratogenic outcomes in humans. The overall summary odds ratio was 1.01 ($\chi^2 = 0.05$, $p = 0.815$) with a 95 percent confidence interval of 0.66–1.55. When the studies were separated according to study type, the summary odds ratio for cohort studies was 0.95 with a 95 percent confidence interval of 0.62–1.45. For case-control studies, the summary odds ratio was 1.27 with a 95 percent confidence interval of 0.83–1.94. The corresponding chi-square values were not statistically significant at the $p = 0.05$ level.

Drug Intell Clin Pharm 1988:*22*:813–24.

META-ANALYSIS has become a popular strategy to use in clarifying the status of therapeutic modalities. The term meta-analysis was introduced in 1976 by Glass to describe the combination and quantitative determination of results from a group of independent research studies.[1] Since that time, a large body of literature applying this concept has been produced, mostly in the fields of psychology and sociology. Several meta-analytic methods have been presented[2] but few have focused on analysis of epidemiological studies. This paper presents one such method. Bendectin is used as an example for this analysis because its potential teratogenic effects have been the subject of a large number of prospective and retrospective epidemiological studies, and because it illustrates many important points of meta-analysis that have not previously been adequately described in the literature.

One area where meta-analysis of epidemiological data may be particularly useful is collating the published data concerning the teratogenicity of pharmacological agents prescribed and ingested during pregnancy. Typically when a clinician or researcher must reach an informed opinion concerning the possibility of teratogenic effects of a given therapeutic modality, he often faces contradicting and sometimes controversial results generated by different studies and study methodologies. In these circumstances, decisions concerning teratogenicity traditionally have been based upon a literature review involving a critical, albeit subjective, assessment of the methodology and data presented, possibly influenced to some extent by personal experience.

It is vital that practicing physicians and their pregnant patients be provided with the best possible estimate of a given compound's safety in pregnancy. Because premarketing studies exclude pregnant women, alternate methodologies must be employed to identify and avoid those agents that are clearly teratogenic and yet not exclude those drugs that are efficacious and not associated with congenital malformations in humans.

An example of the latter was the combination product Bendectin, until its removal from the market in 1983 the only antiemetic approved in the U.S. for nausea and vomiting in pregnancy. Its removal was a direct consequence of negative publicity and financial concerns about litigation and increased insurance premiums. A number of epidemiological studies concluded that Bendectin was not associated with an increased risk of birth defects, and were unable to demonstrate a homogeneous pattern of defects in offspring exposed to the product in utero. The ability of meta-analysis to objectively combine and quantify a potential risk from a number of epidemiological studies would be particularly appealing for the assessment of teratogenic risk.

An article by Sacks et al. criticized published meta-analyses of randomized controlled clinical trials for not addressing all of the important issues when conducting such analyses.[3] Using their recommended format, we present a systematic strategy that can be performed by a clinical researcher to conduct a meta-analysis of epidemiological studies.

Sacks et al. cited six major areas that should be addressed in a meta-analysis: study design, combinability, control of bias, statistical analysis, sensitivity analysis, and application of results.[3] In the present article, each of these areas of concern is addressed with respect to epidemiological studies along with a proposed method of handling problems in that particular area. To provide a more logical flow in this article, the section on control of bias precedes the section on combinability.

It should be noted that meta-analysis is not a single method for the aggregation of research results, but a strategy that can employ many different methods. The common characteristic of these methods is the single overall quantitative statistics used to summarize research results on a particular topic.

STUDY DESIGN

Step 1. Establishment of Protocol

Like any person reviewing a scientific topic, the meta-analyst must state explicitly the question to be addressed by the analysis. This is critical as analytical methods may need to be altered to accommodate different purposes. For example, the objective of a meta-analysis could be (1) to establish an overall relationship between selected patient groups and a factor under consideration, (2) to provide a more definitive answer when discrepant results have been reported, (3) to plan future research studies, or (4) to analyze within- or between-group differences with respect to a factor. The purpose of the present analysis falls into the first category: to determine whether a relationship exists between maternal consumption of Bendectin during pregnancy and subsequent fetal abnormality.

Once the objective is stated, it is important to develop a predetermined protocol or research plan for the meta-analysis. One must state explicitly the inclusion and exclusion criteria as well as the methods to be used. This study involves all research papers published in English in the medical literature that have examined the relationship between first-trimester Bendectin administration in humans and the presence of one or more major malformations as described by Heinonen et al.[4] Bendectin was originally formulated as a combination product consisting of doxylamine succinate (an antihistamine with antinauseant properties), dicyclomine hydrochloride (an antispasmodic), and pyridoxine hydrochloride (vitamin B_6). In 1976, dicyclomine was removed from the formulation in the U.S., and, in July 1978, Bendectin was licensed as a two-ingredient product containing doxylamine and pyridoxine. Because published studies may report on the use of one formulation or the other, or both, we considered a study acceptable if data were presented for doxylamine and dicyclomine together, or for doxylamine alone. In other words, Bendectin administration is defined as the first-trimester administration of either the doxylamine-dicyclomine combination or doxylamine alone. In order to be included in this analysis, a study may be either a case-control or cohort study in design and there must be one group of subjects that was exposed to the drug and a control group that was not exposed to the drug and a control group that was not exposed to the drug. Excluded will be case reports, editorials, reviews, and studies from which data specifically for Bendectin cannot be extracted (i.e., those reporting only results for antinauseants in general). Also excluded will be studies that do not provide sufficient data for analysis. Although important in determining cause and effect, reports dealing with animals are not considered admissible for the present analysis.

Research results will be combined using the procedure of Mantel and Haenszel.[5] A probability level of ≤ 0.05 will be statistically significant for all tests of significance in the analysis.

Step 2. Literature Search

An important requisite for a meta-analysis, as for any literature review, is a thorough literature search. Glass advocates an exhaustive search through published and unpublished sources until all possible articles on the subject have been found. The method of searching for articles should be established a priori and stated in the text of the meta-analysis.

In this study, the database of Bibliographic Retrieval Services was searched using the key words antinauseant, birth defect, fetal abnormality, teratogenicity, malformation, doxylamine, dicyclomine, and the trade names Bendectin, Lenotan, and Debendox. All references from the extracted papers and case reports were investigated. Standard textbooks containing summaries of teratogenicity data, such as those by Schardein, Shepard,[8] and Briggs et al.,[9] were consulted for further undetected references.

Step 3. Range of Patients

In order to judge the validity of conclusions from a meta-analysis and the generalizability of their results, the analyst should state a priori which studies will be included on the basis of their study subjects, both cases and controls. In general, the more narrow the scope, the greater will be the validity at the expense of decreased generalizability. When assessing the teratogenic potential of a given compound using meta-analysis, a number of factors such as age range of patients, primary disease state being treated, severity of disease state, obstetrical history, diet, smoking habits, alcohol intake, concurrent prescription and nonprescription drug use, and socioeconomic status may be important. Because this analysis takes a general approach to the relationship between Bendectin exposure and fetal malformations, data were not specifically stratified for any of these factors.

Step 4. Range of Diagnosis

It is essential that the diagnosis be explicity defined in order to assure combinability of results. The researcher must consider as outcomes the diagnosis of disease or disorder in groups undergoing treatment as well as diagnosis of adverse reactions. This meta-analysis deals with pregnancy, the diagnosis of which is straightforward. However, the definition of the outcome, malformation, as an identification or diagnosis may be subject to some question. When dealing with teratogenicity data, the meta-analysis must consider which of a number of possible outcomes are most relevant for the drug or chemical of interest. For instance, is one interested in all malformations regardless of severity, all major malformations, or a specific defect or syndrome of defects? Should an adverse outcome for a given exposure include stillbirths, therapeutic abortions, surgically correctable minor malformations such as undescended testes and strabismus, or cosmetic outcomes such as birthmarks and changes in pigmentation? As previously mentioned, studies were included in this analysis if they addressed one or more major malformations as outlined by Heinonen et al.[4]

Step 5. Range of Treatments

Often a result may be related to the amount of drug ingested or the duration of chemical exposure. Consequently, the range of treatments used in the primary studies that will be acceptable for a particular meta-analysis must be specified, including the amount taken and time or duration of exposure.

Our analysis accepted all mother/child pairs with ingestion/exposure in utero to any amount of Bendectin during the first trimester of pregnancy. It is possible to perform the analyses on subgroups by stratifying according to level of exposure or time of exposure, provided these data are available in the primary literature.

CONTROL OF BIAS

Step 6. Selection Bias

When determining which of the primary studies will be included in the meta-analysis, Sacks et al. recommend that the judges be blind and base their decision only on the methodology, not the results.[3] For example, the prestige, reputation, or standards for peer review of the journal in which the study is published may alter the perceived value of results. We suggest making a checklist based on the a priori inclusion and exclusion criteria. Table 1 presents a checklist of inclusion criteria for the present analysis.

Step 7. Data-Extraction Bias

Similar to the selection of studies, the collection of data for meta-analysis involves judgment. The potential for this type of bias can be reduced by having different investigators independently extract data from the published reports. Observers can be blinded by photocopying appropriate sections from each paper and removing all identifying statements and titles.

Step 8. Interobserver Agreement

In order to test agreement among observers, reliability measures should be calculated. Cohen has presented a method for determining the degree of agreement between two judges when categorizing any number of items using a nominal scale, called the kappa statistic.[10] Light presented a formula for kappa when there are more than two judges.[11]

Table 1
Criteria for Inclusion and Exclusion of Articles in This Meta-Analysis

		ACCEPTABILITY		
PARAMETER	CRITERION	YES	MAYBE	NO
Presentation	English language			
Subjects	human subjects			
	maternal Bendectin exposure			
	nonexposed control			
Outcomes	outcome = major malformation			

A minimum acceptable kappa value should be agreed upon a priori. This is a matter of judgment, with 0.8 being an arbitrary standard that many consider desirable. Rosenthal presents tables and discusses the determination of effective reliability among judges.[2]

When there is disagreement on either inclusion of papers or data extraction, observers must arrive at a satisfactory solution without compromising the analysis.

Step 9. Source of Support

The source of funding for a study may have a bearing on outcome due to bias in selection or evaluation. As a result, the reader may place a greater or lesser credence on the outcome of a study, depending on its financing.

In the present meta-analysis, eight (47 percent) of the studies were supported by government grants or contracts,[4,12–18] three (18 percent) were reports from research units (support not stated),[19–21] five (29 percent) came from physicians having a university affiliation (study support not stated),[22–26] and only one (6 percent) was sponsored solely by a pharmaceutical manufacturer.[27] One study supported by government contracts also received support from two manufacturers.[4] There was no apparent relationship between the source of funding and findings of the nine studies in this analysis that reported source of funding. This cannot be considered conclusive because almost half of the studies did not provide this information. Any trend toward segregated results (i.e., results in one direction with peer review funding and in the opposite direction with private funding) should be a cause for concern and would warrant close scrutiny of the research methodologies to properly evaluate the relative merits of those studies. In the latter situation, it may be necessary to introduce a weighting scheme or block on some variable to compensate for differences in study methodology if this is identified as a problem.

COMBINABILITY

Step 10. List of Accepted Papers

The research studies to be analyzed should be listed to allow readers to investigate reports more thoroughly. Table 2 lists all Bendectin studies considered admissible for analysis according to the established criteria. Studies are categorized in this table as cohort or case-control. The malformation(s) described, the use of matched controls, and the nature of the study (prospective or retrospective) are also tabulated.

Step 11. Log of Rejected Trials

Rejected papers should be listed along with reasons for rejection. Table 3 lists the Bendectin studies that were rejected from this meta-analysis and the reasons for rejection. It is important to state at this point that rejection of a given paper for meta-analysis is not necessarily a reflection of the methodological or scientific validity of that study, but is simply a function of the previously established inclusion criteria for the analysis. Thus, a study may be methodologically sound but not included, or a study with flawed design may be included in the analysis depending on the nature of the inclusion criteria. In the latter case, the analyst may wish to introduce a weighting scheme to compensate for differences in the design validity.

Table 2
Studies of the Teratogenicity of Bendectin Meeting the Criteria for Meta-Analysis

REF.	AUTHORS	STUDY TYPE	DATA COLLECTION	MALFORMATION DESCRIBED
4	Heinonen et al.	C	P	any major
12	Eskenazi and Bracken	CC	R	any major
13	Fleming et al.	C	P	any major
14	Michaelis et al.	C	P*	any major
15	Milkovich and van der Berg	C	P	"severe"
16	Morelock et al.	C	P	1 major, or 3 or more minor
17	Rothman et al.	CC	R	cardiac
18	Zierler and Rothman	CC	R	cardiac
19	Aselton and Jick	C	R	any major
20	Gibson et al.	C	P	any major
21	Jick et al.	C	R	any major
22	General Practitioner Research Group	C	P	any major
23	Golding et al.	CC	R*	cleft lip/palate
24	Greenberg et al.	CC	R*	any major
25	Newman et al.	C	R*	any major
26	Smithells and Sheppard	C	R	any major
27	Bunde and Bowles	C	R*	any major

* Matched control group
C = cohort; CC = case-control; P = prospective; R = retrospective.

The report of Harron et al. was rejected for several reasons: the authors did not define a group of infants exposed to the drug nor was a control group identified; they estimated the number of exposed fetuses by using the number of prescriptions dispensed and attempted to correlate this with incidences of teratogenic outcomes.[28] The report of Nelson and Forfar was not considered admissible because it reported data for dicyclomine only.[29] The report of Cordero et al.,[30] as well as those of Mitchell et al.,[31,32] were not included in the analysis because they addressed an issue different from the question at hand. These three studies compared Bendectin exposure in malformed newborns having suspected Bendectin-produced anomalies with Bendectin exposure in newborns having other types of malformations. It was presumed that if Bendectin were a teratogen, it would be responsible for production of specific fetal abnormalities or a syndrome of such abnormalities. Suspected abnormalities included oral clefts, cardiac, neural tube, or abdominal fusion defects, pyloric stenosis, and limb reduction defects. This is an example of studies having control groups different from those studies in Table 2, as different issues were addressed in their respective researches. Three additional studies were excluded from analysis for various reasons (Table 3).[33–35]

Table 3
Studies of the Teratogenicity of Bendectin Rejected from Meta-Analysis

REF.	AUTHORS	REASON FOR REJECTION
28	Harron et al.	inadequate selection of groups and poor definition of treatment
29	Nelson and Forfar	reported on dicyclomine only
30	Cordero et al.	compared specific malformations with other malformations
31	Mitchell et al.	
32	Mitchell et al.	
33	Kullander and Kallen	Bendectin not separated from other antinauseants
34	Yerushalmy and Milkovich	
35	Gibson et al.	used animals only

Step 12. Definition of Study Type

In a meta-analysis, articles are normally separated according to type of study. Glass pointed out that a critical requirement of meta-analysis is that the independent variables must be the same.[1,6]

There are two main types of epidemiological studies: cohort and case-control. The outcome of a cohort study is the relative risk; for a case-control study it is an estimate of the relative risk called the odds ratio (OR). With (relatively) unbiased sampling and the rare-disease assumption, the OR is an approximate measure of the risk ratio or relative risk. Because these two types of studies have independent and dependent variables reversed, they were once considered to be noncombinable. However, because they both address the same issue and the outcome measures are mathematically the same (relative risk and odds ratio both calculated as A_iD_i/B_iC_i; Figure 1), it is considered admissible to combine them. To verify this assumption, we recommend that the cohort and case-control studies be analyzed separately and we have done so here. Analyzing the two study types separately was also necessary for illustrative purposes.

Preparation of Data for Statistical Analysis. Data from each study should be entered into a 2 × 2 table as illustrated in Figure 1. Note that n and m represent numbers of subjects in the factor groups and outcome groups, respectively. The subscripts 1 and 0 represent the presence and absence, respectively, of the given

	Outcome		
Factor status	Disease	No disease	Total
Exposure	A	B	n_1
No exposure	C	D	n_0
Total	m_1	m_0	N

Figure 1. Graphic presentation of data from cohort or case-control studies.

outcome or factor. The individual cells of the 2 × 2 table are designated by A_i, B_i, C_i, and D_i.

In some cases it may be necessary to extract only those data that are consistent with the inclusion criteria when constructing the 2 × 2 table for a given study. For example, in this analysis only those data concerning major malformations from the General Practitioner Clinical Trails,[22] and first-trimester drug exposure from Golding et al.[23] were used in preparing the 2 × 2 tables. Smithells and Sheppard provided only the prevalence rate for the defined control group,[26] and therefore the size of that group was conservatively estimated in constructing the table. In addition, only exposures during the first 13 weeks of pregnancy were used in the present analysis.

Table 4 presents 2 × 2 tables from cohort and case-control studies. The cohort studies compared outcomes for Bendectin-exposed fetuses with outcomes for nonexposed fetuses with respect to all major congenital malformations as defined in the inclusion criteria. In these studies, researchers categorized fetuses as Bendectin-exposed or nonexposed, then searched patient records for evidence of fetal malformation. The case-control studies compared Bendectin exposure in malformed and normal fetuses. In these studies, researchers began with live neonates, categorized them as normal or malformed, then either interviewed mothers or searched the records for evidence of Bendectin exposure.

Frequently, it may be of value to break down results even further in order to obtain full information from the data at hand. For example, drug exposure may be stratified by amount of drug ingested or by time (i.e., first trimester of pregnancy vs. other trimesters), or patients may be grouped by age or obstetrical history.

Step 13. Significance Testing of Individual 2 × 2 Tables

After 2 × 2 tables have been constructed, Breslow and Day recommend calculation of the individual significance of studies being analyzed.[36] For that determination, chi-square with Yates' correction is commonly calculated using the formula called the Mantel-Haenszel chi-square:

$$\chi_i^2 = \frac{(N_i - 1)[\,|A_iD_i - B_iC_i| - N_i/2]^2}{n_{1_i} \bullet n_{0_i} \bullet m_{1_i} \bullet m_{0_i}} \quad \text{Eq. 1}$$

where A_i, B_i, C_i, D_i, n_{1i}, n_{0i}, m_{1i}, m_{0i}, and N_i are the values obtained from the individual 2 × 2 tables as defined in the previous section and illustrated in Figure 1. This formula differs from the traditional chi-square in that $N_i - 1$ replaces N_i. Fisher's exact test is appropriate for 2 × 2 tables but may take considerable time to calculate when sample sizes are large, as is often the case in epidemiological studies. In addition, considerable rounding errors may be introduced, depending on the method of calculation. The Mantel-Haenszel chi-square statistic has one degree of freedom, and its significance can be determined by referring to chi-square tables in any statistics text or computerized statistics package.

Table 4 presents the results of significance tests for the reports being analyzed. The cell frequency totals from the cohort and case control studies are presented at the bottom of Table 4. When a 2 × 2 table is constructed from the sums of each of the individual cells, the resulting summary odds ratio (OR_s) (0.54) is significantly less than unity ($\chi^2 = 184.79$; $p < 10^{-8}$). Thus, if a decision were based on this chi-square value, one would conclude not only that Bendectin was not associated with an increased incidence of fetal malformations, but that it was, in fact, protective against such outcomes. This is clearly an inappropriate conclusion. The estimate of variance used in the denominator of the chi-square formula uses N, and because N is very large it makes almost any difference statistically significant. This example illustrates one reason why meta-analysis is advocated over the simple combination of raw data for pooling research results.

Of the 17 studies analyzed, none of the cohort studies was significant. In contrast, a significant association between Bendectin exposure and fetal malformations was identified in two of the five case-control studies. Golding et al. originally reported no association between Bendectin exposure and fetal abnormalities but when the 2 × 2 table was constructed from data for first-trimester exposure only, as required by our criteria, a significant relationship was apparent.[23]

The report of Rothman et al. found a weak but statistically significant association between Bendectin (and other drugs) and some congenital heart defects. That study was not designed to investigate Bendectin per se, but rather the relationship between hormones taken during pregnancy and congenital heart defects in the offspring. A number of nonhormonal agents including ampicillin, codeine, aspirin, and Bendectin were reportedly taken more frequently by the mothers of affected children. Criticism has been directed toward the method with which this information was obtained. Mothers were asked the open-ended question, "Did you take any pills, medicine, or drugs about the time pregnancy began? Please include medicines taken only once or twice as well as medicine taken regularly." Thus, the presentation of the question may have invited major recall bias since mothers with malformed babies were more likely to be concerned with and presumably better able to remember the events of pregnancy (including drug use) than were women whose offspring were not malformed.[17]

A subsequent study which sought to evaluate and remove the possible bias resulting from differential recall of exposure history by obtaining such information from two sources, a telephone questionnaire and obstetrical records, was unable to demonstrate a statistically significant relationship between congenital cardiac abnormalities and maternal ingestion of Bendectin.[18] There are few instances such as this where a potential flaw in research methodology has been identified and the relationship between drug exposure and teratogenicity subsequently reevaluated. This raises the issue of whether results from individual studies should be weighted according to such predetermined criteria as Campbell and Stanley's threats to validity.[37] Significance could then be tested on the weighted data with "better" studies receiving higher weights.

Table 4
Results of Studies Comparing Outcomes of Fetuses Exposed or Not Exposed to Bendectin

		CONGENITAL DEFECT				
REF.	EXPOSURE	YES	NO	TOTAL	CHI-SQUARE	P
4	yes	79	1090	1169	0.13	0.718
	no	3169	45944	49113		
	total	3248	47034	50282		
12	yes	44	78	122	2.67	0.102
	no	659	1634	2293		
	total	703	17121	2415		
13	yes	31	589	620	0.12	0.728
	no	1208	21149	22357		
	total	1239	21738	22977		
14	yes	18	856	874	0.00	1.000
	no	19	855	874		
	total	37	1711	1728		
15	yes	14	614	628	2.80	0.094
	no	343	9234	9577		
	total	357	9848	10205		
16	yes	31	344	375	0.45	0.503
	no	93	1222	1315		
	total	124	1566	1690		
17	yes	24	46	70	3.92	0.048
	no	366	1208	1574		
	total	390	1254	1644		
18	yes	52	121	173	0.13	0.716
	no	240	607	847		
	total	292	728	1020		
19	yes	2	1362	1364	0.00	0.957
	no	4	3886	3890		
	total	6	5248	5254		
20	yes	78	1607	1685	0.38	0.538
	no	245	5526	5771		
	total	323	7133	7456		
21	yes	24	2231	2255	0.20	0.652
	no	56	4526	4582		
	total	80	6757	6837		
22	yes	2	70	72	0.05	0.815
	no	18	571	589		
	total	20	641	661		
23	yes	12	9	21	4.91	0.027
	no	184	398	582		
	total	196	407	603		
24	yes	76	88	164	0.82	0.365
	no	760	748	1508		
	total	836	836	1672		
25	yes	6	1186	1192	2.52	0.113
	no	70	6671	6741		
	total	76	7857	7933		
26	yes	28	1685	1713	0.07	0.793
	no	31	1682	1713		
	total	59	3367	3426		
27	yes	11	2207	2218	2.55	0.110
	no	21	2197	2218		
	total	32	4404	4436		
TOTAL	yes	532	14183	14715	184.79	
	no	7486	108058	115544		
	total	8018	122241	130259		

To some extent, testing for homogeneity of effect can help detect the presence of systematic bias in studies being considered for analysis.

Another problem with this type of analysis is that 17 statistical tests were performed and a level of 0.05 set for significance. This means we are willing to accept an error rate of 1 in 20 in rejecting the null hypothesis when it is true. Since 17 tests were done, there is a strong likelihood that one of the significant results may have been due to chance, and does not represent a true difference between groups. This is called a Type 1 error, or alpha slippage, which can occur whenever a series of statistical tests is performed.

In judging these findings, one must also recall the results from the cohort studies. These studies were also designed to investigate the relationship between Bendectin and dysmorphogenesis. Therefore, one would expect similar results. All cohort studies were nonsignificant, as were three of the case-control studies. Of the remaining two, one was only marginally significant and may have contained flaws due to recall bias. The last result could have been due to alpha slippage.

Therefore, it is acknowledged that differences in statistical significance have emerged among the case-control studies in this analysis, but there is a strong possibility that these findings may be artifacts. Further investigation is required to clarify this finding.

Step 14. Measurement: Calculating Homogeneity of Effects

Prior to determining the OR_s, the proposed quantitative statistic of a meta-analysis of epidemiological data described in Step 15, one may wish to seek some assurance that the studies being considered can indeed be pooled. When a number of studies are performed to test the same hypothesis, results may be expected to vary due to random error. However, a result or set of results may be substantially different from the others, possibly because of a systematic difference in research design, and could skew the interpretation of overall findings. Those studies that produce markedly different findings may need to be identified and investigated to determine whether they can be included in the meta-analysis.

Mantel and Haenszel avoided the issue of nonhomogeneity of effect by claiming that this was not a necessary assumption.[5] When Glass first presented his approach to meta-analysis, his position was that all studies should be included as long as the independent variables were the same. The assumption was that random error would cancel out and that the meta-analysis would converge on the truth.[1,6] This would appear to coincide with the stand of Mantel and Haenszel.[5]

Sacks et al. recommended that a test for homogeneity of effect be performed to detect systematic bias among studies.[3] Mantel et al. warn the analyst to be cautious in selection of a test for homogeneity of effect. They showed that several proposed tests were not suitable, but offered no effective alternative at that time.[38]

Test for Homogeneity. Breslow and Day presented a test for homogeneity using the logit approach that is suitable for any set of risk estimates, including the Mantel-Haenszel OR_s. The test is as follows:

$$\chi^2 = \Sigma(w_i \bullet \ln^2 OR_i) - [(w_i \bullet \ln OR_i)]^2 / \Sigma w_i \qquad \text{Eq. 2}$$

This is a chi-square test that has k − 1 degrees of freedom where k is the number of studies under consideration. OR_i are the individual odds ratios calculated in each study and w_i are the weights representing the reciprocal of the variance for the natural logarithm of the OR estimate:

$$w_i = [1/A_i + 1/B_i + 1/C_i + 1/D_i]^{-1} \qquad \text{Eq. 3}$$

Both the OR_i and w_i are calculated after adding 0.5 to each cell in each of the k 2 × 2 table being tested for homogeneity.[36]

Breslow and Day warn that this test is subject to instability when N_i is small and do not recommend it for general practice such as when testing for homogeneity between strata within a single study.[36] However, because most epidemiological studies have a large number of subjects, there should be little problem when testing homogeneity of effect between studies. Alternate methods exist but often involve extensive calculations that require computer assistance. This method has the advantage of calculation ease.

When cohort and case-control studies are combined, the overall chi-square is 25.19 (degrees of freedom [df] = 16, p = 0.067), suggesting that, overall, the studies are not significantly heterogeneous. However, there is a trend toward heterogeneity.

L'Abbé et al. recommend a graphic method of data display to detect obvious heterogeneity.[39] Figure 2 depicts the plot of the Bendectin risk versus the control risk for all 17 studies included in this analysis. As can be seen, the plotted points cluster around the diagonal line representing a relative risk of 1 for Bendectin. Regression analysis produced an intercept of 0.002 and a slope of 1.184 which was not significantly different from unity (t = 1.69, df = 16, p = 0.111). Two values were identified as outliers, namely those representing the studies of Golding et al.[23] and Greenberg et al.[24] One value was above the diagonal and the other below, indicating opposite effects. As well, case-control studies were all grouped at the extreme end of the distribution. This suggests some possible systematic difference between case-control and cohort studies, and that it may be wise to separate the studies by type and do additional subanalyses.

When analyzed separately, the chi-square value from Breslow and Day's test for homogeneity of effect for cohort studies was 10.11 (df = 11, p = 0.521) and for case-control studies it was 12.60 (df = 4, p = 0.013). One can therefore conclude that the effect sizes of the

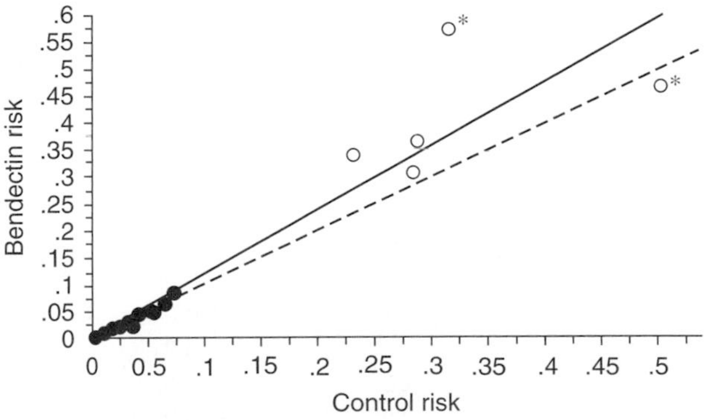

***Figure 2.** Plot of Bendectin risk versus control risk for congenital anomaly reported in the 17 studies included in this meta-analysis. Cohort studies are represented by solid circles and the case-control studies by open circles. The regressed line (solid) has an intercept of 0.002 and a slope of 1.184 which was not significantly different from unity (t = 1.69, df = 16, p = 0.111). The dotted line has a slope of 1 representing a relative risk of 1 for Bendectin, and the asterisks denote two studies that were identified as outliers.*

cohort studies do not exhibit significant heterogeneity, but that the effect sizes of the case-control studies do, and one may consider analyzing the two study types separately. Meta-analysis of both the cohort studies and the case-control studies produced similar results, i.e., they did not demonstrate a statistically significant relationship between Bendectin exposure in the first trimester of pregnancy and fetal malformation. This supports Glass's position that all studies having the same independent variables should be included, and his assumption that random error tends to cancel out.[1,6]

STATISTICAL ANALYSIS

Step 15. Statistical Methods

The important advantage of meta-analysis is that it produces a single overall quantitative measure of the effect of a given treatment on a specified outcome, in this case the effect of drug exposure during pregnancy on malformations in the fetus of that pregnancy. Many summary statistics could be used to describe this overall effect. For example, one could use logistic regression which has several advantages.[36] The calculations, however, are quite complex and most often require computer assistance.

Calculation of the Summary Odds Ratio. One of the most widely used statistics in epidemiology is the Mantel-Haenszel summary odds ratio which serves as a reasonable estimate of the risk ratio for the outcome in question in treated versus untreated subjects. The OR_s may be calculated using the following formula proposed by Mantel and Haenszel.[5]

$$OR_s = \frac{\Sigma A_i D_i / N_i}{\Sigma B_i C_i / N_i} \qquad \text{Eq. 4}$$

The formula weights each $A_i\ D_i$ and $B_i\ C_i$ according to the total number of subjects in that particular study. This weighting scheme produces a result that approximates the importance of the study with respect to precision, as the weights approximate the variance.

For the 17 studies we analyzed, the OR_s was 1.01, or essentially unity, indicating that Bendectin was not associated with an increased risk of teratogenic outcomes. When analyzed separately, the OR_s for cohort studies was 0.95. For case-control studies, OR_s was 1.27 suggesting only a slight association, if any, between Bendectin and teratogenic outcomes. The estimates of relative risk for individual cohort studies and odds ratios for individual case-control studies are found in Tables 5 and 6, respectively. Also included in each table is the OR_s for each study type.

Significance Testing of the Summary Odds Ratio. It is important to test the overall summary statistic of association for its statistical significance. Mantel and Haenszel presented the following chi-square test for this purpose:[5]

$$\chi^2 = [|\Sigma A_i - \Sigma E(A_i)| - 0.5]^2 / \Sigma V(A_i) \qquad \text{Eq. 5}$$

where $E(A_i) = n_1 m_1 / N_i$ and $V(A_i) = n_1 \bullet n_0 \bullet m_1 \bullet m_0 / N_i^2\ (N_i - 1)$. The resulting chi-square has one degree of freedom and provides a two-tailed p value which may be halved for a one-tailed test.

The overall chi-square for this analysis was 0.05 with a corresponding two-tailed p value of 0.815. Strictly speaking, the observed OR_s of 1.01 is not significantly different from unity and one may conclude that Bendectin did not exert a teratogenic effect. The chi-square for cohort studies in this analysis was 0.66 ($p = 0.418$), and one may draw the same conclusion for cohort studies as for all studies combined. For case-control studies, chi-square was 2.71 ($p = 0.100$) indicating that the OR_s of 1.27 is not significantly greater than unity.

Table 5
Risk Ratios and Confidence Intervals for Cohort Studies Comparing Malformation Risk in Fetuses Exposed and Not Exposed to Bendectin

	MALFORMATION RISK			95 PERCENT
REF.	BENDECTIN	CONTROL	RISK RATIO	CONFIDENCE INTERVAL*
4	0.068	0.065	1.05	0.84–1.30
13	0.050	0.054	0.93	0.65–1.31
14	0.021	0.022	0.95	0.50–1.79
15	0.022	0.036	0.62	0.37–1.06
16	0.083	0.071	1.17	0.79–1.73
19	0.001	0.001	1.43	0.26–7.78
20	0.046	0.042	1.09	0.85–1.40
21	0.011	0.012	0.87	0.54–1.40
22	0.028	0.031	0.91	0.22–3.84
25	0.005	0.010	0.48	0.21–1.11
26	0.016	0.018	0.89	0.54–1.51
27	0.005	0.009	0.52	0.25–1.08
TOTAL	0.021	0.027		
Average	0.011	0.014	0.71	
Summary odds ratio			0.95	0.62–1.45

* $CI_i = RR_i \bullet \exp\{\pm 1.96 \bullet [(1-A_i/n_{1_i})/A_i + (1-C_i/n_{0_i})/C_i]^{1/2}\}$ where RR_i = the risk ratio $(A_i/n_{1_i})/(C_i/n_{0_i})$

Table 6
Mantel-Haenszel Estimates of Odds Ratios and Confidence Intervals for Case-Control Studies of Fetuses Exposed or Not Exposed to Bendectin

REF.	AD/N	BC/N	ODDS RATIO (AD/BC)	95 PERCENT CONFIDENCE INTERVAL*
12	29.77	21.28	1.40	0.96–2.05
17	17.64	10.24	1.72	1.04–2.86
18	30.95	28.47	1.09	0.76–1.55
23	7.92	2.75	2.88	1.19–6.96
24	34.00	40.00	0.85	0.62–1.17
TOTAL	78.36	59.99	4.21	
Average odds ratio			1.40	
Summary odds ratio			1.27	0.83–1.94

* $CI_i = (A_iD_i/B_iC_i)\bullet\exp[\pm 1.96\bullet(1/A_i + 1/B_i + 1/C_i + 1/D_i)^{1/2}]$
A = number of malformed infants that had been exposed to Bendectin; B = number of nonmalformed infants that had been exposed to Bendectin; C = number of malformed infants that had not been exposed to Bendectin; D = number of nonmalformed infants that had not been exposed to Bendectin; N = total number of subjects in the study.

Step 16. Statistical Errors

All studies that employ statistical tests select a level of significance that the researchers are willing to accept. The most common level is 0.05, as we have done in this meta-analysis. This means that we are willing to incorrectly reject the null hypothesis five times in 100 when it is in fact true. This presents a problem in that 5 percent of all papers may be statistical artifacts and may not represent actual effects. Thus, meta-analysts need to address this problem of Type 1 errors. Since this analysis included a total of 17 studies, one might expect one study to demonstrate a statistically significant association by chance alone, and the problem of Type 1 errors was not considered great.

A similar problem could exist with Type 2 errors, i.e., failing to find an effect when, in fact, one does exist. This may pose a particular problem when results demonstrate lack of effect (i.e., teratogenicity) or equivalence of two treatments. Each primary study in which there is no statistically significant relationship between the compound and outcome(s) of interest should address the issue of power. Of the 17 studies included in this analysis, 15 found no relationship between first-trimester Bendectin exposure and subsequent major malformations. Of these 15 studies, only 2 gave any consideration to power.

Power Analysis. Orwin has presented a formula which is a simple mathematical manipulation that can be used to determine how many studies of a given effect size are required to bring a calculated effect size to any given value.[40] In order to perform a power analysis, summary statistics must be converted to effect sizes. Unlike statistical significance, which is directly related to sample size, an effect size may be thought of as significance without the influence of sample size. In other words, effect size represents the "true" impact of an intervention. An effect size must be calculated for each study. For a 2 × 2 table, the effect size is calculated from the chi-square value.[41]

$$d_i = [4\chi_i^2/(N_i - \chi_i^2)]^{1/2} \qquad \text{Eq. 6}$$

The sign of d is the same as the sign of $A_iD_i - B_iC_i$. The average d is then determined. Cohen has determined that an effect size d = 0.2 is considered small, 0.5 is medium, and 0.8 is large.[41] The overall effect size d for all 17 studies in the analysis was 0.013; the value of d for cohort studies was –0.014 and for case-control studies d was 0.065. All three are quite low in absolute value and are considered small according to Cohen's criterion.

Orwin's formula is calculated as follows:

$$N_{fs} = N_0\,(d_0 - d_c)/(d_c - d_{fs}) \qquad \text{Eq. 7}$$

where N_{fs} is the number of studies of a given effect size (d_{fs}) required to be added to N_0, the existing number of studies having effect size d_0, to produce an overall effect size of d_c. For our studies,

$$N_{fs} = 17(0.013 - 0.2)/(0.2 - 0.5) = 10.59 \qquad \text{Eq. 8}$$

Therefore, increasing the overall effect size d to 0.2 (i.e., a small effect) would require the addition of 11 studies with effect size d = 0.5 (i.e., a medium effect size). Since none of the published studies produced an effect size as large as 0.5, the largest being only 0.007, it would be highly unlikely that one could find 11 unpublished studies (of similar sample size) having an effect size of 0.5. Similarly 33 studies having d = 0.3, more than triple the largest so far, would be required. This would seem to be a great improbability because such results would undoubtedly have been published. Unfortunately, no statistical test yet exists to precisely determine such a probability, and one must therefore use judgment.

Step 17. Confidence Intervals

The confidence interval (CI) provides more information allowing readers to better evaluate the significance of results than does a test of statistical significance. CI should be provided for each study and, if possible, for the overall summary statistic.

The 95 percent confidence intervals for the relative risk estimates from the individual cohort studies are found in the last column of Table 5, and for the odds ratios of the individual case control studies in the last column of Table 6. It should be noted that the CI are not symmetrical due to the asymmetry of distribution of possible values for the odds ratio. Thus the natural logarithm has been used in an attempt to normalize values.

The CI is used to present a statistic in a manner that allows the reader to interpret its meaning more fully than when presented with only significance values. If the CI contains unity, it means that the risk ratio for patients exposed to Bendectin in the first trimester is not statistically different from the risk for unexposed patients. This is comparable to the chi-square test in Step 15 (equation 5).

Calculation of the 95 Percent Confidence Interval for the Summary Odds Ratio. To determine CI for the OR_s, a problem exists in that this statistic lacks a robust variance estimate.[36] A logical candidate would be the variance estimate used as the denominator in the overall significance test. However, that number represents the total variance, while the OR_s and its CI represent summary statistics for the average study. Thus, to calculate the CI, one would use a proportionate amount of that variance under the assumption that each study contributed a similar proportion toward the total variance. This is a reasonable assumption because the OR_s was calculated using a weighted average based on the variance in each study.[5] Since the calculation of CI involves natural logarithms, the error term used would be the square root of the reciprocal of that variance:

$$\text{Standard error (SE)}_{OR_s} = [\Sigma V(A_i)/k]^{-1/2} \quad \text{Eq. 9}$$

and the confidence interval would be calculated from the following equation:

$$CI(OR_s) = OR_s \bullet \exp\{\pm z \bullet [\Sigma V(A_i)/k]^{-1/2}\} \quad \text{Eq. 10}$$

where k is the number of studies in the analysis.

Thus, for cohort and case-control studies combined, the overall OR_s is 1.01 with a 95 percent confidence interval of 0.66–1.55. When analyzed separately, the OR_s for cohort and case-control studies had 95 percent confidence intervals of 0.62–1.45 and 0.83–1.94, respectively. All three CI contain unity, further confirming that there is no statistically significant relationship between maternal Bendectin exposure during the first trimester of pregnancy and subsequent fetal abnormalities.

Step 18. Subgroup Analyses

Since drug exposure in pregnancy is seldom an isolated phenomenon, analysis of human teratogenicity data may require stratification for a number of factors, depending on the intended focus of the analysis. Such factors may include environmental influences, age, obstetrical history, race, personal habits such as alcohol intake and smoking history, trimester of drug exposure, duration of exposure, quantity consumed, the presence of other disease states, or study design (e.g., prospective vs. retrospective). In addition, the condition for which Bendectin was prescribed, nausea and vomiting of pregnancy, may be a risk factor for adverse outcomes. If one wishes to assess the risk of fetal abnormalities due to Bendectin exposure in a certain subgroup of patients, then 2 × 2 tables would need to be constructed using only those data, provided they exist in the primary literature, and the analysis conducted as described. As an example, we wished to investigate the risk of fetal malformation associated with exposure to the three-component formulation of Bendectin. The appropriate 2 × 2 tables were isolated from the cohort studies[13–15,20,22,25–27] and the overall OR_s calculated to be 0.87 ($\chi^2 = 2.70$, $p = 0.100$) with 95 percent confidence limits of 0.55–1.37. These results are similar to those obtained from analysis of all cohort studies (Table 5).

SENSITIVITY ANALYSIS

Step 19. Quality Assessment

With more subjective methods of literature review, there is a tendency to place less emphasis on those studies that may have flaws in research methodology. Those who are critical of meta-analysis are vehemently opposed to mixing poorly designed studies with well-designed studies, arguing that using insufficiently valid studies falsely inflates results.[42] Glass pointed out that no researcher would advocate poorly designing a study, that one should not ignore existing studies with minor flaws because there are no perfect studies, and that each study does contain some kernel of truth which is of value.[6] Furthermore, he showed that there often appears to be little, if any, relationship between the validity of research design and effect size.[43] As a result, meta-analysts may argue that all studies meeting the a priori inclusion criteria, regardless of their quality, should be included.

If one detected a serious design flaw that may have influenced the overall results, one could perform a sensitivity analysis. This is done by removing that study from the list and recalculating the summary statistics (OR_s, summary chi-square, and CI). If the results do not change markedly, then the study should remain in the analysis as its inclusion tends to increase the generalizability of results. However, if results differ substantially, such as changing from nonsignificant to significant, further analysis is indicated.

On the other hand, Rosenthal[2] and Sacks et al.[3] recommend assessing the rigor of a paper and considering this when making recommendations. One way to deal with this problem is to analyze study design weaknesses according to a set of criteria such as Campbell and Stanley's threats to validity.[36] Thus, primary studies could be assigned a weight according to strengths and weaknesses, and statistics could be recalculated. Rosenthal recommended that this be done by blind observers and that such analysis requires determination of inter-rater reliability.[2] Chalmers et al. have presented a method for determining the quality of controlled randomized clinical trials.[44] For nonrandomized studies, this method would require adaptation.

In this analysis, the possibility that recall bias may have affected the results of the study by Rothman et al.[17] was raised earlier. Removal of this study through sensitivity analysis decreased the OR_s of the case-control studies from 1.27 to 1.14 with a 95 percent confidence interval of 0.76–1.70. The chi-square value was 0.98 ($p = 0.322$). The results of this meta-analysis are insensitive to the results of this particular study, and one would be justified in its inclusion.

Step 20. Publication Bias

Rosenthal identified a tendency in the literature to publish only significant findings. He termed this the "file drawer problem" because this policy results in the accumulation of a number of unpublished studies in researchers' file drawers. He has presented a formula for estimating the significance of the file drawer problem when a meta-analysis produces significant results.[45] However, this formula would be used only when the studies themselves were the variable of interest. In this analysis, we are interested in determining the overall risk for a given patient. Thus Rosenthal's formula would be inappropriate. A reasonable alternative is to use Orwin's formula as discussed in Step 16.[40] Determining the extent of possible publication bias is not unlike power analysis for nonsignificant results. Each provides us with some quantitative measure of the magnitude of the findings, with respect to disproving them, and requires judgment for interpretation. These results may provide some basis for the degree of faith that may be put in the overall summary findings of the meta-analysis.

APPLICATION OF RESULTS

Step 21. Caveats

The results of this meta-analysis confirm the findings of previous subjective reviews of the Bendectin literature: Bendectin is not associated with an increased risk of major malformations in offspring exposed to the product during the first trimester of pregnancy. [46–48] The scope of this analysis is broad in that any major malformation was acceptable for inclusion and, as a consequence, the results generally apply to any first-trimester exposure to the product. One could argue that a causal relationship between Bendectin exposure and a specific malformation or syndrome of malformations may be masked by an endpoint of this magnitude. It is important to state at this point that the meta-analysis alone should not be the sole determinant of whether a particular compound can be used safely in pregnancy. Instead such a decision should be based on all available information—in vitro data, animal teratogenicity testing, studies not included in the present analysis—of which the meta-analysis may only represent analysis—of which the meta-analysis may only represent a relatively minor proportion. In this light, one could refer to those studies which compared Bendectin exposure in offspring with specific malformations with those born with other malformations.[30–32] These studies did not meet the inclusion criteria but are nevertheless important in forming an overall opinion of the safety of Bendectin in pregnancy. None of the in vitro or animal studies was able to demonstrate the existence of a causal relationship, lending further support to the results of this meta-analysis.

Step 22. Economic Impact

The economic and social impact of the lack of relationship between Bendectin ingestion during pregnancy and fetal malformation is complicated and difficult to determine. Bendectin is perhaps the best studied product in pregnancy and is neither currently available nor likely ever to be available to the patients most apt to benefit from it. This is not because of the results of any epidemiological studies but rather because of a decision by the manufacturer to remove the product from the market in reaction to negative publicity and financial concerns resulting from unwarranted litigation costs and increases in insurance premiums. Perhaps the greatest impact of these events is that physicians will be forced to prescribe, and pregnant women to take, medications for which there is not the large amount of teratogenicity data that exists for Bendectin, the ultimate impact of which remains to be seen.

SUMMARY

This article presented a stepwise method for conducting a meta-analysis of epidemiological data. Although it has been applied to teratogenicity studies, it is equally applicable to epidemiological studies in other areas. This method is one of a number of possible approaches, and was presented as the starting point for subsequent modifications and improvements. One area in particular that needs to be addressed more fully is the minimization of data-extraction bias. In addition, more rigid criteria are needed for selecting and rejecting papers as well as for determining reliability measures for intraobserver agreement. A reliable method for determining the quality of a study and a corresponding weighting scheme would also be desirable.

Meta-analysis of Bendectin teratogenicity studies confirmed previous subjective analyses that Bendectin is not associated with teratogenic outcomes in humans, but meta-analysis alone should not be the sole determinant of whether a particular compound can be used safely in pregnancy. Instead, such a decision should be based on all available information, including in vitro data, and animal teratogenicity testing, as well as a good measure of common sense, particularly when considering the temporal relationship between exposure to the agent in question and the outcome of interest.

The authors thank Kristan L'Abbé of the Graduate Department of Community Health and the Departments of Health Administration and Medicine, University of Toronto, for reviewing this manuscript and providing constructive criticism.

REFERENCES

1. GLASS GV. Primary, secondary, and meta-analysis of research. *Educ Res* 1976;5:3-8.
2. ROSENTHAL R. Meta-analytic procedures for social research. Beverly Hills, CA: Sage Publications, 1984.
3. SACKS HS, BERRIER J, REITMAN D, ANCONA-BERK VA, CHALMERS TC. Meta-analyses of randomized controlled trials. *N Engl J Med* 1987;*316*:450-5.
4. HEINONEN OP, SLONE D, SHAPIRO S. Birth defects and drugs in pregnancy. Littleton, MA: PSG Publishing, 1977.
5. MANTEL N, HAENSZEL W. Statistical aspects of the analysis of data from retrospective studies of disease. *JNCI* 1959;22:719-48.
6. GLASS GV. Integrating findings: the meta-analysis of research. *Rev Res Educ* 1978;*5*:351-79.
7. SCHARDEIN JL. Chemically induced birth defects. New York: Marcel Dekker, 1985.
8. SHEPARD TH. Catalog of teratogenic agents. 5th ed. Baltimore: Johns Hopkins University Press, 1986.
9. BRIGGS GG, FREEMAN RK, YAFFE SJ. Drugs in pregnancy and lactation. 2nd ed. Baltimore: Williams and Wilkins, 1986.
10. COHEN J. A coefficient of agreement for nominal scales. *Educ Psychol Meas* 1960;*20*:37-46.
11. LIGHT RJ. Measures of response agreement for qualitative data: some generalizations and alternatives. *Psychol Bull* 1971;76:365-77.
12. ESKENAZI B, BRACKEN M. Bendectin (Debendox) as a risk factor for pyloric stenosis. *Am J Obstet Gynecol* 1982;*144*:919-24.
13. FLEMING DM, KNOX JDE, CROMBIE DL. Debendox in early pregnancy and fetal malformation. *Br Med J* 1981;283:99-101.
14. MICHAELIS J, MICHAELIS H, GLÜCK E, KOLLER S. Prospective study of suspected associations between certain drugs administered during early pregnancy and congenital malformations. *Teratology* 1983;*27*:57-64.
15. MILKOVICH L, VAN DEN BERG BJ. An evaluation of the teratogenicity of certain antinauseant drugs. *Am J Obstet Gynecol* 1976; *125*:244-48.
16. MORELOCK S, HINGSON R, KAYNE H, et al. Bendectin and fetal development: a study at Boston City Hospital. *Am J Obstet Gynecol* 1982; *142*:209-13.
17. ROTHMAN KJ, FYLER DC, GOLDBLATT A, KREIDBERG MB. Exogenous hormones and other drug exposures of children with congenital heart disease. *Am J Epidemiol* 1979;*109*:433-9.
18. ZIERLER S, ROTHMAN KJ. Congenital heart disease in relation to maternal use of Bendectin and other drugs in early pregnancy. *N Engl J Med* 1985;*313*:347-52.
19. ASELTON PJ, JICK H. Additional followup of congenital limb disorders in relation to Bendectin use. *JAMA* 1983;250:33-4.

20. GIBSON GT, COLLEY DP, MCMICHAEL AJ, HARTSHORNE JM. Congenital anomalies in relation to the use of doxylamine/dicyclomine and other antenatal factors. *Med J Aust* 1981;*1*:410-14.
21. JICK H, HOLMES LB, HUNTER JR, MADSEN S, STERGACHIS A. First trimester drug use and congenital disorders. *JAMA* 1981;*246*:343-46.
22. General Practitioner Clinical Trials. Drugs in pregnancy survey. *Practitioner* 1963;191:775-80.
23. GOLDING J, VIVIAN S, BALDWIN JA. Maternal anti-nauseants and clefts of lip and palate. *Hum Toxicol* 1983;2:63-73.
24. GREENBERG G, INMAN WHW, WEATHERALL JAC, ADALSTEIN AM, HASKEY JC. Maternal drug histories and congenital abnormalities. *Br Med J* 1977;2:853-6.
25. NEWMAN NM, CORREY JF, DUDGEON GI. A survey of congenital abnormalities and drug in a private practice. *Aust NZ J Gynaecol* 1977;*17*:156-9.
26. SMITHELLS RW, SHEPPARD S. Teratgenicity testing in humans: a method of demonstrating safety of Bendectin. *Teratology* 1978;*17*:31-6.
27. BUNDE CA, BOWLES DM. A technique for controlled survey of case records. *Curr Ther Res* 1963;*5*:245-8.
28. HARRON DWG, GRIFFITHS K, SHANKS RG. Debendox and congenital malformations in Northern Ireland. *Br Med J* 1980;*281*: 1379-81.
29. NELSON MM, FORFAR JO. Associations between drugs administered during pregnancy and congenital abnormalities of the fetus. *Br Med J* 1971;*i*:523-7.
30. CORDERO JF, OAKLEY GP, GREENBERG F, JAMES LM. Is Bendectin a teratogen? *JAMA* 1981;*245*:2307-10.
31. MITCHELL AA, ROSENBERG L, SHAPIRO S, SLONE D. Birth defects related to Bendectin use in pregnancy. 1. Oral clefts and cardiac defects. *JAMA* 1981;*245*:2311-4.
32. MITCHELL AA, SCHWINGL PJ, ROSENBERG L, LOUIK C, SHAPIRO S. Birth defects in relation to Bendectin use in pregnancy. II. Pyloric stenosis. *Am J Obstet Gynecol* 1983;*147*:737-42.
33. KULLANDER S, KALLEN B. A prospective study of drugs and pregnancy. II. Anti-emetic drugs. *Acta Obstet Gynecol Scand* 1976;55:105-11.
34. YERUSHALMY J, MILKOVICH L. Evaluation of the teratogenic effect of meclizine in man. *Am J Obstet Gynecol* 1965;*93*:553-62.
35. GIBSON JP, STAPLES RE, LARSON EJ, KUHN WL, HOLTKAMP DE, NEWBERNE JW. Teratology and reproduction studies with an antinauseant. *Toxicol Appl Pharmacol* 1968;*13*:439-47.
36. BRESLOW NE, DAY NE. Statistical methods in cancer research. Vol. I. The analysis of case-control studies. IARC Scientific Publications No. 32. Lyon, France: International Agency for Research on Cancer, 1980.
37. CAMPBELL DT, STANLEY JC. Experimental and quasi-experimental designs for research. Boston: Houghton-Mifflin, 1963.
38. MANTEL N, BROWN C, BYAR DP. Tests for homogeneity of effect in an epidemiologic investigation. *Am J Epidemiol* 1977;*106*:125–9.
39. L'ABBÉ KA, DETSKY AS, O'ROURKE K. Meta-analysis in clinical research. *Ann Intern Med* 1987;*107*:224-33.
40. ORWIN RG. A fail-safe N for effect size in meta-analysis. *J Educ Stat* 1983;*8*:157-9.
41. COHEN J. Power analysis for the social sciences. New York: Academic Press, 1977.
42. EYSENCK HJ. An exercise in mega-silliness (letter). *Am Psychol* 1978;*33*:517.
43. GLASS GV, MCGAW B, SMITH ML. Meta-analysis in social research. Beverly Hills, CA: Sage Publications, 1981.
44. CHALMERS TC, SMITH H, BLACKBURN B, et al. A method for assessing the quality of a randomized control trial. *Controlled Clin Trials* 1981;*2*:31-49.
45. ROSENTHAL R. The file drawer problem and tolerance for null results. *Psychol Bull* 1979:*86*:638-41.
46. BRENT RR. The Bendectin saga: another American tragedy. *Teratology* 1983;*27*:283-6.
47. HOLMES LB. Teratogen update: Bendectin. *Teratology* 1983;*27*: 277-81.
48. LEEDER JS, SPIELBERG SP, MACLEOD SM. Bendectin: the wrong way to regulate drug availability. *Can Med Assoc J* 1983;*126*:1085-7.

EXTRACTO

En este articulo se presentan los pasos a seguir para hacer un meta-análisis de estudios epidemiológicos, según las guías más recientes. Este método sistemático es recomendado a aquellos que deseen evaluar estudios epidemiológicos publicados para llegar a un estimado cuantitativo respecto al impacto de un tratamiento. El caso del Bendectin se utiliza como ejemplo ilustrativo. Los meta-analistas deben establecer "a priori" el propósito del análisis y un protocolo completo que deberan seguir fielmente. Los autores presentan métodos que ayuden al investigador a ejecutar cada uno de los 22 pasos en las seis areas mayors, que se utilizan para desarrollar dicho protocolo. Mediante el meta-análisis ilustrativo del Bendectin, se confirmó que el medicamento no está relacionado a efectos teratogénicos en humanos.

LUZ LABRADA

RESUME

La méta-analyse introduite en 1976 par Glass est une technique consistant en l'analyse combinée et quantitative des résultats obtenus de plusieurs études indépendantes. Cette méthode est utilisée beaucoup en sociologie et en psychologie et les auteurs nous présentent ici une application de cette analyse en épidémiologie.

La méta-analyse utilize une approche systématique et est recommandée lorsqu'on veut évaluer des études épidémiologiques parues dans la littérature scentifique de façon à estimer de façon globale l'impact d'un traitement particulier. Le Bendectin est utilisé pour illustrer les différentes étapes d'une méta-analyse.

La première étape de la méta-analyse est de déterminer le sujet exact de l'analyse et d'étblir un protocole précis du plan de recherche. Ce protocole devra par la suite être suivi et les différentes étapes effectuées devront être décrites et compilées.

Pour aider à développer une telle technique de travail, les auteurs présentent et illustrent la méthodologic permettant d'exécuter les 22 étapes necessaries à la méta-analyse dans 6 domaines majeurs soient: le plan de recherche, la combinalité, le contrôle des biais, les analyses statistiques, les analyses de sensibilité et l'application des résultats.

L'illustration de la méta-analyse par lc Bendectin confirme que le Bendectin n'est pas relié à des effets tératogènes chez l'humain.

ANN LAUMIERE

Reprinted from Einarson TR, Leeder JS, Koren G. A method for meta-analysis of epidemiological studies. Drug Intell Clin Pharm. 1988;22:813-24 with permission.

CHAPTER 25

BIAS AGAINST THE NULL HYPOTHESIS IN MATERNAL-FETAL PHARMACOLOGY AND TOXICOLOGY

Gideon Koren

In the context of this review, *bias against the null hypothesis* is defined as the systematic discrimination leading to decreased scientific presentation, peer-reviewed publication, and public dissemination of studies that show no or nonsignificant differences between or among the comparison groups. Examples of common comparisons are the effect of drug A versus drug B and the effect of drug C by contrasting "before" and "after" treatment values.

While clinicians and researchers often intuitively believe that such bias exists, it is routinely very difficult to prove it because of lack of access to source data. The potential detrimental effects of such bias on the advancement of new, balanced scientific knowledge are as difficult to ascertain because misinformation may cause adverse effects that are difficult to measure.

I have chosen the areas of maternal-fetal drug therapy and maternal-fetal toxicology to explore the sources and potential effects of such bias because of the uniqueness of the clinical situation: More than half of all pregnancies are unplanned,[1] leading millions of women every year to unknowingly expose their fetuses to drugs they have been taking. Once such exposures become apparent, high levels of anxiety are exhibited by women, their families, and health professionals in fear of teratogenic effects. These fears often lead women to consider or even to undergo abortions of otherwise-wanted pregnancies. In this context, the existence of epidemiologic studies that show a drug to be safe in pregnancy (and thus not to increase the baseline teratogenic risk of the studied population) is of paramount importance. If bias exists against the presentation and publication of such "negative" studies (i.e., studies that could not reject the null hypothesis), then women and their health professionals are more likely to be swayed by the "positive" studies that might have been published and brought to their attention.

Since the inception of the Motherisk program, a teratology counseling service for women and their health professionals in the Division of Clinical Pharmacology/Toxicology at the Hospital for Sick Children in Toronto, we have been repeatedly surprised by the immediate impact on women of "positive" reports claiming teratogenic effects of various xenobiotic agents, often ignoring a large body of "negative" evidence. After developing[2] and validating[3] tools to quantify women's perception of teratogenic risk, we have shown that women exposed to nonteratogenic agents (e.g., dental x-rays or acetaminophen) assign themselves a 25% risk of major malformations, which is in the range of the known risk of thalidomide.[2] The same women correctly assigned the baseline teratogenic risk in the general population at around 5%.[2] These figures have been tragically supported by unfortunate events that followed the meltdown of the nuclear plant in Chernobyl 10 years ago when pregnant women in Athens, Greece, thousands of miles away from the Ukraines, were erroneously led to believe that they had a substantial teratogenic risk from the radionuclides, leading about half of them to abort their pregnancies.[4]

Several sources of misinformation have been identified by us: Largely distributed books aimed at pregnant women often contain inaccurate and misleading information on teratogenic risk, almost always to alarm rather then to reassure.[2] Unfortunately, we often encounter cases in which physicians are the source of misinformation, suggesting to women that they abort their pregnancies "to be on the safe side." The severe public health impact of such misinformation has led us to initiate research aimed at quantifying the extent of the bias against the null hypothesis and at critically evaluating data coming from other centers. These studies will be briefly described and discussed.

EVIDENCE-BASED CHARACTERIZATION OF THE BIAS

Bias in Presentation in Scientific Meetings

The first mechanism used by medical researchers to publicize new knowledge is presentation in scientific meetings. The Society of Pediatric Research (SPR) annually holds a large meeting at which new data of pregnancy outcome after various intrauterine insults are presented, along with many other types of research topics. With maternal cocaine use achieving epidemic proportions in North America, scores of papers dealing with cocaine effects on neonates have been submitted to the SPR's annual meeting since the early 1980s.[5] The SPR's abstracts, published by the journal *Pediatric Research*, allow a unique and rare opportunity to assess whether bias against the null hypothesis exists because accepted abstracts are published side by side with rejected ones, with the former being denoted by special symbols.[5] Analysis of all abstracts dealing with cocaine in pregnancy revealed that abstracts showing no adverse effects of cocaine had a marginal chance of being accepted for presentation, whereas the majority of those documenting adverse fetal or neonatal effects were accepted.

From The Division of Clinical Pharmacology/Toxicology, Department of Pediatrics and Research Institute, The Hospital for Sick Children, and the Departments of Pediatrics, Pharmacology, Pharmacy, and Medicine, University of Toronto.

Supported in part by grants from the Medical Research Council of Canada, the National Health Research Development Program, Health Canada, Physician Services Inc. (Toronto), and the Motherisk Research Fund.

Based on the Nineteenth Rawls-Palmer Advance in Medicine Lectureship, March 5, 1997, San Diego, Calif., as presented to the American Society for Clinical Pharmacology and Therapeutics.

Received for publication March 25, 1997; accepted March 27, 1997.

Further analysis revealed that the "negative" papers (those showing no adverse effects of cocaine) were overall of superior scientific quality, with more common validation of cocaine use and statistically larger study and control groups of patients.[5] This bias would have led participants in the SPR meetings to obtain a distorted estimation of the teratogenic risk of cocaine. Because such meetings are the first opportunity for practicing physicians to be updated on new knowledge, a bias in the type of information presented to them may have far-reaching effects.

For example, of six abstracts that examined whether maternal cocaine use is associated with the sudden infant death syndrome (SIDS), the two "negative" studies were rejected. In Motherisk we have encountered a perfectly healthy neonate of a cocaine-using mother whose physician put on a home apnea monitor to deal with the risk of SIDS. The single mother in this case could not cope with the instrument and the child was transferred to foster care.[5] To date, with a 10-year retroscope it is evident through large controlled studies that cocaine is not a factor that increases the risk of SIDS[6]; hence the two "negative" SPR reports that were rejected from presentation were scientifically the correct ones.

Bias in Publication in Peer-Reviewed Journals

It may be argued that although the decreased presentation of "negative" studies in scientific meetings is serious, it is mainly peer-reviewed scientific articles that shape the status of new knowledge. In 1991 Easterbrook et al.[7] examined the fate of research projects approved by the Central Oxford Research Ethics Committee from 1984 to 1987.

They confirmed our findings showing that studies with statistically significant results were more likely to be presented in scientific meetings than those with nonsignificant results or "null" results (i.e., the comparison groups are similar). More importantly, "negative" studies had, on average, a 2.3-fold less chance of being published in peer-reviewed journals and, once published, it was in journals with lower citation impact factors. The bias was stronger for observational studies than for interventional protocols. Projects producing "negative" studies had substantially less chance of being further funded than those with "positive" results. The authors reiterated that "conclusions based only on a review of published data should be interpreted cautiously, especially for observational studies. Improved strategies are needed to identify the results of unpublished as well as published studies."[7]

Bias in Media Reporting

With more than 20,000 medical journals, all of us rely unintentionally on electronic media and newspaper reports to be alerted to new medical knowledge. Naturally, when one hears on the news about a new study pertaining to one's scientific interest, one will search, find, and read that article. However, most often such new stories are not in our specific areas of research, and hence even highly sophisticated and critical scientists are "stuck" with what the media have told them. If media reporting is biased against negative data, then clinicians and patients alike will be victims of unbalanced information, stressing the "positive" data.

We have recently compared the rates of newspaper reporting of two studies, one negative[8] and one positive,[9] published back to back in the *Journal of the American Medical Association.* Both studies analyzed an area of public health concern: radiation as a risk for cancer. Seventeen newspapers publishing 19 reports on the two studies were identified. Nine reports were dedicated entirely to the positive study and 10 reports covered both studies. Of importance, none of the reports were dedicated to the negative study only.[10] In reports covering both studies, the mean length of the positive reports was twofold longer than the mean length of the negative reports (354 ± 181 versus 192 ± 178 words; $p = 0.04$). The mean quality score of the positive reports was significantly higher than the score of the negative reports (10.1 ± 3.4 versus 5.9 ± 4.9; $p = 0.02$; quality scores could range from 0 to 12).[10]

THE SYNERGISTIC NEGATIVE EFFECTS OF NEGATIVE RESULTS

The above evidence implies that bias against "negative" results exists at every step of presentation and dissemination of new medical knowledge. A study with "negative" results is less likely to be accepted for presentation in scientific meetings. If the authors try to publish these data in peer-reviewed journals, they are less likely to be successful, and even if they are, publication will likely be in a journal with a lower citation impact. If he or she is lucky enough to publish these data, the chance that the lay media will help disseminate such data is slim.

Although there is no simple way to estimate the cumulative effect of bias in all these steps, there is no doubt that they all act to discourage researchers from publishing "negative" studies, thus creating the *file-drawer effect*, a term coined by Rosenthal[11] for negative studies that remain hidden in the file drawer and are never published.

TESTING THE EFFECT OF MISINFORMATION ON BIAS CREATION

One of the most thorny issues in the area of maternal-fetal toxicology is the potential effects of mild maternal drinking on pregnancy outcome. An estimated 50% of women of reproductive age drink socially in amounts of up to several drinks a week. With half of the pregnancies to date unplanned, this will translate to about one quarter of all fetuses exposed in utero to some alcohol. During the past 3 decades, hundreds of studies have described the numerous detrimental effects of the *fetal alcohol syndrome* and *fetal alcohol effects*, both of which result from heavy maternal drinking during pregnancy. In contrast, a large body of evidence to date has failed to show adverse fetal outcome after mild and rare drinking in the first trimester. In two recent meta-analyses of all available studies, the Motherisk program has failed to show increased fetal risks of mild maternal drinking.[12,13]

Although the message that heavy maternal drinking may cause fetal damage is very important, numerous agencies, public figures, and health professionals extrapolate from it to advise women that even small amounts of alcohol may cause fetal damage. In 1991 the Manitoba Medical Association launched a campaign to increase public awareness regarding the reproductive risks of alcohol.[14] As part of this campaign, a 1-minute video advertisement was produced, and it was aired by several television organizations. We believed this recording to be unduly alarming,[15] specifically because it suggests that even a single drink during pregnancy can cause fetal harm. Therefore we tried to quantify women's perceptions of the teratogenic risk of alcohol and to evaluate whether this videotape could change their attitudes.[16]

We studied 30 nonpregnant adult women from 19 to 52 years of age, 20 of whom were public health professionals and 10 of whom were university students. All were first asked to estimate the amount of maternal alcohol consumption that may cause fetal damage ("even a single drink" or "small amounts every day" or "large amounts every day"). Then they watched the Manitoba videotape and subsequently completed the questionnaire again.

The video contained the following narrative text, accompanied by a view of a fetus frozen in an ice cube that dropped in slow motion into a glass of whisky[14]:

"Your baby . . . Drinking alcohol during pregnancy may cause physical, mental, and behavioral abnormalities in your baby. There is no known safe amount. Regardless of age or race, any drink containing alcohol puts your baby at risk. What you drink your baby drinks. Is there any choice?"

Subsequently there is a view of a pregnant woman being offered a drink to which she answers:

"No thanks, we are not drinking."

Before watching the movie, 21 participants believed that it took one drink per day throughout pregnancy to harm a baby, whereas only seven believed that even a single drink during pregnancy could harm the unborn. After the movie, 19 believed that even one drink during pregnancy could harm the fetus ($p < 0.0001$). No woman changed her view to a less alarming one.[16]

It can be argued that it is safer to err on the conservative side and to advise women that medicinal or recreational drugs are teratogenic even if existing data do not reject the null hypothesis. However, at the end of this information line stand millions of women in the reproductive age group who may decide, on the basis of wrong information, to abort otherwise wanted pregnancies. Although it may be politically incorrect to suggest that low doses of an "evil" such as alcohol can be safe in early pregnancy, the medical community should refrain from political or ideologic considerations when evaluating medical evidence.

THE BENDECTIN SAGA—ANATOMY OF BIAS AND ITS DETRIMENTAL EFFECTS

Bendectin, a combination of the H_1-blocker doxylamine and vitamin B_6, was the most widely prescribed antiemetic for nausea and vomiting of pregnancy in the United States and Canada during the 1960s and 1970s. Because of mounting litigations claiming that the drug caused a variety of unrelated congenital malformations, the drug was withdrawn from the market by its manufacturer in 1983.[17] Two different and independent meta-analyses based on more than 100,000 cases have shown that Bendectin does not increase the rates of malformations in general or of specific defects.[18,19] By 1997 most legal claims have been rejected by the courts in the United States.[17]

The drug is still available in Canada (Diclectin, Duchesnay, Laval, Quebec). In 1989, the *Toronto Star* "discovered" that a drug that was removed from the American market was still available, carrying a headline that read "Drug still on market feared another thalidomide." This prompted the Minister of Health and Welfare to appoint an expert committee, which advised him that the drug is safe and should therefore be unambiguously labeled for morning sickness.[17]

The severe bias against the null hypothesis in this case resulted in the removal of the only U.S. Food and Drug Administration–approved drug for nausea and vomiting in pregnancy, leaving an estimated 2 million pregnant American women each year to experience the natural course of morning sickness. Not surprisingly, then, Neutel and Johansen have shown that the rate of hospitalization of women as a result of severe forms of nausea and vomiting in pregnancy has more than doubled since the removal of Bendectin, carrying direct costs of many millions of dollars every year.[20] The indirect costs and detrimental effects on women's quality of life have not been yet defined. We recently showed that a substantial number of women who are not offered an antiemetic for severe forms of nausea and vomiting in pregnancy choose to abort their otherwise-wanted pregnancies.[21] Because of the common occurrence of nausea and vomiting in pregnancy (50% to 70% of all pregnant women), the bias against the null hypothesis in this case has led to tangible and readily measurable ill effects on the health and well-being of large numbers of women, who remained orphaned from the benefits of pharmacotherapy during a very vulnerable period of their lives.

THE EFFECTS OF THE BIAS ON META-ANALYSIS

The *file-drawer effect* results in an undefined number of "negative" studies that remain unknown to the scientific community.[11] The systematic, quantitative review of studies through meta-analysis is based on the ability to retrieve and analyze all available studies. The fear of bias through missing unpublished "negative" reports has led meta-analysts to add to their design a sensitivity analysis that estimates how many unknown "negative" studies with a given effect size are needed to change a significantly positive odds ratio. For example, if a single additional negative study would nullify a statistically significant odds ratio, then the investigators, as well as their readers, should interpret such result extremely cautiously.

EDUCATIONAL IMPLICATIONS

The notion that "negative" results are not "good news" is not hidden from graduate and postgraduate students. This may lead them to "toil" to get the data to look "positive" through "massage" of data, by forging results, or by highlighting a spurious nonhypothesis-driven "positive" result in the presence of a largely "negative" message. It is of utmost importance for mentors, supervisors, and academic program directors to make their students aware of the existence of bias against the null hypothesis and its attendant risks. Students must understand that the importance of results should not be dependent on their directionality, but rather on the a priori questions that have been asked and the hypothesis that has driven them. Well-designed studies should be planned in a way that their message will be important with either "negative" or "positive" results.

REFERENCES

1. [Anonymous]. Better news on population. Lancet 1992;339:1600.
2. Koren G, Bologa M, Long D, Henderson K, Feldman Y, Shear N. Perception of teratogenic risk by pregnant women exposed to drugs and chemicals in early pregnancy. Am J Obstet Gynecol 1989;160:1190-4.
3. Koren G, Pastuszak A, Pellegrini E. Prevention of unnecessary pregnancy termination by counseling women on drug, chemical and radiation exposure during the first trimester. Teratology 1990;41:657–62.
4. Trichopoulos D, Zavitsanos X, Koutis C, Drogari P. The victims of Chernobyl in Greece: induced abortions after the accident. Br Med J 1987;295:1100.
5. Koren G, Graham K, Shear N, Einarson T. Bias against the null hypothesis: the reproductive hazards of cocaine. Lancet 1982;2:1440-2.
6. Kandall SR, Gaines J, Habel L, Davidson G, Jessop D. Relationship of maternal substance abuse to subsequent sudden infant death syndrome in offspring. J Pediatr 1993;123:120-6.
7. Easterbrook PJ, Berlin JA, Gopalan R, Matthews DR. Publication bias in clinical research. Lancet 1991;337:867-72.
8. Jablon S, Hrubec Z, Boia JD Jr. Cancer in population living near nuclear facilities: a survey of mortality nationwide and incidence in two states. JAMA 1991;265:1403-8.
9. Wing S, Shy CM, Wood JL, Wolf S, Cragle DL, From EL. Mortality among workers at Oak Ridge National Laboratory. JAMA 1991;265:1397-402.
10. Koren G, Klein N. Bias against negative studies in newspaper reports of medical research. JAMA 1991; 266:1824-6.
11. Rosenthal R. The file drawer problem and tolerance for null results. Psychol Bull 1979;86:638-41.
12. Devlin J, Agro K, Trepanier E, Makarechian N, Einarson T, Koren G. The effect of moderate alcohol consumption on spontaneous abortion, still birth and premature birth: a meta-analysis. Biol Neonate [in press].
13. Polygenis D, Wharton S, Malmberg C, Sherman N, Kennedy D, Koren G, et al. Moderate alcohol consumption during pregnancy and fetal malformations; a meta-analysis. Neurotoxicol Teratol [in press].
14. The Manitoba Medical Association. Fetal alcohol syndrome: the preventable birth defect [videotape]. Winnipeg, Manitoba: Manitoba Medical Association, 1991.
15. Koren G. Drinking and pregnancy [letter]. Can Med Assoc J 1991;145:1552.
16. Koren G, Koren T, Gladstone J. Mild maternal drinking and pregnancy outcome: perceived versus true risks. Clin Chim Acta 1996;246:155-62.
17. Orenstein M, Einarson A, Koren G. Bendectin/diclectin for morning sickness: a Canadian follow-up of an American tragedy. Reprod Toxicol 1995;9:1-6.
18. Einarson TR, Leeder JS, Koren G. A method of meta-analysis of epidemiological studies. Drug Inteli Clin Pharm 1988;22:813-24.
19. McKeigne PM, Lamm SH, Linn S, Kutcher JS. Bendectin and birth defects: I: meta-analysis of epidemiologic studies. Teratology 1994;50:27-37.
20. Neutel CI, Johansen HL. Measuring drug effectiveness by default: the case of Bendectin. Can J Publ Health 1995;86:66-70.
21. Mazotta P, Magee L, Koren G. Therapeutic abortions due to severe morning sickness: an unacceptable combination. Can Fam Physician [in press].

CHAPTER 26

BIAS AGAINST THE NULL HYPOTHESIS: THE REPRODUCTIVE HAZARDS OF COCAINE

Gideon Koren, Karen Graham, Heather Shear, and Tom Einarson

Motherisk Programme, Department of Pediatrics, Division of Clinical Pharmacology; Research Institute and Faculty of Pharmacy; and Departments of Pediatrics and Pharmacology, University of Toronto, Toronto, Ontario, Canada

Summary

To examine whether studies showing no adverse effects of cocaine in pregnancy have a different likelihood of being accepted for presentation by a large scientific meeting, all abstracts submitted to the Society of Pediatric Research between 1980 and 1989 were analysed. There were 58 abstracts on fetal outcome after gestational exposure to cocaine. Of the 9 negative abstracts (showing no adverse effect) only 1 (11%) was accepted, whereas 28 of the 49 positive abstracts were accepted (57%). This difference was significant. Negative studies tended to verify cocaine use more often and to have more cocaine and control cases. Of the 8 rejected negative studies and the 21 rejected positive studies, significantly more negative studies verified cocaine use, and predominantly reported cocaine use rather than use of other drugs. This bias against the null hypothesis may lead to distorted estimation of the teratogenic risk of cocaine and thus cause women to terminate their pregnancy unjustifiably.

INTRODUCTION

In biomedical research it can be hard to publish negative results in peer reviewed journals. Although such studies may be perceived as "not news", how can we quantify this impression when the data languish unpublished? Underreporting of safe use of drugs and chemicals in pregnancy may be detrimental. Pregnant women exposed to non-teratogens perceive their teratogenic risk to be in the range of 25%, which is similar to that of thalidomide.[1] After the Chernobyl disaster it was estimated that half of the pregnant women in Greece terminated their pregnancy due to erroneous perception of teratogenic risk.[2]

Because young fecund adults are the greatest recreational users of cocaine, the drug's hazards to the fetus are of concern. The extent and potential severity of such adverse effects are controversial. Intrauterine growth retardation,[3,4] abruptio placenta,[5,6] prematurity,[7,3] sudden infant death syndrome,[8] and neonatal behavioural abnormalities[6,9] have been reported. Interpretation of these results is hampered by clustering of other risk factors in pregnant women who use cocaine, such as use of other drugs of abuse, cigarettes, and alcohol and socioeconomic status.

When counselling pregnant women who have used cocaine we often reveal an unrealistically high perception of teratogenic risk, which often leads to requests for termination. Whilst many of our patients "know" that cocaine use is a serious risk to pregnancy, they are not aware of the controversy and of the many negative reports. We have investigated whether studies showing no adverse effects of cocaine in pregnancy have a different likelihood of being reported by a large scientific organisation than do studies showing adverse effects.

METHODS

All abstracts submitted to the annual meeting of the Society for Pediatric Research are published in the April issue of *Pediatric Research.* Unaccepted abstracts are also published, with those selected for presentation marked with a symbol. We identified all abstracts on cocaine in pregnancy submitted to the meeting between 1980 and 1989. The abstracts were evaluated by a reader who was blinded to the title and to the acceptance symbol. Abstracts that omitted measurements of pregnancy outcome were excluded.

The following items were extracted from each abstract: no effect or adverse pregnancy outcome; verification of cocaine use by history and/or urine analysis; involvement of polydrug users compared with cocaine users only; and inclusion of comparison groups and their size. Accepted and rejected abstracts showing adverse effects (positive) were compared with those showing no adverse effects (negative) by Fisher's exact or t tests for unpaired results as appropriate.

RESULTS

No abstracts on cocaine in pregnancy were submitted before 1985. From a total of 68 abstracts on cocaine use during pregnancy 10 did not report pregnancy outcome measurements (4 were epidemiological, 4 were animal studies, and 2 were analytical). The 58 studies reported various end-points (table I). 49 abstracts were positive and 9 were negative. 28 of the positive abstracts (57%) but only 1 of the negative abstracts (11%) were accepted ($p = 0.013$) (table II).

To examine whether the quality of the negative abstracts was poorer, thus leading to more frequent rejection, we compared them with the positive abstracts (table III). The two groups did not differ significantly in involvement of polydrug users, inclusion of control groups or matched controls, and inclusion of socioeconomic status. Negative studies tended to verify cocaine use in pregnancy more often, although not significantly so. Similarly such studies tended to have more cocaine and control cases.

We also compared the 8 rejected negative with the 21 rejected positive abstracts (table IV). Significantly more negative studies verified cocaine use ($p = 0{\cdot}01$). The negative studies tended to be larger in numbers of cocaine-exposed patients, although not significantly so. Similarly almost all negative studies (7/8) had control groups whereas only 14/21 of the positive rejected studies were controlled (not significant).

Table I
Fetal Outcome Measurements*

OUTCOME MEASUREMENT	NO OF STUDIES	OUTCOME MEASUREMENT	NO OF STUDIES
Birth weight and/or length	24	Necrotising enterocolitis	3
Gestational age	20	Apgar score	3
Head circumference	11	Cardiovascular changes	2
Malformations	9	Auditory response	2
Intracranial haemorrhage	8	Spontaneous abortions	2
Neonatal neurobehavioural examination	6	Pneumogram pattern	2
SIDS	6	Apnoea	2
Neurological abnormalities	5	Sepsis	2
		Death	2
Bayley scale of infants development	3	Obstetric complications	2

* A study could report on more than one variable.
Placental haemorrhage, fetal breathing, neonatal withdrawal, eye vascularity, caesarean section, meconium staining, central-nervous-system structural damage, urinary tract infection, increased cerebral blood flow, pneumothorax, and hyaline membrane disease—1 each.
SIDS = sudden infant death syndrome.

DISCUSSION

Cocaine has gained a wide public reputation of being an "evil drug", because of its link with many illegal activities. The drug is almost "expected" to have adverse effects on the fetus. Indeed, published studies have stressed various adverse fetal outcome measurements.[3-9] However, these effects occurred in women dependent on cocaine and who had a cluster of risk factors, including use of other illicit drugs, heavy alcohol and cigarette consumption, and poor medical follow-up. Attempts to control for these factors are difficult because cocaine users tend to consume more cigarettes and alcohol than those who abuse other drugs.[10,11] Findings from this group have been widely publicised as being applicable to the mild, recreational user of cocaine, who often discontinues use during pregnancy. For example, a newspaper article in Toronto warned women that even one dose of cocaine in pregnancy can harm the baby.[12]

Table II
Abstracts on Fetal Outcome After Cocaine Exposure in Pregnancy

FETAL OUTCOME	ACCEPTED	NOT ACCEPTED	TOTALS
Adverse	28	21	49
Not adverse	1	8	9
Total	29	29	58

Counselling women exposed to cocaine in early pregnancy in Greater Toronto led us to suspect that there is substantial distortion of medical information, which has led many women to terminations even when they were exposed briefly and mildly in early pregnancy.

In the present study we used the rare opportunity created by the Society for Pediatric Research, which publishes not only accepted but also rejected abstracts. Our analysis revealed that the likelihood of a negative study being selected for presentation was negligible, whereas a positive study was likely to be accepted in 57% of cases. It is generally assumed that studies are selected for presentation or publication based on objective scientific criteria. In selecting criteria for this assessment we tried to identify those elements in an abstract that reviewers are likely to use. The data indicated that negative abstracts were similar to or better than positive abstracts. In particular negative abstracts tended to verify cocaine use more frequently, which is probably the most important independent variable in such studies.

The positive abstracts, being a substantially larger group than the negative, are likely to include both scientifically sound and flawed papers. In a comparison of the 21 rejected positive with the 8 rejected negative abstracts, we found the negative studies to be superior in almost every variable studied. This strengthens the suggestion that most negative studies were not rejected because of scientific flaws, but rather because of bias against their non-adverse message. The subconscious message may be that if a study did not detect an adverse effect of cocaine when the common knowledge is that this is a "bad drug", then the study must be flawed.

To study the impact of this bias, consider the association between cocaine use and SIDS. There are published studies to suggest higher rates of SIDS with gestational use of cocaine,[8] although some investigators could not detect such a relation.[13] We found 6 abstracts on SIDS; 3 claimed association with cocaine use and 3 did

Table III
Comparison of Abstracts Showing Adverse Outcome with Those Showing No Adverse Outcome

—	ADVERSE (n = 49)	NON-ADVERSE (n = 9)
Cocaine users		
Predominantly cocaine use	42 *(86%)*	9 *(100%)*
Verification of cocaine use	19 *(39%)*	6 *(67%)*
Sample size	105·5(288.8)*	199·2 (184·7)
Controls		
Used controls	39 *(80%)*	8 *(89%)*
Matched for variables	17 *(35%)*	2 *(22%)*
Sample size	91·1 (198·4)	1767·6 (3622·9)†

* Mean (SD).
† 1 abstract contained 8235 controls; without this abstract the mean sample size and standard deviation for the control non-adverse group would be 150·6 and 269·2, respectively.

Table IV
Comparison of Positive and Negative Abstracts Not Accepted

—	ADVERSE (n = 21)	NON-ADVERSE (n = 8)
Cocaine users		
Predominantly cocaine use	16 *(76%)*	8 *(100%)**
Verification of cocaine use	4 *(19%)*	6 *(75%)†*
Sample size	69·5 (148 4)	222·9(269·0)
Controls		
Used controls	14 *(67%)*	7 *(88%)*
Matched for variables	7 *(33%)*	2 *(25%)*
Sample size	68·8 (124·5)	270(25·9)‡

Adverse *vs* non-adverse: *p = 0 08, †p = 0·01, and ‡p <0·001.

not. 2 of the positive abstracts but none of the negative abstracts were accepted for presentation.

We were recently consulted about a case that highlighted a detrimental effect of this reporting bias. Foster parents brought to the Motherisk Clinic a baby exposed in utero to cocaine, to find out whether he needs to continue to be monitored for apnoea. At birth the attending physician told the natural mother, who was unmarried but wished to keep the child, that there is a high risk for SIDS and therefore the baby should be monitored during sleep for apnoea. Neighbours had complained to a childrens' aid group that the "monitor goes on too frequently", and the child was taken from the natural mother against her will. The history revealed that the child had never had apnoea and was healthy. 1 of the negative abstracts had actually detected a lower frequency of respiratory distress syndrome in children exposed in utero to cocaine than in controls.[14] This paper was not accepted for presentation.

Bias by journals, scientific societies, and funding agencies against negative results may have far-reaching detrimental effects: scientists, realising their slim chance of having such data acknowledged, may be thus discouraged from submitting negative results. Rosenthal[15] identified a tendency of psychology journals to publish only significant findings—the file drawer problem. Even more alarming, this bias may lead scientists to massage or misrepresent data to obtain positive results.[16]

It is the duty of editorial boards, scientific committees, and funding agencies to acknowledge this serious bias and to indicate clearly that research results are not more important if they are positive. Rather importance should be dictated by the relevance of the scientific questions and by the ways they are answered.

This study was supported in part by a grant from Health and Welfare Canada. G. K. is a career scientist of Ontario Ministry of Health and K. G. receives an Ontario Graduate Studies award.

Correspondence should be addressed to G. K., Division of Clinical Pharmacology, Hospital for Sick Children, 555 University Avenue, Toronto, M5G 1X8 Ontario, Canada.

REFERENCES

1. Koren G, Bologa M, Long D, Shear N. Their perception of teratogen risk by pregnant women exposed to drugs and chemicals during the first trimester. *Am J Obstet Gynecol* 1989; **160:** 1190–94.
2. Trichopoulos D, Zavitsanos X, Koutis, C, Drogari P, Proukakis C, Petridov E. The victims of Chernobyl in Greece induced abortions after the accident. *Br Med J* 1987; **295:** 1100
3. Chouteau M, Brickner Namerow P, Leppert P. The effect of cocaine abuse on birth weight and gestational age. *Obstet Gynecol* 1988, **72:** 351–54.
4. Zuckerman B, Frank DA, Hingson R, et al Effect of cocaine use on fetal growth. *N Engl J Med* 1989; **320:** 762–68.
5. Acker D, Sachs BP, Tracey KJ, Wise WE Abruptio placentae associated with cocaine use. *Am J Obstet Gynecol* 1983; **146:**220–21.
6. Chasnoff IJ, Burns WJ, Schnoll SH, Burns KA. Cocaine use in pregnancy. *N Engl J Med* 1985; **313:** 666–69.
7. Oro AS, Dixon SD. Perinatal cocaine and methamphetamine exposure: maternal and neonatal correlates *J Pediatr* 1987; **111:** 571–78.
8. Chasnoff IJ, Burns KA, Burns WJ. Cocaine use in pregnancy perinatal morbidity and mortality. *Neurotoxicolol Teratol* 1987; **9:**291–93.
9. Chasnoff IJ, Griffith DR, MacGregor S, Dirkes K, Burns KA. Temporal patterns of cocaine use in pregnancy. *JAMA* 1989; **261:** 1741.
10. Frank DA, Zuckerman BS, Amaro H, et al Cocaine use during pregnancy. prevalence and correlates. *Pediatrics* 1988; **82:** 888–95.
11. Koren G, Feldman Y, MacLeod SM. Motherisk II: the first year experience in counselling pregnant women on their teratogenic risk. In: Koren G, ed. Maternal fetal toxicology: clinicians' guide New York: Marcel Dekker, 1990: 383–402.
12. Brody J. Babies injured for life by cocaine, study says. *Globe and Mail* Sept 6, 1988.
13. Bauchner H, Zuckerman B, McClain M, Frank D, Fried LE, Hayne H. Risk of sudden infant death syndrome among infants with in utero exposure to cocaine. *J Pediatr* 1988; **113:** 831–34.
14. Maynard EC, Dreyer SA, Oh W. Prenatal cocaine exposure and hyaline membrane disease (HMD) *Pediatr Res* 1989; **24:** 223A.
15. Rosenthal R The file drawer problem and tolerance for null results *Psychol Bull* 1979; **86:** 638–41.
16. Ewing T Thalidomide scientist "guilty of fraud" says committee *Nature* 1988, **336:** 101.

CHAPTER 27

REPORTING BIAS IN RETROSPECTIVE ASCERTAINMENT OF DRUG-INDUCED EMBRYOPATHY

Benjamin Bar-Oz, Myla E. Moretti, Guy Mareels, TonyVan Tittelboom, and Gideon Koren

The rate of congenital malformations after first-trimester exposure to itraconazole was four times higher when ascertained retrospectively than prospectively (13·0 vs 3·2%, p = 0·006). Reporting bias in retrospective studies should be acknowledged in interpretation of such data.

Ethical limitations mean that the vast majority of medicinal drugs are introduced without data in pregnant women.[1] At least 50% of pregnancies are unplanned, so during the postmarketing phase, many women in the early stages of pregnancy may be inadvertently exposed to drugs. As part of the regulatory requirements, manufacturers are expected to collect postmarketing data, including pregnancy outcome data. Typically, these data include reports of pregnancy outcome collected during the postpartum period. Such data are widely used to estimate the safety of drugs for counselling of pregnant women.[1,2] A serious bias in retrospective cohorts could arise if families experiencing adverse pregnancy outcome are more likely to report the outcome than those who had a normal outcome. If this bias occurs, retrospective cohorts would be expected to report higher human teratological risk than really exists, thus distorting the actual rates of these adverse outcomes, and may lead to unfounded fears among pregnant women, their families, and health professional.[3,4] However, the existence of such bias has not been systematically proven or quantified. The objective of this study was to investigate whether the rates of adverse pregnancy outcomes among retrospectively reported pregnancies and prospectively ascertained pregnancies differed.

We used two cohorts of women exposed to the antifungal drug itraconazole during the first trimester of pregnancy. Pregnancies were reported to the international pharmacovigilance department of the manufacturer in Belgium (Janssen Pharmaceutica). The first cohort (retrospective) included all cases of exposure reported after delivery. The second cohort (prospective) included all cases of exposure reported during pregnancy and before pregnancy outcome was known. For both cohorts data included maternal age, gravidity, parity, the dose and duration of itraconazole therapy, and duration of gestation when the drug was taken. Outcome data included rates of livebirth, abortion, and miscarriage, gestational age, birthweight, Apgar scores, and identity of any major malformations. For continuous variables, the two cohorts were compared by means of the unpaired *t* test for normally distributed data and the Mann-Whitney rank-sum test for data that were not distributed normally. Proportions were compared by χ^2 test . The risk ratio of major malformations in the retrospective versus the prospective cohort was calculated with the Mantel-Haenszel method.

Comparison of Retrospective and Prospective Cohorts

	RETROSPECTIVE COHORT (n = 166)	PROSPECTIVE COHORT (n = 198)*	P
Mean (SD) maternal age (years)	29·7 (4·9)	30·1 (5·0)	0·47
Reproductive history†			
Gravidity	1 (1–2)	2 (1–7)	0·25
Parity	1 (0–2)	0 (0–4)	0·55
Outcome			
Livebirth	108	156	0.015 (Livebirth to Fetal death)
Termination of pregnancy	26	15	
Miscarriage	31	25	
Fetal death (>20 weeks)	1	3	
Exposure			
Total daily dose (mg)†	350 (50–600)	200 (50–800)	0·27
Total exposure length in pregnancy (days)†	4 (1–154)	3 (1–9)	0·98
Characteristic of infant			
Gestational age at delivery (weeks)	39·7	40·1	0·1
Birthweight (kg)	3·40	3·44	0·26
Female/male (%)	60:40	51:49	0·37
Apgar at 1 min†	9 (4–10)	9(4–10)	0·47
Apgar at 5 min†	10 (8–10)	10(5–10)	0·37
Major malformations in liveborn/total	14/108	5/156	0·006
Major malformations including terminations	17/111	5/156	<0·001

* Total outcomes 199, since there was one set of twins.
† Median (range); compared by Mann-Whitney test.

In the retrospective cohort, 212 cases were collected; of them, 166 women were confirmed to have used itraconazole at least during the first trimester of pregnancy. In the prospective cohort, 229 cases completed their follow-up and among them 198 were confirmed to have had first-trimester exposure (with one set of twins). Only first-trimester exposures were included in the analysis. An additional 14 cases were lost to follow-up (6% of the total of 243). Maternal characteristics and itraconazole dosing schedule did not differ between the two cohorts (table). Women in the retrospective cohort reported significantly more induced abortions and miscarriages. The distributions of gestational age, birthweight, and Apgar scores in the two groups were similar. Among the children of women in the retrospective cohort, 13·0% (14 of 108) had major malformations (panel), compared with 3·2% (five of 156) among the prospective cohort ($p = 0{\cdot}006$); the risk ratio was 4·04 (95% CI 1·50–10·9). For the analysis including pregnancies that were terminated as well as those ending in livebirths, the risk ratio was 4·78 (1·82–12·6).

Major Malformations Observed

RETROSPECTIVE COHORT	PROSPECTIVE COHORT
Liveborn	**Liveborn**
Undescended testicle	Bilateral retinal detachment, microphthalmos
Congenital dislocation of the hip (two)	Malformation of right hand (dysplasia and missing fingers)
Ventricular septal defect	Pyloric stenosis (requiring surgery)
Hypospadias (requiring surgery)	Congenital dislocation of the hip
Agenesis of fingers and toes	Congenital heart disease, unknown
Congenital heart disease, unknown blindness	
Omphalocele, coccygeal teratoma, anal atresia	
Naevus flammeus on neck and forehead	
Hydronephrosis	
Club foot, microcephalia, intracerebral malformation, unknown	
Trisomy 21	
Kidney reflux	
Aborted fetuses	
Gastroschisis	
Trisomy 21	
Malformation unspecified	

The chances that a major malformation would be reported after first-trimester exposure to itraconazole were four times higher when the woman or her physician filed the report during the post-partum period than when women were followed up prospectively. Differences in the reported rates of birth defects are not likely to be due to biologically important differences between the two cohorts. These data strongly suggest that retrospective cohorts introduce a major reporting bias: women whose children have major birth defects, or their physicians, are more likely to contact the manufacturer to report the outcome, whereas women who have healthy babies are much less motivated to report the outcome. In a matched comparison with women exposed to non-teratogenic drugs, the malformation rate in our prospective cohort was numerically identical to that in the prospective control group (unpublished).

Because data from retrospective cohorts are often the first available, they are used by clinicians to counsel patients. Our findings suggest that retrospective, voluntary reports of birth defects in association with medicinal drugs should be interpreted cautiously owing to a significant reporting bias. This bias can distort the estimate of safety and risk of fetal exposure to these agents.

1 Koren G, Pastuszak A, Ito S. Drugs in pregnancy. *N Engl J Med* 1998; **338:** 1128–37.
2 Koren G, Graham K, Feigenbaum A, Einarson T. Evaluation and counseling of teratogenic risk: the motherisk approach. *J Clin Pharmacol* 1993; **33:** 405–11.
3 Koren G, Bologa M, Long D, Feldman Y, Shear NH. Perception of teratogenic risk by pregnant women exposed to drugs and chemicals during the first trimester. *Am J Obstet Gynecol* 1989; **160:** 1190–94.
4 Koren G, Gladstone D, Robeson C, Robieux I. The perception of teratogenic risk of cocaine. *Teratology* 1992; **46:** 567–71.

Motherisk Program, Division of Clinical Pharmacology and Toxicology, Hospital for Sick Children, Toronto, CIBC Wood Gundy Children's Miracle Foundation, Chair in Child Health Research, University of Toronto, Toronto, Ontario, Canada (B Bar-Oz MD, M E Moretti MS, Prof G Koren MD); **and Janssen Pharmaceutica, Beerse, Belgium** (G Mareels PhD, T Van Tittleboom MD)

Correspondence to: Prof Gideon Koren, Motherisk Program, Division of Clinical Pharmacology, Hospital for Sick Children, 555 University Avenue, Toronto, Ontario, Canada M5G 1X8

SECTION 2

MATERNAL MORBIDITIES

CHAPTER 28

FALL IN MEAN ARTERIAL PRESSURE AND FETAL GROWTH RESTRICTION IN PREGNANCY HYPERTENSION: A META-ANALYSIS

P von Dadelszen, M P Ornstein, S B Bull, A G Logan, G Koren, and L A Magee

Summary

Background. We investigated the relation between fetoplacental growth and the use of oral antihypertensive medication to treat mild-to-moderate pregnancy hypertension.
Methods. The study design was a metaregression analysis of published data from randomised controlled trials. Data from a paper that was regarded as an extreme statistical outliner were excluded from primary analyses. The change in (group) mean arterial pressure (MAP)from enrolment to delivery was compared with indicators of fetoplacental growth.
Findings. Greater mean difference in MAP with antihypertensive therapy was associated with the birth of a higher proportion of small-for-gestational-age (SGA) infants (slope:0·09 [SD 0·03], r^2 = 0·48, p = 0·006, 14 trials) and lower mean birthweight significant after exclusion of data from another paper regarded as an extreme statistical outliner (slope: –14·49 [6·98] r^2 = 0·16, p = 0·049, 27). No relation with mean placental weight was seen (slope –2·01 [1·62], r^2 = 0·15, p = 0·25, 11 trials).
Interpretation. Treatment-induced falls in maternal blood pressure may adversely affect fetal growth. Given the small maternal benefits that are likely to be derived from therapy, new data are urgently needed to elucidate the relative maternal and fetal benefits and risks of oral antihypertensive drug treatment of mild-to-moderate pregnancy hypertension.

Lancet 2000; **355**: 87–92

INTRODUCTION

Hypertension complicates 10% of pregnancies,[1] and is associated with an increase in maternal morbidity and mortality, as well as in perinatal mortality, intrauterine growth restriction, prematurity, and complications of prematurity (such as respiratory distress syndrome).The excess perinatal morbidity and mortality reflect both the fetal syndrome of pre-eclampsia (ie, fetal distress, intrauterine growth restriction) and the consequences of delivery due to deteriorating maternal disease.

The goal of antihypertensive treatment is to improve maternal and perinatal outcomes. Historically, there has been concern that lower blood pressure will reduce the perfusion of the intervillous space of the placenta, which does not autoregulate its blood flow. This is an especial concern in disorders that are associated with placental abnormalities, either a primary defect in placentation[2] (ie, pre-eclampsia) or accelerated placental ageing[3] (eg, chronic hypertension), or both.

As part of a larger meta-analysis of randomised controlled trials of antihypertensive therapy for mild-to-moderate pregnancy hypertension,[4] we found that there was a statistical trend towards an increase in small-for-gestational-age (SGA) infants among women taking antihypertensive therapy, compared with those who took placebo or no therapy (odds ratio 1·31 [95% CI 0·98–1·75], n = 15 trials, 1782 women), irrespective of both underlying type of hypertension and drug class. This treatment effect was, however, inconsistent in both its magnitude and direction. A previous Cochrane review[5] attributed the heterogeneity to the results of the trial by Butters and colleagues[6] that compared long-term atenolol with placebo for chronic hypertension in pregnancy, and found a large increase in SGA infants among atenolol-treated patients. In that small trial, there were two postrandomisation withdrawals from the control group for severe hypertension, leading some,[5] but not all[7] researchers to discount the study's findings and its therapeutic implications. Other explanations for the heterogeneity among treatment trials have not been considered, including the magnitude of treatment-induced falls in maternal blood pressure.

Any effect of antihypertensive therapy on fetal growth is important to clarify, because the likely maternal benefits (ie, a decrease in episodes of blood pressure >160/100–110 mm Hg) are

Departments of Obstetrics and Gynaecology
(P von Dadelszen MRCOG, M P Ornstein MD, L A Magee FRCPC),
Medicine (Prof S B Bull PhD, Prof A G Logan FRCPC, L A Magee), **and Paediatrics** (Prof G Koren MD), **University of Toronto, Toronto, Canada**
Correspondence to: Dr L A Magee, 600 University Avenue, Suite 428, Toronto, Ontario, Canada M5G 1 × 5
(e-mail:laura.magee@utoronto.ca)

small. A reduction in intrauterine growth velocity could certainly lead to premature iatrogenic intervention during pregnancy (resulting in prematurity-related neonatal mortality and morbidity), neurodevelopmental abnormalities (particularly in low-birthweight babies[8]), and, possibly, cardiovascular health problems in later life.[9]

We assessed the relation between the magnitude of antihypertensive-induced falls in maternal blood pressure and fetoplacental growth by metaregression analysis. The controversial data from Butters and colleagues[6] were excluded from the primary analyses. Our study was done within the context of a systematic review of randomised controlled trials of oral antihypertensive drugs to treat mild-to-moderate pregnancy hypertension.

METHODS

As part of a larger meta-analysis,[4] MEDLINE was searched for published randomised controlled trials (1966–97; key words: antihypertensive agents, bedrest, hospitalisation, plasma volume expansion, plasma substitutes, maternal mortality, pregnancy, pregnancy complications, perinatology, neonatology, infant newborn diseases, infant, infant mortality), Excerpta Medica (1989-92) was consulted to identify *Clinical and Experimental Hypertension in Pregnancy* (now *Hypertension in Pregnancy*), which was hand-searched for 1992–97. In addition, we went through the references of retrieved papers, and a standard toxicology text.[10] Titles, abstracts, or photocopies of the methods of retrieved papers were screened and data abstracted independently by two retrievers who corroborated their findings (ie, double-checked their data and resolved disagreement through discussion). The most up-to-date data were abstracted from duplicate publications.

Inclusion criteria were: English/French language, human pregnancy, randomised controlled trial, orally administered drug or non-drug therapy for mild-to-moderate pregnancy hypertension, and assessment of the effectiveness of maternal antihypertensive therapy or perinatal risk, or both. Seemingly inadequate methods of randomisation (eg, randomisation by alternate allocation) were included because most reports failed to describe the method of randomisation adequately. Trials that administered either placebo/no therapy or antihypertensive therapy to controls were included, because our interest was in the treatment-induced change in mean arterial pressure (MAP). Abstracts were excluded. Abstracted data were entered into the Review Manager Software, version 3·1 (UK Cochrane Collaboration, Oxford, UK).

Trials were divided into three types as follows: chronic hypertension treated throughout pregnancy; mild-to-moderate late-onset hypertension (ie, pregnancy-induced hypertension, gestational hypertension, or chronic hypertension treated only later in pregnancy) randomised to either treatment or placebo/no therapy; and late-onset hypertension randomised to one of two active agents.

MAP, defined as diastolic blood pressure + (pulse pressure/3), was chosen as an integrated measure of perfusion pressure. When not reported directly, MAP was calculated from reported systolic and diastolic blood pressure, the validity of this value was checked by use of data from studies that reported all three measurements (ie, MAP, systolic and diastolic blood pressure). For each trial, the change in MAP from trial entry to the last record in pregnancy was calculated from treatment values; this defined mean differences in MAP for each trial. Therefore, a positive difference in MAP reflected a greater fall in MAP in the treatment group than in the control group. Most trials did not report how blood pressure was measured, or specify the Korotkoff phase used to define diastolic blood pressure.

The severity of hypertension was defined by mean at enrolment: mild (MAP 107–113 mm Hg), moderate (MAP 114–129 mm Hg) or severe (MAP ≥130 mm Hg). Both the dose and duration of therapy were found for the groups of treated women and controls. Fetal outcomes of interest were: gestational age at delivery, SGA infants (definition recorded), mean crude birthweight, and mean placental weight.

For quantitative meta-analysis, the summary statistic was the Peto odds ratio (defined as [O-E]/V, where O is the observed number of events, E is the expected number of events, and V is the exact hypergeometric variance of O).[11] Calculations were based on the fixed-effects model, which assumed that between-trial variation in outcome was due to chance alone.

The primary objective of the metaregression was to estimate the association of treatment-induced difference in MAP with measures of fetoplacental growth (ie, SGA infants, birthweight, and placental weight [by mean difference between groups]), by use of summary data from each trial. Other risk factors for poor fetoplacental growth (type of hypertension, type of antihypertensive therapy, and difference between groups in treatment duration) were of secondary interest but could not be included in the regression because of the limited number of trials that reported these endpoints. Nonetheless, before the meta-regression, colinearity between difference in MAP and each of these factors was assessed by non-parametric methods[12] (ie, Spearman's, Mann-Whitney *U* test, or Kruskal-Wallis test, as appropriate). Lack of evidence for colinearity was taken as support that the coefficient for difference in MAP in the regression model would remain the same (or change only slightly) irrespective of what else was included in the model.[12]

The metaregression was done by weighted least-squares regression. The relation between difference in MAP and each of the measures of fetoplacental growth was estimated by Pearson's r^2. A p value <0·05 was considered to be significant. For the SGA outcome, the natural logarithm of the odds ratio for a given trial was used as the dependent variable in the regression.[11] For the continuous outcomes (ie, birthweight and placental weight), the mean difference between treatment groups was used. Each study was weighted in the metaregression to account for the fact that the trials were of different size, and therefore, study-specific effect measures (ie, natural logarithm of the odds ratio or mean differences) were not all measured with equal precision.[12] The weights were determined as inverse of the variance of the study-specific outcome variable.[12] We weighted each data point by multiplying both the independent (ie, difference in MAP) and the dependent variable (eg, natural logarithm of the odds ratio for a given trial for SGA infants) by the square root of the weight.

To be conservative,[13] we omitted the data of Butters and colleagues[6] from the primary analysis. This trial was identified to be a statistical outlier (by our work and by others). However, we also did a sensitivity analysis in which data from the paper by Butters and colleagues were included, and both non-parametric (Spearman's)[12] and parametric (Pearson's *r*) methods were used. Secondary analyses included the relation between other risk factors for poor fetoplacental growth and measures of that growth.

RESULTS

45 randomised controlled trials (41 publications)[14–53] were identified that randomly allocated 3773 women with mild-to-moderate pregnancy hypertension to oral anti-hypertensive treatment. Seven trials (six publications)[6,14–18] randomised women with chronic hypertension to therapy or placebo/no therapy. A further 38 trials randomly allocated women with late-onset hypertension

to antihypertensive therapy or either placebo/no therapy (15 trials),[19–33] or other antihypertensive therapy (23 trials, 20 publications).[34–53]

The drugs used in these trials were: methyldopa (dose range 500–4000 mg/day); β-blockers—acebutolol (400–1200 mg/day), atenolol (50–200 mg/day), labetalol (200–2400 mg/day), metoprolol (50–300 mg/day), oxprenolol (80–640 mg/day), pindolol (10–25 mg/day), propranolol (30–160 mg/day); thiazide diuretics—bendrofluazide (5–10 mg/day), chlorothiazide (1·0 g/day), hydrochlorthiazide (50 mg/day); ketanserin (20–80 mg/day); hydralazine (25–200 mg/day); calcium-channel blockers—isradipine (5 mg/day), nicardipine (600 mg/day), nifedipine (40–120 mg/day), verapamil (360–480 mg/day); and clonidine (150–1200 μg/day). Only the dosing rage was reported for each trial. For drug versus drug trials, β-blockers were always the experimental intervention, and methyldopa was always the control or standard treatment.

In terms of quality, 12 (27%) of 45 randomised controlled trials described adequate allocation concealment, 40 (89%) described successful randomisation by balanced baseline maternal characteristics between groups, and 13 (29%) described adequate outcome-assessment masking. There was no apparent impact of these factors on trial outcomes (data not presented).

No collinearity was detected between mean difference in MAP and either mean difference in treatment duration of antihypertensive therapy (Spearman's ρ = 0·10, p = 0·68, 19 trials) or mean total duration of therapy in the experimental group of antihypertensive versus placebo/no therapy trials (ρ = 0·10, p = 0·84, eight trials). The median (range) duration of therapy for all trials was 8·0 (1·87–27·5) weeks, and all women were treated during the third trimester.

Mean difference in MAP did not differ between trials that enrolled women with chronic hypertension (5·34 [–2·00 to 19·00] mm Hg, six trials) or late-onset hypertension (0·70 [–13·00 to 15·76], p = 0·27, 23 trials). There was a trend towards greater treatment-induced mean difference in MAP among trials that administered placebo/no therapy to controls: β-blockers versus placebo/no therapy (5·93 [1·33–7·99] mm Hg, seven trials), other antihypertensives versus placebo/no therapy (5·02 [–2·00 to 19·00] mm Hg, six trials), β-blocker versus other antihypertensive therapy (1·35 [–13·00 to 15·76] mm Hg, 12 trials), or other antihypertensive versus other antihypertensive (–0·30 [–2·00 to 1·73], p = 0·05, four trials).

15 trials (13 publications)[6,15,16,24,25,27,29,31,35,37,45,46,53] that randomly allocated treatment to 1587 women, described both mean blood pressure control and the proportion of SGA infants. All but five trials defined SGA as birthweight below 10th centile for gestational age, with appropriate tables: three trials (two publications [16,27]) did not define SGA (but the author of one publication[16] with two trials has routinely used below 10th centile for gestational age in other publications), one used below 5th centile for gestational age,[35] and another used below 250 in Usher's curve.[45] Greater treatment-induced mean difference in MAP was associated with a higher proportion of SGA infants (figure 1); results are presented by type of hypertension and treatment of control group for clarity. With the paper by Butters and colleagues[6] excluded, the slope was 0·09 (SE 0·03; r^2 = 0·48, p = 0·006). With the inclusion of the paper by Butters and colleagues,[6] the slope of the linear-regression line was the same by non-parametric analyses (0·09 [0·04], p = 0·01) or parametric analyses (0·09 [0·04], p = 0·065). The latter was not significant, due to expansion of the SE of the regression coefficient.

Analysis according to the type of hypertension was possible only for the late-onset hypertension groups, since there were only three chronic hypertension trials (apart from that of Butters and colleagues). The subgroup results were similar to those overall, whether controls were treated with placebo/no therapy (slope 0·12 [0·05], p = 0·12, five trials) or antihypertensive drug therapy (slope 0·21 [0·07], p = 0·04, six trials). There was no association between mean difference in duration of therapy and the log odds of SGA infants (p = 0·92, ten trials). Mean total treatment duration for treatment group of antihypertensive treatment versus placebo/no therapy trials was also not significantly related to the log odds of an SGA infant (p = 0·30, seven trials).

27 trials (25 publications)[14–16,24,25,27,29–32,35–37,39,41–43,46–48,50–53] randomly allocating treatment to 2305 women, described both mean blood pressure control and mean birthweight. Treatment-induced mean difference in MAP was not significantly associated with lower mean birthweight (figure 2). However, the data point

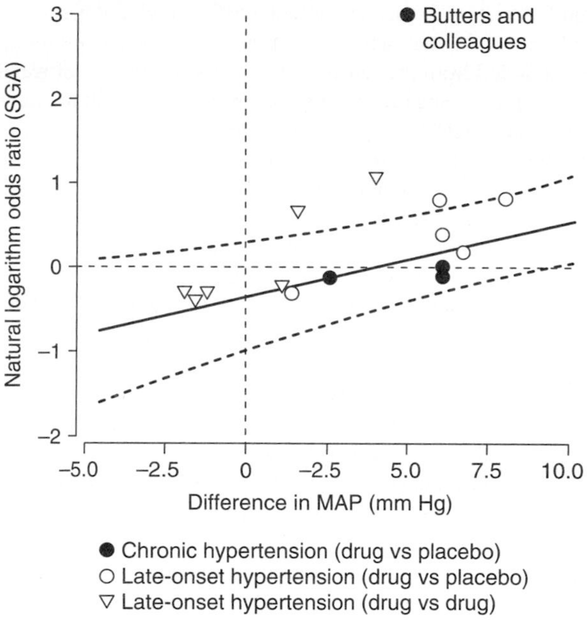

Figure 1. Relation between fall in MAP and proportion of SGA infants.

Spearman's ρ = 0.69 (p = 0.007) without Butters and colleagues' trial,[6] ρ = 0.64 (p = 0.01) with that trial.

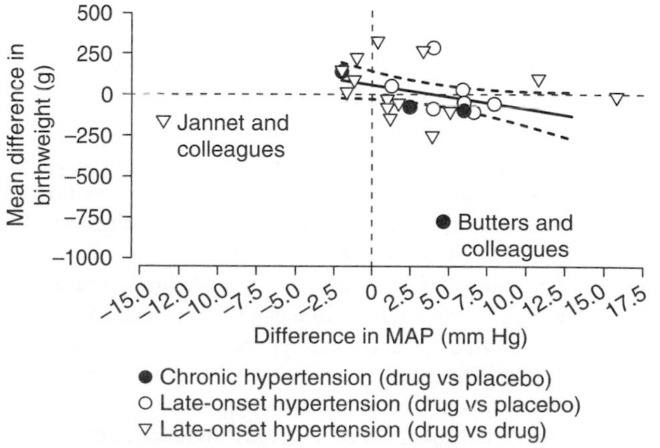

Figure 2. Relation between fall in MAP and low birthweight.

Spearman's ρ = –0.46 (p = 0.021) without both outlier trials;[6,48] ρ = –0.31 (p = 0.122) with both outlier trials; ρ = 0.44 (p = 0.025) without trial of Jannet and colleagues;[48] ρ = 0.30 (p = 0.14) without trial of Butters and colleagues.[6]

from the trial by Jannet and colleagues[48] (which did not report the incidence of SGA infants) was an extreme statistical outlier, and was excluded from the sensitivity analysis. By the use of weighted non-parametric Spearman's regression,[12] a significant relation was demonstrated (slope:–14·49 [6·98], $r^2 = 0{\cdot}16$, $p = 0{\cdot}049$), such that over the range of reported mean difference in MAP, a 10 mm Hg fall in MAP was associated with a 145 g decrease in birthweight. Just 16% of the variation in mean birthweight between groups could be explained by the differential fall in MAP between treatment and control groups, and three trials (two[18,22] in this analysis) reported significant differences in gestational age at delivery. With inclusion of Butters and colleagues' trial[6] (and exclusion of that of Jannet and colleagues[48]), the slope of the linear-regression line did not change by either non-parametric analyses (–14·06 [9·18], p = 0·02) or parametric analyses (–14·06 [9·18], p = 0·14); however, inclusion of Jannet and colleagues (and exclusion of that of Butters and colleagues) shows that the relation was dependent on omitting this trial (slope: –3·84 [6·54], p = 0·14 [non-parametric], p = 0·56 [parametric]). There are no methodological problems in the trial of Jannet and colleagues (women randomly assigned metoprolol or nicardipine) that could explain the marked disparity in its results.

Analysis by type of hypertension and antihypertensive treatment showed non-significant inverse relations between difference in MAP and mean birthweight: chronic hypertension (slope –18·60 [20·91], p = 0·44, five trials), late-onset hypertension with placebo/no therapy of controls (–16·69 [11·66], p = 0·23, six trials), and late-onset hypertension with antihypertensive therapy of controls (–17·47 [15·27], p = 0·27, 14 trials). There was no association between either mean difference in duration of therapy (p = 0·60, 19 trials) or mean total duration of therapy among the treatment group of drugs versus placebo/no therapy trials (p = 0·34, nine trials).

11 trials (ten publications)[14,16,25,31,32,36,41,47,48,50] randomly allocating treatment to 1119 women, reported both mean blood pressure control and mean placental weight. No significant relation was seen between mean difference in MAP and mean placental weight (p = 0·25, 11 trials). Subgroup analysis was possible only for the late-onset hypertension trials that compared two antihypertensive drugs; no significant relation was found (p = 0·47, six trials). There was no significant association between mean difference in duration of therapy and mean placental weight (p = 0·88, nine trials).

DISCUSSION

By meta-analysis, we investigated the apparent heterogeneity of the influence of oral antihypertensive treatment on the odds ratio for delivering an SGA infant. Despite exclusion of the trial[6] by Butters and colleagues, we found a relation between mean treatment-induced falls in MAP and impaired fetal growth, as assessed by birthweight corrected for gestational age (usually defined as <10th centile). This relation could not be explained by type of hypertension, type of antihypertensive agent, or mean duration of therapy, since none of these were related to mean difference in MAP.

A puzzling finding is that antihypertensive therapy was associated with poor fetal growth, whereas the duration of that therapy was not. The mean difference in treatment duration between groups was very small, and could not explain the difference in fetal growth between groups, overall. However, even among placebo/no therapy controlled trials, the mean total duration of therapy did not relate to fetal growth; in this analysis, all women were treated for a median of 10·3 weeks, and a minimum of 3·3 weeks in the third trimester. Possibly antihypertensive treatment during this period of greatest fetal growth velocity is most important.

That antihypertensive therapy may adversely affect intrauterine fetal growth is a clinically important finding. The exclusion of the trial by Butters and colleagues from the analysis increases the clinical impact, given the concerns expressed about this small trial with methodological problems.

No relation between mean difference in MAP and crude mean birthweight was seen, when we excluded only the trial by Butters and colleagues. However, two of the trials in the analysis found a significant difference in gestational age at delivery, which is the most important determinant of birthweight. In addition, the trial by Jannet and colleagues[48] was a statistical outlier in finding a much greater difference in both fall in MAP and birthweight between groups, for reasons that were unexplained by trial design or type of antihypertensive (ie, nicardipine *vs* metoprolol); with exclusion of this trial, we still showed a significant relation between mean difference in MAP and mean birthweight, Over the reported range of fall in MAP, a 10 mm Hg fall was associated with a 145 g decrease in mean birthweight. However, this post-hoc analysis must be viewed with caution. No relation was seen between mean difference in MAP and mean placental weight.

Previously, β-blockers have been singled out as being the class of antihypertensive associated with an increased risk of poor fetal growth.[54] However, the influence of MAP on the odds ratio for SGA infants appeared to be unrelated to the type of antihypertensive treatment. It is unlikely that different classes of antihypertensive medication,with differing modes of pharmacological action, would have consistent fetoplacental toxic effects and, consequently, cause reduced fetal growth. More likely is that the observed effect on fetal growth was related to uteroplacental perfusion abnormalities, but this conjecture remains unproven.

Certainly, vasoactive medication could influence fetal growth. This could be a directly toxic pharmacological effect, affecting metabolism within the fetoplacental unit or the transfer of nutrients across the placenta. Reduced perfusion pressure within the intervillous space could similarly affect both the placenta and the fetus symmetrically, or, in the face of abnormal placentation, differentially; we could neither exclude nor confirm an associated abnormality of placental growth, given that fall in MAP and placental weight were not related. A reduction in intervillous perfusion may also cause sufficient stress to accelerate fetal pulmonary maturation. This mechanism would be consistent with the previously observed treatment-induced decrease in respiratory distress syndrome in a previously published meta-analysis,[5] as well as our previous meta-analysis.[4] Fetuses subjected to in-utero stress are less likely than those without such stress to develop respiratory distress syndrome,[55,56] when delivered in good condition. Although the observed reduction in intrauterine growth velocity may be associated with improved neonatal outcome (ie, respiratory distress syndrome), there are concerns that such an adverse intrauterine environment could both increase the risk of iatrogenic antenatal and intrapartum interventions and lead to an excess of health problems in adulthood.[9]

This metaregression is limited in several ways. This analysis was restricted to published randomised controlled trials, augmented by results published only in the Cochrane reviews after personal communication with the trialists; this leaves analysis open to both publication bias and the file drawer effect. Not all trials reported the covariates of interest (principally blood pressure) or all fetal outcomes of interest (principally, the proportion of SGA infants). Use of averages of covariates measured in the individual patient (eg, difference in MAP) must be done with caution because they may not adequately reflect important between-patient, within-trial differences.[57] The practice of omitting data from trials that are statistical outliers has been recommended by some[13] but not all authorities.[12] Finally, meta-analyses and metaregressions are, by their nature, observational and retrospective. Therefore, they should only be considered hypothesis-generating, and a prelude to a randomised controlled trial.[58]

In summary, the implications of the observed impact of the treatment-induced fall in blood pressure on fetal growth must be considered seriously. Women are unlikely to suffer from either acute or chronic deleterious effects, over the 9 months of pregnancy, from blood pressures that are below 170/110 mm Hg.[59,60] At present, we cannot be sure of the impact that antihypertensive treatment for mild-to-moderate pregnancy hypertension may have on perinatal outcomes. New data from clinical trials are needed.

CONTRIBUTORS

P von Dadelszen, M P Ornstein, and L A Magee were responsible for the data abstraction and statistical analyses (meta-analysis and meta-regression). A G Logan and G Koren aided in the design of the stidy and acted as content experts in the fields of hypertension and perinatal morbidity, respectively. S B Bull aided in the statistical analysis. P von Dadelszen and L A Magee wrote the manuscript.

ACKNOWLEDGMENTS

This work was supported by the Physicians' Services Incorporated and an educational grant from the Department of Medicine,Mount Sinai Hospital, Toronto, Canada. S B Bull and A G Logan are senior scientists of the Samuel Lunenfeld Research Institute of Mount Sinai Hospital, Toronto. G Koren is the CIBC World Market Children's Miracle Foundation Chair in child health research, Hospital for Sick Children, Toronto, Canada.

REFERENCES

1. National High Blood Pressure Education Program Working Group. Report on high blood pressure in pregnancy. *Am J Obstet Gynecol* 1990; **163:** 1691–712.
2. Khong TY, de Wolf F, Robertson WB, Brosens I. Inadequate maternal vascular response to placentation in pregnancies complicated by pre-eclampsia and by small-for-gestational-age infants. *Br J Obstet Gynaecol* 1986; **93:** 1049–59.
3. Zuspan FP, O'Shaughnessy RW. Maternal physiology and diseases: chronic hypertension in pregnancy. In: Pitkin RM, Zlatnik FJ, ed. Yearbook of obstetrics and gynecology. Chicago: Yearbook Medical Publishers, 1979: 11.
4. Magee LA, Ornstein MP, von Dadelszen P. Clinical review: management of mild to moderate pregnancy hypertension. *BMJ* 1999; **318:** 1332–36.
5. Collins R, Duley L. Any antihypertensive therapy for pregnancy hypertension. In: Enkin MW, Keirse MJNC, Renfrew MJ, Neilson JP, eds. Pregnancy and childbirth module. In Cochrane Library review no 04426, Cochrane Collaboration, April 21. Oxford: Update Software, 1994.
6. Butters L, Kennedy S, Rubin PC. Atenolol in essential hypertension during pregnancy. *BMJ* 1990; **301:** 587–89.
7. Redman CWG. Controlled trials of antihypertensive drugs in pregnancy. *Am J Kidney Dis* 1991; **17:** 149–53.
8. Tyson JE, Kennedy K, Broyles S, Rosenfeld CR. The small for gestational age infant: accelerated or delayed pulmonary maturation? Increased or decreased survival? *Pediatrics* 1995; **95:** 534–38.
9. Barker DJ. The Wellcome Lecture, 1994. The fetal origins of adult disease. *Proc R Soc Lond B Biol Sci* 1995; **262:** 37–43.
10. Briggs GG, Freeman RK, Yaffe SK, eds. Drugs in pregnancy and lactation: a reference guide to fetal and neonatal risk, 4th edn. Baltimore: Williams & Wilkins, 1994.
11. Fleiss JL. The statistical basis of meta-analysis. *Stat Method Med Res* 1993; **2:** 121–45.
12. Berlin JA, Antman EM. Advantages and limitations of metaanalytic regressions of clinical trials data. *Online J Curr Clin Trials* 1994; **3** (document no 132).
13. Greenland S. A critical look at some popular meta-analytic methods. *Am J Epidemiol* 1994; **140:** 290–301.
14. Sibai BM, Grossman RA, Grossman HG. Effects of diuretics in plasma volume in pregnancies with long-term hypertension. *Am J Obstet Gynaecol* 1984; **150:** 831–35.
15. Arias F, Zamora J. Antihypertensive treatment and pregnancy outcome in patients with mild chronic hypertension. *Obstet Gynecol* 1978; **53:** 489–94.
16. Sibai BM, Mabie WC, Shamsa F, Villar MA, Anderson GD. A comparison of no medication versus methyldopa or labetalol in chronic hypertension during pregnancy. *Am J Obstet Gynecol* 1990; 162: 960–67.
17. Weitz C, Khouzami V, Maxwell K, Johnson JWC. Treatment of hypertension in pregnancy with methyldopa: a randomized double blind study. *Int J Gynaecol Obstet* 1987; **25:** 35–40.
18. Steyn DW, Odendaal HJ. Randomised controlled trial of ketanserin and aspirin in prevention of pre-eclampsia. *Lancet* 1997; **350:** 1267–71.
19. Menzies DN. Controlled trial of chlorothiazide in treatment of early pre-eclampsia. *BMJ* 1964; **1:** 739–42.
20. Leather HM, Baker P, Humphreys DM, Chadd MA. A controlled trial of hypotensive agents in hypertension in pregnancy. *Lancet* 1968; ii: 488–90.
21. Redman CWG, Beilin LJ, Bonnar J. Ounsted MK. Fetal outcome in trial of antihypertensive treatment in pregnancy. *Lancet* 1976; ii: 753–756.
22. Rubin PC, Butters L, Clark DM, et al. Placebo-controlled trial of atenolol in treatment of pregnancy-associated hypertension. *Lancet* 1983; i: 431–34.
23. Cruickshank DJ, Robertson AA, Campbell DM, MacGillivray I. Maternal obstetric outcome measured in a randomised controlled study of labetalol in the treatment of hypertension in pregnancy. *Clin Exp Hypertens Pregn* 1991; **B10:** 333–44.
24. Pickles CJ, Symonds EM, Broughton Pipkin F. The fetal outcome in a randomized double-blind controlled trial of labetalol versus placebo in pregnancy-induced hypertension. *Br J Obstet Gynaecol* 1989; **96:** 38–43.
25. Sibai BM, Gonzales AR, Mabie WC, Moretti M. A comparison of labetalol plus hospitalization versus hospitalization alone in the management of preeclampsia remote from term. *Obstet Gynecol* 1987; **70:** 323–27.
26. Walker JJ, Crooks A, Erwin L, Calder AA. Labetalol in pregnancy-induced hypertension: fetal and maternal effects. In Reily A, Symonds EM, eds, International Congress Series 591. Amsterdam: Excerpta Medica, 1982: 148–60.
27. Hogstedt S, Lindberg B, Lindeberg S, Ludviksson K. Effect of metoprolol on fetal heart rate patterns during pregnancy and delivery. *Clin Exp Hypertens Pregn* 1984; **B3:** 152.

28. Wichman K, Ryden G, Karlberg BE. A placebo controlled trial of metoprolol in the treatment of hypertension in pregnancy. *Scand J Lab Invest* 1984; **169:** 90–95.
29. Plouin PF, Breart G, Llado J, et al. A randomised comparison of early with consecutive use of antihypertensive drugs in the management of pregnancy-induced hypertension. *Br J Obstet Gynaecol* 1990; **97:** 134–41.
30. Bott-Kanner G, Hirsch M, Friedman S, et al. Antihypertensive therapy in the management of hypertension in pregnancy—a clinical double-blind study of pindolol. *Clin Exp Hypertens Pregn* 1992;**B11:** 207–20.
31. Sibai BM, Barton JR, Akl S, Sarinoglu C, Mercer BM. A randomized prospective comparison of nifedipine and bed rest versus bed rest alone in the management of preeclampsia remote from term. *Am J Obstet Gynecol* 1992; **167:** 879–84.
32. Wide-Swensson DH, Ingemarsson I, Lunell NO, et al. Calcium channel blockade (isradipine) in treatment of hypertension in pregnancy: a randomized placebo-controlled study. *Am J Obstet Gynecol* 1995; **173:** 872–78.
33. Phippard AF, Fischer WE, Horvath JS, et al. Early blood pressure control improves pregnancy outcome in primigravid women with mild hypertension. *Med J Aust* 1991; **154:** 378–82.
34. Lardoux H, Blazquez G, Leperlier E, Gerard J. Essai overt, comparatif, avec tirage au sort pour le traitement de l'HTA gravidique moderée: methyldopa, acebutolol, labetalol. *Arch Mal Coeur* 1988; **81:** (suppl HTA):137–40.
35. Plouin PF, Breart G, Maillard F, Papiernik E, Relier JP, for the Labetalol Methyldopa Study group. Comparison of antihypertensive efficacy and perinatal safety of labetalol and methyldopa in the treatment of hypertension in pregnancy: a randomized controlled trial. *Br J Obstet Gynaecol* 1988; **95:** 868–79.
36. Lamming GD, Broughton Pipkin F, Symonds EM. Comparison of the alpha and beta blocking drug, labetalol, and methyldopa in the treatment of moderate and severe pregnancy-induced hypertension. *Clin Exp Hypertens Pregn* 1980; **A2:** 865–95.
37. Redman CWG. A controlled trial of the treatment of hypertension in pregnancy: labetalol compared with methyldopa. International Congress Series 591 Amsterdam: Excerpta Medica 1978: 101–10.
38. El-Qarmalawi AM, Morsy AH, Al-Fadly A, Obeid A, Hashem M. Labetalol vs methyldopa in the treatment of pregnancy-induced hypertension. *Int J Gynaecol Obstet* 1995; **49:** 125–30.
39. Oumachigui A,Verghese M, Balachander J. A comparative evaluation of metoprolol and methyldopa in the management of pregnancy-induced hypertension. *Ind Heart J* 1992; **44:** 39–41.
40. Gallery EDM, Ross MR, Gyory AZ. Antihypertensive treatment in pregnancy: analysis of different responses to oxprenolol and methyldopa. *BMJ* 1985; **291:** 563–66.
41. Fidler J, Smith V, Fayers P, de Swiet M. Randomised controlled comparative study of methyldopa and oxprenolol in treatment of hypertension in pregnancy. *BMJ* 1983; **286:** 1927–30.
42. Ellenbogen A, Jaschevatzky O, Davidson A, Anderman S, Grunstein S. Management of pregnancy-induced hypertension with pindolol: comparative study with methyldopa. *Int J Gynaecol Onstet* 1986; **24:** 3–7.
43. Livingstone I, Craswell PW, Bevan EB. Propranolol in pregnancy; three year prospective study. *Clin Exp Hypertens Pregn* 1983; **B2:** 341–50.
44. Hjertberg R, Faxelius G, Lagercrantz H. Neonatal adaption in hypertensive pregnancy—a study of labetalol vs hydralazine treatment. *J Perinat Med* 1993; **21:** 69–75.
45. Rosenfeld JB. Antihypertensive therapy in the management of hypertensio in pregnancy—a clinical double-blind study of pindolol. *Clin Exp Hypertens Pregn* 1992; **B11:** 207–20.
46. Paran E, Holzberg G, Mazor M, Zmora E, Insler V. β-adrenergic blocking agents in the treatment of pregnancy-induced hypertension. *Int J Pharmacol Ther* 1995; **33:** 119–23.
47. Montan S, Ingemarsson I, Marsal K, Sjoberg NO. Randomised controlled trial of atenolol and pindolol in human pregnancy: effects on fetal haemodynamics. *BMJ* 1992; **304:** 946–49.
48. Jannet D, Carbonne B, Sebban E, Milliez J. Nicardipine versus metoprolol in the treatment of hypertension during pregnancy: a randomized comparative trial. *Obstet Gynecol* 1994; **84:** 354–59.
49. Marlettini MG, Crippa S, Morelli-Labate AM, Contarini A, Orlandi C. Randomized comparison of calcium antagonists and beta-blockers in the treatment of pregnancy-induced hypertension. *Curr Ther Res* 1990; **45:** 684–94.
50. Montan S, Anandakumar C, Arulkumaran A, Ingemarsson I, Ratnam SS. Randomised controlled trial of methyldopa and israpidine in preeclampsia—effects on uteroplacental and fetal hemodynamics. *J Perinat Med* 1996; **24:** 177–84.
51. Wide-Swensson D, Montan S, Arulkumaran S, Ingemarsson I, Ratnam SS. Effect of methyldopa and isradipine in fetal heart rate pattern assessed by computerized cardiotocography in human pregnancy. *Am J Obstet Gynecol* 1993; **169:** 1581–85.
52. Voto LS, Zin C, Neira J, Lapidus AM, Margulies M. Ketanserin versus α-methyldopa in the treatment of hypertension during pregnancy: a preliminary report. *J Cardiovasc Pharmacol* 1987; **10:** S101–03.
53. Horvath JS, Phippard A, Korda A, Henderson-Smart DJ,Child A, Tiller DJ. Clonidine hydrochloride—a safe and effective antihypertensive agent in pregnancy. *Obstetrics* 1985; **66:** 634–38.
54. Rey E, LeLorier J, Burgess E, Lange IR, Leduc L. Report of Canadian Hypertension Society Consensus Conference: 3. Pharmacologic treatment of hypertensive disorders of pregnancy. *CMAJ* 1997; **157:** 1245–54.
55. Ley D, Wide-Swensson D, Lindroth M, Svenningsen N, Marsal K. Respiratory distress syndrome in infants with impaired intrauterine growth. *Acta Paediatr* 1997; **86:** 1090–96.
56. Cooper PA, Sandler DL, Simchowitz ID, Galpin JS. Effects of sub-optimal intra-uterine growth on preterm infants between 30 and 32 weeks' gestation. *S Afr Med J* 1997; **87:** 314–18.
57. Lau J, Ioannidis JPA, Schmid CH. Quantitative synthesis in systemic reviews. *Ann Intern Med* 1997; **127:** 820–26.
58. Borzak S, Ridker PM. Discordance between meta-analyses and large-scale randomized, controlled trials. *Ann Intern Med* 1995; **123:** 873–77.
59. Sibai BH. Treatment of hypertension in pregnant women. *N Engl J Med* 1996; **335:** 257–65.
60. Redman CWG. Hypertension in pregnancy. In: de Swiet M, ed. Medical disorders in obstetric practice, 3rd edn. Oxford: Blackwell, 1995: 182–25.

CHAPTER 29

PREVALENCE OF DEPRESSION DURING PREGNANCY: SYSTEMATIC REVIEW

Heather A. Bennett, Adrienne Einarson, Anna Taddio, Gideon Koren, and Thomas R. Einarson

Objective. Current estimates of the prevalence of depression during pregnancy vary widely. A more precise estimate is required to identify the level of disease burden and develop strategies for managing depressive disorders. The objective of this study was to estimate the prevalence of depression during pregnancy by trimester, as detected by validated screening instruments (ie, Beck Depression Inventory, Edinburgh Postnatal Depression Score) and structured interviews, and to compare the rates among instruments.

Data Sources. Observational studies and surveys were searched in MEDLINE from 1966, CINAHL from 1982, EMBASE from 1980, and HealthSTAR from 1975.

Methods of Study Selection. A validated study selection/ data extraction form detailed acceptance criteria. Numbers and percentages of depressed patients, by weeks of gestation or trimester, were reported.

Tabulation, Integration, and Results. Two reviewers independently extracted data; a third party resolved disagreement. Two raters assessed quality by using a 12-point checklist. A random effects meta-analytic model produced point estimates and 95% confidence intervals (CIs). Heterogeneity was examined with the χ^2 test (no systematic bias detected). Funnel plots and Begg-Mazumdar test were used to assess publication bias (none found). Of 714 articles identified, 21 (19,284 patients) met the study criteria. Quality scores averaged 62%. Prevalence rates (95% CIs) were 7.4% (2.2, 12.6), 12.8% (10.7, 14.8), and 12.0% (7.4, 16.7) for the first, second, and third trimesters, respectively. Structured interviews found lower rates than the Beck Depression Inventory but not the Edinburgh Postnatal Depression Scale.

Conclusion. Rates of depression, especially during the second and third trimesters of pregnancy, are substantial. Clinical and economic studies to estimate maternal and fetal consequences are needed. (Obstet Gynecol 2004;103: 698–709. © 2004 by The American College of Obstetricians and Gynecologists.)

Depression is widespread and common throughout the world. National population-based studies have used lay-administered interviews to determine the rate of depression within the community. Estimates of the 1-year prevalence of major depressive disorder in adult women have been 7% in Taiwan[1] and Australia,[2] 8% in Santiago, Chile,[3] and 9% in Canada[4] and in Sao Paulo, Brazil.[5] Rates in the United States have ranged from 7% to13%.[6–8] In European countries (ie, the United Kingdom, Belgium, France, Germany, The Netherlands, and Spain), a 6-month prevalence rate of 7% in the total adult population has been reported,[9] and in Italy the prevalence of current depression in the adult population has been estimated at 8%.[10]

Not only are a substantial number of women affected, but there is also a high degree of impairment associated with this disorder. Depression has been identified as a leading cause of disability-adjusted life years (ie, the sum of years of potential life lost due to premature mortality and the years of productive life lost due to disability) for women globally.[11] Without doubt, major depressive disorder represents a major health problem for women of all nationalities.

It is now recognized that hormonal changes associated with the reproductive cycle increase the lifetime risk for affective disorders in a proportion of women.[12] Pregnancy, a major life event accompanied by hormonal changes, can represent a time of increased vulnerability for the onset or return of depression.[13,14] Some women experience their first depressive episode during pregnancy, whereas others with a history of depression are at increased risk for its recurrence, continuation, or exacerbation.[15,16]

From the Faculty of Pharmacy and Department of Medicine, Faculty of Pharmacology, University of Toronto, Ontario, Canada; The Motherisk Program and Department of Pharmacy, The Hospital for Sick Children, Toronto, Ontario, Canada.

Nevertheless, gaps exist in our understanding of this disorder. For instance, estimates of the prevalence of depressive symptoms and major depressive disorder throughout pregnancy have ranged from 8% to 51%[17,18] and from 10% to 17%,[17,19–21] respectively. Such large ranges do not assist our understanding of this disorder.

Valid information on prevalence is of importance because it identifies the level of disease burden on the population and health care system. Strategies for disease management require knowledge of its prevalence throughout all phases of a woman's life.[22] Such knowledge may enable identification of risk factors for depression, optimizing prevention and treatment interventions. A more precise estimate than that afforded by individual small studies is required.

The diagnosis of depression, both in the general population and during pregnancy, is most often based on clinical signs and symptoms as reported by the patient. The essential features of a major depressive episode have been defined by the *Diagnostic and Statistical Manual of Mental Disorders, Fourth Edition.*[23] The standard approach to diagnosis is for a mental health professional to perform a structured clinical interview for *Diagnostic and Statistical Manual of Mental Disorders, Fourth Edition* axis I disorders.[24]

In response to high costs associated with clinician interviews, lay-administered structured interviews and patient self-report questionnaires have been developed. Although not diagnostic, self-report questionnaires are sensitive to depressive symptoms,[25] and cutoff scores have been statistically predetermined to detect respondents likely to have major depression disorder.[26]

Somatic symptoms of pregnancy can be difficult to separate from those of depression. The use of unvalidated questionnaires may result in inaccurate estimations of the prevalence of depression during gestation. Two instruments, the Edinburgh Postnatal Depression Score [27] and the Beck Depression Inventory,[28] have been validated for an obstetric population. In the absence of research that provides clinician diagnoses, results from studies that use screening instruments afford an acceptable measure for the determination of the prevalence of depression during pregnancy.

This study's aim was to derive an overall estimate of the prevalence of depression by trimester of pregnancy, as determined by the Edinburgh Postnatal Depression Scale, the Beck Depression Inventory, and structured clinical interviews, and to compare the rates among instruments.

SOURCES

A comprehensive search of the following databases was performed by combining the key words "preg*," "*natal," "depress*," "psychiatr*," "mood," and "affective." MEDLINE was searched from 1966, EMBASE from 1980, CINAHL from 1982, and HealthSTAR from 1975 to February 2003. A secondary search of the same data-bases, including the Cochrane Library, from 1990 to March 2003 was performed for the key words "EPDS," "BDI," and "pregnancy." This date range was chosen because the earliest validation of screening instruments in pregnant populations was 1990. To avoid bias that may have been incurred as a result of linguistic restrictions, [29] the literature was searched regardless of language of publication. Additionally, researchers in the field were contacted, and a search of the Proquest Digital Dissertations database was performed.

Titles and abstracts of identified studies were assessed for relevance to the topic, and hard copies of appropriate studies were obtained for further evaluation. References from review papers, meta-analyses, and identified studies were assessed to identify additional articles. When data were not presented in an extractable form, attempts were made to contact the corresponding authors of the articles.

STUDY SELECTION

Studies were selected for inclusion based on predefined criteria. Original research in the form of observational cohorts, surveys, and database analyses were considered acceptable for inclusion. Outcomes were to be reported as the number of women depressed as a percentage of the total number of women assessed. In addition, the time of the measurement (ie, weeks of gestation or trimester) was to be reported. Finally, the demographics of patients must have been described.

The population of interest was pregnant women aged more than 17 years. Research based solely on teenaged pregnancies was excluded to avoid bias due to factors specifically related to that population. To eliminate research that relied on selected subgroups (eg, pregnancies complicated by human immunodeficiency virus, study selection was restricted to research on samples of pregnant women recruited through general obstetric and prenatal units and to population surveys. Because rates of depression are correlated with socioeconomic status,[30] publications that examined only women of low socioeconomic status were analyzed separately. The primary outcome of interest was the rate of depression during each trimester of pregnancy, as determined by cutoff scores on the Beck Depression Inventory and the Edinburgh Postnatal Depression Scale and by structured clinical interviews.

A study selection form that detailed the inclusion and exclusion criteria defined above was created. Two independent reviewers tested the form on a random sample (n = 6) of articles that were judged to be typical (acceptable) papers. Clarity, ease of application, and reliability of the form were assessed. Minor modifications, including the reordering of questions and the omission of redundant questions, were made according to the reviewers' recommendations.[31]

Studies were required to meet all inclusion criteria; the presence of any exclusion criteria resulted in rejection from the analysis. In a 2-step process, the same 2 reviewers independently determined whether studies met inclusion criteria. In step 1, each reviewer assessed and categorized abstracts of articles as "included," "unsure," or "rejected." Interrater reliability was estimated by the κ statistic. Discrepancies were resolved by consensus, and a third reviewer adjudicated unresolved disputes; the judgment of the third reviewer was considered final.

Complete articles were obtained for those in the included and unsure categories. The selection process was repeated until all articles were ultimately categorized as included and excluded. Reasons for rejections and exclusions of studies were recorded.

A data-extraction form was designed a priori, and a panel of 3 academic experts assessed its face validation. The feasibility, appropriateness of data, and ease of use was established as described above for study selection. The same 2 reviewers independently extracted data from each article using the data-extraction form. A third party resolved disagreement in the same manner as for study inclusion.

To gain insight into the validity of study design that may affect interpretation of results, we considered the quality of the studies.[32] A qualitative checklist was devised by adapting variables in the NHS Centre for Reviews and Dissemination guidance for undertaking systematic reviews.[33] Because the greatest potential for bias in observational studies may be patient selection,[34] the selection of study participants and attrition rates were assessed based on the following variables: recruitment strategies, inclusion and exclusion criteria, outcome assessment, information on nonresponders and dropouts, and patient demographics. Two independent reviewers performed the assessment and a third party resolved disagreement in the same manner as for study selection. Because it is not clear that study outcomes are correspondingly affected by the same factors as those used in calculating the quality of the study, weighting of the included studies according to the quality score was not performed.[35]

We considered the recruitment strategy adequate if evidence was provided that the sample was a random sample of the study population. The recruitment method should have been stated and sufficient information given on the sampling strategy to enable the reviewers to make such a judgment. If this information was lacking, authors should have presented evidence that the sample was representative of the general population. Similarly, inclusion and exclusion criteria were considered adequate if information was provided in an explicit manner. Reasons for nonparticipation, dropouts, and missing data had to have been reported for these variables to be determined adequate.

All variables were assumed to be of equal importance to the validity of the original research and were weighted equally. Each was assigned a score of 1 if deemed adequate and 0 if deemed inadequate. An index of study quality was obtained by summing the scores of the variables. The maximum possible score attainable was 12.

Comparative trials provide the highest quality data; however, in this analysis, results for single groups (eg, rate of depression equals the number of depressed patients divided by the total number of patients assessed in the study) were considered acceptable. Prevalence was estimated by dividing the number of women identified as depressed by the total number of women remaining in the study at the time of assessment. A stepwise approach was used to summarize and quantify the outcome data of the accepted studies.[36]

A random-effects model for rates [35] was used to combine data. This method of combining results weights by sample size and adjusts for between-study variance, serving to reduce the impact of between-study differences. Analyses were performed for each method of evaluation (ie, self-report versus interview). Studies that explored depression in women of low socioeconomic status were analyzed separately. Each analysis provided a weighted average rate across studies and a 95% confidence interval (CI). Statistical comparisons of rates among trimesters and among methods of determination (ie, instruments) were made using the Kruskal-Wallis test.

Because of variations in the presentation and detection of this disorder, heterogeneity across rates was expected. Before estimation of the meta-analytic rate, a χ^2 test[37] was used to detect heterogeneity among reported rates. This procedure tests the hypothesis that the rates are equal in all studies. Additionally, forest plots were constructed plotting each study point and 95% CI estimate.[38] A forest plot is a graphical display of results from individual studies, allowing visual comparison of trial results and examination of the degree of heterogeneity among studies. In the event of significant heterogeneity, a search was made for moderator variables (ie, to identify possible systematic bias).[35]

Publication bias, which may be a substantial problem in observational studies,[39] was assessed by using funnel plots[40] in which the reported prevalence rates were plotted against sample size. In the absence of publication bias, a symmetrical funnel should be seen. Results from small studies are often prone to random variation and will be dispersed symmetrically around a central overall effect size. As sample size increases, the degree of variation should decrease, producing a symmetrical funnel.[41] We tested the results for significance using the adjusted rank correlation test based on the Kendall τ as proposed by Begg and Mazumdar.[42]

To determine robustness of the results, sensitivity analyses were performed. First, studies deemed to be of low quality (a score of 5 or less) were omitted and data were reanalyzed. Second, studies that used modified screening tools were omitted, and the data were again reanalyzed. Finally, each study was removed in turn and the analysis was rerun. If results differed substantially, further investigations were undertaken.

RESULTS

In total, 714 studies were identified for potential inclusion. Of those, 40 fulfilled all inclusion criteria. A further 19 were excluded because they had inappropriate outcome measures (n = 16), could not be retrieved (n = 1), had inappropriate patient populations (n = 1), and did not examine the appropriate disease state (n = 1). The study selection process is shown in Figure 1. The primary interrater agreement for study inclusion was acceptable ($\kappa = 0.57$, $P < .05$).

Thus, 21 articles fulfilled all criteria and were suitable for inclusion in the analyses. Tables 1 and 2 provide descriptive details of the included studies. The Beck Depression Inventory and the Edinburgh Postnatal Depression Scales were each used in 8 publications. Seven authors reported results from structured interviews. Two authors used both the Beck Depression Inventory and a structured interview to assess depression status. Articles originated from 13 countries, with the United States contributing more studies than any other country (n = 6). Most researchers recruited from urban populations (n = 18); the majority of studies included participants of diverse socioeconomic status (n = 15). The largest study,[43] an epidemiologic survey undertaken in England, screened more than 12,000 patients. Other studies recruited participants through obstetric and pre-natal units and smaller sample sizes (mean 409, range 29–1,489) were reported. Nearly half of the studies (n = 10) were published between 2000 and 2002, possibly reflecting an increasing interest in this topic. Eighteen authors reported participation rates higher than 70%. The mean dropout rate was 12.3% (range 0–25%) and 12.4% (range 0–35%) for the 11 cross-sectional and 10 longitudinal studies, respectively. Mean age of participants was 27.7 (standard deviation [SD] 2.4) years.

The mean quality score of the reports was 7.4 (SD 1.8) of 12, or about 62%. The interrater agreement in scoring with the quality scale was good (r = 0.86, $P < .01$). Disagreement was primarily caused by differences in interpretation, was easily resolved, and consensus was achieved in all cases.

Within each trimester rates displayed heterogeneity, as detected by χ^2 ($P < .05$). Articles that contributed substantially to χ^2 values were examined for the presence of moderator variables. In all studies examined, there were no observable differences among participants with respect to age, socioeconomic status, parity, marital status, or any other reported variable. Therefore, we concluded that differences were not due to systematic differences. Results for all analyses are summarized in Table 3 and displayed in Figure 2. When only a single study was available, individual study results were reported.

The prevalence of depression (95% CI) was 7.4% (2.2, 12.6), 12.8% (10.7, 14.8), and 12.0% (7.4, 16.7) for each trimester, respectively. Overall rates did not differ significantly across trimesters (Kruskal-Wallis test, P = .372). Calculated 95% CIs overlapped substantially.

When rates were compared among the 3 methods (ie, Edinburgh Postnatal Depression Scale, Beck Depression Inventory, and structured interview), a significant difference was found (Kruskal-Wallis test, P = .007). The Dunn post hoc test determined that results differed significantly only between the Beck Depression Inventory and structured interviews (P = .003).

Results of sensitivity analyses that omitted studies with low (5 or less) quality scores and those that had used modified instruments were not appreciably different from the initial results. Similarly, results of analyses that excluded each study in turn were not meaningfully different from the initial results.

Visual examination of funnel plots of studies that examined women throughout the second and third trimesters provided no evidence of publication bias. The number of observations on each side of the meta-analytic average is approximately equal, the spread around the meta-analytic average is about the same, and the shape of the scatter is as expected. The τ correlation coefficient for each plot was not significant ($\tau = -0.02$, $P = .929$ and $\tau = 0.27$, $P = .217$, respectively). The small number of studies identified for the first trimester precluded assessment of publication bias for that period. The funnel plot for studies that examined women during the third trimester of pregnancy is shown in Figure 3.

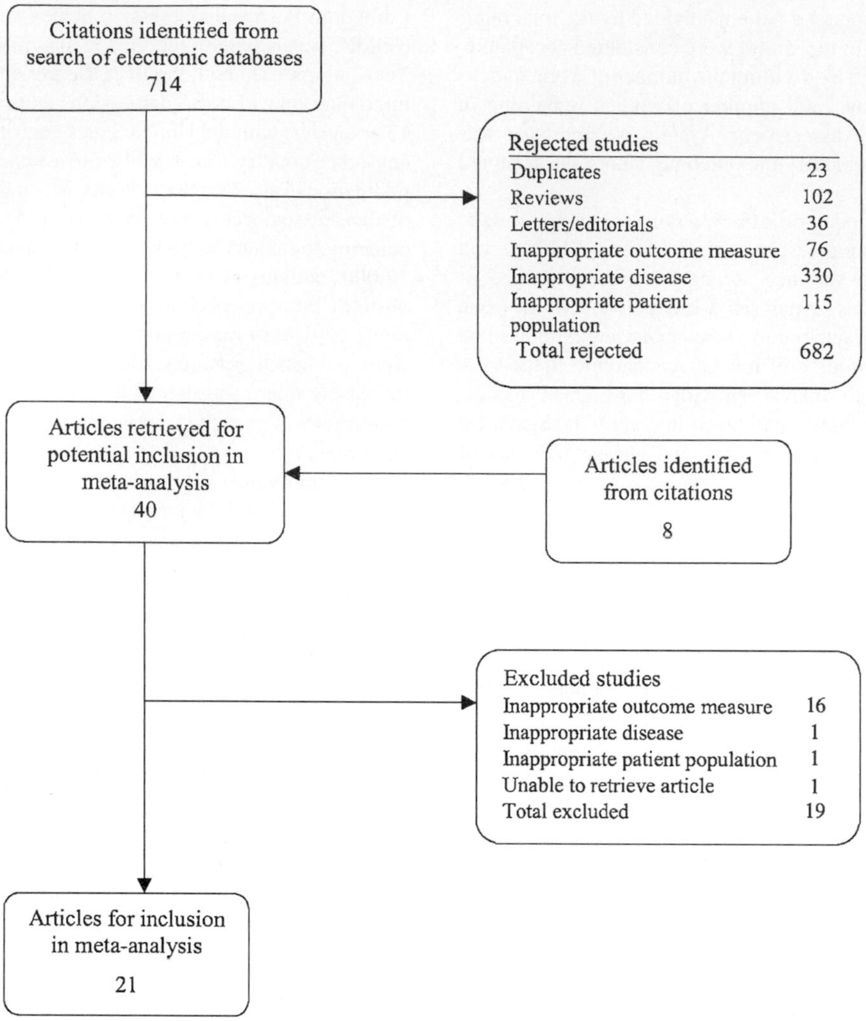

Figure 1. Flow diagram of study selection for inclusion in the meta-analyses.

Bennett. Depression During Pregnancy. Obstet Gynecol 2004.

CONCLUSION

A consideration of this analysis is the heterogeneity observed among study results. Intuitively, the most likely reason for differences in rates is the variety of outcome measures used within the original research. However, when studies were analyzed based on the method of detection of depression heterogeneity remained ($P < .001$).

Alternatively, bias due to the underlying differences inherent in observational studies, for example research from different jurisdictions, may contribute to the heterogeneity. [32] However, O'Hara et al [44] performed a meta-analysis of the prevalence of postpartum depression and reported that the country in which studies were per-formed did not account for the variance in rates. Based on their results, it may be argued that the rate of depression during pregnancy is also unlikely to be influenced by the country of study. Such an assumption would appear to be supported by the convergent rates of major depressive disorder (7–9%) observed in population-based studies of adult female populations in many countries.[1–5,9,10] U.S. estimates, however, have varied between 7.1% and 13%.[6–8] Discrepancies have been reported to be due to methodologic differences.[45] An adjusted estimate of 5.2% for the adult population, compared with 6.5% and 10.1% in the original surveys, has been reported.[45] A third U.S. survey (2001–2002) estimated that 6.6% of adults suffer with major depressive disorder.[46] Although rates for women were not presented separately, it is reasonable to assume that those rates would be similarly downwardly affected. Thus, the revised U.S. prevalence also supports the assumption that the rate of depression during pregnancy is unlikely to be influenced by the country of study.

Another explanation is that the heterogeneity may be due to variation in the underlying risk of patients.[47] Demographics as reported in the original research suggest that patients in each study were comparable. However, not all authors reported on the psychiatric history of the participants. Those with a history of psychiatric disorders would likely score higher on screening instruments. This may in part account for the observed differences between the study outcomes. Unfortunately, because of the limited number of articles included in the analyses, meta-regression to investigate the source of the heterogeneity between studies was not possible. However, it is likely that rates do vary and that these variations are mainly due to chance (ie, sampling error).

Table 1
Details of Studies That Determined the Prevalence of Depression by Self-Report Questionnaire, by Trimester

TRIMESTER	AUTHOR	YEAR PUBLISHED	COUNTRY	INSTRUMENT	CUTOFF SCORE	DEPRESSED (%)	QUALITY SCORE
1	Birndorf et al[70]	2002	United States	BDI	≥ 10	24.6	9
	Pajulo et al[71]	2001	Finland	EPDS	≥ 12	5.3	6
2	Dayan et al[21]	2002	France	EPDS	≥ 15	11.2	7
	Evans et al[43]	2001	England	EPDS	≥ 13	13.9	8
	Gotlib et al[17]	1989	Canada	BDI	≥ 10	21.4	5
	Matthey et al[72]	2000	Australia	BDI	> 9	12.1	9
	Pajulo et al[71]	2001	Finland	EPDS	> 12	8.7	6
	Salamero et al[51]	1994	Spain	BDI	> 15	15.9	3
	Seguin et al[68]	1995	Canada	BDI	> 15	2.2	9
	Seguin et al[68]	1995	Canada	BDI	≥ 10	29.6*	9
3	Bolton et al[73]	1998	England	EPDS	≥ 13	29*	8
	Chung et al[67]	2001	Hong Kong	BDI	≥ 15	8.7	8
	Da Silva et al[69]	1998	Brazil	EPDS	> 13	37.9*	7
	Evans et al[43]	2001	England	EPDS	≥ 13	15.1	8
	Gotlib et al[17]	1989	Canada	BDI	≥ 10	25.8	5
	Johanson et al[19]	2000	England	EPDS	> 14	9.8	7
	Josefsson et al[74]	2001	Sweden	EPDS	≥ 10	17.4	8
	McKee et al[75]	2001	United States	BDI-II	≥ 14	51.4*	9
	O'Heron†	1991	United States	BDI	≥ 16	19.6	6
	Pajulo et al[71]	2001	Finland	EPDS	> 12	7.5	6
	Verdoux et al[76]	2002	France	EPDS	> 12	5	7

BDI = Beck Depression Inventory; EPDS = Edinburgh Postnatal Depression Scale.
Studies of women of low socioeconomic status.
* O'Heron CA. Coping and postpartum depression: an analysis of coping and depression during pregnancy and the puerperium [dissertation].
Saint Louis (MO): University of Missouri; 1991.

Table 2
Details of Studies That Determined the Prevalence of Depression by Structured Interview, by Trimester

TRIMESTER	AUTHOR	YEAR PUBLISHED	COUNTRY	INSTRUMENT	TYPE OF DEPRESSION	DEPRESSED (%)	QUALITY SCORE
1	Affonso et al [57]	1990	United States	SADS-PPG	Major	1.00	9
	Affonso et al [57]	1990	United States	SADS-PPG	Minor	0.50	9
	Areias et al [77]	1996	Portugal	SADS	Minor	3.70	11
	Kitamura et al [78]	1993	Japan	SADS	Minor	10.80	9
2	O'Hara [20]	1986	United States	modified SADS	Major	6.10	8
	Areias et al [77]	1996	Portugal	SADS	Minor	9.30	11
	Gotlib et al [17]	1989	Canada	modified SADS	Minor	79.20	5
	O'Hara [20]	1986	United States	modified SADS	Minor	3.00	8
	Hobfoll et al [66]	1995	United States	RDC	Minor	11.50*	7
	Hobfoll et al [66]	1995	United States	RDC	Major	16.10*	7
3	Affonso et al [57]	1990	United States	SADS-PPG	Minor	0.50	9
	Areias et al [77]	1996	Portugal	SADS	Minor	16.70	11
	Gotlib et al [17]	1989	Canada	modified SADS	Minor	8.10	5
	O'Heron †	1991	United States	SCID	Minor	14.10	6
	Hobfoll et al [66]	1995	United States	RDC	Major	4.20*	7
	Hobfoll et al [66]	1995	United States	RDC	Minor	20.80*	7

SADS-PPG = Schedule for Affective Disorders and Schizophrenia–Pregnancy and Postpartum Guidelines; SADS = Schedule for Affective Disorders and Schizophrenia; SCID = Structured Clinical Interview for DSM-IV Axis I Disorders; RDC = Research Diagnostic Criteria.
* Studies of women of low socioeconomic status
† O'Heron CA. Coping and postpartum depression: an analysis of coping and depression during pregnancy and the puerperium [dissertation].
Saint Louis (MO): University of Missouri; 1991.

Table 3
Summary of Meta-Analytic and Individual Study Results of the Prevalence of Depression During Pregnancy

	PREVALENCE (%)											
		1st TRIMESTER				2nd TRIMESTER				3rd TRIMESTER		
	INSTRUMENT	STUDIES (*n*)	PATIENTS (*n*)	RATE	95 % CONFIDENCE INTERVAL	STUDIES (*n*)	PATIENTS (*n*)	RATE	95 % CONFIDENCE INTERVAL	STUDIES (*n*)	PATIENTS (*n*)	RATE
Interview or questionnaire*	5	528	7.4	2.2, 12.6	10	14,811	12.8	10.7, 14.8	12	16,453	12.0	7.4, 16.7
SA1	5	528	7.4	2.2, 12.6	7	13,245	11.7	9.4, 13.9	10	15,863	11.1	5.9, 16.2
SA2	4	326	9.5	3.2, 15.8	8	14,417	13.7	11.5, 15.8	10	15,956	13.5	10.0,17.0
Validated questionnaires†	2	152	14.2	10.7, 21.7	7	14,363	13.9	11.7,16.1	8	15,810	13.2	9.4,17.1
EPDS ≥ 10	1	95	5.3	2.4, 12.7	3	12,889	11.7	8.8, 14.7	5	14,656	11.1	6.4, 15.9
BDI ≥ 9	1	57	24.6	17.4, 42.5	4	1,474	16.7	12.9, 20.6	3	1,154	17.8	5.5, 30.2
Interview †	3	376	4.9	3.2, 7.7	3	448	9.1	6.5, 11.8	4	643	8.8	1.8, 15.9
Studies of women of low socioeconomic status												
Interview or questionnaire*		No studies identified			2	290	36.9	18.0, 55.8	4	733	35.0	24.3,45.6
Validated questionnaires †		No studies identified			1	98	46.9	40.4, 61.4	3	541	39.2	22.9, 55.5
SA1		No studies identified			1	98	46.9	40.4, 61.4	3	541	39.2	22.9,55.5
EPDS ≥ 10		No studies identified				No studies identified			2	436	29.5	25.2, 33.8
BDI ≥ 9		No studies identified			1	98	46.9	40.4, 61.4	1	105	51.4	41.3,69.2
Interview †		No studies identified			1	192	27.6	22.7,35.7	1	192	25.0	20.2, 32.9

SA1 = sensitivity analysis excluding studies with a low (< 5) quality score; SA2 = sensitivity analysis excluding studies that used modified assessment tools.
* Combined results from structured clinical interviews and self report questionnaires.
† Includes Edinburgh Postnatal Depression Score with a cutoff score ≥ 10, Beck Depression Inventory ≥ 9.

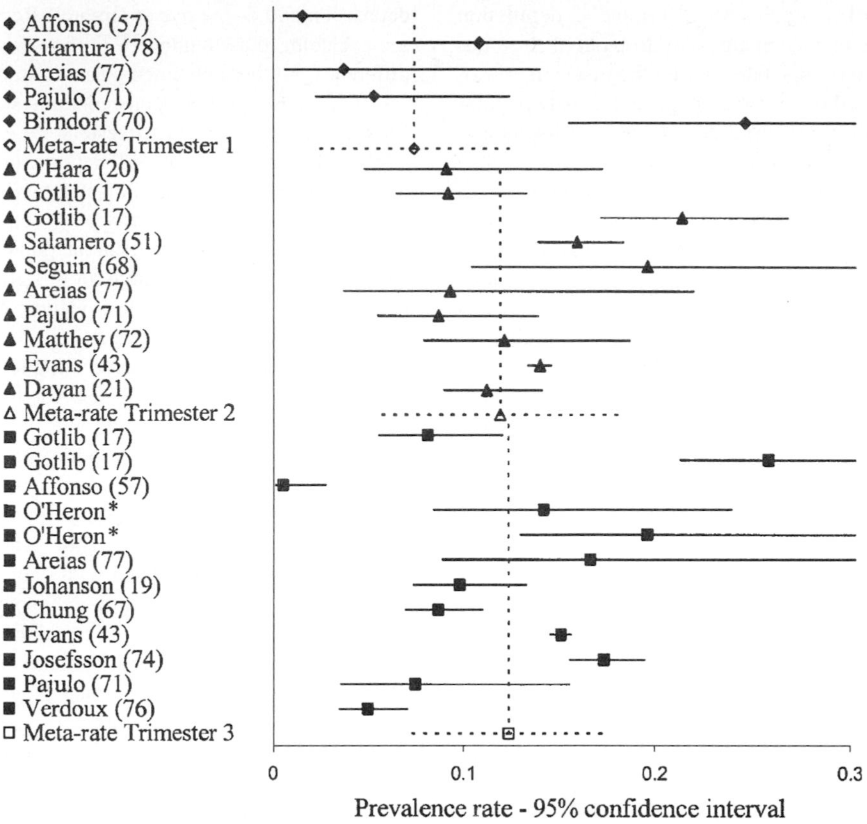

*Figure 2. Forest plot of studies that examined the prevalence of depression during pregnancy, by trimester. *O'Heron CA. Coping and postpartum depression: an analysis of coping and depression during pregnancy and the puerperium [dissertation]. Saint Louis (MO): University of Missouri; 1991.*

Bennett. Depression During Pregnancy. Obstet Gynecol 2004.

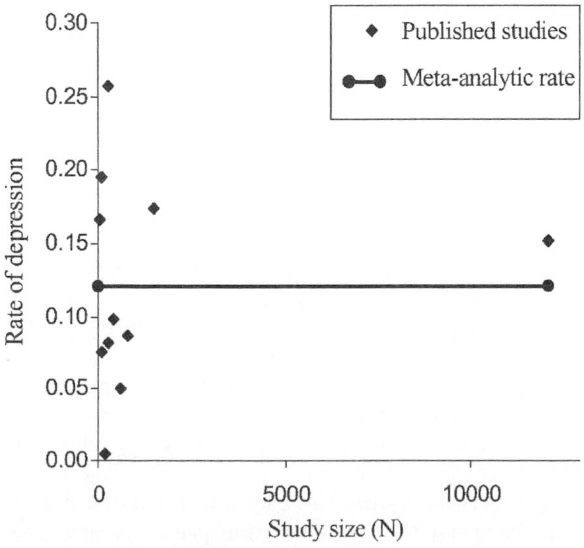

Figure 3. Funnel plot of studies that examined the prevalence of depression during the third trimester of pregnancy.

Bennett. Depression During Pregnancy. Obstet Gynecol 2004.

The lower rate of depression (7.4%) estimated during the first trimester must be interpreted with caution. Few studies were available for that period, and rates have been determined on the basis of small numbers of patients. It may simply be that many women do not seek prenatal care until they are further advanced in their pregnancy, or that depressed women often delay seeking prenatal care.[48] If this is the case, the "true" prevalence of depression for the first trimester may be greater than that estimated in this research.

However, the increased number of women detected as having depressive disorder during the second (12.8%) and third (12.0%) trimesters may have been a result of the greater demands of advancing pregnancy. That is, late-stage pregnancy may be a risk factor for depression. However, that aspect of depression during pregnancy was not addressed in this study and further investigation to determine such an association is required.

Another noteworthy point is that some studies included only participants without a recent history of psychiatric disorder. That criterion may have resulted in the inclusion of "healthy" participants, and thus a conservative prevalence estimate. However, it has been well documented that physicians' rate of recognition of depression during the obstetric period is low.[49,50] Thus, relatively few women may have had such a diagnosis, and the impact of the inclusion criteria may not have affected study participation as previously described.

Considering the evidence presented here, it is likely that the rates estimated by the current analyses, in particular for the first trimester of pregnancy, are conservative. Confirmation of this assumption requires further studies to determine if depression causes women to decline to participate or to drop out of the studies. Nevertheless, in this analysis, rates during the first trimester of pregnancy were similar to those seen in the general female population. Second-trimester and third-trimester rates were substantially higher than that observed in the general female population (7–9%) in all countries that have conducted population-based surveys.

Interestingly, rates determined with the Beck Depression Inventory, but not those determined with the Edinburgh Postnatal Depression Score, were significantly higher than those determined by structured interview. One possible reason for this difference is that the Beck Depression Inventory has a greater number of somatic (physical) items than the Edinburgh Postnatal Depression Score. The importance of those physical items has been assessed in pregnant women in whom a psychiatric illness has not been diagnosed.[51] It was reported that higher scores on the Beck Depression Inventory in populations who have a high incidence of somatic complaints (eg, pregnancy) should not be interpreted as indicators of depression when physical items contribute to the final score. Rather, qualitative analysis of the somatic items is important.

Alternatively, the observed difference between the Beck Depression Inventory and structured interview rates may be an artifact of the self-report measurement method. The positive predictive value of screening instruments is influenced by the prevalence of a disease in the population. That is, the positive predictive value of a test, at a specified cutoff score, will decrease as the prevalence of the disease in the population decreases.[37] We assumed that researchers chose cutoff values appropriate for the population under investigation thus avoiding a decrease in the positive predictive value of the instruments used. Therefore, we included studies that reported cutoff scores for the Edinburgh Postnatal Depression Score from 10 or more to more than 14, and for the Beck Depression Inventory from 9 or more to 16 or more. Despite the variation in scores, there was no correlation between cutoff scores and reported prevalence for either instrument, suggesting that using lower cutoff scores did not necessarily result in an increase in the observed prevalence.

It must be remembered that there are 4 possible outcomes based on the use of screening instruments: true and false positives, and true and false negatives. Individuals identified as "false positives" have been reported to have higher levels of psychopathology than do "true-negative" individuals. Also, many measures of psychosocial dysfunction for false-positive individuals have been found not to significantly differ from those for true-positive individuals.[52] Persons with major depressive disorder experience substantial functional, occupational, and social impairment. Those with subthreshold depressive symptoms, which are less intense and of shorter duration than major depressive disorder, also experience substantial interference in daily functioning which is likely to warrant treatment.[53,54] In fact, it is still unclear whether major depressive disorder is a single clinical disease encompassing an array of symptom levels or whether depressive symptoms are essentially different from clinical depression.[55,56] Thus, the inclusion of such individuals in estimates of prevalence may be clinically important, especially if one is considering the level of disease burden and health-related events on the population and health care system.

Researchers who undertook structured interviews used a number of modified instruments. The specificity and sensitivity of those instruments has not been reported, and the bias, if any, of using them in this population is unknown. This raises important questions regarding the degree to which they accurately and adequately measure depression and depressive symptoms. Results of sensitivity analyses excluding those studies,[17,20,57] however, were not significantly different from those obtained when all studies were included.

For women of low socioeconomic status, meta-analytic rates for the second and third trimesters were 47% and 39%, respectively, when obtained by self-report, and 28% and 25% when determined by structured clinical interviews. The greater prevalence rates observed in this group are consistent with that reported in deprived groups in the general population.[30] However, there were far fewer studies available for this group, and further research is needed. Based on available evidence, we believe these women are likely to experience substantially higher rates of depression than are women of higher socioeconomic status.

Depression increases the risk for the onset of physical and social disability. It is associated with increased medical resource consumption and decreased productivity levels [58] that have an impact not only the on patient but also on family members, friends, employers, and society.[59] Equally important are the outcomes related to the pregnancy itself. For example, depression during pregnancy has been associated with poor health behaviors,[60] risk-taking behavior,[50,60] preeclampsia,[61,62] poor pregnancy outcomes,[63] and an increased risk of progression to postpartum depression.[16,64,65] Recognition and treatment of depression during the obstetric period may not only reduce the risk of immediate adverse outcomes, but it also may be effective in reducing the number of women in whom postnatal depression would otherwise develop.

Several limitations of this analysis warrant mention. First, few authors reported reasons for refusal or dropouts. Thus, results from studies were analyzed using data from completers (ie, per-protocol results). The effect of dropouts on the estimated prevalence is unknown and warrants further examination. It may be expected that when data are collected longitudinally (ie, over the entire pregnancy), higher dropout rates would occur than for studies of cross-sectional design. However, dropout rates for research of longitudinal and cross-sectional design were comparable (mean of 12.4% and 12.3%, respectively). The 4 studies with high dropout rates (20% or higher)[43,66–68] were evenly divided between the 2 types of study design. Therefore, the assumption that the number of dropouts is dependent on study design is unlikely to be relevant to this analysis.

Another explanation is that depression itself resulted in participant withdrawal. Depressed women may have a greater tendency than nondepressed women to discontinue, resulting in an underestimation of the prevalence. Indirect evidence to support such an assumption was provided by Gotlib et al,[17] who reported that as many as 18% of dropouts in that study were depressed. Hence, the reported prevalence in the original studies may have been understated due to the unknown depression status of the women who declined to participate or did not complete the study. For this reason, the prevalence of depression during pregnancy, as estimated in this analysis, may be conservative.

Second, some included studies were not originally designed to collect prevalence data. This may have impacted the reported prevalence. For example, some researchers excluded women who had experienced a previous depressive episode. Such a criterion would likely result in samples being relatively healthy and a subsequent inadequate representation of the "true" demographics of the general population of pregnant women. This may also have resulted in differences in the underlying risk of the participants, accounting for some of the observed heterogeneity among study outcomes.

Third, this analysis did not assess the duration of depressive disorder in this group of patients. Nor was it possible to examine whether the depression was present before pregnancy. Some women may have experienced depression for the entire pregnancy, whereas others may have been depressed for only a portion of that time. To determine such outcomes, individual patient data for each trimester of pregnancy would be required. Those data were not available from the published studies.

Fourth, this research is unable to rule out the possibility of detection bias. Being pregnant and seeking medical care may have resulted in the diagnosis of an existing depression that otherwise would not have been made; ie, the prevalence of depression in the general female population may be underestimated. If this is the case, conclusions based on the comparison between the findings of the current research and rates reported from population-based national studies may be overstated. Finally, because only one study from a developing country (Brazil)[69] was included in this analysis, results may not generalize to less developed regions.

Nonetheless, a consistent picture has emerged, indicating that substantial numbers of women experience depression at some point during pregnancy. What is less clear, however, is the incidence of the disorder. Whether women experience depression on a continued or intermittent basis throughout pregnancy, or in subsequent pregnancies, is unknown. Also, disease severity has not been well documented. The provision of adequate treatment strategies for such a large patient group requires that those questions be answered.

This research systematically evaluated studies that examined the prevalence of depression in pregnant women. It provides a comprehensive estimate of the prevalence of prenatal depression. The rate of depression during the first trimester of pregnancy is similar to that observed in the general female population, whereas the rates during the second and third trimesters are nearly double that rate. Pregnant women of low socioeconomic status appear to have even higher rates of depression than does the general pregnant population. However, more studies using validated instruments are required to support the findings of this research and to provide a quantitative estimate of the difference between various socioeconomic strata of society.

The levels of disability associated with depression during pregnancy were not examined in the present research and are unknown. Further investigation into these matters is warranted. Longitudinal studies to examine maternal and fetal outcomes, and associated clinical and economic consequences, are needed to clarify and quantify the risks of depression during pregnancy.

REFERENCES

1. Liu S, Prince M, Blizard B, Mann A. The prevalence of psychiatric morbidity and its associated factors in general health care in Taiwan. Psychol Med 2002;32:629–37.
2. Australian Institute of Health and Welfare. National health priority areas report. Mental health 1998. Canberra: The Institute; 1999. AIHW Cat. No. PHE 13.
3. Araya R, Rojas G, Fritsch R, Acuna J, Lewis G. Common mental disorders in Santiago, Chile: prevalence and socio-demographic correlates. Br J Psychiatry 2001;178: 228–33.
4. Statistics Canada. Health indicators, volume 2002, no. 1, Depression. Ottawa, (ON): Statistics Canada, CIHI; 2002. Catalogue No: 82-221-XIE.
5. Andrade L, Walters EE, Gentil V, Laurenti R. Prevalence of ICD-10 mental disorders in a catchment area in the city of Sao Paulo, Brazil. Soc Psychiatry Psychiatr Epidemiol 2002;37: 316–25.
6. Regier DA, Narrow WE, Rae DS, Manderscheid RW, Locke BZ, Goodwin FK. The de facto US mental and addictive disorders service system: epidemiologic catchment area prospective 1-year prevalence rates of disorders and services. Arch Gen Psychiatry 1993;50: 85–94.
7. Bland RC. Epidemiology of affective disorders: a review. Can J Psychiatry 1997;42: 367–77.
8. Kessler RC, McGonagle KA, Zhao S, Nelson CB, Hughes M, Eshleman S, et al. Lifetime and 12-month prevalence of DSM-III-R psychiatric disorders in the United States: results from the National Comorbidity Survey. Arch Gen Psychiatry 1994;51: 8–19.
9. Lepine JP, Gastpar M, Mendlewicz J, Tylee A. Depression in the community: the first pan-European study DEPRES (Depression Research in European Society). Int Clin Psychopharmacol 1997;12: 19–29.
10. Berardi D, Leggieri G, Bertti CG, Rucci P, Pezzoli A, Paltrinieri E, et al. Depression in primary care: a nationwide epidemiological survey. Fam Pract 2002;19:397–400.
11. Murray CJ, Lopez AD. Alternative projections of mortality and disability by cause 1990–2020: global burden of disease study. Lancet 1997;349: 1498–504.
12. Parry BL, Newton RP. Chronobiological basis of female-specific mood disorders. Neuropsychopharmacology 2001;25 (5 suppl):S102–8.
13. Wisner KL, Gelenberg AJ, Leonard H, Zarin D, Johanson R, Frank E. Pharmacologic treatment of depression during pregnancy. JAMA 1999;282: 1264–69.
14. Robert E. Treating depression in pregnancy. NEngl J Med 1996;335: 1056–58.
15. Nonacs R, Cohen LS. Depression during pregnancy: diagnosis and treatment options. J Clin Psychiatry 2002;63: 24–30.
16. Burt VK, Stein K. Epidemiology of depression throughout the female life cycle. J Clin Psychiatry 2002;63: 9–15.
17. Gotlib IH, Whiffen VE, Mount JH, Milne K, Cordy NI. Prevalence rates and demographic characteristics associated with depression in pregnancy and the postpartum. J Consult Clin Psychol 1989;57: 269–74.
18. Da Costa D, Larouche J, Dritsa M, Brender W. Psychosocial correlate of prepartum and postpartum depressed mood. J Affect Disord 2000;59: 31–40.
19. Johanson R, Chapman G, Murray D, Johnson I, Cox J. The North Staffordshire Maternity Hospital prospective study of pregnancy-associated depression. J Psychosom Obstet Gynaecol 2000;21: 93–7.
20. O'Hara MW. Social support, life events, and depression during pregnancy and the puerperium. Arch Gen Psychiatry 1986;43: 569–73.
21. Dayan J, Creveuil C, Herlicoviez M, Herbel C, Baranger E, Savoye C, et al. Role of anxiety and depression in the onset of spontaneous preterm labor. Am J Epidemiol 2002;155: 293–301.
22. US Department of Health and Human Services. Breaking ground, breaking through: the strategic plan for mood disorder research of the National Institute of Mental Health. Bethesda (MD): National Institute of Mental Health; 2002.
23. First MB, editor. Diagnostic and statistical manual. 4th ed. Text revision (DSM-IV-TR™, 2000). Washington (DC): American Psychiatric Association; 2000.
24. First MB, Spitzer RL, Gibbon M, Williams JB. User's guide for the structured clinical interview for DSM-IV axis I disorders: clinician version: SCID-I. New York (NY): New York Psychiatric Institute; 2003.
25. US Department of Health and Human Services, Public Health Service, Agency for Health Care Policy and Research. Depression Guideline Panel. Depression in primary care. Volume 1: detection and

diagnosis. Clinical practice guideline no. 5. Rockville (MD): Agency for Health Care Policy and Research; 1993. Publication No. 93–0550.

26. Sharp LK, Lipsky MS. Screening for depression across the lifespan: a review of measures for use in primary care settings. Am Fam Physician 2002;66: 1001–08.
27. Murray D, Cox JL. Screening for depression during pregnancy with the Edinburgh depression scale (EPDS). J Reprod Infant Psychol 1990;8: 99–107.
28. Holcomb WL, Stone LS, Lustman PJ, Gavard JA, Mostello DJ. Screening for depression in pregnancy: characteristics of the Beck Depression Inventory. Obstet Gynecol 1996;88: 1021–5.
29. Gregoire G, Derderian F, Le Lorier J. Selecting the language of the publications included in a meta-analysis: is there a Tower of Babel bias? J Clin Epidemiol 1995;48: 159–63.
30. Gazmararian JA, James SA, Lepkowski JM. Depression in black and white women. The role of marriage and socioeconomic status. Ann Epidemiol 1995;5: 455– 63.
31. Meade MO, Richardson WS. Selecting and appraising studies for a systematic review. Ann Intern Med 1997;127: 531–7.
32. Stroup DF, Berlin JA, Morton SC, Olkin I, Williamson GD, Drummond MD, et al. Meta-analysis of observational studies in epidemiology: a proposal for reporting. JAMA 2000;283: 2008–12.
33. NHS Centre for Reviews and Dissemination. Undertaking systematic reviews of research on effectiveness. 2nd ed. York: York Publishing Services; 2001. CRD Report No. 4.
34. Sterne JA, Gavaghan D, Egger M. Publication and related bias in meta-analysis: power of statistical tests and prevalence in the literature. J Clin Epidemiol 2000;53: 1119 –29.
35. Einarson T. Pharmacoeconomic applications of meta-analysis for single groups using antifungal onychomycosis lacquers as an example. Clin Ther 1997;19: 559–69.
36. Einarson T, Leeder JS, Koren G. A method for meta-analysis of epidemiological studies. Drug Intell Clin Pharm 1988;22: 813–24.
37. Kuzma JW, Bohnenblust SE. Basic statistics for the health sciences. Mountain View (CA): Mayfield Publishing Company; 2001;156–63.
38. Lewis S, Clarke M. Forest plot: trying to see the wood and the trees. BMJ 2001;322: 1479–80.
39. Easterbrook PJ, Berlin JA, Gopalan R, Matthews DR. Publication bias in clinical research. Lancet 1991;337: 867–72.
40. Light RJ, Pillemer DB. Summing up. The science of reviewing research. Cambridge (MA): Harvard University Press; 1984. p. 63–72.
41. Egger M, Smith GD, Schneider M, Minder C. Bias in meta-analysis detected by a simple, graphical test. BMJ 1997;315: 629–34.
42. Begg CB, Mazumdar M. Operating characteristics of a rank correlation test for publication bias. Biometrics 1994; 50: 1088–101.
43. Evans J, Heron J, Francomb H, Oke S, Golding J. Cohort study of depressed mood during pregnancy and after childbirth. BMJ 2001;323: 257–60.
44. O'Hara MW, Swain AM. Rates and risk of postpartum depression: a meta-analysis. Int Rev Psychiatry 1996;8: 37–54.
45. Narrow WE, Rae DS, Robins LN, Regier DA. Revised prevalence estimates of mental disorders in the United States. Arch Gen Psychiatry 2002;59: 115–23.
46. Kessler RC, Berglund P, Demler O, Robert J, Koretz D, Merikangas KR, et al. The epidemiology of major depressive disorder. JAMA 2003;289: 3095–105.
47. Thompson SG, Smith TC, Sharp SJ. Investigation of underlying risk as a source of heterogeneity in meta-analysis. Stat Med 1997;16: 2741–58.
48. Kelly RH, Danielsen B, Golding J, Anders T, Gilbert W, Zatzick DF. Adequacy of prenatal care among women with psychiatric diagnoses giving birth in California in 1994 and 1995. Psychiatr Serv 1999;50: 1584–90.
49. Boyd RC, Pearson JL, Blehar MC. Prevention and treatment of depression in pregnancy and the postpartum period: summary of a maternal depression roundtable: a US perspective. Arch Womens Ment Health 2002;4: 79–82.
50. Kelly RH, Zatzick DF, Anders TF. The detection and treatment of psychiatric disorders and substance use among pregnant women cared for in obstetrics. Am J Psychiatry 2001;158:213–19.
51. Salamero M, Marcos T, Gutierrez F, Rebull E. Factorial study of the BDI in pregnant women. Psychol Med 1994;24: 1031–5.
52. Gotlib IH, Lewinsohn PM, Seeley JR. Symptoms versus a diagnosis of depression: differences in psychosocial functioning. J Consult Clin Psychol 1995;63: 90–100.
53. Coverdale JH, Chervenak FA, Bayer T, McCullough LB. Ethically justified clinically comprehensive guidelines for the management of the depressed pregnant patient. Am J Obstet Gynecol 1996;174: 169–73.
54. Pini S, Perkonnig A, Tansella M, Wittchen H. Prevalence and 12-month outcome of threshold and subthreshold mental disorders in primary care. J Affect Disord 2002;56: 37–48.
55. Judd LL, Akiskal HS, Maser JD, Zeller PJ, Endicott J, Coryell W. A prospective 12-year study of subsyndromal and syndromal depressive symptoms in unipolar major depressive disorders. Arch Gen Psychiatry 1998;55: 694–700.
56. Solomon A, Haaga DA, Arnow BA. Is clinical depression distinct from subthreshold depressive symptoms? A review of the continuity issue in depression research. J Nerv Ment Dis 2001;189: 498–506.
57. Affonso DD, Lovett S, Paul N, Sheptak S. A standardized interview that differentiates pregnancy and postpartum symptoms from perinatal clinical depression. Birth 1990; 17:121–30.
58. Ormel J, VonKorff M, Oldehinkel AJ, Simon G, Tiemens BG, Utson TB. Onset of disability in depressed and non-depressed primary care patients. Psychol Med 1999;29: 847–53.
59. Clark DA. Canadian perspectives on research in depression. Can J Behav Sci 1998;30: 207–12.
60. Zuckerman B, Amaro H, Bauchner H, Cabral H. Depressive symptoms during pregnancy: relationship to poor health behaviors. Am J Obstet Gynecol 1989;160: 1107–11.
61. Paarlberg KM, Vingerhoets JJ, Passchier J, Dekker GA, Van Geijn FP. Psychosocial factors and pregnancy out-come: a review with emphasis on methodological issues. J Psychosom Res 1995;39: 563–95.
62. Kurki T, Hiilesmaa V, Raitasalo R, Mattila H, Ylikorkala O. Depression and anxiety in early pregnancy and risk for preeclampsia. Obstet Gynecol 2000;95: 487–90.
63. US Department of Health and Human Services. Mental health: a report of the surgeon general. Rockville (MD): National Institutes of Health, National Institute of Mental Health; 1999.
64. Chaudron LH, Klein MH, Remington P, Palta M, Allen C, Essex MJ. Predictors, prodromes and incidence of postpartum depression. J Psychosom Obstet Gynaecol 2001;22: 103–12.
65. Stowe ZN, Nemeroff CB. Women at risk for postpartum-onset major depression. Am J Obstet Gynecol 1995;173: 639–45.
66. Hobfoll SE, Ritter C, Lavin J, Hulsizer MR, Cameron RP. Depression prevalence and incidence among inner-city pregnant and postpartum women. J Consult Clin Psychol 1995;63: 445–53.
67. Chung TK, Lau TK, Yip AS, Chiu HF, Lee DT. Antepartum depressive symptomatology is associated with adverse obstetric and neonatal outcomes. Psychosom Med 2001;63: 830–4.
68. Seguin L, Potvin L, St-Denis M, Loiselle J. Chronic stressors, social support, and depression during pregnancy. Obstet Gynecol 1995;85: 583–9.
69. Da Silva VA, Moraes-Santos AR, Carvalho MS, Martins ML, Teixeira NA. Prenatal and postnatal depression among low income Brazilian women. Braz J Med Biol Res 1998;31: 799–804.
70. Birndorf CA, Madden A, Portera L, Leon AC. Psychiatric symptoms, functional impairment, and receptivity toward mental health treatment among obstetrical patients. Int J Psychiatry Med 2001;31: 355–65.
71. Pajulo M, Savonlahti E, Sourander A, Helenius H, Piha J. Antenatal depression, substance dependency and social support. J Affect Disorder 2001;65: 9–17.
72. Matthey S, Barnett B, Ungerer J, Waters B. Paternal and maternal depressed mood during the transition to parenthood. J Affect Disorder 2000;60: 75–85.

73. Bolton HL, Hughes PM, Turton P, Sedgwick P. Incidence and demographic correlates of depressive symptoms during pregnancy in an inner London population. J Psychosom Obstet Gynaecol 1998;19: 202–9.
74. Josefsson A, Berg G, Nordin C, Sydsjo G. Prevalence of depressive symptoms in late pregnancy and postpartum. Acta Obstet Gynecol Scand 2001;80: 251–5.
75. McKee MD, Cunningham D, Jankowksi KR, Luis S. Health-related functional status in pregnancy: relationship to depression and social support in a multi-ethnic population. Obstet Gynecol 2001;97: 988–93.
76. Verdoux H, Sutter AL, Glatigny-Dallay E, Minisini A. Obstetrical complications and the development of postpartum depressive symptoms: a prospective survey of the MATQUID cohort. Acta Psychiatr Scand 2002;106: 212–19.
77. Areias ME, Kumar R, Barros H, Figueiredo E. Comparative incidence of depression in women and men, during pregnancy and after childbirth: validation of the Edinburgh Postnatal Depression Scale in Portuguese mothers. Br J Psychiatry 1996;169: 30–5.
78. Kitamura T, Shima S, Sugawara M, Toda MA. Psychological and social correlates of the onset of affective disorders among pregnant women. Psychol Med 1993;23: 967–75.

Address reprint requests to: Heather A. Bennett, BPharm, Faculty of Pharmacy, University of Toronto, 19 Russell Street, Toronto, ON M5S 2S2, Canada; e-mail: heather.bennett@utoronto.ca.

Received August 21, 2003. Received in revised form November 28, 2003. Accepted December 12, 2003.

Reprinted from Bennett HA, Einarson A, Taddio A, Koren G, Einarson TR. Prevalence of depression during pregnancy: systematic review. Obstet Gynecol. 2004;103:698–709 with permission from Lippincott Williams & Wilkins.

CHAPTER 30

PERINATAL RISKS OF UNTREATED DEPRESSION DURING PREGNANCY

Lori Bonari,[1] Natasha Pinto,[1] Eric Ahn,[1] Adrienne Einarson,[2] Meir Steiner,[3] and Gideon Koren[4]

Manuscript received November 2003, revised, and accepted February 2004.

[1]Graduate student, Motherisk Program, The Hospital for Sick Children and the Department of Pharmacology, University of Toronto, Toronto, Ontario. [2]Associate Director, Motherisk Program, The Hospital for Sick Children, Toronto, Ontario. [3]Professor of Psychiatry, McMaster University, Hamiton, Ontario. [4]Director, Motherisk Program, The Hospital for Sick Children, Toronto, Ontario; Professor, the Department of Pharmacology, University of Toronto. Toronto, Ontario; Ivey Chair in Molecular Toxicology, University of Western Ontario, London, Ontario.

Objective: To review the literature on the perinatal risks involved in untreated depression during pregnancy.

Method: We searched Medline and medical texts for all studies pertaining to this area up to the end of April 2003. Key phrases entered were depression and pregnancy, depression and pregnancy outcome, and depression and untreated pregnancy. We did not include bipolar depression.

Results: While there is wide variability in reported effects, untreated depression during pregnancy appears to carry substantial perinatal risks. These may be direct risks to the fetus and infant or risks secondary to unhealthy maternal behaviours arising from the depression. Recent human data suggest that untreated postpartum depression, not treatment with antidepressants in pregnancy, results in adverse perinatal outcome.

Conclusion: The biological dysregulation caused by gestational depression has not received appropriate attention: most studies focus on the potential but unproven risks of psychotropic medication. No in-depth discussion of the role of psychotherapy is available. Because they are not aware of the potentially catastrophic outcome of untreated maternal depression, this imbalance may lead women suffering from depression to fear teratogenic effects and refuse treatment.

(Can J Psychiatry 2004;49:726–735)

Information on funding and support and author affiliations appears at the end of the article.

Clinical Implications

- This review reveals some potential risks of untreated depression during pregnancy, with possibly significant implications for practice and further research.
- Clinicians and women themselves need to be educated about the perils of unchecked depression in pregnancy so that they can make truly informed treatment decisions.
- Considering the high prevalence of depression, antenatal treatment might prevent some adverse pregnancy outcomes. However, neither psychotherapy nor pharmacotherapy can be offered if most women are undiagnosed.

Limitations

- The psychiatry literature offers relatively little information on untreated depression during pregnancy.
- This review focused only on the hypothalamo–pituitary–adrenal axis to investigate the etiology of depression.

Key Words: untreated depression, pregnancy outcome, perinatal development, etiology, prevalence, hypothalamo–pituitary–adrenal axis

Traditionally, pregnancy has been thought of as a period of well-being and happiness. The pregnancy state itself has been thought to protect women from depression (1,2). However, women of child-bearing age frequently suffer from major depression (3,4). Lifetime depression risk estimates in community-derived samples have varied between 10% and 25% of pregnant women (5–7). Two recent studies that screened obstetric patients at random for depressive symptoms found that 20% of patients actually met criteria for a diagnosis of depression (8,9). Antepartum depression is also common in women with a history of depressive illness, such that some researchers now believe pregnancy to be a risk factor for a mood disorder in those with such a history (10–12).

Despite the prevalence of depression during pregnancy and the growing body of literature associated with its treatment, whether pharmacologic or otherwise, large numbers of women are untreated. A 2003 study by Marcus and others found that 1 in 5 pregnant women experience depression but that few seek treatment (12). This large study of 3472 pregnant obstetric clinic patients revealed both underdiagnosis and undertreatment of depression during pregnancy: 20% of obstetric patients scored high on the Centre for Epidemiologic Studies Depression Scale (CESD). Although CESD scores do not by themselves diagnose clinical depression, only 13.8% of these women were receiving any form of mental health care. The remaining 86.2% of women with depressive symptoms were not receiving any treatment at all (defined as medication, psychotherapy, or counselling). Over one-half of the women in the study had been taking medications for depression and had stopped once they conceived. These results are similar to another 2003 study, which found a 20% depression rate in random screening for depression among pregnant women in a hospital obstetric setting (9). In that study, fewer than 21% of the women with depression were receiving treatment. The Marcus and others study concluded that the stigma of having depression during pregnancy may prevent women from seeking active treatment—women may feel guilty for suffering during what is supposed to be a happy period (12). In this review, our objective

Address for correspondence: Dr G Koren, The Motherisk Program, Hospital for Sick Children, 555 University Avenue, Toronto, ON M5G 1X8
e-mail: gkoren@sickkids.ca

was to summarize the state of knowledge about depression during pregnancy. We focused on some of the major consequences of untreated maternal depression.

METHODS

We searched Medline and medical texts for studies pertaining to depression during pregnancy published up to the end of April 2003. We included the MeSH phrases depression and pregnancy, depression and pregnancy outcome, and depression and untreated and pregnancy. We reviewed only English-language papers. We restricted the review to original human and animal studies and did not consider case reports or letters to the editor. We excluded studies dealing with bipolar depression.

ETIOLOGY OF POOR PREGNANCY OUTCOME IN DEPRESSION PATIENTS

Depression has been recognized as a disease that affects fetal health (13). Although both psychological and biological explanations have been proposed, hormonal hypotheses have received the most attention. Depression has been associated with hypothalamo–pituitary–adrenal (HPA) axis hyperactivity. Maternal stress, anxiety, or depression, which are regulated by peptides derived from the activated HPA axis (14–19), are all thought to influence birth outcome. This increased HPA-axis activity may directly affect fetal growth. Maternal depression may not only activate the mother's HPA axis; it may in turn cause an increase in the release of corticotropin-releasing hormone (CRH) from the placenta via the actions of catecholamines and cortisol. CRH may also influence the timing and onset of delivery, which could explain why women suffering from depression show higher rates of premature labour (16,17). Animal studies have found that stress during pregnancy is associated with dysfunction of the HPA axis and subsequent abnormal development of fetal tissue (10,18,20). An alternate hypothesis asserts that depression alters excretion of vasoactive hormones and neuroendocrine transmitters, which then induce vascular changes in a pregnant woman (21).

To support the HPA-axis hypothesis of depression's impact on pregnancy, the relation between mood changes and obstetric experience and alterations in plasma cortisol, betaendorphin, and CRH were examined in 97 women (18). Plasma levels of these hormones were obtained throughout pregnancy, at delivery, and postpartum. Mood disturbance rates were highest at 38 weeks' gestation, while plasma hormone levels rose throughout the pregnancy and peaked before labour. Cortisol, beta-endorphin, and CRH climbed significantly throughout the pregnancy and were highly correlated to one another. Those women with the highest clinical depression scores were given significantly more pain relief during labour. This may also be related to endorphin levels, which rise throughout pregnancy and fall dramatically during delivery. In line with previous studies, higher rates of mood disturbance were found in the late antenatal period than in the postnatal period; this correlated with hormone levels, which peaked in late pregnancy and fell postpartum (18). These data suggest a role for CRH and the HPA axis in the interaction between antenatal mood states and obstetric events.

Although the existing literature suggests various ways in which hormonal deviations may affect pregnant women, much remains unclear in regard to defining the mechanisms by which depression adversely affects pregnancy outcome.

RISKS OF UNTREATED DEPRESSION DURING PREGNANCY

While conflicting studies exist that either stress or dispute the significance of obstetric complications in women with depression (22,23), it is well recognized that there is maternal morbidity and mortality associated with untreated mental conditions (24–28), including suicide attempts (37). Most researchers have found that untreated depression may have associated obstetric complications and puerperal pathologies (3,13,17,21,29–36). It has been suggested that mental illness may affect a pregnancy by affecting the mother's emotional state. The prevalent idea is that psychopathological symptoms during pregnancy have physiological consequences for the fetus. Gestational hypertension and subsequent preeclampsia have also been linked to mothers with untreated depression during pregnancy (15,21). Untreated depression during pregnancy has been associated with such adverse outcomes as spontaneous abortion (37), bleeding during gestation (38), increased uterine artery resistance (39), low Apgar scores (36), admission to a neonatal care unit (13), neonatal growth retardation (13,40,41), spontaneous early labour (42,43), fetal death (36), low birth weight in babies (15,17,34,38,44), babies small for their gestational age (34,38,41), perinatal and birth complications (15,38,45), preterm deliveries (13,17,35,42,43,46), and high cortisol levels in offspring at birth (40,47).

Depression has also been linked to such operative deliveries as cesarean section or vaginal instrumental (13) and to a subjective description of labour as more painful and therefore more commonly needing epidural analgesia (18,48). Physiology aside, studies have found that mental illness can affect a mother's functional status, her ability to obtain prenatal care, and her ability to avoid unhealthy behaviour. Women suffering from depression are more likely to smoke or use alcohol or other substances, which may confound pregnancy outcome (49). In this review, we discuss all the above outcomes more thoroughly.

One of the most obvious concerns regarding untreated depression during pregnancy is worsening of the condition itself, which may lead to suicide ideation or attempts. Untreated antenatal depression may be associated with a 50% to 62% risk of a postpartum episode and a worsening of the psychiatric condition (50,51). Termination of pregnancy on psychiatric grounds is common (52,53). According to the National Depressive and Manic-Depressive Association consensus statement on the undertreatment of depression, 15% of women who do not treat their depression during pregnancy attempt suicide (54,55), while 50% to 62% continue to suffer from depression in the postpartum period (55). Suicide attempts during pregnancy have been described (54,56). It has been estimated that depression may be responsible for 30 000 to 35 000 suicides yearly in North America (55).

PRETERM DELIVERY AND GROWTH RETARDATION

It has been proposed that psychopathology during pregnancy adversely affects the uterine environment and therefore affects fetal outcome (51). Steer and others found elevated risks for preterm delivery (<37 weeks), low birth weight (< 2500 g), and babies small for their gestational age (<10th percentile) among women who had scores of 21 or more on the Beck Depression Inventory (BDI) and who were not receiving active treatment (34). These researchers also regressed the BDI scores of 389 pregnant women to indicators of poor pregnancy outcome. Among these women, the

Table 1
Summary of Depression in Pregnancy Studies

STUDY	SAMPLE SIZE	STUDY DESIGN	ENDPOINTS
Chung and others (13)	959	Prospective observational study	Perinatal risks of depression in late pregnancy: increased risk of epidural analgesia RR = 2.56 (95%CI, 1.24 to 5.30) operative deliveries RR = 2.28 (95%CI, 1.15 to 4.53) admission to neonatal care unit RR = 2.18 (95%CI, 1.02 to 4.66).
Paarlberg and others (58)	399	Prospective study	Statistically significant maternal psychosocial risk factors associated with increased risk of low birth weight: depressive mood in the first trimester OR 1.12 (95% CI, 1.01 to 1.24) low subjective severity rating of daily stressors in the first trimester OR 0.41 (95%CI, 0.17 to 0.97).
Lou and others (32)	70 cases, 50 control subjects	Prospective study	Birth weight and head circumference significantly affected by stress and smoking. Stress was a significant determinant of small head circumference.
Steer and others (34)	712	Prospective cohort study	In adult women, with each increase in the Beck Depression Inventory, risk of a poor outcome rose 5% to 7% ($P < 0.05$): risk of low birth weight <2500 g 3.97 (95%CI, 3.80 to 4.15) risk of preterm delivery <37 weeks 3.39 (95%CI, 3.24 to 3.56) risk of having a small-for-gestational-age infant at 10th percentile 3.02 (95%CI, 2.88 to 3.17).
Dayan and others (42)	634	Cohort study	Depression in women with prepregnancy body mass index below 19 was positively associated with outcome OR 6.9 (95%CI, 1.8 to 26.2). Trait anxiety in women and a history of preterm labour OR 4.8 (95%CI, 1.1 to 20.4). State anxiety in women and vaginal bleeding OR 3.6 (95%CI, 0.9 to 14.7).
Field and others (40)	166	Prospective cohort study	Women experiencing high anger and concomitant high scores on depression and anxiety scales had fetuses that were more active and had growth delays. Fetuses had high prenatal cortisol and adrenaline and low dopamine and serotonin levels, similar to their mothers. Newborns had disorganized sleep patterns and performed less than optimally on the Brazelton Neonatal Behavior Assessment Scale.
Hoffman and others (41)	666	Prospective cohort study	Among women with lower occupational status, every unit increase on the CESD was associated with a reduction of 9.1 g (95%CI, –16.0 to –2.3) in gestational-age-adjusted birth weight.
Zuckerman and others (49)	1014	Prospective cohort study	Maternal depressive symptoms were associated with the following: increased life stress ($P < 0.001$) decreased social support ($P < 0.001$) poor weight gain ($P < 0.01$) use of cigarettes ($P < 0.001$), alcohol ($P < 0.001$), and cocaine ($P < 0.05$).
Allister and others (59)	10 cases, 10 control subjects	Prospective cohort study	Women with untreated depression had the following: fetuses with an elevated baseline FHR and a 3.5-fold delay in return to baseline FHR after vibroacoustic stimulus presentation significantly higher anxiety levels.
Bergant others (60)	36 cases, 36 control subjects	Prospective cohort study	A psychosomatic investigation showed that patients with recurrent abortion were significantly more satisfied with their quality of life where leisure time, financial situation, and occupation was concerned, compared with control subjects. Those who had spontaneous abortions owing to a physical disorder had longer relationships with partners and more frequent miscarriages. Eighteen women had successful pregnancy outcomes within 2 years after recurrent miscarriage. These women were significantly younger and had fewer physically related abortions, compared with the 18 women who were still childless. "Psychological factors seem to be of subordinate importance as a cause for recurrent spontaneous abortion," while physical abnormalities in the reproductive system have a more important effect on the success of a future pregnancy.

(Continued)

Table 1
Summary of Depression in Pregnancy Studies *(Continued)*

STUDY	SAMPLE SIZE	STUDY DESIGN	ENDPOINTS
Bosquet and others (66)	48 cases, 62 control subjects	Interventional study	Maternal depressive symptoms, and maternal state of mind with regard to attachment as associated with mother and child behaviours: greater coherence of mind was associated with a more positive outcome (r^2 change = 0.08, $P = 0.05$) preoccupied tendencies were repeatedly adversely associated with outcome in the control group depression in mothers as measured by the CESD tended to be associated with hostility in the intervention group (r^2 change = 0.11, $P = 0.05$).
Nulman and others (69)	86 cases, 36 control subjects	Prospective study	Exposure to tricyclic antidepressants or fluoxetine throughout gestation did not adversely affect global IQ, language development, or behaviour of preschool and early school children. Maternal duration of depression was significantly and negatively associated with IQ ($P = 0.05$; 95%CI, –32.94 to –0.40). Language was negatively associated with number of episodes of maternal depression after delivery ($P = 0.01$; 95%CI, –0.51 to –0.06).
Sugiura-Ogasawara and others (62)	61	Prospective study	Baseline depressive symptoms were significantly associated with subsequent miscarriage in 10 (22%) of 45 patients with recurrent miscarriages ($P = 0.004$).
Zax and others (36)	337	Prospective cohort study	Women with neurotic depression had children with lower Apgar scores and experienced more fetal deaths.
Maki and others (70)	12 059	Cohort study	Association of maternal depression and criminality in offspring was as follows: for male offspring involved in nonviolent crimes, OR 1.4 (95%CI, 1.0 to 1.9) for violent offenders, OR 1.6 (95%CI, 1.1 to 2.4) for female offspring involved in nonviolent crimes, OR 1.7 (95% CI, 0.9 to 3.3) for violent crimes, OR 0.6 (95%CI, 0.1 to 6.0).
Hammen and others (71)	816	Cohort study	Children aged 15 years of mothers with depression were twice as likely to be diagnosed with depression, compared with children of never-depressed mothers (20.1% vs 10.2%, $\chi^2 = 14.05$, $P < 0.001$). Exposure to maternal depression at any period in the first 10 years equally predicted youth depression if the mother had depression only once (19% vs 10%, $\chi^2 = 6.83$, $P < 0.001$).
Kelly and others (31)	186	Questionnaires and medical records review	Of the women receiving prenatal care,70 (38%) met screening criteria for psychiatric disorders or substance use. Symptoms were recorded in 43%of the charts, diagnoses in 18%, evaluations in 35%, and treatments in only 23%.
Preti and others (38)	41 pairs	Prospective case–control study	Babies of women with depression were more likely than those of control subjects to be small for their gestational age (22 vs 1, $\chi^2 = 4.34$, $P = 0.03$). Cases were significantly more likely than control subjects to have suffered at least 1 obstetric complication (85% vs 60%, $\chi^2 = 5.03$, $P = 0.02$). Bleeding during gestation was seen significantly more among cases than control subjects (observed for 4 cases and no control subjects).
Teixeira and others (39)	100	Cohort study	Uterine artery resistance index was significantly associated with both Spielberger state anxiety ($r = 0.31$, $P < 0.002$) and trait anxiety scores ($r = 0.28$, $P < 0.005$). Women with state anxiety scores > 40 ($n = 15$) had higher mean uterine resistance index than those with scores ≤ 40 (mean difference with mean resistance index 24%, 95%CI, 12% to 38%, $P < 0.0001$).
Orr and others (43)	1399	Prospective study	Spontaneous preterm birth occurred among 12.7% of those with a CESD score in the upper 10th percentile and among 8.0% of those with a lower score (RR = 1.59). Adjusted OR for an elevated CESD score was 1.96 (95%CI, 1.04 to 3.72).
Mahomed and others (48)	189	Prospective cohort study	Stress hormone levels were associated with maternal anxiety, depression, self-esteem scores, and changes associated with mothers' labour experience and pain:

Table 1
Summary of Depression in Pregnancy Studies *(Continued)*

STUDY	SAMPLE SIZE	STUDY DESIGN	ENDPOINTS
			patients who were distressed and required analgesia had higher cortisol levels women who described a more positive labour experience at 24 hours had higher cortisol levels There were no significant correlations between psychological test scores and stress hormone levels labour pain at the time and a more positive recollected labour experience were associated with high cortisol levels.
Josefsson and others (50)	1558	Longitudinal study	Prevalence of depressive symptoms during the following periods: late pregnancy, 17% in the maternity ward, 18% 6 to 8 weeks postnatally, 13% 6 months postnatally, 13%. Correlation between antenatal and postnatal depressive symptoms was $r = 0.50$ ($P < 0.0001$).
Appleby and others (54)	76 cases	Retrospective study based on population data	Standardized mortality ratio for postnatal suicide was 0.17. Stillbirth was associated with a rate 6 times that in all women after childbirth.
Evans and others (51)	9028	Longitudinal cohort	Depression scores higher at 32 weeks gestational age than 8 weeks and 8 months postpartum
Hostetter and others (57)	34	Prospective cohort	Twenty-two of 34 subjects required an increase in their daily dose of medication to maintain euthymia. Increased dosage occurred at mean 27.1, SD 7.1 weeks.
Arck and others (61)	94	Prospective cohort	Significantly higher numbers of MCT+, CD8+ T cells, and TNF-K+ cells per mm^2 tissue were observed in deciduas of women with high stress scores.
O'Connor and others (67)	7144	Retrospective cohort	Postnatal depression at 8 weeks (OR 2.27; 95%CI, 1.55 to 3.31) and 8 months (OR 1.68; 95%CI, 1.12 to 2.54) was associated with children's behavioural problems.
Erickson and others (30)	717	Questionnaire	Psychological variables showed differences between multigravidae and primigravidae in birth complications.
Wadhwa and others (35)	90	Prospective cohort	Increased prenatal life-event stress was associated with a decrease in birth weight (OR 1.32). Each unit increase of anxiety was associated with 3-day decrease in gestational age at birth.
Michel-Wolfromm and others (37)	60	Observational case series (no statistics performed)	No proof of solely psychological cause for spontaneous abortion.
Ashman and others (47)	74	Prospective cohort	Children with increased levels of internalizing symptoms whose mothers had a history of depression showed elevated baseline cortisol levels.
D'Alfonso and others (3)	64	Questionnaire	This study suggests that any woman can develop moderate-to-strong symptoms of depression during pregnancy.
Kurki and others (21)	623	Prospective cohort	Anxiety or depression, or both, were associated with increased risk (OR 3.1; 95%CI, 1.4 to 6.9) for preeclampsia.
Perkin and others (22)	1515	Prospective cohort	Perinatal depression and anxiety were unrelated to or weakly associated with obstetric complications.
Kent and others (23)	96	Prospective cohort	No association was found between resistance index and anxiety scores.
Frank and others (28)	128	Randomized controlled trial	Imipramine hydrochloride has a significant prophylactic effect when maintained at an average dosage of 200 mg daily.
Smith and others (18)	97	Prospective study	This study suggests a role for circulating corticotropin-releasing hormone in the regulation of maternal cortisol secretion. It also finds a relationship between maternal postnatal mood states and beta endorphin and between antenatal mood states and obstetric events

OR = odds ratio; RR = relative risk; CESD = Centre for Epidemiology Depression Scale; FHR = fetal heart rate risk of a poor outcome rose 5% to 7% ($P < 0.05$) for each point by which the BDI total score increased (34). In other studies, prenatal stress and depression have been similarly significantly associated with lower infant birth weight and gestational age at birth (34,35,44,57,58). A recent study of women with lower socioeconomic status found depression to be associated with restricted fetal growth and babies small for their gestational age (41). A clear association has been found between increased hypothalamic, pituitary, and placental hormones and the occurrence of preterm labour (42,46). Recent studies have suggested that maternal depression is linked with smaller head circumference and lower Apgar scores in offspring (10,32,36). Of growing concern is the effect of perinatal depression on fetoplacental integrity and fetal CNS development (59).

PREECLAMPSIA

Studies have also investigated the link between depression and preeclampsia. Defined as blood pressure higher than 140/100 mm Hg and proteinuria, preeclampsia is a serious pregnancy complication. Strenuous work, depression, and anxiety may increase the risk for this condition, whereas the stress of daily living has not been associated with it. Kurki and colleagues studied 623 nulliparous Finnish women at low risk for preeclampsia. All women had a healthy first trimester and were then tested with standard Beck Depression and Anxiety scales at a median 12 weeks (21). Depression was detected in 30% of the women, which matches with the known prevalence of depression during pregnancy in the Finnish population (21). Anxiety was detected in 16%, and proteinuric preeclampsia was detected in 4.5%. Depression was associated with an increased risk for preeclampsia (odds ratio 2.5; 95%CI, 1.2 to 5.3), as was anxiety. However, this risk did not increase with higher BDI scores. Multiple logistic regression found depression to be associated with 2.5-fold increased risk for preeclampsia and either depression or anxiety to be associated with a 3.1-fold increased risk for this condition. Depression and anxiety may be harmful through an altered excretion of vasoactive hormones and other neuroendocrine transmitters. This may in turn cause vasoconstriction and uterine artery resistance and, therefore, elevate blood pressure (17,21).

SPONTANEOUS ABORTION

Several studies have suggested that depression may be a risk factor for spontaneous abortion (29,37,60,61). Stress and hormones associated with depression, such as CRH and adrenocorticotrophic hormone (ACTH), may interact with T cells or mast cells to produce changes in cytokine production. Because a balance in the nervous and endocrine systems is required to maintain pregnancy, the imbalance caused by depression may be abortogenic (29,61,62). Miscarriage has been hypothesized to be caused by a Th1–Th2 cytokine imbalance, which is suspected to be influenced by psychological factors. Cytokines may play protective roles during pregnancy, and a shift in their relative amounts is thought to activate coagulation, lead to vasculitis, and affect maternal blood supply to the embryo, thereby producing ischemic autoamputation and miscarriage.

Psychological influences on the endocrine and immune systems have been examined, suggesting that a pregnant woman's psychological state can mediate pregnancy outcome through these body systems (15). While women who experience recurrent spontaneous abortions may present with psychological disorders, whether depression is a causal factor in abortion or whether it is a result is under debate. Several published studies have shown that emotional distress may be associated with recurrent spontaneous abortions and reproductive failure (37,62). Conversely, other studies failed to show such association (60). In a recent study, "women's neuroticism" and current depressive symptoms were found to be negatively correlated with natural killer-cell activity, which is thought to predict miscarriage. Studies have even suggested that pre- and periconceptional psychological state may affect the number of oocytes retrieved and fertilized, as well as a woman's pregnancy and delivery outcome (13). A study by Sugiura-Ogasawara and others examined whether psychosocial factors influence subsequent miscarriages in women experiencing spontaneous recurrent abortions. Women with a history of 2 or more miscarriages and no live births received a mental status assessment according to the Symptom Checklist-90-Revised (SCL-90-R) psychopathology scale. Data were then examined to see whether women's personality traits (including depression) could predict subsequent miscarriage. Twenty-two percent of participants miscarried, and the miscarriage rate was positively associated with current depression ($P = 0.004$), neuroticism, interpersonal sensitivity, and psychosis. Only depression showed a statistically significant predictive value for miscarriage. Since it is widely accepted that acute and chronic stress can affect the immune system, this study suggests that the chronic stress of depression may be associated with altered immune system factors, which may affect pregnancy viability (62).

FETAL PHYSIOLOGY

Ultrasonography has been used to suggest that the fetus of a mother suffering from depression spends more time in sleep and exhibits less body movement than the fetus of a mother without depression (13). A similar study using ultrasonography suggested that maternal depression may affect fetal heart rate response to vibroacoustic stimulation (59). This test produces cardio acceleration typical of a healthy fetus and is commonly used to assess fetal well-being. In women with untreated depression, there was a delayed fetal response to a vibroacoustic stimulus applied to the maternal abdomen. In women with depressed BDI scores, fetal heart rate response was reduced. According to the investigators, this could signal alterations in the internal hormonal environment that have implications for postnatal information processing (59).

MATERNAL HEALTH-RELATED BEHAVIOUR

It has also been postulated that depression may lead to unhealthy behaviours that can indirectly affect obstetric outcome: depression can manifest in unhealthy lifestyle and coping behaviours during pregnancy; these may then mediate birth outcome (15,49). Mental illness may also cause cognitive distortions that affect decision-making capacities; it may therefore be associated with poor attendance at antenatal clinics and substance abuse (49,63). Zuckerman and colleagues found a significant association between depressive symptoms during pregnancy and the use of cigarettes, alcohol, and cocaine (49). Pregnant women with depression are more likely to lack volition to follow physician care regimes. They may not be as well nourished, show affected capacity to make decisions, and suffer from reduced sleep; they may also engage in more unhealthy behaviours than women who do not suffer from depression.

Women with depression may suffer from problems in social function, emotional withdrawal, and excessive concern regarding their future ability to parent (15). They may report excessive worry about pregnancy and are less likely to regularly attend obstetrical visits or have regular ultrasounds. Because they tend to present with diminished appetite, they therefore have lower-than-normal weight gain throughout pregnancy. They may also demonstrate poor self-care and lack of compliance with prenatal care. Conversely, women without depression are more likely to be proactive about health care in pregnancy (15). Women with depression tend to use prenatal vitamins less often than women without depression and to be less informed about the value of folic acid (49). Women suffering from depression show lack of initiative and motivation to seek help, as well as a negative perception regarding any potential benefit of obstetric services (49,64). These behaviours may all increase the risk for adverse pregnancy outcome. Severe depression also carries the risk of self-injurious, psychotic, impulsive, and harmful behaviours. If left untreated, depression during pregnancy has been known to deteriorate into acute forms of other psychiatric disturbances (4).

PERINATAL DEVELOPMENT

Stress during pregnancy has a suggested association with delayed developmental milestones in offspring (as well as with clinging, crying, hyperactivity, low frustration threshold, unsocial behaviour, schizophrenia, and attention-deficit hyperactivity disorder) (46). Depression during pregnancy is currently being studied in this context (65).

NEONATAL NEUROBEHAVIOURAL EFFECTS

Following birth, depression in women may be associated with reduced attachment, reduced parent–child bonding, and delays in offsprings' cognitive and emotional development (10,66–68). Lower language achievements and long-term behavioural problems may also be seen in some children whose mothers suffered from depression (66). Mothers suffering from depression report inability to carry out maternal duties far more often than do their counterparts without depression, and their infants show irritability, hostility, and erratic sleep (40), as well as an enhanced stress response (66). Infants whose mothers suffer from depression have been found to have reduced brain electrical activity across the left frontal lobe, a region of the brain associated with such positive emotions as joy. A review by Wisner and others argued that untreated depression is associated with inconsolability and excessive crying of offspring at birth (65). Maternal state of mind may powerfully affect parenting behaviour, even immediately following birth. It has also been speculated that, owing to disruptions in the caretaking environment, children of mothers with depression are at increased risk for internalizing problems (65). Such children reported more internalizing symptoms on the Dominic Interactive questionnaire, a pediatric DSM-III-R mental disorders scale (47). In a study by Nulman and colleagues, postpartum maternal depression —not the use of fluoxetine or tricyclic antidepressants during pregnancy—predicted lower cognitive and language development in preschool offspring (69).

INFANT STRESS HORMONE LEVELS

One study investigated the stress hormone levels of children whose mothers suffered from depression (47). The hypothesis underlying this study was that disruptions in early caretaking could have long-term repercussions for the HPA axis, which mediates stress response. Salivary cortisol levels were measured in offspring of mothers with and without depression. These samples were taken after arrival at the laboratory, after a laboratory stressor, and during a normal day outside the laboratory. Offspring of mothers with depression showed elevated baseline cortisol levels as well as elevated response to the stressor. In response to a fear-potentiated paradigm, children of mothers with depression had a higher cortisol elevation. This study concluded that maternal depression in the first 2 years of life may be associated with high cortisol levels in offspring. That elevated cortisol is found in children of mothers suffering from depression has also been noted in another study (40). These findings suggest increased baseline stress and decreased coping with stressors that present in the child's life.

PSYCHOPATHOLOGY IN OFFSPRING

In other studies, children of mothers suffering from depression showed an increased risk of behavioural and emotional problems, including affective disorders. A 2003 study has also suggested a significant association with criminality in offspring of mothers with antenatal untreated depression (70). Further, studies have found that these children are 6 times more likely to develop depression than are children of mothers without depression, suggesting that genetic susceptibility has a role, in addition to environment (71).

CONCLUSION

The biological dysregulation that occurs in depression may not be ideal for pregnancy. Despite this, most studies tend to focus on the risks to obstetric outcome of psychotropic medications, rather than on the risks of untreated depression. Very few studies consider nonpharmacologic therapy during pregnancy. This imbalance may lead women who suffer from depression to refuse treatment because they fear teratogenic effects. They are not aware that they potentially put their pregnancy and their baby at risk, especially when so few receive psychotherapy. When patients refuse treatment during pregnancy, we recommend that they be monitored to assess for such possible adverse outcomes as suicidal tendencies, deteriorating social functions, psychosis, and inability to comply with obstetrical evaluations (5). Given the potential impact of antenatal mental disturbances on maternal and infant outcomes, pregnant women require further psychiatric evaluation and treatment within the obstetrical sector. The perinatal period can become a critical time to screen for and identify depression, since pregnant women have increased contact with health services. Finally, when making clinical decisions, clinicians should weigh the growing body of literature suggesting potential adverse effects of untreated depression during pregnancy against the literature that has failed to find risks associated with in utero antidepressant exposure.

FUNDING AND SUPPORT

Lori Bonari was supported by a grant from the Ontario Graduate Scholarship and the Hospital for Sick Children Research Training Competition. The study was supported by a grant from the Council of Ontario Women's Health.

REFERENCES

1. [Anonymous]. Pregnancy depression. Lancet 1984;2(8396):206.
2. Buist A. Managing depression in pregnancy. Aust Fam Physician 2000;29:663–7.
3. D'Alfonso A, Iovenitti P, Casacchia M, Carta G. Disturbances of humour in postpartum: our experience. Clin Exp Obstet Gynecol 2002;29:207–11.
4. Stocky A, Lynch J. Acute psychiatric disturbance in pregnancy and the puerperium. Baillieres Best Pract Res Clin Obstet Gynaecol 2000; 14(1):73–87.
5. Wisner KL, Zarin DA, Holmboe ES, Appelbaum PS, Gelenberg AJ, Leonard HL, and others. Risk-benefit decision making for treatment of depression during pregnancy. Am J Psychiatry 2000;157:1933–1940.
6. Llewellyn AM, Stowe ZN, Nemeroff CB. Depression during pregnancy and the puerperium. J Clin Psychiatry 1997;58 (Suppl 15):26–32.
7. Kessler, McGonagle KA, Swartz M. Sex and depression in the National Comorbidity Survey I: lifetime prevalence, chronicity and recurrence. J Affect Disord 1993;29:85–96.
8. Birndorf CA, Madden A, Portera L, Leon AC. Psychiatric symptoms, functional impairment, and receptivity toward mental health treatment among obstetrical patients. Int J Psychiatry Med 2001;355–65.
9. Scholle SH, Haskett RF, Hanusa BH, Pincus HA, Kupfer DJ. Addressing depression in obstetrics/gynecology practice. Gen Hosp Psychiatry 2003,25(2):83–90.
10. Nonacs R, Cohen LS. Depression during pregnancy: diagnosis and treatment options. J Clin Psychiatry 2002;63(7):24–30.
11. Altshuler LL, Hendrick V, Cohen LS. Course of mood and anxiety disorders during pregnancy and the postpartum period. J Clin Psychiatry 1998;59 (Suppl 2):29–33.
12. Marcus SM, Flynn HA, Blow FC, Barry KL. Depressive symptoms among pregnant women screened in obstetrics settings. J Womens Health (Larchmont) 2003;12:373–80.
13. Chung TK, Lau TK, Yip AS, Chiu HF, Lee DT. Antepartum depressive symptomatology is associated with adverse obstetric and neonatal outcomes. Psychosom Med 2001;63:830–4.
14. Chrousos GP, Torpy DJ, Gold PW. Interactions between the hypothalamicpituitary-adrenal axis and the female reproductive system: clinical implications. Ann Intern Med 1998;129:229–40.
15. Paarlberg KM, Vingerhoets AJ, Passchier J, Dekker GA, van Geijn HP. Psychosocial factors and pregnancy outcome: a review with emphasis on methodological issues. J Psychosom Res 1995;39:563–95.
16. Sandman CA, Wadhwa PD, Dunkel-Schetter C, Chicz-DeMet A, Belman J, Porto M, and others. Psychobiological influences of stress and HPA regulation on the human fetus and infant birth outcomes. Ann N Y Acad Sci 1994;739:198–210.
17. Sandman CA, Wadhwa PD, Chicz-DeMet A, Dunkel-Schetter C, Porto M. Maternal stress, HPA activity, and fetal/infant outcome. Ann N Y Acad Sci 1997;814:266–75.
18. Smith R, Cubis J, Brinsmead M, Lewin T, Singh B, Owens P, and others. Mood changes, obstetric experience and alterations in plasma cortisol, beta-endorphin and corticotrophin releasing hormone during pregnancy and the puerperium. J Psychosom Res 1990;34 (1):53–69.
19. Wadhwa PD, Dunkel-Schetter C, Chicz-DeMet A, Porto M, Sandman CA. Prenatal psychosocial factors and the neuroendocrine axis in human pregnancy. Psychosom Med 1996;58:432–46.
20. Dorn LD, Susman EJ, Petersen AC. Cortisol reactivity and anxiety and depression in pregnant adolescents: a longitudinal perspective. Psychoneuroendocrinology 1993;18:219–39.
21. Kurki T, Hiilesmaa V, Raitasalo R, Mattila H, Ylikorkala O. Depression and anxiety in early pregnancy and risk for preeclampsia. Obstet Gynecol 2000;95:487–90.
22. Perkin MR, Bland JM, Peacock JL, Anderson HR. The effect of anxiety and depression during pregnancy on obstetric complications. Br J Obstet Gynaecol 1993;100:629–34.
23. Kent A, Hughes P, Ormerod L, Jones G, Thilaganathan B. Uterine artery resistance and anxiety in the second trimester of pregnancy. Ultrasound Obstet Gynecol 2002;19:177–9.
24. [Anonymous]. American Psychiatric Association: practice guildeline for major depressive disorder in adults. Am J Psychiatry 1993; 150(Suppl 1):1–26.
25. [Anonymous]. Health Indicators. Volume 2002, no 1. Depression. Ottawa (ON): Statistics Canada; 2002. Catalogue no 82-221-XIE.
26. Altshuler LL, Cohen LS, Moline ML, Kahn DA, Carpenter D, Docherty JP. The expert consensus guideline series. Treatment of depression in women. Postgrad Med 2001;(Special No):1–107.
27. Angst J, Baastrup P, Grof P, Hippius H, Poldinger W, Weis P. The course of monopolar depression and bipolar psychoses. Psychiatr Neurol Neurochir 1973;76:489–500.
28. Frank E, Kupfer DJ, Perel JM, Cornes C, Jarrett DB, Mallinger AG, and others. Three year outcomes for maintenance therapies in recurrent depression. Arch Gen Psychiatry 1990;47:1093–9.
29. Arck PC. Stress and pregnancy: loss of immune mediators, hormones and neurotransmitters. Am J Reprod Immunol 2001;46:117–23.
30. Erickson MT. The influence of health factors on psychological variables predicting complications of pregnancy, labor and delivery. J Psychosom Res 1976;20(1):21–24.
31. Kelly R, Zatzick D, Anders T. The detection and treatment of psychiatric disorders and substance use among pregnant women cared for in obstetrics. Am J Psychiatry 2001;158:213–9.
32. Lou HC, Hansen D, Nordentoft M, Pryds O, Jensen F, Nim J, and others. Prenatal stressors of human life affect fetal brain development. Dev Med Child Neurol 1994;36:826–32.
33. Orr ST, Miller CA. Maternal depressive symptoms and the risk of poor pregnancy outcome. Review of the literature and preliminary findings. Epidemiol Rev 1995;17:165–71.
34. Steer RA, Scholl TO, Hediger ML, Fischer RL. Self-reported depression and negative pregnancy outcomes. J Clin Epidemiol 1992; 45:1093–9.
35. Wadhwa PD, Sandman CA, Porto M, Dunkel-Schetter C, Garite TJ. The association between prenatal stress and infant birth weight and gestational age at birth: a prospective investigation. Am J Obstet Gynecol 1993;169:858–65.
36. Zax M, Sameroff AJ, Babigian HM. Birth outcomes in the offspring of mentally disordered women. Am J Orthopsychiatry 1977;47:218–30.
37. Michel-Wolfromm H. The psychological factor in spontaneous abortion. J Psychosom Res 1968;12(1):67–71.
38. Preti A, Cardascia L, Zen T, Pellizzari P, Marchetti M, Favaretto G, and others. Obstetric complications in patients with depression—a population-based case-control study. J Affect Disord 2000;61:101–6.

39. Teixeira JM, Fisk NM, Glover V. Association between maternal anxiety in pregnancy and increased uterine artery resistance index: cohort based study. BMJ 1999;318:153–7.
40. Field T, Diego M, Hernandez-Reif M, Salman F, Schanberg S, Kuhn C, and others. Prenatal anger effects on the fetus and neonate. J Obstet Gynaecol 2002;22:260–6.
41. Hoffman S, Hatch MC. Depressive symptomatology during pregnancy: evidence for an association with decreased fetal growth in pregnancies of lower social class women. Health Psychol 2000;19:535–43.
42. Dayan J, Creveuil C, Herlicoviez M, Herbel C, Baranger E, Savoye C, and others. Role of anxiety and depression in the onset of spontaneous preterm labor. Am J Epidemiol 2002;155:293–301.
43. Orr ST, James SA, Blackmore PC. Maternal prenatal depressive symptoms and spontaneous preterm births among African-American women in Baltimore, Maryland. Am J Epidemiol 2002;156:797–802.
44. McAnarney ER, Stevens-Simon C. Maternal psychological stress/depression and low birth weight. Is there a relationship? Am J Dis Child 1990;144:789–92.
45. Cohler BJ, Gallant DH, Grunebaum HU, Weiss JL, Gamer E. Pregnancy and birth complications among mentally ill and well mothers and their children. Soc Biol 1975;22:269–78.
46. Weinstock M. Alterations induced by gestational stress in brain morphology and behaviour of the offspring. Prog Neurobiol 2001; 65:427–51.
47. Ashman SB, Dawson G, Panagiotides H, Yamada E, Wilkins CW. Stress hormone levels of children of depressed mothers. Dev Psychopathol 2002;14:333–49.
48. Mahomed K, Gulmezoglu AM, Nikodem VC, Wolman WL, Chalmers BE, Hofmeyr GJ. Labor experience, maternal mood and cortisol and catecholamine levels in low-risk primiparous women. J Psychosom Obstet Gynaecol 1995;16:181–6.
49. Zuckerman B, Amaro H, Bauchner H, Cabral H. Depressive symptoms during pregnancy: relationship to poor health behaviors. Am J Obstet Gynecol 1989;160:1107–11.
50. Josefsson A, Berg G, Nordin C, Sydsjo G. Prevalence of depressive symptoms in late pregnancy and postpartum. Acta Obstet Gynecol Scand 2001;80:251–5.
51. Evans J, Heron J, Francomb H, Oke S, Golding J. Cohort study of depressed mood during pregnancy and after childbirth. BMJ 2001;323:257 60.
52. Kenyon FE. Termination of pregnancy on psychiatric grounds: a comparative study of 61 cases. Br J Med Psychol 1969;42:243–54.
53. Krener P, Treat JN, Hansen RL. Research in pregnancy and mental illness: testing old wives' hypotheses. J Psychosom Obstet Gynaecol 1993;14:163–83.
54. Appleby L. Suicide during pregnancy and in the first postnatal year. BMJ 1991;302:137–40.
55. Hirschfeld RM, Keller MB, Panico S, Arons BS, Barlow D, Davidoff F, and others. The National Depressive and Manic-Depressive Association consensus statement on the undertreatment of depression. JAMA 1997;277:333–40.
56. Kleiner GJ, Greston WM. Suicide during pregnancy. In: Cherry SH, Merkatz IR, editors. Complications of pregnancy: medical, surgical, psychosocial and perinatal. Volume 4. 4th ed. Philadelphia (PA): Williams & Wilkins; 1991. p 269–89.
57. Hostetter A, Stowe ZN, Strader JR Jr, McLaughlin E, Llewellyn A. Dose of selective serotonin uptake inhibitors across pregnancy: clinical implications. Depress Anxiety 2000;11(2):51–7.
58. Paarlberg KM, Vingerhoets AJ, Passchier J, Dekker GA, Heinen AG, van Geijn HP. Psychosocial predictors of low birthweight: a prospective study. Br J Obstet Gynaecol 1999;106:834–41.
59. Allister L, Lester BM, Carr S, Liu J. The effects of maternal depression on fetal heart rate response to vibroacoustic stimulation. Dev Neuropsychol 2001;20:639–51.
60. Bergant AM, Reinstadler K, Moncayo HE, Solder E, Heim K, Ulmer H, and others. Spontaneous abortion and psychosomatics. A prospective study on the impact of psychological factors as a cause for recurrent spontaneous abortion. Hum Reprod 1997;12:1106–10.
61. Arck PC, Rose M, Hertwig K, Hagen E, Hildebrandt M, Klapp BF. Stress and immune mediators in miscarriage. Hum Reprod 2001;16: 1505–11.
62. Sugiura-Ogasawara M, Furukawa TA, Nakano Y, Hori S, Aoki K, Kitamura T. Depression as a potential causal factor in subsequent miscarriage in recurrent spontaneous aborters. Hum Reprod 2002; 17:2580–84.
63. Marcus SM, Barry KL, Flynn HA, Blow FC. [Improving detection, prevention and treatment of depression and substance abuse in childbearing women: critical variables in pregnancy and pre-pregnancy planning, 1998.] Located at University of Michigan Clinical Ventures, Faculty Group Practice.
64. Coverdale JH, Chervenak FA, McCullough LB, Bayer T. Ethically justified clinically comprehensive guidelines for the management of the depressed pregnant patient. Am J Obstet Gynecol 1996; 174):169–73.
65. Wisner KL, Gelenberg AJ, Leonard H, Zarin D, Frank E. Pharmacologic treatment of depression during pregnancy. JAMA 1999;282:1264–9.
66. Bosquet M, Egeland B. Associations among maternal depressive symptomatology, state of mind and parent and child behaviors: implications for attachment-based interventions. Attach Hum Dev 2001;3:173–99.
67. O'Connor TG, Heron J, Glover V. Antenatal anxiety predicts child behavioral/emotional problems independently of postnatal depression. J Am Acad Child Adolesc Psychiatry 2002;41:1470–7.
68. Weinberg MK, Tronick EZ. The impact of maternal psychiatric illness on infant development. J Clin Psychiatry 1998;59(Suppl 2):53–61.
69. Nulman I, Rovet J, Stewart DE, Wolpin J, Pace-Asciak P, Shuhaiber S, and others. Child development following exposure to tricyclic antidepressants or fluoxetine throughout fetal life: a prospective, controlled study. Am J Psychiatry 2002;159:1889–95.
70. Maki P, Veijola J, Rasanen P, Joukamaa M, Valonen P, Jokelainen J, and others. Criminality in the offspring of antenatally depressed mothers: a 33-year follow-up of the Northern Finland 1966 birth cohort. J Affect Disord 2003;74:273–8.
71. Hammen C, Brennan PA. Severity, chronicity, and timing of maternal depression and risk for adolescent offspring diagnoses in a community sample. Arch Gen Psychiatry 2003;60:253–8.

CHAPTER 31

MALFORMATION RATES IN CHILDREN OF WOMEN WITH UNTREATED EPILEPSY: A META-ANALYSIS

Shawn Fried,[1] *Eran Kozer,*[1,2,3] *Irena Nulman,*[1,2,3] *Thomas R. Einarson,*[1,2] *and Gideon Koren*[1,2,3]

[1] *University of Toronto, Toronto, Ontario, Canada,* [2]*The Motherisk Program, Toronto, Ontario, Canada and* [3]*Division of Clinical Pharmacology/Toxicology, The Hospital for Sick Children, Toronto, Ontario, Canada*

Abstract

Background. It is widely quoted that women with epilepsy have a higher than baseline risk for giving birth to a child with malformations, independent of the effects of antiepileptic drugs.

Objective. To determine, based on available evidence, if epilepsy *per se* represents a teratogenic risk. To systematically review all studies investigating the occurrence of major malformation rates among children of treated or untreated women with epilepsy and non-exposed controls who do not have epilepsy.

Methods. A meta-analysis, using a random effects model, was conducted of all cohort and case-control studies reporting malformation rates in children of women with epilepsy exposed or unexposed to antiepileptic drugs compared with that of children of nonepileptic women. Medline (1966–2001), EMBASE, the Cochrane database as well as REPROTOX (an information system on environmental hazards to human reproduction and development) databases were accessed.

Results. We found ten studies reporting results of untreated epilepsy (n = 400) and their non-epileptic healthy controls (n = 2492). Nine out of ten studies also reported results on 1443 patients exposed to antiepileptic drugs and their 2526 unexposed healthy controls. The risk for congenital malformations in the offspring of women with untreated epilepsy was not higher than among nonepileptic controls (odds ratio [OR] = 1.92; 95% CI 0.92–4.00). There was evidence of publication bias, thus with bias removed the OR was 0.99 (95% CI 0.49–2.01). In contrast, the offspring of epileptic women who received antiepileptic drugs had higher incidences of malformation than controls (OR 3.26; 95% CI 2.15–4.93).

Conclusion. Our study does not support the commonly held view that epilepsy *per se* represents a teratogenic risk. Our study suggests that this view is the result of a publication bias, with several small (<100 participants) positive studies leading to a premature conclusion.

It is estimated that one million women of childbearing age currently have a diagnosis of epilepsy in the US[1] and women with epilepsy account for 0.5% of all pregnancies.[2] Mounting evidence suggests that over the past decade there has been an increase in perinatal risks, associated with pregnant women who have epilepsy, for both mother and child.[3] All commonly used antiepileptic drugs have been associated with an increased risk for major malformations in both animal and human studies.

It has been speculated that a genetic predisposition of the mother's epilepsy results in the susceptibility to anticonvulsant-related teratogenicity.[4] The frequency and severity of seizures can also play a role in causing an adverse outcome. There is a widely cited view that epilepsy *per se* may contribute to an adverse outcome.[5] A potential interaction between genetic and environmental components makes it difficult to attribute an adverse outcome to any single factor.[6,7]

While some studies have suggested a characteristic pattern of anomalies resulting from antiepileptic drug therapy during pregnancy,[8,9] others have implicated epilepsy itself as an associative factor in the occurrence of malformations.[10,11] Although a role for epilepsy in teratogenicity has been suggested, conflicting results have made it difficult to counsel patients and their families when they are planning pregnancy.

In order to better define the extent to which epilepsy contributes to the development of congenital malformations, we systematically reviewed the literature and conducted a meta-analysis of all studies that investigated the rates of malformations among offspring of untreated pregnant women with epilepsy compared with those of treated epileptic women and nonepileptic controls.

METHODS

Data Sources and Study Selection

A search of the literature was conducted for studies reporting the association of untreated epilepsy with pregnancy outcome. The following OVID (4.3.0) databases (and relevant segment dates) were searched electronically by a professional librarian: Medline (1966–2001), EMBASE, the Cochrane database as well as REPROTOX (an information system on environmental hazards to human reproduction and development) [key words were: malformations, epilepsy, pregnancy, antiepileptic drugs, untreated epilepsy]. Teratology text references, the references in the bibliographies of all the included studies and review articles that were identified by the search strategy were searched manually. Controlled human population studies, both cohort and case control, in all languages were selected.

Objective

The objective was to determine if epilepsy *per se* represents a teratogenic risk, using available evidence. To systematically review all studies reporting on major malformation rates among children of treated or untreated women with epilepsy and non-exposed controls.

Inclusion Criteria

The inclusion criteria in this meta-analysis were studies that reported pregnancy outcomes for women with epilepsy (defined

Study	Women with epilepsy not receiving treatment (n/N)	Women without epilepsy [control] (n/N)	Weight (%)	OR (95% CI random)
Holmes et al.[13]	0/98	6/508	6.5	0.39 (0.02–7.02)
Spiedel and Meadow[14]	0/59	6/448	6.5	0.57 (0.03–10.29)
Jick and Terris[15]	0/67	4/594	6.3	0.97 (0.05–18.25)
Holmes et al.[16]	3/57	3/57	20.0	1.00 (0.19–5.18)
Koch et al.[11]	2/18	4/66	17.0	1.94 (0.33–11.54)
Koch et al.[17]	2/25	1/25	8.9	2.09 (0.18–24.62)
Fedrick[18]	1/18	9/649	12.0	4.18 (0.50–34.90)
Koch et al.[19]	2/20	1/43	8.9	4.67 (0.40–54.80)
Van der Pol et al.[20]	2/22	1/55	9.0	5.40 (0.46–62.87)
Fabris et al.[21]	1/16	0/47	5.1	9.19 (0.36–237.49)
Total (95% CI)	13/400	35/2492	100.0	1.92 (0.92–4.00)

Test for heterogeneity chi-square = 5.34, df = 9, p = 0.8
Test for overall effect z = 1.74, p = 0.08

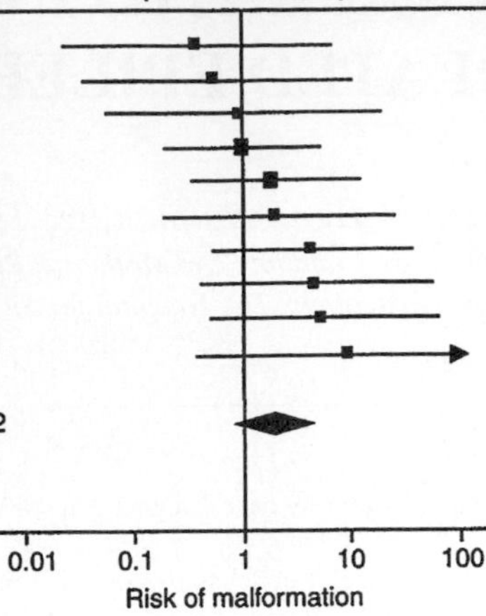

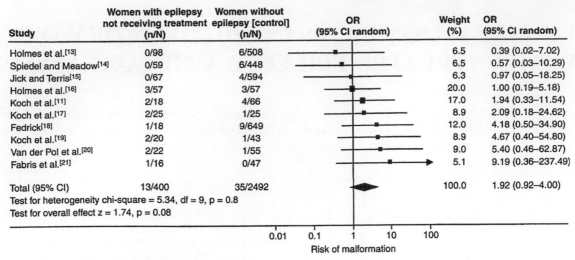

Figure 1. Major malformations in offspring of women with untreated epilepsy and healthy controls. n = number of offspring with malformations; N = total number of offspring; OR = odds ratio.

using the International League Against Epilepsy criteria)[12] who were untreated with antiepileptic drugs and included comparison groups comprising children of women without epilepsy and not exposed to antiepileptic drugs.

Convulsive disorders due to other aetiologies (e.g. post-traumatic) were not included. When data were available, genetic disorders (e.g. chromosomal abnormalities and disorders due to single gene mutation) and positional deformity or deformations (e.g. congenital dislocation of hip) were not considered to be major malformations.

Exclusion criteria consisted of non-controlled studies, studies reporting on women exposed to other known teratogens or diseases, and papers not separating treated from untreated patients with epilepsy.

One reviewer screened all the abstracts, titles, and, if necessary, full reports for inclusion in this review. Based on this preliminary screening, studies were chosen for detailed review by two reviewers who applied the selection criteria and decided independently which studies should be included in the final analysis. In cases of disagreement between the two reviewers, the decision was made based on the assessment of a third reviewer. There was no blinding of authors or results. When multiple studies reported data for the same populations or subpopulations, only the study reporting the more comprehensive data was included.

Data Extraction and Synthesis

Using structured data collection forms, two reviewers extracted data independently and entered it into 2 × 2 tables. Discrepancies were resolved by discussion. All data entries were double-checked manually.

We used the Cochrane Review Manager software (Revman 4.1) to calculate the pooled odds ratio (OR) and 95% CI, assuming a random-effects model.

Two analyses were conducted. The first compared the rates of malformations in offspring of women with epilepsy who did not take antiepileptic drugs during the first trimester with those in offspring of controls who did not have epilepsy. The second compared the rates of malformations in children of women who had epilepsy and were treated with antiepileptic drugs with the rates in children of controls who did not have epilepsy.

Study	Women with epilepsy receiving antiepileptic drugs (n/N)	Women without epilepsy [control] (n/N)	Weight (%)	OR (95% CI random)
Koch et al.[11]	6/70	4/66	10.0	1.45 (0.39–5.40)
Koch et al.[17]	8/116	5/116	13.0	1.64 (0.52–5.18)
Koch et al.[19]	6/89	1/43	3.7	3.04 (0.35–26.05)
Van der Pol et al.[20]	2/35	1/55	2.9	3.27 (0.29–37.52)
Fedrick[18]	8/165	9/649	18.3	3.62 (1.38–9.54)
Spiedel and Meadow[14]	17/324	6/448	19.3	4.08 (1.59–10.46)
Holmes et al.[13]	16/316	6/508	19.0	4.46 (1.73–11.53)
Jick and Terris[15]	9/297	4/594	12.2	4.61 (1.41–15.09)
Fabris et al.[21]	1/31	0/47	1.6	4.67 (0.18–118.44)
Total (95% CI)	73/1443	36/2526	100.0	3.26 (2.15–4.93)

Test for heterogeneity chi-square = 3.88, df = 8, p = 0.87
Test for overall effect z = 5.59, p < 0.00001

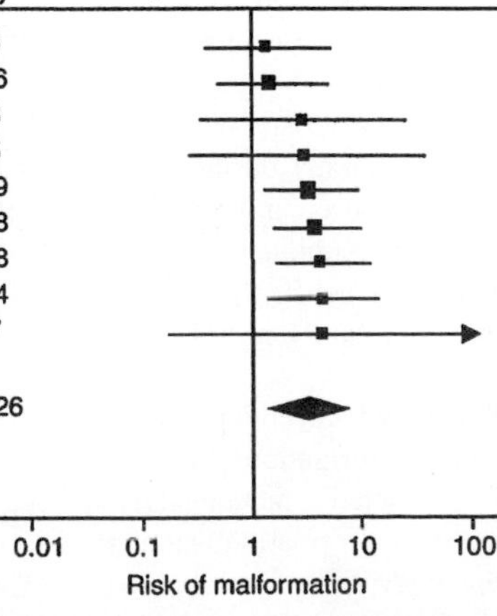

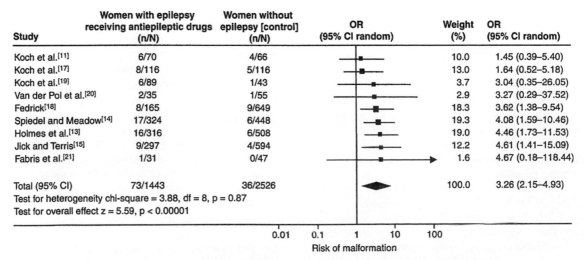

Figure 2. Major malformations in offspring of epileptic mothers treated with antiepileptic drugs and in healthy controls. n = number of offspring with malformations; N = total number of offspring; OR = odds ratio.

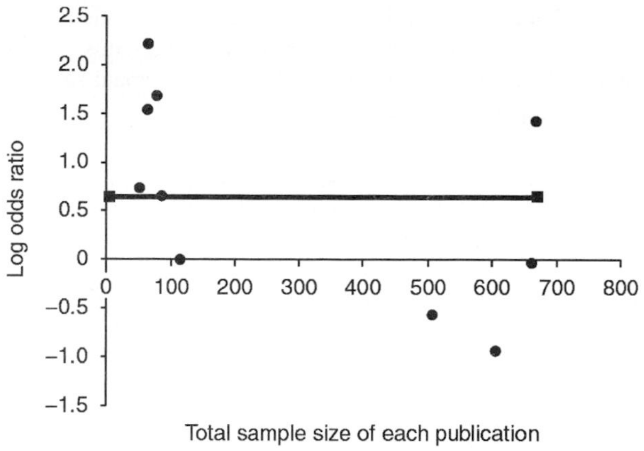

Figure 3. Funnel plot of publications[11,13-21] (included in this meta-analysis) that compared major malformations in offspring of untreated women with epilepsy with that of offspring of women without epilepsy. The solid black line represents the pooled odds ratio.

RESULTS

The search generated 2615 titles, of which 287 abstracts in all languages were selected for further analysis. A total of 74 articles were selected for complete review. Ten of these studies met the inclusion criteria and were included in the analysis, including five prospective cohort studies, four case control studies and one study using both prospective and retrospective design.[11,13-21] Sixty-four studies were excluded. The list of excluded papers can be provided by the authors. We included ten studies reporting the results of untreated epilepsy (n = 400) and their non-epileptic healthy controls (n = 2492). Nine out of ten studies also reported on 1443 pregnancies of women exposed to antiepileptic drugs and 2526 healthy non-epileptic unexposed women. The difference in the number of controls is due to matching.

The risk for congenital malformations in the offspring of women with untreated epilepsy was not higher than that in the offspring of controls who did not have epilepsy (OR 1.92; 95% CI 0.92–4.00) [figure 1]. The studies were not heterogeneous (p for heterogeneity = 0.80). In contrast, the offspring of women treated with antiepileptic drugs had a significantly higher incidence of major malformations than the offspring who did not have epilepsy (OR 3.26; 95% CI 2.15–4.93) [figure 2]. The studies were not heterogeneous (p for heterogeneity = 0.87).

Funnel plots of the data were made, with sample size plotted against the natural log of each OR. Figure 3 reveals the possibility of publication bias, since there were no small studies with negative results. We then adjusted the plot by inserting pseudo-values representing unpublished studies of equal size but opposite results for those studies with a sample size of <100. Figure 4 depicts the funnel plot of the adjusted data. The summary OR decreased to 0.99 (95% CI 0.49–2.01) from 1.92 (95% CI 0.92–4.00), suggesting that there really is no difference in malformations in children of untreated women with epilepsy versus children of women without epilepsy. On the other hand, the plot for treated mothers (not shown) showed no such publication bias.

Sensitivity analyses revealed no significant differences between cohort and case control studies for comparisons of the offspring of antiepileptic drug-treated epileptic women with the offspring of nonepileptic controls and comparisons of the offspring of untreated women with epilepsy with the offspring of nonepileptic controls.

Our study had a power of 78% to detect a significant (α error rate = 0.05) difference in the rate of malformations between untreated epileptic women and nonepileptic control. A total of 54 more studies of average size including 15 505 more patients would be needed to show such effect to be significant.

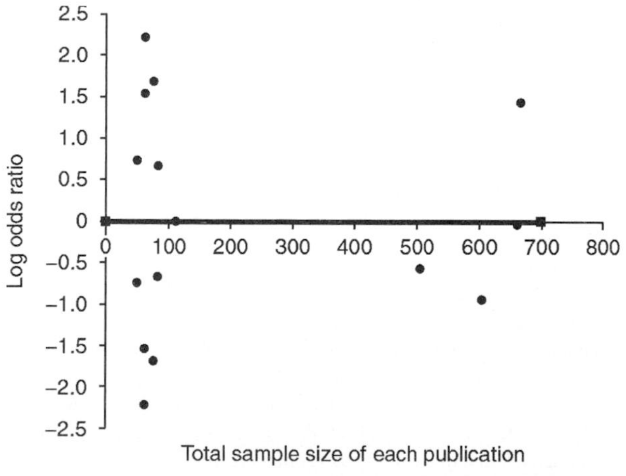

Figure 4. Adjusted funnel plot after removal of the possibility of publication bias of publications[11,13-21] (included in this meta-analysis) that compared major malformations in offspring of untreated women with epilepsy with that of offspring of women without epilepsy. The plot was adjusted by inserting pseudo-values representing unpublished studies of equal size but opposite results for those studies with <100 participants. The solid black line represents the pooled odds ratio.

DISCUSSION

Our findings did not confirm an increase in rates of major malformations among children of untreated epileptic women compared with that among children of nonepileptic controls. This information is reassuring for women with epilepsy who do not need to take antiepileptic drugs. It is also important for women with specific types of epilepsy and their physicians, who may choose to discontinue antiepileptic drugs during the first trimester in order to reduce the risks of major malformations. The teratogenic risk associated with antiepileptic drugs appears to be 4–8%, approximately 2–3 times greater than the general obstetric population.[22] Presently there is no consensus regarding which anticonvulsant drug is the safest for the patient's unborn child. Moreover, a number of factors exist that may affect the teratogenic potential of an antiepileptic medication, such as the number of co-administered drugs, drug dose, time of exposure, pharmacokinetics and differences in metabolism.[23,24] However, with increased severity of epilepsy, there is usually an increase in drug dose, and more common use of polytherapy.

The majority of selected studies did not report the type, duration, or severity of epilepsy. Furthermore, information about clinical indications for treatment discontinuation and seizure-free periods was not reported by the majority of studies. Another potential shortcoming of our study is its inability to account for the effects of seizures during pregnancy. Seizure frequency has been shown to increase by 17–37% during gestation.[25,26] Several mechanisms have been attributed to an increase in seizure activity including pregnancy-induced changes in antiepileptic drug pharmacokinetics, increased stress, higher levels of estrogen and drug regimen adherence problems. The occurrence of status epilepticus may result in fetal death in a substantial number of cases, as well as pose the risk for maternal death.[27]

Untreated epileptic women who are pregnant may represent those having a less severe form of epilepsy with lower frequencies of seizures and hence lower frequencies of malformations are observed in their offspring.[7] This hypothesis is supported by the fact that women treated with polytherapy may have more severe forms of epilepsy.[23]

On the other hand, women with untreated epilepsy may not necessarily have milder forms of the disorder. Other forms (e.g. temporal lobe) may be equally severe, but do not result in tonic-clonic seizures, and may be tolerable in the mother without harming the fetus. The present study was unable to determine whether that was the case because of incomplete reporting of the exact nature of the epilepsy by the original authors. Equally important, it will be critical to assess the potential role of paternal epilepsy in future studies.

The funnel plot presented in figure 3 clearly shows that small studies (e.g. with <100 participants) were all positive, (e.g. showing an association between maternal epilepsy and increased malformation rate). It is very important to address such bias, and this is done by including in the analysis 'mirror image' results plotted on the 'negative' side. Such analyses, correcting for the bias produced by small sample size, further balances the overall result of the whole group of studies.

Another potential difficulty is bias against publications of negative trials (the 'file drawer' syndrome). However, in this particular case, unpublished negative cohorts, if they exist, would strengthen the result of a lack of effect of untreated epilepsy on malformation rates of offspring.

In conclusion, our study does not support the commonly held view that epilepsy *per se* represents a risk for increased congenital malformations. We suggest that the current literature on the topic suffers from publication bias, which produces distortion. More studies are needed to control for the type, severity, and frequency of seizure disorders on teratogenic risk.

ACKNOWLEDGEMENTS

Supported in part by Novartis, Barcelona, Spain. Eran Koser was supported by a Fellowship from the Research Training Center, The Hospital for Sick Children, Toronto, Ontario, Canada and Dr Gideon Koren is a senior scientist of the Canadian Institute for Health Research. The authors have no conflicts of interest directly relevant to the content of this manuscript.

REFERENCES

1. Devinsky O, Yerby M. Women with epilepsy: reproduction and effects of pregnancy on epilepsy. Neurol Clin 1994;12:479-495.
2. Yerby MS. Pregnancy and epilepsy. Epilepsia 1991; 32 Suppl. 6: s51-9.
3. Martin PJ, Millac PAH. Pregnancy, epilepsy, management and outcome: a 10-year perspective. Seizure 1993; 2: 277-80.
4. Janz D. On major malformations and minor anomalies in the offspring of parents with epilepsy: review of the literature. In: Janz D, Dam M, Richens A, et al., editors. Epilepsy, pregnancy, and the child. New York: Raven Press, 1982: 211-22.
5. Majewski F, Steger M, Richter B, et al. The teratogenicity of hydantoins and barbiturates in humans, with considerations on the etiology of malformations and cerebral disturbances in the children of epileptic parents. Int J Biol Res Pregnancy 1981; 2 (1): 37-45.
6. Dansky LV, Finnell RH. Parental epilepsy, anticonvulsant drugs, and reproductive outcome: epidemiologic and experimental findings spanning three decades. 2: human studies. Reprod Toxicol 1991; 5 (4): 301-35.
7. Nulman I, Laslo D, Koren G. Treatment of epilepsy in pregnancy. Drugs 1999; 57 (4): 535-44.
8. Jones KL, Lacro RV, Johnson K, et al. Patterns of malformations in the children of women treated with carbamazepine during pregnancy. N Engl J Med 1989;320:1661-6.
9. Clayton-Smith J, Donnai D. Fetal valproate syndrome. J Med Genet 1995; 32: 724-7.
10. Nulman I, Scolnik D, Chitayat D, et al. Findings in children exposed in utero to phenytoin and carbamazepine monotherapy: independent effects of epilepsy medications. Am J Med Genet 1997; 68: 18-24.
11. Koch S, Gopfert-Geyer I, Jager-Roman E, et al. Antiepileptika wahrend der schwangerschaft. Dtsch Med Wochenschr 1983; 108: 250-7.
12. International League Against Epilepsy, Commission on Classification and Terminology of the International League Against Epilepsy. Proposal for revised classification of epilepsies and epileptic syndromes. Epilepsia 1990; 30: 389-99.
13. Holmes LB, Harvey EA, Coull BA, et al. The teratogenicity of anticonvulsant drugs. N Engl J Med 2001; 344:1132-8.
14. Spiedel BD, Meadow SR. Maternal epilepsy and abnormalities of the fetus and newborn. Lancet 1972; 21: 839-43.
15. Jick SS, Terris BZ. Anticonvulsants and congenital malformations. Pharmacotherapy 1997; 17: 561-4.
16. Holmes LB, Rosenberger PB, Harvey EA, et al. Intelligence and physical features of children of women with epilepsy. Teratology 2000; 61: 196-202.
17. Koch S, Losche G, Jager-Roman E, et al. Major and minor birth malformations and antiepileptic drugs. Neurology 1992;42 Suppl. 5:83-8.
18. Fedrick J. Epilepsy and pregnancy: a report from the Oxford Record Linkage Study. BMJ 1973; 2: 442-8.
19. Koch S, Hartmann A, Jager-Roman E, et al. Major malformations in children of epileptic parents: due to epilepsy or its therapy? In: Janz D, Dam M, Richens A, et al., editors. Epilepsy, pregnancy and the child. New York: Raven Press, 1982: 313-5.
20. Van der Pol MC, Hadders-Algra M, Huisjes HJ, et al. Antiepileptic medication in pregnancy: late effects on the children's central nervous system development. Am J Obstet Gynecol 1991; 164: 121-8.
21. Fabris C, Licata D, Stasiowska B, et al. Il neonato da madre epilettica: rischio malformativo ed auxologico. Pediatr Med Chir 1989; 11: 27-32.
22. Yerby M. Pregnancy, teratogenesis and epilepsy. Neurol Clin 1994; 12: 749-71.
23. Kaneko S, Otani K, Fukushima J, et al. Teratogenicity of antiepileptic drugs: analysis of possible risk factors. Epilepsia 1988; 29: 459-67.
24. Kaneko S, Fukushima Y, Sato T, et al. Teratogenicity of antiepileptic drugs: a prospective study. Jpn J Psychiatry Neurol 1986; 40: 447-50.
25. Byrne B. Epilepsy and pregnancy. Ir Med J 1997; 90: 173-4.
26. Lopes-Cendes I, Andermann E, Candes F, et al. Risk factors for changes in seizure frequency during pregnancy of epileptic women: a cohort study [abstract]. Epilepsia 1992; 33 Suppl. 3: 57.
27. Donaldson JO. Neurologic disorders of pregnancy. In: Reece EA, Hobbins JC, Mahoney MJ, et al., editors. Medicine of the fetus and mother. Philadelphia (PA): JB Lippincott, 1992: 1097-102.

Correspondence and offprints: Dr *Gideon Koren*, Division of Clinical Pharmacology, The Hospital for Sick Children, 555 University Avenue, Toronto, ON, M5G 1X8, Canada. E-mail: gkoren@sickkids.ca

Reprinted from Fried S, Kozer E, Nulman I, Einarson TR, Koren G. Malformation rates in children of women with untreated epilepsy: a meta-analysis. Drug Saf 2004;27:197-202 with permission from Wolters Kluwer Health.

CHAPTER 32

PREGNANCY OUTCOME FOLLOWING NON-OBSTETRIC SURGICAL INTERVENTION

Raanan Cohen-Kerem,[a] Craig Railton,[a] Dana Oren,[a] Michael Lishner,[b] and Gideon Koren[a]

[a]*Motherisk Program, Division of Clinical Pharmacology and Toxicology, Department of Pediatrics, University of Toronto, Hospital for Sick Children, 555 University Ave., Toronto, Ontario, Canada M5G 1X8*

[b]*Department of Medicine A, Meir Hospital, Kfar-Saba, Israel*

Manuscript received August 16, 2004; revised manuscript March 15, 2005

Abstract

Objective. To evaluate the effects of non-obstetric surgical procedures on maternal and fetal outcome.
Methods. A systematic review of all English language literature.
Results. Fifty-four papers met the inclusion criteria. The overall number of patients reported was 12,452. Reported maternal death was rare at .006%. The miscarriage rate was 5.8%; however, this number is difficult to interpret since matched controls were not available. The rate of elective termination of pregnancy following non-obstetric surgery was 1.3%. The rate of premature labor induced by non-obstetric surgical intervention was 3.5% and this was noted specifically following appendectomy versus other types of interventions ($P < .001$). A total of 2.5% of pregnancies resulted in fetal loss. The prematurity rate was 8.2%. The rate of major birth defects among women who underwent non-obstetric surgical intervention in the first trimester was 3.9%. Sub-analysis of papers reporting on appendectomy during pregnancy revealed a high rate (4.6%) of surgery-induced labor. Fetal loss associated with appendectomy was 2.6%; however, this rate was increased when peritonitis was present (10.9%).
Conclusions. Modern surgical and anesthesia techniques appear to diminish the rate of maternal death. Surgery in the first trimester does not appear to increase major birth defects and should not be delayed when indicated. Acute appendicitis with peritonitis is associated with higher risk to the mother and fetus.

Keywords: Pregnancy; Surgery; Pregnancy outcome; Fetus

We systematically reviewed the English literature to determine the effect of non-obstetrical surgical procedures on pregnancy outcome. While more than 8000 urgent surgical procedures are performed each year in pregnant patients [1], the fetal risks have not been critically evaluated. Our goal is to provide the surgeons up-to-date accurate information for decision making in such cases.

METHODS

Data Sources

A literature search was performed using MEDLINE and Cochrane Controlled Trials Register databases for the years 1966–2002. All of the titles of papers on non-obstetric surgical intervention during pregnancy were considered. Combination of Medical Subject Headings (MeSH) terms (*pregnancy outcome, pregnancy complications, and surgical procedures*) in an "explode" mode was used as search strategy. MeSH terms specific for different non-obstetrical surgical procedures (*appendectomy, cholecystectomy, and laparoscopy*) combined with pregnancy were also used. All titles and abstracts published in the English literature were evaluated, excluding animal studies, comments, letters, editorials, and reviews. References from the retrieved articles and those that were rejected were scanned as well in order to identify further papers.

Study Selection

Each article was evaluated according to the preset inclusion criteria. These included studies reporting any surgical intervention, urgent or elective, under anesthesia (regional or general) during pregnancy, performed at any trimester of pregnancy, and reporting pregnancy outcome measurements. All types of study design were considered, although studies had to report a series of at least 10 patients to be included. Studies reporting minor interventions or obstetric procedures (eg, skin excisions, chorionic villi sampling, amniocentesis) under local anesthesia during pregnancy were excluded. Papers discussing procedures such as cesarean delivery, fetal surgery, and dilation and curettage were excluded as well. Studies reporting women exposed to known teratogens (eg, chemotherapy or radiotherapy for malignancy) were excluded. Among papers that reported on the same group of patients, only the most recent and updated one was considered to prevent duplication of data.

Data Gathering

The quality of the papers was evaluated with respect to study design, number of patients, and whether confounders affecting pregnancy outcome were considered. Data regarding the underlying condition and the indication for the surgical procedure were collected. Pregnancy outcome measurements such as miscarriage, voluntary termination due to surgical intervention in pregnancy, cesaean delivery, or delivery induced by the preceding surgery were retrieved as well. Fetal and newborn outcome such as fetal loss, prematurity, malformations, and post-delivery complication were recorded. Maternal complications following surgical intervention and underlying condition were also collected.

Data Analysis

Data were collected and tallied in tabular form. We found high variability among studies in terms of indication for surgery, surgical approach, different anesthetic methods, and improved care for the neonate in the recent years. Meta-analysis was judged to be inappropriate. Therefore, critical synthesis of reasonably similar studies was performed.

RESULTS

The literature search resulted in 4052 titles that were scanned for relevance according to the preset inclusion criteria. Fifty-four articles matched our inclusion criteria and were included in the systematic review; 52 were retrospective cohorts or case series, 1 was a prospective cohort, and 1 described a case-control study (Table 1). Four publications were based on patients' registry data. Thirty-five (65%) publications were published since 1990. Most of the publications focused on acute abdominal conditions requiring urgent or semi-urgent surgical intervention (eg, appendicitis). Only 1 paper focused on thyroidectomy during pregnancy, mainly for malignancy, where decision making could be made electively. Table 2 delineates the studies according to the surgical procedure. In most of the papers, pregnancy outcome was a secondary end point. The focus of most papers was on the surgical aspects of diagnosis and measures associated with the underlying acute medical conditions that required urgent surgical intervention during pregnancy.

Reported Patients

The overall number of patients reported in articles based on patients' registries was 12,452; however, overlap of patients was noted in papers originating in the Swedish Registry [2–4]; therefore, each was addressed individually to avoid data duplication. The total number of patients reported excluding the Swedish Registry was 4473 (this number includes 2565 patients reported from the Manitoba Health Insurance records [5].

Fifteen papers did not report the trimester of pregnancy when the surgical intervention took place. The total number of patients reported by trimesters was 1387: 411 patients in the first trimester, 688 in the second, and 288 patients in the third trimester.

Maternal Death

Maternal complications following surgical procedure during pregnancy were not reported consistently among the reviewed studies. Only 1 maternal death of a woman undergoing laparoscopic cholecystectomy due to intra-abdominal hemorrhage 2 weeks postoperatively during the 20th week of pregnancy was reported [6]. This corresponds to a maternal death rate of .006%.

Miscarriages

The overall number of reported miscarriages was 236, which is 5.8% of all reported patients who underwent a surgical intervention throughout their pregnancy. In papers that specified trimester of pregnancy, the rate of miscarriages was 10.5% (n = 43) of the pregnant women who were exposed to surgical intervention in the first trimester. Although the rate of miscarriages according to the reviewed papers was not high, it would be very difficult to evaluate this value in the lack of a control group collected in a similar manner but without surgery. The reported patients were exposed to the surgical procedures at various points in their gestational ages, and thus their chances for a naturally occurring abortion, not associated with surgery, would be highly variable as well. Therefore those rates should not be over-interpreted.

Elective Termination

From the studies reporting on elective termination following a surgical procedure, 1.3% (n = 23) of women elected to terminate. The rationale for termination was not specified in most papers.

Delivery Induced by Surgical Procedure

The rate of delivery induced by the surgical intervention, whether the etiology for that was the procedure itself or the underlying condition was 3.5% (79/2282). This adverse outcome was prevalent in studies reporting on appendectomy in pregnancy. Fewer cases dealing with medical conditions other then appendicitis reported on surgery-induced labor (73/1559 vs. 6/723, $P < .001$).

FETAL OUTCOME

Fetal Death

A total of 2.5% (n = 45) of pregnancies resulted in fetal loss. This number does not include studies based on patients' registries. A total of 1.8% (n = 99) of deaths of 5405 cases were reported by the Swedish registry [2]. Later, the same group reported 14 cases of fetal death among 778 (1.8%) patients from the Swedish Registry undergoing appendectomy during pregnancy [3]. Obviously, based on the same database, an overlap exists between the 2 populations. Reedy, based on the Swedish registry as well, reported a rate of .8% (30/3704) of fetal death cases [4].

Prematurity

The prematurity rate in the reviewed articles was 8.2% (597/7313). This rate includes patients from registries.

Major Birth Defects

The rate of major birth defects concluded from the reviewed studies was 2.0% (194/9878). The calculation was based on all studies, excluding late reviews of the Swedish Registry [3,4] to avoid data overlap. From studies that reported on patients per trimester and major birth defects, the rate of major malformation among patients who underwent a surgical procedure during the first trimester was 3.9% (105/2663).

Appendectomy in Pregnancy

Since appendicitis is more of a homogenous surgical condition, we conducted a sub-analysis of the previous parameters with respect to appendectomy. All papers were retrospective series except for 1 paper based on the Swedish Registry [3]. None of these papers addressed confounders (Table 1).

Data summary for parameters on outcome following appendectomy are presented in Table 3. A unique feature of appendectomy is

Table 1
Characteristics of the Included Publications with the Retrieved Data

FIRST AUTHOR AND YEAR OF PUBLICATION	PROCEDURE	STUDY DESIGN	N (TRIMESTERS: 1,2,3)	PREGNANCY OUTCOME			FETAL OUTCOME			MATERNAL MORTALITY
				SA	TA	SURGERY INDUCED DELIVERY	DEATH	PREMATURITY	MM	
Finch 1974 [17]	Appendectomy	Retro. series	56 (16,25,15)	0	0	0	4	2	0	0
Mohammed 1975 [18]	Appendectomy	Retro. series	20 (12,6,2)	2	0	0	1	2	0	0
Cunningham 1975 [19]	Appendectomy	Retro. series	34 (10,16,8)	2	0	NA	1	3	0	0
Townsend 1976 [31]	Appendectomy	Retro. series	29 (3,14,7)	1	1	1	2	2	0	0
Gomez 1979 [32]	Appendectomy	Retro. series	35 (9,17,9)	NA	NA	1	0	3	0	0
Punnonen 1979 [33]	Appendectomy	Retro. series	24 (2,14,8)	0	0	2	1	1	0	0
Frisenda 1979 [34]	Appendectomy	Retro. series	37 (10,16,11)	1	0	0	0	1	0	0
Farquharson 1980 [20]	Appendectomy	Retro. series	25 (9,13,3)	NA	NA	1	1	4	0	0
McComb 1980 [35]	Appendectomy	Retro. series	19 (3,9,7)	1	NA	NA	1	3	0	0
Horowitz 1985* [21]	Appendectomy	Retro. series	10 (1,9,0)	1	0	1	3	1	0	0
Doberneck 1985 [36]	Appendectomy	Retro. series	29 (9,14,6)	0	2	3	0	3	0	0
Bailey 1986 [22]	Appendectomy	Retro. series	41 (NA)	1	NA	NA	1	0	1	0
Liang 1989 [23]	Appendectomy	Retro. series	24 (6,12,6)	0	0	3	0	5	0	0
Tamir 1990† [24]	Appendectomy	Retro. series	77 (27,37,13)	2	7	4	0	23	0	0
Mazze 1991 [3]	Appendectomy	Retro. registry	778 (272,400,106)	NA	NA	39	14	57	18	NA
Halvorsen 1992‡ [37]	Appendectomy	Retro. series	12 (0,6,6)	0	0	0	1	2	0	0
To 1995§ [38]	Appendectomy	Retro. series	34 (13,13,8)	5	0	4	0	5	0	0
Al-Mulhim 1996 [25]	Appendectomy	Retro. series	49 (10,31,8)	3	0	7	7	3	0	0
Andersen 1999 [39]	Appendectomy	Retro. series	56 (12,28,16)	4	0	2	1	4	0	0
Hee 1999¶ [26]	Appendectomy	Retro. series	117 (28,67,22)	4	2	0	NA	2	NA	0
Mourad 2000 [27]	Appendectomy	Retro. series	67 (17,27,23)	0	0	1	0	3	0	0
Tracey 2000 [28]	Appendectomy	Retro. series	22 (5,6,11)	0	0	1	0	5	0	0
Sakhri 2001 [29]	Appendectomy	Retro. series	23 (2,6,15)	0	0	0	1	3	0	0
Hsu 2001 [30]	Appendectomy	Retro. series	35 (1,19,5)	0	3	3	1	0	0	0
Hill 1975 [40]	Cholecystect.	Retro. series	20 (NA)	1	1	0	1	0	0	0
Dixon 1987 [41]	Cholecystect.	Retro. series	18 (3,14,1)	0	2	0	0	1	0	0
Swisher 1994 [42]	Cholecystect.	Retro. series	16 (5,11,0)	0	0	0	0	2	0	0
Davis 1995 [43]	Cholecystect.	Retro. series	19 (4,10,5)	0	0	0	0	5	0	0
Steinbroook 1996 [44]	Cholecystect.	Retro. series	10 (NA)	0	0	0	0	0	0	0
Barone 1999 [6]	Cholecystect.	Retro. series	46 (NA)	0	0	1	2	1	1	1
Cosenza 1999 [45]	Cholecystect.	Retro. series	32 (8,22,2)	1	2	0	1	1	0	0
Daradkeh 1999 [46]	Cholecystect.	Retro. series	16 (2,10,4)	0	0	0	0	0	0	0
Muench 2001 [47]	Cholecystect.	Retro. series	14 (NA)	0	0	0	0	1	0	0
Curet 1996 [8]	Laparoscopy	Case control	34 (15,19,0)	0	0	0	0	0	0	0
Amos 1996 [48]	Laparoscopy	Retro. series	12 (NA)	2	0	0	4	0	0	0
Reedy 1997 [4]	Laparoscopy	Retro. registry	3,704 (NA)	NA	NA	NA	30	NA	173	NA

(*Continued*)

Table 1
Characteristics of the Included Publications with the Retrieved Data (*Continued*)

FIRST AUTHOR AND YEAR OF PUBLICATION	PROCEDURE	STUDY DESIGN	N (TRIMESTERS: 1,2,3)	PREGNANCY OUTCOME			FETAL OUTCOME			MATERNAL MORTALITY
				SA	TA	SURGERY INDUCED DELIVERY	DEATH	PREMATURITY	MM	
Conron 1998 [9]	Laparoscopy	Retro. series	21 (12,0,9)	1	0	0	1	1	0	0
Akira 1999 [10]	Laparoscopy	Retro. series	35 (NA)	1	0	NA	1	0	0	0
Andreoli 1999 [11]	Laparoscopy	Retro. series	18 (4,11,3)	0	0	0	0	1	0	0
Affleck 1999 [12]	Laparoscopy	Retro. series	98 (NA)	0	0	NA	0	11	0	0
Lyass 2001 [13]	Laparoscopy	Pros. cohort	22 (7,8,7)	0	0	0	0	0	0	0
Rojansky 2002 [14]	Laparoscopy	Retro. series	37 (NA)	2	1	0	0	3	2	0
Hess 1988 [49]	Adnexal	Retro. series	54 (9,41,4)	5	1	0	0	3	0	0
Platek 1995 [50]	Adnexal	Retro. series	19 (NA)	1	0	0	0	0	0	0
Soriano 1999 [51]	Adnexal	Retro. series	93 (64,29,0)	7	NA	0	0	8	3	0
Moore 1999 [52]	Adnexal	Retro. series	14 (0,9,0)	0	0	0	1	3	0	0
Usui 2000 [53]	Adnexal	Retro. series	60 (NA)	2	0	0	3	7	2	0
Hamilton 1968 [54]	Thyroidectomy	Retro. series	24 (5,18,1)	0	0	0	0	1	0	0
Duncan 1986 [5]	Various	Retro. registry	2565 (NA)	181	NA	NA	NA	NA	82	NA
Mazze 1989 [2]	Various	Retro. registry	5405 (2252,1881,1272)	NA	NA	NA	99	423	102	NA
Kort 1993 [55]	Various	Retro. series	78 (0,36,42)	NA	0	NA	3	17	0	0
El-Amin 1998 [56]	Various	Retro. series	41 (NA)	2	0	NA	0	5	0	0
Gerstenfeld 2000 [57]	Various	Retro. series	106 (53,52,1)	2	NA	1	2	11	NA	0
Visser 2001 [58]	Various	Retro. series	76 (NA)	NA	1	4	0	12	1	0

MM = major malformations; NA = not available (information is missing or not clear); Pros = prospective; Retro = retrospective.

* Horowitz et al reported on 12 patients; however, 2 patients were operated on at the puerperium.

† The study by Tamir reported on 84 patients; however, only 77 were eligible for pregnancy outcome analysis; 7 patients were diagnosed at the puerperium.

‡ Halvorsen et al reported on a group of 16 patients; however, the report considers only those who were diagnosed with acute appendicitis.

§ To et al reported on a group of 38 patients; however, 4 patients were treated in the postpartum period, and therefore only 34 were considered for analysis.

¶ Missing data on several patients; information on preterm termination is not available for 5 of 11 patients.

Table 2
The Included Publications (N = 54) According to the Surgical Procedure at Focus

SURGICAL PROCEDURE	NO. OF PUBLICATIONS
Appendectomy*	24
Cholecystectomy*	9
Laparoscopy†	9
Adnexal mass	5
Miscellaneous	7

* Papers that were focusing on 1 type of condition managed either by laparotomy or laparoscopy.

† Papers discussing laparoscopic procedures focusing on more than 1 type of intervention (eg, laparoscopic appendectomy and laparoscopic cholecystectomy).

an apparently high rate of surgery-induced delivery (4.6% or 73/1559). There appears to be a difference between the rate of surgery-induced labor when appendicitis is compared to other medical conditions (73/1559 vs. 6/723, $P < .001$). The fetal loss rate for appendectomy during pregnancy was 2.6% (40/1559) versus 1.2% (56/4485) for other surgical procedures during pregnancy ($P < .001$). The fetal loss rate was 10.9% when peritonitis was present.

COMMENTS

The need for non-obstetric surgery in pregnancy has been estimated to be .12% [1]. This translates to 8000 cases in the United States every year. Estimation of the effect that general anesthesia and surgical intervention have on reproductive risk among these patients is critical in evaluating therapeutic choices.

The available world literature includes more than 10,000 patients in 54 studies. The main focus of these articles was not maternal and fetal outcome but mainly diagnosis, surgical management, or the effects of anesthesia. The wide variability of surgical indication and anesthetic technique and article focus made the comparison and combination of these articles difficult. There was also very little information on other possible confounders of pregnancy outcome such as maternal age, lifestyle, underlying condition, and drugs. For these reasons we felt that meta-analysis of the articles would not be meaningful. Yet, systematic review of these papers does allow several observations:

Table 3
Pregnancy Outcome Measures for Studies Reporting on Appendectomy During Pregnancy

OUTCOME MEASURE	n	N	%
Miscarriages	27	815	3.0
Elective termination	15	755	2.0
Surgery induced delivery	73	1559	4.7
Fetal loss	40	1536	2.6
Fetal loss in patients with perforated appendix	18	182	10.9
Prematurity	137	1653	8.3
Major birth defects	18	464*	3.9

* Only for patients who were operated on during the first trimester.

Maternal Outcomes

There was inconsistent reporting of maternal outcomes in the papers. The report of 1 death in approximately 12,542 procedures (.006%) implies that the risk of death is extremely low. This rate is lower than one would expect based on traditional teaching. However, it is possible given the nature of the published papers that some bias against reporting deaths occurred. It seems that concerns over possible maternal death due to anesthesia and surgery alone are not a reason to delay prompt treatment of the underlying surgical condition.

Miscarriage is a big concern for both patient and physician. The overall rate of 5.8% for miscarriage/fetal death for all trimesters and the rate of 10.5% for first trimester patients certainly is concerning. However, the lack of control groups for the patients makes these results difficult to interpret. One cannot separate the contribution of surgery and anesthesia from the underlying medical condition.

Elective termination occurred in 1.3% of women. The reasons for termination of pregnancy were not given. One could speculate that it may be due to fears about possible teratogenicity of anesthetics or concerns over fetal hypoxia. We did note that there appears to be a trend in reporting increased rates of elective termination since 1990. It is not readily apparent why this may be the case. Possible reasons would include improved reporting of outcomes, changes in societal attitudes, or even legal code changes.

The rate of premature delivery induced by the surgical intervention or underlying condition was 3.5% and was only reported in cases of appendectomy. This will be discussed further under the appendectomy section.

Fetal Outcomes

The fetal loss rate was 2.5% in non-registry studies and ranged from .8% to 1.8% in registry studies. Interpretation is limited by the lack of a suitable control groups. Premature birth occurred in 8.2% of cases. Improvements in neonatal care have occurred with time and it makes comparison of results across years impossible. Premature labor that might have resulted in fetal loss in 1985 may not have the same outcome today. We noted that the fetal loss rate in studies on appendectomy appeared higher.

The rate of major birth defects in the studies reviewed was 2.0%, excluding late reviews of the Swedish registry data. The rate of major birth defects in patients undergoing surgery during the first trimester was 3.9%. This rate is slightly higher than the expected rate of 1% to 3% for major birth defects in the general population [7]. None of the individual studies showed that the increased rate of birth defects was statistically significant.

Laparoscopic versus Open Procedures

We identified 9 studies that focused on laparoscopic surgery during pregnancy. None of the studies came to the conclusion that laparoscopic procedures were harmful to the mother or fetus. In general, the most common conclusion was that laparoscopic surgery was safe and may benefit with the patient when compared to open procedures [8–14].

Appendectomy in Pregnancy

Appendectomy is probably the most frequently performed non-obstetrical surgical procedure in pregnancy [15,16]. We noted differences in the data for this medical condition when compared to others.

The rate of premature delivery for patients with appendicitis was statistically higher when compared to other medical conditions ($P < .001$). Including registry data, the fetal loss rate for patients undergoing appendectomy was significantly greater than the fetal loss rate ($P < .001$) for patients undergoing other surgical procedures during pregnancy. The already high fetal loss rate during appendicitis increases to 10.9% when peritonitis is present. It appears from these simple comparisons that the effects of acute appendicitis and surgery on the patient are more severe and different from other acute conditions requiring surgery during pregnancy. Most papers on appendectomy concluded that there is worse maternal and fetal outcome if peritonitis develops and encouraged prompt diagnosis and treatment of this condition [17–30].

SUMMARY

We identified 54 papers that provided maternal and fetal outcome data for review. Although maternal death is rare (<1/10,000), it can occur. There appears to be no difference between open and laparoscopic procedures. Premature labor and fetal loss are the most common undesired consequences, especially if acute appendicitis is present. Acute appendicitis has significantly more severe effects on the maternal and fetal outcome particularly if peritonitis develops when compared to other acute surgical conditions during pregnancy.

Based on our review of the literature, we came to the following conclusions:

- Using modern surgical and anesthetic techniques, the risk of maternal death appears to be very low.
- Surgery and general anesthesia do not appear to be major risk factors for spontaneous abortion.
- The rate of elective termination appears to be in the range of the general population.
- Non-obstetric surgical procedures do not increase the risk for major birth defects. Hence, urgent surgical procedures should be performed when needed.
- Acute appendicitis, especially when accompanied by peritonitis, appears to be genuine risk for surgery-induced labor or fetal loss.

This review and analysis underscores our lack of knowledge in this area and points out a critical need for better data, with details not only on surgical condition, the anesthetic and surgical techniques, but also careful attention to confounders such as the underlying maternal condition and its management, smoking, alcohol consumption, socioeconomic status, and many others.

ACKNOWLEDGMENT

GK holds the Ivey Chair in Molecular Toxicology, University of Western Ontario.

REFERENCES

[1] Jenkins TM, Mackey SF, Benzoni EM, et al. Non-obstetric surgery during gestation: risk factors for lower birthweight. Aust N Z J Obstet Gynaecol 2003;43:27–31.

[2] Mazze RI, Kallen B: Reproductive outcome after anesthesia and operation during pregnancy: a registry study of 5405 cases. Am J Obstet Gynecol 1989;161:1178–85.

[3] Mazze RI, Kallen B: Appendectomy during pregnancy: a Swedish registry study of 778 cases. Obstet Gynecol 1991;77:835–40.

[4] Reedy MB, Kallen B, Kuehl TJ: Laparoscopy during pregnancy: a study of five fetal outcome parameters with use of the Swedish Health Registry. Am J Obstet Gynecol 1997;177:673–9.

[5] Duncan PG, Pope WD, Cohen MM, et al. Fetal risk of anesthesia and surgery during pregnancy. Anesthesiology 1986;64:790–4.

[6] Barone JE, Bears S, Chen S, et al. Outcome study of cholecystectomy during pregnancy. Am J Surg 1999;177:232–6.

[7] Heinonen OP, Slone D, Shapiro S: *Birth Defects and Drugs in Pregnancy*. Littleton, MA: Publishing Sciences Group; 1977.

[8] Curet MJ, Allen D, Josloff RK, et al. Arch Surg 1996;131:546–50.

[9] Conron RW Jr, Abbruzzi K, Cochrane SO, et al. Laparoscopic procedures in pregnancy. Am Surg 1999;65:259–63.

[10] Akira S, Yamanaka A, Ishihara T, et al. Gasless laparoscopic ovarian cystectomy during pregnancy: comparison with laparotomy. Am J Obstet Gynecol 1999;180:t-7.

[11] Andreoli M, Sayegh SK, Hoefer R, et al. Laparoscopic cholecystectomy for recurrent gallstone pancreatitis during pregnancy. South Med J 1996;89:1114–5.

[12] Affleck DG, Handrahan DL, Egger MJ, et al. The laparoscopic management of appendicitis and cholelithiasis during pregnancy. Am J Surg 1999;178:523–9.

[13] Lyass S, Pikarsky A, Eisenberg VH, et al. Is laparoscopic appendectomy safe in pregnant women? Surg Endosc 2001;15:377–9.

[14] Rojansky N, Shushan A, Fatum M: Laparoscopy versus laparotomy in pregnancy: a comparative study. J Am Assoc Gynecol Laparosc 2002;9:108–10.

[15] McGee TM. Acute appendicitis in pregnancy. Aust N Z J Obstet Gynaecol 1989;29:378–85.

[16] Mourad J, Elliott JP, Erickson L, et al. Appendicitis in pregnancy: new information that contradicts long-held clinical beliefs. Am J Obstet Gynecol 2000;182:1027–9.

[17] Finch DR, Lee E: Acute appendicitis complicating pregnancy in the Oxford region. Br J Surg 1974;61:129–32.

[18] Mohammed JA, Oxorn H: Appendicitis in pregnancy. CMAJ 1975; 112:1187–8.

[19] Cunningham FG, McCubbin JH: Appendicitis complicating pregnancy. Obstet Gynecol 1975;45:415–20.

[20] Farquharson RG: Acute appendicitis in pregnancy. Scott Med J 1980; 25:36–8.

[21] Horowitz MD, Gomez GA, Santiesteban R, et al. Acute appendicitis during pregnancy. Diagnosis and management. Arch Surg 1985;120: 1362–7.

[22] Bailey LE, Finley RK Jr, Miller SF, et al. Acute appendicitis during pregnancy. Am Surg 1986;52:218–21.

[23] Liang CC, Hsieh TT, Chang SD: Appendicitis during pregnancy. Changgeng Yi Xue Za Zhi 1989;12:208–14.

[24] Tamir IL, Bongard FS, Klein SR: Acute appendicitis in the pregnant patient. Am J Surg 1990;160:571–5.

[25] Al Mulhim AA: Acute appendicitis in pregnancy. A review of 52 cases. Int Surg 1996;81:295–7.

[26] Hee P, Viktrup L: The diagnosis of appendicitis during pregnancy and maternal and fetal outcome after appendectomy. Int J Gynaecol Obstet 1999;65:129–35.

[27] Mourad J, Elliott JP, Erickson L, et al. Appendicitis in pregnancy: new information that contradicts long-held clinical beliefs. Am J Obstet Gynecol 2000;182:1027–9.

[28] Tracey M, Fletcher HS: Appendicitis in pregnancy. Am Surg 2000; 66:555–9.
[29] Sakhri J, Youssef S, Ben Letaifa D, et al. Acute appendicitis during pregnancy. Tunisie Medicale 2001;79:521–5.
[30] Hsu YP, Chen RJ, Fang JF, et al. Acute appendicitis during pregnancy: a clinical assessment. Chang Gung Med J 2001;24:245–50.
[31] Townsend JM, Greiss FC: Appendictiis in pregnancy. South Med J 1976;69:1161–3.
[32] Gomez A, Wood M: Acute appendicitis during pregnancy. Am J Surg 1979;137:180–3.
[33] Punnonen R, Aho AJ, Gronroos M, et al. Appendicectomy during pregnancy. Acta Chir Scand 1979;145:555–8.
[34] Frisenda R, Roty AR Jr, Kilway JB, et al. Acute appendicitis during pregnancy. Am Surg 1979;45:503–6.
[35] McComb P, Laimon H: Appendicitis complicating pregnancy. Can J Surg 1980;23:92–4.
[36] Doberneck RC: Appendectomy during pregnancy. Am Surg 1985;51:265–8.
[37] Halvorsen AC, Brandt B, Andreasen JJ: Acute appendicitis in pregnancy: complications and subsequent management. Eur J Surg 1992; 158:603–6.
[38] To WW, Ngai CS, Ma HK: Pregnancies complicated by acute appendicitis. Aust N Z J Surg 1995;65:799–803.
[39] Andersen B, Nielsen TF: Appendicitis in pregnancy: diagnosis, management and complications. Acta Obstet Gynecol Scand 1999;78:758–62.
[40] Hill LM, Johnson CE, Lee RA: Cholecystectomy in pregnancy. Obstet Gynecol 1975;46:291–3.
[41] Dixon NP, Faddis DM, Silberman H: Aggressive management of cholecystitis during pregnancy. Am J Surg 1987;154:292–4.
[42] Swisher SG, Schmit PJ, Hunt KK, et al. Biliary disease during pregnancy. Am J Surg 1994;168:576–9.
[43] Davis A, Katz VL, Cox R: Gallbladder disease in pregnancy. J Reprod Med 1995;40:759–62.
[44] Steinbrook RA, Brooks DC, Datta S: Laparoscopic cholecystectomy during pregnancy. Review of anesthetic management, surgical considerations. Surg Endosc 1996;10:511–5.
[45] Cosenza CA, Saffari B, Jabbour N, et al. Surgical management of biliary gallstone disease during pregnancy. Am J Surg 1999;178:545–8.
[46] Daradkeh S, Sumrein I, Daoud F, et al. Management of gallbladder stones during pregnancy: conservative treatment or laparoscopic cholecystectomy? Hepatogastroenterology 1999;46:3074–6.
[47] Muench J, Albrink M, Serafini F, et al. Delay in treatment of biliary disease during pregnancy increases morbidity and can be avoided with safe laparoscopic cholecystectomy. Am Surg 2001;67:539–42.
[48] Amos JD, Schorr SJ, Norman PF, et al. Laparoscopic surgery during pregnancy. Am J Surg 1996;171:435–7.
[49] Hess LW, Peaceman A, O'Brien WF, et al. Adnexal mass occurring with intrauterine pregnancy: report of fifty-four patients requiring laparotomy for definitive management. Am J Obstet Gynecol 1988; 158:1029–34.
[50] Platek DN, Henderson CE, Goldberg GL: The management of a persistent adnexal mass in pregnancy. Am J Obstet Gynecol 1995; 173:1236–40.
[51]. Soriano D, Yefet Y, Seidman DS, et al. Laparoscopy versus laparotomy in the management of adnexal masses during pregnancy. Fertil Steril 1999;71:955–60.
[52] Moore RD, Smith WG: Laparoscopic management of adnexal masses in pregnant women. J Reprod Med 1999;44:97–100.
[53] Usui R, Minakami H, Kosuge S, et al. A retrospective survey of clinical, pathologic, and prognostic features of adnexal masses operated on during pregnancy. J Obstet Gynaecol Res 2000;26:89–93.
[54] Hamilton NT, Paterson PJ, Breidahl HD: Thyroidectomy during pregnancy. Med J Aust 1968;1:431–3.
[55] Kort B, Katz VL, Watson WJ: The effect of nonobstetric operation during pregnancy. Surg Gynecol Obstet 1993;177:371–6.
[56] El Amin AM, Yahia Al-Shehri M, Zaki ZM, et al. Acute abdomen in pregnancy. Int J Gynaecol Obstet 1998;62:31–6.
[57] Gerstenfeld TS, Chang DT, Pliego AR, et al. Nonobstetrical abdominal surgery during pregnancy in Women's Hospital. J Matern Fetal Med 2000;9:170–2.
[58] Visser BC, Glasgow RE, Mulvihill KK, et al. Safety and timing of nonobstetric abdominal surgery in pregnancy. Dig Surg 2001;18: 409–17.

CHAPTER 33

MATERNAL HYPERTHERMIA AND THE RISK FOR NEURAL TUBE DEFECTS IN OFFSPRING: SYSTEMATIC REVIEW AND META-ANALYSIS

Myla E. Moretti, Benjamin Bar-Oz,† Shawn Fried,* and Gideon Koren**

Background. In animals, excessive core body temperatures have been documented to cause malformations; neural tube defects (NTDs) are among the most frequently reported. In humans, data are inconclusive and often conflicting. The objective of our report is to determine the risk for neural tube defects associated with maternal hyperthermia in early pregnancy

Methods. We conducted a systematic review and meta-analysis to evaluate available evidence on this topic in humans. MEDLINE, EMBASE, references from published reports, and biologic abstracts from meetings were searched for relevant studies. Reviewers evaluated all the retrieved articles and extracted the relevant data. Individual and summary odds ratios and relative risks were calculated using the Mantel–Haenszel method.

Results. Fifteen studies, reporting on 1,719 cases and 37,898 non-cases, were included in the meta-analysis. The overall odds ratio for neural tube defects associated with maternal hyperthermia was 1.92 (95% confidence interval = 1.61–2.29). When analyzed separately, the 9 case-control studies had an odds ratio of 1.93 (1.53–2.42). The summary relative risk for the 6 cohort studies was 1.95 (1.30 –2.92).

Conclusions. Maternal hyperthermia in early pregnancy is associated with increased risk for neural tube defects and may be a human teratogen.

(*Epidemiology* 2005;16: 216–219)

Nearly 100 years ago, scientists discovered that malformations could be induced in various animal species by exposing the mother to high core body temperatures during critical periods of gestation.[1] Although a number of teratologic outcomes were produced, including fetal loss and various malformations, the brain was particularly sensitive.[2,3] In humans, an elevated core body temperature can occur with fever caused by viral or bacterial illnesses. In addition, extreme exercise, saunas, hot tubs, heated beds, and electric blankets may all lead to increased body temperatures. Presently, there is no consensus as to the role of hyperthermia during pregnancy in causing malformations in humans. Many of the available studies are inconclusive due to insufficient sample size.

A fever can be of varying duration, as with exposure to other potential teratogens. A fever may be recognized and treated with antipyretics or it may remain unidentified or untreated. Serious illnesses accompanied by fevers (eg, malaria) may be associated with poor nutritional intake by the mother, which itself may be associated with poor pregnancy outcome. The infectious agent itself may be teratogenic (such as rubella, varicella or cytomegalovirus). The literature on the effects of maternal hyperthermia has investigated various outcomes, including pregnancy loss and specific malformations. Our objective was to investigate the association between maternal hyperthermia in early pregnancy and the risk for risk for neural tube defects (NTDs). We chose this outcome because there are a substantial number of published studies on this association, and because it is an outcome for which animal data lend biologic plausibility.

METHODS

We searched MEDLINE and EMBASE to locate articles in any language in 1966 through August 2003. In addition, the reference sections from articles retrieved from the original database searches were inspected for additional publications. Published meeting abstracts and proceedings were also searched between 1980 and February 2003 for studies in progress or studies not published in the peer reviewed literature. The keywords "pregnancy," "pregnancy outcome," "birth defect," "teratogen," and "congenital abnormalities" were searched. The intersection of this search with articles retrieved by using the keyword "hyperthermia" generated the final set of articles retrieved for evaluation.

Two investigators familiar with clinical study design acted as reviewers, selecting studies for inclusion in the meta-analysis based on preset inclusion criteria and following a standardized checklist (Appendix 1, available with the electronic version of this article). Reviewers received only the Methods sections; they were unaware of the authors' and journal names, and year of publication. Studies were excluded if they were not performed in humans, did not report pregnancy outcome, did not specifically extract information on neural tube defects, reported on fewer than 5 subjects, did not have a control group, were not cohort or case–control studies, or did not report hyperthermia exposure occurring in the first trimester. Hyperthermia or fever was included if it was either internal (such as maternal fever caused by illness) or external (exposures to hot tubs, heated beds, saunas or electric blankets). Each reviewer listed the reason for exclusion.

The reviewers were then given the Results section of each of the included papers, with identifying information removed.

Submitted 21 October 2003; final version accepted 22 November 2004.
From the *The Motherisk Program, The Hospital for Sick Children, Toronto, Canada; †Department of Neonatology, Hadassah Medical Center, Jerusalem, Israel.
B.B.O. received a Research Fellowship Award from The Hospital for Sick Children's Research Institute
G.K. is a Senior Scientist of the Canadian Institutes for Health Research.
Supplemental material for this article is available with the online version of the journal at www.epidem.com
Correspondence: Myla Moretti, Assistant Director, Motherisk Program, The Hospital for Sick Children, 555 University Avenue, Toronto, Ontario M5G 1X8, Canada. E-mail: momrisk@sickkids.ca.

ISSN: 1044-3983/05/1602-0216
DOI: 10.1097/01.ede.0000152903.55579.15

Reviewers extracted the relevant data from the text and tables, and entered these numbers into 2 × 2 tables. The following neural tube defects were included: anencephaly, spina bifida, encephalocele, myelomeningocele, exencephaly, myeloschisis, iniencephaly, and craniorachischisis. Studies were included if they reported the total number of NTDs, even if the numbers of specific NTDs were not specified. Internal hyperthermia was defined as documented maternal fever (either receiving treatment or not) or documentation of maternal illnesses know to be associated with fever ("febrile illnesses") in the first trimester of pregnancy. External hyperthermia was defined as exposure to at least 15 minutes of high temperature exposure via hot tub, sauna, electric blanket or heated waterbed in the first trimester of pregnancy.

Each reviewer extracted the data independently. For studies about which there was disagreement on inclusion or data extraction, the reviewers discussed the rationale for their choices and came to consensus. The extracted data were entered into Cochrane's Review Manager (version 4.1, Ox-ford: Cochrane Collaboration). For summaries that included case-control studies, we calculated individual and summary odds ratios (ORs) and 95% confidence intervals (CIs) by the Mantel-Haenszel method. For cohort studies we used the relative risk (RR) and 95% CI. Included studies were tested for heterogeneity using the χ^2 test. Publication bias was assessed by visual examination of the funnel plot (effect size versus log study size) and by the trim-and-fill method of Duval and Tweedie.[4,5]

RESULTS

Initially, 42 studies were identified and presented to the reviewers for possible inclusion. Of these, we subsequently excluded 24 articles because they did not meet the inclusion criteria or because the Methods and Results sections did not provide sufficient information. For example, a study from a Japanese group [6] was excluded because it described a retrospective cohort with no control group. Another study[7] reported sauna use in all cases and all controls and focused on comparing habits of sauna use in the 2 groups. One study[8] was excluded because the report did not give the total number of prospectively collected subjects but rather described only the affected cases in detail. An additional 3 studies were excluded because they were publication of duplicate data.[9–11] A full list of excluded articles is available from the authors (Appendix 2, available with the electronic version of this article).

Details regarding the 15 included studies are shown in Table 1. [12–26] There were 9 case–control studies, with a total of 1601 NTD cases and 5149 controls. The overall OR was 1.93 (95% CI = 1.53–2.42) for NTDs associated with maternal hyperthermia exposure (Fig. 1). There were 6 prospective cohort studies reporting on 8,798 exposed infants and 24,069 unexposed infants, yielding an overall RR of 1.95 (CI = 1.30 –2.92) (Fig. 2). When combined, the overall OR of all 15 studies was 1.92 (CI = 1.61-2.29). The χ^2 test for heterogeneity was 13.14 ($df = 13$; $P = 0.44$), with no statistical evidence for heterogeneity. One cohort study [24] did not contribute to the summary rates because there were no NTDs detected, and thus the individual RR/OR could not be estimated. Findings did not vary by year of publication. Some publications reported on other potential sources for variation in findings (eg, maternal characteristics, degree of fever and folate intake). However, there were not sufficient data to conduct secondary analysis on these parameters. A funnel plot arrangement of the results was asymmetric, suggesting the presence of publication bias. The adjusted odds ratio (using the trim-and-fill method) was 1.86 (95% CI = 1.54–2.24).

DISCUSSION

Hyperthermia was the first environmental teratogen identified by scientists in animal models. Even so, there has not been a consensus

Table 1
Studies Included in Meta-Analysis of Maternal Hyperthermia and NTDs

FIRST AUTHOR, YEAR	NO. SUBJECTS	HEAT SOURCE: TYPE	HEAT SOURCE: DEFINITION
Retrospective case-control studies			
Chance, 1978 [12]	43 NTD; 63 normal controls	Internal	Fever ≥38.9°C
Halperin, 1978 [13]	45 NTD; 48 normal controls	Internal and external	"High fever" or sauna 43°C
Miller, 1978 [14]	63 NTD; 64 normal controls	Internal and External	≥38.9°C fever for ≥1 day, or very hot sauna ≥15 min
Fisher, 1981 [15]	17 NTD; 17 Down syndrome controls	Internal	Fever >38.9°C
Shiota, 1982 [16]	113 NTD; 113 normal controls	Internal	"Febrile illness"
Dlugosz, 1992 [17]	224 NTD; 224 normal controls	Internal	"High fever"
Lynberg, 1994 [18]	385 NTD; 3647 malformed controls	Internal	
Shaw, 1998 [19]	504 NTD; 509 normal controls	Internal	"Febrile illnesses"
Shaw, 2002 [20]	252 NTD; 464 normal controls	Internal	At least 37.8°C
Prospective cohort studies			
Coffey, 1959 [21]	656 hyperthermia; 658 control	Internal	"Influenza"
McDonald, 1961 [22]	148 fever; 3103 control	Internal	Febrile illnesses and infections
Klienebrecht, 1979 [23]	2302 fever; 2501 control	Internal	"Febrile illness" or "influenza"
Little, 1991 [24]	55 fever; 54 control	Internal	Fever 38.4°C for ≥24 h
Milunsky, 1992 [25]	5,566 fever; 17,188 controls	Internal and external	Fever 37.8°C or "use of hot tub, sauna, or electric blanket"
Chambers, 1998 [26]	71 hyperthermia; 265 controls	Internal	Fever ≥38.9°C for ≥24 h

First Author	No. Exposed/ No. Cases	No. Exposed/ No. Controls	Weight %	Odds Ratio (95% CI)
Chance[12]	3/43	0/63	0.6	11 (0.55-220)
Halperin[13]	3/45	1/48	1.0	3.4 (0.34-34)
Miller[14]	7/63	0/64	0.6	17 (0.96-310)
Fisher[15]	4/17	0/17	0.6	12 (0.58-236)
Shiota[16]	16/113	7/113	5.7	2.5 (0.99-6.3)
Dlugosz[17]	16/224	15/224	8.8	1.1 (0.52-2.2)
Lynberg[18]	42/340	282/3647	29.5	1.7 (1.2-2.4)
Shaw[19]	137/504	82/509	34.3	1.9 (1.4-2.6)
Shaw[20]	43/252	38/464	19.0	2.3 (1.4-3.7)
Total	**271/1601**	**425/5149**	**100.0**	**1.93 (1.53-2.42)**

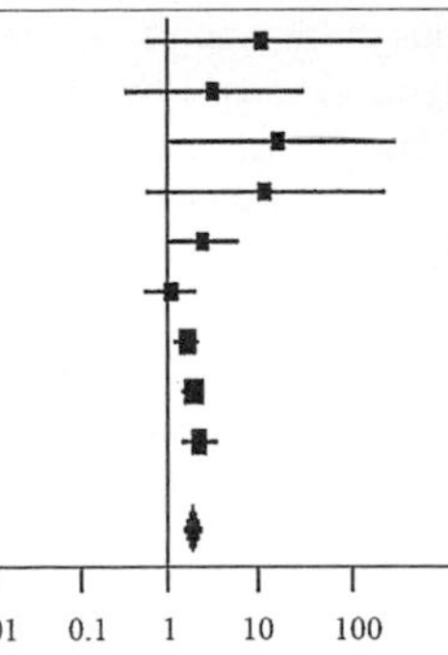

Figure 1. Individual and summary odds ratios for case–control studies of maternal hyperthermia and NTDs.

about its effect in humans. In animals, one can deliver precise amount of hyperthermia in terms of timing, length, and degree. Evaluation of exposure in humans has been substantially more complicated. In humans, hyperthermia is often associated with an infectious disease that may pose a risk to the fetus both in terms of the pathogen itself and through other changes in maternal well being and nutritional status.

We focused on NTDs because this was the endpoint of most human studies on pregnancy outcomes after exposure to hyperthermia. Most studies were conducted before the association between risk for NTD and low folate intake was established and, therefore, data on daily folate or blood levels of this vitamin were not included. Four studies made note of maternal use of multivitamins or folic acid specifically. [18-20,25] In 2 of these publications,[18,19] elevated risks for NTD persisted even after adjusting for maternal multivitamin use; in the more recent article by Shaw et al,[20] the ORs for the association of hyperthermia with NTDs were somewhat lower among vitamin users but still elevated. In contrast, Milunsky et al [25] showed that only hot tub use affected NTD risk after controlling for folic acid, while the risks for NTD following maternal fever, sauna or electric blanket use in pregnancy were minimal.

In the analysis reported here, the heat source for most studies was influenza or other febrile illnesses. However, a similar increased risk was found in studies where hyperthermia was due to exposure to external heat sources (eg, Milunsky et al[25]). These studies suggest that, as in the animal data, it is core body temperature and not confounding effects of viral infections that cause NTDs. Of note, Lynberg et al [18] reported that influenza was associated with an increased risk for NTDs, whereas other febrile illnesses did not appear to increase the NTD risk after adjusting for confounders. Only 3 studies reported on outcome after both internal fever and external hyperthermia[13,14,25]; however, the sample size was very small in 2 of these studies,[13,14] and in the third,[25] internal and external heat sources were not separated.

There was some indication of a dose response. Milunsky et al[25] reported that risks were higher among women who had exposure to more than one heat source, and Chambers et al[26] found all cases of NTDs were in the high-fever group. Even so, given the limited data addressing specific details of magnitude and duration of the exposures, it remains unclear whether the hyperthermia itself or the maternal illness was the cause of the teratogenic outcomes.

Several studies explicitly reported the pharmacologic treatment of the maternal fevers,[14,16,18,19,26] although data were rarely presented in a way we could include in our analysis. Lynberg et al [18] found that ORs for NTDs were increased if medications were taken, whereas Shaw et al[19] reported that use of medications decreased risks for NTD. We found very similar effects in case–control and cohort studies, lending further credibility to the observed association. The studies were statistically homogeneous, suggesting that pooling the data is appropriate.

One of the concerns regarding meta-analysis is the combination of studies with a range of quality. As suggested originally by Glass [27,28] and confirmed by us,[29] the quality of the study does not appear to affect the directional of the results. However, there are too few empiric observations to support such generalizations.

Publication bias also was a concern in meta-analysis. Arranging the results in a funnel plot should produce an inverted funnel if publication bias is not present. In this case the funnel plot

First Author	No. Cases/ No. Exposed	No Cases/ No. Not Exposed	Weight %	Relative Risk (95% CI)
Coffey[21]	17/656	5/658	16.7	3.4 (1.3-9.2)
McDonald[22]	1/148	15/3103	4.0	1.4 (0.2-11)
Klienebrecht[23]	17/2302	12/2801	30.1	1.7 (0.8-3.6)
Little[24]	0/55	0/54	0.0	Not Estimable
Milunsky[25]	17/5566	32/17188	47.4	1.6 (0.9-3.0)
Chambers[26]	2/71	0/265	1.8	18 (0.9-380)
Total (95%CI)	**54/8798**	**64/24069**	**100.0**	**1.95 (1.30-2.92)**

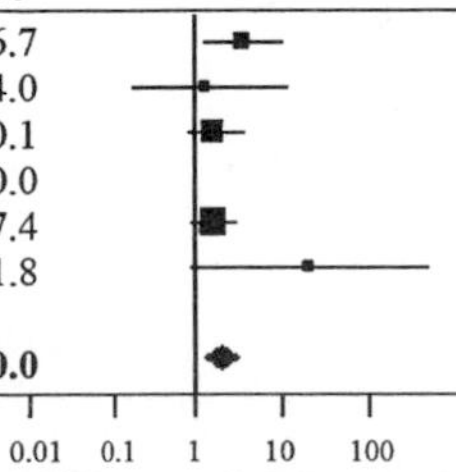

Figure 2. Individual and summary relative risks for prospective cohort studies of maternal hyperthermia and NTDs.

was not symmetrical, with the lower left quadrant absent, suggesting a deficit of smaller negative studies. Among the methods for quantifying the degree of asymmetry (and thus publication bias) the most widely used is the trim–and-fill method proposed by Duval and Tweedie.[4,5] In this analysis the assessment did not change the direction or significance of the results, suggesting that publication bias is not an important factor in these results.

In the studies reviewed here, hyperthermia met many of the criteria for a human teratogen as established by Shepard.[30] The exposures occurred at a critical time in prenatal development; only studies that defined exposures in the first trimester were included in our meta-analysis. The findings were consistent across epidemiologic studies of high quality. Despite the fact that some of the studies did not control for confounders or biases, all studies showed the same directional of risk. Finally, as described earlier, similar consistent findings have been shown in animals, which lends biologic plausibility to teratogenic causality. To strengthen the evidence for causality, future studies should attempt to define exposures with more detail and precision, while incorporating measures of folate intake to correct for this potential effect modifier.

REFERENCES

1. Warkany J. Teratogen update: hyperthermia. *Teratology.* 1986;33: 365–371.
2. Edwards MJ. Congenital defects in guinea pigs: prenatal retardation of brain growth of guinea pigs following hyperthermia during gestation. *Teratology.* 1969;2:329 –336.
3. Edwards MJ. Congenital defects in guinea pigs: fetal resorptions, abortions, and malformations following induced hyperthermia during early gestation. *Teratology.* 1969;2:313–328.
4. Duval S, Tweedie R. Trim and fill: a simple funnel-plot-based method of testing and adjusting for publication bias in meta-analysis. *Biometrics.* 2000;56:455– 463.
5. Duval S, Tweedie R. A nonparametric "trim and fill" method of accounting for publication bias in meta-analysis. *J Am Stat Assoc.* 2000;95:89 –98.
6. Hirayama Y, Suzuki H, Arima M. Maternal hyperthermia during pregnancy in severely multi-disabled children [Japanese]. *No To Hattatsu.* 1992;24:559 –564.
7. Saxen L, Holmberg PC, Nurminen M, Kuosma E. Sauna and congenital defects. *Teratology.* 1982;25:309 –313.
8. Smith DW, Clarren SK, Harvey MA. Hyperthermia as a possible teratogenic agent. *J Pediatr.* 1978;92: 878–883.
9. Layde PM, Edmonds LD, Erickson JD. Maternal fever and neural tube defects. *Teratology.* 1980;21:105–108.
10. Erickson JD. Risk factors for birth defects: data from the Atlanta Birth Defects Case-Control Study. *Teratology.* 1991;43:41–51.
11. Botto LD, Erickson JD, Mulinare J, Lynberg MC, Liu Y. Maternal fever, multivitamin use, and selected birth defects: evidence of interaction? *Epidemiology.* 2002;13:485– 488.
12. Chance PF, Smith DW. Hyperthermia and meningomyelocele and anencephaly (letter). *Lancet.* 1978;1:769 –770.
13. Halperin LR, Wilroy RSJr. Maternal hyperthermia and neural-tube defects (letter). *Lancet.* 1978;2:212–213.
14. Miller P, Smith DW, Shepard TH. Maternal hyperthermia as a possible cause of anencephaly. *Lancet.* 1978;1:519 –521.
15. Fisher NL, Smith DW. Occipital encephalocele and early gestational hyperthermia. *Pediatrics.* 1981;68:480 –483.
16. Shiota K. Neural tube defects and maternal hyperthermia in early pregnancy: epidemiology in a human embryo population. *Am J Med Genet.* 1982;12:281–288.
17. Dlugosz L, Vena J, Byers T, Sever L, Bracken M, Marshall E. Congenital defects and electric bed heating in New York State: a register-based case-control study. *Am J Epidemiol.* 1992;135: 1000–1011.
18. Lynberg MC, Khoury MJ, Lu X, Cocian T. Maternal flu, fever, and the risk of neural tube defects: a population- based case-control study. *Am J Epidemiol.* 1994;140: 244 –255.
19. Shaw GM, Todoroff K, Velie EM, Lammer EJ. Maternal illness, including fever and medication use as risk factors for neural tube defects. *Teratology.* 1998;57:1–7.
20. Shaw GM, Nelson V, Carmichael SL, Lammer EJ, Finnell RH, Rosenquist TH. Maternal periconceptional vitamins: interactions with selected factors and congenital anomalies? *Epidemiology.* 2002;13:625– 630.
21. Coffey VP, Jessop WJE. Maternal influenza and congenital deformities: A prospective study. *Lancet.* 1959;2:935–938.
22. McDonald AD. Maternal health in early pregnancy and congenital defect. *Br J Prev Soc Med.* 1961;15:154 –166.
23. Kleinebrecht J, Michaelis H, Michaelis J, Koller S. Fever in pregnancy and congenital anomalies (letter). *Lancet.* 1979;1:1403.
24. Little BB, Ghali FE, Snell LM, Knoll KA, Johnston W, Gilstrap LC III. Is hyperthermia teratogenic in the human? *Am J Perinatol.* 1991;8:185–189.
25. Milunsky A, Ulcickas M, Rothman KJ, Willett W, Jick SS, Jick H. Maternal heat exposure and neural tube defects. *JAMA.* 1992;268:882– 885.
26. Chambers CD, Johnson KA, Dick LM, Felix RJ, Jones KL. Maternal fever and birth outcome: a prospective study. *Teratology.* 1998;58: 251–257.
27. Glass GV. Primary, secondary, and meta-analysis of research. *Educ Res.* 1976;5:3– 8.
28. Glass GV. Integrating findings: the meta-analysis of research. *Rev Res Educ.* 1978;5:351–79.
29. Seto A, Einarson T, Koren G. Pregnancy outcome following first trimester exposure to antihistamines: meta-analysis. *Am J Perinatol.* 1997;14:119 –124.
30. Shepard. TH. *Catalog of Teratogenic Agents.* 10th ed. Baltimore: Johns Hopkins University Press; 2001.

CHAPTER 34

RISK OF VARICELLA INFECTION DURING LATE PREGNANCY

Gideon Koren

Abstract

Question. I have a patient who contracted varicella at 26 weeks' gestation. She is very concerned and would consider termination if it were earlier in the pregnancy. What are the current predictions of risk for her fetus?
Answer. Based on review of all available studies, we could not detect a single case of congenital varicella syndrome in the third trimester of pregnancy (0/208), as compared with 5/645 (0.78%) in the first and 9/592 (1.52%) in the second trimester ($P < .01$ third vs first and second). You can reassure your patient.

Résumé

Question. L'une de mes patientes a contracté la varicelle à sa 26ᵉ semaine de gestation. Elle s'inquiète beaucoup et envisagerait un avortement si la grossesse n'était pas si avancée. Quelles sont les prédictions actuelles de risque pour son fœtus?
Réponse. En nous fondant sur toutes les études à notre disposition, nous n'avons pas pu cerner un seul cas du syndrome de la varicelle congénitale durant le troisième trimestre de la grossesse (0/208), par rapport à 5/645 (0,78%) durant le premier trimestre et 9/592 (1,52%) durant le deuxième trimestre (P< ,01 au troisième par rapport au premier et au deuxième). Vous pouvez rassurer votre patiente.

The varicella virus is teratogenic in humans. It results in serious and debilitating symptoms that include limb-shortening defects and eye and brain malformations.[1] Usually, seronegative women contract the virus from young children at home or at work (eg, teachers and caretakers). Typical of many rare syndromes, the morphologic pathology of congenital varicella syndrome (CVS) has been described in case reports.[1] Only during the last decade have several large epidemiologic studies directly investigated the incidence of CVS among exposed fetuses.

We systematically reviewed all cohort studies to quantify the incidence of CVS in order to counsel pregnant women exposed to varicella. We searched MEDLINE, EMBASE, and textbooks on infection during pregnancy and lactation. Methods sections of identified papers were reviewed to select all cohort studies that described an overall number of pregnant women contracting varicella and the number of children exhibiting CVS. Varicella infection could be confirmed by clinical appearance or serologic changes or both. Alkalay et al[1] have described criteria for CVS.

> Do you have questions about the safety of drugs, chemicals, radiation, or infections in women who are pregnant or breastfeeding? We invite you to submit them to the Motherisk Program by fax at (416) 813–7562; they will be addressed in future Motherisk Updates.Published Motherisk Updates are available on the College of Family Physicians of Canada website **(www.cfpc.ca)**. Some articles are published in *The Motherisk Newsletter* and on the Motherisk website **(www.motherisk.org)** also.

Motherisk questions are prepared by the **Motherisk Team** *at the Hospital for Sick Children in Toronto, Ont.* **Dr Koren,** *a Senior Scientist at the Canadian Institutes for Health Research and Director of the Motherisk Program, is supported by the Research Leadership for Better Pharmacotherapy during Pregnancy and Lactation and, in part, by a grant from the Canadian Institutes for Health Research.*

Excluded from the analysis were case reports, case series, editorials, and reviews, as were cohort studies describing women contracting herpes zoster (shingles) rather than varicella. Overall rate of CVS was calculated by pooling data in all studies. No attempt was made to weight the data. Rates of CVS were compared by trimester of exposure using Fisher's exact test, as were rates among those receiving varicella zoster immune globulin (VZIG) versus others.

Between 1958 and 2002, 10 cohort studies[2-11] calculated the overall incidence of CVS among 2002 motherchild pairs (Table 1[2-11]). Seven studies also calculated incidence for each trimester of pregnancy. Overall rate of CVS was 14/2021 (0.7%) (95% confidence interval [CI] 0 to 5). The rate was 5/645 (0.78%) for first-trimester exposure, 9/592 (1.52%) for second-trimester exposure, and 0/208 (0%) for third-trimester exposure. The third-trimester rate was lower than the first- and second-trimester rates ($P < .01$). The trend toward higher rates in the second trimester than the first trimester (odds ratio 1.9) was not statistically significant ($P = .19$). Enders et al[8] described 92 women who received VZIG to prevent CVS; none of their babies contracted CVS, but nine among the 731 who did not receive VZIG did.

Based on 2021 available cases in 10 studies, incidence of CVS has been calculated at 0.7% with a trend toward more cases during the second trimester. It appears that CVS does not afflict fetuses during the third trimester. At present, seronegative women who have been in contact with someone with varicella are advised to take VZIG, which can be given by either intramuscular or intravenous injection.[12]

While the biologic plausibility of this treatment comes from favorable results in ameliorating or preventing clinical varicella in immunocompromised or otherwise healthy patients, no controlled studies show that VZIG prevents CVS. Our analysis reveals that the rate of CVS among 92 VZIG-treated mothers tended to be lower than among untreated mothers.[8] Because of the rarity of varicella infection in pregnancy in general and of CVS in particular, it is unlikely that a randomized controlled prospective study will have

Table 1
Incidence of Congenital Varicella Syndrome in Cohort Studies

STUDY	FIRST TRIMESTER	SECOND TRIMESTER	THIRD TRIMESTER	OVERALL (%)
Siegal,[4] 1973	1/27	0/32	0/76	1/135 (0.74)
Paryani and Arvin,[5] 1986	1/11	0/11	0/19	1/41 (2.43)
Balducci et al,[6] 1992	0/35			0/35 (0)
Pasturszak et al,[7] 1994	1/86	0/30		1/116 (0.86)
Enders et al,[8] 1994	1/236	7/351		9/823 (1.09)
Jones et al,[9] 1994	1/110	1/46	0/13	2/169 (1.18)
Harger et al,[11] 2002	0/140	1/122	0/100	1/362 (0.28)
Hill,[2] 1958				0/30 (0)
Manson,[3] 1962				0/288 (0)
Figueroa-Damian and Arredondo-Garcia,[10] 1997				0/22 (0)
Mean (%)	5/645 (0.78)	9/592 (1.52)	0/208 (0)	14/2021 (0.7)*

* Not all studies classified data by trimester. Hence the sum of cases of first plus second plus third trimester is lower than the "overall" number.

sufficient power to show a favourable effect of VZIG. Moreover, with VZIG being labeled for varicella infection in pregnancy, it is unlikely that ethics review boards will approve such a study.

With the recent introduction of a varicella vaccine,[13] it is likely that rates of seronegativity among women of reproductive age will gradually decrease, and hence incidence of CVS will likely decrease. While the overall rate of CVS among seronegative women exposed to the virus appears to be low, a 0.7% rate of CVS implies a substantially increased risk of major malformations above the 1% to 3% risk in the general population. For comparison, the rate of positive Down syndrome among women aged 35 is 1/350 (0.3%).

REFERENCES

1. Alkalay AL, Pomerance JJ, Rimoin DL. Fetal varicella syndrome. *J Pediatr* 1987;111:320-3.
2. Hill AB. Virus diseases in pregnancy and congenital defects. *Br J Prev Soc Med* 1958;12:1-7.
3. Manson J. *Rubella and other virus infections during pregnancy. Reports on public health and medical subjects No. 101.* Toronto, Ont: Ministry of Health; 1962.
4. Siegal M. Congenital malformations following chickenpox, measles, mumps and hepatitis. *JAMA* 1973;226:1521-4.
5. Paryani SG, Arvin AM. Intrauterine infection with varicella zoster virus after maternal varicella. *N Engl J Med* 1986;314(24):1542-6.
6. Balducci J, Rodis JF, Rosengren S, Vintzilosa M, Spiney G, Vosseller C. Pregnancy outcome following first trimester varicella infection. *Obstet Gynecol* 1992;79:5-6.
7. Pasturszak A, Levy M, Schick B, Zuber C, Feldman M, Gladstone J, et al. Outcome after maternal varicella infection in the first 20 weeks of pregnancy. *N Engl J Med* 1994;330:901-5.
8. Enders G, Miller E, Craddock Watson J, Bolley I, Ridenhelg M. Consequences of varicella and herpes zoster in pregnancy. *Lancet* 1994;343:1548-51.
9. Jones KL, Johnson KA, Chambers CD. Offspring of women infected with varicella during pregnancy: a prospective study. *Teratology* 1994;49:29-32.
10. Figueroa-Damian R, Arredondo-Garcia JL. Patient outcome of pregnancy complicated with varicella infection during the first twenty weeks of gestation. *Am J Perinatol* 1997;14:401-4.
11. Harger JH, Ernest JM, Thurman GR, Moawad A, Thom E, Landon MB, et al. Frequency of congenital varicella syndrome in a prospective cohort of 347 pregnant women. *Obstet Gynecol* 2002;100:260-5.
12. Koren G, Money D, Boucher M, Aoki F, Petric M, Innocencion G, et al. Serum concentrations, efficacy, and safety of a new, intravenously administered varicella zoster immune globulin in pregnant women. *J Clin Pharmacol* 2002;42:267-74.
13. Gershon AA. Varicella vaccine: rare serious problems—but the benefits still outweigh the risks. *J Infect Dis* 2003;188:945-7.

Reprinted from Koren G. Risk of varicella infection during late pregnancy. Can Fam Physician 2003;49:1445-6 with permission.

SECTION 3

ALCOHOL, CAFFEINE, COCAINE AND ENVIRONMENTAL EXPOSURE

CHAPTER 35

ASSOCIATION BETWEEN MODERATE ALCOHOL CONSUMPTION DURING PREGNANCY AND SPONTANEOUS ABORTION, STILLBIRTH AND PREMATURE BIRTH: A META-ANALYSIS

Niloufar Makarechian,[1] Karen Agro,[1] John Devlin,[1] Eric Trepanier,[1] Gideon Koren,[2,3] and Thomas R. Einarson[1,2]

[1]Faculty of Pharmacy, University of Toronto; [2]Motherisk Program, The Hospital for Sick Children; [3]Division of Clinical Pharmacology and Toxicology, The Hospital for Sick Children, and Department of Pharmacology, University of Toronto, Toronto, Ontario

---

N Makarechian, K Agro, J Devlin, E Trepanier, G Koren, TR Einarson. Association between moderate alcohol consumption during pregnancy and spontaneous abortion, stillbirth and premature birth: A meta-analysis. Can J Clin Pharmacol 1998;5(3):169–176.

Objective. To examine the effect of moderate alcohol consumption during pregnancy on the risk of spontaneous abortion, stillbirth and premature birth.
Data Sources. A structured MEDLINE search from 1966 to December 1993 using the key words 'alcoholic beverage' or 'alcohol drinking', 'pregnancy outcome' or 'pregnancy complication' and 'analytic studies (epidemiologic)'; a structured search of PsycLit from 1974 to 1994 using the keywords 'alcohol abuse', 'alcohol drinking attitudes', 'alcohol drinking patterns', 'alcohol intoxication', 'alcoholic beverage' or 'alcoholism' and 'pregnancy', 'prenatal', 'neonatal development' or 'neonatal development'; and a bibliographic search of selected review articles.
Study Selection. Case-control or cohort studies of pregnant human subjects that included a moderate alcohol consumption group defined as consumption of more than two alcoholic drinks per week up to and including two drinks per day and an abstained group defined as consumption of two or fewer alcoholic drinks per week (alcoholic drink defined as 15 mL or 10 g of absolute alcohol), and that examined the outcome of spontaneous abortion, stillbirth or premature birth.
Data Extraction. Two independent reviewers assessed the methodological quality of each study and abstracted data. The heterogeneity of individual study odds ratios was assessed, and data were pooled using a random effects model.
Results. Eight studies were included in the analysis. The trials had a mean methodological quality score of 0.74 (range 0.67 to 0.83, maximum 1.0). Heterogeneity existed among the individual odds ratios for spontaneous abortion (P=0.007). Significant heterogeneity did not exist for the other outcomes. For the pooled outcomes, the odds ratio for spontaneous abortion was 1.35 (95% CI 1.09 to 1.67), the odds ratio for stillbirth was 0.65 (CI 0.46 to 0.91) and the odds ratio for premature birth was 0.95 (CI 0.79 to 1.15).
Conclusions. Moderate maternal alcohol consumption is associated with an increased risk of spontaneous abortion and a decreased risk of stillbirth, and has no effect on premature birth.

Key Words: *Alcohol, Neonatal development, Premature birth, Spontaneous abortion, Stillbirth*

Association entre une consommation modérée d'alcool pendant la grossesse et l'avortement spontané, la mortinatalité et la naissance prématurée: une méta-analyse
Objectif. Examiner l'effet d'une consommation modérée d'alcool pendant la grossesse sur le risque d'avortement spontané, de mortinatalité et de naissance prématurée.
Sources Des Données. Une recherche structurée sur *MEDLINE* de 1966 à décembre 1993 faisant appel aux mots-clés «alcoholic beverage (boisson alcoolisée)» ou «alcohol drinking (consommation d'alcool)», «pregnancy outcome (effets sur la grossesse)» ou «pregnancy complication (complications de la grossesse)» et «analytic studies (études analytiques/épidémiologiques)»; une recherche structurée de *PsycLit* de 1974 à 1994 faisant appel aux mots-clés «alcohol abuse (abus d'alcool)», «alcohol drinking attitudes (comportements relatifs à la consommation d'alcool)», «alcohol drinking patterns (schémas de consommation d'alcool)», «alcohol intoxication (intoxication alcoolique)», «alcoholic beverage (boissons alcoolisées)» ou «alcoholism (alcoolisme)» et «pregnancy (grossesse)», «prenatal (prénatal)» ou «neonatal development (développement néonatal)»; et une recherche bibliographique d'articles de synthèse choisis.
Sélection Des Articles. Les études cas/témoins ou les études de cohortes de femmes enceintes qui incluaient un groupe consommant modérément de l'alcool défini comme une consommation de plus de deux boissons alcoolisées par semaine jusqu' à deux boissons alcoolisées par jour et un groupe abstinent défini comme une consommation de deux ou moins de deux boissons alcoolisées par semaine, et qui examinaient les résultats concernant les avortements spontanés, la mortinatalité et les naissances prématurées.
Extraction Des Données. Deux réviseurs indépendants ont évalués la qualité méthodologique de chaque étude et des données extraites. L'hétérogénéité des risques relatifs des études individuelles a été évaluée, et les données ont été regroupées selon un modèle d'effets aléatoires.

Résultats. Huit études ont été incluses dans l'analyse. Les essais démontraient un score moyen de qualité méthodologique de 0,74 (fourchette de 0,67 à 0,83, maximum de 1,0). Une hétérogénéité existait parmi les risques relatifs individuels concernant l'avortement spontané (P=0,007). Une hétérogénéité significative n'existait pas pour les autres résultats. Pour les résultats regroupés, les risques relatifs pour l'avortement spontané était de 1,35 (IC 95%, 1,09-1,67), pour la mortinatalité de 0,65 (IC 0,46-0,91) et pour la naissance prématurée de 0,95 (IC 0,79-1,15).

Conclusions. Une consommation modérée d'alcool est associée à un risque accru d'avortement spontané et à une diminution du risqué de mortinatalité, et n'a aucun effet en ce qui concerne le risque de naissance prématurée.

Since the discovery of the teratogenicity of ethanol, there has been extensive discussion in both the medical literature and the popular press regarding the effects of maternal drinking on the fetus. At the Hospital for Sick Children's Motherisk Program in Toronto, Ontario, approximately 10% of the 140 telephone calls received daily pertain to the use of alcohol in pregnancy (data on file at Motherisk). Many callers are concerned about the moderate levels of alcohol that they consumed before knowing that they were pregnant. Callers frequently associate ethanol ingestion in any amount with an increased risk of an adverse pregnancy outcome. Although the fetal alcohol syndrome typifies the effects of alcohol on the offspring of mothers who drink excessive amounts of alcohol during pregnancy (1), including intrauterine growth retardation, stillbirth and prematurity, the effect of moderate alcohol consumption on various pregnancy outcomes remains unclear.

Despite the large number of observational studies investigating the effects of moderate alcohol consumption during pregnancy on various maternal and neonatal outcomes, the results of these studies have been inconsistent. A meta-analysis of controlled studies published in the medical literature was conducted to quantify the effect of moderate maternal alcohol consumption on pregnancy outcomes.

The purpose of this meta-analysis was to determine the effect of moderate alcohol consumption during pregnancy on the risk of spontaneous abortion, stillbirth and premature birth.

MATERIALS AND METHODS

A computerized search was conducted to identify studies examining the relationship between moderate alcohol consumption during pregnancy, and fetal and maternal outcomes. The medical literature published between January 1966 and December 1993 was searched using the bibliographic database of the National Library of Medicine (MEDLINE) with the keywords 'alcoholic beverage' or 'alcohol drinking', 'pregnancy outcome' or 'pregnancy complication', and 'analytic studies (epidemiologic)'. The psychology literature was searched using the Silver Platter bibliographic database PsycLit I (1974 to 1986) and PsycLit II (1987 to 1994) with the keywords 'alcohol abuse', 'alcohol drinking attitudes', 'alcohol drinking patterns', 'alcohol intoxication', 'alcoholic beverage' or 'alcoholism', and 'pregnancy', 'prenatal', 'neonatal development' or 'neonatal disorders'. Both searches were limited to human subjects. Selected review articles (2–8) and a widely used teratology textbook (9) were also examined to ensure that all relevant articles were included in the analysis.

Inclusion criteria for studies in the analysis were inclusion of pregnant human females; inclusion of subjects who consumed moderate amounts of alcohol, defined as more than two alcoholic drinks per week up to and including two drinks per day (alcoholic drink defined as 15 mL or 10 g of absolute alcohol); case-control or cohort studies; and inclusion of an abstainer or low consumption group ('low consumption' defined as consumption of up to and including two alcoholic drinks per week). Studies in which moderate alcohol levels could not be separated from other alcohol amounts; case reports, editorials and reviews; and studies that did not provide sufficient data for analysis were excluded from the analysis.

The Methods section of each study was examined independently by at least two authors of the present paper using the inclusion and exclusion criteria. To avoid bias, the reviewers were blinded to the names of the journal and authors, and to the results, by removing all identifying statements. If the two reviewers did not agree, a third author served as adjudicator. In the event that the Methods section did not provide sufficient information by which to make a decision, the complete article was reviewed for the absent information, and reasons for exclusion were identified.

The following definitions were used in the meta-analysis. Spontaneous abortion was defined as expulsion of an embryo or fetus from the uterus before the stage of viability (10) (approximately 20 weeks' gestation); stillbirth was defined as the birth of an infant who shows no evidence of life after birth (10); and premature birth was defined as delivery at less than 37 weeks' gestation.

The quality of the individual studies included in the meta-analysis was assessed. Quality assessment scales for cohort and case-control studies included in the analysis were adapted from Hartzema (11) (Appendix 1). Inter-rater agreement among the four authors in this analysis was calculated. Inter-rater reliability for the quality scores of all items was determined by calculating the effective reliability (12). Spearman's pairwise ρ was calculated for the four raters for a random sample of 10 articles meeting the inclusion criteria. The mean ρ was calculated and corrected for attenuation by using the Spearman-Brown prophecy formula (12). An effective reliability value of 0.8 or higher was considered evidence of acceptable agreement among the raters. After inter-rater agreement was established, the remaining studies included in the analysis were divided among the authors and independently assessed.

Data from each study were extracted independently by at least two authors. Differences in data extraction were mediated by a third author and resolved by consensus. Data from each study were entered into a 2×2 table.

The Q statistic for homogeneity of effect was calculated to determine the appropriateness of combining the studies. Relative risk and odds ratios (ORs) were calculated for cohort and case-control studies, respectively. The significance of individual studies was determined by calculating the 95% CI. The risk ratios for stillbirth, spontaneous abortion and premature delivery associated with moderate maternal alcohol consumption were estimated by calculating a summary OR for each outcome according to the method of Mantel and Haenszel (13). The 95% CI for the summary OR was calculated according to the method proposed by Miettinen (14). Sensitivity analyses determined whether combining case-control and cohort studies affected the results. $P \leq 0.05$ was deemed significant for all statistical tests.

Correspondence: Dr TR Einarson, Faculty of Pharmacy, University of Toronto, 19 Russel Street, Toronto, Ontario M5S 2S2. Telephone 416–978–6212, fax 416–978–8511, e-mail 76766.72@compuserve.com
Accepted for publication December 3, 1997

RESULTS

The literature search produced approximately 500 articles published between 1966 and 1993, of which 210 appeared relevant upon initial inspection. Fifty-seven articles met the objectives (15-71); however, only eight studies met all of the inclusion criteria and were included in the meta-analysis (Table 1). Forty-nine studies were excluded for the reasons outlines in Table 2.

Quality Assessment

The effective reliability of quality assessment between the raters was 0.90. There was no correlation between the quality scores and the odd ratios for any of the three outcomes examined. The quality assessment scores for the eight studies included in the meta-analysis are presented in Table 3.

Spontaneous Abortion

Three studies included in the meta-analysis examined the relationship between moderate alcohol consumption and the incidence of spontaneous abortion (Table 4) – two case-control studies (15,18) and one cohort study (29). Overall, the summary OR was 1.35 (95% CI 1.09 to 1.67). χ^2 for the test for homogeneity of effect was 9.84 (degrees of freedom [df]=2, P=0.007), indicating that heterogeneity existed among the studies. One study had an OR inconsistent with that of the other two and was identified as the outlier (29). Removal of the outlier resulted in a χ^2 value of 1.36 (df=1, P=0.244), suggesting that the two remaining studies were not heterogeneous. Removal of the outlier did not substantially alter the summary OR (OR=1.51, 95% CI 1.20 to 1.89).

Stillbirth

Three studies examining the relationship between moderate alcohol consumption and stillbirth were included in the analysis (Table 5) – two cohort studies (29,52) and one case-control study (43). The value for the homogeneity of effect suggested that, overall, the

Table 1
Studies Included in the Meta-Analysis

AUTHOR, YEAR (REFERENCE)	STUDY TYPE	OUTCOME EVALUATED
Kline et al, 1980 (15)	Case-control	Spontaneous abortion
Windham et al, 1992 (18)	Case-control	Spontaneous abortion
Walpole et al, 1989 (29)	Cohort	Spontaneous abortion, stillbirth
Little and Weinberg, 1993 (43)	Case-control	Stillbirth
EUROMAC, 1992 (47)	Cohort	Premature birth
Verkerk et al, 1993 (48)	Cohort	Premature birth
Marbury et al, 1983 (52)	Cohort	Stillbirth, premature birth
Berkowitz et al, 1982 (67)	Case-control	Premature birth

Table 2
Studies Rejected from the Meta-Analysis

REASON FOR REJECTION	STUDY, YEAR (REFERENCE)
Alcohol drinking groups not delineated according to definition used in meta-analysis	Smith et al, 1986 21)
	Shiono et al, 1986 (17)
	Coles et al, 1991 (27)
	Brown et al, 1991 (28)
	Graham et al, 1988 (31)
	Coles et al, 1987 (56)
	Russell et al, 1988 (70)
	Harlap et al, 1980 (71)
	Haste et al, 1991 (69)
Insufficient numbers of subjects to evaluate specified outcome	Mehl et al, 1993 (20)
	Ioffe et al, 1987 (60)
	Barr et al, 1990 (68)
	Landesman-Dwyer et al, 1981 (26)
	Streissguth et al, 1986 (32)
	Parazzini et al, 1990 (40)
	Streissguth et al, 1984 (44)
	Raymond and Mills, 1993 (19)
Alcohol intake not correlated directly with outcomes	Day et al, 1991 (25)
	Hingson et al, 1982 (38)
	Gibson et al, 1983 (49)
	Tennes et al, 1980 (54)
	Peacock et al, 1991 (63)
Unable to extract data as presented	Mills et al, 1987 (39)
	Little et al, 1977 (51)
	Olsen et al, 1983 (66)
	Walpole et al, 1990 (64)
	Westney et al, 1991 (24)
	Lumley et al, 1985 (46)
Outcomes addressed in meta-analysis not examined	Ioffe et al, 1990 (23)
	Walpole et al, 1991 (30)
	Jacobson et al, 1993 (33)
	Staisey and Fried, 1983 (34)
	Day et al, 1990 (35)
	O'Connor et al, 1987 (36)
	Borges et al, 1993 (37)
	Landesman-Dwyer et al, 1978 (41)
	Streissguth et al, 1980 (59)
	Hanson et al, 1978 (45)
	Richardson et al, 1989 (55)
	Martin et al, 1977 (58)
	Sulaiman et al, 1988 (61)
	Forrest et al, 1991 (62)
	Kline et al, 1987 (65)
	Russell et al, 1991 (16)
	Rossett et al, 1983 (22)
	Brooke et al, 1989 (53)
	Forest et al, 1991 (62)
	Streissguth et al, 1983 (42)
	Silva et al, 1981 (50)
	Greene et al, 1990 (57)

Table 3
Quality Assessment Scores for Articles Included in the Meta-Analysis

AUTHOR, YEAR (REFERENCE)	QUALITY SCORE (%)
Kline et al, 1980 (15)	74*
Windham et al, 1992 (18)	71
Walpole et al, 1989 (29)	72
Little et al, 1993 (43)	78
EUROMAC, 1992 (47)	78
Verkerk et al, 1993 (48)	67
Marbury et al, 1983 (52)	72
Berkowitz et al, 1982 (67)	83

* Mean score from the four judges

studies were not heterogeneous (χ^2=2.22, df=2, P=0.330). The summary OR was 0.65 (95% CI 0.46 to 0.91). The cohort and case-control studies underwent sensitivity analysis separately. The case-control study had an OR of 0.57 (95% CI 0.38 to 0.85). Removal of this study from the analysis resulted in a summary OR of 0.99 (95% CI 0.48 to 2.02), indicating that the results were unstable to the sensitivity analysis.

Premature Birth

Four studies that examined the relationship between moderate alcohol consumption and premature birth were included in the analysis (Table 6) – three cohort studies (47,48,52) and one case-control study (67). When the studies were combined, the χ^2 value for homogeneity of effect was 7.32 (df = 3, P = 0.062), suggesting that, overall, the studies were not significantly heterogeneous. The summary OR for all the studies was 0.95 (95% CI 0.79 to 1.15). When the case-control study was not included in the sensitivity analysis, the summary OR and 95% CI were not altered substantially (OR=0.96, 95% CI 0.79 to 1.17).

DISCUSSION

The present meta-analysis estimated the effect of moderate maternal alcohol consumption on three pregnancy outcomes: spontaneous abortion, stillbirth and premature birth. Moderate alcohol consumption was defined as consumption of more than two drinks per week up to and including two drinks per day. An alcoholic drink was defined as 15 mL or 10 g of absolute alcohol.

An accurate measure of alcohol consumption is critical in determining the relationship between maternal alcohol consumption and reproductive outcomes. Accurately measuring alcohol consumption is difficult because most studies employ self-reporting by women. It is thus difficult to ascertain whether the women's reported average intake is truly indicative of their consumption. During pregnancy, even moderate drinkers may under-report their alcohol consumption (72). This may be attributed to the stigma associated with drinking alcohol during pregnancy. In addition, retrospective reporting of alcohol consumption introduces a potential recall bias into studies because women experiencing an adverse reproductive outcome may be more likely to recall the amount of alcohol that they ingested.

Another major problem that is encountered when determining the amount of alcohol consumed is that most data are reported as average daily intake. This method 'homogenizes patterns of use' because it does not allow for the separation of the effects of different patterns of alcohol use (73). For example, a study may report alcohol consumption as one drink per day, when in fact the mother had consumed seven drinks in one day and had abstained from drinking during the remainder of the week.

A final problem encountered in assessing alcohol consumption is the lack of consistency in the definition of moderate alcohol consumption in various studies. This variability made data extraction difficult and resulted in the exclusion of numerous studies from the analysis.

Confounding variables can have a substantial impact on study results. Variables such as smoking, marijuana and caffeine use, maternal age, education, socioeconomic and employment status, maternal weight and parity all have potential reproductive consequences. Although many of the studies relied on statistical methods to control for these effects, the studies in our meta-analysis did not adjust for the same confounders.

Table 4
Number of Spontaneous Abortions in Moderate Alcohol and Control Groups

		SPONTANEOUS ABORTION					
REFERENCE	GROUP	YES	NO	TOTAL	ODDS RATIO	95% CI	STUDY TYPE
15	Moderate alcohol	151	107	258	1.65	1.25 to 2.18	Case-control
	Control	441	516	957			
	Total	592	623	1215			
18	Moderate alcohol	40	73	113	1.23	0.82 to 1.85	Case-control
	Control	386	869	1255			
	Total	426	942	1368			
29	Moderate alcohol	10	255	265	0.46	0.22 to 0.99	Cohort
	Control	24	284	308			
	Total	34	539	573			
	Combined	1052	2104	3156	1.35	1.09 to 1.67	
	All case-control	1018	1565	2583	1.51	1.20 to 1.89	

Table 5
Number of Stillbirths in Moderate Alcohol and Control Groups

		STILL BIRTH					
REFERENCE	GROUP	YES	NO	TOTAL	ODDS RATIO	95% CI	STUDY TYPE
29	Moderate alcohol	6	259	265	1.40	0.042 to 4.65	Cohort
	Control	5	303	308			
	Total	11	562	573			
43	Moderate alcohol	31	123	154	0.57	0.38 to 0.85	Case-control
	Control	1070	2426	3496			
	Total	1101	2549	3650			
52	Moderate alcohol	5	1014	1019	0.82	0.33 to 2.03	Cohort
	Control	68	11,261	11,329			
	Total	73	12,275	12,348			
	Combined	1185	15,386	16,571	0.65	0.46 to 0.91	
	All case-control	84	12,837	12,921	0.99	0.48 to 2.02	

Further limitations of our study relate to the outcomes assessed in this meta-analysis. Spontaneous abortion reports may not be accurate. Women may report a spontaneous abortion when in fact a therapeutic abortion has occurred. Alternatively, a spontaneous abortion may occur without the mother's knowledge if it occurred sufficiently early in the pregnancy. The overall OR for stillbirth initially suggested a negative association with maternal alcohol consumption. This result did not hold true after sensitivity analysis.

The relatively small number of studies addressing the end-point of stillbirth further limits our ability to come to a definite conclusion. Furthermore, the studies were either case-control or cohort, which may explain the instability of some of the results.

A number of issues need to be addressed. The instability of the stillbirth results rendered the results inconclusive and suggests that future studies examining this outcome are required. Our meta-analysis evaluated only three pregnancy outcomes. Various fetal outcomes must be assessed with respect to maternal alcohol consumption. These outcomes include congenital malformations; indicators of intrauterine growth such as birth weight, length and head circumference; and cognitive and neurobehavioural disorders.

These data have helped to solidify the advice that Motherisk gives to the 10% of women who call about the effects of moderate alcohol consumption and who typically drank socially before realizing that conception had occurred. Such callers are told that, based on all available data, and assuming that drinking has discontinued, they do not have an increased risk of spontaneous abortion, stillbirth or premature birth. Such advice may be of special importance to women who had such adverse effects in previous pregnancies.

Table 6
Number of Premature Births in Moderate Alcohol and Control Groups

		PREMATURE BIRTH					
REFERENCE	GROUP	YES	NO	TOTAL	ODDS RATIO	95% CI	STUDY TYPE
47	Moderate alcohol	62	1143	1205	1.34	0.99 to 1.81	Cohort
	Control	161	3976	4137			
	Total	223	5119	5342			
48	Moderate alcohol	7	162	169	0.86	0.37 to 2.03	Cohort
	Control	25	499	524			
	Total	32	661	693			
52	Moderate alcohol	61	958	1019	0.78	0.60 to 1.02	Cohort
	Control	857	10,472	11,329			
	Total	918	11,430	12,348			
67	Moderate alcohol	8	17	25	0.79	0.32 to 1.91	Case-control
	Control	77	129	206			
	Total	85	146	231			
	Combined	1258	17,356	18,614	0.95	0.79 to 1.15	
	All cohort	1173	17,210	18,383	0.96	0.79 to 1.17	

APPENDIX 1

Evaluation criteria for the quality of cohort studies

1. Is the sample (abstainer and alcohol-exposed groups) demographically homogeneous (ie, matching on variables after assignment to groups or by logistic regression or demonstrated in a table with demographic data)?
2. Was alcohol consumption equally ascertained throughout sample? (Look for recall bias and provide one point per confirmation method.)
3. Was the same screening method used to measure outcomes for the entire sample?
4. Were the outcomes uniformly classified throughout the sample? (Were definitions of outcomes provided?)
5. Dropout rates and characteristics of dropouts in both groups should be accounted for and comparable.
6. Is the cohort representative of the population using alcohol? (Score 0 if all of one demographic group, for example low socioeconomic status; score 1 if demographically representative of the population but a small sample size; score 2 if characteristics of a 1 score but sample is large.)
7. Cohorts should be followed from the beginning of pregnancy. (Score 2 if specifically defined as the first prenatal visit to a physician.)
8. Appropriateness of statistics (P value and CI). Dichotomous variable: Odds ratio with logistic regression is as suitable as matching. Continuous variable: *t* test (for two groups) or ANOVA (for more than two groups) with P value or CI.
9. Are objectives and conclusions related to alcohol exposure? (Did the investigators relate the conclusions to the objectives studied?)

APPENDIX 2

Evaluation criteria for the quality of case-control studies

1. Was there a defined selection method for cases and controls?
2. Was alcohol exposure ascertained in both groups? A score of 1 is the maximum possible for case-controls unless the investigators started with children possessing the same outcome and then questioned the mothers about alcohol use. If this was the case, all mothers should exhibit the same recall bias.
3. Data collection should be structured, eg, questionnaire (score 1) and the investigator blinded to the outcomes (score 1). A score of 2 is only possible if both criteria are met.
4. Time of alcohol exposure should be confirmed. (For malformation, drinking must have occurred in the first trimester.)
5. Unbiased exclusion criteria provided for cases and controls.
6. Same level of outcome screening for cases and controls. (Score 1 if the mother was interviewed or the chart was examined; score 2 if the mother was interviewed and the chart was examined.)
7. Are cases and controls homogeneous with respect to demographics? For example, matching on variables or by logistic regression or demonstrated in a table with demographic data.
8. Appropriateness of statistics (P value and CI). Dichotomous variable: Odds ratio with logistic regression is as suitable as matching. Continuous variable: *t* test (for two groups) or ANOVA (for more than two groups) with P value or CI.
9. Are objectives and conclusions related to alcohol exposure? Did the investigators relate the conclusions to the objectives studied?

REFERENCES

1. Verkerk PH. The impact of alcohol misclassification on the relationship between alcohol and pregnancy outcomes. Int J Epidemiol 1992;21:S33-7.
2. Forrest F, Florey CD. The relation between maternal alcohol consumption and child development: the epidemiological evidence. J Public Health Med 1991;13:247-55.
3. Brien JF, Smith GN. Effects of alcohol (ethanol) on the fetus. J Dev Physiol 1991;15:21-32.
4. Forrest F, Florey CD, Taylor D. Maternal alcohol consumption and child development. Int J Epidemiol 1992;21:S17-23.
5. Tittmar HG. What's the harm in just a drink? Alcohol Alcohol 1990;25:287-91.
6. Coles CD. Impact of prenatal alcohol exposure on the newborn and the child. Clin Obstet Gynecol 1993;36:255-266.
7. Robles N, Day NL. Recall of alcohol consumption during pregnancy. J Stud Alcohol 1990;51:403-7.
8. West JR, Goodlett CR, Brandt JP. New approaches to research on the long-term consequences of prenatal exposure to alcohol. Alcohol Clin Exp Res 1990;14:684-9.
9. Briggs GG, Reeman RK, Yaffe SJ. A Reference Guide to Fetal and Neonatal Risk: Drugs in Pregnancy and Lactation, 4th edn. Baltimore: Williams and Wilkins, 1994.
10. Stedman's Illustrated Medical Dictionary, 24th edn. Baltimore: Williams and Wilkins, 1982.
11. Hartzema AG. Guide to interpreting and evaluating the phramacoepidemiologic literature. Ann Pharmacother 1992;26:96-8.
12. Rosenthal R. Meta-analytic Procedures for Social Research. Beverly Hills: Sage Publications, 1984.
13. Mantel N, Haenszel W. Statistical aspects of the analysis of data from retrospective studies of disease. J Natl Cancer Inst 1959;22: 719-48.
14. Miettinen O. Estimability and estimation in case-referent studies. Am J Epidemiol 1976;103:226-35.
15. Kline J, Shrout P, Stein Z, Susser M, Warburton D. Drinking during pregnancy and spontaneous abortion. Lancet 1980;2:176-80.
16. Russell M, Czarnecki DM, Cowan R, McPherson E, Mudar PJ. Measures of maternal alcohol use as predictors of development in early childhood. Alcohol Clin Exp Res 1991;15:991-1000.
17. Shiono PH, Klebanoff MA, Rhoads GG. Smoking and drinking during pregnancy. Their effects on preterm birth. JAMA 1986;255:82-4.
18. Windham GC, Fenster L, Swan SH. Moderate maternal and paternal alcohol consumption and the risk of spontaneous abortion. Epidemiology 1992;3:364-70.
19. Raymond EG, Mills JL. Placental abruption. Maternal risk factors and associated fetal conditions. Acta Obstet Gynecol Scand 1993;72:633-9.
20. Mehl LE, Manchanda S. Use of chaos theory and complex systems modeling to study alcohol effects on fetal condition. Comput Biomed Res 1993;26:424-48.
21. Smith LE, Coles CD, Lancaster J, Fernhoff PM, Falek A. The effect of volume and duration of prenatal ethanol exposure on neonatal physical and behavioral development. Neurobehav Toxicol Teratol 1986;8:375-81.
22. Rosett HL, Weiner L, Lee A, Zuckerman B, Dooling E, Oppenheimer E. Patterns of alcohol consumption and fetal development. Obstet Gynecol 1983;61:539-46.

23. Ioffe S, Chernick V. Prediction of subsequent motor and mental retardation in newborn infants exposed to alcohol in utero by computerized EEG analysis. Neuropediatrics 1990;21:11-7.
24. Westney L, Bruney R, Ross B, Clark JF, Rajguru S, Ahluwalia B. Evidence that gonadal hormone levels in amniotic fluid are decreased in males born to alcohol users in humans. Alcohol Alcohol 1991;26:403-7.
25. Day NL, Robles N, Richardson G, et al. The effects of prenatal alcohol use on the growth of children at three years of age. Alcohol Clin Exp Res 1991;15:67-71.
26. Landesman-Dwyer S, Ragozin AS, Little RE. Behavioral correlates of prenatal alcohol exposure: a four-year follow-up study. Neurobehav Toxicol Teratol 1981;3:187-93.
27. Coles CD, Brown RT, Smith IE, Platzman KA, Erickson S, Falek A. Effects of prenatal alcohol exposure at school age: I. Physical and cognitive development. Neurotoxicol Teratol 1991;13:357-67.
28. Brown RT, Coles CD, Smith IE, et al. Effects of prenatal alcohol exposure at school age: II. Attention and behavior. Neurotoxicol Teratol 1991;13:369-76.
29. Walpole I, Zubrick S, Pontre J. Confounding variables in studying the effects of maternal alcohol consumption before and during pregnancy. J Epidemiol Community Health 1989;43:153-61.
30. Walpole I, Zubrick S, Pontre J, Lawrence C. Low to moderate maternal alcohol use before and during pregnancy, and neurobehavioral outcome in the newborn infant. Dev Med Child Neurol 1991;33:875-883.
31. Graham JM Jr, Hanson JW, Darby BL, Barr HM, Streissguth AP. Independent dysmorphology evaluations at birth and 4 years of age for children exposed to varying amounts of alcohol in utero. Pediatrics 1988;81:772-8.
32. Streissguth AP, Barr HM, Sampson PD, Parrish-Johnson JC, Kirchner GL, Martin DC. Attention, distraction and reaction time at age 7 years and prenatal alcohol exposure. Neurobehav Toxicol Teratol 1986;8:717-25.
33. Jacobson JL, Jacobson SW, Sokol RJ, Martier SS, Ager JW, Kaplan-Estrin MG. Teratogenic effects of alcohol on infant development. Alcohol Clin Exp Res 1993;17:174-84.
34. Staisey NL, Fried PA. Relationships between moderate maternal alcohol consumption during pregnancy and infant neurological development. J Stud Alcohol 1983;44:262-70.
35. Day NL, Richardson G, Robles N, et al. Effect of prenatal alcohol exposure on growth and morphology of offspring at 8 months of age. Pediatrics 1990;85:748-52.
36. O'Connor MJ, Sigman M, Brill N. Disorganization of attachment in relation to maternal alcohol consumption. J Consult Clin Psychol 1987;55:831-6.
37. Borges G, Lopez-Cervantes M, Medina-Mora ME, Tapia-Conyer R, Garrido F. Alcohol consumption, low birth weight and preterm delivery in the National Addiction Survey (Mexico). Int J Addict 1993;28:355-68.
38. Hingson R, Alpert JJ, Day N, et al. Effects of maternal drinking and marijuana use on fetal growth and development. Pediatrics 1982;70:539-46.
39. Mills JL, Graubard BI. Is moderate drinking during pregnancy associated with an increased risk for malformations? Pediatrics 1987;80:309-14.
40. Parazzini F, Bocciolone L, La Vecchia C, Negri E, Fedele L. Maternal and paternal moderate daily alcohol consumption and unexplained miscarriages. Br J Obstet Gynaecol 1990;97:618-22.
41. Landesman-Dwyer S, Keller LS, Streissguth AP. Naturalistic observations of newborns: Effects of maternal alcohol intake. Alcohol Clin Exp Res 1978;2:171-7.
42. Streissguth AP, Barr HM, Martin DC. Maternal alcohol: use and neonatal habituation assessed with the Brazelton scale. Child Dev 1983;54:1109-18.
43. Little RE, Weinberg CR. Risk factors for antepartum and intrapartum stillbirth. Am J Epidemiol 1993;137:1177-89.
44. Streissguth AP, Martin DC, Barr HM, et al. Intrauterine alcohol and nicotine exposure: Attention and reaction time in 4-year-old children. Dev Psychol 1984;20:533-41.
45. Hanson JW, Streissguth AP, Smith DW. The effects of moderate alcohol consumption during pregnancy on fetal growth and morphogenesis. J Pediatr 1978;92:457-60.
46. Lumley J, Correy JF, Newman NM, Curran JT. Cigarette smoking, alcohol consumption and fetal outcome in Tasmania 1981-82. Aust NZ J Obstet Gynaecol 1985;25:33-40.
47. EUROMAC. A European concerted action: maternal alcohol consumption and its relation to the outcome of pregnancy and child development at 18 months. Int J Epidemiol 1992; (Suppl 1):S1-87.
48. Verkerk PH, van Noord-Zaadstra BM, Florey CD, de Jonge GA, Verloove-Vanhorick SP. The effect of moderate maternal alcohol consumption on birth weight and gestational age in a low risk population. Early Hum Dev 1993;32:121-9.
49. Gibson GT, Baghurst PA, Colley DP. Maternal alcohol, tobacco and cannabis consumption and the outcome of pregnancy. Aust NZ J Obstet Gynaecol 1983;23:15-9.
50. Silva VA, Laranjeira RR, Dolnikoff M, Grinfeld H, Masur J. Alcohol consumption during pregnancy and newborn outcome: A study in Brazil. Neurobehav Toxicol Teratol 1981;3:169-72.
51. Little RE. Moderate alcohol use during pregnancy and decrease in infant birth weight. Am J Public Health 1977;67:1154-6.
52. Marbury MC, Linn S, Monson R, Schoenbaum S, Stubblefield PG, Ryan KJ. The association of alcohol consumption with outcome of pregnancy. Am J Public Health 1983;73:1165-8.
53. Brooke OG, Anderson HR, Bland JM, Peacock JL, Stewart CM. Effects on birth weight of smoking, alcohol, caffeine, socioeconomic factors, and psychosocial stress. BMJ 1989;298:795-801.
54. Tennes K, Blackard C. Maternal alcohol consumption, birth weight, and minor physical anomalies. Am J Obstet Gynecol 1980;138:774-80.
55. Richardson GA, Day NL, Taylor PM. The effect of prenatal alcohol, marijuana, and tobacco exposure on neonatal behavior. Infant Behav Dev 1989;12:199-209.
56. Coles CD, Smith IE, Falek A. Prenatal alcohol exposure and infant behavior: immediate effects and implications for later development. Adv Alcohol Subst Abuse 1987;6:87-104.
57. Greene T, Ernhart CB, Martier S, Sokol R, Ager J. Prenatal alcohol exposure and language development. Alcohol Clin Exp Res 1990;14:937-45.
58. Martin J, Martin DC, Lund CA, Streissguth AP. Maternal alcohol ingestion and cigarette smoking and their effects on newborn conditioning. Alcohol Clin Exp Res 1977;1:243-7.
59. Streissguth AP, Barr HM, Martin DC, Herman CS. Effects of maternal alcohol, nicotine, and caffeine use during pregnancy on infant mental and motor development. Alcohol Clin Exp Res 1980;4:152-64.
60. Ioffe S, Chernick V. Maternal alcohol ingestion and incidence of respiratory distress syndrome. Am J Obstet Gynecol 1987;156:1231-5.
61. Sulaiman ND, Florey CD, Taylor DJ, Ogston SA. Alcohol consumption in Dundee primigravidas and its effects on outcome of pregnancy. BMJ 1988;296:1500-3.
62. Forrest F, Florey CD, Taylor D, McPherson F, Young JA. Reported social consumption during pregnancy and infants' development at 18 months. BMJ 1991;303:22-6.
63. Peacock JL, Bland M, Anderson HR. Effects on birth weight of alcohol and caffeine consumption in smoking women. J Epidemiol Community Health 1991;45:159-63.
64. Walpole I, Zubrick S, Pontre J. Is there a fetal effect with low to moderate alcohol use before or during pregnancy. J Epidemiol Community Health 1990;44:297-301.
65. Kline J, Stein Z, Hutzler M. Cigarettes, alcohol, marijuana: varying associations with birthweight. Int J Epidemiol 1987;16:44-51.
66. Olsen J, Rachootin P, Schiodt AV. Alcohol use, conception time, and birth weight. J Epidemiol Community Health 1983;37:63-5.

67. Berkowitz GS, Holford TR, Berkowitz RL. Effects of cigarette smoking, alcohol, coffee, and tea consumption on pre-term delivery. Early Hum Dev 1982;7:239-50.
68. Barr HM, Darby BL, Streissguth AP, et al. Prenatal exposure to alcohol, caffeine tobacco and aspirin: effects on fine and gross motor performance. Dev Psychol 1990;26:339-49.
69. Haste FM, Anderson HR, Brooke OG, Bland JM, Peacock JL. The effects of smoking and drinking on the anthropometric measurements of neonates. Paediatr Perinat Epidemiol 1991;5:83-92.
70. Russell M, Skinner JB. Early measures of maternal alcohol misuse as predictors of adverse pregnancy outcomes. Alcohol Clin Exp Res 1988;12:824-30.
71. Harlap S, Shiono PH. Alcohol, smoking, and incidence of spontaneous abortion in the first and second trimester. Lancet 1980;2:173-77.
72. Larroque B. Alcohol and the fetus. Int J Epdemiol 1992;21(Suppl 1):S8-16.
73. Day NL. Comments on 'Abstaining for foetal health'. Br J Addict 1991;86:1057-61.

Reprinted from Makarechian N, Agro K, Devlin J, Trepanier E, Koren G, Einarson TR. Association between moderate alcohol consumption and spontaneous abortion, stillbirth and premature birth: a meta-analysis. Can J Clin Pharmacol. 1998;5:170-76 with permission.

CHAPTER 36

MODERATE ALCOHOL CONSUMPTION DURING PREGNANCY AND THE INCIDENCE OF FETAL MALFORMATIONS: A META-ANALYSIS

Dimitris Polygenis, Sean Wharton,* Christine Malmberg,* Nagwa Sherman,* Debbie Kennedy,† Gideon Koren,† and Thomas R. Einarson‡*

**Doctor of Pharmacy Program, Faculty of Pharmacy, The University of Toronto, Toronto, Ontario,Canada*

†The Motherisk Program, The Division of Clinical Pharmacology and Toxicology, Department of Pediatrics and The Research Institute, The Hospital for Sick Children Toronto and The Department of Pharmacology, The University of Toronto, Toronto, Ontario, Canada

‡Faculty of Pharmacy, The University of Toronto, Toronto, Ontario, Canada

Received 22 July 1996; Accepted 25 June 1997

POLYGENIS, D., S. WHARTON, C. MALMBERG, N. SHERMAN, D. KENNEDY, G. KOREN AND T. R. EINARSON. *Moderate alcohol consumption during pregnancy and the incidence of fetal malformations: A meta-analysis.* NEUROTOXICOL TERATOL 20(1) 61–67. 1998.—To determine whether there is an association between moderate alcohol consumption in the first trimester of pregnancy and increased risk of fetal malformations, we conducted a literature search using Medline (1966-present), PsycLit (1974–1995), and EMBASE (1988–1995). The following inclusion criteria were used to select the studies to be evaluated: 1) pregnant women; 2) moderate alcohol consumption (>2 drinks/week to 2 drinks/day); 3) case-control or cohort studies; 4) presence of an abstainer group (0 to 2 drinks/wk); 5) outcome measures include major or minor malformations; 6) papers published in the English language. The exclusion criteria were: 1) studies in which moderate alcohol consumption could not be confirmed; 2) case reports, and editorials. The Methods section of each study was examined independently by two blinded investigators with a third investigator settling any disagreement. The number of malformations in the abstainer and moderate alcohol consuming groups in two by two tables. Out of 24 studies which met the inclusion criteria, only seven had extractable data. The included studies evaluated 130,810 pregnancy outcomes, with 24,007 in the moderate alcohol group and 106,803 in the control group. An overall Mantel-Haenszel odds ratio showed that the relative risk for fetal malformations was 1.01 with 95% confidence limits of 0.94 to 1.08 and a chi-square for homogeneity of 8.26 ($p = 0.220$). Quality of the studies did not correlate with their showing negative or positive association. Moderate alcohol consumption during the first trimester of pregnancy is not associated with increased risk of fetal malformations.

Moderate alcohol Pregnancy Meta-analysis Fetal malformations

DESCRIPTIONS of deleterious effects of alcohol consumption on the fetus have appeared early in history, although the first scientific study documenting alcohol's harmful effects was not published until 1968 (70). Fetal Alcohol Syndrome (FAS), characterized by pre- and post-natal growth retardation, facial dysmorphology, and central nervous system (CNS) dysfunction, was recognized in 1973 as a consequence of chronic alcohol exposure during pregnancy (31). Since then, major and minor malformations, spontaneous abortion, and decreased birth weight have been among the many reported consequences of heavy alcohol use during pregnancy (1,70). In contradistinction to these reports, the effects of moderate alcohol consumption, defined as less than two drinks per day, on fetal malformations remains unclear.

The National Institute of Drug Abuse Survey has recently documented that moderate drinking during pregnancy is common in the western world (45). An American study (61) found that 25% of pregnant women had drunk an alcoholic beverage in the previous month.

Many studies have assessed moderate drinking in pregnancy, reporting conflicting results for the same neonatal outcomes. Our recent meta-analysis has investigated the relationship between moderate alcohol consumption during pregnancy and incidence of spontaneous abortions, stillbirths, and premature birth (14) showing a 35% increase in rates of spontaneous abortion with no effect on incidence of stillbirths and premature births. To date, there has not been a comprehensive analysis addressing the consequences of moderate alcohol consumption on fetal malformations. Consequently, clinicians have difficulty in counselling women on the risk of moderate alcohol consumption in pregnancy. Because half of the pregnancies in North America are unplanned, many women, often unknowingly, extend drinking into the first trimester of their pregnancy as is reflected by the 10% of daily inquiries to the MotherRisk Program concerning alcohol consumption in pregnancy (44).

The inconsistency in the medical literature concerning the effect of maternal alcohol exposure on the fetus is partially due to poorly defined study samples and outcome parameters, inadequate research design, difficulty in controlling for confounding factors, and inappropriate statistics (66,70). Specifically, problems arise in quantifying and defining moderate alcohol consumption and in the inaccurate use of terms such as malformation, anomaly, birth defect, dysmorphic, deformation, and dysplasia (74,77).

The technique of meta-analysis provides a method to assess and resolve conflict in the literature. This technique utilizes well-defined, objective criteria in selecting and evaluating data from a range of studies to increase statistical power (55). The objective of the present analysis is to determine whether there is an association between moderate alcohol consumption in the first trimester of pregnancy and fetal malformations.

METHOD

The relationship between moderate alcohol consumption during pregnancy and occurrence of malformations in the offspring was performed by comparing groups comprised of mothers consuming moderate alcohol amounts, to control groups consisting of abstainers.

Definitions

The abstainer group was comprised of subjects who consumed up to, and including two alcoholic drinks per week, whereas the moderate alcohol consumption group incorporated individuals with an alcohol intake of greater than two drinks per week, and up to and including two drinks per day. One alcoholic drink was defined as containing 15 ml, 0.5 oz. or 14 g of absolute alcohol. Offspring were considered to have a malformation if they had any of the conditions or defects as defined by Heinonen, Slone, and Shapiro (28), exhibiting structural and functional defects at or soon after birth, which have a major impact on the life of the child or those that have to be corrected surgically. An important feature of our analysis was that both study and control groups had to have a similar definition and inclusion of malformations. In some studies the malformations were obtained from the medical records [e.g., (41)] whereas in other cases offspring were independently assessed by study personnel [e.g., (48)]. A prerequisite for this analysis was that the exposed and unexposed group had to be analyzed in an identical way.

Search Strategy

A computerized literature search was conducted using several data bases including MEDLINE (1966–1995), Embase (1988–1995), PsycLit I (1974–1986), and PsycLit II (1987–mid-1995). Articles examining the relationship between moderate alcohol consumption during pregnancy and the occurrence of malformations were identified using the following keywords: "alcohol and pregnancy outcome," "alcohol drinking," and the text words "alcohol" and "pregnancy."

Study Selection

The following inclusion criteria were applied to the studies extracted by the literature search: 1) pregnant women; 2) moderate alcohol consumption as defined above; 3) case control or cohort studies; 4) presence of an abstainer group as previously defined; 5) data pertaining to malformations; 6) studies in the English language. The exclusion criteria were: 1) studies in which moderate alcohol consumption, as defined above, could not be separated from other alcohol consumption patterns; and 2) case reports, editorials, and reviews.

The Methods section of each study was examined independently by two investigators to select appropriate studies. The inclusion and exclusion criteria were applied to each article and the results of this assessment recorded on a score sheet (Appendix 1). To limit bias throughout this process, the investigators were blinded to the journal name, authors, and the results by removing all identifying statements and by reviewing only the Methods section. In the event that agreement could not be reached between the two investigators, a third investigator was consulted. If the Methods section failed to provide sufficient information by which to make a decision, the complete article was reviewed for missing information.

Data Extraction

Data extraction was performed on each study by two investigators using a standardized form for dichotomous variables. Each author reviewed all the studies that met the inclusion criteria and a consensus was reached. In the case of disagreement, the study would pass on to a third author for independent assessment; however, this was not necessary because a consensus was reached on all data extracted. All data extracted were entered into standardized 2×2 tables illustrating the number of malformations and nonmalformations in the alcohol- and nonalcohol-consuming groups.

Statistical Methods

Odds ratios and 95% confidence intervals for significance were calculated for both case control and cohort studies. An overall Mantel–Haenszel relative risk ratio was calculated with a 95% confidence interval as described by Miettinen (42). A chi-square for heterogeneity of outcome and for homogeneity of samples was also performed. A level of 0.05 (p) was considered significant. Sensitivity analyses based on differences in study design, results, and sample size were performed to evaluate any possible changes in the risk. As well, a power analysis was performed to identify the validity of the conclusions.

Quality Assessment

Quality assessment was performed on all studies accepted for analysis based on criteria adapted from Hartzema (27) (Appendix 2). Two investigators evaluated all the articles for quality and a consensus was reached in all instances.

RESULTS

Over 500 articles were published between 1966 and 1995 on the subject of alcohol and pregnancy outcome. Of these, 61 were identified as relevant for study (2–11,13,15–26,29,30,32–41,43,46–52, 54,56–60,62–65,67–69,71–73,75,76). This initial decision was made by looking at the title of the study and the abstract. Twenty-four studies met our inclusion criteria. Only 7 of the 24 studies were used in the analysis due to problems with data extraction. These problems consisted of inadequate reporting of raw data, inadequate delineation of alcohol consumption, lack of an abstainer group, and failure to define the trimester in which drinking took place.

A total of seven studies (8,39,41,43,48,56,63) were combined that examined the relationship between moderate alcohol consumption and fetal malformations (Table 1). Six (8,39,41,43,48,56) of the studies were cohort and one was a case control (63). The odds ratio (OR) for major malformations among the moderate alcohol users was of 1.01 and a 95% confidence interval (CI) of 0.94 to 1.08. The chi-squared (χ^2) for homogeneity yielded a value of 8.26 ($p = 0.220$) confirming that the studies, both case control and cohort, can be combined for analysis. The OR of 1.01 indicates that there is no increased risk of fetal malformations associated with maternal moderate alcohol consumption.

Table 1
Results of Studies Comparing Incidence of Fetal Malformations in Mothers with Mode Consumption

			CONGENTIAL DEFECT				
REF.	TYPE OF STUDY	EXPOSURE	YES	NO	TOTAL	OR	95% CI
McDonald et al. (41)	Case-control	Yes	166	7191	7357	1.05	0.69–1.23
		No	1701	77279	78980		
		Total	1867	84470	86337		
Davis et al. (8)	Cohort	Yes	4	474	478	9.09	0.49–1.69
		No	0	479	479		
		Total	4	953	957		
Silva et al. (63)	Cohort	Yes	5	63	68	2.3	0.43–12.32
		No	2	58	60		
		Total	7	121	128		
Rossett et al. (56)	Cohort	Yes	4	158	162	0.37	0.12–1.11
		No	17	247	264		
		Total	21	405	426		
Ouellete et al. (48)	Cohort	Yes	18	110	128	1.59	0.76–3.34
		No	14	136	150		
		Total	32	246	278		
Mills et al. (43)	Cohort	Yes	1187	14108	15295	0.99	0.91–1.08
		No	1336	15778	17114		
		Total	2523	29886	32409		
Lumley et al. (39)	Cohort	Yes	14	505	519	1.13	0.66–1.96
		No	233	9523	9756		
		Total	247	10028	10275		

OR = odds ratio, CI = confidence interval.

Sensitivity Analysis

The largest and most recent study (41) represented 66% of the total sample. This study had an OR of 1.05 (95% CI 0.89–1.23). A sensitivity analysis with or without this study was performed to identify the impact of its large sample size on the results. Excluding this study resulted in an OR of 1.00 (95% CI 0.92–1.08) for the remaining six studies. The χ^2 for homogeneity was 7.99 (p = 0.157). Removal of this study did not have an effect on the conclusions and the remaining studies were still homogenous.

Three of the seven studies (39,41,43) made up 99% of the total sample. When these studies were removed the resulting OR was 1.20 for the remaining four (95% CI 0.71–2.02). However, these remaining studies (8,48,56,63) only represented 1% of the total number of pregnancy outcomes. One study (8) in this group had an OR of 9.09 (95% CI 0.49–169.40). This study was further analyzed as the OR differed from all other studies. There were no malformations in the abstainer group or the heavy alcohol consumption group. However, the moderate group had four malformations. Although this study was not significant in terms of risk, further investigation found that birth weight was also included with the group of malformations, possibly skewing the results. Based on these results alone, it would appear that the higher incidence of malformations in this one group may be due to chance or the influence of birth weight. Another study (63) had found a trend toward increased risk of malformations in the alcohol-exposed group (OR 2.30; 95% CI 0.43–12.33). However, it examined women of low socioeconomic class and poor nutritional intake, potentially increasing the risk of malformation. Without this study and the previous one mentioned the overall OR (two studies) becomes 1.00 (95% CI 0.93–1.08) with a χ^2 of 4.97 (p = 0.174).

Cornfield's method for power yielded a Z-score of 26.0 (99.99%). This result ensures that there is no difference between the two study groups.

Quality Assessment

All of the studies used in the statistical analysis were evaluated in terms of quality to assess whether quality of the study affected its results being positive or negative. This analysis revealed no correlation between quality scores and the negativity (i.e., no association with fetal malformations) or positivity of the results.

DISCUSSION

Whereas heavy alcohol consumption by pregnant women has been shown to cause distinct and serious fetal pathology (12,39), the effects of moderate alcohol consumption still remain unclear. This meta-analysis has attempted to assess whether there is a measurable risk of fetal malformations due to moderate alcohol consumption during pregnancy. With more than 20,000 exposed babies we found no increased risk resulting from moderate alcohol consumption defined as less than two drinks per day during the first trimester. These results are not intended to justify drinking during pregnancy. However, because half of the pregnancies in North America are unplanned, millions of women each year consume moderate amounts of alcohol before realizing they have conceived. Our experience in the Motherisk Program indicates that these women experience high levels of anxiety due to misinformation and extrapolation from data on Fetal Alcohol Syndrome in heavy drinkers. A variety of organizations warn women against drinking in pregnancy and stress that any amount can be teratogenic. For example, the Manitoba Medical Association stated in a televised campaign that even one drink can harm the unborn baby. We have recently documented that such campaigns can change women's perceptions in a misleading way. The present meta-analysis is the first attempt to combine all available fetal safety data following mild to moderate drinking during embryogenesis. This meta-analysis had several limitations, primarily due to the variability in methodology and interpretation of studies on fetal abnormalities and maternal alcohol exposure. Most of these studies are limited by the self-reporting of alcohol use. This method is used to obtain data on alcohol consumption and often underestimates true intake. Problems with self-reporting include underreporting and recall bias (53,66). Underreporting may be a consequence of the stigma associated with drinking during pregnancy. On the other hand, recall bias is the inability to remember accurate time and amount of alcohol, primarily due to the delay between actual consumption and timing of the interview (53). Such difficulties in accurately quantifying alcohol intake is an inherent limitation of most studies. Our study may be limited due to the need to exclude 16 studies due to difficulty in data extraction; this can be explained by the lack of a standardized alcohol consumption scale and the inability to isolate treatment and control groups in accordance with our definition of moderate alcohol consumption. Further difficulties in collecting data from these studies arise as a result of the inconsistency within the medical literature regarding the definition of malformation. Our study used the comprehensive definition delineated by Heinonen, Slone, and Shapiro in their large collaborative project (44). This strict application of the definition resulted in the exclusion of several studies; however, it increases the validity of the results.

Further difficulties inherent in fetal outcome involve the introduction of confounding variables that may concomitantly affect the fetus. Because these studies deal with human subjects, we cannot negate the relative contribution of smoking, other drug use, and socioeconomic status. Because women who drink in pregnancy tend to cluster other reproductive risk factors, our negative association indicates that drinking up to two drinks a day is not associated with major malformations despite potential presence of other risk factors.

CONCLUSION

This meta-analysis suggests that moderate alcohol consumption in the first trimester of pregnancy does not increase the risk of major malformations. Women consuming these amounts before finding out they have conceived should not be misinformed to believe they have a higher than normal teratogenic risk. Such false alarm may lead many of them to consider termination of otherwise-wanted pregnancies.

REFERENCES

1. Abel, E. L.; Sokol, R. J.: Maternal and fetal characteristics affecting alcohol's teratogenicity. Neurobehav. Toxicol. Teratol. 8:329–334; 1986.
2. Alpert, J. J.; Day, N.; Dooling, E.; Hingson, R.; Oppenheimer, E.; Rosett, H. L.; Weiner, L.; Zuckerman, B.: Maternal alcohol consumption and newborn assessment: Methodology of the Boston city hospital prospective study. Neurobehav. Toxicol. Teratol. 3:195–201; 1981.
3. Aro. T.: Maternal diseases, alcohol consumption and smoking during pregnancy associated with reduction limb defects. Early Hum. Dev. 9:49–57; 1983.
4. Autti, Ramo I.; Granstrom, M. L.: The psychomotor development during the first year of life of infants exposed to intrauterine alcohol of various duration. Fetal alcohol and development. Neuropediatrics 22:59–64; 1991.
5. Beattie, J. O.; Day, R. E.; Cockburn, F.; Garg, R. A.: Alcohol and the fetus in the west of Scotland. Br. Med. J. 284:17–20; 1983.
6. Coles, C. D.; Smith, I.; Fernhoff, P. M.; Falek, A.: Neonatal neurobehavioral characteristics as correlates or maternal alcohol use during gestation. Alcohol. Clin. Exp. Res. 9:454–460; 1985.
7. Correy, J. F.; Newman, N.; Collins, J. A.; Burrows, E. A.; Burrows, R. F.; Curran, T. J.: Use of prescription drugs in the first trimester and congenital malformations. Aust. NZ J. Obstet. Gynaecol. 31:340–344; 1991.
8. Davis, P. J. M.; Partridge, J. W.; Storrs, C. N.: Alcohol consumption in pregnancy. How much is safe? Arch. Dis. Child 57:940–943; 1982.
9. Day, N. L.; Jasperse, D.; Richardson, G.; Robles, N.; Sambamoorthi, U.; Taylor, P.; Scher, M.; Cornelius, M.: Prenatal exposure to alcohol: Effect on infant growth and morphologic characteristics. Pediatrics 84:536–547; 1989.
10. Day, N. L.; Richardson, G.; Robles, N.; Sambamoorthi, U.; Taylor, P.; Scher, M.; Stoffer, D.; Jasperse, D.; Cornelius, M.: Effect of prenatal alcohol exposure on growth and morphology of offspring at 8 months of age. Pediatrics 85:748–752; 1990.
11. Day, N. L.; Richardson, G. A.; Geva, D.; Robles, N.: Alcohol, marijuana, and tobacco: Effects of prenatal exposure on offspring growth and morphology at age six. Alcohol. Clin. Exp. Res. 18:786–794; 1994.
12. Day, N.: Comments on 'abstaining for foetal health.' Br. J. Addict. 86:1057–1061; 1991.
13. Deisher, R. W.; Litchfield, C.; Hope, K.: Birth outcomes of prostituting adolescents. J. Adolesc. Health 12:528–533; 1991.
14. Devlin, J.; Trepanier, E.; Agro, K.; Makerechian, N.; Koren, G.; Einarson, T. R.: The relationship between moderate alcohol consumption during pregnancy and spontaneous abortion, stillbirth, premature birth and birth weight: A meta analysis. Proceedings of the 1995 meeting of the Canadian Pharmacoepidemiology Forum.
15. du V Florey, C.; Taylor, D.; Bolumar, F.; Izarugaza, I.; Kaminski, M.; Van Noord Zaadstra, B.; Dode, J.: A European concerted action: maternal alcohol consumption and its relation to the outcome of pregnancy and child development at 18 months. Int. J. Epidemiol. 21:S1–S87; 1992.
16. Ernhart, C. B.; Sokol, R. J.; Martier, S.; Moron, P.; Nadler, D.; Ager, J. W.; Wolf. A.: Alcohol teratogenicity in the human: A detailed assessment of specificity, critical period, and threshold. Am. J. Obstet. Gynecol. 156:33–39; 1987.
17. Ernhart, C. B.; Sokol, R. J.; Ager, J. W.; Morrow Tlucak, M.; Martier, S.: Alcohol related birth defects: Assessing the risk. Ann. NY Acad. Sci. 562:159–172; 1989.
18. Ernhart, C. B.; Wolf, A. W.; Pinn, P. L.; Sokol, R. J.; Kennard, M. J.; Filipovich, H. F.: Alcohol related birth defects: Syndromal anomalies, intrauterine growth retardation, and neonatal behavioral assessment. Alcohol. Clin. Exp. Res. 9:447–453; 1985.
19. Flores Huerta, S.; Hernandez Montes, H.; Argote, R. M.; Villalpando, S.: Effects of ethanol consumption during pregnancy and lactation on the outcome and postnatal growth of the offspring. Ann. Nutr. Metab. 36:121–128; 1992.

20. Forrest, F.; Florey, C. D.; Taylor, D.; McPherson, F.; Young, J. A.: Reported social alcohol consumption during pregnancy and infants' development at 18 months. Br. Med. J. 303:22–26; 1991.
21. Godel, J. C.; Pabst, H. F.; Hodges, P. E.; Johnson, K. E.; Froese, G. J.; Joffres, M. R.: Smoking and caffeine and alcohol intake during pregnancy in a northern population: Effects on fetal growth. Can. Med. Assoc. J. 147:181–188; 1992.
22. Graham, J. M.; Hanson, J. W.; Darby, B. L.; Barr, H. M.; Streissguth, A. P.: Independent dysmorphology evaluations at birth and 4 years of age for children exposed to varying amounts of alcohol in utero. Pediatrics 81:722–778; 1988.
23. Grisso, J. A.; Roman, E.; Inskip, H.; Beral, V.; Donovan, J.: Alcohol consumption and outcome of pregnancy. J. Epidemiol. Commun. Health 38:232–235; 1984.
24. Halliday, H. L.; Reid, M. M.; McClure, G.: Results of heavy drinking in pregnancy. Br. J. Obstet. Gynaecol. 89:892–895; 1982.
25. Halmesmaki, E.; Raivio, K.; Ylikorkala. O.: A possible association between maternal drinking and fetal clubfoot [abstract]. N. Engl. J. Med. 312:790; 1985.
26. Hanson, J. W.; Streissguth, P.; Smith, D. W.: The effects of moderate alcohol consumption during pregnancy on fetal growth and morphogenesis. J. Pediatr. 92:457–460; 1978.
27. Hartzema, A. G.: Guide to interpreting and evaluating the pharmacoepidemiologic literature. Ann. Pharmacother. 26:96–98; 1992.
28. Heinonen, O.; Slone, D.; Shapiro, S.: Birth defects and drugs in pregnancy; maternal drug exposure and congenital malformations. Boston, MA: Littleton; 1976.
29. Hollstedt, C.; Dahlgren, L.; Rydberg, U.: Outcome of pregnancy in women treated at an alcohol clinic. Acta Psychiatr. Scand. 67:236–248;1983.
30. Jacobson, J. L.; Jacobson, S. W.; Sokol, R. J.; Martier, S. S.; Ager, J. W.; Kaplan Estrin, M. G.: Teratogenic effects of alcohol on infant development. Alcohol. Clin. Exp. Res. 17:174–183; 1993.
31. Jones, K. L.; Smith, D. W.; Ulleland, C. N.; Streissguth, A. P.: Pattern of malformation in offspring of chronic alcoholic mothers. Lancet i:1267–1271; 1973.
32. Kaminski, M.; Franc, M.; Lebouvier, M.; Mazaubrun, C. D.; Rumeau Rouquette, C.: Moderate alcohol use and pregnancy outcome. Neurobehav. Toxicol. Teratol. 3:173–181; 1981.
33. Kaminski, M.; Rumeau, C.; Schwartz, D.: Alcohol consumption in pregnant women and the outcome of pregnancy. Alcohol. Clin. Exp Res. 2:155–163; 1978.
34. Koide, T.; Saito, Y.; Sakamoto, T.; Murao, S.: Peripartal cardiomyopathy in Japan. A critical reappraisal of the concept. Jpn. Heart J. 13:488–501; 1972.
35. Larsson, G.: Prevention of fetal alcohol effects. Acta Obstet. Gynecol. Scand. 62:171–178; 1983.
36. Lazzaroni, F.; Bonassi, S.; Magnani, M.; Calvi, A.; Repetto, E.; Serra, G.; Podesta, F.; Pearce, N.: Moderate maternal drinking and outcome of pregnancy. Eur. J. Epidemiol. 9:599–606; 1993.
37. Little, R. E.; Asker, R. L.; Simon, P. D.; Renwick, J. H.: Fetal growth and moderate drinking in early pregnancy. Am. J. Epidemiol. 123:270–278; 1986.
38. Little, R. E.; Streissguth, A. P.: Drinking during pregnancy in alcoholic women. Alcohol. Clin. Exp. Res. 2:179–183; 1978.
39. Lumley, J.; Correy, J. F.; Newman, N. M.; Curran, J. T.: Cigarette smoking, alcohol consumption and fetal outcome in Tasmania 1981–82. Aust. N Z J. Obstet. Gynaecol. 25:33–40; 1985.
40. Mau, G.: Moderate alcohol consumption during pregnancy and child development. Eur. J. Pediatr. 133:233–237; 1980.
41. McDonald, A, D.; Armstrong, B. G.; Sloan, M.: Cigarette, alcohol, and coffee consumption and congenital defects. Am. J. Public Health 82:91–93; 1992.
42. Miettinen, O.: Estimability and estimation in case-referrent studies. Am. J. Epidemiol. 103:226–235; 1976.
43. Mills, J. L., Graubard, B. I.: is moderate drinking during pregnancy associated with an increased risk for malformations? Pediatrics 80:309–314; 1987.
44. MotherRisk Clinic Statistics: Motherisk Program, The Hospital for Sick Children, Toronto.
45. National Institute on Drug Abuse: National Household Survey on Drug Abuse: 1990 Population Estimates. DHHS Pub. No. (ADM) 91–1732. Washington, DC: Supt. Of Docs., U.S. Govt. Print. Off., 1991.
46. O'Connor, M. J.; Brill, N. J.; Sigman, M.: Alcohol use in primiparous women older than 30 years of age: Relation to infant development. Pediatrics 78:444–450; 1986.
47. Olsen, J.: The association between birth weight, placenta weight, pregnancy duration, subfecundity, and child development. Scand. J. Soc. Med. 22:213–218; 1994.
48. Ouellette, E. M.; Rosett, H. L.; Rosman, P.; Weiner, L.: Adverse effects on offspring of maternal alcohol abuse during pregnancy. N. Eng. J. Med. 297:528–530; 1977.
49. Plant, M. L.; Plant, M. A.: Family alcohol problems among pregnant women: Links with maternal substance use and birth abnormalities. Dev. Med. Child Neurol. 28:649–654; 1986.
50. Plant, M. L.; Plant, M. A.: Maternal use of alcohol and other drugs during pregnancy and birth abnormalities: Further results from a prospective study.Alcohol Alcohol. 23:229–233; 1988.
51. Plant, M. L.: Alcohol consumption during pregnancy: Baseline data from a Scottish prospective study. Br. J. Addict. 79:207–214; 1984.
52. Plant, M. L.: Drinking amongst pregnant women: some initial results from a prospective study.Alcohol Alcohol. 19:153–157; 1984.
53. Robles, N.; Day, N. L.: Recall of alcohol consumption during pregnancy. J. Stud. Alcohol 51:403–407; 1990.
54. Roeleveld, N.; Vingerhoets, E.; Zielhuis, G. A.; Gabreels, F.: Mental retardation associated with parental smoking and alcohol consumption before, during, and after pregnancy. Prev. Med. 21:110–119; 1992.
55. Rosenthal, R.: Meta-analytic procedures for social research. Beverly Hills: Sage; 1984.
56. Rosett, H. L.; Weiner, L.; Lee, A.; Zuckerman, B.; Dooling, E.; Oppenheimer, E.: Patterns of alcohol consumption and fetal development. Obstet. Gynecol. 61:539–546; 1983.
57. Rostand, A.; Kaminski, M.; Lelong, N.; Dehaene, P.; Delestret, I.; Klein, Bertrand, C.; Querleu, D.; Crepin, G.: Alcohol use in pregnancy craniofacial features, and fetal growth. J. Epidemiol. Commun. Health 44:302–306; 1990.
58. Rubin, D.; Krasilnikoff, P. A.; Leventhal, J. M.; Berget, A.; Weile, B.: Cigarette smoking and alcohol consumption during pregnancy by Danish women and their spouses a potential source of fetal morbidity. Am. J. Drug Alcohol Abuse 14:405–417; 1988.
59. Russell, M.; Skinner, J. B.: Early measures of maternal alcohol misuse as predictors of adverse pregnancy outcomes. Alcohol. Clin. Exp. Res. 12:824–830; 1988.
60. Saxen, I.: Epidemiology of cleft lip and palate. An attempt to rule out chance correlation. Br. J. Prev. Soc. Med. 29:103–110; 1975.
61. Serdula, M.; Williamson, D.; Kendrick, J.; Anda, R.; Byers, T.: Trends in alcohol consumption by pregnant women 1985–1988. JAMA 265:876–879; 1991.
62. Shiono, P. H.; Klebanoff, M. A.; Rhoads, G. G.: Smoking and drinking during pregnancy. JAMA 255:82–84; 1986.
63. Silva, A. V.; Laranjeira, R. R.; Dolnikoff, M.; Grinfeld, H.; Masur, J.: Alcohol consumption during pregnancy and newborn outcome: A study in Brazil. Neurobehav. Toxicol. Teratol. 3:169–172; 1981.
64. Sokol, R. J.;Miller, S. I.; Debanne, S.; Golden, N.; Collins, G.; Kaplan, J.; Martier, S.: The Cleveland NIAAA prospective alcohol pregnancy study: The first year. Neurobehav. Toxicol. Teratol. 3:203–209; 1981.
65. Staisey, N. L.; Fried, P. A.: Relationships between moderate maternal alcohol consumption during pregnancy and infant neurological development. J. Stud. Alcohol 44:262–270; 1983.
66. Streissguth, P.: Summary and recommendations: Epidemiologic and human studies on alcohol and pregnancy. Neurobehav. Toxicol. 3:241–242; 1981.
67. Streissguth, A. P.; Martin, D. C.; Martin, J. C.; Barr, H. M.: The Seattle longitudinal prospective study on alcohol and pregnancy. Neurobehav. Toxicol. Teratol. 3:223–233; 1981.

68. Streissguth, A. P.; Barr, H. M.; Martin, D. C.: Offspring effects and pregnancy complications related to self reported maternal alcohol use. Dev. Pharmacol. Ther. 5:21–32; 1982.
69. Sulaiman, N. D.; du V Florey, C.; Taylor, D. J.; Ogston, S. A.: Alcohol consumption in Dundee primigravidas and its effects on outcome of pregnancy. Br. Med. J. 296:1500–1503; 1988.
70. Taylor, D. J.: Pregnancy alcohol consumption. Fetal Maternal Med. Rev. 5:121–135; 1993.
71. Taylor, C. L.; Jones, K. L.; Jones, M. C.; Kaplan, G. W.: Incidence of renal anomalies in children prenatally exposed to ethanol. Pediatrics 94:209–212; 1994.
72. Tennes, K.; Blackard, C.: Maternal alcohol consumption, birth weight, and minor physical anomalies. Am. J. Obstet. Gynecol. 138:774–780; 1980.
73. Tikkannen, J.; Heinonen, O. P.: Risk factors for ventricular septal defect in Finland. Public Health 105:99–112; 1991.
74. Verkerk, P. H.: The impact of alcohol misclassification on the relationship between alcohol and pregnancy outcome. Int. J. Epidemiol. 21:S33–S37; 1992.
75. Walpole, I.; Zubrick, S.; Pontre, J.: Is there a fetal effect with low to moderate alcohol use before or during pregnancy? J. Epidemiol. Commun. Health 44:297–301; 1990.
76. Werler, M. M.; Lammer, E. J.; Rosenberg, L.; Mitchell, A. A.: Maternal alcohol use in relation to selected birth defects. Am. J. Epidemiol. 134:691–698; 1991.
77. Wright, J. T.; Barrison, I.; Toplis, P. J.; Waterson, J.: Alcohol and the fetus. Br. J. Hosp. Med. March: 260–266; 1983.

APPENDIX 1

CRITERIA FOR ACCEPTANCE OF STUDY INTO META-ANALYSIS

Article Code Number: ——————

Reviewer Number:——————

SELECTION CRITERIA		
INCLUSION	Yes	No
1) Does the study deal with pregnant human females?		
2) Was alcohol consumption 0–2 drinks/day (or grams or mL equivalency)		
3) Was it a case control or cohort study?		
4) Is there a control group that was not exposed to alcohol?		
5) Is the measured outcome of fetal malformations as defined in Appendix A?		
EXCLUSION		
1) Can you separate the data on 2 drinks alone in a 2 drinks and greater study?		
2) Is it a case report, editorial, or review study?		
3) Does the study provide sufficient data for analysis?		
4) Does the study deal with Fetal-Alcohol-Syndrome or binge drinking?		
COMMENTS:		
ACCEPT:		

APPENDIX 2A

EVALUATION CRITERIA FOR THE QUALITY OF CASE CONTROL STUDIES

CRITERIA	SCORE	MAX
1 Was there a defined selection method for cases and controls?		1
2 Was alcohol exposure ascertained in both groups?		1
3 Data collection should be structured and the investigator blinded to the outcomes.		2
4 Time of alcohol exposure should be confirmed.		1
5 Unbiased exclusion criteria provided for cases and control.		1
6 Same level of outcome screening for cases and controls. Score 2 if the mother was interviewed and the chart was examined.		2
7 Are cases and controls homogenous with respect to demographics?		1
8 Appropriate use of statistics (p-value and CI)		1
9 Are objectives and conclusion related to alcohol exposure?		1
TOTAL		11

APPENDIX 2B
EVALUATION CRITERIA FOR THE QUALITY OF COHORT STUDIES

CRITERIA	SCORE	MAX
1 Is the sample demographically homogenous?		1
2 Was alcohol consumption equally ascertained throughout sample?		1
3 Was the same screening method used to measure outcome for the entire sample?		1
4 Were the outcomes uniformly classified throughout sample?		1
5 Drop out rates and characteristics of drop outs in both groups should be accounted for and comparable.		1
6 Is the cohort representative of the population using alcohol and is the sample size large?		2
7 Cohorts should be followed from the beginning of pregnancy. Score 2 if defined as first prenatal visit to physician.		2
8 Appropriateness of statistics.		1
9 Are objectives and conclusion related to alcohol exposure?		1
TOTAL		11

CHAPTER 37

THE ROLE OF ACETALDEHYDE IN PREGNANCY OUTCOME AFTER PRENATAL ALCOHOL EXPOSURE

Marjie L. Hard, Thomas R. Einarson,† and Gideon Koren**

**Division of Clinical Pharmacology and Toxicology and †Faculty of Pharmacy, University of Toronto and Department of Pediatrics, The Hospital For Sick Children, Toronto, Ontario, Canada*

Summary

It is not known why some heavy-drinking women give birth to children with alcohol-related birth defects (ARBD) whereas other do not. The objective of this study was to determine whether the frequency of elevated maternal blood acetaldehyde levels among alcoholics is in the range of ARBD among alcoholic women. MEDLINE was searched from 1980 to 2000 using the key words acetaldehyde, pharmacokinetics, and alcoholism for controlled trials reporting blood or breath acetaldehyde levels in alcoholics and nonalcoholics. Separately, using the key words fetal alcohol syndrome, epidemiology, prevalence, incidence, and frequency, articles were identified reporting ARBD incidences among the offspring of heavy drinkers. Of 23 articles reporting acetaldehyde levels in alcoholics, four met the inclusion criteria. Forty-three studies reported on the rate of ARBD in heavy drinkers, and 14 were accepted. Thirty-four percent of heavy drinkers had a child with ARBD, and 43% of chronic alcoholics had high acetaldehyde levels. The similar frequencies of high acetaldehyde levels among alcoholics and the rates of ARBD among alcoholic women provide epidemiologic support to the hypothesis that acetaldehyde may play a major role in the cause of ARBD.

Key Words: Acetaldehyde—Epidemiology—Fetal alcohol Syndrome—Incidence.

The worldwide incidence of fetal alcohol syndrome among the general population has been estimated as 0.97 per 1000 live births. This rate increases to about 4.3% when considering only the heavy-drinking population (two or more drinks per day or five or more drinks per occasion, or a clinical diagnosis of alcohol abuse) (1). The observation that not all heavy drinkers will have a child affected adversely by prenatal alcohol abuse (2) raises the need to identify the sources of this variability.

Some researchers have suggested that acetaldehyde may be the causative agent in alcohol-related birth defects (ARBD). It is the first oxidation product of ethanol and a highly toxic substance. It is known to bind covalently to a number of proteins and enzymes (3,4) and to impair mitochondrial function (5,6). Extensive evidence exists to implicate acetaldehyde in the development of liver disease secondary to chronic alcohol abuse (7,8); however, its role in the development of fetal alcohol syndrome remains unclear.

Numerous animal models have shown that both ethanol and acetaldehyde are teratogens, but the relative role played by each remains controversial (9–15). For example, coadministration of ethanol and pyrazole, a potent alcohol dehydrogenase (ADH) inhibitor, to maternal mice resulted in an increase in the number of malformations produced in their offspring, suggesting that it is ethanol rather than acetaldehyde that is damaging the fetus (9). Conversely, it has also been shown that concurrent administration of the aldehyde dehydrogenase (ALDH) inhibitor cyanamide potentiates the teratogenic effects of alcohol, implying that sustained acetaldehyde levels are responsible for the adverse fetal effects (11).

Chronic alcoholism results in increased ethanol elimination rates and decreased gastric first-past metabolism (16–19). Despite these changes, peak blood alcohol levels do not differ significantly between alcoholics and nonalcoholics (19–22). In contrast, acetaldehyde levels are elevated only in some alcoholics (8,21,23), reaching as high as 100 μmol/L (24,25), compared with very low levels (<5 μmol/L) in nonalcoholics and in most alcoholics (Table 1). In a small study, alcoholic women who gave birth to children with fetal alcohol syndrome had a tendency toward higher acetaldehyde concentrations than alcoholic women who had normal children (26,27). It has also been shown that concentrations of hemoglobin-acetaldehyde adducts were significantly higher among alcoholic women who delivered children with fetal alcohol effects compared with alcoholics who delivered healthy children (28). These studies suggest that acetaldehyde may play a determinant role in the extent and variability of fetal damage.

In the current study we wished to explore the potential role of maternal pharmacokinetic variability as a mechanism for variability in fetal damage. Ethanol itself has very low variability in peak levels because it is distributed into the extracellular fluid, which is very similar among subjects. This similarity is the basis for the wide medicolegal use of breath-alcohol concentration as an estimate for the number of drinks consumed. In contrast, blood acetaldehyde concentrations have been shown to be higher in some chronic alcoholics compared with most alcoholics and nonalcoholics. Hence, it was the purpose of this investigation to determine whether the frequency of high acetaldehyde levels corresponds to the reported rates of ARBD by comparing the incidence of elevated acetaldehyde levels among alcoholics to the incidence of ARBD among heavy drinkers. If the rates were similar, it would lend epidemiologic support to the causative role of acetaldehyde in ARBD.

METHODS

A search was conducted for all controlled trials that reported acetaldehyde levels among alcoholics, using the key words acetaldehyde, alcoholism, ethanol, and pharmacokinetics in MEDLINE from 1980 to the present. When references were found that reported acetaldehyde levels in alcoholics in comparison to nonalcoholics, PubMed was used to locate all related articles. Studies were excluded if artifactual formation of acetaldehyde was evident and not corrected for, if the number of subjects

Table 1
Comparison of Acetaldehyde Levels in Alcoholics and Controls

REFERENCE	ALCOHOLIC ACETALDEHYDE (μmol)	NONALCOHOLIC ACETALDEHYDE (μmol)
Eriksson (1980)*	<2	<2
Lindros (1980)	5–100	<0.5
Maring (1983)*	2–14	<2
Nuutinen (1984)	0.1–14	<2
Hesselbrock (1985)†	21.43	15.81
Shaskan (1985)†	14.4 (2.6)	4.3 (0.9)
Lucas (1986)	3.12 (0.65)	1.67 (0.12)
DiPadova (1987)	1.89 (0.08)	0.68 (0.21)
DiPadova (1987)*	1.03 (0.08)	0.68 (0.21)
Panés (1992)	0.05–5	<0.5

Ranges, means and means (±SE) are reported.
* Abstinent alcoholics.
† Breath acetaldehyde in alcoholic and nonalcoholic nonsmokers (ng/L).

exhibiting elevated acetaldehyde levels could not be determined, and if the alcoholics had been abstinent before the study. Studies that had inadequate control groups (i.e., subjects who drank more than the equivalent of 30 g absolute alcohol per week) were also excluded. Finally, our criteria did not allow for inclusion of studies that measured in vitro acetaldehyde formation in blood taken from alcoholics after the addition of ethanol. Studies were included if they allowed us to extract information about the number of alcoholics who had high (>2 μmol/L) blood or breath acetaldehyde levels compared with nonalcoholic controls. Studies were required to use analytic methods that would minimize artifactual acetaldehyde formation. Examples of acceptable methods for acetaldehyde determination include the improved perchloric acid (PCA) method and the isotonic semicarbazide method.

We used the term fetal alcohol syndrome under the MEDLINE subheading epidemiology to locate articles reporting the incidence of ARBD among heavy drinkers from 1967 to 2000. PubMed was also searched using key words such as fetal alcohol syndrome, epidemiology, incidence, prevalence, and frequency. Heavy drinkers were considered to be subjects who consumed an average of two or more drinks per day or had a clinical diagnosis of alcoholism. We excluded studies that reported an incidence of ARBD among the general population or in light to moderate drinkers (two or fewer drinks per day) and articles in which the amount of alcohol consumed was not defined or in which it could not be determined how many of the affected offspring had been born to heavy drinkers. Articles that did not give a diagnosis of fetal alcohol syndrome or fetal alcohol effects or describe the presence of malformations consistent with ARBD were not included. Studies were not accepted if fetal alcohol syndrome and not fetal alcohol effects were identified, or if a prenatal effect of alcohol was measured by a single parameter such as birth weight. Prospective and retrospective studies were included when it could be determined how many pregnancies of heavy-drinking women resulted in fetal alcohol syndrome, fetal alcohol effects, or abnormalities or malformations consistent with a prenatal effect of alcohol.

One author (M.L.H.) retrieved the relevant articles and two judges assessed the acceptability of those papers. If disagreement occurred, the rationale for inclusion or exclusion of a paper would be set forth and a consensus would be achieved. Data extraction was done in a similar fashion. From each study, we identified the number of alcoholics having elevated acetaldehyde levels relative to controls and the number of alcoholics having a child with ARBD.

Incidence rates were combined across studies according to the method described by Einarson (29). Between-study variance (Q), meta-analytic average across trials, standard error, and 95% confidence intervals were calculated and compared for overlap for the incidences of high acetaldehyde levels and ARBD among alcoholics.

RESULTS

Incidence of Elevated Acetaldehyde Levels Among Alcoholic Subjects

Our search for publications dealing with acetaldehyde levels in alcoholics yielded 212 citations, of which 25 were found to contain relevant information. Articles were excluded on the basis of artifactual formation of acetaldehyde (20,22,30), in six we could not determine how many alcoholics (20,22,30), in six we could not determine how many alcoholics had high acetaldehyde levels (31–36), in two the alcoholics had been abstinent before the study (37,38), and in four the acetaldehyde levels were measured in vitro (39–42). Matthewson et al. (43) allowed control subjects to drink as much as 100 g absolute alcohol per day, so that study was excluded. The report by Nuutinen et al. (24) was excluded because data from eight of the nine subjects had already been used in a previous report (25); thus, it was a duplicate study. Four further papers were excluded because acetaldehyde levels were reported in alcoholics in the presence of an ALDH inhibitor (44–47).

Four studies matched our inclusion criteria (21,23,25,48), where we could determine how many of the alcoholic subjects had high blood acetaldehyde concentrations (see Table 2). Data were collected from a total of 54 alcoholics and 26 controls.

The summary meta-analytic average rate was 43% (95% confidence interval [$CI_{95\%}$], 21–65%). As shown in Table 2, the test for homogeneity was significant ($Q = 11.05$, $df = 3$, $p < 0.025$). The study by Nuutinen et al. (21) contributed the most to the chi-square value. When that study was removed from the analysis, the average rate became 54% ($CI_{95\%}$, 28–79%) and Q was not significant ($Q = 3.82$, $df = 2$, $p < 0.15$). Heterogeneity of the sample may be due to differences in liver disease state, possible differences in nutritional status of the alcoholics, or chance random error.

Table 2
Fraction of Alcoholics with Elevated Acetaldehyde Levels

REFERENCE	N	ELEVATED ACETALDEHYDE (%)
Lindros (1980)	9	4 (44)
Nuutinen (1983)	13	2 (15)
Takase (1990)	19	11 (58)
Panés (1992)	25	14 (56)
Rate (±SE) (%)		43% (11%)
$CI_{95\%}$		21–65
Q*		11.05†

* Homogeneity chi-square.
† $P < 0.025$, $df = 3$.
($CI_{95\%}$, 95% confidence interval; Q*, between-study variance.

Incidence of Alcohol-Related Birth Defects in the Offspring of Alcoholic Women

Our search of the epidemiology literature on fetal alcohol syndrome yielded 173 citations from MEDLINE and 370 citations from PubMed. Forty-three prospective and retrospective studies were obtained that reported on fetal outcome in the drinking population. Studies that reported the incidence of ARBD among the general population (49–60), in individuals who had two or fewer drinks daily (61–63), or where the amount of alcohol consumed could not be determined (64) were excluded. Four articles were excluded because we could not determine how many of the affected offspring were born to heavy drinkers (65–68). Eight studies were not included because a diagnosis of fetal alcohol syndrome and fetal alcohol effects was not given, malformations or abnormalities were not identified to be consistent with a prenatal effect of alcohol, or a prenatal alcohol effect was assessed by a single parameter (69–76). One study was not included because only cases of fetal alcohol syndrome were reported (77).

Fourteen of the citations matched our inclusion criteria (Table 3), and three separate analyses were performed. In the first analysis, 11 studies in which the authors had explicitly diagnosed offspring as having fetal alcohol syndrome and fetal alcohol effects were used (78–88). A meta-analytic average of 30% with a $CI_{95\%}$ of 17–43% was found ($Q = 234.9$, $df = 10$, $p < 0.001$). In a second analysis (n = 13), two additional studies were included that reported the presence of abnormalities and/or major malformations among the offspring of heavy drinkers that were consistent with a prenatal effect of alcohol without diagnoses of fetal alcohol syndrome or fetal alcohol effects (89,90); this yielded an average of 34% with a $CI_{95\%}$ of 21–47% ($Q = 313.2$, $df = 12$, $p < 0.001$). One more study, in which fetal alcohol syndrome or effects were produced in the offspring of alcoholic subjects who had multiple births (91), was included in the third analysis (n = 14), recognizing the increased risk for producing a child affected by prenatal alcohol exposure with advanced maternal age. This analysis resulted in an overall meta-analytic average of 34% with a $CI_{95\%}$ of 21–47% ($Q = 313.2$, $df = 13$, $p < 0.001$). The results of each analysis did not differ significantly, and heterogeneity of the sample was detected. The lack of homogeneity may have arisen from factors that are thought to influence fetal outcome after in utero alcohol exposure, such as differences in maternal drinking patterns, socioeconomic status, and maternal malnutrition. The diagnosticians' ability to diagnose ARBD and differences resulting from random variability may have also contributed to the heterogeneity.

Table 3
Proportion of Heavy Drinkers to have Offspring with an Alcohol-Related Birth Defect

REFERENCE	N	ARBD (%)
Jones (1974)	19	6(32)
Ouellette (1977)*	42	29(69)
Hanson (1978)	70	9(13)
Olegard (1979)	21	14(67)
Sokol (1980)*	42	16(38)
Silva (1981)	26	6(23)
Larsson (1983a)	89	2(2.2)
Larsson (1983b)	39	2(5.1)
Iosub (1985)†	92	30(33)
Robinson (1987)	54	14(26)
Halmesmaki (1988)	59	41(71)
Rostand (1990)	51	15(29)
Autti-Ramo (1992)	51	29(57)
Maillard (1999)	44	12(27)
Rate (±SE)‡		34%(7%)
$CI_{95\%}$		21% to 47%
Q§		313.2‖

* References that were included in the second analysis.
† Additional reference that was also used in the third analysis.
‡ Only the results from the analysis of all the references listed in the table are reported. Rates of 30% (7%) and 34% (7%) were obtained for the first and second analysis, respectively and are not significantly different from the third analysis.
§ Homogeneity χ^2.
‖ $P < 0.001$.
$CI_{95\%}$, 95% confidence interval; Q, between-study variance.

The 43% incidence rate of high acetaldehyde levels in alcoholics did not differ significantly from the 34% incidence rate for the offspring of heavy drinkers to be affected by ARBD. The 95% confidence intervals (ie, 21–65% ad 21–47%, respectively) overlapped completely.

DISCUSSION

Under normal conditions, when ethanol is oxidized, acetaldehyde is not detectable in peripheral or arterial blood, but it may become elevated under certain conditions, including genotypic ALDH deficiency, treatment with an ALDH inhibitor, and chronic alcoholism (92,93). Elevated acetaldehyde levels may occur in chronic alcoholism as a result of enhanced oxidation of ethanol resulting from induction of CYP2E1 and a concomitant reduction in ALDH activity.

In this study, we determined that the proportion of alcoholics who have elevated acetaldehyde levels is 43% ($CI_{95\%}$, 21–65%). The studies included in this analysis all used valid and acceptable methods for acetaldehyde determination. The isotonic semicarbazide (21,25) and the improved PCA methods (21,23) were used, along with a procedure for correction of artifactual acetaldehyde formation in three of the four studies. Panés et al. (48) used a polyethylene glycol-sodium azide solution instead of PCA for protein precipitation, which has previously been shown to produce no artifactual formation (94). However, according to Eriksson and Fukunaga (93), this method still must be evaluated for the need for correction of artifactual acetaldehyde.

The demographics of the subjects included in the analysis for determining the incidence of high acetaldehyde levels were similar. All subjects were 31–59 years of age with at least a 10-year drinking history, with the exception of one subject in the study by Nuutinen et al. (21) who had been drinking for only 3–4 years. The upper limit of the age of the subjects exceeds a woman's fertile age. It seems possible that with advancing age, and thus increased duration of alcohol consumption, there is a greater potential for liver damage and possibly elevated acetaldehyde levels. Therefore, our results may be an overestimate for women of child-bearing age, although none of the studies indicated that higher acetaldehyde levels were found in older subjects. If our results are an overestimate for women of child-bearing age, then the true value may be even closer to the rate of children with ARBD born to alcoholic women.

The doses of ethanol given in each study yielded similar peak blood ethanol concentrations (30–35 mmol/L). Associated liver injury was reported in all studies, but the severity of liver injury was variable between subjects. The nutritional status of subjects was reported only by Nuutinen et al. (21) as being poor. The subjects in the study by Takase et al. (23) were of Japanese descent, but those who had the atypical ALDH genotype were not included. Therefore, the lack of homogeneity in the proportions of patients having high acetaldehyde levels found among the studies of alcoholics may have been caused by nutritional differences among alcoholics and differences in liver disease status among subjects. When the study by Nuutinen et al. was removed from the analysis, homogeneity was achieved. Because of the small sample size, the results of that study probably did not reflect the actual population parameter.

Alcoholic liver disease may be a precursor for high acetaldehyde levels (23,33,39,43) that may result from a disease-induced reduction in ALDH (24,38,95,96) and may be reversible after a period of abstinence (43,45). The reversibility of ALDH activity in alcoholic liver disease, however, is probably dependent on the severity of liver damage (39,45). Differences in the severity of liver lesions may explain why some studies found normalization of acetaldehyde levels after a period of abstinence (31,37) but others did not (38,39). The heterogeneity of the results of the studies included in our analysis may therefore be explained by differences in liver dysfunction. Lindros et al. (25) reported fatty changes in six and increased transaminases in five of eight alcoholics tested. Nuutinen et al. (21) reported cirrhosis in 1 subject and slight to severe fatty degeneration in 5 of 13 subjects. Alcoholic liver disease was reported in all of the 19 alcoholics (7 with cirrhosis and 12 with fibrosis) in the study by Takase et al. (23) and in all but 4 of the 25 subjects (4 with steatosis, 4 with fibrosis, 7 with hepatitis, and 6 with cirrhosis) in the study by Panés et al. (48). The effect of the study by Nuutinen et al. in creating the overall heterogeneity may have been because only about half of the subjects included had liver dysfunction related to alcoholism, but in the other studies most of the subjects had damage to the liver. At present, data on liver complications among women bearing children with ARBD are not available. In a follow-up study of women who bore children with ARBD, almost 20% of the women who could be located had died several years after the birth of the child (97). Although the cause of death was not reported, liver insufficiency is a common cause of death among alcoholics.

The data concerning the incidence of ARBD among heavy drinkers were combined in three separate analyses. Including studies that did not provide a diagnosis of fetal alcohol syndrome or effects but described the presence of malformations consistent with ARBD had no significant effect on the estimated incidence of ARBD among heavy drinkers ($30 \pm 7\%$ vs. $34 \pm 7\%$). Including one study in which each subject bore more than one child (91) also had no effect on the calculated incidence of ARBD among heavy drinkers ($34 \pm 7\%$).

All the patients examined in the studies of ARBD included in this analysis were similar with respect to the information that could be extracted. All subjects met the minimum criteria used for heavy drinking (two or more drinks daily or five drinks per occasion, or a diagnosis of alcohol abuse); however, differences in the average alcohol consumption between studies may have contributed to the heterogeneity. For example, the heavy drinkers in the study by Ouellette et al. (90) consumed more alcohol than in the studies by Silva et al. (80), Rostand et al. (87), and Maillard et al. (88), which may explain the twofold difference in the incidence of ARBD reported. It has been well established that low socioeconomic status is a risk factor for ARBD, and it was found that the three studies that had "average" (84,85) and "middle class and well-educated" subjects (82) reported the lowest incidence of ARBD. Because not every study reported the average alcohol consumption and the socioeconomic status of the subjects, we cannot determine whether these parameters actually had an effect on our results; therefore, we assume that differences were due to sampling.

Other factors that may have contributed to the heterogeneity include random variation in the population, differences in criteria used to diagnose fetal alcohol syndrome and effects, genetic differences among populations, and differences in the diagnosticians' astuteness for making the diagnosis.

The incidence of ARBD may be artificially high among certain ethnic groups because of some ethnic facial features, such as epicanthal folds and a depressed nasal bridge, that are consistent with the facial characteristics of fetal alcohol syndrome. The studies that were included here that included subjects of African American, Native Indian, Puerto Rican, Brazilian, and Asian descent (78–80,88,89,91) did not report incidences of ARBD that were unexpectedly high and did not contribute to the heterogeneity.

In conclusion, there is a concordance between the percentage of high blood acetaldehyde among alcoholics and the rates of ARBD among children of alcoholic women. This lends epidemiologic support to the hypothesis that acetaldehyde may play a causative role in ARBD. We would like to hypothesize that because alcoholic liver disease may produce high acetaldehyde levels, women who have offspring affected by prenatal alcohol exposure may be alcoholics with damaged livers. These hypotheses should be tested through an appropriately powered, prospective study where both maternal acetaldehyde levels and fetal outcome can be examined.

ACKNOWLEDGEMENT

This work was supported by a grant from the Canadian Institute of Health Research. Gideon Koren is a Senior Scientist of the Canadian Institute of Health Research. Marjie Hard is a recipient of a graduate studentship from the Research Institute, The Hospital for Sick Children.

REFERENCES

1. Abel EL. An update on incidence of FAS: FAS is not an equal-opportunity birth defect. *Neurotoxicol Teratol* 1995;17:437–43.
2. Smith DW, Jones KL, Hanson JW. Perspectives on the cause and frequency of the fetal alcohol syndrome. *Ann NY Acad Sci.* 1976; 273:138–9.
3. Mauch TJ, Donohue TM Jr, Zetterman RK, et al. Covalent binding of acetaldehyde selectively inhibits the catalytic activity of lysine-dependent enzymes. *Hepatology* 1986;6:263–9.
4. Tuma DJ, Sorrell MF. Functional consequences of acetaldehyde binding to proteins. *Alcohol Alcoholism* 1987;Suppl 1:61–6.
5. Matsuzaki S, Lieber CS. Increased susceptibility of hepatic mitochondria to the toxicity of acetaldehyde after chronic ethanol consumption. *Biochem Biophys Res Commun* 1977;75:1059–65.
6. Cederbaum AI, Lieber CS, Rubin E. The effect of acetaldehyde on mitochondrial function. *Arch Biochem Biophys* 1974;161:36–9.
7. Peters TJ, Ward RJ. Role of acetaldehyde in the pathogenesis of alcoholic liver disease. *Mol Aspects Med* 1988;10:179–90.

8. Li CJ, Nanji, AA, Siakotos AN, Lin RC. Acetaldehyde-modified and 4-hydroxynonenal-modified proteins in the livers of rats with alcoholic liver disease. *Hepatology* 1997;26:650–7.
9. Ukita K, Fukui Y, Shiota K. Effects of prenatal alcohol exposure in mice: influence of an ADH inhibitor and a chronic inhalation study. *Reprod Toxicol* 1993;7:273–81.
10. Ledig M. Tholey G, Kopp P, Mandel P. An experimental study of fetal alcohol syndrome in the rat: biochemical modifications in brain and liver. *Alcohol Alcoholism* 1989;24:231–40.
11. Ali F, Persaud TV. Mechanisms of fetal alcohol effects: role of acetaldehyde. *Exp Pathol* 1988;33:17–21.
12. Sanchis R, Sancho-Tello M, Chirivella M, et al. The role of maternal alcohol damage on ethanol teratogenicity in the rat. *Teratology* 1987;36:199–208.
13. Hillbom ME, Sarviharju MS, Lindros KO. Potentiation of ethanol toxicity by cyanamide in relation to acetaldehyde accumulation. *Toxicol Appl Pharmacol* 1983;70:133–9.
14. Sreenathan RN, Padmanabhan R, Singh S. Teratogenic effects of acetaldehyde in the rat. *Drug Alcohol Depend* 1982;9:339–50.
15. Sreenathan RN, Singh S, Padmanabhan R. Effect of acetaldehyde on skeletogenesis in rats. *Drug Alcohol Depend* 1984;14:165–74.
16. Nuutinen H, Lindros K, Hekali P, Salaspuro M. Elevated blood acetate as indicator of fast ethanol elimination in chronic alcoholics. *Alcohol* 1985;2:623–6.
17. Ueno Y, Adachi J, Imamichi H, et al. Effect of the cytochrome P-45IIE1 genotype on ethanol elimination rate in alcoholics and control subjects. *Alcohol Clin Exp Res* 1996;20:17–21A.
18. Frezza M, Di Padova C, Pozzato et al. High blood alcohol levels in women. The role of decreased gastric alcohol dehydrogenase activity and first-pass metabolism. *N Engl J Med* 1990;322:95–9.
19. DiPadova C, Worner TM, Julkunen RJ, Lieber CS. Effects of fasting and chronic alcohol consumption on the first-pass metabolism of ethanol. *Gastroenterology* 1987;92:1169–73.
20. Adachi J, Mizoi Y, Fukunaga T, et al. Comparative study on ethanol elimination and blood acetaldehyde between alcoholics and control subjects. *Alcohol Clin Exp Res* 1989;13:601–4.
21. Nuutinen HU, Salaspuro MP, Valle M, Lindros KO. Blood acetaldehyde concentration gradient between hepatic and antecubital venous blood in ethanol-intoxicated alcoholics and controls. *Eur J Clin Invest* 1984;14;306–11.
22. Palmer KR, Jenkins WJ. Impaired acetaldehyde oxidation in alcoholics. *Gut* 1982;23:729–33.
23. Takase S, Yasuhara M, Takada A, Ueshima Y. Changes in blood acetaldehyde levels after ethanol administration in alcoholics. *Alcohol* 1990;7:37–41.
24. Nuutinen HH, Lindros KO, Salaspuro M. Determinants of blood acetaldehyde level during ethanol oxidation in chronic alcoholics. *Alcohol Clin Exp Res* 1983;7:163–8.
25. Lindros KO, Stowell A. Pikkarainen P, Salaspuro M. Elevated blood acetaldehyde in alcoholics with accelerated ethanol elimination. *Pharmacol Biochem Behav* 1980;13(Suppl 1):119–24.
26. Veghelyi PV, Osztovics M. The alcohol syndromes: The intrarecombigenic effect of acetaldehyde. *Experientia* 1978;34:195–6.
27. Veghelyi PV. Fetal abnormality ad maternal ethanol metabolism [letter]. *Lancet* 1983;2:53–4.
28. Niemela O, Halmesmaki E, Ylikorkala O. Hemoglobin-acetaldehyde adducts are elevated in women carrying alcohol-damaged fetuses. *Alcohol Clin Exp Res* 1991;15:1007–10.
29. Einarson TR, Pharmacoeconomic applications of meta-analysis for single groups using antifungal onychomycosis lacquers as an example. *Clin Ther* 1997;19:559–69.
30. Harada S, Agarwal DP, Goedde HW, Takagi S. Blood ethanol and acetaldehyde levels in Japanese alcoholics and controls. *Pharmacol Biochem Behav* 1983;18(suppl 1):139–40.
31. DiPadova C, Worner TM, Lieber CS. Effect of abstinence on the blood acetaldehyde response to a test dose of alcohol in alcoholics. *Alcohol Clin Exp Res* 1987;11:559–61.
32. Peters TJ, Ward RJ, Rideout J, Lim CK. Blood acetaldehyde and ethanol levels in alcoholism. *Prog Clin Biol Res* 1987;241:215–30.
33. Cobden I, Matthewson K, Carr WP, et al. Effect of ethanol challenge on serum glycoproteins in alcoholic and nonalcoholic liver disease. *Alcohol Alcoholism* 1987;22:257–63.
34. Lucas D, Menez JF, Berthou F, et al. Determination of free acetaldehyde in blood as the dinitrophenylhydrazone derivative by high-performance liquid chromatography. *J Chromatogr* 1986;382:57–66.
35. Shaskan EG, Dolinsky ZS. Elevated endogenous breath acetaldehyde levels among abusers of alcohol and cigarettes. *Prog Neuropsychopharmacol Biol Psychiatry* 1985;9:267–72.
36. Hesselbrock VM, Shaskan EG. Endogenous breath acetaldehyde levels among alcoholic and non-alcoholic probands: effect of alcohol use and smoking. *Prog Neuropsychopharmacol Biol Psychiatry* 1985; 9:259–65.
37. Eriksson CJ, Peachey JE. Lack of difference in blood acetaldehyde of alcoholics and controls after ethanol ingestion. *Pharmacol Biochem Behav* 1980;13(suppl 1):101–5.
38. Maring JA, Weigand K, Brenner HD, Von Wartburg JP. Aldehyde oxidizing capacity of erythrocytes in normal and alcoholic individuals. *Pharmacol Biochem Behav* 1983;18(suppl 1):135–8.
39. Uppal R, Rosman A, Hernandez R, et al. Effects of liver disease on red blood cell acetaldehyde in alcoholics and non-alcoholics. *Alcohol Alcoholism* 1991;Supp 1:323–6.
40. Hernandez-Munoz R, Ma XL, Baraona E, Lieber CS. Member of acetaldehyde measurement with minimal artifactual formation in red blood cells and plasma of actively drinking subjects with alcoholism. *J Lab Clin Med* 1992;120:35–41.
41. Baraona E, Di Padova C, Tabasco J, Lieber CS. Red blood cells: a new major modality for acetaldehyde transport from liver to other tissues. *Life Sci* 1987;40:253–8.
42. Peterson CM, Polizzi CM. Improved method for acetaldehyde in plasma and hemoglobin-associated acetaldehyde: results in teetotaler and alcoholics reporting for treatment. *Alcohol* 1987;4: 477–80.
43. Matthewson K, Al Mardini H, Barlett K, Record CO. Impaired acetaldehyde metabolism in patients with noon-alcoholic liver disorders. *Gut* 1986;27:756–64.
44. Brien JF, Peachey JE, Loomis CW. Calcium carbimide–ethanol interaction. *Clin Pharmacol Ther* 1980;27:426–33.
45. Wicht F, Fisch HU, Nelles J, et al. Divergence of ethanol and acetaldehyde kinetics and of the disulfiram–alcohol reaction between subjects with and without alcoholic liver disease. *Alcohol Clin Exp Res* 1995;19:356–61.
46. Peachey JE, Brien JF, Zilm DH, et al. The calcium cyanamide–ethanol interaction in man. Effects of repeated ethanol administration. *J Stud Alcohol* 1981;42:208–16.
47. Helander A, Lowenmo C, Johansson M. Distribution of acetaldehyde in human blood: effects of ethanol and treatment with disulfiram. *Alcohol Alcoholism* 1993;28:461–8.
48. Panés J, Caballeria J, Guitart R, et al. Determinants of ethanol and acetaldehyde metabolism in chronic alcoholics. *Alcohol Clin Exp Res* 1992;17:48–53.
49. Sampson PD, Streissguth AP, Bookstein FL, et al. Incidence of fetal alcohol syndrome and prevalence of alcohol-related neurodevelopmental disorder. *Teratology* 1997;56:317–26.
50. Tanka H. Fetal alcohol syndrome: a Japanese perspective. *Ann Med* 1998;302:21–26.
51. Leversha AM, Marks RE. The prevalence of fetal alcohol syndrome in New Zealand. *NZ Med J* 1995;108:502–5.
52. Cadle RG, Dawson T, Hall BD. The prevalence of genetic disorders, birth defects and syndromes in central and eastern Kentucky. *J Ky Med Assoc* 1996;94:237–41.
53. Williams RJ, Odaibo FS, McGee JM. Incidence of fetal alcohol syndrome in northeastern Manitoba. *Can J Public Health* 1999;90:192–4.
54. Habbick BF, Nanson JL, Snyder RE, et al. Fetal alcohol syndrome in Saskatchewan: unchanged incidence in a 20-year period. *Can J Public Health* 1996;87:204–7.

55. Miller LA, Shaikh T, Stanton C, et al. Surveillance for fetal alcohol syndrome in Colorado. *Public Health Rep* 1995;110:690–7.
56. Mena M, Casanueva V, Fernandez E, et al. Fetal alcohol syndrome at schools for mentally handicapped children in Concepcion, Chile. *Bull Pan Am Health Organ* 1986;20:157–69.
57. Egeland GM, Perham-Hester KA, Hook EB. Use of capture-recapture analyses in fetal alcohol syndrome surveillance in Alaska. *Am J Epidemiol* 1995;141:335–41.
58. Palmer C. Fetal alcohol effects–incidence and understanding in the Cape [letter]. *S Afr Med J* 1985;68:779–80.
59. Sokol RJ, Martier S, Ager J, et al. Fetal alcohol syndrome (FAS): new definition, new prospective sample, same etiology [abstract]. *Alcohol Clin Exp Res* 2000;17:260.
60. Abel EL, Sokol RJ. A revised conservative estimate of the incidence of FAS and its economic impact. *Alcohol Clin Exp Res* 1991;15:514–24.
61. Fried PA, O'Connell CM. A comparison of the effects of prenatal exposure to tobacco, alcohol, cannabis and caffeine on birth size and subsequent growth. *Neurotoxicol Teratol* 1987;9:79–85.
62. Gibson GT, Baghurst PA, Colley DP. Maternal alcohol, tobacco and cannabis consumption and the outcome of pregnancy. *Aust NZ J Obster Gynaecol* 1983;23:15–9.
63. Walpole I, Zubrick S, Pontre J. Is there a fetal effect with low to moderate alcohol use before or during pregnancy? *J Epidemiol Community Health* 1990;44:297–301.
64. May PA, Hymbaugh KJ, Aase JM, Samet JM. Epidemiology of fetal alcohol syndrome among American Indians of the Southwest. *Soc Biol* 1983;30:374–87.
65. Vitez M, Koranyi G, Gonczy E, et al. A semiquantitative score system for epidemiology studies of fetal alcohol syndrome. *Am J Epidemiol* 1984;119:301–8.
66. Hingson R, Alpert JJ, Day N, et al. Effects of maternal drinking and marijuana use on fetal growth and development. *Pediatrics* 1982;70:539–46.
67. Day NL, Jasperse D, Richardson G, et al. Prenatal exposure to alcohol: effect on infant growth and morphologic characteristics. *Pediatrics* 1989;84:536–41.
68. Stoler JM, Holmes LB. Under-recognition of prenatal alcohol effects in infants of known alcohol-abusing women. *J Pediatr* 1999;135:430–6.
69. Kaminski M, Franc M, Lebouvier M, et al. Moderate alcohol use and pregnancy outcome. *Neurobehav Toxicol Teratol* 1981;3:173–81.
70. Primatesta P, Del Corno G, Bonazzi MC, Waters WE. Alcohol and pregnancy: an international comparison. *J Public Health Med* 1993;15:69–76.
71. Lumley J, Correy JF, Newman NM, Curran JT. Cigarette smoking, alcohol consumption and fetal outcome in Tasmania 1981–82. *Aust NZ J Obstet Gynaecol* 1985;25:33–40.
72. Verkerk PH, Noord-Zaadstra BM, Florey CD, et al. The effect of moderate maternal alcohol consumption on birth weight and gestational age in a low-risk population. *Early Hum Dev* 1993;32:121–9.
73. Wright JT, Waterson EJ, Barrison IG, et al. Alcohol consumption, pregnancy, and low birthweight. *Lancet* 1983;1:663–5.
74. Abel EL, Hanningan JH. "J-shaped" relationship between drinking during pregnancy and birth weight: reanalysis of prospective epidemiological data. *Alcohol Alcoholism* 1995;30:345–55.
75. Little RE, Streissguth AP, Barr HM, Herman CS. Decreased birth weight in infants of alcoholic women who abstained during pregnancy. *J Pediatr* 1980;96:974–7.
76. Russell M. Intrauterine growth in infants born to women with alcohol-related psychiatric diagnoses. *Alcohol Clin Exp Res* 1977; 1:225–31.
77. Sokol RJ, Ager J, Martier S, et al. Significant determinants of susceptibility to alcohol teratogenicity. *Ann NY Acad Sci* 1986; 477:87–102.
78. Jones KL, Smith DW, Streissguth AP, Myrianthopoulos NC. Outcome in offspring of chronic alcoholic women. *Lancet* 1974;1:1076–8.
79. Robinson GC, Conry JL, Conry RF. Clinical profile and prevalence of fetal alcohol syndrome in an isolated community in British Columbia. *Can Med Assoc J* 1987;137:203–7.
80. Silva VA, Laranjeira RR, Dolnikoff M, et al. Alcohol consumption during pregnancy and newborn outcome: a study in Brazil. *Neurobehav Toxicol Teratol* 1981;3:169–72.
81. Olegard R, Sabel KG, Aronsson M, et al. Effects on the child of alcohol abuse during pregnancy. Retrospective and prospective studies. *Acta Paediatr Scand Suppl* 1979;275:112–21.
82. Hanson JW, Streissguth AP, Smith DW. The effects of moderate alcohol consumption during pregnancy on fetal growth and morphogenesis. *J Pediatr* 1978;92:457–60.
83. Autti-Ramo I, Gaily E, Granstrom ML. Dysmorphic feature in offspring of alcoholic mothers. *Arch Dis Child* 1992;67:712–16.
84. Larsson G. Prevention of fetal alcohol effects. An antenatal program for early detection of pregnancies at risk. *Acta Obstet Gynecol Scand* 1983;62:171–8.
85. Larsson G, Ottenblad C, Hagenfeldt L, et al. Evaluation of serum gamma-glutamyl transferase as a screening method for excessive alcohol consumption during pregnancy. *Am J Obstet Gynecol* 1983;147:654–7.
86. Halmesmaki E. Alcohol counselling of 85 pregnant problem drinkers: effect on drinking and fetal outcome. *Br J Obstet Gynaecol* 1988;95:243–7.
87. Rostand A, Kaminski M, Lelong N, et al. Alcohol use in pregnancy, craniofacial features, and fetal growth. *J Epidemiol Community Health* 1990;44:302–6.
88. Maillard T, Lamblin D, Lessure JF, Fourmaintraux A. Incidence of fetal alcohol syndrome on the southern part of Reunion Island (France). *Teratology* 1999;60:51–52.
89. Sokol RJ, Miller SI, Reed G. Alcohol abuse during pregnancy: an epidemiologic study. *Alcohol Clin Exp Res* 1980;4:135–45.
90. Ouellette EM, Rosett HL, Rosman NP, Weiner L. Adverse effects on offspring of maternal alcohol abuse during pregnancy. *N Engl J Med* 1977;297:528–30.
91. Iosub S, Fuchs M, Bingol N, et al. Incidence of major congenital malformations in offspring of alcoholics and polydrug abusers. *Alcohol* 1985;2:521–3.
92. Eriksson CJ. Human blood acetaldehyde concentration during ethanol oxidation (update 1982). *Pharmacol Biochem Behav* 1983;18(Suppl 1):141–50.
93. Eriksson CJ, Fukunaga T. Human blood acetaldehyde (update 1992). *Alcohol Alcoholism* 1993;2(Supp):9–25.
94. DeMaster EG, Redfern B, Weir K, et al. Elimination of artifactual acetaldehyde in the measurement of human blood acetaldehyde by the use of polyethylene glycol and sodium azide: normal blood acetaldehyde levels in the dog and human after ethanol. *Alcohol Clin Exp Res* 1983;7:436–42.
95. Thomas M, Halsall S, Peters TJ. Role of hepatic acetaldehyde dehydrogenase in alcoholism: demonstration of persistent reduction of cytosolic activity in abstaining patients. *Lancet* 1982;2:1057–8.
96. Palmer KR, Jenkins WJ. Aldehyde dehydrogenase in alcoholic subjects. *Hepatology* 1985;5:260–3.
97. Astley SJ, Bailey D, Talbot C, Clarren SK. Fetal alcohol syndrome primary prevention through FAS diagnosis: I. Identification of high-risk birth mothers through the diagnosis of their children. *Alcohol Alcoholism* 2000;35:499–508.

CHAPTER 38

MODERATE TO HEAVY CAFFEINE CONSUMPTION DURING PREGNANCY AND RELATIONSHIP TO SPONTANEOUS ABORTION AND ABNORMAL FETAL GROWTH: A META-ANALYSIS

Olavo Fernandes, Mona Sabharwal,* Tom Smiley,* Anne Pastuszak,† Gideon Koren,† and Thomas Einarson*†‡*

**Doctor of Pharmacy Program, Faculty of Pharmacy, University of Toronto;† The Motherisk Program, The Division of Clinical Pharmacology and Toxicology, Department of Pediatrics and Research, The Hospital for Sick Children; and ‡Department of Health Administration, Faculty of Medicine, University of Toronto, Toronto, Canada*

Abstract

The objective was to determine the association of moderate to heavy caffeine consumption during pregnancy on spontaneous abortion and birth weight in humans. Data sources used included a computerized literature search of MEDLINE (1966–July 1996); EMBASE (1988–November 1996); Psychlit I (1974–1986); Psychlit II (1987–1996); CINAHL (1982–May 1996) and manual search of bibliographies of pertinent articles. Inclusion criteria were: English language research articles; pregnant human females; case control or cohort design; documented quantity of caffeine consumption during pregnancy; control group with minimal or no caffeine consumption (0 to 150 mg caffeine/d); documented data regarding spontaneous abortion and/or fetal growth. The exclusion criteria were: case reports; editorials; review papers. The methods section of each study was examined independently by two blinded investigators with a third investigator adjudicating disagreements. Two independent investigators extracted data onto a standardized form. A third investigator adjudicated discrepancies. We compared a caffeine-exposed group (> 150 mg/d) and controls (0 to 150 mg/d), using Mantel–Haenszel pooling. Of the 32 studies meeting inclusion criteria, 12 had extractable data (6 for spontaneous abortion, 7 for low birth weight, 1 common study). Mantel–Haenszel odds ratio ($CI_{95\%}$) was 1.36 (1.29–1.45) for spontaneous abortion in 42,988 pregnancies. The overall risk ratio was 1.51 (1.39–1.63) for low birthweight (<2500 g) in 64,268 pregnancies. Control for cofounders such as maternal age, smoking, and ethanol use was not possible. We concluded that there is a small but statistically significant increase in the risks for spontaneous abortion and low birthweight babies in pregnant women consuming > 150 mg caffeine per d. A possible contribution to these results of maternal age, smoking, ethanol use, or other confounders could not be excluded. (c) 1998 Elsevier Science Inc.

Keywords: caffeine; pregnancy; spontaneous abortion; congenital malformations.

INTRODUCTION

In 1980, the United States Food and Drug Administration issued a warning regarding the use of caffeine during pregnancy (1). While conclusions about human teratogenicity could not be definite at that time, the FDA suggested that as a precautionary measure, pregnant women should be advised to avoid or limit their consumption of food or drugs containing caffeine. Due to the large worldwide consumption of caffeinated beverages (e.g., coffee, tea, cola) it is important to know whether such a warning is actually warranted. Should caffeine consumption during pregnancy be linked to adverse effects such as spontaneous abortion or fetal growth retardation, that finding would have important implications for public health. Furthermore, the potential impact of that association is underscored by the fact that low birth weight is associated with high mortality and morbidity in neonates.

Caffeine clearance from the body is essentially unchanged during the first trimester of pregnancy. However, a significant delay in elimination occurs in the second and third trimester, as the half life of caffeine extends to 10.5 h from a normal half life of 2.5 to 4.5 h in the nonpregnant woman (2). Caffeine is known to readily cross the placenta. Substantial quantities pass into the amniotic fluid, umbilical cord blood, and the urine and plasma of neonates. In addition, the human fetus and neonate have low levels of the enzymes necessary for caffeine metabolism.

Several mechanisms for caffeine to produce adverse outcomes have been postulated. For example, caffeine increases cellular cyclic adenosine monophosphate (cAMP) through phosphodiesterase inhibition. The rise in cAMP may interfere with fetal cell growth and development (3).

Animal studies of caffeine and pregnancy outcomes have reported considerable variability in results. Some studies have suggested a link between caffeine and teratogenesis, fetal resorption, and decreased fetal weight (4,5). An increase in the malformation rate, specifically cleft palate and ectrodactyly, was demonstrated in rats and mice at caffeine doses of 100 mg/kg/d or more (5). This effect was not seen at doses of 50 mg/kg/d. It is important to note that humans ingest caffeine at significantly lower doses of 1.7 to 4.5 mg/kg/d (5).

Epidemiologic studies have produced incomplete or conflicting results concerning the effects of caffeine exposure during pregnancy. To date, we are unaware of a formal meta-analysis quantifying the potential risks. Therefore, the present meta-analysis was conducted to determine the association of moderate to heavy caffeine consumption during pregnancy on spontaneous abortion and birth weight in humans.

Address correspondence to Dr. Koren at the Hospital For Sick Children, 555 University Avenue, Toronto, ON, M5G 1X8 Canada.

Received 24 *October* 1997; *Final revision received* 1 *April* 1998; *Accepted* 4 *April* 1998.

MATERIALS AND METHODS

Original research studies investigating the effects of moderate to heavy caffeine consumption during pregnancy on spontaneous abortion and fetal growth in humans were examined using meta-analysis based on methods described by Einarson et al. (6). *Spontaneous abortion* was defined for this analysis as expulsion from the uterus of products of conception before the fetus is viable (approximately 20 weeks of gestation). Included in the definition were fetal loss, fetal death, and miscarriage. *Fetal growth* was defined by standard measures that included birth weight, birth weight for gestational age, birth weight by percentile, body length, and head circumference. *Low birth weight* was defined as birth weight less than 2500 g and intrauterine growth retardation (IUGR) was defined as birth weight less than the tenth percentile for gestational age (7).

Values for *caffeine content* of beverages and foods were recorded as defined by the caffeine content in milligrams outlined in each individual study. If the caffeine content was not presented in milligrams (mg), then the following standard conversions were used: one cup of coffee was equivalent to 74 mg of caffeine and one cup of tea was equivalent to 27 mg of caffeine (8). Due to the nature of caffeine consumption, a group of pregnant women with absolute non-exposure to caffeine is difficult to find. We recognize that the term *control group* has several different meanings in epidemiology. For the purposes of this meta-analysis, the *control* was defined as a group exposed to minimal or no caffeine (0 to 150 mg caffeine/d). *Moderate caffeine consumption* was defined as 151 to 300 mg caffeine/d and *heavy caffeine consumption* was >300 mg caffeine/d.

Search Strategy

A computerized literature search was completed using the following databases: MEDLINE (1966–December 1996); EMBASE (1988–November 1996); Psychlit I (1974–1986) and Psychlit II (1987–1996); CINAHL (1982–May 1996). Articles examining the relationship between caffeine consumption and pregnancy were identified using the search terms "pregnancy and caffeine" along with "pregnancy outcome and caffeine." Search terms were initially kept as broad as possible in order to ensure that articles that were not indexed strictly by the desired outcomes (i.e., spontaneous abortion and fetal growth) were not missed. All abstracts retrieved from the computer search were independently reviewed by at least two investigators to identify articles relating to the desired outcomes. Additional references were identified from bibliographies of retrieved articles and selected reviews (4,5,9,10).

Study Selection

An independent review was conducted by removing all identifiers and having two investigators independently evaluate the methods sections of all retrieved articles using a checklist of the inclusion and exclusion criteria. The inclusion criteria for the meta-analysis were: English language articles; pregnant human females; case control or cohort design; caffeine exposure during pregnancy; documented quantity of caffeine consumption; control group with minimal or no caffeine consumption (0 to 150 mg caffeine/d); and documented data regarding spontaneous abortion and/or fetal growth. Case reports or case series, editorials, and review articles were excluded. Reviewers were blinded to journal names, author names and study results. In the event that agreement could not be reached between the two reviewers or if sufficient information was not provided in the methods sections, a third investigator was consulted who served as the adjudicator. If the adjudicator could not reach a decision based on the methods section alone, the entire paper was reviewed by all judges.

Data Extraction

Data extraction was performed on all included articles independently by two investigators who were blinded to the journal and authors' names. Data were extracted using a standardized form that recorded study characteristics, sample characteristics, caffeine content stratification, confounding factors, and outcome results in both caffeine and control groups. Extracted quantitative data for spontaneous abortion and fetal growth were entered in 2×2 tables for control and caffeine groups. Data extraction forms were reviewed for agreement by a third investigator, who conducted an individual assessment of the study if there was a disagreement in values or information.

Statistical Methods

Odds ratios were calculated for individual case control studies and risk ratios were calculated for individual cohort studies along with associated 95% confidence intervals. A combined Mantel–Haenszel odds ratio (11) was calculated for each outcome comparison and an overall 95% confidence interval was calculated by the method described by Miettinen (12). In the event that all the combined studies were cohort studies, an overall Mantel–Haenszel relative risk ratio was calculated. A Q value (χ^2) and P-value for homogeneity of samples was calculated using standard statistical methods. A level of $P < 0.05$ (two-tailed) was considered significant for all statistical tests. For each outcome, the main analysis comprised of a comparison of a caffeine exposure group (> 150 mg caffeine/d) to a control group (0 to 150 mg caffeine/d). Subgroup and sensitivity analyses were performed to investigate comparisons among moderate, heavy, control, and zero caffeine consumption levels; research design (i.e., cohort and case control studies); the effect of large studies; and the effect of adding studies that did not meet the meta-analysis caffeine content stratification criteria to identify and evaluate possible changes to odds ratios and relative risk ratios.

RESULTS

Study Selection

Over 275 abstracts of articles dealing with caffeine exposure in pregnancy published between 1966 and 1996 were identified by the initial search strategy. Upon examination of these abstracts and review articles, 32 papers were identified as potentially eligible and were entered into the study selection process (13–44). After the blinded independent study selection process, 21 articles (13–33) met the inclusion criteria and were potentially eligible for the meta-analysis. Interobserver agreement was 87% after the initial application of the inclusion criteria. However, full consensus was reached after adjudication. The data extraction process was performed on the 21 articles. During this process, an additional nine studies were studies were excluded. Table 1 outlines excluded studies and reasons for rejection. A total of 12 studies were accepted into the analysis process (six studies for the spontaneous abortion outcome (16,17,27,29–31) and seven studies (19–23,30,32) for the fetal growth outcome, which includes one study (30) that was accepted for both outcome. At this time, two additional studies (23,30) were excluded from the main analysis and used only for

Table 1
Excluded Studies and Reasons for Rejection

Barr et al. (35) Pastore and Savitz (37) Peacock et al. (42) Rosenberg et al. (36) Wisborg et al. (44)	Do not contain desired outcomes as defined by our inclusion criteria
Fried and O'Connell (34) Godel et al. (41) Kline et al. (40) Larroque et al. (38)	Control group not identified as defined by our inclusion criteria
Shu et al. (26) Watkinson and Fried (13) Wilcox et al. (28)	Data not combinable according to our caffeine stratification criteria (rejected on attempt to extract data)
Barr and Streissguth (14) Munoz et al. (43) Peacock et al. (25) Vandenberg (39) Weathersbee et al. (15)	Data not extractable
Beaulac-Baillargeon and Desrosiers (18) Desrosiers (18) Furuhashi et al. (33) Olsen et al. (24)	Control group not defined by study

sensitivity analyses since their caffeine stratification did not meet the exact caffeine stratification definitions for combinability. Tables 2 and 3 summarize characteristics of accepted studies.

Spontaneous Abortion

Table 4 presents odds ratios and risk ratios for individual studies for spontaneous abortion. In the main analysis, comparing spontaneous abortions in the caffeine exposure group (>150 mg caffeine/d) to the control group, a total of five studies (16,17,27,29,31) were included (three cohort and two case control studies) involving a total of 42,889 patients. The combined odds ratio ($CI_{95\%}$) was 1.36 (1.29–1.45) with Q = 21.21 ($P < 0.001$) for heterogeneity of outcome. Table 5 outlines the type and results of sensitivity analysis, which did not greatly alter the odds ratio. However, the removal of one study (31) greatly improved the homogeneity of the analysis (Q = 3.52, $P < 0.318$). Due to caffeine stratification of the accepted studies, a comparison of the control to "zero" caffeine consumption was not possible.

Fetal Growth

All seven accepted studies measured fetal growth according to low birth weight (<2500 g). Two of those studies also evaluated intrauterine growth retardation (IUGR). Table 6 outlines individual odds ratios and risk ratios for individual studies used in the low birth weight outcome comparison. In the main analysis, comparing low birth weight babies in the caffeine exposure group (>150 mg caffeine/d) to the control group, a total of five studies (19–22,32) were included (all cohort designs) involving a total of 64,268 patients (Table 7). The combined relative risk was 1.51 (1.39–1.63) with Q = 8.72 ($P = 0.068$) for heterogeneity of outcome. Table 7 outlines the type and results of sensitivity analysis, which did not greatly alter the summary relative risk. Further subgroup analyses on the low birth weight outcome are also displayed in Table 7. The risk ratios ($CI_{95\%}$) for comparisons of moderate caffeine consumption to control was 1.33 (1.21–1.47), 1.81 (1.61–2.04) comparing heavy caffeine consumption to control, and 1.38 (1.20–1.60) comparing heavy caffeine consumption to moderate caffeine consumption. A risk ratio of 1.06 (1.00–1.13) resulted from our comparison of the control to "zero" caffeine consumption. As this risk ratio included unity, it validated our choice of control group (0 to 150 mg caffeine/d). A combined risk ratio of 1.56 (1.34–1.82) was calculated for two studies (19,21) that investigated IUGR, which supports our data for low birth weight.

DISCUSSION

Epidemiologic studies involving caffeine consumption by pregnant women have resulted in differing results concerning adverse fetal outcomes. This meta-analysis was designed to examine the risk of spontaneous abortion and fetal growth retardation, as these two outcomes are sources of significant morbidity, mortality, and societal burden in terms of costs.

Table 2
Relationship Between Caffeine Exposure and Spontaneous Abortion: Summary of Study Characteristics

ARTICLE	STUDY DESIGN	*n*	SOURCES OF CAFFEINE IDENTIFIED	CAFFEINE CONVERSION FACTORS (mg/cup UNLESS SPECIFIED)
Armstrong et al. (17)	cohort, retrospective	35,848	coffee	not specified
Dominguez-Rojas et al. (31)	cohort, retrospective	691	coffee	coffee: 140
Fenster et al. (27)	case control, retrospective	852 cases 1618 controls	coffee, tea, cola	coffee: 107; tea: 34; cola: 47 mg/can
Infante-Rivard et al. (29)	case control, retrospective	331 cases 993 controls	coffee, tea, cola	coffee: 107; tea: 34; cola: 47 mg/can
Mills et al. (30)	cohort, prospective	423	coffee, tea, cola, cocoa, medications	coffee: 100; tea: 40; cocoa: 30; cola: 40 mg/can; decaffeinated coffee: 1.5

Table 3
Relationship Between Caffeine Exposure and Fetal Growth: Summary of Study Characteristics

ARTICLE	STUDY DESIGN	*n*	SOURCES OF CAFFEINE IDENTIFIED	CAFFEINE CONVERSION FACTORS (mg/cup UNLESS SPECIFIED)
Caan and Goldhaber (23)	case control, retrospective	131 cases 136 controls	coffee, tea, cola,	not specified
Fenster et al. (21)	cohort, retrospective	1,230	coffee, tea, cola,	coffee: 107; tea: 34; cola: 47 mg/can;
Fortier et al. (19)	cohort, retrospective	7,025	coffee, tea, cola, chocolate	coffee: filtered or percolated 109 mg; instant 74 mg; expresso 168 mg; tea: bag 49 leaves or instant 30 mg; cola: 29 mg; chocolate: 56 mg
Linn et al. (32)	cohort, retrospective	12,205	coffee, tea	not specified
Martin and Bracken (20)	cohort, prospective	3,891	coffee, tea, cola, medications	coffee: 107 mg; tea: 34; cola: 47 mg/serving
McDonald et al. (22)	cohort, retrospective	40,445	coffee	not specified
Mills et al. (30)	cohort, prospective	423	coffee, tea, cola, cocoa, medications	coffee: 100; tea: 40; cola: 40 mg/can; cocoa: 30 mg; decaffeinated coffee: 1.5

Table 4
Results of Individual Studies Comparing Spontaneous Abortions in Caffeine Exposure (>150 Caffeine mg/d) to Control Groups (0 to 150 Caffeine mg/d)

	CAFFEINE EXPOSURE >150 mg/d		CONTROLS		
ARTICLE	SPONTANEOUS ABORTION	NO SPONTANEOUS ABORTION	SPONTANEOUS ABORTION	NO SPONTANEOUS ABORTION	OR/RR (95% CI)
Armstrong et al. (17)	1,577	4,564	6,183	23,524	RR = 1.23 (1.18–1.29)
Dominguez-Rojas et al. (31)	146	329	23	193	RR = 2.89 (1.92–4.35)
Fenster et al. (27)	152	256	455	1,028	OR = 1.34 (1.07–1.69)
Infante-Rivard et al. (29)	92	186	239	807	OR = 1.67 (1.25–2.22)
Mills et al. (30)[a]	43	291	16	70	RR = 1.44 (0.86–2.44)
Srisuphan and Bracken (16)	27	852	41	2,215	RR = 1.69 (1.05–2.73)
Summary odds ratio					OR = 1.36 (1.29–1.45)

OR/RR = odds/risk ratio calculated with the Mantel-Haenszel formula; 95% CI = 95% confidence interval for odds ratio.
[a] not included in summary odds ratio as study's caffeine stratification of groups did not meet the exact caffeine stratification definitions or combinability in the meta-analysis (assumptions made to test data as a sensitivity analysis as described in Methods).

Table 5
Combined Results of Studies Comparing Spontaneous Abortion in Caffeine Exposure (>150 mg Caffeine/d) to Control Groups (0 to 150 mg Caffeine/d)

				TEST FOR HOMOGENEITY		
ANALYSIS	*n*	SUMMARY RATIO	95% CI	Q	DF	*P*
Primary analysis (Studies 16, 17, 27, 29, 31)	42,889	OR = 1.36	1.29–1.45	21.21	4	<0.001
Cohort studies only	39,674	RR = 1.26	1.20–1.33	13.52	2	0.001
Case control studies only	3,215	OR = 1.46	1.22–1.74	1.36	1	0.244
Sensitivity: removing study #17		OR = 1.69	1.45–1.98	14.48	3	0.002
Sensitivity: adding in study #30		OR = 1.37	1.29–1.45	21.38	5	<0.001
Sensitivity: removing outlier study #31		OR = 1.33	1.26–1.42	3.52	3	0.318

DF = degrees of freedom.

Table 6
Results of Individual Studies Comparing Low Birth Weight Caffeine Exposure (>150 mg Caffeine/d) to Control Groups (0 to 150 mg Caffeine/d)

	CAFFEINE EXPOSURE >150 mg/d		CONTROLS		
ARTICLE	LBW	BIRTH WEIGHT >2500 g	LBW	BIRTH WEIGHT >2500 g	OR/RR (95% CI)
Caan, Goldhaber (23)†[a]	34	27	96	108	OR = 1.42 (0.79–2.52)
Fenster et al. (21)	26	217	61	926	RR = 1.73 (1.12–2.68)
Fortier et al. (19)	79	1,156	242	5,251	RR = 1.45 (1.14–1.86)
Linn et al. (32)	116	1,152	839	10,098	RR = 1.19 (0.99–1.49)
Martin and Bracken (20)	32	987	38	2,603	RR = 2.18 (1.37–3.47)
McDonald et al. (22)	455	5,001	1,837	33,152	RR = 1.59 (1.44–1.75)
Mills et al. (30)[a]	5	82	16	320	RR = 1.21 (0.46–3.20)
Summary odds ratio					OR = 1.51 (1.39–1.63)

OR/RR = odds/risk ratio from individual studies; 95% CI = 95% confidence interval for odds ratio. LBW = low birth weight defined as birth weight < 2500 g.

[a] not included in summary odds ratio as study's caffeine stratification of groups did not meet the exact caffeine stratification definitions for combinability in the meta-analysis (assumptions made to test data as a sensitivity analysis as described in Methods).

This meta-analysis indicates a modest but statistically significant relationship between moderate to heavy caffeine consumption in pregnancy and the risk for spontaneous abortion and low birth weight. In order to reasonably assess the implications of these findings, the results of subgroup and sensitivity analyses must be examined along with the limitations of the accepted studies.

Defining an appropriate reference group was a challenge in this analysis. Most of the studies did not explicitly differentiate low-exposed and unexposed groups. The control group (0 to 150 mg caffeine/d) was chosen based on the large number of studies that utilized this categorization as "light" caffeine users (<150 mg/d). Results of the sensitivity analysis comparing "zero" caffeine intake to the control group (0 to 150 mg/d) validated the assumption that less than 150 mg of caffeine consumption per d constituted an appropriate control group for our meta-analyses. Srisuphan et al. (16) reported similar findings in their research, which explored caffeine consumption and the risk of spontaneous abortion. They postulated a possible "threshold effect" of around 150 mg/d, reasoning that intake below this level would not be enough caffeine to affect the fetus in terms of cell growth, cell division, or utero-placental circulation.

Spontaneous Abortion

The analysis indicates a small but significant relationship between moderate to heavy caffeine consumption and the risk for spontaneous

Table 7
Combined Results of Studies Examining Low Birth Weight

		SUMMARY		HOMOGENEITY		
ANALYSIS	*n*	RATIO	95% CI	Q	DF	*P*
Primary analysis (Studies 19–22, 32)[a]	64,268	RR = 1.51	1.39–1.63	8.72	4	0.068
Sensitivity: removing study #22		RR = 1.38	1.20–1.57	6.53	3	0.088
Sensitivity: adding study #30		RR = 1.50	1.39–1.63	8.91	5	0.113
Sensitivity: adding study #23		OR = 1.55	1.42–1.69	9.55	5	0.089
Combined results comparing LBW in moderate[b] caffeine exposure to control[c] group (19–22, 32)	61,374	RR = 1.33	1.21–1.47	6.97	4	0.137
Combined results analysis comparing LBW in heavy[d] caffeine exposure to control[c] group (19–22, 32)	58,013	RR = 1.81	1.61–2.04	10.98	4	0.029
Combined results analysis comparing LBW in heavy[d] caffeine exposure to moderate[b] group (19–22, 32)	9,221	RR = 1.38	1.20–1.60	2.76	4	0.598
Combined results analysis comparing LBW in "zero"[e] caffeine exposure to control [c] group (19–22, 32)	82,640	RR = 1.06	1.00–1.13	3.07	4	0.546

LBW = low birth weight defined as birth weight <2500 g.

[a] Main analysis compares caffeine exposure (>150 mg/d) to control group.

[b] 150 to 300 mg caffeine/d

[c] 0 to 150 mg caffeine/d.

[d] >300 mg caffeine/d.

[e] Groups designated as having no caffeine intake.

abortion. The study by Armstrong and colleagues (17) contributed heavily to the sample size of this analysis. When that study was removed from the main analysis (Table 5), the odds ratio increased to 1.69 (95% CI, 1.45–1.98). The overall analysis for spontaneous abortion exhibited a large degree of heterogeneity ($Q = 21.21$, $P < 0.001$). We identified the study by Dominguez-Rojas and coworkers (31) as an outlier by examining its contribution to the variance of Q for homogeneity. We performed a sensitivity analysis to determine the effect of this study on both homogeneity and the summary odds ratio. After its removal, the summary odds ratio was reduced slightly to 1.31, and the heterogeneity statistics became nonsignificant ($Q = 3.52$, $P = 0.318$). That study was analyzed to determine a possible explanation for its divergent results. The study had been conducted in Madrid, Spain and espresso coffee was the most common form of caffeine consumption reported. This coffee was found to contain about 140 mg caffeine/cup, which is almost twice as strong as a cup of coffee consumed in North America (8). When examining the results of the expectant mothers who had consumed more than 420 mg caffeine per d, it was found that 61 out of 87 (71%) pregnancies resulted in spontaneous abortion. In comparison, the study by Armstrong et al. (17), conducted in Montreal, Canada, investigated a group of women who had consumed over 700 mg of caffeine/d in the form of regular coffee. The rate of spontaneous abortion in those women was 30.9%. It is interesting to note the difference in the concentration of caffeine in the two studies and the resultant rates of spontaneous abortion. It may be that the consumption of beverages containing highly concentrated caffeine over short periods has a more significant effect on fetal development than conventional beverage consumption, or that espresso coffee has other unmeasured ingredients that may also be contributing to outcomes. These theories warrant consideration in future research.

In summary, the sensitivity and subgroup analyses performed within the spontaneous abortion analysis indicated that no group of studies (cohort or case control) or individual investigation influenced, to any degree, the overall main analysis of the summary odds ratio. The study by Dominguez-Rojas and coworkers (31) contributed to the heterogeneity of the analysis, however, the change in summary odds ratio was negligible, and nonheterogeneity was achieved when that study was removed from the analysis.

Low Birth Weight

The risk ratio calculated for the main analysis of studies (control versus > 150 mg caffeine/d) was 1.51 (1.43–1.69). The study by McDonald et al. (22) was substantially larger than the others. Upon removal of that study from the main analysis for low birth weight, the relative risk was reduced to 1.38 (1.20–1.57). Adding the study by Mills and colleagues (30) or Caan and Goldhaber (23), which used different controls and consumption groups than our criteria, had virtually no effect on the outcome of the summary risk ratio or confidence intervals calculated in the main analysis (Table 7).

In order to explore a possible dose–effect relation-ship between caffeine consumption and risk of outcome, we calculated summary risk ratios for control versus moderate (150 to 300 mg caffeine/d) and control versus heavy (>300 mg caffeine/d) groups. These increasing ratios suggest an increased risk of low birth weight neonates in relation to the amount of caffeine consumed above 150 mg/d.

Finally, two studies (19,21) were combined that defined IUGR as birth weight less than the tenth percentile for gestational age, to determine whether there was an association. The summary risk ratio calculated by combining these two studies was almost identical to the overall analysis for low birth weight, thus supporting our original findings.

Study Limitations

When combining studies addressing the reproductive risks of caffeine, one has to acknowledge the limitations inherent to this research.

Measurement of Caffeine

All of the studies that were accepted into the meta-analyses depended on the recall of the mother or expectant mother with regards to her level and sources of caffeine consumption. Ability to accurately recall and report the amount of caffeine ingested partly depends on whether the research was done prospectively or retrospectively. To study this type of recall bias, Fenster et al. (45) tested the recall of women who had been asked to report their caffeine consumption six months earlier. They showed that the women were able to reproduce their answers from six months earlier, within 1 cup of coffee, 77% of the time. As presented in Tables 2 and 3, four of the five studies in each of the two overall meta-analysis groups were researched retrospectively. Although recall bias may be a source of error in estimation, Fenster et al. showed that a habitual beverage such as coffee (which was the main source of caffeine in all studies) is often consumed in daily patterns that may not be very difficult to predict.

A second possible type of error introduced into the issue of caffeine measurement is encountered upon estimating the amount of

Table 8
Potential Confounders as Identified by Included Studies

1. Smoking
2. Alcohol
3. Maternal age
4. Cannabis
5. Previous abortion
6. Gravidity
7. Parity
8. Employment status
9. Education
10. Body type
11. Infection
12. Family history
13. Race
14. Drug use
15. Married status
16. Menarcheal age
17. Prior gynecologic surgery
18. Interval from previous pregnancy less than 6 months
19. Pregnancy induced hypertension
20. Uterine abnormality
21. Previous stillbirth
22. Insurance coverage
23. Use of tap water
24. Nausea during pregnancy
25. Weight extremes
26. Hours of physical activity/week
27. Previous low birth weight newborn
28. Previous preterm births
29. Weight gain in pregnancy

Table 9
Comparison of Confounding Factors of Accepted Spontaneous Abortion Studies

STUDY	CONFOUNDERS IDENTIFIED[a]	REPORTED RR/OR (95% CI)	ADJUSTED RR/OR (95% CI)	COMMENTS
Armstrong et al. (17)	1,2,3,5,6,8,9,13	OR = 1.17 (1.03–1.32) for zero vs. 375–675 mg caffeine consumption	not reported	After adjusting for confounders, reported risk of spontaneous abortion increases by factor of 1.017 per cup of coffee consumed per day ($P = 0.01$)
Dominguez-Rojas et al. (31)	1,2,3,5,15,16	RR = 1.87 (1.12–3.14) for 141–280 mg, RR = 5.15 (2.70–9.82) for 291–420 mg, RR = 20.47 (10.85–38.65) for >420 mg	OR = 2.20 (1.22–3.96) for 141–280 mg, OR = 4.81 (2.28–10.14) for 291–420 mg, OR = 5.43 (7.34–32.43) for >420 mg	Outlier study (see discussion) Spanish hospital workers Expresso coffee (160 mg/cup)
Fenster et al. (27)	1,2,3,5,6,8,9,13, 15,21,22,23,24	OR = 1.24 (0.90–1.71) 151–300 mg, OR = 1.55 (1.04–2.31) >300 mg	OR = 1.17 (0.84–1.62) 151-300 mg, OR = 1.22 (0.8–1.87) >300 mg	55% increased likelihood of heavy caffeine consumption for cases as compared to controls (association increases with dose)
Infante-Rivard et al. (29)	1,2,3,6,9,19,20	not reported	OR = 1.95 (1.29–2.93) for 0–48 vs 163–321 mg caffeine	Pattern of increased risk for fetal loss with increasing quantity of caffeine intake OR increased by a factor of 1.22 for each 100 mg caffeine intake per day.
Mills et al. (30)	1,2,3,5,6,7,8,9, 11,12,13,14	not stated	OR = 1.15 (0.89–1.49)	Study used for sensitivity purposes only
Srisuphan and Bracken (16)	1,2,3,4,5,6,7, 13,16,17,18	RR = 1.95 [P (for significance) = .07 for control] (1–150 mg vs >150 mg	RR = 1.73; P (for significance) = 0.03	Positive association between caffeine use and smoking
Wilcox et al. (28)	1,2,3,4,5,6,9,10	RR = 2.4 (0.80–7.00) control vs >150 mg	N/A	Sample too small ($n = 171$) for extensive multivariate analysis

[a] See Table 8 for confounder numbering scheme.

caffeine contained in specific servings. Most studies utilized an educated "guess" by taking averages of various analyzed samples obtained from their study population. In order to examine the variation in caffeine content of beverages, conversion factors used for estimating caffeine content in each study are presented in Tables 2 and 3.

A third potential error involving caffeine intake estimation involves the lack of identification of all sources of caffeine consumed. Tables 2 and 3 summarize the sources of caffeine included in each study. Varying protocols exist, with three studies taking only coffee into account in their estimation of consumption. Although coffee is the most common source of caffeine, this systematic error would generally lead to a degree of underestimation of caffeine use. It is assumed that this underestimation would occur to the same extent in the control and caffeine consumption groups.

Combinability of Results

In order to perform a meta-analysis of studies one needs data that can be validly combined. Some studies were excluded on the basis of stratifications of caffeine consumption that differed from those used in the meta-analysis. Furthermore, additional studies were excluded because they lacked valid controls.

A formal quality assessment was not performed on individual studies. However, the inclusion/exclusion criteria, along with a systematic data extraction process, served as an inherent quality assessment mechanism.

Undetected Spontaneous Abortions

Wilcox and associates (28) showed that approximately 25% of biochemically detected pregnancies ended before being clinically detected. One might assume that early loss of pregnancy would follow the patterns of late spontaneous abortion among the various stratifications of caffeine consumption. The extent to which this assumption is valid determines the amount of error introduced into the meta-analysis.

Confounders

Various confounding factors were identified in the accepted articles (Table 8). Tables 9 and 10 illustrate how individual studies handled

Table 10
Comparison of Confounding Factors of Accepted Fetal Growth Studies

STUDY	CONFOUNDERS IDENTIFIED[a]	REPORTED RR/OR (95% CI)	REPORTED ADJUSTED RR/OR (95% CI)	COMMENTS
Caan et al. (23)	1,2,3,6,13,29	OR = 2.30 (CI not stated) for zero vs > 300 mg caffeine consumption per day	OR = 3.53 (1.05–11.81) for zero vs > 300 mg caffeine consumption per day	Case control study. Small study size.
Fenster et al. (21)	1,2,3,5,7,8,9,13, 15,19,21,22	OR = 2.36 (1.17–4.93) for zero vs >300 mg/d caffeine consumption (LBW)	OR = 2.05 (0.86–4.88) zero vs. >300 mg caffeine consumption (LBW)	Reported OR adjusted for age, parity, race, hypertension, cigarette, and alcohol consumption.
Fortier et al. (19)	1,2,3,7,8,9,15, 21,25,26,27,28	OR = 1.86 for 0–10 mg vs 151–300 mg in IUGR (CI not stated)	OR = 1.4 (1.05–1.85) for 0–10 mg vs 151–300 mg in IUGR	OR for IUGR were for full term births.
Linn et al. (32)	1,2,3,5,6,7,8,9, 13,15,21,25	OR = 1.45 for > 300 mg vs control (CI not stated)	OR = 1.17 (0.85–1.61) for control vs > 300 mg	Frequency of smoking was over 3 times greater in coffee drinkers 300 mg/d
Martin and Bracken (20)	1,2,3,4,5,7,8, 13,15,21,25,29	RR = 4.0 (1.9–8.6) for zero vs > 300 mg/d	RR = 4.6 (2.0–10.5) for zero consumption vs > 300 mg/d	Analysis included term births only RR actually increased after adjusting for confounders
McDonald et al. (22)	1,2,3,5,6,7,8, 9,13	not stated as crude OR (estimated by logistic regression in next column)	OR = 1.34 (1.10–1.65) for low birth weight adjusted for gestational age; zero vs 375–750 mg per d	Women who drank > 10 cups of coffee per day OR = 1.43 (1.02–2.02).
Mills et al. (30)	1,2,3,5,6,7,8,9, 11,12,13,14	not stated	not stated	Birth weight percentile was lower in caffeine users after adjustment. *P* (for significance) = 0.06

[a] See Table 8 for confounder numbering scheme.

the important issue of confounders and how they have adjusted risk ratios accordingly. The most important common confounders appear to be concurrent smoking, alcohol use, maternal age over 35, and previous spontaneous abortion. Most other confounding factors would be equally distributed among the various stratifications of caffeine consumption. However, levels of smoking, alcohol use, and maternal age have been shown to have a positive correlation with levels of caffeine consumption (9). Certainly, adjustment for these confounders by multivariate analysis would be a desirable component to interpreting the influence of confounders on summary ratios. Unfortunately, due to the nature of data presentation in the individual studies, adjustment for these confounders was not possible. For example, when these studies reported the number of spontaneous abortions in caffeine- exposed and non-exposed groups, they did not specifically delineate the number of smokers in each caffeine stratification group. Consequently, we were unable to adjust the overall summary ratios for either outcome of the meta-analysis for smoking or any of the other confounders.

Risk of spontaneous abortion increases as the quantity of cigarettes smoked/d increases (9). In most of the five studies in the main analysis for spontaneous abortion, the odds ratios were not altered significantly even after the researchers adjusted for smoking and other confounders (as reported in each study). It would have been interesting to have been able to quantify the interrelationship between caffeine and smoking on spontaneous abortion.

The issue of smoking as a confounder in the fetal growth analysis is an interesting one. It has been postulated that the negative effects of caffeine on fetal growth occur in the third trimester, as this is the time when the greatest rate of growth occurs (5). Nicotine is known to increase the rate of metabolism of caffeine in humans. Pregnant women have only one-third the capacity to metabolize caffeine in the third trimester of pregnancy (2). This reduction, combined with the fact that the fetus is unable to metabolize caffeine, is thought to be an important contributing factor in the proposed fetal growth retardation. The issue is complex because smoking is known to retard fetal growth by a different mechanism (9). Our accepted studies illustrate these conflicting results as two of the studies (20,23) actually showed higher risk ratios for the relationship of caffeine consumption with low birth weight after adjustment for smoking. In direct contrast to this observation, the study by Fortier and colleagues (19) showed that the risks from caffeine consumption and smoking were more than additive in their contributions to the risk of fetal growth retardation. Although the results of any particular study involved in the analyses were not significantly altered by adjustment for confounders, it should be noted that the summary effect of the confounder may have inflated the results of the meta-analyses.

Our results suggest a small but statistically significant increase in the risks for spontaneous abortion and for low birth weight babies in pregnant women consuming more than 150 mg of caffeine per d. Pregnant women should be encouraged to be aware of dietary caffeine intake and to consume less than 150 mg of caffeine/d from all sources throughout pregnancy. Future research should include reliable methods of caffeine measurement, standardized control and caffeine exposure groups, and a standard approach to control for confounders.

REFERENCES

1. Goyan JE. Food and Drug Administration news release no.P80–36. Washington, DC: September 1980;4.
2. Knutti R, Rothweiler H, Schlatter C. The effect of pregnancy on the pharmacokinetics of caffeine. Arch Toxicol. 1982; 5(Suppl):187–92.
3. Weathersbee PS, Lodge R. Caffeine: its direct and indirect influence on reproduction. J Reprod Med. 1977;19:55–63.
4. Thayer PS, Palm PE. A current assessment of the mutagenic and teratogenic effects of caffeine. CRC Crit Rev Toxicol. 1975;3:345.
5. Wilson JG, Scott WJ. The teratogenic potential of caffeine in laboratory animals. In: Dews PB, ed. Caffeine: perspectives from recent research. Berlin: Springer-Verlag; 1984:165–87.
6. Einarson TR, Leeder JS, Koren G. A method for meta-analysis of epidemiologic studies. Drug Intell Clin Pharm. 1988;22:813–24.
7. Arbuckle TE, Sherman GJ. An analysis of birth weight by gestational age in Canada. Can Med Assoc J. 1989;140:157–60, 165.
8. Gilbert RM, Marshman JA, Schwieder M, Berg R. Caffeine content of beverages as consumed. Can Med Assoc J. 1976;114:205–8.
9. Golding J. Reproduction and caffeine consumption—a literature review. Early Hum Dev. 1995;43:1–14.
10. Martin JC. An overview: maternal nicotine and caffeine consumption and offspring outcome. Neurobehav Toxicol Teratol. 1982;4: 421–7.
11. Mantel N, Haenszel W. Statistical aspects of the analysis of data from retrospective studies of disease. J Natl Cancer Inst. 1959;22: 719–48.
12. Miettinen O. Estimability and estimation in case-referent studies. Am J Epidemiol. 1976;103:226–35.
13. Watkinson B, Fried PA. Maternal caffeine use before, during and after pregnancy and effects upon offspring. Neurobehav Toxicol Teratol. 1985;7:9–17.
14. Barr HM, Streissguth AP. Caffeine use during pregnancy and child outcome: a seven year prospective study. Neurotoxicol Teratol. 1991;13:441–448.
15. Weathersbee PS, Olsen LK, Lodge JR. Caffeine in pregnancy. Postgrad Med. 1977;62:64–9.
16. Srisuphan W, Bracken M. Caffeine consumption during pregnancy and association with late spontaneous abortion. Am J Obstet Gynecol. 1986;154:14–20.
17. Armstrong BG, McDonald AD, Sloan M. Cigarette, alcohol, and coffee consumption and spontaneous abortion. Am J Public Health. 1992;82:85–7.
18. Beaulac-Baillargeon L, Desrosiers C. Caffeine-cigarette interaction on fetal growth. Am J Obstet Gynecol. 1987;157:1236–40.
19. Fortier I, Marcoux S, Beaulac-Baillargeon L. Relation of caffeine intake during pregnancy to intrauterine growth retardation and preterm birth. Am J Epidemiol. 1993;137:931–40.
20. Martin TR, Bracken M. The association between low birth weight and caffeine consumption during pregnancy. Am J Epidemiol. 1987;126: 813–21.
21. Fenster L, Eskenazi B, Windham GC, Swan SH. Caffeine consumption during pregnancy and fetal growth. J Public Health. 1991;81: 458–61.
22. McDonald AD, Armstrong BG, Sloan M. Cigarette, alcohol, and coffee consumption and prematurity. Am J Public Health. 1992: 87–90.
23. Caan BJ, Goldhaber MK. Caffeinated beverages and low birth-weight: a case-control study. Am J Public Health. 1989;79:1299–1300.
24. Olsen J, Overvad K, Frische G. Coffee consumption, birthweight and reproductive failures. Epidemiology. 1991;2:370–374.
25. Peacock JL, Bland JM, Anderson HR. Effects on birthweight of alcohol and caffeine consumption in smoking women. J Epidemiol Community Health. 1991;45:159–63.
26. Shu XO, Hatch MC, Mills J, Clemens J, Susser M. Maternal smoking, alcohol drinking, caffeine consumption, and fetal growth: results from a prospective study. Epidemiology. 1995;6:115–20.
27. Fenster L, Eskenazi B, Windham GC, Swan SH. Caffeine consumption during pregnancy and spontaneous abortion. Epidemiology. 1991;2:168–74.
28. Wilcox AJ, Weinberg CR, Baird DD. Risk factors for early pregnancy loss. Epidemiology. 1990;1:382–5.
29. Infante-Rivard C, Fernandez A, Gautheir R, David M, Rivard GE. Fetal loss associated with caffeine intake before and during pregnancy. JAMA. 1993;270:2940–3.
30. Mills JL, Holmes LB, Aarons JH, et al. Moderate caffeine use and the risk of spontaneous abortion and intrauterine growth retardation. JAMA. 1993;269:593–7.
31. Dominguez-Rojas V, Juanes-Pardo JR, Astasio-Arbiza P, Ortega-Molina P, Gordillo-Florenico E. Spontaneous abortion in a hospital population: are tobacco and coffee intake risk factors? Eur J Epidemiol. 1994;10:665–8.
32. Linn S, Schoenbaum SC, Monson RR, Rosner B, Stubblefield PG, Ryan KJ. No association between coffee consumption and adverse outcomes of pregnancy. N Engl J Med. 1982;306:141–5.
33. Furuhashi N, Sato S, Suzuki M, Hiruta M, Tanaka M, Takahashi. Effects of caffeine ingestion during pregnancy. Gynecol Obstet Invest. 1985;19:187–91.
34. Fried PA, O'Connell. A comparison of the effects of prenatal exposure to tobacco, alcohol, cannabis and caffeine on birth size and subsequent growth. Neurotoxicol Teratol. 1987;9:79–85.
35. Barr HM, Streissguth AP, Martin DC, Herman CS. Infant size at eight months of age: relationship to maternal use of alcohol, nicotine, and caffeine during pregnancy. Pediatrics. 1984;74:336–41.
36. Rosenberg L, Mitchell AA, Shapiro S, Slone D. Selected birth defects in relation to caffeine-containing beverages. JAMA. 1982; 247:1429–32.
37. Pastore LM, Savitz DA. Case-control study of caffeinated beverages and preterm delivery. Am J Epidemiol. 1995;141:61–9.
38. Laroque B, Kaminski M, Lelong N, Subtil D, Dehaene P. Effects on birth weight of alcohol and caffeine consumption during pregnancy. Am J Epidemiol. 1993;137:941–50.
39. Van den berg BJ. Epidemiologic observations of prematurity: effects of tobacco, coffee, and alcohol. In: Reed DM, Stanley FJ, eds. The epidemiology of prematurity. Baltimore: Urban and Schwarzenberg Inc.; 1977:157–76.
40. Kline J, Levine B, Silverman J, et al. Caffeine and spontaneous abortion of known karotype. Epidemiology. 1991;2:409–17.
41. Godel JC, Pabst HF, Hodges PE, Johnson KE, Froese GJ, Joffres MR. Smoking and caffeine and alcohol intake during pregnancy in a northern population: effect on fetal growth. Can Med Assoc J. 1992;147:181–8.
42. Peacock JL, Bland JM, Anderson HR. Preterm delivery: effects of socioeconomic factors, psychological stress, smoking, alcohol, and caffeine. BMJ. 1995;311:531–6.
43. Muñoz LM, Lönnerdal B, Keen CL, Dewey KG. Coffee consumption as a factor in iron deficiency anemia among pregnant women and their infants in Costa Rica. Am J Clin Nutr. 1988;48:645–51.
44. Wisborg K, Henriken TB, Hedegaard M, Secher NJ. Smoking during pregnancy and preterm birth. Br J Obstet Gynaecol. 1996;103:800–5.
45. Fenster L, Swan SH, Windham GC, Neutra RR. Assessment of reporting consistency in a case-control study of spontaneous abortions. Am J Epidemiol. 1991;133:477–88.

CHAPTER 39

FETAL EFFECTS OF COCAINE: AN UPDATED META-ANALYSIS

Antonio Addis,[a] Myla E. Moretti,[b] Fayyazuddin Ahmed Syed,[b] Thomas R. Einarson,[c] and Gideon Koren[b]

[a]*Centro per la Valutazione della Efficacia della Assistenza Sanitaria, Modena, Italy*

[b]*Motherisk Program, Division of Clinical Pharmacology, The Hospital for Sick Children, Toronto, Canada*

[c]*Faculty of Pharmacy, University of Toronto, Toronto, Canada*

Received 24 October 2000; received in revised form 5 January 2001; accepted 18 February 2001

Abstract

Background. A very large number of women in the reproductive age group consume cocaine, leading to grave concerns regarding the long term health of millions of children after in utero exposure. The results of controlled studies have been contradictory, leading to confusion, and, possible, misinformation and misperception of teratogenic risk.

Objective. To systematically review available data on pregnancy outcome when the mother consumed cocaine.

Methods. A meta-analysis of all epidemiologic studies based on a priori criteria was conducted. Comparisons of adverse events in subgroups of exposed vs. unexposed children were performed. Analyses were based on several exposure groups: mainly cocaine, cocaine plus polydrug, polydrug but no cocaine, and drug free.

Results. Thirty three studies met our inclusion criteria. For all end points of interest (rates of major malformations, low birth weight, prematurity, placental abruption, premature rupture of membrane [PROM], and mean birth weight, length and head circumference), cocaine-exposed infants had higher risks than children of women not exposed to any drug. However, most of these adverse effects were nullified when cocaine exposed children were compared to children exposed to polydrug but no cocaine. Only the risk of placental abruption and premature rupture of membranes were statistically associated with cocaine use itself.

Conclusions. Many of the perinatal adverse effects commonly attributed to cocaine may be caused by the multiple confounders that can occur in a cocaine using mother. Only the risk for placental abruption and PROM could be statistically related to cocaine. For other adverse effects, additional studies will be needed to ensure adequate statistical power.

Keywords: Pregnancy; Meta-analysis; Cocaine; Fetal effects

INTRODUCTION

The high prevalence of cocaine use has become a major health concern during pregnancy. Cocaine crosses the human placenta, with varying proportions absorbed by the placenta, suggesting that the placenta may offer a degree of protection to some fetuses after bolus administration [1]. Cocaine is a CNS stimulant with effects thought to be due to its sympathomimetic-driven fetal, uterine, or maternal vasoconstriction and hypertension leading to infarcts or hemorrhages at any time during gestation and in any structure. This feature may explain the variability of clinical effects attributed to cocaine use. A typical well-defined "fetal cocaine syndrome" has not been identified [2]; however, exposure to cocaine during pregnancy has been associated with shorter gestation, premature delivery, abruptio placenta, and other maternal and neonatal adverse effects. In the past, congenital malformations of almost every system have been reported leading many clinicians to believe that the drug is teratogenic [3]. Reports of fetal cocaine effects have been controversial and it has been difficult to elucidate these effects, because interpretation of the results is hampered by the fact that cocaine use is commonly accompanied by confounding factors such as concomitant use of cigarettes and other recreational drugs, including heroin, cannabis, methadone, and others, all of which may affect pregnancy outcome by themselves.

Our original systematic review and meta-analysis in 1991 [4] suggested that cocaine exposure during pregnancy is not a major risk for malformation (except for the genito-urinary tract). When cocaine users were compared to women not consuming any drugs of abuse, a variety of risks emerged. Yet when we compared pregnancy and neonatal outcomes in children of cocaine consumers with polydrug consumers, the increased risk for most of the adverse outcomes was nullified. A major issue at that stage was the relatively small number of studies for each adverse end point. Since 1989 (the last year included in our previous meta-analysis), however, scores of studies on cocaine exposure during pregnancy have been published. Hence, the present meta-analysis has allowed us to separate the exposure data into several comparisons:

(1) between all combinations of exposures that involve cocaine use during pregnancy (cocaine alone, polydrug including cocaine, polydrug not including cocaine);
(2) between the different methodologies used to determine exposure (urine analysis, maternal interview, chart review).

The aim of this updated meta-analysis was to arrive at an overall quantitative estimate of the effect of cocaine use on pregnancy outcome and potential pregnancy complications, with a substantially increased power.

METHODS

Data Sources

The medical literature published between January 1989 and December 1997 was searched for papers dealing with the outcome of pregnancy following gestational cocaine exposure. The literature

Table 1
Results of Search on Cocaine Use During Pregnancy

TYPE OF STUDY	NO.
Case Reports/Case Series	80
Letters	43
Editorials	22
Reviews and Commentaries	87
Studies not reporting fetal or pregnancy outcomes	127
In vitro studies/placenta perfusion	39
Outcomes beyond the scope of this meta analysis	54
Studies without control group	19
Cocaine users not separated from other drugs	12
Studies included in the meta-analysis	*33*
Total	525

search was performed in the MEDLINE and EMBASE bibliographic databases. A search strategy using a combination of "*pregnancy* " or "*abnormalities drug induced* " and "*cocaine* " keywords (MeSH) was used. All references in the retrieved articles were screened for further papers. From all the references we excluded the non-english papers, comments, letters, editorials, and reviews (Table 1). However, the references from these excluded publications were also scanned for other studies not quoted by the databases. All studies considered in the previous meta-analysis were retrieved and resubmitted to the inclusion or exclusion process.

Study Selection

Searches were reviewed or completed independently and in duplicate. Investigators were blinded as to the name of the journal, the authors of the paper, the hospital or site of the study, and the funding agency supporting the study. This blinding was accomplished by removing all identifying statements and titles prior to photocopying the papers for review by another investigator. Without this identification, the prestige, reputation, or standards of the journal or author could not interfere with the selection or analysis of articles. Although, theoretically, journals have a typeset style that could identify them, the junior investigator who conducted blinding of the papers was not familiar with the different styles. The criteria for inclusion of papers in this analysis were: human exposure to any amount of cocaine during any or all trimesters of pregnancy, as evidenced by drug history or urine test, and report of outcome of pregnancy or fetal development. Only case-control or cohort studies with at least one control group were included. Use of other drugs is common among cocaine users and was not an exclusion criterion. Case reports, reviews, editorials, and letters were excluded from the analysis but retrieved and followed up for further papers. The Methods section of each paper was evaluated using a scoring sheet, prepared a priori, which listed these inclusion criteria. Studies fulfilling all inclusion criteria were accepted for analysis. Successfully included studies were read and information was extracted using a standardized data extraction form. The information collected included the size and selection of cocaine and control groups, and the pregnancy and fetal outcome measurements studied. Studies were analyzed separately according to various exposure groups, namely:

(a) pregnant women exposed to cocaine alone, compared to drug free controls;
(b) pregnant women exposed to cocaine plus any other drugs of abuse (e.g. heroin, methadone, marijuana, LSD, amphetamines) compared to drug free controls; alcohol and cigarettes were not considered drugs of abuse in this case
(c) pregnant women exposed to cocaine alone compared to cocaine plus other drugs or abuse;
(d) pregnant women exposed to cocaine alone versus other drug addictions (and no cocaine);
(e) pregnant women exposed to cocaine plus other drugs versus other drug addictions (and no cocaine).

To avoid duplication of results, after data extraction we examined data results of included studies with a cross analysis of author groups.

The outcomes considered were related to maternal and neonatal health, namely major malformations, low birth weight, prematurity, premature rupture of membranes (PROM), abruptio placenta, meconium, gestational age, head circumference, birth weight and birth length. Studies examining only certain subtypes of malformations or studies with unspecified addictions were excluded from the analysis.

Data Analysis

All controlled studies were pooled together and weighted to calculate the relative risk (RR) and 95% confidence interval ($CI_{95\%}$) using a random effect model [5]. For outcomes measured in a continuous scale (i.e. head circumference, birth weight, length, gestational age), weighted mean differences were calculated, also using in this case, the random effect model. χ^2 tests for heterogeneity were also performed for all outcomes of interest in this analysis.

Sensitivity analyses were performed on the study methodol ogy (by excluding retrospective analysis) and according to the method used to identify cocaine users (by excluding studies that use chart review or maternal interview methologies). These analyses were performed with the aim of assessing the impact of identification bias in the study population.

RESULTS

More than 600 scientific references were considered because they deal with the human effects of cocaine used during pregnancy, with an exponential growth in number of papers published in recent years. Of these, 516 studies were retrieved and, based on a review of their methods sections, only 36 studies met the inclusion criteria for this analysis. Of these 36 studies, 3 studies [6,7,8] were excluded after a more detailed analysis because in these studies there were multiple exposures in more than 10% of cases in all groups and because it was not possible to identify the different outcomes according to single or multiple exposures. Table 1 lists the types and number of rejected studies. Studies were excluded because they were case reports (80), editorials (22), letters (43), reviews or commentaries (87), studies without fetal or pregnancy outcomes (127), in vitro studies or placenta perfusions (39), studies with outcomes not within the scope of this meta-analysis (54), studies without a control group (19), or studies where cocaine users had been not separated from users of other drugs (12) (For full list see appendix). Table 2 highlights the characteristics of the 33 included studies. Exposure was mainly ascertained through urine or meconium analysis (73%) or by chart review and/or maternal interview (27% of the studies), while outcome was mainly confirmed

Table 2
Characteristics of Studies Included in the Meta-Aanalysis

REFERENCE	OUTCOMES	STUDY GROUPS (SAMPLE SIZE)	STUDY TYPE	DATA COLLECTION
1. Bateman 1993 (16)	Birth defects Low birth weight Prematurity Abruptio Gestational Age Head circumference Weight Length	Cocaine Alone (361) Drug Free (387)	Cohort prospective	Urine analysis Chart review
2. Bingol 1987 (12)	Birth defects Head circumference Weight Length	Cocaine Alone (50) Drug Free (340) Polydrugs With Cocaine (110)	Cohort retrospective	Interview of the mother Chart review
3. Chasnoff 1985 (17)	Birth defects Abruptio placenta Head circumference Weight Length	Cocaine Alone (12) Drug Free (15) Polydrugs With Cocaine (12) Polydrugs No Cocaine (15)	Cohort prospective	Urine analysis
4. Chasnoff 1987 (18)	Birth defects Prematurity Weight Head circumference Length	Polydrugs With Cocaine (52) Polydrugs No Cocaine (73)	Cohort prospective	Urine analysis, Chart review
5. Chasnoff 1988 (19)	Birth defects Low birth weight Prematurity Abruptio placenta Weight Head circumference	Cocaine Alone (53) Drug Free (40)	Cohort prospective	Urine analysis
6. Chavez 1989 (20)	Birth defects	Cocaine Alone (1063) Drug Free (8326)	Case control retrospective	Chart review Interview of the mother
7. Chazotte 1991 (21)	Low birth weight Gestational Age Weight	Cocaine Alone (42) Drug Free (42)	Cohort prospective	Urine analysis
8. Cherukuri 1988 (22)	Birth defects Low birth weight Prematurity PROM Gestational Age Head circumference Weight Length	Cocaine Alone (55) Drug Free (55)	Cohort retrospective	Interview of the mother Chart review
9. Chouteau 1988 (23)	Low birth weight Prematurity	Cocaine Alone (124) Drug Free (218)	Cohort retrospective	Urine analysis
10. Cohen 1991 (13)	Low birth weight Prematurity Gestational Age Weight	Cocaine Alone (56) Drug Free (166) Polydrugs With Cocaine	Cohort retrospective	Urine analysis
11. Eyler 1994 (24)	Birth defects Low birth weight Prematurity Abruptio placenta Gestational Age Weight	Cocaine Alone (168) Drug Free (168)	Cohort retrospective	Chart review
12. Fulroth 1989 (25)	Prematurity Meconium	Cocaine Alone (35) Drug Free (1021) Polydrugs No Cocaine (35)	Cohort prospective	Urine analysis Chart review

(*Continued*)

Table 2
Characteristics of Studies Included in the Meta-Analysis (*Continued*)

REFERENCE	OUTCOMES	STUDY GROUPS (SAMPLE SIZE)	STUDY TYPE	DATA COLLECTION
13. Galanter 1992 (26)	PROM Abruptio placenta Meconium	Polydrugs With Cocaine (51) Polydrugs No Cocaine (350)	Cohort prospective	Urine analysis
14. Gillogley 1990 (27)	Birth defects Low birth weight Prematurity PROM Abruptio placenta Weight Length	Cocaine Alone (139) Drug Free (293) Polydrugs With Cocaine (35) Polydrugs No Cocaine (125)	Cohort retrospective	Urine analysis, Chart review
15. Hadeed 1989 (28)	Birth defects Low birth weight Prematurity Abruptio placenta Head circumference Weight Length	Cocaine Alone (56) Drug Free (56)	Cohort prospective	Urine analysis
16. Isenberg 1987 (29)	Weight	Cocaine Alone (13) Drug Free (36)	Cohort prospective	Urine analysis
17. Keith 1989 (30)	Low birth weight Prematurity PROM Abruptio placenta Gestational Age Weight	Cocaine Alone (63) Drug Free (123) Polydrugs With Cocaine (137) Polydrugs No Cocaine (27)	Cohort retrospective	Chart review
18. Kelley 1991 (14)	Low birth weight Prematurity Abruptio placenta Gestational Age Head Circumference Weight Length	Cocaine Alone (30) Drug Free (30)	Cohort retrospective	Chart review
19. Kistin 1996 (31)	Birth defects Low birth weight Abruptio placenta Prematurity	Cocaine Alone (64) Drug Free (13,043)	Cohort retrospective	Urine analysis Chart review
20. Little 1989 (32)	Birth defects Meconium	Polydrugs With Cocaine (53) Drug Free (100)	Cohort prospective	Interview of the mother Chart review
21. McCalla 1991 (33)	PROM Abruptio placenta	Cocaine Alone (128) Drug Free (983)	Cross sectional study	Urine analysis
22. MacGregor 1987 (34)	Low birth weight Prematurity Abruptio placenta Gestational Age Weight	Cocaine Alone (24) Drug Free (70) Polydrugs With Cocaine (46)	Cohort prospective	Chart review
23. Mastrogiannis 1990 (35)	Abruptio placenta PROM Meconium	Cocaine Alone (40) Drug Free (46)	Cohort retrospective	Urine analysis
24. Matera 1990 (36)	PROM Abruptio placenta	Cocaine Alone (51) Drug Free (350) Polydrugs No Cocaine (65)	Cohort prospective	Urine analysis
25. Nair 1994 (37)	Low birth weight Weight Length	Polydrugs With Cocaine (55) Polydrugs No Cocaine (86)	Cohort prospective	Meconium analysis

(*Continued*)

Table 2
Characteristics of Studies Included in the Meta-Analysis (*Continued*)

REFERENCE	OUTCOMES	STUDY GROUPS (SAMPLE SIZE)	STUDY TYPE	DATA COLLECTION
26. Neerhof 1989 (10)	Birth defects Prematurity Abruptio placenta Gestational Age Weight	Cocaine Alone (113) Drug Free (88) Polydrugs With Cocaine (24)	Cohort prospective	Urine analysis
27. Richardson 1991 (11)	Low birth weight	Polydrugs With Cocaine (34) Drug Free (590)	Cohort prospective	Interview of the mother
28. Rosengren 1993 (38)	Low birth weight Prematurity Abruptio placenta PROM Weight Length	Cocaine Alone (21) Drug Free (600)	Cohort prospective	Meconium analysis
29. Ryan 1987 (39)	Prematurity Gestational Age Head circumference Weight Length	Drug Free (50) Polydrugs With Cocaine (50) Polydrugs No Cocaine (50)	Cohort prospective	Urine analysis Chart review
30. Singer 1994 (40)	Low birth weight Prematurity Gestational Age Weight Length	Cocaine Alone (100) Drug Free (100)	Cohort retrospective	Urine analysis, interview of the mother
31. Sprauve 1997 (41)	Birth defect Low birth weight prematurity Abruptio placenta	Cocaine Alone (483) Drug Free (3158)	Cohort retrospective	Urine analysis
32. Stafford 1994 (42)	Birth defects	Cocaine Alone (40) Drug Free (40)	Cohort prospective	Urine analysis
33. Zuckerman 1989 (43)	Birth defects Gestational Age Head circumference Weight Length	Drug Free (1010) Polydrugs With Cocaine (114) Polydrugs No Cocaine (202)	Cohort prospective	Urine analysis, Chart review

using physician examination or record examination. The studies reported pregnancy and neonatal outcomes of 4184 women exposed to cocaine during pregnancy. Nineteen percent of these were also exposed to others drugs (i.e. heroin, methadone, marijuana). The outcomes were compared with 31,544 drug free pregnancy controls and with 963 women exposed to other addictions but not cocaine. There were no new papers, published after our last meta-analysis, that reported outcome of meconium staining and as such, that outcome is not reported in the results here.

Major Malformations (Fig. 1)

The teratogenic potential of cocaine was investigated in 16 (47%) of included studies. Major malformations were those described by Heinonen et al., [9]. Comparing women for whom cocaine was the only drug of abuse in pregnancy with drug free controls, the pooled relative risk was significantly elevated (RR: 1.70, $CI_{95\%}$ 1.12–2.60). Six studies reported the number of malformed children after exposure during pregnancy to cocaine plus others addictions (heroin, marijuana, methadone, etc). The pooled relative risk was also significant in this case (RR: 2.10; $CI_{95\%}$ 1.42–3.09). The significance disappeared when the risk for major malformations was analyzed in women exposed to cocaine alone compared to women exposed to cocaine plus other addictions. When we used women exposed to polydrugs without cocaine as the control, we were not able to identify a significant risk for major malformations in the women exposed to cocaine alone or to polydrugs with cocaine. A test for heterogeneity showed that all studies detected an effect size of similar magnitude and direction with the exception of the comparison between cocaine alone versus polydrugs with cocaine exposures. In this case, a single study was responsible for the heterogeneity [10]. When that study was removed, the heterogeneity test was no longer significant.

Low Birth Weight (Fig. 2)

Of the included studies, 18 (54%) reported data on the number newborns with low birth weight after cocaine exposure. The rate of low birth weight was defined as the number of live births weighing less then 2,500 *g*. As in the previous analysis, mothers exposed to

Comparison: Cocaine vs Drug Free

Study	Relative Risk (95%CI Random)	Weight %	RR (95%CI Random)	Year
Chasnoff (85)		3.0	2.46 [0.25, 24.22]	85
Bingol		9.1	4.86 [1.60, 14.72]	87
Cherukuri		2.8	0.49 [0.05, 5.26]	88
Hadeed		2.2	1.00 [0.06, 15.60]	89
Chavez		12.2	2.49 [1.07, 5.82]	89
Chasnoff (89)		3.7	6.96 [0.92, 52.77]	89
Neerhof		5.4	1.95 [0.39, 9.80]	89
Gillogley		8.4	1.05 [0.32, 3.44]	90
Elateman		5.5	1.37 [0.28, 6.75]	93
Stafford		5.8	3.00 [0.64, 13.98]	94
Eyler		12.6	1.44 [0.63, 3.29]	94
Kistin		13.4	2.13 [0.99, 4.58]	96
Sprauve		15.9	0.63 [0.34, 1.16]	97
Total (95%CI)		**100.0**	**1.70 [1.11, 2.60]**	

Comparison: Polydrugs with Cocaine vs Drug Free

Study	Relative Risk (95%CI Random)	Weight %	RR (95%CI Random)	Year
Chasnoff (85)		2.1	1.33 [0.09, 19.23]	85
Bingol		11.9	2.21 [0.72, 6.82]	87
Neerhof		6.1	9.17 [1.89, 44.35]	89
Zuckerman		60.5	1.75 [1.06, 2.89]	89
Little		15.8	2.83 [1.06, 7.52]	89
Gillogley		3.6	1.05 [0.13, 8.12]	90
Total (95%CI)		**100.0**	**2.10 [1.42, 3.09]**	

Comparison: Cocaine vs Poly Drugs with Cocaine

Study	Relative Risk (95%CI Random)	Weight %	RR (95%CI Random)	Year
Chasnoff (85)		18.8	2.00 [0.21, 19.23]	85
Bingol		30.6	2.20 [0.67, 7.26]	87
Neerhof		31.0	0.21 [0.07, 0.68]	89
Gillogley		19.7	1.01 [0.12, 8.73]	90
Total (95%CI)		**100.0**	**0.90 [0.23, 3.43]**	

Comparison: Cocaine vs Poly Drugs without Cocaine

Study	Relative Risk (95%CI Random)	Weight %	RR (95%CI Random)	Year
Chasnoff (85)		47.6	2.46 [0.25, 24.22]	85
Gillogley		52.4	3.60 [0.41, 31.76]	90
Total (95%CI)		**100.0**	**3.00 [0.62, 14.54]**	

Comparison: Polydrugs with Cocaine vs Polydrugs without Cocaine

Study	Relative Risk (95%CI Random)	Weight %	RR (95%CI Random)	Year
Chasnoff (85)		8.0	1.33 [0.09, 19.23]	85
Chasnoff (87)		32.2	0.51 [0.16, 1.59]	87
Zuckerman		59.8	1.58 [0.84, 2.97]	89
Total (95%CI)		**100.0**	**1.08 [0.49, 2.38]**	

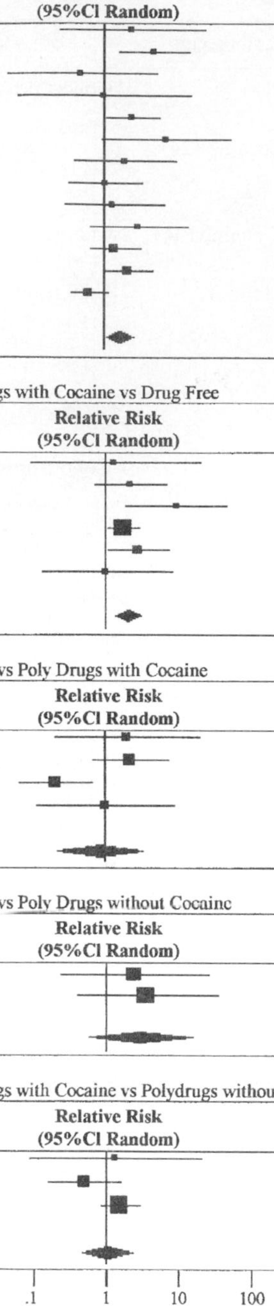

Figure 1. Major Malformations.

cocaine alone or to polydrugs with cocaine show a significant pooled relative risk of low birth weight when compared to a drug free control (RR: 2.85, $CI_{95\%}$ 2.28–3.56 and 4.28, $CI_{95\%}$ 2.47–7.43, respectively). When we used as controls the mothers exposed to polydrugs with or without cocaine, the significance disappeared. Results were homogeneous in three comparisons (cocaine alone versus polydrug with and without cocaine; and polydrug with cocaine versus polydrug without cocaine). The test for heterogeneity was positive in the first two comparisons with drug free controls (cocaine alone and polydrug with cocaine). However, in the comparison of cocaine plus polydrugs versus drug free controls, the heterogeneity was due to a single study [11]. When this study was removed, the heterogeneity disappeared. In the first comparison of cocaine alone versus drug free, use of only prospective studies in which urine analysis was used to identify cocaine users, resulted in homogeneity.

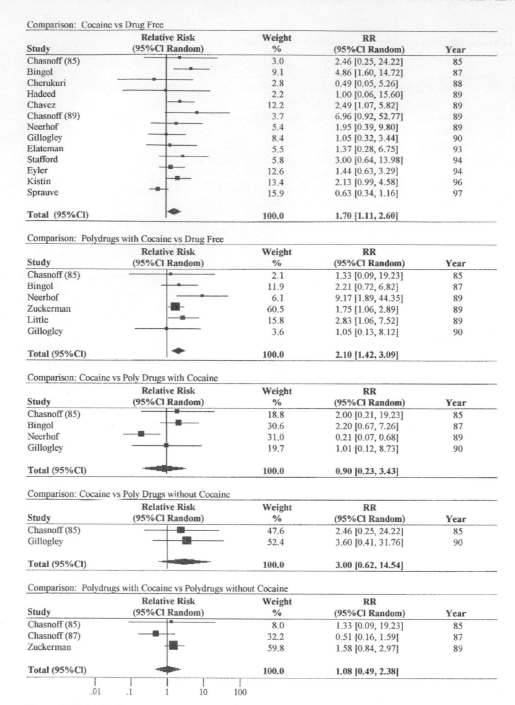

Birth Weight (Fig. 3)

Similar trends are shown for the data on the rate of low birth weight. Use of cocaine during pregnancy (alone or with polydrugs) was associated with the risk of a weighted average birth weight reduction of from 495 g to 512 g. When pregnant women exposed

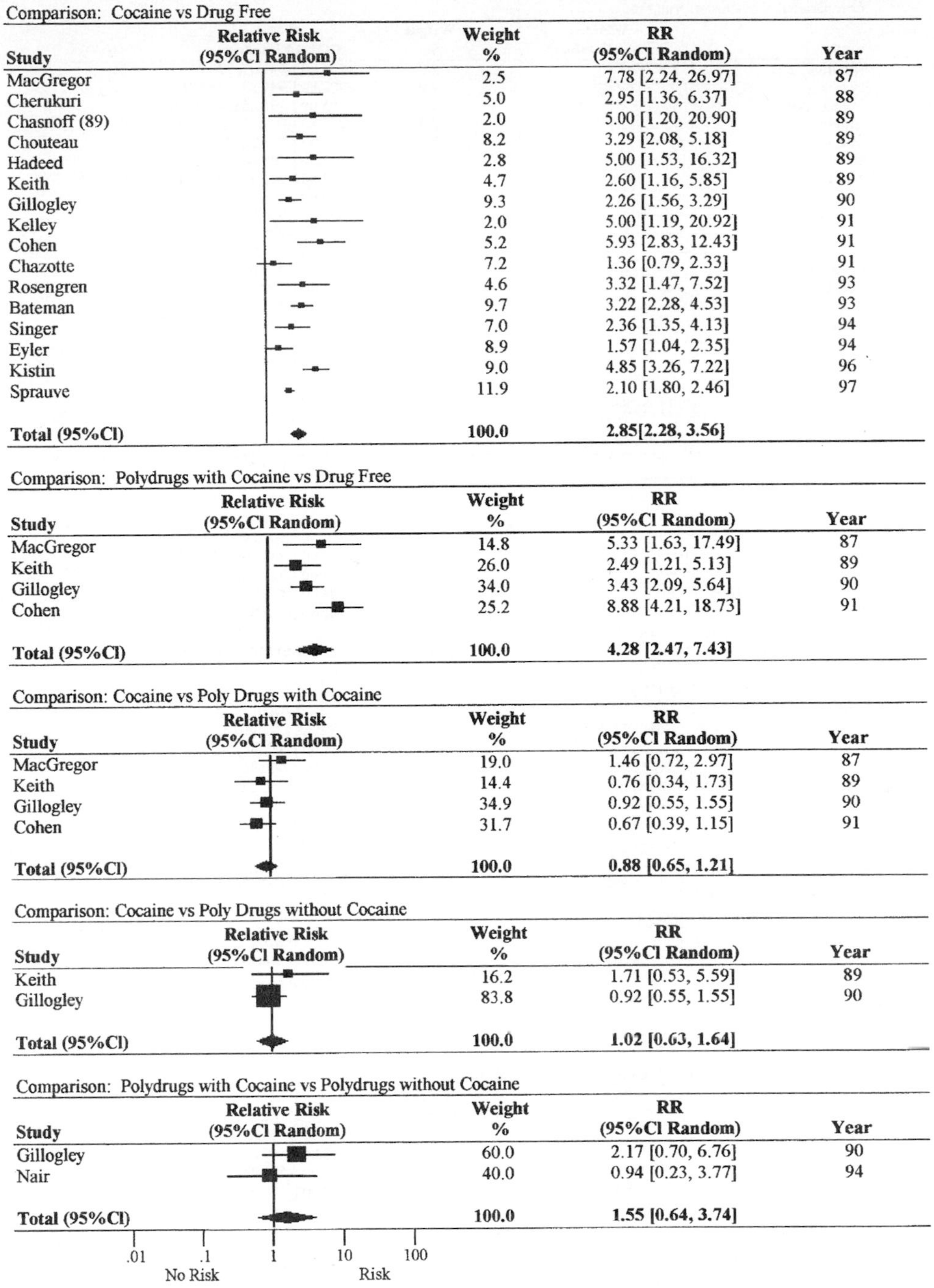

Comparison: Cocaine vs Drug Free

Study	Weight %	RR (95%CI Random)	Year
MacGregor	2.5	7.78 [2.24, 26.97]	87
Cherukuri	5.0	2.95 [1.36, 6.37]	88
Chasnoff (89)	2.0	5.00 [1.20, 20.90]	89
Chouteau	8.2	3.29 [2.08, 5.18]	89
Hadeed	2.8	5.00 [1.53, 16.32]	89
Keith	4.7	2.60 [1.16, 5.85]	89
Gillogley	9.3	2.26 [1.56, 3.29]	90
Kelley	2.0	5.00 [1.19, 20.92]	91
Cohen	5.2	5.93 [2.83, 12.43]	91
Chazotte	7.2	1.36 [0.79, 2.33]	91
Rosengren	4.6	3.32 [1.47, 7.52]	93
Bateman	9.7	3.22 [2.28, 4.53]	93
Singer	7.0	2.36 [1.35, 4.13]	94
Eyler	8.9	1.57 [1.04, 2.35]	94
Kistin	9.0	4.85 [3.26, 7.22]	96
Sprauve	11.9	2.10 [1.80, 2.46]	97
Total (95%CI)	**100.0**	**2.85[2.28, 3.56]**	

Comparison: Polydrugs with Cocaine vs Drug Free

Study	Weight %	RR (95%CI Random)	Year
MacGregor	14.8	5.33 [1.63, 17.49]	87
Keith	26.0	2.49 [1.21, 5.13]	89
Gillogley	34.0	3.43 [2.09, 5.64]	90
Cohen	25.2	8.88 [4.21, 18.73]	91
Total (95%CI)	**100.0**	**4.28 [2.47, 7.43]**	

Comparison: Cocaine vs Poly Drugs with Cocaine

Study	Weight %	RR (95%CI Random)	Year
MacGregor	19.0	1.46 [0.72, 2.97]	87
Keith	14.4	0.76 [0.34, 1.73]	89
Gillogley	34.9	0.92 [0.55, 1.55]	90
Cohen	31.7	0.67 [0.39, 1.15]	91
Total (95%CI)	**100.0**	**0.88 [0.65, 1.21]**	

Comparison: Cocaine vs Poly Drugs without Cocaine

Study	Weight %	RR (95%CI Random)	Year
Keith	16.2	1.71 [0.53, 5.59]	89
Gillogley	83.8	0.92 [0.55, 1.55]	90
Total (95%CI)	**100.0**	**1.02 [0.63, 1.64]**	

Comparison: Polydrugs with Cocaine vs Polydrugs without Cocaine

Study	Weight %	RR (95%CI Random)	Year
Gillogley	60.0	2.17 [0.70, 6.76]	90
Nair	40.0	0.94 [0.23, 3.77]	94
Total (95%CI)	**100.0**	**1.55 [0.64, 3.74]**	

Figure 2. Low Birthweight (<2,500 g).

to polydrugs with or without cocaine were used as controls the significant birth weight reduction disappeared. Regarding the combinability of the included studies reporting birth weight after cocaine exposure, the comparisons of cocaine alone or with polydrugs versus drug free control was homogeneous after the exclusion of outliers, Bingol [12] and Cohen [13], respectively. All other comparisons were homogeneous.

Birth Length (Fig. 4)

Consistent with the data on birth weight, use of cocaine (alone or in combinations with polydrugs) during pregnancy was associated with the risk of a weighted average birth length reduction of from 2.17 to 2.57 cm. Using as controls mothers exposed to polydrugs with or without cocaine, there was no difference in birth length of newborns exposed to cocaine (with or without polydrugs) during pregnancy. All comparisons were homogeneous with the exception of cocaine alone versus drug free controls where one outlier [14] caused the heterogeneity.

Prematurity (Fig. 5)

Prematurity was defined as a live birth before 37 weeks of gestation. Pregnant women exposed to cocaine alone or to cocaine plus

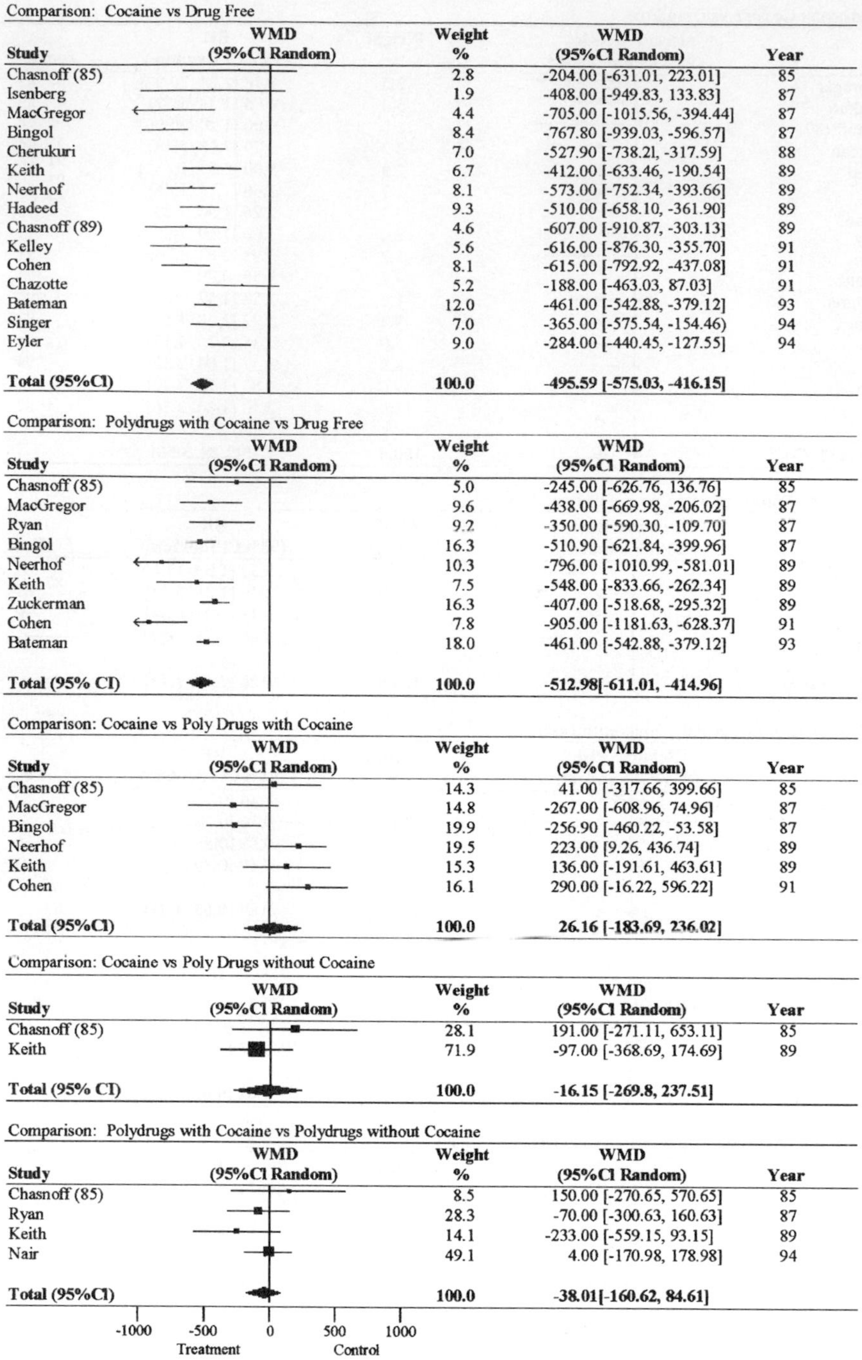

Comparison: Cocaine vs Drug Free
Study | WMD (95%CI Random) | Weight % | WMD (95%CI Random) | Year
Chasnoff (85) 2.8 -204.00 [-631.01, 223.01] 85
Isenberg 1.9 -408.00 [-949.83, 133.83] 87
MacGregor 4.4 -705.00 [-1015.56, -394.44] 87
Bingol 8.4 -767.80 [-939.03, -596.57] 87
Cherukuri 7.0 -527.90 [-738.21, -317.59] 88
Keith 6.7 -412.00 [-633.46, -190.54] 89
Neerhof 8.1 -573.00 [-752.34, -393.66] 89
Hadeed 9.3 -510.00 [-658.10, -361.90] 89
Chasnoff (89) 4.6 -607.00 [-910.87, -303.13] 89
Kelley 5.6 -616.00 [-876.30, -355.70] 91
Cohen 8.1 -615.00 [-792.92, -437.08] 91
Chazotte 5.2 -188.00 [-463.03, 87.03] 91
Bateman 12.0 -461.00 [-542.88, -379.12] 93
Singer 7.0 -365.00 [-575.54, -154.46) 94
Eyler 9.0 -284.00 [-440.45, -127.55] 94
Total (95%CI) 100.0 -495.59 [-575.03, -416.15]
Comparison: Polydrugs with Cocaine vs Drug Free
Study | WMD (95%CI Random) | Weight % | WMD (95%CI Random) | Year
Chasnoff (85) 5.0 -245.00 [-626.76, 136.76] 85
MacGregor 9.6 -438.00 [-669.98, -206.02] 87
Ryan 9.2 -350.00 [-590.30, -109.70] 87
Bingol 16.3 -510.90 [-621.84, -399.96] 87
Neerhof 10.3 -796.00 [-1010.99, -581.01] 89
Keith 7.5 -548.00 [-833.66, -262.34] 89
Zuckerman 16.3 -407.00 [-518.68, -295.32] 89
Cohen 7.8 -905.00 [-1181.63, -628.37] 91
Bateman 18.0 -461.00 [-542.88, -379.12] 93
Total (95% CI) 100.0 -512.98[-611.01, -414.96]
Comparison: Cocaine vs Poly Drugs with Cocaine
Study | WMD (95%CI Random) | Weight % | WMD (95%CI Random) | Year
Chasnoff (85) 14.3 41.00 [-317.66, 399.66] 85
MacGregor 14.8 -267.00 [-608.96, 74.96] 87
Bingol 19.9 -256.90 [-460.22, -53.58] 87
Neerhof 19.5 223.00 [9.26, 436.74] 89
Keith 15.3 136.00 [-191.61, 463.61] 89
Cohen 16.1 290.00 [-16.22, 596.22] 91
Total (95%CI) 100.0 26.16 [-183.69, 236.02]
Comparison: Cocaine vs Poly Drugs without Cocaine
Study | WMD (95%CI Random) | Weight % | WMD (95%CI Random) | Year
Chasnoff (85) 28.1 191.00 [-271.11, 653.11] 85
Keith 71.9 -97.00 [-368.69, 174.69] 89
Total (95% CI) 100.0 -16.15 [-269.8, 237.51]
Comparison: Polydrugs with Cocaine vs Polydrugs without Cocaine
Study | WMD (95%CI Random) | Weight % | WMD (95%CI Random) | Year
Chasnoff (85) 8.5 150.00 [-270.65, 570.65] 85
Ryan 28.3 -70.00 [-300.63, 160.63] 87
Keith 14.1 -233.00 [-559.15, 93.15] 89
Nair 49.1 4.00 [-170.98, 178.98] 94
Total (95%CI) 100.0 -38.01[-160.62, 84.61]
-1000 -500 0 500 1000
Treatment Control

Figure 3. Birthweight.

polydrugs had a higher risk of preterm delivery (RR: 2.48 $CI_{95\%}$ 2.02–3.06 and 3.19 $CI_{95\%}$ 2.30–4.41, respectively) than did drug free controls. Comparing mothers exposed to cocaine alone versus polydrugs with cocaine or mothers with cocaine and polydrug exposure versus polydrugs without cocaine did not result in a significant risk for prematurity. When mothers exposed to cocaine alone were compared with the group of mothers exposed to polydrugs without cocaine we notice again a significant risk of prematurity (RR: 1.72 $CI_{95\%}$ 1.19–2.52). All comparisons were homogeneous with the exception of the first comparison cocaine alone versus drug free control). This comparison became homogeneous when only prospective studies with identification of cocaine users by urine or meconium analysis were considered.

Gestational Age (Fig. 6)

The analysis of a continuous variable like gestational age confirmed the findings on prematurity after cocaine exposure during pregnancy. There was a significant reduction of the gestational age when we compare the mothers exposed to cocaine (alone or with other drugs) versus drug free control groups. Mothers using cocaine alone did not have a significant reduction of gestational

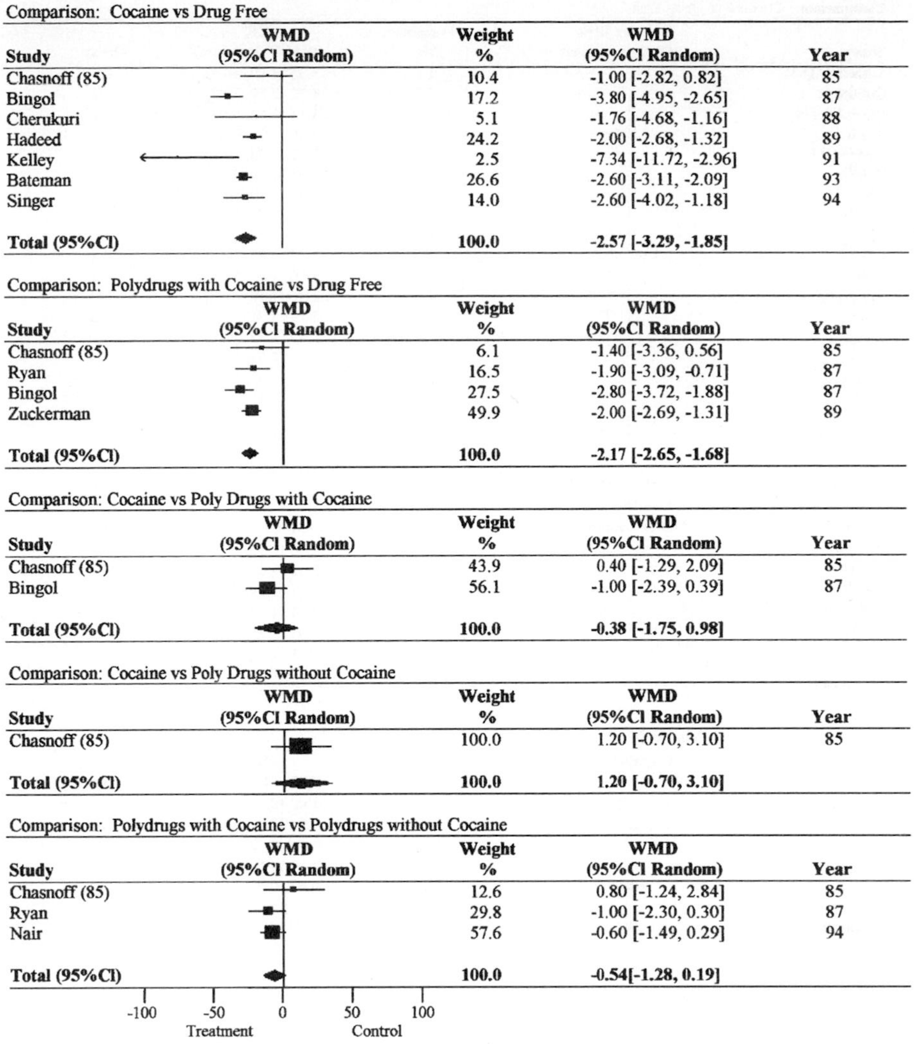
Comparison: Cocaine vs Drug Free
Study
WMD (95%CI Random)
Weight %
WMD (95%CI Random)
Year
Chasnoff (85) 10.4 -1.00 [-2.82, 0.82] 85
Bingol 17.2 -3.80 [-4.95, -2.65] 87
Cherukuri 5.1 -1.76 [-4.68, -1.16] 88
Hadeed 24.2 -2.00 [-2.68, -1.32] 89
Kelley 2.5 -7.34 [-11.72, -2.96] 91
Bateman 26.6 -2.60 [-3.11, -2.09] 93
Singer 14.0 -2.60 [-4.02, -1.18] 94
Total (95%CI) 100.0 -2.57 [-3.29, -1.85]
Comparison: Polydrugs with Cocaine vs Drug Free
Chasnoff (85) 6.1 -1.40 [-3.36, 0.56] 85
Ryan 16.5 -1.90 [-3.09, -0.71] 87
Bingol 27.5 -2.80 [-3.72, -1.88] 87
Zuckerman 49.9 -2.00 [-2.69, -1.31] 89
Total (95%CI) 100.0 -2.17 [-2.65, -1.68]
Comparison: Cocaine vs Poly Drugs with Cocaine
Chasnoff (85) 43.9 0.40 [-1.29, 2.09] 85
Bingol 56.1 -1.00 [-2.39, 0.39] 87
Total (95%CI) 100.0 -0.38 [-1.75, 0.98]
Comparison: Cocaine vs Poly Drugs without Cocaine
Chasnoff (85) 100.0 1.20 [-0.70, 3.10] 85
Total (95%CI) 100.0 1.20 [-0.70, 3.10]
Comparison: Polydrugs with Cocaine vs Polydrugs without Cocaine
Chasnoff (85) 12.6 0.80 [-1.24, 2.84] 85
Ryan 29.8 -1.00 [-2.30, 0.30] 87
Nair 57.6 -0.60 [-1.49, 0.29] 94
Total (95%CI) 100.0 -0.54[-1.28, 0.19]
-100 -50 0 50 100
Treatment
Control

Figure 4. Birth length.

age when compared with women exposed to polydrugs with cocaine. Similar results were found for polydrugs with cocaine exposure versus polydrugs without cocaine exposure. Of the included studies, only one reported the data on gestational age comparing women exposed to cocaine alone versus polydrugs without cocaine. After the exclusion of one outlier in the comparison of cocaine with polydrugs versus drug free control all comparisons were homogeneous.

Abruptio Placenta (Fig. 7)

Of the included studies, 17 reported data on abruptio placenta after cocaine exposure. The risk for this pregnancy complication was significant when we considered the studies that compared mothers exposed to cocaine alone or in combination with other addictions versus drug free controls or versus exposure to polydrugs but not cocaine. No risk of abruptio placenta was noted when we considered mothers exposed to cocaine alone versus women exposed to cocaine plus other drugs. The pooled risk for abruptio placenta was higher in studies comparing cocaine alone or with polydrugs versus polydrugs without cocaine. All comparisons were homogeneous.

Premature Rupture of Membrane (PROM) (Fig. 8)

This analysis included 8 studies. The pooled relative risk for PROM was significantly higher for pregnant women exposed to cocaine alone or with polydrugs compared to drug free controls or to polydrugs but not cocaine. The only comparison not found to be significant was cocaine alone versus polydrugs with cocaine. In all comparisons, the test for heterogeneity showed that all studies detected an effect size of similar magnitude and direction.

Head Circumference (Fig. 9)

Ten studies reported measurements of head circumference in children exposed to cocaine during pregnancy. Cocaine use (alone or with polydrugs) during pregnancy was associated with a significant risk of reduction of head circumference in the newborns. Cocaine alone or with other addictions did not lead to a significant reduction

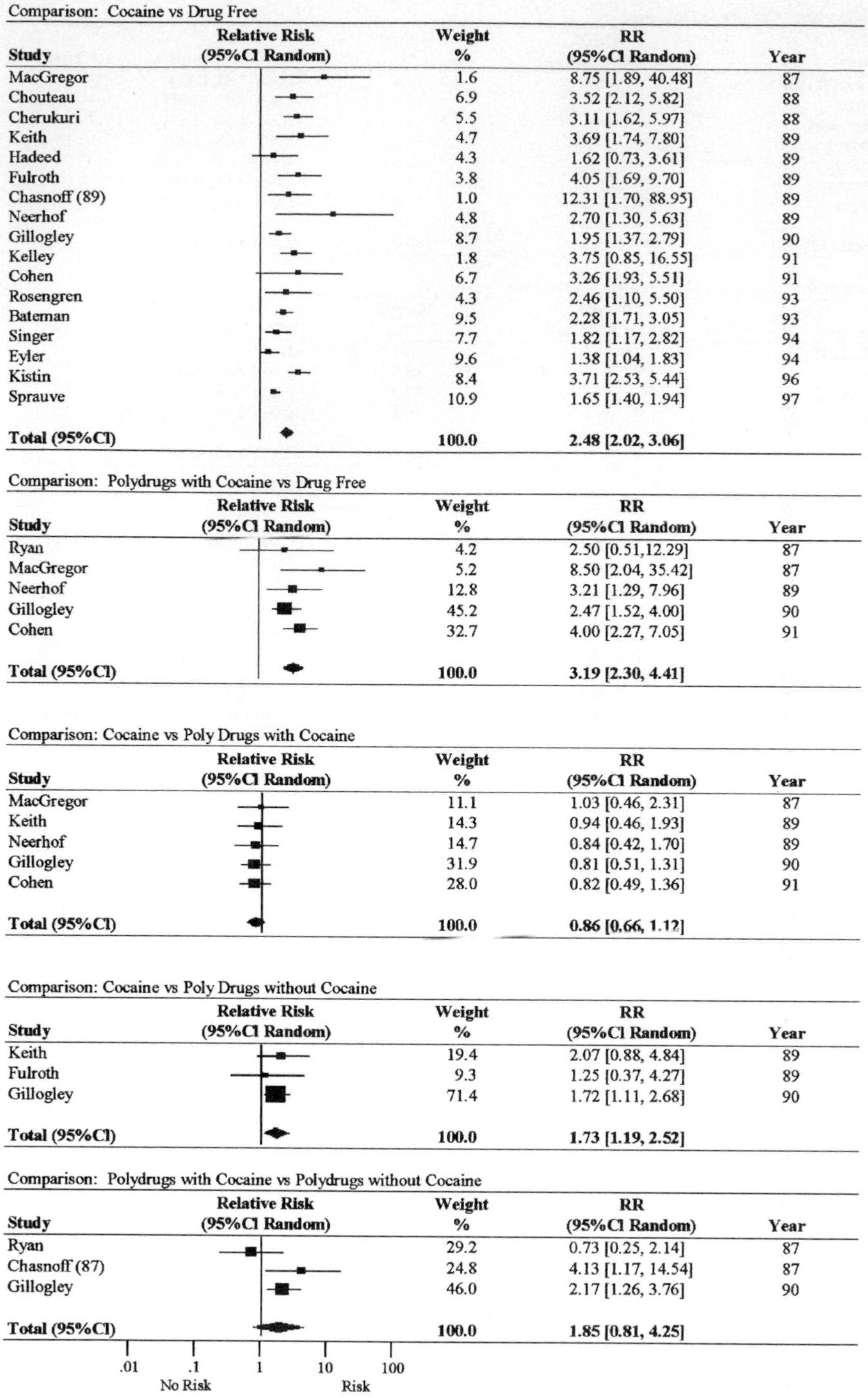

Comparison: Cocaine vs Drug Free
Study
Relative Risk (95%CI Random)
Weight %
RR (95%CI Random)
Year
MacGregor 1.6 8.75 [1.89, 40.48] 87
Chouteau 6.9 3.52 [2.12, 5.82] 88
Cherukuri 5.5 3.11 [1.62, 5.97] 88
Keith 4.7 3.69 [1.74, 7.80] 89
Hadeed 4.3 1.62 [0.73, 3.61] 89
Fulroth 3.8 4.05 [1.69, 9.70] 89
Chasnoff (89) 1.0 12.31 [1.70, 88.95] 89
Neerhof 4.8 2.70 [1.30, 5.63] 89
Gillogley 8.7 1.95 [1.37. 2.79] 90
Kelley 1.8 3.75 [0.85, 16.55] 91
Cohen 6.7 3.26 [1.93, 5.51] 91
Rosengren 4.3 2.46 [1.10, 5.50] 93
Bateman 9.5 2.28 [1.71, 3.05] 93
Singer 7.7 1.82 [1.17, 2.82] 94
Eyler 9.6 1.38 [1.04, 1.83] 94
Kistin 8.4 3.71 [2.53, 5.44] 96
Sprauve 10.9 1.65 [1.40, 1.94] 97
Total (95%CI) 100.0 2.48 [2.02, 3.06]
Comparison: Polydrugs with Cocaine vs Drug Free
Study
Relative Risk (95%CI Random)
Weight %
RR (95%CI Random)
Year
Ryan 4.2 2.50 [0.51,12.29] 87
MacGregor 5.2 8.50 [2.04, 35.42] 87
Neerhof 12.8 3.21 [1.29, 7.96] 89
Gillogley 45.2 2.47 [1.52, 4.00] 90
Cohen 32.7 4.00 [2.27, 7.05] 91
Total (95%CI) 100.0 3.19 [2.30, 4.41]
Comparison: Cocaine vs Poly Drugs with Cocaine
Study
Relative Risk (95%CI Random)
Weight %
RR (95%CI Random)
Year
MacGregor 11.1 1.03 [0.46, 2.31] 87
Keith 14.3 0.94 [0.46, 1.93] 89
Neerhof 14.7 0.84 [0.42, 1.70] 89
Gillogley 31.9 0.81 [0.51, 1.31] 90
Cohen 28.0 0.82 [0.49, 1.36] 91
Total (95%CI) 100.0 0.86 [0.66, 1.12]
Comparison: Cocaine vs Poly Drugs without Cocaine
Study
Relative Risk (95%CI Random)
Weight %
RR (95%CI Random)
Year
Keith 19.4 2.07 [0.88, 4.84] 89
Fulroth 9.3 1.25 [0.37, 4.27] 89
Gillogley 71.4 1.72 [1.11, 2.68] 90
Total (95%CI) 100.0 1.73 [1.19, 2.52]
Comparison: Polydrugs with Cocaine vs Polydrugs without Cocaine
Study
Relative Risk (95%CI Random)
Weight %
RR (95%CI Random)
Year
Ryan 29.2 0.73 [0.25, 2.14] 87
Chasnoff (87) 24.8 4.13 [1.17, 14.54] 87
Gillogley 46.0 2.17 [1.26, 3.76] 90
Total (95%CI) 100.0 1.85 [0.81, 4.25]
.01
.1
1
10
100
No Risk
Risk

Figure 5. Prematurity (<37 weeks).

of head circumference when compared to polydrug (but not cocaine) exposure. All these comparisons were found to be homogeneous. Only two studies had data eligible for the comparison between exposure to cocaine alone versus cocaine with polydrugs, and showed no significant reduction of head circumference. Finally, only one study reported data comparing head circumference after cocaine alone versus polydrugs with no cocaine. No significant risk was detected in this last comparison.

Sensitivity Analysis

Both retrospective analyses and studies identifying exposure by maternal interview or chart extraction may result in bias as to the correct exposure type. For this reason a secondary analysis was performed, excluding all retrospective studies and analyses where the identification of cocaine exposure was done by chart extraction or maternal interview. After the exclusion of those studies, the risk

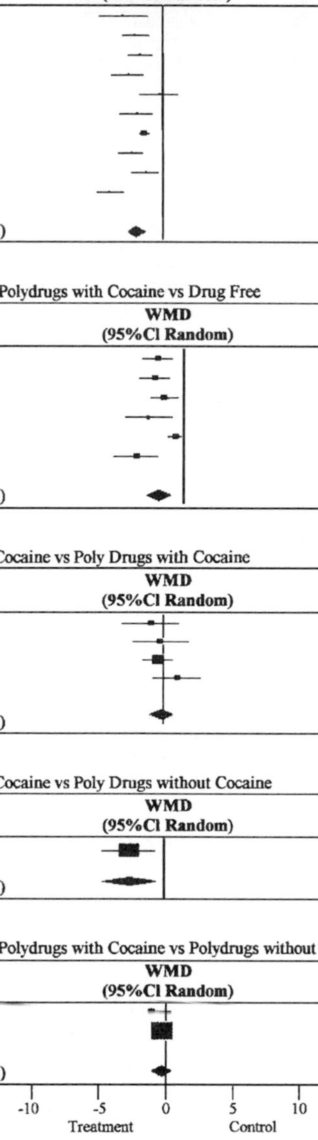

Comparison: Cocaine vs Drug Free

Study	Weight %	WMD (95%CI Random)	Year
MacGregor	5.9	-2.70 [-4.44, -0.96]	87
Cherukuri	10.5	-1.82 [-2.76, -0.881	88
Neerhof	11.2	-1.50 [-2.34, -0.66]	89
Keith	8.9	-2.40 [-3.58, -1.22]	89
Chazotte	7.6	-0.20 [-1.59, 1.19]	91
Kelley	9.2	-1.78 [-2.91, -0.65]	91
Bateman	14.6	-1.20 [-1.54, -0.86]	93
Cohen	11.1	-2.20 [-3.07, -1.33]	94
Eyler	10.7	-1.20 [-2.11, -0.29]	94
Singer	10.3	-3.60 [-4.57, -2.63]	94
Total (95%CI)	**100.0**	**-1.83[-2.36, -1.29]**	

Comparison: Polydrugs with Cocaine vs Drug Free

Study	Weight %	WMD (95%CI Random)	Year
Ryan	17.3	-1.70 [-2.73, -0.67]	87
MacGregor	17.2	-1.90 [-2.94, -0.86]	87
Neerhof	17.8	-1.20 [-2.18, -0.22]	89
Keith	12.3	-2.30 [-3.91, -0.69]	89
Zuckerman	22.4	-0.50 [-0.94, -0.06]	89
Cohen	13.0	-3.20 [-4.72, -1.68]	94
Total (95%CI)	**100.0**	**-1.65 [-2.46, -0.84]**	

Comparison: Cocaine vs Poly Drugs with Cocaine

Study	Weight %	WMD (95%CI Random)	Year
MacGregor	15.4	-0.80 [-2.72, 1.12]	87
Keith	15.5	-0.10 [-2.01, 1.81]	89
Neerhof	48.6	-0.30 [-1.38, 0.78]	89
Cohen	20.4	1.00 [-0.67, 2.67]	94
Total (95%CI)	**100.0**	**-0.08 [-0.83, 0.67]**	

Comparison: Cocaine vs Poly Drugs without Cocaine

Study	Weight %	WMD (95%CI Random)	Year
Keith	100.0	-2.40 [-4.21, -0.59]	89
Total (95%CI)	**100.0**	**-2.40 [-4.21, -0.59]**	

Comparison: Polydrugs with Cocaine vs Polydrugs without Cocaine

Study	Weight %	WMD (95%CI Random)	Year
Ryan	18.9	-0.90 [-2.26, 0.46]	87
Zuckerman	81.1	-0.10 [-0.66, 0.46]	89
Total (95%CI)	**100.0**	**-0.25 [-0.86, 0.36]**	

Figure 6. Gestational Age.

of major malformation was still significantly higher in mothers exposed to cocaine than in drug free controls (RR: 2.43, $CI_{95\%}$ 1.09–4.93) but was not significant in the comparison of pregnancy with cocaine alone versus polydrugs without cocaine exposures. Using the same exclusion criteria, we recalculated the relative risk or weighted average of: low birth weight (RR: 2.82, $CI_{95\%}$ 1.72–4.64), birth weight deficit (weighted average: –485 g $CI_{95\%}$ –550.8 g, –379.9 g), birth length deficit (weighted average: –2.18 cm $CI_{95\%}$ –2.84, –1.52 cm), prematurity (RR: 2.44 $CI_{95\%}$ 1.90–3.12), gestational age deficit (weighted average: –1.24 weeks, $CI_{95\%}$ –1.61, –0.8 weeks), abruptio placentae (RR: 5.89 $CI_{95\%}$ 1.90–3.12), PROM (RR: 1.58 $CI_{95\%}$ 1–2.51), and head circumference deficit (weighted average –1.7 cm $CI_{95\%}$ –2.0, –1.35 cm) in women exposed to cocaine alone versus drug free control. In none of these comparisons with cocaine versus drug free controls did the significance disappear. The same sensitivity analysis did not change the nonsignificant relative risk of cocaine alone versus polydrug/no cocaine for other endpoints (data not shown).

DISCUSSION

Because very large numbers of women in the reproductive age group consume cocaine, there are serious concerns regarding the long term health of millions of children exposed in utero to this recreational drug [2]. An issue widely recognized by researchers and clinicians is that, in addition to cocaine, many other risk factors occur and may adversely affect infants exposed in utero to cocaine. These include other drugs of abuse and cigarettes, alcohol, poor prenatal care, single motherhood, and poverty, to mention a few [2,15]. Any attempt to separate the effects of cocaine from other drugs of abuse must, therefore address the role of the various confounders.

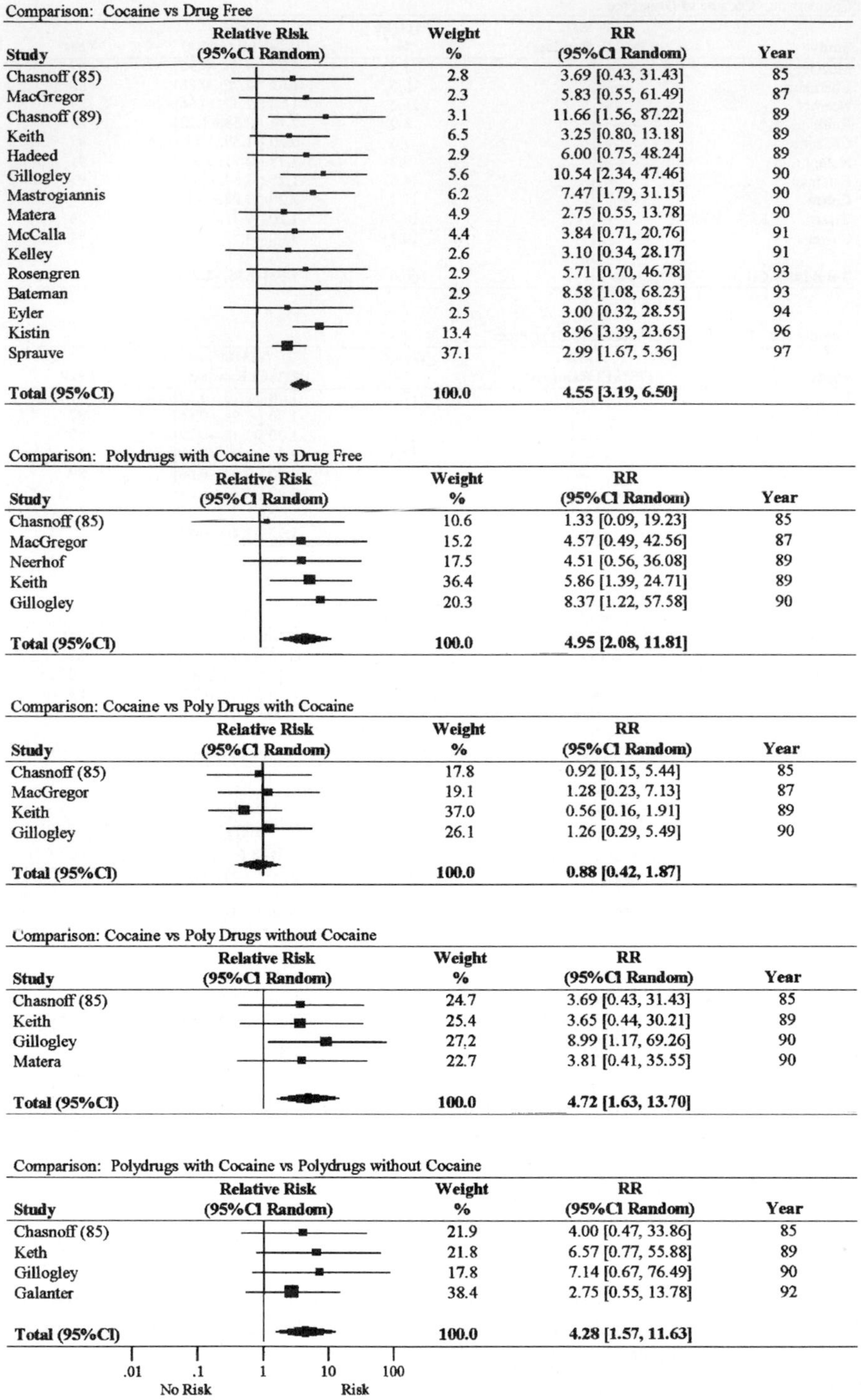

Comparison: Cocaine vs Drug Free

Study	Weight %	RR (95%CI Random)	Year
Chasnoff (85)	2.8	3.69 [0.43, 31.43]	85
MacGregor	2.3	5.83 [0.55, 61.49]	87
Chasnoff (89)	3.1	11.66 [1.56, 87.22]	89
Keith	6.5	3.25 [0.80, 13.18]	89
Hadeed	2.9	6.00 [0.75, 48.24]	89
Gillogley	5.6	10.54 [2.34, 47.46]	90
Mastrogiannis	6.2	7.47 [1.79, 31.15]	90
Matera	4.9	2.75 [0.55, 13.78]	90
McCalla	4.4	3.84 [0.71, 20.76]	91
Kelley	2.6	3.10 [0.34, 28.17]	91
Rosengren	2.9	5.71 [0.70, 46.78]	93
Bateman	2.9	8.58 [1.08, 68.23]	93
Eyler	2.5	3.00 [0.32, 28.55]	94
Kistin	13.4	8.96 [3.39, 23.65]	96
Sprauve	37.1	2.99 [1.67, 5.36]	97
Total (95%CI)	**100.0**	**4.55 [3.19, 6.50]**	

Comparison: Polydrugs with Cocaine vs Drug Free

Study	Weight %	RR (95%CI Random)	Year
Chasnoff (85)	10.6	1.33 [0.09, 19.23]	85
MacGregor	15.2	4.57 [0.49, 42.56]	87
Neerhof	17.5	4.51 [0.56, 36.08]	89
Keith	36.4	5.86 [1.39, 24.71]	89
Gillogley	20.3	8.37 [1.22, 57.58]	90
Total (95%CI)	**100.0**	**4.95 [2.08, 11.81]**	

Comparison: Cocaine vs Poly Drugs with Cocaine

Study	Weight %	RR (95%CI Random)	Year
Chasnoff (85)	17.8	0.92 [0.15, 5.44]	85
MacGregor	19.1	1.28 [0.23, 7.13]	87
Keith	37.0	0.56 [0.16, 1.91]	89
Gillogley	26.1	1.26 [0.29, 5.49]	90
Total (95%CI)	**100.0**	**0.88 [0.42, 1.87]**	

Comparison: Cocaine vs Poly Drugs without Cocaine

Study	Weight %	RR (95%CI Random)	Year
Chasnoff (85)	24.7	3.69 [0.43, 31.43]	85
Keith	25.4	3.65 [0.44, 30.21]	89
Gillogley	27.2	8.99 [1.17, 69.26]	90
Matera	22.7	3.81 [0.41, 35.55]	90
Total (95%CI)	**100.0**	**4.72 [1.63, 13.70]**	

Comparison: Polydrugs with Cocaine vs Polydrugs without Cocaine

Study	Weight %	RR (95%CI Random)	Year
Chasnoff (85)	21.9	4.00 [0.47, 33.86]	85
Keth	21.8	6.57 [0.77, 55.88]	89
Gillogley	17.8	7.14 [0.67, 76.49]	90
Galanter	38.4	2.75 [0.55, 13.78]	92
Total (95%CI)	**100.0**	**4.28 [1.57, 11.63]**	

Figure 7. Abruptio Placenta.

In our original meta-analysis, performed a decade ago [4], there was often insufficient statistical power to address differences between cocaine exposed fetuses and controls. Due to the tremendous volume of research published during the last ten years, we had the opportunity to address several important adverse effects widely attributed to cocaine. Yes, for several endpoints, statistical power is still an issue.

There are potential weaknesses in meta-analysis of observational studies dealing with cocaine, where many other aspects of women's life may affect outcome. Studies differ in the method and time of ascertainment of major malformations. By separating studies into those where women were exposed mainly to cocaine, to cocaine plus other drugs, mostly to other drugs, or were drug free, we have attempted to partially control for some of the confounding factors mentioned above, known to adversely affect infants. However, one cannot safely ascertain that the distribution of potential confounders is similar across exposure groups. It is possible that, for example, women who use cocaine only smoke cigarettes

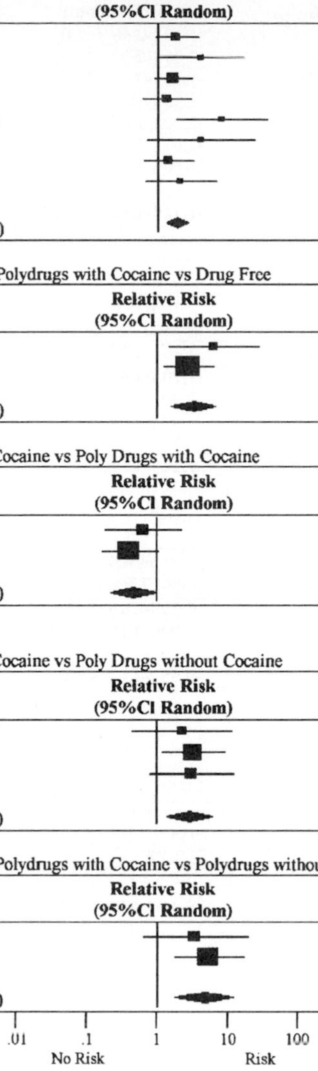

Comparison: Cocaine vs Drug Free

Study	Relative Risk (95%CI Random)	Weight %	RR (95%CI Random)	Year
Cherukuri		20.2	1.80 [0.91, 3.54]	88
Keith		5.2	3.90 [1.01, 15.10]	89
Gillogley		25.5	1.63 [0.89, 2.97]	90
Matera		16.4	1.33 [0.63, 2.84]	90
Mastrogiannis		4.7	7.47 [1.79, 31.15]	90
McCalla		3.4	3.84 [0.71, 20.76]	91
Galanter		16.5	1.39 [0.65, 2.95]	92
Rosengren		8.0	2.04 [0.69, 6.05]	93
Total (95%CI)		**100.0**	**1.85 [1.35, 2.52]**	

Comparison: Polydrugs with Cocaine vs Drug Free

Study	Relative Risk (95%CI Random)	Weight %	RR (95%CI Random)	Year
Keith		22.5	5.86 [1.39, 24.71]	89
Gillogley		77.5	2.66 [1.23, 5.78]	90
Total (95%CI)		**100.0**	**3.18 [1.61, 6.29]**	

Comparison: Cocaine vs Poly Drugs with Cocaine

Study	Relative Risk (95%CI Random)	Weight %	RR (95%CI Random)	Year
Keith		34.2	0.67 [0.20, 2.18]	89
Gillogley		65.8	0.45 [0.19, 1.05]	90
Total (95%CI)		**100.0**	**0.51 [0.26, 1.03]**	

Comparison: Cocaine vs Poly Drugs without Cocaine

Study	Relative Risk (95%CI Random)	Weight %	RR (95%CI Random)	Year
Keith		20.0	2.19 [0.46, 10.37]	89
Gillogley		51.6	3.06 [1.16, 8.04]	90
Matera		28.5	2.97 [0.81, 10.93]	90
Total (95%CI)		**100.0**	**2.84 [1.42, 5.68]**	

Comparison: Polydrugs with Cocaine vs Polydrugs without Cocaine

Study	Relative Risk (95%CI Random)	Weight %	RR (95%CI Random)	Year
Keith		30.7	3.29 [0.64, 16.79]	89
Gillogley		69.3	5.00 [1.69, 14.79]	90
Total (95%CI)		**100.0**	**4.40 [1.78, 10.85]**	

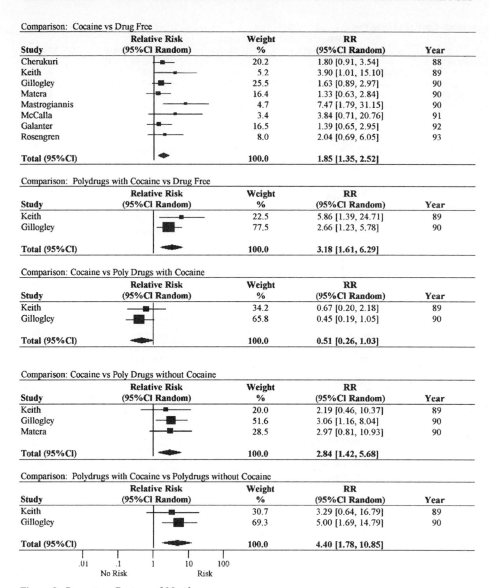

Figure 8. Premature Repture of Membranes.

and drink ethanol differently than women consuming cocaine plus other drugs.

The rates of major malformations among children of cocaine users are significantly higher than among drug free women. However, when these babies are compared to those exposed to other drugs of abuse, the effect size is not significant, suggesting that the various confounders, also occurring in polydrug/no cocaine users, are responsible for this effect. An identical trend has emerged for other endpoints, including gestational age, birth weight, birth length, and head circumference as well as the rates of prematurity and low birth weight. However, these findings may also be interpreted differently. It is impossible from the available data to apportion the risk of cocaine vs the confounders. It is possible for example, that both in the "cocaine only" and "cocaine plus polydrug," most of the risk is caused by cocaine. Also, one does not know that the distribution of confounders is similar between these two types of users. There is however, a large body of evidence showing that polydrug users have all the confounders cocaine users have, thus assisting in estimating the risk conferred by cocaine itself.

The two adverse effects measured by this systematic review that appeared to be significantly associated with cocaine itself are the rates of abruptio placenta and premature rupture of membranes. In both cases, cocaine users had higher risks for these adverse events than women consuming other drugs of abuse. These results are different from those in our original analysis [4], where there was insufficient power to prove placental abruption as directly associated with cocaine. It is possible that other associations will emerge as significant with more studies and higher statistical power (e,g., major malformations in cocaine vs. polydrug no-cocaine; RR 3.0, $CI_{95\%}$ 0.62–14.54, which did not reach significance, possibly because only two studies were available).

It is important to note that the analysis of major malformations cannot address specific malformations that may be directly related to cocaine exposure. Equally important, this analysis did not include reports of neurobehavioral endpoints, which are currently the focus of much research and clinical attention. A separate systematic review will be needed to address long term brain development in these children.

Comparison: Cocaine vs Drug Free

Study	WMD (95%CI Random)	Weight %	WMD (95%CI Random)	Year
Chasnoff (85)		2.2	-1.10 [-2.48, 0.28]	85
Bingol		14.0	-2.00 [-2.55, -1.45]	87
Cherukuri		6.3	-1.90 [-2.72, -1.08]	88
Chasnoff (89)		5.2	-1.90 [-2.80. -1.00]	89
Hadeed		21.3	-2.00 [-2.45, -1.55]	89
Kelley		2.1	-2.07 [-3.50, -0.64]	91
Bateman		49.0	-1.50 [-1.79, -1.21]	93
Total (95%CI)		**100.0**	**-1.72 [-1.93, -1.52]**	

Comparison: Polydrugs with Cocaine vs Drug Free

Study	WMD (95%CI Random)	Weight %	WMD (95%CI Random)	Year
Chasnoff (85)		6.4	-1.20 [-2.35, -0.05]	85
Ryan		9.6	-1.50 [-2.44, -0.56]	87
Zuckerman		48.3	-1.30 [-1.72, -0.88]	87
Bingol		35.7	-1.00 [-1.49, -0.51]	87
Total (95%CI)		**100.0**	**-1.21 [-1.51, -0.91]**	

Comparison: Cocaine vs Poly Drugs with Cocaine

Study	WMD (95%CI Random)	Weight %	WMD (95%CI Random)	Year
Chasnoff (85)		38.0	0.10 [-1.16, 1.36]	85
Bingol		62.0	-1.00 [-1.69, -0.31]	87
Total (95%CI)		**100.0**	**-0.58 [-1.63, 0.46]**	

Comparison: Cocaine vs Poly Drugs without Cocaine

Study	WMD (95%CI Random)	Weight %	WMD (95%CI Random)	Year
Chasnoff (85)		100.0	0.50 [-1.05, 2.05]	85
Total (95%CI)		**100.0**	**0.50 [-1.05, 2.05]**	

Comparison: Polydrugs with Cocaine vs Polydrugs without Cocaine

Study	WMD (95%CI Random)	Weight %	WMD (95%CI Random)	Year
Chasnoff (85)		9.4	0.40 [-0.95, 1.75]	85
Zuckerman		36.6	-0.40 [-0.91, 0.11]	87
Ryan		21.4	-0.70 [-1.51, 0.11]	87
Nair		32.6	0.20 [-0.37, 0.77]	94
Total (95%CI)		**100.0**	**-0.19 [-0.64, 0.25]**	

-4 -2 0 2 4

Treatment Control

Figure 9. Head Circumference.

REFERENCES

[1] Simone C, Derewlany LO, Koren G. Cocaine transfer across a cocaine exposed placental cotyledon perfused in vitro. Life Sci 1995; 57:PL137-PL140.

[2] Volpe JJ. Effect of cocaine use on the fetus. New Engl J Med 1992;327:399–407.

[3] Koren G. Cocaine and the human fetus: the concept of teratophilia. Neurotoxicol Teratol. 1993;15:301–4; discussion 311–2.

[4] Lutiger B, Graham K, Einarson TR, Koren G. Relationship between gestational cocaine use and pregnancy outcome: a meta-analysis. Teratology 1991;44:405–14.

[5] DerSimonian R, Laird N. Meta-analysis in clinical trials. Controlled Clinical Trials 1986;7:177–188.

[6] Forman R, Klein J, Meta D, Barks J, Greenwald M, Koren G. Maternal and neonatal characteristics following exposure to cocaine in Toronto. Reproductive Toxicology 1993;7:619–22.

[7] Handler A, Kistin N, Davis F, Ferre C. Cocaine use during pregnancy: perinatal outcomes. American Journal of Epidemiology 1991;133:818–25.

[8] Spence MR, Williams R, DiGregorio GJ, Kirby-McDonnell A, Polansky M. The relationship between recent cocaine use and pregnancy outcome. Obstet Gynecol 1991;78:326–9.

[9] Heinonen OP, Slone D, Shapiro S. Birth Defects and Drugs in Pregnancy. 1977.

[10] Neerhof MG, MacGregor SN, Retzky SS, Sullivan TP. Cocaine abuse during pregnancy: peripartum prevalence and perinatal outcome. American Journal of Obstetrics & Gynecology 1989;161: 633–8.

[11] Richardson GA, Day NL. Maternal and neonatal effects of moderate cocaine use during pregnancy. Neurotoxicol Teratol 1991;13: 455–60.

[12] Bingol N, Fuchs M, Diaz V, Stone R, Gromisch D. Teratogenicity of cocaine in humans. J Pediatr 1987;110:93–6.

[13] Cohen HR, Green JR, Crombleholme WR. Peripartum cocaine use: estimating risk of adverse pregnancy outcome. Int J Gynaecol Obstet 1991;35:51–4.

[14] Kelley SJ, Walsh JH, Thompson K. Birth outcomes, health problems, and neglect with prenatal exposure to cocaine. Pediatric Nursing 1991;17:130–6.

[15] Graham K, Koren G. Characteristics of pregnant women exposed to cocaine in Toronto between 1985 and 1990. Canadian Medical Association Journal 1991;144: 563–8.

[16] Bateman DA, Ng SK, Hansen CA, Heagarty MC. The effects of intrauterine cocaine exposure in newborns. Am J Pub Health 1993; 83:190–3.

[17] Chasnoff IJ, Burns W, Schnoll SH, Burns KA. Cocaine use in pregnancy. New Engl J Med 1985;313:666–9.

[18] Chasnoff IJ, Burns KA, Burns W. Cocaine use in pregnancy;perinatal morbidity and mortality. Neurotoxicol Teratol 1987;161: 291–3.

[19] Chasnoff IJ, Chisum GM, Kaplan WE. Maternal cocaine use and genitourinary tract malformation. Teratology 1988;37:201–4.

[20] Chavez GF, Mulinare J, Cordero JF. Maternal cocaine use during early pregnancy as a risk factor for congenital urogenital anomalies. JAMA 1989;262:795–8.

[21] Chazotte C, Forman L, Gandhi J. Heart rate patterns in fetuses exposed to cocaine. Obstet Gynecol 1991;78:323–5.

[22] Cherukuri R, Minkoff H., Feldman J, Parekh A, Glass L. A cohort study of alkaloidal cocaine ("crack") in pregnancy. Obstet Gynecol 1988;72:147–151.

[23] Chouteau M, Namerow, PB, Leppert, P. The effects of cocaine abuse on birth weight and gestational age. Obstet Gynecol 1988;72:351–4.

[24] Eyler FD, Behnke M, Conlon M, Woods NS, Frentzen B. Prenatal cocaine use: a comparison of neonates matched on maternal risk factors. Neurotoxicol Teratol 1994;16:81–7.

[25] Fulroth R, Phillips B, Durand DJ. Perinatal outcome of infants exposed to cocaine and/or heroin in utero. Am J Dis Child 1989;143: 905–10.

[26] Galanter M, Egelko S, De Leon G, Rohrs C, Franco H. Crack/cocaine abusers in the general hospital: assessment, and initiation of care. American Journal of Psychiatry. 1992;149:810–15.

[27] Gillogley KM, Evans AT, Hansen RL, Samuels SJ, Batra KK. The perinatal impact of cocaine, amphetamine, and opiate use detected by universal intrapartum screening. American Journal of Obstetrics & Gynecology 1990;163:1535–42.

[28] Hadeed AJ, Siegel SR. Maternal cocaine use during pregnancy: effect on the newborn infant. Pediatrics 1989;84:205–10.

[29] Isenberg S, Spierer A, Inkelis S. Ocular signs of cocaine intoxication in neonates. American Journal of Ophthamology 1987;103:211–14.

[30] Keith LG, MacGregor S, Friedell S, Rosner M, Chasnoff IJ, Sciarra J. Substance abuse in pregnany women: Recent experience at the Perinatal Center for Chemical Dependence of Northwestern Memorial Hospital. Obstet Gynecol 1999;73:715–20.

[31] Kistin N, Handler A, Davis F, Ferre C. Cocaine and cigarettes: a comparison of risks. Paediatr Perinat Epidemiol 1996;10:269–78.

[32] Little BB, Snell LM, Klein VR, Gilstrap LCI. Cocaine abuse during pregnancy: maternal and fetal implications. Obstet Gynecol 1989; 73:157–60.

[33] McCalla S, Minkoff HL, Feldman J, et al. The biologic and social consequences of perinatal cocaine use in an inner-city population: results of an anonymous cross-sectional study. American Journal of Obstetrics & Gynecology 1991;164:625–30.

[34] MacGregor S, Keith LG, Chasnoff IJ, et al. Cocaine use during pregnancy: adverse perinatal outcome. American Journal of Obstetrics & Gynecology 1987;157: 686–90.

[35] Mastrogiannis DS, Decavalas GO, Verma U, Tejani N. Perinatal outcome after recent cocaine usage. Obstet Gynecol 1990;76: 8–11.

[36] Matera C, Warren WB, Moomjy M, Fink DJ, Fox HE. Prevalence of use of cocaine and other substances in an obstetric population. American Journal of Obstetrics & Gynecology 1990;163:797–801.

[37] Nair P, Rothblum S, Hebel R. Neonatal outcome in infants with evidence of fetal exposure to opiates, cocaine, and cannabinoids. Clinical Pediatrics 1994;33:280–5.

[38] Rosengren SS, Longobucco DB, Bernstein BA, et al. Meconium testing for cocaine metabolite: prevalence, perceptions, and pitfalls. American Journal of Obstetrics & Gynecology 1993;168: 1449–56.

[39] Ryan L, Ehrlich S, Finnegan L. Cocaine abuse in pregnancy. Neurotoxicol Teratol 1987;9:295–9.

[40] Singer L, Arendt R, Song LY, Warshawsky E, Kliegman R. Direct and indirect interactions of cocaine with childbirth outcomes. Archives of Pediatrics & Adolescent Medicine 1994;148:959–64.

[41] Sprauve ME, Lindsay MK, Herbert S, Gravew W. Adverse perinatal outcome in parturients who use crack cocaine. Obstet Gynecol 1997; 89:674–8.

[42] Stafford JR, Jr., Rosen TS, Zaider M, Merriam JC. Prenatal cocaine exposure and the development of the human eye. Ophthalmology 1994;101:301–8.

[43] Zuckerman B, Frank DA, Hingson R, et al. Effects of maternal marijuana and cocaine use on fetal growth. New Engl J Med 1989;320:762–8.

APPENDIX. REJECTED STUDIES

Case reports/case series (n = 80)

Abramowicz, 1991 [1]; Apple, 1990 [2]; Bakht, 1990 [3]; Beltran, 1995 [4]; Brown, Jr., 1993 [5]; Burkett, 1990 [6]; Carlan, 1991 [7]; Cohen, 1991 [8]; Collins, 1989 [9]; Deolivcira, 1991 [10]; Dollberg, 1989 [11]; Dominguez, 1991 [12]; Evelyn, 1992 [13]; Geggel, 1989 [14]: George, 1995 [15]; Gieron-Korthals, 1994 [16]; Gomez-Anson, 1994 [17]; Gonsoulin, 1990 [18]; Good, 1992 [19]; Green-field, 1991 [20]; Greenland, 1989 [21]; Hall, 1992 [22]; Hannig, 1991 [23]; Harris, 1993 [24]; Hepper, 1995 [25]; Ho, 1994 [26]; Hoeger, 1996 [27]; Hoyme, 1990 [28]; Hsu, 1992 [29]; Iriye, 1994 [30]; Iriye, 1995 [31]; Jack, 1990 [32]; Jasnosz, 1994 [33]; Jawahar, 1997 [34]; Johnson, 1995 [35]; Kankirawatana, 1993 [36]; Kapur, 1991 [37]; Lampley 1996 [38]; Lessick, 1991 [39]; Lezcano, 1994 [40]; Liu, 1992 [41]; Martinez, 1994 [42]; Meeker, 1990 [43]; Mendelson, 1992 [44]; Mercado, 1989 [45]; Miller, 1990 [46]; Mishra, 1995 [47]; Mittleman, (1989b) [48]; Moen, 1993 [49]; Moriya, 1995 [50]; Murphy, 1993 [51]; Nolte, 1991 [52]; Nyirjesy, 1993 [53]; Okoruwa, 1995 [54]; Ostrea, Jr., 1994 [55]; Perlow, 1990 [56]; Peters, 1992 [57]; Porat, 1991 [58]; Potter, 1994 [59]; Rais-Bahrami, 1990 [60]; Reznik, 1989 [61]; Robin, 1994 [62]; Sarpong, 1992 [63]; Seballos, 1994 [64]; Sheinbaum, 1992 [65]; Sims, 1989 [66]; Singer, 1995 [67]; Skopp, 1997 [68]; Spinazzola, 1992 [69]; Spires, 1989 [70]; Spital, 1991 [71]; Streissguth, 1991 [72]; Sturner, 1991 [73]; Sumner, 1993 [74]; Sztulman, 1990 [75]; Thatcher, 1989 [76]; Towers, 1993 [77]; van den Anker, 1993 [78]; Viscarello, 1992 [79]; Wilson, 1993 [80].

Editorials (n = 22)

Alexander, 1991 [81]; Amoury, 1993 [82]; Anonymous, 1990 a [83]; Anonymous, 1991a [84]; Baxley, 1990 [85]; Brouhard, 1994 [86]; Chasnoff, 1989a [87]; Fantel, 1990 [88]; Heagarty, 1990 [89]; Howard, 1995 [90]; Jentzen, 1993 [91]; Jos, 1995 [92]; Kearney, 1995 [93]; Konkol, (1994a) [94]; Lewis, 1989 [95]; Lone, 1991 [96]; Neuspiel, 1993b [97]; Nora, 1990 [98]; Plessinger, 1993 [99]; Salamy, 1990 [100]; Tudehope, 1989 [101]; Zuckerman, 1994 [102].

Letters (n = 43)

Abdeljaber, 1990 [103]; Ahmed, 1989 [104]; Anonymous, 1990 [105]; Bays, 1991 [106]; Carraccio, 1994 [107]; Chavkin, 1990 [108]; Cottler, 1992 [109]; DiGregorio, 1993 [110]; Downing, 1991 [111]; Fogarty, 1991 [112]; Friedman, 1995 [113]; Goldin, 1989 [114]; Good, 1994 115]; Graham, 1989a [116]; Gratacos, 1993 [117]; Hansen, 1990 [118]; Herschman, 1991 [119]; Hunt, 1990 [120]; Jerome, 1995 [121]; Kain, 1992 [122]; Levy, 1993 [123]; Maynard, 1990 [124]; Miele, 1992 [125]; Mittleman, (1989a) [126]; Moore, 1993 [127]; Morfesis, 1994 [128]; Neuspiel, 1992a [129]; Neuspiel, 1992 [130]; Neuspiel, 1995 [131]; Nucci, 1994 [132]; Page, 1992 [133]; Petrulis, 1992 [134]; Racine, 1994 [135]; Sackoff, 1992 [136]; Shaw, 1991 [137]; Sher, 1989 [138]; Stephens, 1989 [139]; Sugarman, 1995 [140]; Tabor, 1990 [141]; Thorp, Jr. 1991 [142]; van den Anker, 1991 [143]; van den Anker, 1992 [144];Yang, 1995 [145].

Reviews and commentaries (n = 87)

Abel, 1991 [146]; Adams, 1990 [147]; Anonymous, 1989a [148]; Anonymous, 1993 [149]; Aronson, 1990 [150]; Berger, 1990 [151]; Brent, 1994 [152]; Buehler, 1995 [153]; Buehler, 1996 [154]; Byrne, 1992 [155]; Chan, 1997 [156]; Chao, 1996 [157]; Chasnoff, 1989b [158]; Chasnoff, 1993 [159]; Chavkin,1993 [160]; Church, 1993 [161]; Coles, 1992 [162]; Coles, 1993 [163]; Cornish, 1996 [164]; Day, (1993a) [165]; Day, 1993b [166]; Dixon, 1989 [167]; Dow Edwards, 1991 [168]; Dow-Edwards,1993 [169]; Dumas, 1992 [170]; Dungy-Poythress, 1995 [171]; Elhassani, 1990 [172]; Ellen, 1993 [173]; Fantel, 1993 [174]; Ferner, 1993 [175]; Finnegan, 1994 [176]; Frank, 1993 [177]; Garcia, 1990 [178]; Gaskill, 1992 [179]; Giacoia, 1990 [180]; Gintautiene, 1990 [181]; Goldstein, 1990 [182]; Goodwin, 1990 [183]; Grossman, 1993 [184]; Horger, 1990 [185]; Janke, 1990 [186]; Johnson, 1992 [187]; Kaltenbach, 1994 [188]; Kandall, 1991 [189]; Karmel, 1991 [190]; Keller, 1993 [191]; Kenner, 1997 [192]; Khoury, 1991 [193]; Klitsch, 1994 [194]; Knisely, 1991 [195]; Koren, 1989 [196]; Koren, 1993 [197]; Landry, 1996 [198]; Lauder, 1991 [199]; Lewis, 1991 [200]; Litt, 1997 [201]; Lunsford, 1995 [202]; Lutiger, 1991 [203]; Martin, 1992a [204]; Martin, (1992b) [205]; Meyer, 1996 [206]; Miller, 1994 [207]; Miller, 1997 [208]; Murphey, 1993 [209]; Neuspiel, (1993a) [210]; Ostrea, 1992 [211]; Pokorni, 1996 [212]; Richardson, 1993 [213]; Richardson, 1996 [214]; Ripple, 1992 [215]; Rizk, 1996 [216]; Sexson, 1993 [217]; Shepard, 1993 [218]; Slade, 1993 [219]; Spear, 1993 [220]; Sprauve, 1996 [221]; Strauss, 1997 [222]; Sun, 1997 [223]; Swadi, 1993 [224]; Szeto, 1991 [225]; Warner, 1997 [226] Webster, 1993 [227]; Westdorp, 1995 [228]; Wightman, 1991 [229]; Wootton, 1994 [230]; Zuckerman, 1992 [231]; Zuckerman, 1991 [232].

Studies not reporting fetal or pregnancy outcomes (n = 127)

Abusada, 1993 [233]; Alemi, 1996 [234]; Alemi, 1996 [235]; Alemi, 1996 [236]; Amaro, 1990 [237]; Anonymous, (1990 c) [238]; Anonymous, 1996 [239]; Archie, 1997 [240]; Ball, 1997 [241]; Bauchner, 1990 [242]; Behnke, 1997 [243]; Bendersky, 1996 [244]; Berenson, 1991 [245]; Billman, 1996 [246]; Browne, 1992 [247]; Browne, 1994 [248]; Brunader, 1991 [249]; Burke, 1993 [250]; Callahan, 1992 [251]; Cartwright, 1991 [252]; Casanova, 1994 [253]; Chasnoff, 1990 [254]; Charpentier, 1996 [255]; Condie, 1989 [256]; Cornelius, 1993 [257];Cornelius, 1994 [258]; Czeizel, 1990 [259]; de Feo, 1995 [260]; Delaney-Black, 1996 [261]; DePetrillo, 1995 [262]; DeVane, 1991 [263]; DiGregorio, 1994 [264]; Dudish, 1996 [265]; Egelko, 1996 [266]; Elk, 1994 [267]; Elk, 1995 [268]; Ellerbrock, 1995 [269]; Emery, 1995 [270]; Fetters, 1996 [271]; Forman, 1992 [272]; Forman, 1994 [273]; Frank, 1992 [274]; Galanter, 1992 [275]; Gillmore, 1992 [276]; Graham, 1989b [277]; Graham, 1991 [278]; Grant, 1994 [279]; Gomez, 1996 [280]; Hall, 1996 [281]; Hawley, 1995 [282]; Heller, 1996 [283]; Henderson, 1989 [284]; Henderson, 1997 [285]; Hurd, 1991 [286]; Hurt, 1996 [287]; Hurt, (1997a) [288]; Hurt, 1997b [289]; Hutchins, 1997 [290]; Ingersoll, 1996 [291]; Jacobson, 1991 [292]; Jacobson, 1996 [293]; Jain, 1993 [294]; Johnson, 1997 [295]; Joyce, 1995 [296]; Kain, 1995 [297]; Karmel, 1996 [298]; Killeen, 1995 [299]; Klein, 1992 [300]; Klein, 1994 [301]; Kline, 1997 [302]; Konkol, 1994b [303]; Koren, 1992a [304]; Koren, 1992b [305]; Koren, 1992c [306]; Land, 1990 [307]; Lindsay, 1990 [308]; Lanehart, 1994 [309]; Lauria, 1997 [310]; Lindsay, 1991 [311]; Lindsay, 1992 [312]; Lindsay, 1997 [313]; Little, 1990 [314]; Marques, 1993 [315]; Martin, 1996 [316]; Martinez Crespo, 1994 [317]; Mayes, 1996 [318]; McCalla, 1992 [319]; McFarlin, 1996 [320]; Miller, 1993 [321]; Minkoff, 1990 [322]; Moore, 1996 [323]; Moriya, 1994 [324]; Moser, 1993 [325]; Napiorkowski, 1996 [326]; Neuspiel, (1993c) [327]; O'Connor, 1997 [328]; Peeke, 1994 [329]; Pelham, 1992 [330]; Phibbs, 1991 [331]; Polzin, 1991 [332]; Quinn, 1992 [333]; Reddin, 1991 [334]; Regalado, 1996 [335]; Richardson, 1996a [214]; Richardson, 1996b [336]; Rico, 1990 [337]; Rodriguez, 1996 [338]; Rogers, 1991 [339]; Rosenkranz, 1990 [340]; Ruiz, 1994 [341]; Ryan, 1994 [342]; Scafidi, 1996 [343]; Schutzman, 1991 [344]; Singer, 1997 [345]; Smith, 1989 [346]; Strano-Rossi, 1996 [347]; Svikis, 1997 [348]; Tronick, 1996 [349]; Ursitti, 1997 [350]; Vega, 1997 [351]; Wasserman, 1993 [352]; Weeman, 1995 [353]; Weese-Mayer, 1991 [354]; Welch, 1993 [355]; Wingert, 1994 [356]; Zimmerman, 1994 [357]; Zuckerman, 1989a [358].

In vitro studies/placenta perfusion (n = 39)

Ahmed, 1990 [359]; Ahmed, 1991 [360]; Bailey, 1994 [361]; Bailey, 1996 [362]; Cejtin, 1990 [363]; Chiarotti, [364]; Cook, 1996 [365]; Dicke, 1993 [366]; Dicke, 1994 [367]; Gilbert, 1990 [368]; Harker, 1994 [369]; Hurd, 1993 [370]; Johnson, 1996 [371]; Krishna, 1993 [372]; Malek, 1995 [373]; Miller, 1996 [374]; Mirochnick, 1997 [375]; Monga, 1993 [376]; Monga, 1994 [377]; Moore, 1992 [378]; Oyler, 1996 [379]; Prasad, 1994 [380]; Ramamoorthy, (1993a) [381]; Ramamoorthy, (1993b) [382]; Ramamoorthy, 1995 [383]; Richards, 1990 [384]; Roby, 1996 [385]; Roe, 1990 [386]; Saraf, 1995 [387]; Schenker, 1993 [388]; Simone, (1994b) [389]; Simone, 1996 [390]; Simone, 1997 [391]; Smith, 1992 [392]; Smith, 1995 [393]; Sosnoff, 1996 [394];

Sternfeld, 1997 [395]; Wang, 1996 [396]; Winecker, 1997 [397]; Yelian, 1994 [398].

Outcomes beyond the scope of this meta-analysis (n = 54)

Ahluwalia, 1992 [399]; Anonymous, 1989b [400]; Anonymous, 1990b [401]; Anonymous, 1990d [402]; Anonymous, 1991b [403]; Bhushan, 1994 [404]; Burkhead, 1995 [405]; Calhoun, 1991 [406]; Chen, 1991 [407]; Chiu, 1990 [408]; Cohen, 1991 [409]; Cohen, 1994 [410]; Coles, 1992 [411]; Cordero, 1990 [412]; Cotton, 1994 [413]; Curry, 1995 [414]; Dixon, 1989 [415]; Durand, 1990 [416]; Dusick, 1993 [417]; Johnson, 1992 [418]; Frank, 1990 [419]; Fritz, 1993 [420]; Gingras, 1994 [421]; Gottbrath-Flaherty, 1995 [422]; Handler, 1991 [423]; Handler, 1994 [424]; Hanlon-Lundberg, 1996 [425]; Harris, 1992 [426]; Harsham, 1994 [427]; Hoskins, 1991 [428]; Hume, Jr., 1994 [429]; Hurt, 1995; [430]; Jacobson, 1994 [431]; Kandall, 1993 [432]; Legido, 1992 [433]; Lopez, 1995 [434]; Lounsbury, 1989 [435]; Miller, Jr., 1995 [436]; Mirochnick, 1995 [437]; Needlman, 1993 [438]; Neuspiel, 1991 [439]; Neuspiel, 1994 [440]; Nulman, 1994 [441]; Prichep, 1995 [442]; Richardson, 1991 [443]; Richardson, 1994 [444]; Rodning, 1989 [445]; Rodriguez, 1993 [446]; Schneider, 1992 [447]; Skolnick, 1990 [448]; Singer, 1994 [449]; vande Bor, 1990 [450]; Wehbeh, 1995 [451]; Yawn, 1994 [452].

Studies without control group (n = 19)

Beeram, 1993 [453]; Beltran, 1994 [454]; Burkett, 1994 [455]; Chasnoff, (1989c) [456]; Fries, 1993 [457]; Hofkosh, 1995 [458]; Horn, 1992 [459]; Howard, 1995 [460]; Hume, Jr., 1989 [461]; Knight, 1994 [462]; Kramer, 1990 [463]; Link, 1991 [464]; McCalla, 1995 [465]; Ney, 1990 [466]; Racine, 1993 [467]; Rosenstein, 1990 [468]; Slutsker, 1993 [469]; Smit, 1994 [470]; Weathers, 1993 [471].

Cocaine users not separated from other drugs (n = 12)

Doberczak, 1991 [472]; Feldman, 1992 [473]; Forman, 1993 [474]; Handler, 1991 [423]; Hawthorne, 1993 [475]; Hernandez, 1992 [476]; Kaye, 1989 [477]; Nanda, 1990 [478]; Samuels, 1993 [479]; Spence, 1991 [480]; van Baar, 1994 [481]; Van Baar, 1990 [482].

REFERENCES. REJECTED STUDIES

[1] Abramowicz JS, Sherer, DM, Woods, JR, Jr. Acute transient thrombocytopenia associated with cocaine abuse in pregnancy. Obstet Gynecol 1991;78:499–501.

[2] Apple FS, Roe SJ. Cocaine-associated fetal death in utero. J Anal Toxicol 1990;14:259–60.

[3] Bakht FR, Kirshon B, Baker T, Cotton DB. Postpartum cardiovascular complications after bromocriptine and cocaine use. American Journal of Obstetrics & Gynecology 1990;162:1065–6.

[4] Beltran RS, Coker SB. Transient dystonia of infancy, a result of intrauterine cocaine exposure? Pediatr Neurol 1995;12:354–6.

[5] Brown RE, Jr, Galford, R. Postoperative Ischemia after cocaine ingestion. Journal of the Arkansas Medical Society 1993;89: 589–94.

[6] Burkett G, Bandstra, ES, Cohen, J, Steele B, Palow D. Cocainerelated maternal death. American Journal of Obstetrics & Gynecology 1990;163:40–1.

[7] Carlan SJ, Stromquist, C, Angel, JL, Harris M, O'Brien, WF. Cocaine and indomethacin: fetal anuria, neonatal edema, and gastrointestinal bleeding. Obstet Gynecol 1991;78:501–3.

[8] Cohen LS, Sabbagha RE, Keith LG, Chasnoff IJ. Doppler umbilical velocimetry in women with polydrug abuse including cocaine. Int J Gynaecol Obstet 1991;36:287–90.

[9] Collins E, Hardwick RJ, Jeffery H. Perinatal cocaine intoxication. Medical Journal of Australia 1989;150:331–2, 334.

[10] Deoliveira IJ, Cratty BJ. Survey of ten infants exposed prenatally to maternal cocaine use. International Journal of Rehabilitation Research 1991;14:265–6.

[11] Dollberg S, Armon Y, Gur I, Litt R, Gale R. Hyponatremia in a neonate of a cocaine abusing mother. Journal of Toxicology-Clinical Toxicology 1989;27:287–92.

[12] Dominguez R, Aguirre Vila-Coro A, Slopis JM, Bohan TP. Brain and ocular abnormalities in infants with in utero exposure to cocaine and other street drugs [see comments]. Am J Dis Child 1991;145: 688–95.

[13] Evelyn AC, Fine PM. Effects of AIDS, cocaine, and family violence on children in out of home care. Nebraska Medical Journal 1992; 77:245–52.

[14] Geggel RL, McInerny J, Estes NA. Transient neonatal ventricular tachycardia associated with maternal cocaine use. American Journal of Cardiology 1989;63:383–4.

[15] George K, Smith JF, Curet LB. Doppler velocimetry and fetal heart rate pattern observations in acute cocaine intoxication. A case report. Journal of Reproductive Medicine 1995;40:65–7.

[16] Gieron-Korthals MA, Helal A, Martinez CR. Expanding spectrum of cocaine induced central nervous system malformations. Brain & Development 1994;16:253–6.

[17] Gomez-Anson B, Ramsey RG. Pachygyria in a neonate with prenatal cocaine exposure: MR features. Journal of Computer Assisted Tomography 1994;18:637–9.

[18] Gonsoulin W, Borge D, Moise KJ, Jr. Rupture of unscarred uterus in primigravid woman in association with cocaine abuse. American Journal of Obstetrics & Gynecology 1990;163:526–7.

[19] Good WV, Ferriero DM, Golabi M, Kobori JA. Abnormalities of the visual system in infants exposed to cocaine. Ophthalmology 1992; 99:341–6.

[20] Greenfield SP, Rutigliano E, Steinhardt G, Elder JS. Genitourinary tract malformations and maternal cocaine abuse. Urology 1991;37: 455–9.

[21] Greenland VC, Delke I, Minkoff HL. Vaginally administered cocaine overdose in a pregnant woman. Obstet Gynecol 1989;74: 476–7.

[22] Hall TR, Zaninovic A, Lewin D, Barrett C, Boechat MI. Neonatal intestinal ischemia with bowel perforation: an in utero complication of maternal cocaine abuse. AJR American Journal of Roentgenology 1992;158:1303–4.

[23] Hannig VL, Phillips JA. Maternal cocaine abuse and fetal anomalies: evidence for teratogenic effects of cocaine. South Med J 1991;84:498–9.

[24] Harris SR, Osborn JA, Weinberg J, Loock C, Junaid K. Effects of prenatal alcohol exposure on neuromotor and cognitive development during early childhood: A series of case reports. Phys Ther 1993;73:608–17.

[25] Hepper PG. Human fetal behaviour and maternal cocaine use: a longitudinal study. Neurotoxicology 1995;16:139–43.

[26] Ho J, Afshani E, Stapleton FB. Renal vascular abnormalities associated with prenatal cocaine exposure. Clinical Pediatrics 1994;33: 155–6.

[27] Hoeger PH, Haupt G, Hoelzle E. Acute multifocal skin necrosis: synergism between invasive streptococcal infection and cocaineinduced tissue ischaemia? Acta Dermato-Venereologica 1996;76:239–41.

[28] Hoyme HE, Jones KL, Dixon SD, et al. Prenatal cocaine exposure and fetal vascular disruption. Pediatrics 1990;85:743–7.

[29] Hsu CD, Chen S, Feng TI, Johnson TR. Rupture of uterine scar with extensive maternal bladder laceration after cocaine abuse. American Journal of Obstetrics & Gynecology 1992;167:129–30.

[30] Iriye BK, Bristow RE, Hsu CD, Bruni R, Johnson TR. Uterine rupture associated with recent antepartum cocaine abuse. Obstet Gynecol 1994;83:840–1.

[31] Iriye BK, Asrat T, Adashek JA, Carr MH. Intraventricular haemorrhage and maternal brain death associated with antepartum cocaine abuse. British Journal of Obstetrics & Gynaecology 1995;102:68–9.

[32] Jack BW, Davis S, Culpepper L, Hunt VR. Cocaine abuse in maternal-child health care [clinical conference]. Journal of Family Practice 1990;31:477–8, 481–2, 485–8.

[33] Jasnosz KM, Hermansen MC, Snider C, Sang K. Congenital complete absence (bilateral agenesis) of the diaphragm: a rare variant of congenital diaphragmatic hernia. American Journal of Perinatology 1994;11:340–3.

[34] Jawahar D, Leo PJ, Anandarao M, Pachter BR. Cocaine-associated intestinal gangrene in a pregnant woman. American Journal of Emergency Medicine 1997;15:510–12.

[35] Johnson MO, Lobo ML. Case study of the home health management of a child with congenital anomalies associated with prenatal cocaine abuse. Journal of Pediatric Nursing 1995;10:375–82.

[36] Kankirawatana P, Tennison MB, D'Cruz O, Greenwood RS. Mobius syndrome in infant exposed to cocaine in utero. Pediatr Neurol 1993;9:71–2.

[37] Kapur RP, Shaw CM, Shepard TH. Brain hemorrhages in cocaine-exposed human fetuses. Teratology 1991;44:11–18.

[38] Lampley EC, Williams S, Myers SA. Cocaine-associated rhabdomyolysis causing renal failure in pregnancy. Obstet Gynecol 1996;87:804–6.

[39] Lessick M, Vasa R, Israel J. Severe manifestations of oculoauriculovertebral spectrum in a cocaine exposed infant. Journal of Medical Genetics 1991;28:803–4.

[40] Lezcano L, Antia DE, Sahdev S, Jhaveri M. Crossed renal ectopia associated with maternal alkaloid cocaine abuse: a case report. Journal of Perinatology 1994;14:230–3.

[41] Liu SS, Forrester RM, Murphy GS, Chen K, Glassenberg R. Anaesthetic management of a parturient with myocardial infarction related to cocaine use. Canadian Journal of Anaesthesia 1992;39: 858–61.

[42] Martinez JM, Fortuny A, Comas C, et al. Body stalk anomaly associated with maternal cocaine abuse. Prenatal Diagnosis 1994; 14:669–72.

[43] Meeker JE, Reynolds PC. Fetal and newborn death associated with maternal cocaine use. J Anal Toxicol 1990;14:379–82.

[44] Mendelson MA, Chandler J. Postpartum cardiomyopathy associated with maternal cocaine abuse. American Journal of Cardiology 1992; 70:1092–4.

[45] Mercado A, Johnson G, Jr., Calver D, Sokol RJ. Cocaine, pregnancy, and postpartum intracerebral hemorrhage. Obstet Gynecol 1989;73:467–8.

[46] Miller BM, Rosario PG, Prakash K, Patel HK, Gerst PH. Neonatal intestinal perforation: the "crack" connection. American Journal of Gastroenterology 1990;85:767–9.

[47] Mishra A, Landzberg BR, Parente JT. Uterine rupture in association with alkaloidal ("crack") cocaine abuse. American Journal of Obstetrics & Gynecology 1995;173:243–4.

[48] Mittleman RE, Cofino JC, Hearn WL. Tissue distribution of cocaine in a pregnant woman [published erratum appears in J Forensic Sci 1989 Jul;34(4):807]. Journal of Forensic Sciences 1989;34:481–6.

[49] Moen MD, Caliendo MJ, Marshall W, Uhler ML. Hepatic rupture in pregnancy associated with cocaine use. Obstet Gynecol 1993;82: 687–9.

[50] Moriya F, Chan KM, Noguchi TT, Parnassus WN. Detection of drugs-of-abuse in meconium of a stillborn baby and in stool of a deceased 41-day-old infant. Journal of Forensic Sciences 1995;40: 505–8.

[51] Murphy JLJ. Hypertension and pulmonary oedema associated with ketamine administration in a patient with a history of substance abuse. Canadian Journal of Anaesthesia 1993;40:160–4.

[52] Nolte KB. Cocaine, fetal loss, and the role of the forensic pathologist. Journal of Forensic Sciences 1991;36:926–9.

[53] Nyirjesy P, Kamnani AJ, Scharf ML, Suh B. Fulminant tuberculosis complicating pregnancy in a patient infected with the human immunodeficiency virus. Journal of Maternal-Fetal Medicine 1993;2:75–8.

[54] Okoruwa E, Shah R, Gerdes K. Apnea and vomiting in an infant due to cocaine exposure. Iowa Medicine 1995;85:449–50.

[55] Ostrea EM, Jr., Romero A, Knapp DK, Ostrea AR, Lucena JE, Utarnachitt RB. Postmortem drug analysis of meconium in early-gestation human fetuses exposed to cocaine: clinical implications. J Pediatr 1994;124:477–9.

[56] Perlow JH, Schlossberg DL, Strassner HT. Intrapartum cocaine use. A case report. Journal of Reproductive Medicine 1990;35:978–80.

[57] Peters AJ, Abrams RM, Burchfield DJ, Gilmore RL. Seizures in a fetal lamb after cocaine exposure: a case report. Epilepsia 1992;33: 1001–4.

[58] Porat R, Brodsky N. Cocaine: a risk factor for necrotizing enterocolitis. Journal of Perinatology 1991;11:30–2.

[59] Potter S, Klein J, Valiante G, et al. Maternal cocaine use without evidence of fetal exposure. J Pediatr 1994;125:652–4.

[60] Rais-Bahrami K, Naqvi M. Hydranencephaly and maternal cocaine use: a case report. Clinical Pediatrics 1990;29:729–30.

[61] Reznik VM, Anderson J, Griswold WR, Segall ML, Murphy JL, Mendoza SA. Successful fibrinolytic treatment of arterial thrombosis and hypertension in a cocaine-exposed neonate. Pediatrics 1989; 84:735–8.

[62] Robin NH, Zackai EH. Unusual craniofacial dysmorphia due to prenatal alcohol and cocaine exposure. Teratology 1994;50: 160–4.

[63] Sarpong S, Headings V. Sirenomelia accompanying exposure of the embryo to cocaine. South Med J 1992;85:545–7.

[64] Seballos RJ, Mendel SG, Mirmiran-Yazdy A, Khoury W, Marshall JB. Sarcoid cardiomyopathy precipitated by pregnancy with cocaine complications. Chest 1994;105:303–5.

[65] Sheinbaum KA, Badell A. Physiatric management of two neonates with limb deficiencies and prenatal cocaine exposure. Archives of Physical Medicine & Rehabilitation 1992;73:385–8.

[66] Sims ME, Walther FJ. Neonatal ultrasound casebook. Antenatal brain injury and maternal cocaine use. Journal of Perinatology 1989; 9:349–50.

[67] Singer L, Arendt R, Minnes S, Farkas K, Yamashita T, Kliegman R. Increased psychological distress in post-partum, cocaine-using mothers. Journal of Substance Abuse 1995;7:165–74.

[68] Skopp G, Potsch L. A case report on drug screening of nail clippings to detect prenatal drug exposure. Therapeutic Drug Monitoring 1997;19:386–9.

[69] Spinazzola R, Kenigsberg K, Usmani SS, Harper RG. Neonatal gastrointestinal complications of maternal cocaine abuse. New York State Journal of Medicine 1992;92:22–3.

[70] Spires MC, Gordon EF, Choudhuri M, Maldonado E, Chan R. Intracranial (i.c.) hemorrhage in a neonate following prenatal cocaine exposure. Pediatr Neurol 1989;5:324–6.

[71] Spital A, Greenwell R. Severe hyperkalemia during magnesium sulfate therapy in two pregnant drug abusers. South Med J 1991;84:919–21.

[72] Streissguth AP, Grant, TM, Barr, HM, et al. Cocaine and the use of alcohol and other drugs during pregnancy. American Journal of Obstetrics & Gynecology 1991;164:1239–43.
[73] Sturner WQ, Sweeney KG, Callery RT, Haley NR. Cocaine babies: the scourge of the '90s. Journal of Forensic Sciences 1991;36:34–9.
[74] Sumner GS, Mandoki MW, Matthews-Ferrari K. A psychiatric population of prenatally cocaine-exposed children. Journal of the American Academy of Child & Adolescent Psychiatry 1993;32: 1003–6.
[75] Sztulman L, Ducey JJ, Tancer ML. Intrapartum, intranasal cocaine use, and acute fetal distress. A case report. Journal of Reproductive Medicine 1990;35:917–18.
[76] Thatcher SS, Corfman R, Grosso J, Silverman DG, DeCherney AH. Cocaine use and acute rupture of ectopic pregnancies. Obstet Gynecol 1989;74:478–9.
[77] Towers CV, Pircon RA, Nageotte MP, Porto M, Garite TJ. Cocaine intoxication presenting as preeclampsia and eclampsia. Obstet Gynecol 1993;81:545–7.
[78] van den Anker JN, Van Vught EE, Zandwijken GRJ, Cohen Overbeek TE, Lindhout D. Severe limb abnormalities: Analysis of a cluster of five cases born during a period of 45 days. Am J Med Gen 1993;45:659–67.
[79] Viscarello RR, Ferguson DD, Nores J, Hobbins JC. Limb-body wall complex associated with cocaine abuse: further evidence of cocaine's teratogenicity. Obstet Gynecol 1992;80:523–6.
[80] Wilson BE, Hobbs WN. Cocaine toxicity in glycogen storage disease [letter]. Western Journal of Medicine 1993;159:508–9.
[81] Alexander LL. Fetal addiction: health problem or criminal offense? [editorial]. Journal of the National Medical Association 1991;83: 663.
[82] Amoury RA. Necrotizing enterocolitis: A continuing problem in the neonate. World J Surg 1993;17:363–73.
[83] Anonymous. American Academy of Pediatrics Committee on Substance Abuse: Drug-exposed infants. Pediatrics 1990;86:639–642.
[84] Anonymous. Alternative case-finding methods in a crack-related syphilis epidemic–Philadelphia. MMWR - Morbidity & Mortality Weekly Report 1991;40:77–80.
[85] Baxley EG. Cocaine abuse in pregnancy–a myriad of unanswered questions [editorial]. Journal - South Carolina Medical Association 1990;86:555–6.
[86] Brouhard BH. Cocaine ingestion and abnormalities of the urinary tract [editorial; comment]. Clinical Pediatrics 1994;33:157–8.
[87] Chasnoff IJ. Cocaine and pregnancy–implications for the child [editorial]. Western Journal of Medicine 1989;150:456–8.
[88] Fantel AG, Shepard TH. Prenatal cocaine exposure [editorial]. Reproductive Toxicology 1990;4:83.
[89] Heagarty MC. Crack cocaine. A new danger for children [editorial]. Am J Dis Child 1990;144:756–7.
[90] Howard BJ, O'Donnell, KJ. What is important about a study of within-group differences of 'cocaine babies'? [editorial]. Archives of Pediatrics & Adolescent Medicine 1995;149:663–4.
[91] Jentzen J. Medical complications of cocaine abuse [editorial]. American Journal of Clinical Pathology 1993;100:475–6.
[92] Jos PH, Marshall MF, Perlmutter M. The Charleston policy on cocaine use during pregnancy: a cautionary tale. Journal of Law, Medicine & Ethics 1995;23:120–8.
[93] Kearney MH, Murphy S, Irwin K, Rosenbaum M. Salvaging self: a grounded theory of pregnancy on crack cocaine. Nursing Research 1995;44:208–213.
[94] Konkol RJ. Is there a cocaine baby syndrome? [editorial]. Journal of Child Neurology 1994;9:225–6.
[95] Lewis KD, Bennett B, Schmeder NH. The care of infants menaced by cocaine abuse. MCN; American Journal of Maternal Child Nursing 1989;14:324–9.
[96] Lone P. Silencing crack addiction. MCN American Journal of Maternal Child Nursing 1991;16:202–5.
[97] Neuspiel DR. On pejorative labeling of cocaine exposed children [editorial]. Journal of Substance Abuse Treatment 1993;10:407.
[98] Nora JG. Perinatal cocaine use: maternal, fetal, and neonatal effects. Neonatal Network 1990;9:45–52.
[99] Plessinger MA, Woods JRJ. Maternal, placental, and fetal pathophysiology of cocaine exposure during pregnancy. Clin Obstet Gynecol. 1993;36:267–8.
[100] Salamy A, Eldredge L, Anderson J, Bull D. Brain-stem transmission time in infants exposed to cocaine in utero. J Pediatr 1990; 117:627–9.
[101] Tudehope DI. Perinatal cocaine intoxication: a precaution [editorial]. Medical Journal of Australia 1989;150:290–1.
[102] Zuckerman B, Frank DA. Prenatal cocaine exposure: nine years later [editorial; comment]. J Pediatr 1994;124:731–3.
[103] Abdeljaber M, Nolan, BM, Schork, MA. Maternal cocaine use during pregnancy: effect on the newborn infant [letter; comment]. Pediatrics 1990;85:630.
[104] Ahmed MS, Spong, CY, Geringer, JL, Mou, SM, Maulik, D. Prospective study on cocaine use prior to delivery. JAMA 1989;262:1880.
[105] Anonymous. Effects of maternal marijuana and cocaine use on fetal growth [letter; comment]. New Engl J Med 1989;321:979.
[106] Bays J. Fetal vascular disruption with prenatal exposure to cocaine or methamphetamine [letter; comment]. Pediatrics 1991;87:416–18.
[107] Carraccio C, Papadimitriou J, Feinberg P. Subcutaneous (s.c.) fat necrosis of the newborn: link to maternal use of cocaine during pregnancy [letter]. Clinical Pediatrics 1994;33:317–18.
[108] Chavkin W, Kandall SR. Between a "rock" and a hard place: perinatal drug abuse. Pediatrics 1990;85:223–5.
[109] Cottler LB, Compton WM. Re: "Cocaine use during pregnancy: perinatal outcomes" [letter; comment]. American Journal of Epidemiology 1992;135:1425–7.
[110] DiGregorio GJ, Barbieri EJ, Ferko AP, Ruch EK. Prevalence of cocaethylene in the hair of pregnant women [letter]. J Anal Toxicol 1993;17:445–6.
[111] Downing GJ, Horner SR, Kilbride HW. Characteristics of perinatal cocaine-exposed infants with necrotizing enterocolitis [letter]. Am J Dis Child 1991;145:26–7.
[112] Fogarty ME. Re: 'A review of the literature on cocaine abuse in pregnancy' [letter; comment]. Nursing Research.;40:235-, 1991.
[113] Friedman EH. Neurobiology of cocaine binging in pregnancy [letter; comment]. American Journal of Obstetrics & Gynecology 1995;172:1322–3.
[114] Goldin K. Cocaine abuse in pregnancy [letter; comment]. JAMA 1989;262:771.
[115] Good WV, Ferriero D. Ocular effects of prenatal cocaine exposure [letter; comment]. Ophthalmology 1994;101:1321; discussion 132–1321; discussion 132.
[116] Graham K, Koren G. Maternal cocaine use and risk of sudden infant death [letter; comment]. J Pediatr 1989;115:333.
[117] Gratacos E, Torres PJ, Antolin E. Use of cocaine during pregnancy [letter]. New Engl J Med 1993;329:667.
[118] Hansen RL. Diagnosis, treatment, and follow-up of newborns addicted to cocaine. Western Journal of Medicine 1990;153:646.
[119] Herschman Z, Aaron C. Prolongation of cocaine effect [letter; comment]. Anesthesiology 1991;74:631–2.
[120] Hunt CE. Respiratory pattern abnormalities and prenatal cocaine exposure [letter]. Am J Dis Child 1990;144:138–9.
[121] Jerome L. Adopted children exposed to cocaine in utero: confounding factors [letter; comment]. Canadian Medical Association Journal 1995;152:1187–8.
[122] Kain ZN, Kain, TS, Scarpelli, EM. Effect of cocaine use on the fetus [letter; comment]. New Engl J Med 1992;327:1393–4.
[123] Levy M. Is cocaine a risk factor to necrotizing enterocolitis? [letter]. Clinical Pediatrics 1993;32:700–1.
[124] Maynard EC. Maternal abuse of cocaine and heroin [letter; comment]. Am J Dis Child 1990;144:520–1.
[125] Miele NF. Controversial costs of cocaine: [letter; comment]. JAMA. 1992;267:507; discussion 507–507; discussion 508.

[126] Mittleman RE, Cofino, J, Hearn, WL. Addendum on "Cocaine in a Pregnant Woman" [letter]. Journal of Forensic Sciences 1989;34:807.

[127] Moore CM, Brown S, Negrusz A, Tebbett I, Meyer W, Jain L. Determination of cocaine and its major metabolite, benzoylecgonine, in amniotic fluid, umbilical cord blood, umbilical cord tissue, and neonatal urine: a case study [letter]. J Anal Toxicol 1993;17:62.

[128] Morfesis FA. Association between newborn birth weight and prenatal care for cocaine users [letter; comment]. JAMA 1994;271:1161.

[129] Neuspiel DR. Cocaine-associated abnormalities may not be causally related [letter; comment]. Am J Dis Child 1992;146:278–9.

[130] Neuspiel DR, Hamel SC. Neurobehavioral sequelae of fetal cocaine exposure [letter; comment]. J Pediatr 1992;120:661–2.

[131] Neuspiel DR. Screening neonates for intrauterine cocaine exposure [letter; comment]. J Pediatr 1995;126:323–4.

[132] Nucci P, Brancato R. Ocular effects of prenatal cocaine exposure [letter; comment]. Ophthalmology. 1994;101:1321; discussion 132–1321; discussion 132.

[133] Page D. Controversial costs of cocaine [letter; comment]. JAMA. 1992;267:507; discussion 507–507; discussion 508.

[134] Petrulis AS. Hypertension in pregnancy [letter; comment]. New Engl J Med 1992;327:733.

[135] Racine AD, Joyce TJ, Anderson R. The association between prenatal care and birth weight among women exposed to cocaine in New York City: a correction. JAMA 1994;271:1161–2.

[136] Sackoff J, Kline J, Kinney A, Grunebaum A. Cocaine use in obstetric patients underreported [letter]. Am J Pub Health 1992; 82:1043.

[137] Shaw GM, Malcoe LH, Lammer EJ, Swan SH. Maternal use of cocaine during pregnancy and congenital cardiac anomalies [letter]. J Pediatr 1991;118:167–8.

[138] Sher J. Women and crack addiction [letter]. Journal of the American Medical Womens Association 1989;44:166.

[139] Stephens BG. Fetal development and cocaine [letter]. American Journal of Forensic Medicine & Pathology 1989;10:268–9.

[140] Sugarman K, Herman M. Crack cocaine and HIV in the inner city [letter; comment]. New Engl J Med. 1995;332:1233; discussion 1234–5.

[141] Tabor BL, Saffici A. Cocaine effects on fetal behavioral state [letter; comment]. American Journal of Obstetrics & Gynecology 1990;163:1364–5.

[142] Thorp JM, Jr. Cocaine abuse is associated with abruptio placentae and decreased birth weight, but not shorter labor [letter; comment]. Obstet Gynecol 1991;77:807–8.

[143] van den Anker JN, Cohen-Overbeek, TE, Wladimiroff JW, Sauer PJ. Prenatal diagnosis of limb-reduction defects due to maternal cocaine use [letter]. Lancet 1991;338:1332.

[144] van den Anker JN, and Sauer, PJ. Effect of cocaine use on the fetus [letter; comment]. New Engl J Med 1992;327:1394.

[145] Yang YQ, Lee MP, Schenken RS, Henderson GI, Schenker S, Johnson RF. Effects of binding on human transplacental transfer of cocaine [letter; comment]. American Journal of Obstetrics & Gynecology 1995;172:720–2.

[146] Abel EL. The future of cocaine babies: primary care and early intervention. Journal of Pediatric Health Care 1991;5:321–3.

[147] Adams C, Eyler FD, Behnke M. Nursing intervention with mothers who are substance abusers. Journal of Perinatal & Neonatal Nursing 1990;3:43–52.

[148] Anonymous. Urogenital anomalies in the offspring of women using cocaine during early pregnancy–Atlanta, 1968–1980;MMWR-Morbidity & Mortality Weekly Report:1989;38:536–541.

[149] Anonymous. Cocaine in pregnancy. ACOG Committee Opinion: Committee on Obstetrics: Maternal and Fetal Medicine Number 114–September 1992 (replaces no. 81, March 1980). Int J Gynaecol Obstet. 1993;41:102–105.

[150] Aronson RA, Hunt LH. Cocaine use during pregnancy: implications for physicians. Wisconsin Medical Journal 1990;89:105–10.

[151] Berger CS, Sorensen L, Gendler B, Fitzsimmons J. Cocaine and pregnancy: a challenge for health care providers. Health & Social Work 1990;15:310–16.

[152] Brent RL, Beckman, DA. The contribution of environmental teratogens to embryonic and fetal loss. Clin Obstet Gynecol 1994;37: 646–70.

[153] Buehler BA. Cocaine: how dangerous is it during pregnancy? Nebraska Medical Journal 1995;80:116–17.

[154] Buehler BA, Conover B, Andres RL. Teratogenic potential of cocaine. [Review]. Seminars in Perinatology 1996;20:93–8.

[155] Byrne MW, Lerner HM. Communicating with addicted women in labor. MCN; American Journal of Maternal Child Nursing 1992;17: 22–6.

[156] Chan L, Pham H, Reece EA. Pneumothorax in pregnancy associated with cocaine use. [Review]. American Journal of Perinatology 1997;14:385–8.

[157] Chao CR. Cardiovascular effects of cocaine during pregnancy. [Review]. Seminars in Perinatology 1996;20:107–14.

[158] Chasnoff IJ. Drug use in pregnancy. New York State Journal of Medicine 1989;89:255.

[159] Chasnoff IJ. Missing pieces of the puzzle [comment]. Neurotoxicol Teratol. 1993;15:287–8; discussion 311–2.

[160] Chavkin W, Paone, D, Friedmann P, Wilets I. Reframing the debate: toward effective treatment for inner city drug-abusing mothers. Bulletin of the New York Academy of Medicine 1993;70: 50–68.

[161] Church MW. Does cocaine cause birth defects? Neurotoxicol Teratol 1993;15:289; discussion 311–289; discussion 312.

[162] Coles CD. Discussion: Measurement issues in the study of effects of substance abuse in pregnancy. NIDA Research Monograph 1992; 117:248–58.

[163] Coles CD. Saying "goodbye" to the "crack baby" [comment]. Neurotoxicol Teratol 1993;15:290–2; discussion 1993:311–2.

[164] Cornish JW, O'Brien CP. Crack cocaine abuse: an epidemic with many public health consequences. [Review]. Annual Review of Public Health 1996;17:259–73.

[165] Day NL, Cottreau CM, Richardson GA. The epidemiology of alcohol, marijuana, and cocaine use among women of childbearing age and pregnant women. Clin Obstet Gynecol 1993;36: 232–45.

[166] Day NL, Richardson GA. Cocaine use and crack babies: science, the media, and miscommunication [comment]. Neurotoxicol Teratol. 1993;15:293–4; discussion 11–2.

[167] Dixon SD. Effects of transplacental exposure to cocaine and methamphetamine on the neonate. Western Journal of Medicine 1989;150:436–42.

[168] Dow-Edwards DL. Cocaine effects on fetal development: A comparison of clinical and animal research findings. Neurotoxicol Teratol 1991;13:347–52.

[169] Dow-Edwards D. The puzzle of cocaine's effects following maternal use during pregnancy: still unsolved [comment]. Neurotoxicol Teratol. 1993;15:295–6; discussion 311–2.

[170] Dumas L. Assessing the cocaine-addicted mother: guidelines for the initial visit. Home Healthcare Nurse 1992;10:12–18.

[171] Dungy-Poythress LJ. Cocaine effects on pregnancy and infant outcome: do we really know how bad it is? Journal of the Association for Academic Minority Physicians 1995;6:46–50.

[172] Elhassani SB. Cocaine use and effect: a major perinatal risk factor in the nineteen nineties. Journal - South Carolina Medical Association 1990;86:532–5.

[173] Ellen L, Brock MD. Perinatal cocaine abuse as a public health problem. Ceskoslovenska Pediatrie 1993;48:249–51.

[174] Fantel AG. Puzzle of cocaine's effects following maternal use during pregnancy: are there reconcilable differences? [comment]. Neurotoxicol Teratol 1993;15:297; discussion 311–297; discussion 312.

[175] Ferner RE. Adverse drug reaction bulletin. Adv Drug React Bull 1993;161:607–10.

[176] Finnegan LP. The teratogenicity of the drugs of abuse: A symposium. Drug Acohol Depend 1994;36:81.

[177] Frank DA, Zuckerman, BS. Children exposed to cocaine prenatally: pieces of the puzzle [comment]. Neurotoxicol Teratol. 1993;15: 298–300; discussion 311–312.

[178] Garcia SA. Birth penalty: societal responses to perinatal chemical dependence. Journal of Clinical Ethics. 1990;1:135–40; discussion 140–5.

[179] Gaskill SJ. The spectrum of radiologic abnormalities in the neonatal CNS [comment]. Ajnr: American Journal of Neuroradiology 1992;13:1272–1272.

[180] Giacoia GP. Cocaine babies in Oklahoma. Journal - Oklahoma State Medical Association 1990;83:64–7.

[181] Gintautiene K, Longmore W, Abadir AR, et al. Cocaine-induced deaths in pediatric population. Proceedings of the Western Pharmacology Society 1990;33: 247–8.

[182] Goldstein FJ. Toxicity of cocaine. Compendium 1990;11:710, 712, 714–716.

[183] Goodwin FK. From the Alcohol, Drug Abuse, and Mental Health Administration. JAMA 1990;263:1610–1610.

[184] Grossman J, Schottenfeld, RS, Viscarello, R, Pakes, J. Cocaine abuse during pregnancy. NIDA Research Monograph 1993;132:302.

[185] Horger EO, Brown SB, Condon CM. Cocaine in pregnancy: confronting the problem. Journal - South Carolina Medical Association 1990;86:527–31.

[186] Janke JR. Prenatal cocaine use. Effects on perinatal outcome. Journal of Nurse-Midwifery 1990;35:74–7.

[187] Johnson E. From the Alcohol, Drug Abuse, and Mental Health Administration. JAMA 1992;268:854.

[188] Kaltenbach KA. Effects of in-utero opiate exposure: New paradigms for old questions. Drug Acohol Depend 1994;36:83–7.

[189] Kandall SR, Gaines, J. Maternal substance use and subsequent sudden infant death syndrome (SIDS) in offspring. Neurotoxicol Teratol 1991;13:235–40.

[190] Karmel BZ, Gardner JM, Magnano CL. Neurofunctional consequences of in utero cocaine exposure. NIDA Research Monograph 1991;105:535–6.

[191] Keller S, Niebyl J. Cocaine abuse in a high risk obstetrical population. Iowa Medicine 1993;83:153–5.

[192] Kenner C, D'Apolito K. Outcomes for children exposed to drugs in utero. [Review]. Journal of Obstetric, Gynecologic, & Neonatal Nursing 1997;26:595–603.

[193] Khoury MJ, James LM, Lynberg MC. Quantitative analysis of associations between birth defects and suspected human teratogens. Am J Med Gen 1991;40:500–5.

[194] Klitsch M. Prenatal exposure to tobacco, alcohol or other drugs found for more than one in 10 California newborns. Fam Plann Perspect 1994;26:95–6.

[195] Knisely JS, Spear ER, Green DJ, Christmas JT, Schnoll SH. Substance abuse patterns in pregnant women. NIDA Research Monograph 1991;105:280–1.

[196] Koren G, Graham K, Shear H, Einarson T. Bias against the null hypothesis: the reproductive hazards of cocaine. Lancet 1989;2:1440–2.

[197] Koren G. Cocaine and the human fetus: the concept of teratophilia [comment]. Neurotoxicol Teratol. 1993;15:301–4; discussion 311–2.

[198] Landry SH, Whitney JA. The impact of prenatal cocaine exposure: studies of the developing infant. [Review]. Seminars in Perinatology 1996;20:99–106.

[199] Lauder JM. Discussion: Neuroteratology of cocaine - Relationship to developing monoamine systems. NIDA Research Monograph 1991;114:233–247.

[200] Lewis KD. Pathophysiology of prenatal drug-exposure: in utero, in the newborn, in childhood, and in agencies. Journal of Pediatric Nursing 1991;6:185–90.

[201] Litt J, McNeil M. Biological markers and social differentiation: crack babies and the construction of the dangerous mother. [Review]. Health Care for Women International 1997;18:31–41.

[202] Lunsford BK. Pregnancy and cocaine: a charge to nurses. Kansas Nurse 1995;70:8–9.

[203] Lutiger B, Graham K, Einarson TR, Koren G. Relationship between gestational cocaine use and pregnancy outcome: a meta-analysis. Teratology 1991;44:405–14.

[204] Martin ML, Khoury MJ. Cocaine and single ventricle: a population study. Teratology 1992;46:267–70.

[205] Martin ML, Khoury MJ, Cordero JF, Waters GD. Trends in rates of multiple vascular disruption defects, Atlanta, 1968–1989;is there evidence of a cocaine teratogenic epidemic? Teratology:1992;45: 647–653.

[206] Meyer JS, Shearman LP, Collins LM. Monoamine transporters and the neurobehavioral teratology of cocaine. [Review]. Pharmacol Biochem Behav 1996;55: 585–93.

[207] Miller WHJ, Cox SM, Harbison V, Campbell BA. Urine drug screens for drug abuse in pregnancy: Problems and pitfalls. Womens Health Issues 1994;4:152–5.

[208] Miller H. Prenatal cocaine exposure and mother-infant interaction: implications for occupational therapy intervention. [Review]. American Journal of Occupational Therapy 1997;51:119–131.

[209] Murphey LJ, Olsen GD, Konkol RJ. Quantitation of benzoylnorecgonine and other cocaine metabolites in meconium by highperformance liquid chromatography (HPLC). Journal of Chromatography 1993;613:330–5.

[210] Neuspiel DR. Cocaine and the fetus: mythology of severe risk [comment]. Neurotoxicol Teratol. 1993;15:305–6; discussion 311–2.

[211] Ostrea EM, Jr. Detection of prenatal drug exposure in the pregnant woman and her newborn infant. NIDA Research Monograph 1992; 117:61–79.

[212] Pokorni JL, Stanga J. Serving infants and families affected by maternal cocaine abuse: Part 1. [Review]. Pediatric Nursing 1996;22:439–42.

[213] Richardson GA, Day NL, McGauhey PJ. The impact of prenatal marijuana and cocaine use on the infant and child. Clin Obstet Gynecol 1993;36:302–18.

[214] Richardson GA, Hamel SC, Goldschmidt L, Day NL. The effects of prenatal cocaine use on neonatal neurobehavioral status. Neurotoxicol Teratol 1996;18:519–28.

[215] Ripple MG, Goldberger BA, Caplan YH, Blitzer MG, Schwartz S. Detection of cocaine and its metabolites in human amniotic fluid. J Anal Toxicol 1992;16:328–31.

[216] Rizk B, Atterbury JL, Groome LJ. Reproductive risks of cocaine. [Review]. Human Reproduction Update 1996;2:43–55.

[217] Sexson WR. Cocaine: a neonatal perspective. International Journal of the Addictions. 1993;28:585–98.

[218] Shepard TH. Nutritional aspects of embryonic CNS development: In vitro and animal studies. Introduction to part I. Annals of the New York Academy of Sciences 1993;678:1–7.

[219] Slade PH. Legislative and community response to cocaine use in pregnancy. Florida Nurse 1993;41:8, 13.

[220] Spear LP. Missing pieces of the puzzle complicate conclusions about cocaine's neurobehavioral toxicity in clinical populations: importance of animal models [comment]. Neurotoxicol Teratol. 1993;15:307–9; discussion 311–2.

[221] Sprauve ME. Substance abuse and HIV pregnancy. [Review]. Clin Obstet Gynecol 1996;39:316–32.

[222] Strauss RS. Effects of the intrauterine environment on childhood growth. [Review]. British Medical Bulletin 1997;53:81–95.

[223] Sun WY, Chen W. The impact of maternal cocaine use on neonates in socioeconomic disadvantaged population. [Review]. Journal of Drug Education 1997;27:389–96.

[224] Swadi H. Adolescent substance misuse. Current Opinions in Psychiatry 1993;6:511–15.

[225] Szeto HH. Discussion: Methodological issues in controlled studies on effects of prenatal drugs. NIDA Research Monograph.;1991;114: 37–44.

[226] Warner EA, Kosten TR, O'Connor PG. Pharmacotherapy for opioid and cocaine abuse. [Review]. Medical Clinics of North America 1997;81:909–25.

[227] Webster WS, Brown Woodman PDC, Richi, HE. Birth defect - Causes and myths. Today's Life Sci 1993;5:10–19.

[228] Westdorp EJ, Salomone JA, Roberts DK, McIntyre MK, Watson WA. Validation of a rapid urine screening assay for cocaine use among pregnant emergency patients. Academic Emergency Medicine 1995;2:795–8.

[229] Wightman MJ. Criteria for placement decisions with cocaine-exposed infants. Child Welfare 1991;70:653–63.

[230] Wootton J, Miller SI. Cocaine: a review. Pediatrics in Review 1994;15:89–92.

[231] Zuckerman B, Frank DA. "Crack kids": not broken [comment]. Pediatrics 1992;89:337–9.

[232] Zuckerman B. Selected methodologic issues in investigations of prenatal effects of cocaine: Lessons from the past [Review]. NIDA Research Monograph 1991;114: 45–54.

[233] Abusada GM, Abukhalaf IK, Alford DD, et al. Solid-phase extraction and GC/MS quantitation of cocaine, ecgonine methyl ester, benzoylecgonine, and cocaethylene from meconium, whole blood, and plasma. J Anal Toxicol 1993;17:353–8.

[234] Alemi F, Stephens RC. Computer services for patients. Description of systems and summary of findings. Medical Carc 1996;34:OS1-OS9.

[235] Alemi F, Stephens, RC, Javalghi, RG, Dyches, H, Butts, J, Ghadiri, AA randomized trial of a telecommunications network for pregnant women who use cocaine. Medical Care;34:OS10–O1996:S20.

[236] Alemi F, Stephens, RC, Muise, K, Dyches, H, Mosavel, M, Butts, J. Educating patients at home. Community Health Rap Medical Care 1996;34:OS21-OS31.

[237] Amaro H, Fried LE, Cabral H, Zuckerman B. Violence during pregnancy and substance use. Am J Pub Health 1990;80:575–9.

[238] Anonymous. Statewide prevalence of cocaine use during the perinatal period. Rhode Island Medical Journal 1990;73:272.

[239] Anonymous. Population-based prevalence of perinatal exposure to cocaine–Georgia, 1994. MMWR - Morbidity & Mortality Weekly Report. 1996;45: 887–891.

[240] Archie CL, Anderson MM, Gruber EL. Positive smoking history as a preliminary screening device for substance use in pregnant adolescents. Journal of Pediatric & Adolescent Gynecology 1997;10: 13–17.

[241] Ball SA, Schottenfeld RS. A five-factor model of personality, and addiction, psychiatric, and AIDS risk severity in pregnant, and postpartum cocaine misusers. Substance Use & Misuse 1997;32: 25–41.

[242] Bauchner H, Zuckerman B. Cocaine, sudden infant death syndrome, and home monitoring [editorial]. J Pediatr1990;117: 904–6.

[243] Behnke M, Eyler FD, Conlon M, Casanova OQ, Woods NS. How fetal cocaine exposure increases neonatal hospital costs. Pediatrics 1997;99:204–8.

[244] Bendersky M, Alessandri S, Gilbert P, Lewis M. Characteristics of pregnant substance abusers in two cities in the northeast. Am J Drug Alcohol Abuse 1996;22:349–62.

[245] Berenson AB, Stiglich NJ, Wilkinson GS, Anderson GD. Drug abuse and other risk factors for physical abuse in pregnancy among white non-Hispanic, black, and Hispanic women. American Journal of Obstetrics & Gynecology 1991;164:1491–9.

[246] Billman DO, Nemeth PB, Heimler R, Sasidharan P. Prenatal cocaine/polydrug exposure: effect of race on outcome. Journal of Perinatology 1996;16:366–9.

[247] Browne SP, Tebbett IR, Moore CM, Dusick A, Covert R, Yee GT. Analysis of meconium for cocaine in neonates. Journal of Chromatography 1992;575:158–161.

[248] Browne S, Moore C, Negrusz A, Tebbett I, Covert R, Dusick A. Detection of cocaine, norcocaine, and cocaethylene in the meconium of premature neonates. Journal of Forensic Sciences 1994;39: 1515–19.

[249] Brunader RE, Brunader JA, Kugler JP. Prevalence of cocaine and marijuana use among pregnant women in a military health care setting. Journal of the American Board of Family Practice 1991;4: 395–8.

[250] Burke MS, Roth D. Anonymous cocaine screening in a private obstetric population. Obstet Gynecol 1993;81:354–6.

[251] Callahan CM, Grant TM, Phipps P, et al. Measurement of gestational cocaine exposure: sensitivity of infants' hair, meconium, and urine [published erratum appears in J Pediatr 1992 Jul;121(1):156]. J Pediatr. 1992;120:763–8.

[252] Cartwright PS, Schorge JO, McLaughlin FJ. Epidemiologic characteristics of drug use during pregnancy: experience in a Nashville hospital. South Med J 1991;84:867–70.

[253] Casanova OQ, Lombardero N, Behnke M, Eyler FD, Conlon M, Bertholf RL. Detection of cocaine exposure in the neonate. Analyses of urine, meconium, and amniotic fluid from mothers and infants exposed to cocaine. Archives of Pathology & Laboratory Medicine 1994;118:988–93.

[254] Chasnoff IJ, Landress HJ, Barrett ME. The prevalence of illicit-drug or alcohol use during pregnancy and discrepancies in mandatory reporting in Pinellas County, Florida. New Engl J Med 1990;322: 1202–6.

[255] Charpentier PA, Schottenfeld RS. A database model for studies of cocaine-dependent pregnant women, and their families. NIDA Research Monograph 1996;166:242–53.

[256] Condie RG, Brown SS, Akhter MI, Sheehan TMT, Porter L. Antenatal urinary screening for drugs of addiction: Usefulness of sideroom testing? British Journal of Addiction 1989;84:1543–5.

[257] Cornelius MD, Day NL, Cornelius JR, Geva D, Taylor PM, Richardson GA. Drinking patterns and correlates of drinking among pregnant teenagers. Alcohol Clin Exp Res 1993;17:290–4.

[258] Cornelius MD, Richardson GA, Day NL, Cornelius JR, Geva D, Taylor PM. A comparison of prenatal drinking in two recent samples of adolescents, and adults. J Stud Alcohol 1994;55:412–19.

[259] Czeizel A, Racz J. Evaluation of drug intake during pregnancy in the Hungarian Case-Control Surveillance of Congenital Anomalies. Teratology 1990;42:505–12.

[260] de Feo MR, Del Priore D, Mecarelli O. Prenatal cocaine: seizure susceptibility in rat offspring. Pharmacological Research 1995;31: 137–41.

[261] Delaney-Black V, Covington C, Ostrea EJ, et al. Prenatal cocaine and neonatal outcome: evaluation of dose-response relationship. Pediatrics 1996;98:735–40.

[262] DePetrillo PB, Rice JM. Methadone dosing and pregnancy: impact on program compliance. International Journal of the Addictions 1995;30:207–17.

[263] DeVane CL. Pharmacokinetic correlates of fetal drug exposure. NIDA Research Monograph 1991;114:18–36.

[264] DiGregorio GJ, Ferko, AP, Barbieri, EJ, et al. Determination of cocaine usage in pregnant women by a urinary EMIT drug screen and GC-MS analyses. J Anal Toxicol 1994;18:247–50.

[265] Dudish SA, Hatsukami DK. Gender differences in crack users who are research volunteers. Drug Acohol Depend 1996;42:55–63.

[266] Egelko S, Galanter M, Edwards H, Marinelli K. Treatment of perinatal cocaine addiction: use of the modified therapeutic community. Am J Drug Alcohol Abuse 1996;22:185–202.

[267] Elk R, Schmitz J, Manfredi L, Rhoades H, Andres R, Grabowski J. Cessation of cocaine use during pregnancy: a preliminary comparison. Addictive Behaviors 1994;19:697–702.

[268] Elk R, Schmitz J, Spiga R, Rhoades H, Andres R, Grabowski J. Behavioral treatment of cocaine-dependent pregnant women and TB- exposed patients. Addictive Behaviors 1995;20:533–42.

[269] Ellerbrock TV, Harrington PE, Bush TJ, Schoenfisch SA, Oxtoby MJ, Witte JJ. Risk of human immunodeficiency virus infection among pregnant crack cocaine users in a rural community. Obstet Gynecol 1995;86:400–4.

[270] Emery CL, Morway, LF Chung-Park M, Wyatt-Ashmead J, Sawady J, Beddow TD. The Kleihauer-Betke test. Clinical utility, indication, and correlation in patients with placental abruption and cocaine use. Archives of Pathology & Laboratory Medicine 1995;119:1032–7.

[271] Fetters L, Tronick EZ. Neuromotor development of cocaine-exposed and control infants from birth through 15 months: poor and poorer performance. Pediatrics 1996;98:938–43.
[272] Forman R, Schneiderman J, Klein J, Graham K, Greenwald M, Koren G. Accumulation of cocaine in maternal and fetal hair; the dose response curve. Life Sci 1992;50:1333–41.
[273] Forman R, Klein J, Barks J, et al. Prevalence of fetal exposure to cocaine in Toronto, 1990–1991; Clinical & Investigative Medicine - Medecine Cliniqueet Experimentale:1994;17:206–211.
[274] Frank DA, Bauchner H, Zuckerman BS, Fried L. Cocaine and marijuana use during pregnancy by women intending and not intending to breast-feed [see omments]. Journal of the American Dietetic Association 1992;92:215–17.
[275] Galanter M, Egelko S, De Leon G, Rohrs C, Franco H. Crack/cocaine abusers in the general hospital: assessment, and initiation of care. American Journal of Psychiatry 1992;149: 810–15.
[276] Gillmore MR, Butler SS, Lohr MJ, Gilchrist L. Substance use and other factors associated with risky sexual behavior among pregnant adolescents. Fam Plann Perspect 1992;24:255–61.
[277] Graham K, Koren G, Klein J, Schneiderman J, Greenwald M. Determination of gestational cocaine exposure by hair analysis. JAMA 1989;262:3328–30.
[278] Graham K, Koren G. Characteristics of pregnant women exposed to cocaine in Toronto between 1985 and 1990. Canadian Medical Association Journal 1991;144: 563–8.
[279] Grant T, Brown Z, Callahan C, Barr H, Streissguth AP. Cocaine exposure during pregnancy: improving assessment with radioimmunoassay of maternal hair. Obstet Gynecol 1994;83:524–31.
[280] Gomez MP, Bain RM, Major C, Gray H, Read SE. Characteristics of HIV-infected pregnant women in the Bahamas. Journal of Acquired Immune Deficiency Syndromes & Human Retrovirology 1996;12:400–5.
[281] Hall CW, Rouse, BD. Teenagers' knowledge about prenatal exposure to cocaine. Perceptual, Motor Skills 83:1226–, 1996.
[282] Hawley TL, Halle TG, Drasin RE, Thomas NG. Children of addicted mothers: effects of the 'crack epidemic' on the caregiving environment and the development of preschoolers. American Journal of Orthopsychiatry 1995;65:364–79.
[283] Heller MC, Sobel M, Tanaka-Matsumi J. A functional analysis of verbal interactions of drug-exposed children, and their mothers: the utility of sequential analysis. Journal of Clinical Psychology. 1996;52:687–97.
[284] Henderson CE, Terribile S, Keefe D, Merkatz IR. Cardiac screening for pregnant intravenous drug abusers. American Journal of Perinatology 1989;6:397–9.
[285] Henderson LO, Powell MK, Hannon WH, et al. An evaluation of the use of dried blood spots from newborn screening for monitoring the prevalence of cocaine use among childbearing women. Biochemical & Molecular Medicine 1997;61:143–51.
[286] Hurd WW, Smith AJ, Gauvin JM, Hayashi RH. Cocaine blocks extraneuronal uptake of norepinephrine by the pregnant human uterus. Obstet Gynecol 1991;78:249–53.
[287] Hurt H, Brodsky NL, Betancourt L, Braitman LE, Belsky J, Giannetta J. Play behavior in toddlers with in utero cocaine exposure: a prospective, masked, controlled study. Journal of Developmental & Behavioral Pediatrics 1996;17:373–9.
[288] Hurt H, Malmud, E, Betancourt L, Braitman LE, Brodsky NL, Giannetta J. Children with in utero cocaine exposure do not differ from control subjects on intelligence testing. Archives of Pediatrics & Adolescent Medicine 1997;151:1237–41.
[289] Hurt H, Malmud, E, Betancourt L, Brodsky NL, Giannetta J. A prospective evaluation of early language development in children with in utero cocaine exposure, and in control subjects. J Pediatr 1997;130:310–12.
[290] Hutchins E, DiPietro J. Psychosocial risk factors associated with cocaine use during pregnancy: a case-control study. Obstet Gynecol 1997;90:142–7.
[291] Ingersoll K, Dawson K, Haller D. Family functioning of perinatal substance abusers in treatment. Journal of Psychoactive Drugs 1996;28:61–71.
[292] Jacobson SW, Jacobson JL, Sokol RJ, Martier SS, Ager JW, Kaplan MG. Maternal recall of alcohol, cocaine, and marijuana use during pregnancy. Neurotoxicol Teratol 1991;13:535–40.
[293] Jacobson SW, Jacobson JL, Sokol RJ, Martier SS, Chiodo LM. New evidence for neurobehavioral effects of in utero cocaine exposure. J Pediatr 1996;129:581–90.
[294] Jain L, Meyer W, Moore C, Tebbett I, Gauthier D, Vidyasagar D. Detection of fetal cocaine exposure by analysis of amniotic fluid. Obstet Gynecol 1993;81:787–90.
[295] Johnson JM, Seikel JA, Madison CL, Foose SM, Rinard KD. Standardized test performance of children with a history of prenatal exposure to multiple drugs/cocaine. Journal of Communication Disorders 1997;30:45–72.
[296] Joyce T, Racine AD, McCalla S, Wehbeh H. The impact of prenatal exposure to cocaine on newborn costs and length of stay. Health Services Research 1995;30:341–58.
[297] Kain ZN, Mayes LC, Pakes J, Rosenbaum SH, Schottenfeld R. Thrombocytopenia in pregnant women who use cocaine. American Journal of Obstetrics & Gynecology 1995;173:885–90.
[298] Karmel BZ, Gardner JM, Freedland RL. Arousal-modulated attention at four months as a function of intrauterine cocaine exposure and central nervous system injury. Journal of Pediatric Psychology 1996;21:821–32.
[299] Killeen TK, Brady KT, Thevos A. Addiction severity, psychopathology and treatment compliance in cocaine-dependent mothers. Journal of Addictive Diseases 1995;14:75–84.
[300] Klein J, Greenwald M, Becker L, Koren G. Fetal distribution of cocaine: case analysis. Pediatric Pathology 1992;12:463–8.
[301] Klein J, Forman R, Eliopoulos C, Koren G. A method for simultaneous measurement of cocaine, and nicotine in neonatal hair. Therapeutic Drug Monitoring 1994;16:67–70.
[302] Kline J, Ng SK, Schittini M, Levin B, Susser M. Cocaine use during pregnancy: sensitive detection by hair assay. Am J Pub Health 1997;87:352–8.
[303] Konkol RJ, Tikofsky RS, Wells R, et al. Normal high-resolution cerebral 99 mTc-HMPAO SPECT scans in symptomatic neonates exposed to cocaine. Journal of Child Neurology 1994;9:278–83.
[304] Koren G, Gladstone D, Robeson C, Robieux I. The perception of teratogenic risk of cocaine. Teratology 1992;46:567–71.
[305] Koren G, Graham K. Cocaine in pregnancy: analysis of fetal risk. Vet Hum Tox 1992;34:263–4.
[306] Koren G, Klein J, Forman R, Graham K. Hair analysis of cocaine: differentiation between systemic exposure and external contamination. Journal of Clinical Pharmacology 1992;32:671–5.
[307] Land DB, Kushner R. Drug abuse during pregnancy in an inner-city hospital: Prevalence and patterns. Journal of the American Osteopathic Association 1990;90:421–6.
[308] Lindsay MK, Peterson HB, Taylor EB, Blunt M, Willis S, Klein L. Routine human immunodeficiency virus infection screening of women requesting induced first-trimester abortion in an inner- city population. Obstet Gynecol 1990;76:347–50.
[309] Lanehart RE, Clark HB, Kratochvil D, Rollings JP, Fidora AF. Case management of pregnant and parenting female crack and polydrug abusers. Journal of Substance Abuse 1994;6:441–8.
[310] Lauria MR, Qureshi F, Jacques SM, et al. Meconium drug screening of stillborn infants: a feasibility study. Fetal Diagn Ther 1997;12: 248–51.
[311] Lindsay MK, Feng TI, Peterson HB, Slade BA, Willis S, Klein L. Routine human immunodeficiency virus infection screening in unregistered and registered inner-city parturients. Obstet Gynecol 1991;77:599–603.
[312] Lindsay MK, Peterson HB, Boring J, Gramling J, Willis S, Klein L. Crack cocaine: a risk factor for human immunodeficiency virus infection type 1 among inner-city parturients. Obstet Gynecol 1992;80:981–4.

[313] Lindsay MK, Carmichael S, Peterson H, Risby J, Williams H, Klein L. Correlation between self-reported cocaine use and urine toxicology in an inner-city prenatal population. Journal of the National Medical Association 1997;89:57–60.

[314] Little BB, Snell LM, Gilstrap LCI, Johnston WL. Patterns of multiple substance abuse during pregnancy: Implications for mother and fetus. South Med J 1990;83: 507–9.

[315] Marques PR, Tippetts AS, Branch DG. Cocaine in the hair of mother-infant pairs: quantitative analysis and correlations with urine measures and self-report. Am J Drug Alcohol Abuse 1993;19:159–75.

[316] Martin JC, Barr HM, Martin DC, Streissguth AP. Neonatal neurobehavioral outcome following prenatal exposure to cocaine. Neurotoxicol Teratol 1996;18:617–25.

[317] Martinez Crespo JM, Antolin E, Comas C, et al. The prevalence of cocaine abuse during pregnancy in Barcelona. Eur J Obstet Gynecol Reprod Biol 1994;56:165–7.

[318] Mayes LC, Carroll KM. Neonatal withdrawal syndrome in infants exposed to cocaine and methadone. Substance Use & Misuse 1996;31:241–53.

[319] McCalla S, Minkoff HL, Feldman J, Glass L, Valencia G. Predictors of cocaine use in pregnancy. Obstet Gynecol 1992;79:641–4.

[320] McFarlin BL, Bottoms SF. Maternal syphilis: the next pregnancy. American Journal of Perinatology 1996;13:513–518.

[321] Miller WHJ, Resnick MP. Comorbidity in pregnant patients in a psychiatric inpatient setting. Am J Drug Alcohol Abuse 1993;19: 177–185.

[322] Minkoff HL, McCalla S, Delke I, Stevens R, Salwen M, Feldman J. The relationship of cocaine use to syphilis and human immunodeficiency virus infections among inner city parturient women. American Journal of Obstetrics & Gynecology 1990;163:521–6.

[323] Moore C, Dempsey D, Deitermann D, Lewis D, Leikin J. Fetal cocaine exposure: analysis of vernix caseosa. J Anal Toxicol 1996; 20:509–11.

[324] Moriya F, Chan KM, Noguchi TT, Wu PYK. Testing for drugs of abuse in meconium of newborn infants. J Anal Toxicol 1994;18: 41–5.

[325] Moser JM, Jones VH, Kuthy ML. Use of cocaine during the immediate prepartum period by childbearing women in Ohio. American Journal of Preventive Medicine 1993;9:85–91.

[326] Napiorkowski B, Lester BM, Freier MC, et al. Effects of in utero substance exposure on infant neurobehavior. Pediatrics 1996;98:71–5.

[327] Neuspiel DR, Zingman TM, Templeton VH, DiStabile P, Drucker E. Custody of cocaine-exposed newborns: determinants of discharge decisions. Am J Pub Health 1993;83:1726–9.

[328] O'Connor TA, Bondurant HH, Siddiqui J. Targeted perinatal drug screening in a rural population. Journal of Maternal-Fetal Medicine 1997;6:108–10.

[329] Peeke HVS, Dark KA, Salamy A, Salfi M, Shah, SN. Cocaine exposure prebreeding to weaning: Maternal and offspring effects. Pharmacol Biochem Behav 1994;48:403–10.

[330] Pelham TL, DeJong AR. Nationwide practices for screening and reporting prenatal cocaine abuse: a survey of teaching programs. Child Abuse & Neglect 1992;16:763–70.

[331] Phibbs CS, Bateman DA, Schwartz RM. The neonatal costs of maternal cocaine use [see comments]. JAMA 1991;266:1521–6.

[332] Polzin WJ, Kopelman JN, Brady K, Read JA. Screening for illicit drug use in a military obstetric population. Obstet Gynecol 1991;78:600–1.

[333] Quinn AO, Van Mullem C, Sturino K, Broekhuizen F. A multiinstitutional analysis of perinatal cocaine use. Wisconsin Medical Journal. 1992;91:296–9.

[334] Reddin P, Schlimmer B, Mitchell C. Cocaine and pregnant women: a hospital study. Iowa Medicine 1991;81:374–6.

[335] Regalado MG, Schechtman VL, Del Angel AP, Bean, XD. Cardiac and respiratory patterns during sleep in cocaine-exposed neonates. Early Human Development 1996;44:187–200.

[336] Richardson GA, Conroy ML, Day NL. Prenatal cocaine exposure: effects on the development of school-age children. Neurotoxicol Teratol 1996;18:627–34.

[337] Rico H, Costales C, Cabranes JA, Escudero M. Lower serum osteocalcin levels in pregnant drug uses and their newborns at the time of delivery. Obstet Gynecol 1990;75:998–1000.

[338] Rodriguez EM, Mofenson LM, Chang BH, et al. Association of maternal drug use during pregnancy with maternal HIV culture positivity and perinatal HIV transmission. AIDS 1996;10:273–82.

[339] Rogers C, Hall J, Muto J. Findings in newborns of cocaine-abusing mothers. Journal of Forensic Sciences 1991;36:1074–8.

[340] Rosenkranz HS, Klopman G. The carcinogenic potential of cocaine. Cancer Letters 1990;52:243–6.

[341] Ruiz P, Cleary T, Nassiri M, Steele B. Human T lymphocyte subpopulation, and NK cell alterations in persons exposed to cocaine. Clinical Immunology & Immunopathology. 1994;70:245–50.

[342] Ryan RM, Wagner CL, Schultz JM, et al. Meconium analysis for improved identification of infants exposed to cocaine in utero [see comments]. J Pediatr 1994;125:435–40.

[343] Scafidi FA, Field TM, Wheeden A, et al. Cocaine-exposed preterm neonates show behavioral and hormonal differences. Pediatrics 1996;97:851–5.

[344] Schutzman DL, Frankenfield-Chernicoff M, Clatterbaugh HE, Singer J. Incidence of intrauterine cocaine exposure in a suburban setting. Pediatrics 1991;88: 825–7.

[345] Singer L, Arendt R, Farkas K, Minnes S, Huang J, Yamashita T. Relationship of prenatal cocaine exposure and maternal postpartum psychological distress to child developmental outcome. Development & Psychopathology 1997;9:473–89.

[346] Smith IE, Moss-Wells S, Moeti R, Coles CD. Characteristics of non-referred cocaine abusing mothers. NIDA Research Monograph 1989;95:330.

[347] Strano-Rossi S, Chiarotti M, Fiori A, Auriti C, Seganti G. Cocaine abuse in pregnancy: its evaluation through hair analysis of pathological new-borns. Life Sci 1996;59:1909–15.

[348] Svikis DS, Lee JH, Haug NA, Stitzer ML. Attendance incentives for outpatient treatment: effects in methadone- and nonmethadone-maintained pregnant drug dependent women. Drug Acohol Depend 1997;48:33–41.

[349] Tronick EZ, Frank DA, Cabral H, Mirochnick M, Zuckerman B. Late dose-response effects of prenatal cocaine exposure on newborn neurobehavioral performance. Pediatrics 1996;98:76–83.

[350] Ursitti F, Klein J, Koren G. Clinical utilization of the neonatal hair test for cocaine: a four-year experience in Toronto. Biology of the Neonate 1997;72:345–51.

[351] Vega WA, Kolody B, Porter P, Noble A. Effects of age on perinatal substance abuse among whites and African Americans. Am J Drug Alcohol Abuse 1997;23:431–51.

[352] Wasserman DR, Leventhal JM. Maltreatment of children born to cocaine-dependent mothers. Am J Dis Child 1993;147:1324–8.

[353] Weeman JM, Zanetos MA, DeVoe SJ. Intensive surveillance for cocaine use in obstetric patients. Am J Drug Alcohol Abuse 1995; 21:233–9.

[354] Weese-Mayer DE, Klemka-Walden LM, Chan MK, Gingras JL. Effects of prenatal cocaine exposure on perinatal morbidity and postnatal growth in the rabbit. Developmental Pharmacology & Therapeutics 1991;16:221–30.

[355] Welch E, Fleming LE, Peyser I, Greenfield W, Steele BW, Bandstra ES. Rapid cocaine screening of urine in a newborn nursery. J Pediatr 1993;123:468–70.

[356] Wingert WE, Feldman MS, Kim MH, Noble L, Hand I, Yoon JJ. A comparison of meconium, maternal urine, and neonatal urine for detection of maternal drug use during pregnancy. Journal of Forensic Sciences. 1994;39:150–8.

[357] Zimmerman EF, Potturi RB, Resnick E, Fisher JE. Role of oxygen free radicals in cocaine-induced vascular disruption in mice. Teratology 1994;49:192–201.

[358] Zuckerman B, Amaro H, Cabral H. Validity of self-reporting of marijuana and cocaine use among pregnant adolescents. J Pediatr 1989;115:812–815.

[359] Ahmed MS, Zhou DH, Maulik D, Eldefrawi ME. Characterization of a cocaine binding protein in human placenta. Life Sci 1990;46:553–561.

[360] Ahmed MS, Zhou D, Schoof T, et al. Illicit drug use during pregnancy: effects of opiates and cocaine on human placenta. NIDA Research Monograph 1991;105:278–9.

[361] Bailey DN. Studies of cocaethylene (ethylcocaine) formation by human tissues in vitro. J Anal Toxicol 1994;18:13–15.

[362] Bailey DN. Cocaine and cocaethylene binding to human tissues: a preliminary study. Therapeutic Drug Monitoring 1996;18:280–3.

[363] Cejtin HE, Parsons MT, Wilson L, Jr. Cocaine use and its effect on umbilical artery prostacyclin production. Prostaglandins 1990;40:249–57.

[364] Chiarotti M, Strano-Rossi S, Offidani C, Fiori A. Evaluation of cocaine use during pregnancy through toxicological analysis of hair. J Anal Toxicol 1996;20:555–8.

[365] Cook JL, Randall CL. Cocaine does not affect prostacyclin, thromboxane or prostaglandin E production in human umbilical veins. Drug Acohol Depend 1996;41: 113–118.

[366] Dicke JM, Verges DK, Polakoski KL. Cocaine inhibits alanine uptake by human placental microvillous membrane vesicles. American Journal of Obstetrics & Gynecology 1993;169:515–521.

[367] Dicke JM, Verges DK, Polakoski KL. The effects of cocaine on neutral amino acid uptake by human placental basal membrane vesicles. American Journal of Obstetrics & Gynecology 1994;171:485–91.

[368] Gilbert WM, Lafferty CM, Benirschke K, Resnik R. Lack of specific placental abnormality associated with cocaine use. American Journal of Obstetrics & Gynecology 1990;163:998–9.

[369] Harker CT, Bowman CJ, Taylor LMJ, Porter JM. Cooling augments human saphenous vein reactivity to electrical stimulation. J Cardiovasc Pharmacol 1994;23:453–7.

[370] Hurd WW, Gauvin JM, Dombrowski MP, Hayashi RH. Cocaine selectively inhibits β-adrenergic receptor binding in pregnant human myometrium. American Journal of Obstetrics & Gynecology 1993;169:644–9.

[371] Johnson TR, Knisely JS, Christmas JT, Schnoll SH, Ruddy S. Changes in immunologic cell surface markers during cocaine withdrawal in pregnant women. Brain, Behavior, & Immunity 1996;10: 324–336.

[372] Krishna RB, Levitz M, Dancis J. Transfer of cocaine by the perfused human placenta: the effect of binding to serum proteins. American Journal of Obstetrics & Gynecology 1993;169:1418–23.

[373] Malek A, Ivy D, Blann E, Mattison DR. Impact of cocaine on human placental function using an in vitro perfusion system. Journal of Pharmacological & Toxicological Methods 1995;33:213–219.

[374] Miller SR, Middaugh LD, Boggan WO, Patrick KS. Cocaine concentrations in fetal C57BL/6 mouse brain relative to maternal brain and plasma [published erratum appears in Neurotoxicol Teratol 1997 Jan-Feb;19(1):75]. Neurotoxicol Teratol. 1996;18:645–649.

[375] Mirochnick M, Meyer J, Frank DA, Cabral H, Tronick EZ, Zuckerman B. Elevated plasma norepinephrine after in utero exposure to cocaine and marijuana. Pediatrics 1997;99:555–9.

[376] Monga M, Weisbrodt NW, Andres RL, Sanborn BM. The acute effect of cocaine exposure on pregnant human myometrial contractile activity. American Journal of Obstetrics & Gynecology 1993;169:782–5.

[377] Monga M, Chmielowiec S, Andres RL, Troyer, LR, Parisi VM. Cocaine alters placental production of thromboxane and prostacyclin. American Journal of Obstetrics & Gynecology 1994;171:965–9.

[378] Moore C, Browne S, Tebbett I, Negrusz A, Meyer W, Jain L. Determination of cocaine and benzoylecgonine in human amniotic fluid using high flow solid-phase extraction columns and HPLC. Forensic Sci Int 1992;56:177–181.

[379] Oyler J, Darwin WD, Preston KL, Suess P, Cone EJ. Cocaine disposition in meconium from newborns of cocaine-abusing mothers and urine of adult drug users. J Anal Toxicol 1996;20:453–62.

[380] Prasad PD, Leibach FH, Mahesh VB, Ganapathy V. Human placenta as a target organ for cocaine action: interaction of cocaine with the placental serotonin transporter. Placenta 1994;15:267–278.

[381] Ramamoorthy S, Bauman AL, Moore KR, et al. Antidepressant- and cocaine-sensitive human serotonin transporter: molecular cloning, expression, and chromosomal localization. Proceedings of the National Academy of Sciences of the United States of America 1993;90:2542–6.

[382] Ramamoorthy S, Prasad PD, Kulanthaivel P, Leibach FH, Blakely RD, Ganapathy V. Expression of a cocaine-sensitive norepinephrine transporter in the human placental syncytiotrophoblast. Biochemistry 1993;32:1346–53.

[383] Ramamoorthy JD, Ramamoorthy S, Mahesh VB, Leibach FH, Ganapathy V. Cocaine-sensitive σ-receptor, and its interaction with steroid hormones in the human placental syncytiotrophoblast, and in choriocarcinoma cells. Endocrinology 1995;136:924–32.

[384] Richards IS, Kulkarni AP, Bremner WF. Cocaine-induced arrhythmia in human foetal myocardium in vitro: possible mechanism for foetal death in utero. Pharmacology & Toxicology 1990;66:150–4.

[385] Roby PV, Glenn CM, Watkins SL, et al. Association of elevated umbilical cord blood creatine kinase and myoglobin levels with the presence of cocaine metabolites in maternal urine. American Journal of Perinatology 1996;13:453–5.

[386] Roe DA, Little BB, Bawdon RE, Gilstrap LC. Metabolism of cocaine by human placentas: implications for fetal exposure. American Journal of Obstetrics & Gynecology 1990;163:715–18.

[387] Saraf HA, Dombrowski MP, Leach KC, Hurd WW. Characterization of the effect of cocaine on catecholamine uptake by pregnant myometrium. Obstet Gynecol 1995;85:93–6.

[388] Schenker S, Yang Y, Johnson RF, et al. The transfer of cocaine and its metabolites across the term human placenta. Clinical Pharmacology & Therapeutics 1993;53:329–39.

[389] Simone C, Derewlany LO, Oskamp M, Knie B, Koren G. Transfer of cocaine and benzoylecgonine across the perfused human placental cotyledon. American Journal of Obstetrics & Gynecology 1994; 170:1404–10.

[390] Simone C, Byrne BM, Derewlany LO, Koren, G. Cocaine inhibits hCG secretion by the human term placental cotyledon perfused in vitro. Life Sci 1996;58:L-6.

[391] Simone C, Byrne BM, Derewlany LO, Oskamp M, Koren G. The transfer, of cocaethylene across the human term placental cotyledon perfused in vitro. Reproductive Toxicology 1997;11:215–219.

[392] Smith IE, Dent DZ, Coles CD, Falek A. A comparison study of treated, and untreated pregnant, and postpartum cocaine-abusing women. Journal of Substance Abuse Treatment. 1992;9:343–8.

[393] Smith YR, Dombrowski MP, Leach KC, Hurd WW. Decrease in myometrial β-adrenergic receptors with prenatal cocaine use. Obstet Gynecol 1995;85:357–360.

[394] Sosnoff CS, Ann Q, Bernert JTJ, et al. Analysis of benzoylecgonine in dried blood spots by liquid chromatography–atmospheric pressure chemical ionization tandem mass spectrometry. J Anal Toxicol 1996;20:179–184.

[395] Sternfeld M, Rachmilewitz J, Loewenstein-Lichtenstein Y, et al. Normal and atypical butyrylcholinesterases in placental development, function, and malfunction. Cellular & Molecular Neurobiology 1997;17:315–332.

[396] Wang FL, Dombrowski MP, Hurd WW. Cocaine and β-adrenergic receptor function in pregnant myometrium. American Journal of Obstetrics & Gynecology 1996;175:1651–3.

[397] Winecker RE, Goldberger BA, Tebbett I, et al. Detection of cocaine and its metabolites in amniotic fluid and umbilical cord tissue. J Anal Toxicol 1997;21:97–104.

[398] Yelian FD, Sacco AG, Ginsburg KA, Doerr PA, Armant DR. The effects of in vitro cocaine exposure on human sperm motility, intracellular calcium, and oocyte penetration. Fertil Steril 1994;61: 915–921.

[399] Ahluwalia BS, Clark JF, Westney LS, Smith DM, James M, Rajguru S. Amniotic fluid and umbilical artery levels of sex hormones and prostaglandins in human cocaine users. Reproductive Toxicology 1992;6:57–62.
[400] Anonymous. Caring for cocaine's mothers and babies. Naacog Newsletter 1989;16:1,4–6.
[401] Anonymous. Learning handicaps linked to drug exposure [news]. Ohio Medicine 1990;86:14.
[402] AnonymousA tragedy unfolds. Iowa Medicine 1990;80:282.
[403] Anonymous. Drug abuse and HIV infection [news]. Fam Plann Perspect 1991;23:4–5.
[404] Bhushan V, Ng S, Spiller D, Gang H, Inamdar S. Detecting children's passive exposure to cocaine and marijuana. Am J Pub Health 1994;84:675–6.
[405] Burkhead JM, Eriksen NL, Blanco JD. Cocaine use in pregnancy and the risk of intraamniotic infection. Journal of Reproductive Medicine 1995;40:198–200.
[406] Calhoun BC, Watson PT. The cost of maternal cocaine abuse: I. Perinatal cost. Obstet Gynecol 1991;78:731–4.
[407] Chen C, Duara S, Silva Neto G, et al. Respiratory instability in neonates with in utero exposure to cocaine. J Pediatr 1991;119: 111–113.
[408] Chiu TT, Vaughn AJ, Carzoli RP. Hospital costs for cocaine-exposed infants. Journal of the Florida Medical Association 1990;77:897–900.
[409] Cohen HR, Green JR, Crombleholme WR. Peripartum cocaine use: estimating risk of adverse pregnancy outcome. Int J Gynaecol Obstet 1991;35:51–4.
[410] Cohen HL, Sloves JH, Laungani S, Glass L, DeMarinis P. Neurosonographic findings in full-term infants born to maternal cocaine abusers: visualization of subependymal and periventricular cysts. Journal of Clinical Ultrasound 1994;22:327–33.
[411] Coles CD, Platzman KA, Smith I, James ME, Falek A. Effects of cocaine and alcohol use in pregnancy on neonatal growth and neurobehavioral status. Neurotoxicol Teratol 1992;14:23–33.
[412] Cordero L, Custard M. Effects of maternal cocaine abuse on perinatal and infant outcome. Ohio Medicine 1990;86:410–412.
[413] Cotton P. Smoking cigarettes may do developing fetus more harm than ingesting cocaine, some experts say [news]. JAMA 1994;271: 576–7.
[414] Curry M. Cocaine use in pregnancy. Modern Midwife 1995;5:28–9.
[415] Dixon SD, Bejar R. Echoencephalographic findings in neonates associated with maternal cocaine and methamphetamine use: incidence and clinical correlates. J Pediatr 1989;115:770–8.
[416] Durand DJ, Espinoza AM, Nickerson BG. Association between prenatal cocaine exposure and sudden infant death syndrome. J Pediatr 1990;117:909–911.
[417] Dusick AM, Covert RF, Schreiber MD, et al. Risk of i.c. hemorrhage and other adverse outcomes after cocaine exposure in a cohort of 323 very low birth weight infants. J Pediatr 1993;122:438–445.
[418] Johnson EM. From the Alcohol, Drug Abuse, and Mental Health Administration. JAMA 1992;268:447.
[419] Frank DA, Bauchner H, Parker S, et al. Neonatal body proportionality and body composition after in utero exposure to cocaine and marijuana. J Pediatr 1990;117:622–6.
[420] Fritz P, Galanter M, Lifshutz H, Egelko S. Developmental risk factors in postpartum women with urine tests positive for cocaine. Am J Drug Alcohol Abuse 1993;19:187–197.
[421] Gingras JL, Muelenaer A, Dalley LB, O'Donnell KJ. Prenatal cocaine exposure alters postnatal hypoxic arousal responses and hypercarbic ventilatory responses but not pneumocardiograms in prenatally cocaine-exposed term infants. Pediatric Pulmonology 1994; 18:13–20.
[422] Gottbrath-Flaherty EK, Agrawal R, Thaker V, Patel D, Ghai K. Urinary tract infections in cocaine-exposed infants. Journal of Perinatology 1995;15:203–7.
[423] Handler A, Kistin N, Davis F, Ferre C. Cocaine use during pregnancy: perinatal outcomes. American Journal of Epidemiology 1991;133:818–25.
[424] Handler AS, Mason ED, Rosenberg DL, Davis FG. The relationship between exposure during pregnancy to cigarette smoking and cocaine use and placenta previa. American Journal of Obstetrics & Gynecology 1994;170:884–9.
[425] Hanlon-Lundberg KM, Williams M, Rhim T, Covert RF, Mittendorf R, Holt JA. Accelerated fetal lung maturity profiles and maternal cocaine exposure. Obstet Gynecol 1996;87:128–132.
[426] Harris EF, Friend GW, Tolley EA. Enhanced prevalence of ankyloglossia with maternal cocaine use. Cleft Palate-Craniofacial Journal 1992;29:72–6.
[427] Harsham J, Keller JH, Disbrow D. Growth patterns of infants exposed to cocaine and other drugs in utero [published erratum appears in J Am Diet Assoc 1994 Nov;94(11):1254]. Journal of the American Dietetic Association. 1994;94:999–1007.
[428] Hoskins IA, Friedman DM, Frieden FJ, Ordorica SA, Young BK. Relationship between antepartum cocaine abuse, abnormal umbilical artery Doppler velocimetry, and placental abruption. Obstet Gynecol 1991;78:279–282.
[429] Hume RF, Jr., Gingras JL, Martin LS, Hertzberg BS, O'Donnell K, Killam AP. Ultrasound diagnosis of fetal anomalies associated with in utero cocaine exposure: further support for cocaine-induced vascular disruption teratogenesis. Fetal Diagn Ther 1994;9:239–245.
[430] Hurt H, Brodsky NL, Betancourt L, Braitman LE, Malmud E, Giannetta J. Cocaine-exposed children: follow-up through 30 months. Journal of Developmental & Behavioral Pediatrics. 1995;16:29–35.
[431] Jacobson JL, Jacobson SW, Sokol RJ. Effects of prenatal exposure to alcohol, smoking, and illicit drugs on postpartum somatic growth. Alcohol Clin Exp Res 1994;18:317–23.
[432] Kandall SR, Gaines J, Habel L, Davidson G, Jessop D. Relationship of maternal substance abuse to subsequent sudden infant death syndrome in offspring. J Pediatr 1993;123:120–6.
[433] Legido A, Clancy RR, Spitzer AR, Finnegan LP. Electroencephalographic and behavioral-state studies in infants of cocaine-addicted mothers. Am J Dis Child 1992;146:748–752.
[434] Lopez SL, Taeusch HW, Findlay RD, Walther FJ. Time of onset of necrotizing enterocolitis in newborn infants with known prenatal cocaine exposure. Clinical Pediatrics 1995;34:424–9.
[435] Lounsbury B, Lifshitz M, Wilson GS. In utero exposure to cocaine and the risk of SIDS. NIDA Research Monograph 1989;95:352.
[436] Miller JM, Jr., Boudreaux MC, Regan FA. A case-control study of cocaine use in pregnancy. American Journal of Obstetrics & Gynecology 1995;172:180–5.
[437] Mirochnick M, Frank DA, Cabral H, Turner A, Zuckerman B. Relation between meconium concentration of the cocaine metabolite benzoylecgonine and fetal growth. J Pediatr 1995;126:636–8.
[438] Needlman R, Zuckerman B, Anderson GM, Mirochnick M, Cohen DJ. Cerebrospinal fluid monoamine precursors and metabolites in human neonates following in utero cocaine exposure: a preliminary study. Pediatrics 1993;92:55–60.
[439] Neuspiel DR, Hamel SC, Hochberg E, Greene J, Campbell D. Maternal cocaine use and infant behavior. Neurotoxicol Teratol 1991;13:229–33.
[440] Neuspiel DR, Markowitz M, Drucker E. Intrauterine cocaine, lead, and nicotine exposure and fetal growth. Am J Pub Health 1994;84:1492–5.
[441] Nulman I, Rovet J, Altmann D, Bradley C, Einarson T, Koren G. Neurodevelopment of adopted children exposed in utero to cocaine. Canadian Medical Association Journal 1994;151:1591–7.
[442] Prichep LS, Kowalik SC, Alper K, de Jesus C. Quantitative EEG characteristics of children exposed in utero to cocaine. Clinical Electroencephalography 1995;26:166–72.
[443] Richardson GA, Day NL. Maternal and neonatal effects of moderate cocaine use during pregnancy. Neurotoxicol Teratol 1991;13:455–60.

[444] Richardson GA, Day NL. Detrimental effects of prenatal cocaine exposure: illusion or reality? Journal of the American Academy of Child & Adolescent Psychiatry 1994;33:28–34.

[445] Rodning C, Beckwith L, Howard J. Prenatal exposure to drugs: Behavioral distortions reflecting CNS impairment? Neurotoxicology 1989;10:629–34.

[446] Rodriguez EM. Maternal cocaine use harms infants more than HIV infection [news]. American Family Physician 1993;48:319.

[447] Schneider JW, Chasnoff IJ. Motor assessment of cocaine/polydrug exposed infants at age 4 months. Neurotoxicol Teratol 1992;14: 97–101.

[448] Skolnick A. Cocaine use in pregnancy: physicians urged to look for problem where they least expect it [news]. JAMA 1990;264:306, 309.

[449] Singer LT, Yamashita TS, Hawkins S, Cairns D, Baley J, Kliegman R. Increased incidence of intraventricular hemorrhage and developmental delay in cocaine-exposed, very low birth weight infants [see comments]. J Pediatr 1994;124:765–71.

[450] van de Bor M, Walther FJ, Ebrahimi M. Decreased cardiac output in infants of mothers who abused cocaine. Pediatrics 1990;85:30–2.

[451] Wehbeh H, Matthews RP, McCalla S, Feldman J, Minkoff HL. The effect of recent cocaine use on the progress of labor. American Journal of Obstetrics & Gynecology 1995;172:1014–18.

[452] Yawn BP, Thompson LR, Lupo VR, Googins MK, Yawn RA. Prenatal drug use in Minneapolis-St Paul, Minn. A 4-year trend. Archives of Family Medicine 1994;3:520–7.

[453] Beeram MR, Abedin M, Shoroye A, Jayam-Trouth A, Young M, Reid Y. Occurrence of craniosynostosis in neonates exposed to cocaine and tobacco in utero. Journal of the National Medical Association 1993;85:865–8.

[454] Beltran R, Bell T, Fisher S, Ros S. Utility of laboratory screening in cocaine-exposed infants. Clinical Pediatrics 1994;33:683–5.

[455] Burkett G, Yasin, SY, Palow D, LaVoie L, Martinez M. Patterns of cocaine binging: effect on pregnancy [see comments]. American Journal of Obstetrics & Gynecology. 1994;171:372–8; discussion 378.

[456] Chasnoff IJ, Griffith DR. Cocaine: clinical studies of pregnancy, and the newborn. Annals of the New York Academy of Sciences. 1989; 562:260–6.

[457] Fries MH, Kuller JA, Norton ME, et al. Facial features of infants exposed prenatally to cocaine. Teratology 1993;48:413–420.

[458] Hofkosh D, Pringle JL, Wald HP, Switala J, Hinderliter SA, Hamel SC. Early interactions between drug-involved mothers and infants. Within-group differences. Archives of Pediatrics & Adolescent Medicine 1995;149:665–72.

[459] Horn PT. Persistent hypertension after prenatal cocaine exposure. J Pediatr 1992;121:288–291.

[460] Howard J, Beckwith L, Espinosa M, Tyler R. Development of infants born to cocaine-abusing women: biologic/maternal influences. Neurotoxicol Teratol 1995;17: 403–11.

[461] Hume RF, Jr., O'Donnell KJ, Stanger CL, Killam AP, Gingras JL. In utero cocaine exposure: observations of fetal behavioral state may predict neonatal outcome [see comments]. American Journal of Obstetrics & Gynecology 1989;161:685–690.

[462] Knight EM, James, H, Edwards, CH, et al. Relationships of serum illicit drug concentrations during pregnancy to maternal nutritional status. Journal of Nutrition 1994;124:973S–980S.

[463] Kramer LD, Locke GE, Ogunyemi A, Nelson L. Neonatal cocainerelated seizures. Journal of Child Neurology 1990;5:60–4.

[464] Link EA, Weese-Mayer DW, Bryd SE. Magnetic resonance imaging in infants exposed to cocaine prenatally: a preliminary report. Clinical Pediatrics 1991;30:506–8.

[465] McCalla S, Feldman, J, Webbeh, H, Ahmadi, R, Minkoff, HL. Changes in perinatal cocaine use in an inner-city hospital, 1988 to 1992;Am J Pub Health: 1995;85: 1695–1697.

[466] Ney JA, Dooley SL, Keith LG, Chasnoff IJ, Socol ML. The prevalence of substance abuse in patients with suspected preterm labor. American Journal of Obstetrics & Gynecology 1990;162:1562–7.

[467] Racine A, Joyce, T, Anderson R. The association between prenatal care and birth weight among women exposed to cocaine in New York City [published erratum appears in JAMA 1994 Apr 20; 271(15):1161–2]. JAMA. 1993;270:1581–1586.

[468] Rosenstein BJ, Wheeler JS, Heid PL. Congenital renal abnormalities in infants with in utero cocaine exposure. Journal of Urology 1990;144:110–12.

[469] Slutsker L, Smith R, Higginson, G, Fleming D. Recognizing illicit drug use by pregnant women: Reports from Oregon birth attendants. Am J Pub Health 1993;83:61–4.

[470] Smit BJ, Boer K, van Huis AM, Lie-A-Ling IS, Schmidt SC. Cocaine use in pregnancy in Amsterdam. Acta Paed Supp 1994;404:32–5.

[471] Weathers WT, Crane MM, Sauvain KJ, Blackhurst DW. Cocaine use in women from a defined population: prevalence at delivery and effects on growth in infants. Pediatrics 1993;91:350–4.

[472] Doberczak TM, Kandall SR, Wilets I. Neonatal opiate abstinence syndrome in term and preterm infants. J Pediatr 1991;118:933–7.

[473] Feldman J, Minkoff HL, McCalla S, Salwen M. A cohort study of the impact of perinatal drug use on prematurity in an Inner-city population. Am J Pub Health 1992;82:726–8.

[474] Forman R, Klein J, Meta D, Barks J, Greenwald M, Koren G. Maternal and neonatal characteristics following exposure to cocaine in Toronto. Reproductive Toxicology 1993;7:619–622.

[475] Hawthorne JL, Maier RC. Drug abuse in an obstetric population of a midsized city. South Med J 1993;86:1334–8.

[476] Hernandez JT, Hoffman L, Weavil S, Cvejin S, Prange AJ, Jr. The effect of drug exposure on thyroid hormone levels of newborns. Biochemical Medicine & Metabolic Biology 1992;48:255–62.

[477] Kaye K, Elkind L, Goldberg D, Tytun A. Birth outcomes for infants of drug abusing mothers. New York State Journal of Medicine 1989;89:256–61.

[478] Nanda D, Feldman J, Delke I, Chintalapally S, Minkoff H. Syphilis among parturients at an inner city hospital: association with cocaine use and implications for congenital syphilis rates. New York State Journal of Medicine 1990;90:488–90.

[479] Samuels P, Steinfeld JD, Braitman LE, Rhoa MF, Cines DB, McCrae KR. Plasma concentration of endothelin-1 in women with cocaine- associated pregnancy complications. American Journal of Obstetrics & Gynecology 1993;168:528–33.

[480] Spence MR, Williams R, DiGregorio GJ, Kirby-McDonnell A, Polansky M. The relationship between recent cocaine use and pregnancy outcome. Obstet Gynecol 1991;78:326–9.

[481] van Baar AL, Soepatmi S, Gunning WB, Akkerhuis GW. Development after prenatal exposure to cocaine, heroin and methadone. Acta Paed Supp 1994;404:40–6.

[482] Van Baar A. Development of infants of drug dependent mothers. J Child Psychol Psychiatry Allied Discip 1990;31:911–20.

CHAPTER 40

PREGNANCY OUTCOME FOLLOWING MATERNAL ORGANIC SOLVENT EXPOSURE: A META-ANALYSIS OF EPIDEMIOLOGIC STUDIES

Kristen I. McMartin,[1] Merry Chu,[1] Ernest Kopecky,[1] Thomas R. Einarson,[1,2] and Gideon Koren[1,2,3]*

Background. Evidence of fetal damage or demise from occupational organic solvent levels that are not toxic to the pregnant woman is inconsistent in the medical literature. The risk for major malformations and spontaneous abortion from maternal inhalation of organic solvent exposure during pregnancy was summarized using meta-analysis.

Methods. Medline, Toxline, and Dissertation Abstracts databases were searched to locate all research papers published in any language from 1966 to 1994. Included were studies that were case-control or cohort in design and indicated first trimester (or up to 20 weeks gestation for spontaneous abortion) maternal solvent exposure. A summary odds ratio (ORs) with 95% confidence intervals (CI) was calculated from research results combined by the Mantel-Haenszel method.

Results. In total, 559 studies were obtained from the literature search. Five studies for each outcome of interest qualified for inclusion in the analysis. The ORs for major malformations from five studies (n = 7,036 patients) was 1.64 (CI 1.16–2.30) and for spontaneous abortion from five studies (n = 2,899 patients) was 1.25 (CI 0.99–1.58).

Conclusions. Maternal occupational exposure to organic solvents is associated with a tendency toward an increased risk for spontaneous abortion and additional studies may affect the trend. There is a statistically significant association with major malformations which warrants further investigation. *Am. J. Ind. Med.* 34:288–292, 1998.

Keywords: meta-analysis; solvents; pregnancy; major malformation; spontaneous abortion

INTRODUCTION

Organic solvents are a structurally diverse group of low molecular weight liquids that are able to dissolve other organic substances. Chemicals in the solvent class include aliphatic hydrocarbons (mineral spirits, varnish, kerosene), aromatic hydrocarbons (benzene, toluene, xylene), halogenated hydrocarbons (carbon tetrachloride, trichloroethylene), aliphatic alcohols (methanol), glycols (ethylene glycol), and glycol ethers (methoxyethanol) [Schardein, 1985]. Fuels are a mixture of various hydrocarbons. They are generally ubiquitous in industrialized society, both at work and in the home. They may be encountered as individual agents or in complex mixtures such as gasoline. Incidental exposures may include vapors from gasoline, lighter fluid, spot removers, aerosol sprays, and/or paints. These short duration and low level exposures may often go undetected. More serious exposures occur mainly in industrial or laboratory settings during manufacturing and processing operations such as dry cleaning, regularly working with paint removers, thinners, floor and tile cleaners, glue, and as laboratory reagents. Gasoline or glue sniffing, albeit not occurring in the occupational setting, is another source of exposure to organic solvents during pregnancy.

Counseling pregnant women who are occupationally exposed to numerous chemicals (mostly organic solvents) is problematic because it is difficult to estimate the predominant chemicals and their by-products. Even after identifying the more toxic agents, it is still difficult to asses the circumstances of exposure; for many chemicals, one can measure neither airborne nor blood levels. Smelling organic solvents is not indicative of a significant exposure, as the olfactory nerve can detect levels as low as several parts per million, which is not necessarily associated with toxicity. As an example, the odor threshold of toluene is 0.8 parts per million, whereas the TLV-TWA (threshold limit value–time weighted average) is 100 parts per million. In addition, reproductive information on many individual solvents is at best sparse, either limited to animal studies or nonexistent.

Many organic solvents are teratogenic and embryotoxic in laboratory animals, depending on the specific solvent, dose, route of administration, and particular animal species [Schardein, 1985]. The various malformations described include hydrocephaly, exencephaly, skeletal defects, cardiovascular abnormalities, and blood changes. Also, some studies suggest poor fetal development and neurodevelopmental deficits. In a portion of these studies, exposure levels were high enough to induce maternal toxicity.

Organic solvents are a diverse, complex group and because exposure usually involves more than one agent and different circumstances, adequate human epidemiological studies are difficult to interpret. Many studies are subject to recall and response bias and are not always controlled for other risk factors such as age, smoking, ethanol, and concurrent drug ingestion. It is difficult to prove or quantify the suspicion that organic solvents are a reproductive hazard. One may even expect that a ubiquitous exposure to

[1]The Motherisk Program, Division of Clinical Pharmacology and Toxicology, The Department of Pediatrics and The Research Institute, The Hospital for Sick Children, Toronto, Canada

[2]Faculty of Pharmacy, University of Toronto, Toronto, Canada

[3]Departments of Pediatrics, Pharmacology and Medicine, University of Toronto, Toronto, Canada

Contract grant sponsor: Imperial Oil Limited, Toronto, Ontario, Canada

*Correspondence to: Dr. Gideon Koren, Division of Clinical Pharmacology and Toxicology, The Hospital for Sick Children, Toronto, Ontario M5G 1X8, Canada. E-mail: pharmtox@sickkids.on.ca

Accepted 6 April 1998

solvents would by chance alone be associated with an increase in birth defects or spontaneous abortions, which may differ from one study to another. While fetal toxicity is biologically sensible in cases of intoxicated mothers, evidence of fetal damage from levels that are not toxic to the mother is scanty, inconsistent, or missing.

The tool used to analyze the literature for an overall summary of risk between in utero inhalation exposure to organic solvents and adverse pregnancy outcome is meta-analysis. Our meta-analysis aimed at two outcomes of interest—major malformations and spontaneous abortion.

METHODS

A literature search was conducted to collect studies for the meta-analysis. Using Medline, Toxline, and Dissertation Abstracts databases spanning 1966–1994, literature was identified concerning the problem. In addition, colleagues were consulted (regarding unpublished studies) whose area of interest is in occupational exposure and reproductive toxicology. All references from the extracted papers and case reports were investigated. Standard textbooks containing summaries of teratogenicity data were consulted for further undetected references. Key words employed for database searching included: pregnancy, organic solvent, chemical, occupational exposure, adverse fetal outcome, malformation, congenital abnormalities, birth defect, teratogen, abortion, and spontaneous abortion.

The Methods section from each article was selected out and identifying markers of the study, such as author name, institution, journal title, and year, were removed to minimize bias in selecting articles for analysis. The non-identifiable articles were stapled to a data collection sheet and presented to two reviewers for selection into analysis according to preestablished inclusion criteria. Inclusion criteria consisted of human studies of any language: 1) case control or cohort study in design; 2) maternal inhalation occupational organic solvent exposure; 3) outcome was a major malformation as defined by Heinonen [1977] and/or spontaneous abortion (≤20 weeks) as defined by Cunningham et al. [1989]; and 4) first trimester pregnancy exposure. Exclusion criteria consisted of animal studies, non-inhalation exposure, case reports, letters, editorials, review articles, and studies that did not permit extraction of data from 2 × 2 tables. The inclusion of the articles was agreed upon by consensus by independent reviewers and reasons for exclusion were identified. Data from each study were also extracted independently by reviewers. Data were entered into 2 × 2 tables. For subgroup analysis, we also identified and analyzed cohort and case-control studies specifically involving solvent exposure. Major malformations were defined as malformations which were either potentially life threatening or a major cosmetic defect [Heinonen, 1977]. Spontaneous abortion was defined as the spontaneous termination of pregnancy before 20 weeks gestation based on the date of the first day of the last normal menses [Cunningham et al., 1989].

After the data were entered in 2 × 2 tables, risk ratios (RR) for cohort studies and odds ratios (OR) for case-control studies were calculated. To determine the significance of individual studies, χ^2 and 95% confidence intervals (CI) were calculated. To obtain an estimate of the risk ratio for major malformations in exposed vs. unexposed infants, an overall summary OR was calculated by the method of Mantel-Haenszel. A 95% CI was calculated using the method described by Miettinen. The equations and methods of these analyses have been described by Einarson et al. [1988]. Homogeneity was calculated using chi-square. Power analysis and the extent of publication bias were estimated using Orwin's formula [Einarson et al., 1988].

RESULTS

The literature search yielded 559 articles. Of these, 549 were rejected for various reasons, including: animal studies (298), case reports/series (28), review articles (58), editorials (13), duplicate articles (10), not relevant (62), malformation not specified (29), spontaneous abortion not defined (31), unable to extract data (4), no indication of timing of exposure (16). Five papers were included in the major malformation analysis (Table I) and five papers were included in the spontaneous abortion analysis (Table II).

Malformations

Five studies describing results from organic solvent exposure were identified (Table III). The summary OR obtained was 1.64 (95% CI: 1.16–2.30). The test for homogeneity yielded a chi-square of 2.98 (df = 4, P = 0.56). When studies were analyzed separately according to study type, the chi-square value from Breslow and Day's test for homogeneity of effect for cohort studies was 0.52 (df = 1, P = 0.47) and for case control studies it was 0.01 (df = 2, P = 0.99). Meta-analysis of both the cohort studies and case-control studies produced similar results, i.e., they demonstrate a statistically significant relationship between organic solvent exposure in the first trimester of pregnancy and fetal malformation. The summary OR for cohort studies was 1.73 (95% CI: 0.74–4.08) and 1.62 (95% CI: 1.12–2.35) for case-control studies. A subanalysis was performed that excluded unpublished studies from the summary OR. After removing Lemasters [1983], the summary statistic was 1.54 (1.07–2.21).

The file drawer issue can be examined using Orwin's formula (similar to power analysis). The power analysis as suggested by Orwin yielded an average effect size for five studies: Cohen's d = 0.071, the value of d for cohort studies was 0.064 and for case control studies it was 0.076. All three are low in absolute value and are considered small according to Cohen's criterion. According to Orwin's formula, decreasing the overall effect size to 0.05 (small effect) would require the addition of two studies with an effect size d = 0.001 (small effect size).

Table I
Studies of Teratogenicity of Organic Solvents Meeting Criteria for Meta-Analysis

AUTHORS	STUDY TYPE	DATA COLLECTION	MALFORMATION DESCRIBED
Axelsson et al.	C	R	"serious malformations"
Tikkanen et al.	CC	R	cardiac malformations
Holmberg et al.	CC	R	CNS, oral clefts, musculoskeletal, cardiac defects
Cordier et al.	CC	R	"major malformations"
Lemasters	C	R	"major malformations"

CC = Case control. C = Cohort. R = Retrospective.

Table II
Studies of Spontaneous Abortion of Organic Solvents Meeting Criteria for Meta-Analysis

AUTHORS	STUDY TYPE	DATA COLLECTION
Windham et al.	CC	R
Lipscomb et al.	C	R
Shenker et al.	C	P
Pinney	C	R
Eskenazi et al.	C	P

CC = Case control. C = Cohort. R = Retrospective. P = Prospective.

Spontaneous Abortion

Five papers describing results from organic solvent exposure were identified (Table IV). The summary OR obtained was 1.25 (95% CI: 0.99–1.58). The test for homogeneity yielded a chi-square = 4.88 (df = 4, P = 0.300). When studies were analyzed separately according to study type, the chi-square value from Breslow and Day's test for homogeneity of effect for cohort studies was 4.20 (df = 3, P = 0.241). Meta-analysis of both cohort and case-control studies produced similar results, i.e., they do not demonstrate a statistically significant relationship between organic solvent exposure in pregnancy and spontaneous abortion. The summary OR for cohort studies was 1.39 (95% CI: 0.95–2.04) and 1.17 (95% CI: 0.87–1.58) for case control studies. A subanalysis was performed that excluded unpublished studies from the summary OR. By removing Pinney [1990], the summary statistic was 1.31 (1.01–1.69) and by excluding Schenker et al. [1992] from the analysis, the summary statistic was 1.22 (0.96–1.55). Removing both unpublished studies yielded an OR of 1.27 (0.97–1.66). Power analysis suggests that an additional one study with a similar effect size would make the summary OR of 1.25 significant.

Table III
Results of Studies Comparing Outcomes of Fetuses Exposed or Not Exposed to Organic Solvents

			CONGENITAL DEFECT		
REFERENCE	EXPOSURE		YES	NO	TOTAL
Axelsson et al.	Organic solvents	yes	3	489	492
		no	4	492	496
		total	7	981	988
Tikkanen et al.	Organic solvents	yes	23	26	49
		no	546	1,026	1,572
		total	569	1,052	1,621
Holmberg et al.	Organic solvent	yes	11	7	18
		no	1,464	1,438	2,902
		total	1,475	1,475	2,950
Cordier et al.	Organic solvents	yes	29	22	51
		no	234	285	519
		total	263	307	570
Lemasters	Styrene	yes	4	68	72
		no	13	822	835
		total	17	890	907
Total		yes	70	612	682
		no	2,261	4,100	6,354
		total	2,331	4,712	7,036

Table IV
Results of Studies Comparing Outcomes of Fetuses Exposed or Not Exposed to Organic Solvents

			SPONTANEOUS ABORTION		
REFERENCE	EXPOSURE		YES	NO	TOTAL
Windham et al.	Any solvent product	yes	89	160	249
		no	272	575	847
		total	361	735	1,096
Lipscomb et al.	Organic solvent	yes	10	39	49
		no	87	854	941
		total	97	893	990
Schenker et al.	Organic solvents	yes	12	8	20
		no	16	21	37
		total	28	29	57
Pinney	Organic solvents	yes	35	228	263
		no	25	166	191
		total	60	394	454
Eskenazi et al.	Organic solvents	yes	4	97	101
		no	7	194	201
		total	11	291	302
Total		yes	150	532	682
		no	407	1,810	2,217
		total	557	2,342	2,899

DISCUSSION

While estimates for clinically recognized spontaneous abortions as a proportion of all pregnancies vary, the proportion of spontaneous abortions narrowly range from 9–15% in different populations [Lindbohm, 1991]. The variation depends not only on the characteristics of the population but also on the methodology used in studies, for example, the selection of the study population, the source of pregnancy data, and the definition of spontaneous abortion [Lindbohm, 1991].

Evidence of fetal damage or demise from organic solvent levels that are not toxic to the pregnant women is inconsistent in the medical literature. The risk for major malformations and spontaneous abortion from maternal inhalation organic solvent exposure during pregnancy was summarized using meta-analysis. Besides being more objective than the traditional methods of literature review, it has the ability to pool research results from various studies, thereby increasing the statistical strength/power of the analysis. This is especially useful in epidemiologic studies such as cohort studies or case control studies, since very often large numbers of subjects are required in order for any problem to be significantly addressed. This is particularly true for teratogenic studies, where the frequencies of malformation are often very low.

Five studies were included in the spontaneous abortion analysis. The overall ORs of 1.25 indicates that maternal inhalation occupational exposure to organic solvents is associated with a tendency toward a small increased risk for spontaneous abortion. The addition of one study of similar effect size would have rendered this trend statistically significant. Removing the two unpublished studies from the analysis further demonstrates a tendency toward a small increased risk for spontaneous abortion (1.27 (0.97–1.66)).

When studies were analyzed according to study type the summary OR for cohort studies was 1.39 (95% CI: 0.95–2.04). For the case control study the summary OR was 1.18 (95% CI: 0.87–1.58). Their combinability seems justified on the basis of the lack of finding heterogeneity among the results.

This article addresses the use of organic solvents in pregnancy. Organic solvent is a very broad term that includes many classes of chemicals. There may still exist rates of abortion higher than the value reported with certain groups of solvents. However, a detailed analysis of classes of solvents is in order to incriminate a particular solvent. Not all of the studies have examined the same groups of solvents in terms of both extent and range of solvents as well as frequency and duration of exposure. Hence it would be very difficult to obtain any clear estimate of risk for a given solvent, given the limited number of studies available.

To improve further studies of this type, a call for better reporting (in particular, to industrial hygiene assessment) in articles is in order, as it is difficult to judge the "representativeness" of a summary effect if the populations being pooled seem to be heterogeneous.

In this meta-analysis, major malformations were defined by Heinonen [1977] as "potentially life threatening or a major cosmetic defect." In the general population there is a 1–3% baseline risk for major malformations. Estimate incidence via cohort studies indicated two studies with a total of seven malformations in 564 exposures, or 1.2% rate of malformations, which falls within the baseline risk for major malformations.

Five studies were included in the malformation analysis. Study size ranged from 570 to 2,950. The overall summary OR was 1.64 (95% CI: 1.16–2.30), which indicates that maternal inhalation occupational exposure to organic solvents is associated with an increased risk for major malformations. Tests for homogeneity showed a relatively homogeneous group of studies. When studies were analyzed according to study type, the summary OR for cohort studies was 1.73 (95% CI: 0.74–4.08). The summary OR for case control studies was 1.62 (95% CI: 1.12–2.35). Their combinability remains justified on the basis of the lack of finding heterogeneity among the results. Removing the unpublished study from the analysis again demonstrated a statistically significant result (1.54 (1.07–2.21)).

Publication bias is the tendency for statistically significant studies to be submitted and accepted for publication in preference to studies that do not produce statistical significance. This may be the case for solvent exposure and major malformations. Determining the extent of possible publication bias is not unlike power analysis for nonsignificant results. Each provides some quantitative measure of the magnitude of the findings with respect to disproving them and requires judgment for interpretation. A formula for estimating the significance of the file drawer problem when a meta-analysis produces significant results would be Orwin's formula, as discussed for the previous power analysis.

There are some considerations to bear in mind when interpreting results of the malformation and spontaneous abortion meta-analysis:

1. Environmental exposure in pregnancy is seldom an isolated phenomenon; therefore, analysis of human teratogenicity data may require stratification for a number of factors, depending on the intended focus of the analysis.
2. Organic solvents belong to many classes of chemicals. Not all of the studies have examined the exact same groups of solvents in terms of both extent and range of solvents as well as frequency and duration of exposure.
3. The malformations listed in each of the papers seems to reflect a diverse range of anomalies. One might expect to notice a particular trend in malformations between studies; however, this does not appear to be the case.

Our review of the literature reveals that to the best of our knowledge there are no studies that prospectively examine occupational exposure to organic solvents during pregnancy and pregnancy outcome with regard to malformations as the primary objective. Because of the potential implications of this review to a large number of women of reproductive age occupationally exposed to organic solvents, it will be important to verify this cumulative risk estimate by a prospective study. Similarly, it is prudent to minimize women's exposure to organic solvents by ensuring appropriate ventilation systems and protective equipment.

REFERENCES

Axelsson G, Liutz C, Rylander R (1984): Exposure to solvents and outcome of pregnancy in university laboratory employees. Br J Ind Med 41:305–312.

Cordier S, Ha MC, Ayme S, Goujard J (1992): Maternal occupational exposure and congenital malformations. Scand J Work Environ Health 18:11–17.

Cunningham FG, McDonald PC, Gant N (1989): Abortion. In Cunningham FG, McDonald PC, Gant N (eds): "Williams Obstetrics. 18th Ed." Norwalk, CT: Appleton and Lange, pp 489–509.

Einarson TR, Leeder JS, Koren G (1988): A method for meta-analysis of epidemiologic studies. Drug Intell Clin Pharm 22:813–824.

Eskenazi B, Bracken MB, Holford TR, Crady J (1988): Exposure to organic solvents and hypertensive disorders of pregnancy. Am J Ind Med 14:177–188.

Heinonen O (1977): Major malformations. In Heinonen O: "Birth Defects and Drugs in Pregnancy." Littleton, MA: PSG Publishing, pp 65–81.

Holmberg PC, Kurpa K, Riala R, Rantala K, Kuosma E (1986): Solvent exposure and birth defects: An epidemiologic survey. Prog Clin Biol Res 220:179–185.

Lemasters GK (1983): "An Epidemiological Study of Pregnant Workers in the Reinforced Plastics Industry Assessing Outcomes Associated with Live Births." Cincinnati, OH: University of Cincinnati Press.

Lindbohm ML (1991): "Parental Occupational Exposure and Spontaneous Abortion." Tampere, Finland: University of Tampere.

Lipscomb JA, Fenster L, Wrensch M, Shusterman D, Swan S (1991): Pregnancy outcomes in women potentially exposed to occupational solvents and women working in the electronics industry. J Occup Med 33:597–604.

Pinney SM (1990): "An Epidemiological Study of Spontaneous Abortions and Stillbirths on Semiconductor Employees." Cincinnati, OH: University of Cincinnati Press.

Schardein J (1985): Industrial solvents. In Schardein J (ed): "Chemically Induced Birth Defects." New York: Marcel Dekker, pp 645–658.

Schenker MB, Gold EB, Beaumont JJ, Eskenazi B, Hammond SK, Lasley BL, McCurdy SA, Samuels SJ, Saiki CL, Swan SH (1992): "Final Report to the Semiconductor Industry Association. Epidemiologic Study of Reproductive and Other Health Effects Among Workers Employed in the Manufacture of Semiconductors." University of California at Davis.

Tikkanen J, Heinonen O (1988): Cardiovascular malformations and organic solvent exposure during pregnancy in Finland. Am J Ind Med 14:1–8.

Windham GC, Shusterman D, Swan SH, Fenster L, Eskenazi B (1991): Exposure to organic solvents and adverse pregnancy outcome. Am J Ind Med 20:241–259.

Reprinted from McMartin KI, Chu M, Kopecky E, Einarson TR, Koren G. Pregnancy outcome following maternal organic solvent exposure: a meta-analysis of epidemiologic studies. Am J Ind Med 1998;34:288–92 with permission.

SECTION 4

USE OF VITAMINS, CONTRACEPTIVES AND THERAPEUTIC DRUGS

CHAPTER 41

PRENATAL MULTIVITAMIN SUPPLEMENTATION AND RATES OF CONGENITAL ANOMALIES: A META-ANALYSIS

Y. Ingrid Goh,[1,2] *Enkelejd Bollano,*[2] *Thomas R. Einarson,*[1,2] *and Gideon Koren*[1–5]

[1]*Department of Pharmaceutical Sciences, University of Toronto, Toronto ON* [2]*The Motherisk Program, Division of Clinical Pharmacology/Toxicology, The Hospital for Sick Children, Toronto ON* [3]*Faculty of Medicine, University of Toronto, Toronto ON* [4]*Ivey Chair in Molecular Toxicology, University of Western Ontario, London ON* [5]*Department of Medicine, University of Western Ontario, London ON*

Abstract

Background. The use of folic acid-fortified multivitamin supplements has long been associated with decreasing the risk of neural tube defects. Several studies have also proposed the effectiveness of these supplements in preventing other birth defects; however, such effects have never been systematically examined.
Objective. We conducted a systematic review and meta-analysis to evaluate the protective effect of folic acid-fortified multivitamin supplements on other congenital anomalies.
Methods. We searched Medline, PubMed, EMBASE, Toxline, Healthstar, and Cochrane databases for studies describing the outcome of pregnancies in women using multivitamin supplements that were published in all languages from January 1966 to July 2005. The references from all collected articles were reviewed for additional articles. Two independent reviewers who were blinded to the source and identity of the articles extracted data based on predetermined inclusion and exclusion criteria. Using a random effects model, rates of congenital anomalies in babies born to women who were taking multivitamin supplements were compared with rates in the offspring of controls who were not.
Results. From the initial search, 92 studies were identified; 41 of these met the inclusion criteria. Use of multivitamin supplements provided consistent protection against neural tube defects (random effects odds ratio [OR] 0.67, 95% confidence intervals [95% CI] 0.58–0.77 in case control studies; OR 0.52, 95% CI 0.39–0.69 in cohort and randomized controlled studies), cardiovascular defects (OR 0.78, 95% CI 0.67–0.92 in case control studies; OR 0.61, 95% CI 0.40–0.92 in cohort and randomized controlled studies), and limb defects (OR 0.48, 95% CI 0.30–0.76 in case control studies; OR 0.57, 95% CI 0.38–0.85 in cohort and randomized controlled studies). For cleft palate, case control studies showed OR 0.76 (95% CI 0.62–0.93), and cohort and randomized controlled studies showed OR 0.42 (95% CI 0.06–2.84); for oral cleft with or without cleft palate, case control studies showed OR 0.63 (95% CI 0.54–0.73), and cohort and randomized controlled studies showed OR 0.58 (95% CI 0.28–1.19); for urinary tract anomalies, case control studies showed OR 0.48 (95% CI 0.30–0.76), and cohort and randomized controlled studies showed OR 0.68 (95% CI 0.35–1.31); and for congenital hydrocephalus case control studies showed OR 0.37 (95% CI 0.24–0.56), and cohort and randomized controlled studies showed OR 1.54 (95% CI 0.53–4.50). No effects were shown in preventing Down syndrome, pyloric stenosis, undescended testis, or hypospadias.
Conclusion. Maternal consumption of folic acid-containing prenatal multivitamins is associated with decreased risk for several congenital anomalies, not only neural tube defects. These data have major public health implications, because until now fortification of only folic acid has been encouraged. This approach should be reconsidered.

Key Words: Prenatal multivitamins, congenital anomalies, meta-analysis
Competing Interests: None declared.
Received on May 26, 2006
Accepted on June 5, 2006

Résumé

Contexte. L'utilisation de suppléments multivitaminiques fortifiés à l'acide folique est depuis longtemps associée à la baisse du risque d'anomalies du tube neural. Plusieurs études ont également proposé l'efficacité de ces suppléments pour la prévention d'autres anomalies congénitales; cependant, ces effets n'ont jamais fait l'objet d'un examen systématique.
Objectif. Nous avons mené un examen et une méta-analyse systématiques afin d'évaluer l'effet protecteur des suppléments multivitaminiques fortifiés à l'acide folique sur d'autres anomalies congénitales.

Méthodes. Nous avons mené des recherches dans les bases de données Medline, PubMed, EMBASE, Toxline, Healthstar et Cochrane afin d'y recenser les études (qui ont été publiées, toutes langues confondues, entre janvier 1966 et juillet 2005) décrivant les issues de grossesse chez les femmes qui ont utilisé des suppléments multivitaminiques. Les références de tous les articles recensés ont fait l'objet d'une analyse afin d'y trouver des articles additionnels. Deux analystes indépendants, n'ayant pas été mis au courant de la source ni de l'identité des articles en question, ont procédé à l'extraction de données en fonction de critères d'inclusion et d'exclusion prédéterminés. Les taux d'anomalies congénitales chez les enfants nés de femmes ayant pris des suppléments multivitaminiques ont été comparés, au moyen d'un modèle à effets aléatoires, à ceux de témoins n'en ayant pas pris.

Résultats. La recherche initiale a permis l'identification de 92 études; 41 d'entre elles ont satisfait aux critères d'inclusion. L'utilisation de suppléments multivitaminiques a offert une protection uniforme contre les anomalies du tube neural (rapport de cotes des effets aléatoires [RC], 0,67, intervalles de confiance [IC] à 95 %, 0,58–0,77, dans les études cas-témoins; RC, 0,52, IC à 95 %, 0,39–0,69, dans les études de cohorte et les essais comparatifs randomisés), les anomalies cardiovasculaires (RC, 0,78, IC à 95 %, 0,67–0,92, dans les études cas-témoins; RC, 0,61, IC à 95 %, 0,40–0,92, dans les études de cohorte et les essais comparatifs randomisés) et les anomalies affectant les membres (RC, 0,48, IC à 95 %, 0,30–0,76, dans les études cas-témoins; RC, 0,57, IC à 95 %, 0,38–0,85, dans les études de cohorte et les essais comparatifs randomisés). Dans le cas de la fente palatine, les études cas-témoins ont indiqué un RC de 0,76 (IC à 95 %, 0,62–0,93) et les études de cohorte et les essais comparatifs randomisés ont indiqué un RC de 0,42 (IC à 95 %, 0,06–2,84); dans le cas de la fente orale avec ou sans fente palatine, les études cas-témoins ont indiqué un RC de 0,63 (IC à 95 %, 0,54–0,73) et les études de cohorte et les essais comparatifs randomisés ont indiqué un RC de 0,58 (IC à 95 %, 0,28–1,19); dans le cas des anomalies du tractus urinaire, les études cas-témoins ont indiqué un RC à 0,48 (IC à 95 %, 0,30–0,76) et les études de cohorte et les essais comparatifs randomisés ont indiqué un RC de 0,68 (IC à 95 %, 0,35–1,31); et dans le cas de l'hydrocéphalie congénitale, les études cas-témoins ont indiqué un RC de 0,37 (IC à 95 %, 0,24–0,56) et les études de cohorte et les essais comparatifs randomisés ont indiqué un RC de 1,54 (IC à 95 %, 0,53–4,50). Aucun effet préventif n'a été constaté en ce qui concerne le syndrome de Down, la sténose du pylore, la cryptorchidie ou l'hypospadias.

Conclusion. La consommation de multivitamines prénatales contenant de l'acide folique par la mère est associée à une baisse non seulement du risque d'anomalies du tube neural, mais également de celui d'anomalies congénitales graves. Ces données entraînent d'importantes conséquences en matière de santé publique puisque, jusqu'à présent, seule la fortification à l'acide folique a été favorisée. Cette approche devrait être remise en question.

J Obstet Gynaecol Can 2006;28(8):680–689

INTRODUCTION

One in 33 children born in Canada and the United States has a birth defect.[1,2] In 2005, it was estimated that about 150 000 babies are born in North America each year with a birth defect.[3] The burden of illness and the economic cost of birth defects are extremely high.[4,5] More than a decade ago, the preventative role of maternal folate supplementation on the occurrence and the recurrence of neural tube defects was documented in several studies.[6,7,8] Subsequently, preconceptional fortification with folic acid has been shown to reduce the rates of neural tube defects in North America.[9]

During the last decade, several studies have suggested that folic acid-fortified multivitamins may also prevent other congenital anomalies.[10] Botto et al. suggested, on the basis of several studies, that there was a decreased risk for orofacial clefts, limb deficiencies, and cardiovascular abnormalities in babies whose mothers received multivitamin supplementation.[11] To date, however, no systematic review has been conducted to examine existing evidence for the potential of folic acid-containing multivitamins to decrease the risk of congenital anomalies other than neural tube defects. The objective of the present study was to conduct a meta-analysis of studies comparing rates of congenital malformation among women taking vitamin supplements with the rates in controls.

METHODS

We conducted a search of existing studies that focused on pre- and periconceptional maternal ingestion of multivitamins and the rates of malformation in the offspring. The outcome of interest was congenital malformations. All original research articles using randomized controlled trial, case control, or cohort studies were included. All selected articles contained reports of maternal intake of multivitamins during pregnancy, a control group, and raw data describing rates of healthy and malformed children. Articles that did not report usage of multivitamins during pregnancy, articles that focused on specific vitamins, articles describing mothers exposed to other known teratogens, review articles, letters to the editor, and data reports from abstracts or meetings were excluded.

Articles were searched using the terms "multivitamin," "pregnancy," and "malformation" in Medline (January 1966–July 2005), PubMed (1950–July 2005), EMBASE (January 1980–July 2005), Toxline (January 1960–July 2005), Healthstar (January 1966–July 2005), and Cochrane database in all languages. The references from all collected articles were reviewed to locate other original studies.

Two reviewers blinded to authors' names, institution, and journal title assessed all of the articles collected using the selection criteria described above. Data were extracted from these articles to collection forms in 2 x 2 tables. In cases of discrepancy between the reviewers that were not resolved by discussion, the article in question was reviewed by a third blinded reviewer. The odds ratios and 95% confidence intervals were calculated for each study using Review Manager 4.2.7 (2004, The Cochrane Collaboration). Homogeneity among effects was tested by calculating chi-square.

RESULTS

Ninety-two articles were compiled from initial searches of the databases and reference review. Forty-one studies were eligible for the meta-analysis based on the inclusion and exclusion criteria.[12–53] There were 27 case control studies, four randomized control trials, and 10 cohort studies. Fifty-one articles were excluded because they did not report malformation rates, focused specifically on folic acid, did not contain a control group, were review articles, or contained data that were identical to previous studies by the same authors. The use of multivitamin supplementation by the mothers from before the time of conception was associated with a consistent protective effect against neural tube defects (odds ratio [OR] 0.67, 95% confidence interval [CI] 0.58–0.77 in case control studies; OR 0.52, 95% CI 0.39–0.69 in cohort and randomized controlled studies), cardiovascular defects (OR 0.78, 95% CI 0.67–0.92 in case control studies; OR 0.61, 95% CI 0.40–0.92 in cohort and randomized controlled studies), and limb defects

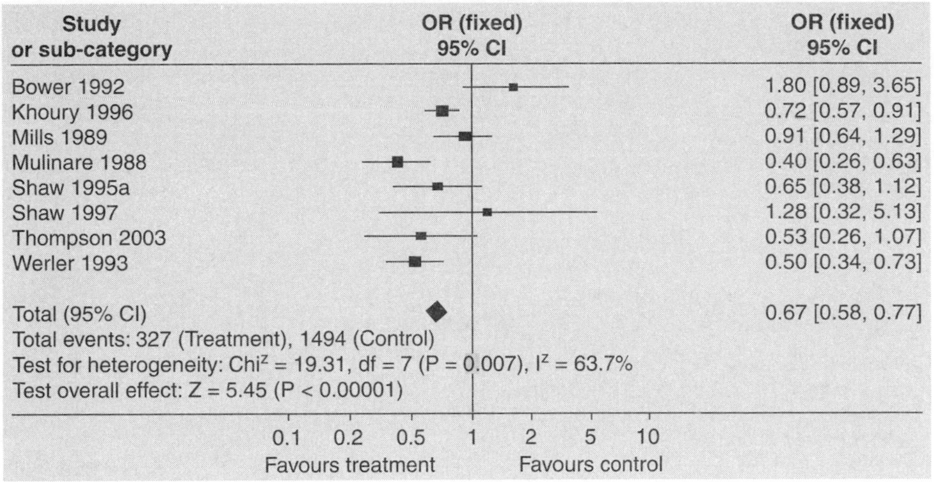

NTD: neural tube defects; OR: odds ratio; CI: confidence interval.

Figure 1. Maternal multivitamin consumption before and in first trimester of pregnancy and risk of NTD in their children (case control studies).

(OR 0.48, 95% CI 0.30–0.76 in case control studies; OR 0.57, 95% CI 0.38–0.85 in cohort and randomized controlled studies). Multivitamin supplementation beginning before pregnancy showed a less consistent protective effect against cleft palate (OR 0.76, 95% CI 0.62–0.93 in case control studies; OR 0.42, 95% CI 0.06–2.84 in cohort and randomized controlled studies), oral cleft with or without cleft palate (OR 0.63, 95% CI 0.54–0.73 in case control studies; OR 0.58, 95% CI 0.28–1.19 in cohort and randomized controlled studies), urinary tract anomalies (OR 0.48, 95% CI 0.30–0.76 in case control studies; OR 0.68, 95% CI 0.35–1.31 in cohort and randomized controlled studies), and congenital hydrocephalus (OR 0.37, 95% CI 0.24–0.56 in case control studies; OR 1.54, 95% CI 0.53–4.50 in cohort and randomized controlled studies) (Figures 1–14). In addition, women who began supplementation in the first trimester after learning of the pregnancy showed a protective effect for neural tube defects (OR 0.80, 95% CI 0.72–0.89) (Figure 15). There was no heterogeneity among the studies.

In contrast, multivitamin supplementation was not associated with a protective effect for Down syndrome (OR 0.56, 95% CI 0.26–1.19 in cohort and randomized controlled studies), congenital pyloric stenosis (OR 1.10, 95% CI 0.79–1.53 in case control studies; OR 0.20, 95% CI 0.02–1.68 in cohort and randomized controlled studies), undescended testis (OR 0.81, 95% CI 0.40–1.64 in cohort studies), and hypospadias (OR 0.44, 95% CI 0.13–1.43 in cohort and randomized controlled studies).

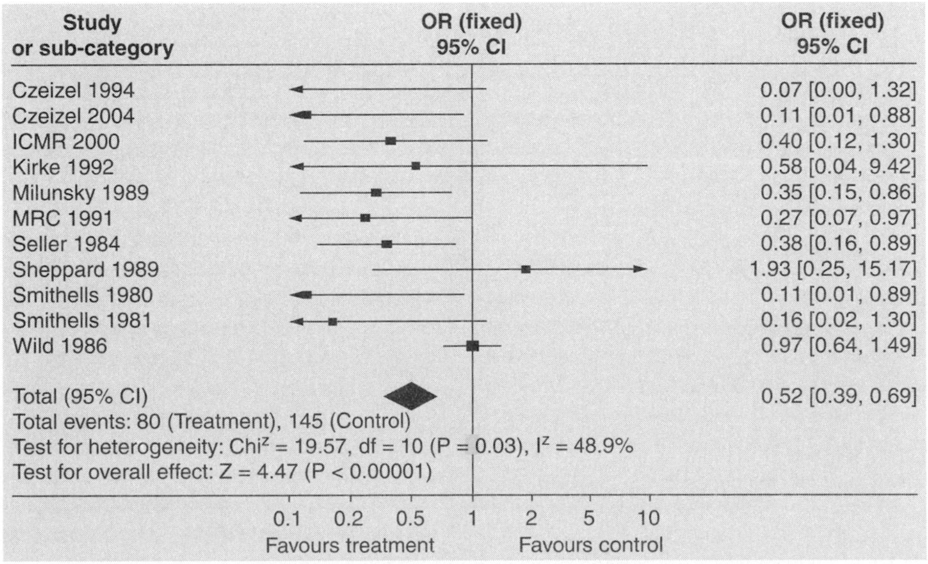

NTD: neural tube defects; RCT: randomized controlled trials; OR: odds ratio; CI: confidence interval.

Figure 2. Maternal multivitamin consumption before and in first trimester of pregnancy and risk of NTD in their children (cohort and RCT studies).

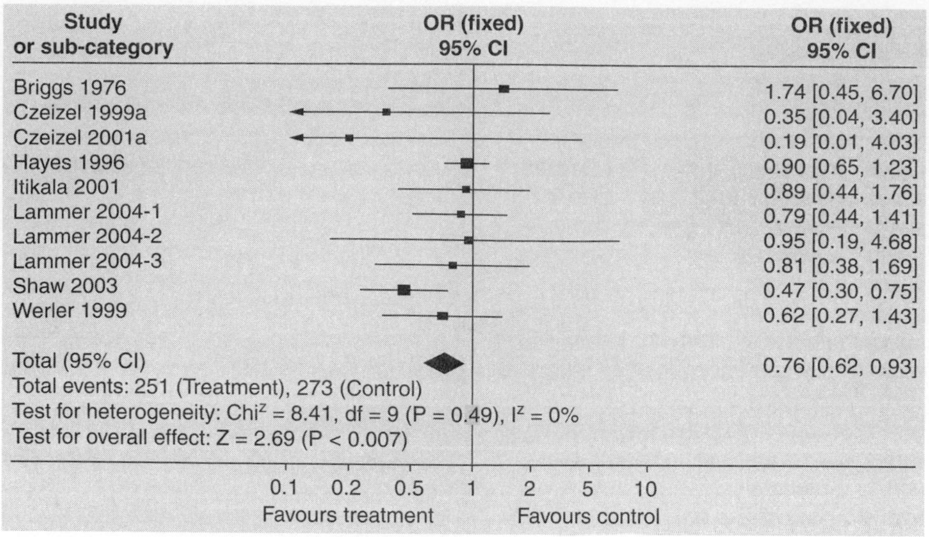

OR: odds ratio; CI: confidence interval.

***Figure 3.** Maternal multivitamin consumption before and in first trimester of pregnancy and risk of cleft palate in their children (case control studies).*

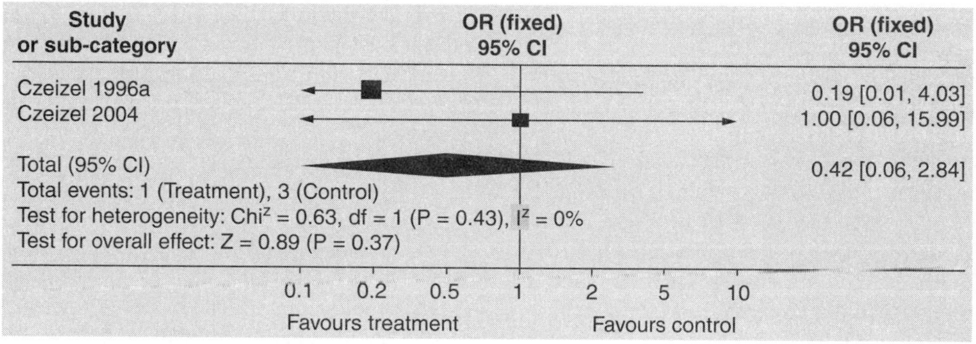

RCT: randomized controlled trials; OR: odds ratio; CI: confidence interval.

***Figure 4.** Maternal multivitamin consumption before and in first trimester of pregnancy and risk of cleft palate in their children (cohort and RCT studies).*

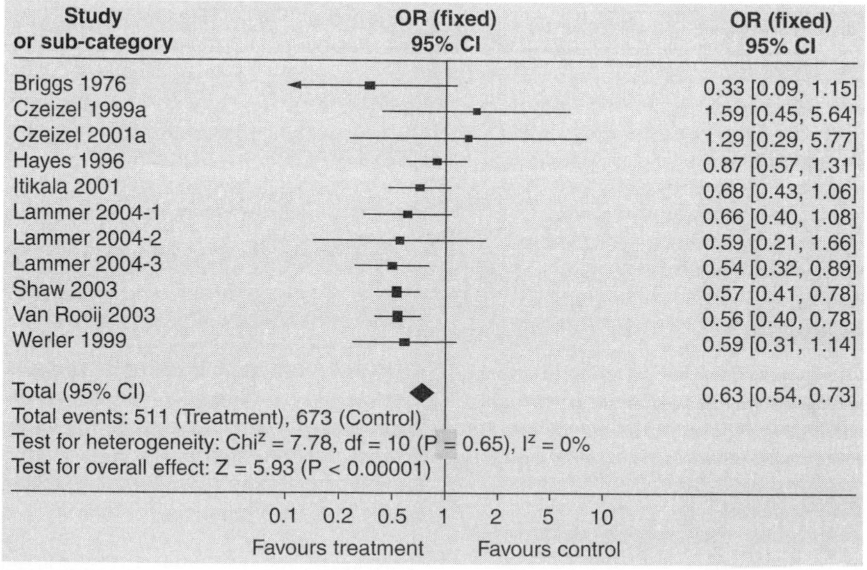

OR: odds ratio; CI: confidence interval.

***Figure 5.** Maternal multivitamin consumption before and in first trimester of pregnancy and risk of cleft lip with or without palate in their children (case control studies).*

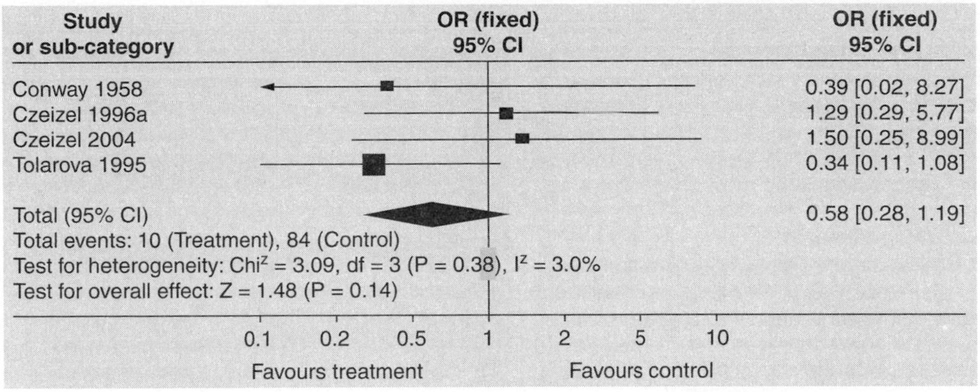

RCT: randomized controlled trials; OR: odds ratio; CI: confidence interval.

Figure 6. Maternal multivitamin consumption before and in first trimester of pregnancy and risk of cleft lip with or without palate in their children (cohort and RCT studies).

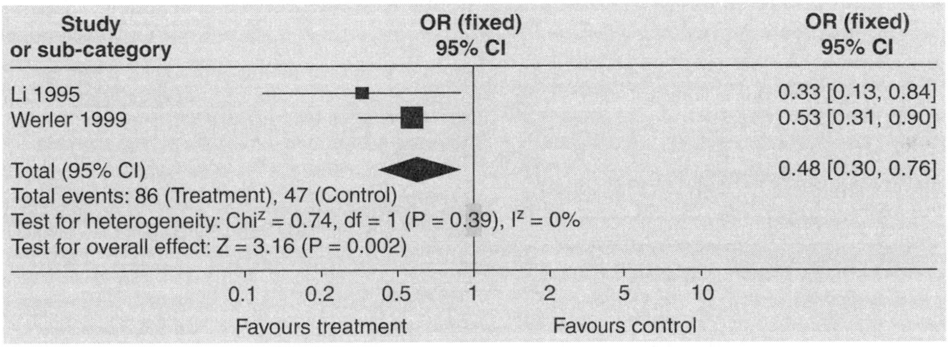

OR: odds ratio; CI: confidence interval.

Figure 7. Maternal multivitamin consumption before and in first trimester of pregnancy and risk of urinary tract anomalies in their children (case control studies).

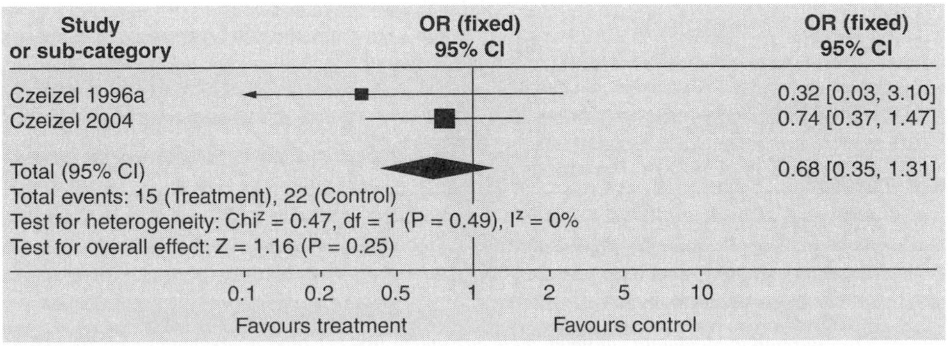

RCT: randomized controlled trials; OR: odds ratio; CI: confidence interval.

Figure 8. Maternal multivitamin consumption before and in first trimester of pregnancy and risk of urinary tract anomalies in their children (cohort and RCT studies).

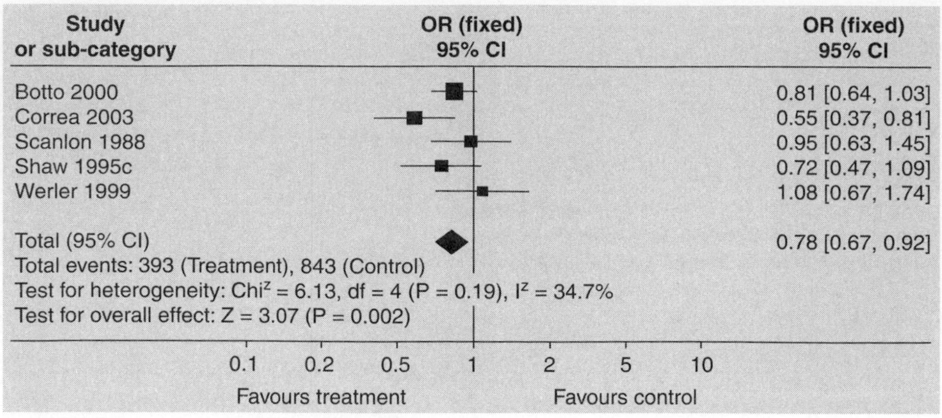

OR: odds ratio; CI: confidence interval.

Figure 9. ***Maternal multivitamin consumption before and in first trimester of pregnancy and risk of cardiovascular defects in their children (case control studies).***

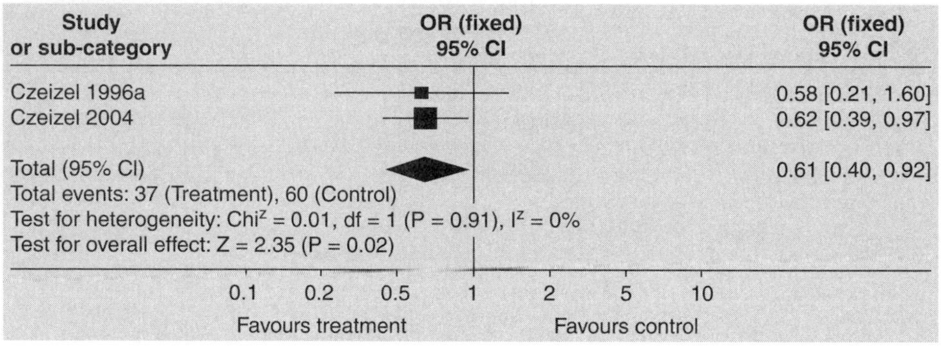

RCT: randomized controlled trials; OR: odds ratio; CI: confidence interval.

Figure 10. ***Maternal multivitamin consumption before and in first trimester of pregnancy and risk of cardiovascular defects in their children (cohort and RCT studies).***

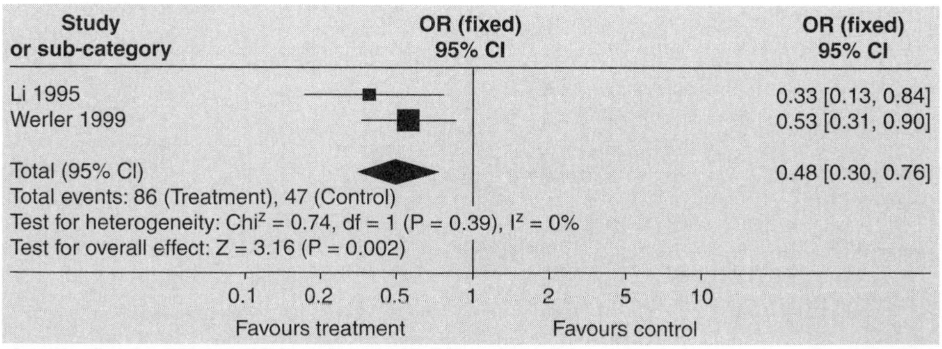

OR: odds ratio; CI: confidence interval.

Figure 11. ***Maternal multivitamin consumption before and in first trimester of pregnancy and risk of limb defects in their children (case control studies).***

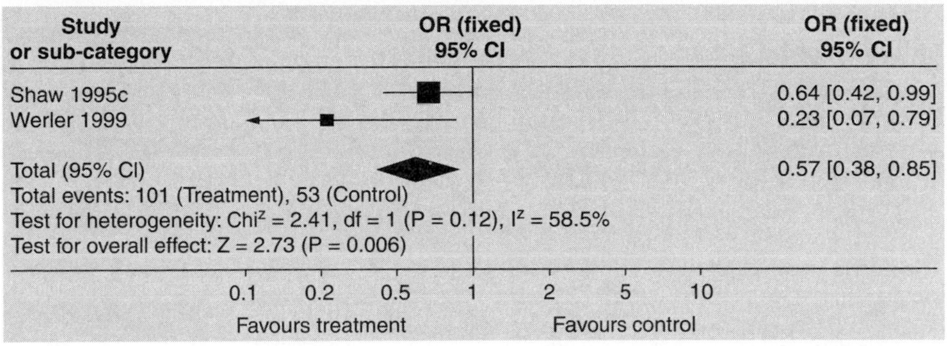

RCT: randomized controlled trials; OR: odds ratio; CI: confidence interval.

Figure 12. Maternal multivitamin consumption before and in first trimester of pregnancy and risk of limb defects in their children (cohort and RCT studies).

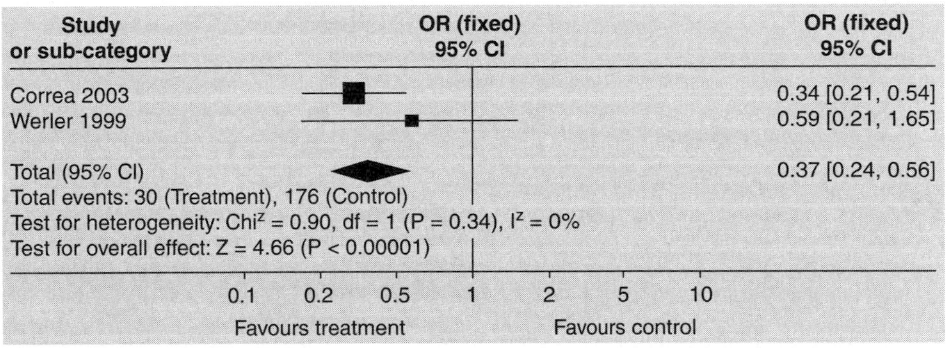

OR: odds ratio; CI: confidence interval.

Figure 13. Maternal multivitamin consumption before and in first trimester of pregnancy and risk of congenital hydrocephalus in their children (case control studies).

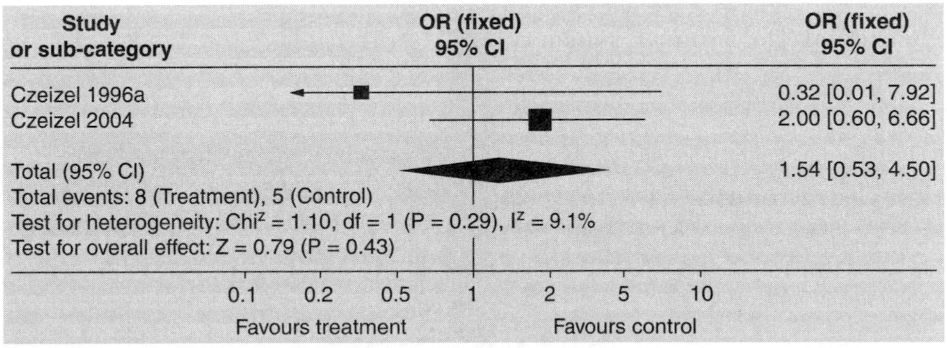

RCT: randomized controlled trials; OR: odds ratio; CI: confidence interval.

Figure 14. Maternal multivitamin consumption before and in first trimester of pregnancy and risk of congenital hydrocephalus in their children (cohort and RCT studies).

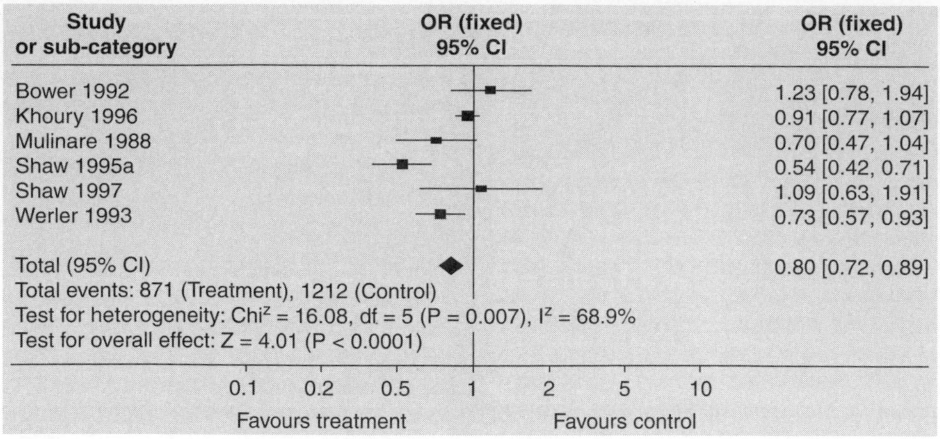
Study
or sub-category
OR (fixed)
95% CI
OR (fixed)
95% CI
Bower 1992
1.23 [0.78, 1.94]
Khoury 1996
0.91 [0.77, 1.07]
Mulinare 1988
0.70 [0.47, 1.04]
Shaw 1995a
0.54 [0.42, 0.71]
Shaw 1997
1.09 [0.63, 1.91]
Werler 1993
0.73 [0.57, 0.93]
Total (95% CI)
0.80 [0.72, 0.89]
Total events: 871 (Treatment), 1212 (Control)
Test for heterogeneity: Chi² = 16.08, df = 5 (P = 0.007), I² = 68.9%
Test for overall effect: Z = 4.01 (P < 0.0001)
0.1
0.2
0.5
1
2
5
10
Favours treatment
Favours control

NTD: neural tube defects; OR: odds ratio; CI: confidence interval.

Figure 15. Maternal multivitamin consumption in first trimester of pregnancy and risk of NTD in their children (case control studies).

DISCUSSION

The present meta-analysis confirms initial impressions that the use of multivitamins fortified with folic acid by women before conception and continuing through the first trimester is associated with a decrease in several serious major malformations. To our knowledge, this is the first systematic review and meta-analysis to examine and document these protective effects.

The majority of the studies included in the meta-analysis were case control studies, although there were also several randomized controlled trials and cohort studies. Not surprisingly, case control studies are more sensitive in showing significant effects for preventing specific malformations than cohort or randomized studies. The observation that all the studies for the majority of endpoints were statistically homogenous lends credibility to the documented effects. There was heterogeneity in the case control studies and cohort studies examining neural tube defects (8 and 11 studies, respectively). Exclusion of one small case control study (Bower and Stanley[17]) and one small cohort study (Sheppard et al.[45]), each of which showed no protective effect, renders the results homogeneous without changing the overall effect size. Moreover, we could not detect a publication bias by employing the funnel plot. Our study, however, is limited by the fact that multivitamin supplements in differing studies may have varied in their composition.

Presently, there are widely publicized recommendations by various authorities for women to supplement with folate at daily doses of at least 0.4mg (4 mg for women at higher risk) to reduce the risk of delivering a child with neural tube defects. In many centres women are advised to begin taking prenatal vitamin supplements when they decide to attempt to conceive, merely to allow them sufficient folate supplementation. It is currently impossible to discern whether folic acid or other vitamins are critical in the prevention of other birth defects.

Only a fraction of women currently take prenatal vitamin supplements at the time of conception, partly because one half of all pregnancies are unplanned. Serious consideration should be given to fortification of flour or other food staples with other vitamins in addition to folate. With increased surveillance of changes in malformation rates as a result of folate fortification, and subsequently larger cohorts, it will be possible to determine whether folate fortification itself is capable of protecting against birth defects other than neural tube defects.

CONCLUSION

The results of the present meta-analysis support the use of prenatal multivitamin preparations containing folic acid to reduce the incidence of several congenital anomalies, including neural tube defects, cardiovascular anomalies, oral cleft, urinary tract anomalies, congenital hydrocephalus, and limb defects. Randomized trials will be necessary to prove which specific vitamin(s) render protective effects.

ACKNOWLEDGEMENTS

Supported by grants from the Canadian Institutes of Health Research and the Research Leadership for Better Pharmacotherapy During Pregnancy and Lactation.

REFERENCES

1. Canadian Perinatal Surveillance System, Congenital Anomalies in Canada: A Perinatal Health Report, 2002. Available at: http://www.phac-aspc.gc.ca/publicat/cac-acc02/pdf/cac2002_e.pdf. Accessed September 1, 2005.
2. Department of Health and Human Services, Centers for Disease and Control Prevention. Available at:http://www.cdc.gov/node.do/id/0900f3ec8000dffe. Accessed September 1, 2005.
3. March of Dimes, Birth Defects. Available at: http://www.marchofdimes.com/pnhec/4439_1206.asp. Accessed September 1, 2005.
4. Kinsman SL, Doehring MC. The cost of preventable conditions in adults with spina bifida. Eur J Pediatr Surg 1996; Suppl 1:17–20.
5. Hunt O, Burden D, Hepper P, Johnston C. The psychosocial effects of cleft lip and palate: a systematic review. Eur J Orthod 2005; 27(3):274–85.

6. Laurence KM, Carter CO, David PA. Major central nervous system malformations in South Wales. II. Pregnancy factors, seasonal variation, and social class effects. Br J Prev Soc Med 1968;22(4): 212–22.
7. Smithells RW, Sheppard S, Schorah CJ, Seller MJ, Nevin NC, Harris R, et al. Possible prevention of neural-tube defects by periconceptional vitamin supplementation. Lancet 1980;1(8164):339–40.
8. Laurence KM, James N, Miller MH, Tennant GB, Campbell H. Double-blind randomised controlled trial of folate treatment before conception to prevent recurrence of neural-tube defects. Br Med J (Clin Res Ed) 1981;282(6275):1509–11.
9. Mills JL, Signore C. Neural tube defect rates before and after food fortification with folic acid. Birth Defects Res A Clin Mol Teratol 2004; 70(11):844–5.
10. Czeizel AE. Periconceptional folic acid containing multivitamin supplementation. Eur J Obstet Gynecol Reprod Biol 1998;78(2): 151–161.
11. Botto LD, Olney RS, Erickson JD. Vitamin supplements and the risk for congenital anomalies other than neural tube defects. Am J Med Genet C Semin Med Genet 2004;125(1):12–21.
12. Botto LD, Khoury MJ, Mulinare J, Erickson JD. Periconceptional multivitamin use and the occurrence of conotruncal heart defects: results from a population-based, case control study. Pediatrics 1996; 98(5):911–7.
13. Botto LD, Mulinare J, Erickson JD. Occurrence of congenital heart defects in relation to maternal mulitivitamin use. Am J Epidemiol 2000;151(9):878–84.
14. Botto LD, Lynberg MC, Erickson JD. Congenital heart defects, maternal febrile illness, and multivitamin use: a population-based study. Epidemiology 2001;12(5):485–90.
15. Botto LD, Mulinare J, Erickson JD. Occurrence of omphalocele in relation to maternal multivitamin use: a population-based study. Pediatrics 2002;109(5):904–8.
16. Botto LD, Mulinare J, Yang Q, Liu Y, Erickson JD. Autosomal trisomy and maternal use of multivitamin supplements. Am J Med Genet A 2004; 125(2):113–6.
17. Bower C, Stanley FJ. Periconceptional vitamin supplementation and neural tube defects; evidence from a case control study in Western Australia and a review of recent publications. J Epidemiol Community Health 1992;46(2):157–61.
18. Briggs RM. Vitamin supplementation as a possible factor in the incidence of cleft lip/palate deformities in humans. Clin Plast Surg 1976;(4):647–52.
19. Correa A, Botto L, Liu Y, Mulinare J, Erickson JD. Do multivitamin supplements attenuate the risk for diabetes-associated birth defects? Pediatrics 2003; (5 Part 2):1146–51.
20. Czeizel AE, Prevention of the first occurrence of neural-tube defects by periconceptional vitamin supplementation. N Engl J Med 1992;327(26):1832–5.
21. Czeizel AE. Prevention of congenital abnormalities by periconceptional multivitamin supplementation. BMJ 1993; 306(6893):1645–8.
22. Czeizel AE, Dudas I, Metneki J. Pregnancy outcomes in a randomised controlled trial of periconceptional multivitamin supplementation. Final report. Arch Gynecol Obstet 1994;255(3):131–9.
23. Czeizel AE. Reduction of urinary tract and cardiovascular defects by periconceptional multivitamin supplementation. Am J Med Genet 1996;62(2):179–83.
24. Czeizel AE, Timar L, Sarkozi A. Dose-dependent effect of folic acid on the prevention of orofacial clefts. Pediatrics 1999;104(6):e66.
25. Czeizel AE. Folic acid and human malformations: misunderstandings. Reprod Toxicol 2001;15(4):441–4.
26. Czeizel AE, Dobo M, Vargha P. Hungarian cohort-controlled trial of periconceptional multivitamin supplementation shows a reduction in certain congenital abnormalities. Birth Defects Res A Clin Mol Teratol 2004;(11):853–61.
27. Hayes C, Werler MM, Willett WC, Mitchell AA. Case control study of periconceptional folic acid supplementation and oral clefts. Am J Epidemiol 1996;143(12):1229–34.
28. Itikala PR, Watkins ML, Mulinare J, Moore CA, Liu Y. Maternal multivitamin use and orofacial clefts in offspring. Teratology 2001; 63(2):79–86.
29. Central Technical Co-ordinating Unit, ICMRCentral Technical Co-ordinating Unit, ICMR. Multicentric study of efficacy of periconceptional folic acid containing vitamin supplementation in prevention of open neural tube defects from India. Indian J Med Res 2000;112: 206–11.
30. Khoury MJ, Shaw GM, Moore CA, Lammer EJ, Mulinare J. Does periconceptional multivitamin use reduce the risk of neural tube defects associated with other birth defects? data from two population-based case control studies. Am J Med Genet 1996;61(1):30–6.
31. Kirke PN, Daly LE, Elwood JH. A randomised trial of low dose folic acid to prevent neural tube defects. The Irish Vitamin Study Group. Arch Dis Child 1992;67(12):1442–6.
32. Li DK, Daling JR, Mueller BA, Hickok DE, Fantel AG, Weiss NS. Periconceptional multivitamin use in relation to the risk of congenital urinary tract anomalies. Epidemiology 1995;6(3):212–8.
33. Loffredo LC, Souza JM, Freitas JA, Mossey PA. Oral clefts and vitamin supplementation. Cleft Palate Craniofac J 2001;38(1):76–83.
34. Mills JL, Rhoads GG, Simpson JL, Cunningham GC, Conley MR, Lassman MR, et al. The absence of a relation between the periconceptional use of vitamins and neural-tube defects. National Institute of Child Health and Human Development Neural Tube Defects Study Group. N Engl J Med 1989;321(7):430–5.
35. Milunsky A, Jick H, Jick SS, Bruell CL, MacLaughlin DS, Rothman KJ, et al. Multivitamin/folic acid supplementation in early pregnancy reduces the prevalence of neural tube defects. JAMA 1989;262(20): 2847–52.
36. [No authors listed] Prevention of neural tube defects: results of the Medical Research Council Vitamin Study. MRC Vitamin Study Research Group. Lancet 1991; 338(8760):131–7
37. Mulinare J, Cordero JF, Erickson JD, Berry RJ. Periconceptional use of multivitamins and the occurrence of neural tube defects. JAMA 1988;260(21):3141–5.
38. Scanlon KS, Ferencz C, Loffredo CA, Wilson PD, Correa-Villasenor A, Khoury MJ, et al. Preconceptional folate intake and malformations of the cardiac outflow tract. Baltimore-Washington Infant Study Group. Epidemiology 1998;9(1):95–8.
39. Seller MJ, Nevin NC. Periconceptional vitamin supplementation and the prevention of neural tube defects in south-east England and Northern Ireland. J Med Genet 1984;21(5):325–30.
40. Shaw GM, O'Malley CD, Wasserman CR, Tolarova MM, Lammer EJ. Maternal periconceptional use of multivitamins and reduced risk for conotruncal heart defects and limb deficiencies among offspring. Am J Med Genet 1995;59(4):536–45.
41. Shaw GM, Schaffer D, Velie EM, Morland K, Harris JA. Periconceptional vitamin use, dietary folate, and the occurrence of neural tube defects. Epidemiology 1995;6(3):219–26.
42. Shaw GM, Lammer EJ, Wasserman CR, O'Malley CD, Tolarova MM. Risks of orofacial clefts in children born to women using multivitamins containing folic acid periconceptionally. Lancet 1995;346 (8972):393–6.
43. Shaw GM, Velie EM, Wasserman CR. Risk for neural tube defect-affected pregnancies among women of Mexican descent and white women in California. Am J Public Health 1997;87(9):1467–71.
44. Shaw GM, Zhu H, Lammer EJ, Yang W, Finnell RH. Genetic variation of infant reduced folate carrier (A80G) and risk of orofacial and conotruncal heart defects. Am J Epidemiol 2003; 158(8):747–52
45. Sheppard S, Nevin NC, Seller MJ, Wild J, Smithells RW, Read AP, et al. Neural tube defect recurrence after 'partial' vitamin supplementation. J Med Genet 1989;26(5):326–9.
46. Smithells RW, Sheppard S, Schorah CJ, Seller MJ, Nevin NC, Harris R, et al. Possible prevention of neural-tube defects by periconceptional vitamin supplementation. Lancet 1980;1(8164):339–340.
47. Smithells RW, Sheppard S, Schorah CJ, Seller MJ, Nevin NC, Harris R, et al. Apparent prevention of neural tube defects by periconceptional vitamin supplementation. Arch Dis Child 1981;56(12):911–8.

48. Thompson SJ, Torres ME, Stevenson RE, Dean JH, Best RG. Periconceptional multivitamin folic acid use, dietary folate, total folate and risk of neural tube defects in South Carolina. Ann Epidemiol 2003;13(6):412–8.
49. Tolarova M, Harris J. Reduced recurrence of orofacial clefts after periconceptional supplementation with high-dose folic acid and multivitamins. Teratology 1995;51(2):71–8.
50. van Rooij IA, Vermeij-Keers C, Kluijtmans LA, Ocke MC, Zielhuis GA, Goorhuis-Brouwer SM, et al. Does the interaction between maternal folate intake and the methylenetetrahydrofolate reductase polymorphisms affect the risk of cleft lip with or without cleft palate? Am J Epidemiol 2003;157(7):583–91.
51. Werler MM, Shapiro S, Mitchell AA. Periconceptional folic acid exposure and risk of occurrent neural tube defects. JAMA 1993;269(10):1257–61.
52. Werler MM, Hayes C, Louik C, Shapiro S, Mitchell AA. Multivitamin supplementation and risk of birth defects. Am J Epidemiol 1999;150(7):675–82.
53. Wild J, Read AP, Sheppard S, Seller MJ, Smithells RW, Nevin NC, et al. Recurrent neural tube defects, risk factors and vitamins. Arch Dis Child 1986;61(5):440–4.

CHAPTER 42

MATERNAL SPERMICIDE USE AND ADVERSE REPRODUCTIVE OUTCOME: A META-ANALYSIS

Thomas R. Einarson,[a] Gideon Koren,[b] David Mattice, and Cim Schechter-Tsafriri[c†]*

A meta-analysis was performed to determine whether the literature provides evidence that periconceptual or postconceptual maternal use of spermicides is detrimental to the developing fetus. Nine studies that investigated teratogenicity met the inclusion criteria. The Mantel-Haenszel summary odds ratio was 1.02 (95% confidence interval = 0.78 to 1.32). The χ^2 analyses was 0.10 for significance from unity ($p = 0.748$) and 8.73 for homogeneity of effects ($p = 0.365$). Studies comparing specific abnormalities with other abnormalities also indicated no association (odds ratio = 0.96; 95% confidence interval = 0.72 to 0.28). Studies investigating other adverse events (spontaneous abortion, stillbirth, reduced fetal weight, prematurity, or increased incidence of female births) showed similar negative results. Cohen's *d,* the overall effect size as determined by Tukey's jackknife method, was –0.001 (95% confidence interval = –0.018 to 0.017). These results indicate that maternal use of spermicides is not associated with adverse fetal outcomes. Meta-analysis adds quantitative support for conclusions from traditional reviews of the subject. (AM J OBSTET GYNECOL 1990; 162:655–60.)

Key words: Teratogenicity, stillbirth, fetal loss, vaginal spermicides, statistical aggregation

Since the thalidomide tragedy during the 1950s, much concern has been directed toward the teratogenic potential of drugs and other types of chemical exposure. It is essential that accurate information of this type be available for practitioners and their pregnant patients. It is equally important that information regarding the safety of drugs in pregnancy be available. Often pregnancy may be terminated because of a decision that is based on incomplete or inaccurate data.

The literature has contained several reports associating spermicides with adverse fetal outcomes. This has led to much comment and litigation, particularly in the United States. Huggins et al.[1] have postulated that three possible mechanisms of action could exist if spermicides were teratogenic. These mechanisms are as follows: (1) the spermicide could be absorbed through the vaginal wall before conception and produce damage to the ovum, (2) sperm could be damaged, but not inactivated, by the spermicide and subsequently could fertilize the ovum, and (3) the spermicide could be absorbed after fertilization and produce direct damage to the embryo. A fourth possibility suggested by Bracken and Vita[2] was that sperm may transport spermicide to the ovum where the spermicide could cause interference with maternal genetic material.

However, conflicting results have been presented in the literature. One statistical method for obtaining an overall quantitative estimate of the effect of a drug on reproduction, especially when conflict exists, is meta-analysis.[3] This technique has been widely used in such cases and is gaining increased popularity in the medical field. The objective of this study was to quantify the relationship between maternal use of spermicides in humans and subsequent adverse fetal outcomes using meta-analysis. A second objective was to familiarize physicians and scientists who deal with reproductive toxicity with this new approach to data analysis.

From the MotheRisk Program, Hospital for Sick Children, and the Faculty of Pharmacy and Departments of Pediatrics and Health Administration, Faculty of Medicine, University of Toronto,[a] the MotheRisk Program, Division of Clinical Pharmacology, Department of Pediatrics, Hospital for Sick Children, Toronto,[b] and the Department of Immunology, McMaster University, Hamilton.[c]

Received for publication January 23, 1989, revised September 22, 1989; accepted October 17, 1989.

*Career Scientist. Ontario Ministry of Health.

† Medical Research Council Summer Student.

6/1/17473

PROTOCOL FOR THE META-ANALYSIS

The first adverse outcome investigated was teratogenicity. Any study that dealt with the delivery of a live infant was considered acceptable for the analysis, but notation was made of how the study controlled for variables that could have been related to adverse outcomes. These variables included maternal age, smoking, alcohol use, drug abuse, socioeconomic status, exposure to industrial or commercial teratogens, and use of prescription or nonprescription drugs.

Any study that described human vaginal use of a nonmercurial spermicide with or without a diaphragm was considered acceptable. All pharmaceutical forms of spermicide were admissible, including foams, jellies, and creams. Spermicide use at the time of conception must have been determined by the original researchers. In addition, spermicide use during the first trimester of pregnancy was examined separately.

Included as fetal abnormalities were any adverse outcome as described by Heinonen et al.,[4] including major or minor malformations, neoplasms, undescended testes, and chromsomal aberrations. Abnormal outcomes must have been diagnosed at birth or within 1 year of birth. Excluded were cases of stillbirth, spontaneous abortion, termination of pregnancy, animal studies, spermicide use in nonpregnant patients, or studies in which exposure was not determined.

Exposed cases must have been compared with a nonexposed control group. All research papers published in English between 1960 and 1987 that addressed the topic were examined, and both cohort and case-control studies were accepted. Excluded were reviews, editorials, case reports, and studies from which sufficient information could not be extracted for analysis.

Research results were combined by means of the method of Mantel and Haenszel.[5] The level accepted for significance of statistical tests was 0.05.

LITERATURE SEARCH

The data base of Bibliographic Retrieval Services was searched with the key words spermicides, birth defects, fetal abnormalities, teratogenicity, malformation, nonoxynol, octoxynol, contraceptives, foam, jelly, cream, and diaphragm. All references from extracted papers were investigated. Standard textbooks that summarized teratogenicity, such as those by Schardein,[6] Shepard,[7] and Briggs et al.,[8] were consulted.

SELECTION OF ACCEPTABLE STUDIES

As recommended by Sacks et al.,[9] potential papers were extracted from the literature, photocopied, and all identifying marks were removed. A reviewer who was not involved in the analysis itself was given only the Methods section of each study and the selection criteria and was asked to evaluate each paper for inclusion into this analysis. Studies were marked as accepted or rejected with reasons for rejection. A second reviewer performed an unblinded evaluation while being unaware of the results from the blinded reviewer. The same papers were selected by both reviewers, with one exception. The blinded reviewer had one inclusion that did not meet the criteria because that study dealt with animals. On discussion that study was excluded, thus resulting in complete agreement.

Table I lists the papers that were accepted by the reviewers. There were nine studies that met the inclusion criteria, including five cohort studies and four case-control studies. All studies used statistical techniques (e.g., multiple regression) to control for possible confounding variables, such as maternal age, smoking, alcohol use, drug abuse, and socioeconomic status.

Table II presents those studies that were rejected and the reasons for rejection. Three studies were rejected because they failed to demonstrate that subjects were actually exposed to spermicides. The study by Jick et al. caused substantial concern after publication because its odds ratio was 2.26 (95% confidence interval, 1.27 to 4.01). However, those authors did not establish exposure to spermicides at conception but determined the prescription of spermicides approximately 9 months before delivery. Consequently that study did not meet our inclusion criteria. The study by Porter et al.[19] found no malformations in similarly identified "exposed" infants. Exposure could not be discerned from the study by Smith et al. because the authors were vague in their description of how exposure was determined. The studies by Louik et al. and Cordero and Layde were excluded from the analysis because the authors did not compare malformed infants with normal infants, but compared a group that had specified malformations with a group with other malformations. Thus independent variables differed from those of the inclusion criteria. Poland and Strobino et al. did not investigate live births but compared abortuses for abnormalities; consequently those studies were also excluded from the primary analysis.

Table II
Studies Rejected from the Meta-Analysis of Teratogenicity and Reasons for Rejection

REASON FOR REJECTION	AUTHORS
Outcome variable not teratogenicity	Harlap et al.,[17] Jick et al.[18] Porter et al.,[19] School et al.[20] Strobino et al.
Dealt with abortus only	Poland, Strobino et al.
Compared groups of malformed infants	Louik et al., Cordero and Layde
Exposure not established	Jick et al., Smith et al. Porter et al.[19]
Insufficient data for analysis (spermicides and intrauterine contraceptive devices combined)	Vessey et al.
Animals only	Abrutyn et al., Buttar, Chvapil et al., Long et al., Saad et al.
Preliminary data only; full report published subsequently by Shapiro et al.[15]	Heinonen et al.[4]

Table I
Results from Studies Investigating the Relationship Between Maternal Use of Spermicides and Teratogenic Outcomes

			95% CONFIDENCE LIMITS			
AUTHORS	STUDY TYPE	ODDS RATIO	LOWER	UPPER	χ^2	*P*
Bracken and Vita[2]	Case-control	1.24	0.85	1.81	1.05	0.306
Huggins et al.[1]	Cohort	1.40	0.48	4.09	0.12	0.728
Linn et al.[10]	Cohort	0.85	0.68	1.06	1.88	0.170
Mills et al.[11]	Cohort	1.05	0.94	1.18	0.59	0.443
Mills et al.[12]	Cohort	0.65	0.35	1.20	1.29	0.207
Polednak et al.[13]	Case-control, matched pairs	0.91	0.62	1.33	0.15	0.700
Rothman[14]	Case-control	1.34	0.93	1.94	2.07	0.151
Shapiro et al.[15]	Cohort	1.04	0.72	1.50	0.02	0.901
Warburton et al.[16]	Case-control	0.95	0.53	1.69	0.00	0.967
Overall		1.02	0.78	1.32	0.10	0.748

Sacks et al.[9] suggested that the support given to the research group by an interested body could be a source of bias. In this series of papers on spermicides, however, only one had any mention of support from the pharmaceutical industry. The report by Shapiro et al.[15] was partially founded by a pharmaceutical company, but it also had federal government support. All of the remaining studies were supported by government or foundation grants, contracts, or both. Therefore there was considered to be little chance of bias because of source of support.

COMBINABILITY OF DATA

Sacks et al.[9] recommended that tests be performed to ensure combinability of data across studies. Lack of homogeneity could suggest systematic bias that could influence results. Breslow and Day suggested calculation of χ^2 for each 2 × 2 table analyzed and for homogeneity of odds ratios. Table I presents individual χ^2 values, none of which was significant. Homogeneity of effects was investigated with the formula presented by Breslow and Day, χ^2 was 8.74 ($df = 8$, $p = 0.365$), thus showing that the odds ratios were not significantly heterogeneous.

L'Abbe et al. suggested that values be plotted on a graph to examine linearity. As can be seen in Fig. 1, the data from this analysis may be appropriately represented by a straight line that has the equation $Y = -0.004 + 1.107X$ ($F = 386.16$; $df = 1, 7$; $p < 0.001$, $r^2 = 0.982$). Thus, from these two tests, it was considered that studies in this analysis could be reasonably combined.

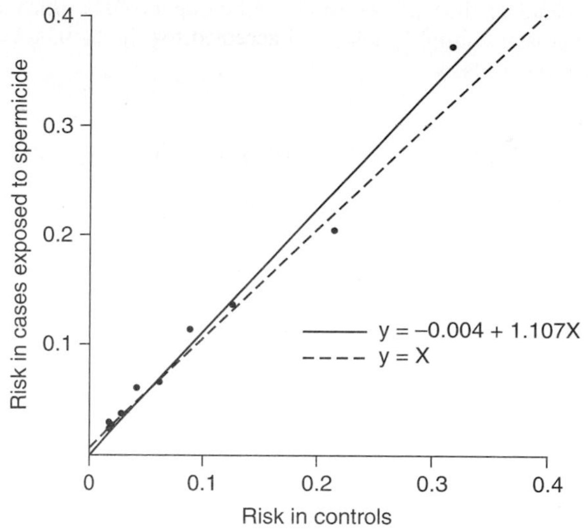

Fig. 1. Homogeneity of results from studies that examined the relationship between maternal spermicide use and teratogenicity.

STATISTICAL ANALYSIS

The Mantel-Haenszel[5] summary odds ratio was 1.02 with a 95% confidence interval from 0.78 to 1.32. Because the interval contained unity, the evidence appears to be against a relationship between maternal use of spermicides and subsequent fetal abnormality. The corresponding Mantel-Haenszel[5] χ^2 for significance of summary odds ratio was 0.10 ($df = 1$, $p = 0.748$).

To examine the power of these findings, Cohen's d was calculated as a measure of effect for each study and was then averaged. The average overall effect size was 0.0085, which would be considered very small. When weighted according to sample size, the overall average d was –0.0013. According to Orwin's formula, it would take 6 studies (averaging 10.415 subjects), each with an effect size of 0.5, or 18 studies with effect sizes of 0.3, to raise this value to 0.2, which Cohen would describe as "small." To achieve an effect size of 0.5 with a total of 10,000 subjects (assuming 5000 in each group) would require an odds ratio of approximately 9.2 if the malformation rate was 2% in control subjects (the usual rate in normal subjects). A malformation rate of 10% (as found here) would require an odds ratio of 3.7. None of the acceptable published studies achieved such a high ratio. Therefore one can be reasonably certain that the results of this analysis are robust.

SUBGROUP ANALYSIS

Five of the studies in this analysis were cohort studies and four were case control studies. The overall odds ratio for cohort studies was 0.99 (95% confidence interval = 0.80 to 1.23) and 1.12 (95% confidence interval = 0.74 to 1.69) for case-control studies. The distribution of odds ratios was not significantly different for the two study types (Mann-Whitney U = 12, $p = 0.624$).

Some studies identified exposure to spermicides as periconceptual, during the first trimester (after the last menstrual period), or any time during pregnancy. Table III presents results

Table III
Results from Studies Investigating the Relationship Between Maternal use of Spermicides at Various Times During Pregnancy and Teratogenic Outcomes

	PERICONCEPTION			FIRST TRIMESTER			ANY TIME DURING PREGNANCY		
AUTHORS	OR	LL	UL	OR	LL	UL	OR	LL	UL
Bracken and Vita[2]	1.24	0.85	1.81	1.00	0.63	1.57			
Huggins et al.[1]							1.40	0.48	4.09
Linn et al.[10]							0.85	0.68	1.06
Mills et al.[11]	1.05	0.94	1.18	1.02	0.86	1.20			
Mills et al.[12]	0.76	0.36	1.61	0.65	0.35	1.20			
Polednak et al.[13]	0.91	0.62	1.33	0.97	0.62	1.53			
Rothman[14]	1.34	0.92	1.93						
Shapiro et al.[15]							1.04	0.72	1.50
Warburton et al.[16]	0.95	0.53	1.69						
Overall	1.06	0.86	1.40	0.98	0.74	1.30	0.91	0.66	1.25

OR, Odds ratio; *LL*, lower limit of 95% Taylor series confidence interval; *UL*, upper limit of 95% Taylor series confidence interval.

according to time of exposure. All summary odds ratios were very close to unity, which was included in all of the 95% confidence intervals.

OTHER TERATOGENICITY EVIDENCE

Meta-analysis is a method of quantifying the literature on a given topic within the confines of the established criteria. Other evidence must not be ignored in formation of an overall opinion. Two studies compared specific malformations with other types of malformations in newborns exposed to spermicides. Table IV summarizes the results of those studies that show that spermicide use was not associated with proposed specific malformations.

Another type of investigation compared malformations in aborted fetuses exposed and not exposed to spermicides. Table V summarizes results that indicate lack of support for the existence of a significant relationship.

OTHER ADVERSE OUTCOMES

Several authors examined the relationship of spermicide use and adverse events other than malformations. These outcomes included fetal loss, stillbirth, low birth weight, preterm delivery, and high female sex ratio (Table VI). As in all other analyses, the 95% confidence intervals contained unity.

Because several outcomes were measured, it was considered appropriate to combine the data to quantify the overall relationship between spermicide exposure and adverse outcomes. Glass presented an example that used Tukey's jackknife method; that method adjusts for multiple related outcomes from studies and determines an overall effect size.

First, results must be convered to Cohen's *d*. Data from 2 × 2 tables may be easily converted with the formula: $d = [4X^2/(N - X^2)]^{1/2}$. This formula is derived by combining formulas from Cohen (pp. 23 and 223). Similarly, the results of a *t* test can be converted with the formula presented by Rosenthal: $d = 2t/(df)^{1/2}$.

Table VII summarizes the effect sizes from all studies that meet the inclusion criteria that reported the adverse impact of spermicides on pregnancy. When combined with Tukey's jackknife method, the overall effect size was –0.001 (95% confidence interval = –0.018 to 0.017). The evidence again confirms lack of relationship between spermicides and adverse reproductive effects.

Table IV
Results from Studies Comparing Specific Malformations with Other Types of Malformations in Fetuses Exposed to Spermicides

AUTHORS	STUDY TYPE	ODDS RATIO	95% CONFIDENCE LIMITS LOWER	UPPER
Louik et al.	Case-control	1.24	0.85	1.18
Cordero and Layde	Case-control	0.95	0.44	3.32
Overall		1.02	0.64	1.62

Table V
Results from Studies Comparing Malformations in Aborted Fetuses Exposed and Not Exposed to Spermicides

AUTHORS	ODDS RATIO	95% CONFIDENCE LIMITS LOWER	UPPER
Poland	1.04	0.29	3.73
Strobino et al.	1.03	0.81	1.31
Overall	1.03	0.46	2.33

COMMENT

Because the spontaneous rates of adverse reproductive effects arc very low, most studies that attempt to establish a relationship between a potential teratogen and outcome fail to recruit enough cases to reach an adequate level of statistical power. Physicians and scientists who try to determine whether a drug or chemical is a potential human teratogen must often decide which of the studies that present opposing results is more credible.

Meta-analysis allows combination of data from different studies, thus achieving appropriate statistical power that may not be present in any of the single studies. The main criticism against the method is that "good" studies may be combined with "bad" studies with each receiving equal weight. However, when performed appropriately the problem dissipates. The process of using a blinded reviewer who must include or exclude studies according to preset criteria should address such methodologic issues.

For example, the controversial study by Jick et al. that prompted multimillion dollar legal suits against the spermicide manufacturer was excluded from this analysis because exposure to the drug at the time of conception was not proved. Those authors used a computer to identify cases of malformed infants and linked them to mothers for whom spermicides had been prescribed during the 600 days before delivery or abortion. One of the authors of that study later declared that many of the mothers of malformed children had discontinued spermicide use long before conception. For the same reason, another of the authors stated that "In retrospect, I believe our article should never have been published."

In the litigious atmosphere that surrounds health care today, it is crucial to develop and crystallize scientific tools powerful enough to disqualify the devastating effects of invalid cases presented to a jury. Classically, the studies presented by the plaintiff (generally parents of a malformed child) must stand against conflicting studies by the defendant (generally a pharmaceutical manufacturer, a physician, or both). Lawyers, judges, or physicians cannot be expected to be able to evaluate single studies in isolation from the statistical context of all available evidence. Meta-analysis is the only approach that combines such data and derives an overall estimate of risk.

The MotheRisk Program in Toronto is an information and consultation service for women exposed to drugs, chemicals, radiation, and infections during pregnancy and lactation. Because the program deals with 40 cases per day, it is cssential that accurate estimates of reproductive risk be determined for hundreds of xenobiotics. Because more than half of the patients who seek consultation have already been exposed to the drug in

Table VI
Summary of Studies Reporting the Relationship Between Maternal Spermicide Use and Adverse Fetal Events Other than Malformations

			LIMITS OF 95% CONFIDENCE INTERVAL	
OUTCOME	AUTHORS	ODDS RATIO	LOWER	UPPER
Fetal loss	Harlap et al.[17]	1.00	0.82	1.23
	Huggins et al.[1]	1.03	0.64	1.65
	Mills et al.[12]	1.01	0.87	1.27
	Scholl et al.[20]	0.80	0.40	1.59
	Overall	1.00	0.77	1.30
Stillbirth	Huggins et al.[1]	0.48	0.10	2.41
Birth weight	Mills et al.[12]	0.85	0.70	1.03
	Polednak et al.[13]	NA*	NA*	NA*
Preterm	Mills et al.[12]	0.90	0.79	1.02
Sex ratio	Mills et al.[12]	0.97	0.90	1.05
	Polednak et al.[13]	1.29	0.95	1.76

NA, Not available.

* Results were reported as weight means: exposed newborn infants were larger (3393.0 ± 437.22 gm) than control infants (3348.6 ± 505.70 gm), $t = -1.25$, $df = 923$, $p = 0.212$; therefore the odds ratio is less than unity.

question before pregnancy is confirmed, the advice "not to be used in pregnancy" is irrelevant. Rather, such patients need to know whether their exposure involves increased reproductive risk. Such information is essential to decide whether to continue or terminate the pregnancy.

The use of meta-analysis to combine data appears to be an important approach to assessment of available studies. Beyond the inherent advantages of meta-analysis, it forces the reviewer to closely evaluate the methodology and results from each study to determine acceptability for inclusion. The value of the use of blinded reviewers is self-evident.

The meta-analysis in this study has shown that maternal use of spermicides is not associated with fetal malformations or any other reported abnormal fetal outcomes. It is hoped that these results, on the basis of all available studies, will help stop the flood of unnecessary and unfounded litigations. Furthermore, it is hoped that this approach will become the standard for evaluation of reproductive outcome after exposure to drugs, chemicals, radiation, or infections in pregnancy.

Table VII
Net Adverse Impact of Spermicides on Pregnancy When Different Adverse Outcomes Are Combined Using Tukey's Jackknife Method

AUTHORS	OUTCOME	ODDS RATIO	COHEN'S D	"PSEUDO" D
Bracken and Vita[2]	Malformation	1.24	0.031	0.020
Harlap et al.[17]	Fetal loss	1.00	0.001	0.004
Huggins et al.[3]	Malformation	1.40	0.030	
	Fetal loss	1.03	0.001	
	Stillbirth	0.48	–0.048	–0.016
Linn et al.[10]	Malformation	0.85	–0.025	–0.010
Mills et al.[11]	Malformation	1.05	0.012	0.010
Mills et al.[12]	Malformation	0.65	–0.020	
	Fetal loss	1.01	0.001	
	Female sex ratio	0.97	–0.011	
	Preterm birth	0.90	–0.025	
	Birth weight	0.85	–0.026	–0.071
Polednak et al.[13]	Malformation	0.91	–0.020	
	Female sex ratio	1.29	0.099	
	Birth weight	NA	–0.082	–0.002
Rothman[14]	Malformation	1.34	0.071	0.041
Scholl et al.[20]	Fetal loss	0.80	–0.054	
	Female sex ratio	1.62	0.216	0.007
Shapiro et al.	Malformation	1.04	0.001	0.004
Warburton et al.[16]	Malformation	0.95	–0.003	0.002
Overall (average)				–0.001*

* 95% Confidence interval = –0.018 to 0.017.

REFERENCES

1. Huggins G, Vessey M, Flavel R, Yeates D, McPherson K. Vaginal spermicides and outcome of pregnancy: findings in a large cohort study. Contraception 1982:25:219-30.
2. Bracken MB, Vita K. Frequency of non-hormonal contraception around conception and association with congenital malformations in offspring. Am J Epidemiol 1983;117:281-91.
3. Einarson TR, Leeder JS, Koren G. A method for meta-analysis of epidemiologic studies. Drug Intell Clin Pharm 1988;22:813-24.
4. Heinonen OP, Slone D, Shapiro S. Birth defects in pregnancy. Littleton, Mass: PSG, 1977.
5. Mantel N, Haenszel W. Statistical aspects of the analysis of data from retrospective studies of disease. JNCI 1959;22:719-48.
6. Schardein JL. Chemically induced birth defects. New York: Marcel Dekker, 1985.
7. Shepard TH. Catalog of teratogenic agents. 5th ed. Baltimore: Johns Hopkins University Press. 1986.
8. Briggs GG, Freeman RK, Yaffe SJ. Drugs in pregnancy and lactation. 2nd ed. Baltimore: Williams & Wilkins, 1986.
9. Sacks HS, Berrier J, Reitman D, Ancona-Berk VA, Chalmers TC. Meta-analyses of randomized controlled trials. N Engl J Med 1987;316:450-5.
10. Linn S, Schoenbaum SC, Monson RR, Rosner B, Stubblefield PG, Ryan KJ. Lack of association between contraceptive usage and congenital malformations in offspring. AM J OBSTET GYNECOL 1983;147:923-8.
11. Mills JL, Harley EE, Reed GF, Berendes HW. Are spermicides teratogenic? JAMA 1982;248:2148-51.
12. Mills JL, Reed GF, Nugent RP, Harley EE, Berendes HW. Are there adverse effects of periconceptional spermicide use? Fertil Steril 1985;43:442-6.
13. Polednak AP, Janerich DT, Glebatis DM. Birth weight and birth defects in relation to maternal spermicide use. Teratology 1982; 26:27-38.
14. Rothman KJ. Spermicide use and Down's syndrome. Am J Public Health 1982;72:399-401.
15. Shapiro S, Slone D, Heinonen OP, et al. Birth defects and vaginal spermicides. JAMA 1982;247:2381-4.
16. Warburton D, Neugut RH, Lustenberger A, Nicholas AG, Kline J. Lack of association between spermicide use and trisomy. N Engl J Med 1987;317:478-82.
17. Harlap S, Shiono PH, Ramcharan S. Spontaneous foetal losses in women using different contraceptives around the time of conception. Int J Epidemiol 1980;9:49-56.
18. Jick H, Shiota K, Shepard TH, et al. Vaginal spermicides and miscarriages seen primarily in the emergency room. Teratogenesis Carcinog Mutagen 1982;2:205-10.
19. Porter JB, Hunter-Mitchell J, Jick H, Walker AM. Drugs and stillbirth. Am J Public Health 1986;76:1428-31.
20. Scholl TO, Sobel E. Tanfer K, Soefer EF, Saidman B. Effects of vaginal spermicides on pregnancy outcome. Fam Plann Perspect 1983;15:244;249-50.

A complete list of references is available from the authors on request.

CHAPTER 43

EVIDENCE-BASED VIEW OF SAFETY AND EFFECTIVENESS OF PHARMACOLOGIC THERAPY FOR NAUSEA AND VOMITING OF PREGNANCY (NVP)

Laura A. Magee,[a] Paolo Mazzotta,[b] and Gideon Koren[b]

Objective. Our goal was to review the safety and effectiveness of available antiemetics for treatment of nausea and vomiting of pregnancy.
Study Design. We performed a quantitative and qualitative overview of observational controlled studies for drug safety in pregnancy and randomized controlled trials for drug effectiveness for nausea and vomiting in pregnancy.
Results. All of the following are safe and effective for treatment of varying degrees of nausea and vomiting in pregnancy: Bendectin/Diclectin (doxylamine, pyridoxine, dicyclomine), antihistamine (H_1) blockers, and phenothiazines; however, the magnitude of effect, particularly for phenothiazines, is in question and may differ among individual agents. Pyridoxine and vitamin B_{12} are safe and may be effective. Metoclopramide, droperidol, and ondansetron may be effective, but safety data are insufficient to recommend them as first-line agents. Corticosteroids may not be as beneficial as first thought, and there may be a small teratogenic risk. The relative effectiveness of various agents is largely unknown.
Conclusion. Many medications, particularly H_1-antagonists and phenothiazines, are safe and effective for treatment of varying degrees of NVP. (Am J Obstet Gynecol 2002;186:S256-61.)

Key words: Nausea and vomiting of pregnancy, anti-emetic therapy, antihistamines, pyridoxine dopamine antagonists, serotonin antagonists, corticosteroids

Nausea and vomiting of pregnancy (NVP) affects 50% to 80% of pregnant women to some degree.[1-2] Symptoms are usually limited to 7 to 12 weeks' gestation, although fewer than 1% of women develop "hyperemesis gravidarum," characterized by severe physical symptoms or medical complications. The diagnosis of NVP is confirmed by symptoms that are self-limited, usually to early pregnancy, but definitely to pregnancy itself. NVP is likely to be multifactorial and remains a diagnosis of exclusion after other potential etiologies have been ruled out.

Because NVP is rarely life-threatening, antiemetic therapy is aimed at improving the quality of women's lives. The choice of antiemetics is based on knowledge of physiologic pathways mediating vomiting and drug effectiveness data from nonpregnant patients. Candidate drugs include antagonists to histamine, acetylcholine, dopamine and serotonin (5-HT_3) receptors located in the chemoreceptor trigger zone, vestibular apparatus, and visceral afferents.

No evidence-based guidelines exist for the management of NVP. Most reviews and editorials[3-5] advise that antiemetic therapy be instituted only when women are unable to maintain hydration, nutrition, or both. Traditionally, dietary and lifestyle changes have been the mainstay of treatment, and there is little reason to question the assumption that dietary recommendations are safe. There are no clinical trials demonstrating their effectiveness, but most women find such an approach at least somewhat useful.[6] Dietary and lifestyle modifications are covered elsewhere in this issue, as are nonpharmacologic approaches that many women regard as safe options.[7, 8] This review will focus on the safety and effectiveness of pharmacologic therapy.

From the Department of Specialized Women's Health, BC Women's Hospital and Health Centre, the Department of Medicine, University of British Columbia,[a] and the Department of Clinical Pharmacology, The Hospital for Sick Children, University of Toronto.[b]

THE DRUGS REVIEWED

Antihistamines (H_1 Blockers)

There are many histamine antagonists; however, only the following have been indicated for nausea and vomiting: buclizine, cyclizine, dimenhydrinate, diphenhydramine, doxylamine, hydroxyzine, and meclizine. Doxylamine, with or without pyridoxine, will be covered elsewhere in this supplement.[9]

A wide body of evidence suggests that H_1 receptor antagonists (eg, dimenhydrinate, diphenhydramine, hydroxyzine, etc) have no human teratogenic potential.[10, 11] The safety of antihistamines (including doxylamine) in pregnancy was confirmed by a recent meta-analysis that reviewed 24 controlled studies, published between 1960 and 1991 and involving more than 200,000 first trimester exposures; first trimester exposure to antihistamines revealed a slightly lower risk for major/minor malformations (pooled OR = 0.76 [95% CI 0.60,0.94]).[12]

A summary of 7 controlled trials examining the effectiveness of various antihistamines for NVP is outlined in Figure 1.[13-18] Pooled data indicate that antihistamines are effective in reducing vomiting in pregnant patients (relative risk [RR] = 0.34 [95% CI 0.27,0.43]), but the studies are not homogeneous (2 = 28.88 with 6 df).[19] Neither study design nor outcome definitions explained this heterogeneity. The variety of histamine antagonists used is the most plausible explanation, but could not be confirmed given the variety of antihistamines used within studies and the lack of consistent outcome reporting by type of antihistamine exposure.

Anticholinergics

Only dicyclomine and scopolamine are used for treatment of nausea and vomiting in the nonpregnant population. The meta-analysis of Bendectin/Debendox failed to demonstrate an increased risk associated with the combination of dicyclomine/doxylamine/

pyridoxine.[20] In addition, a prospective cohort study could not detect malformations, as compared with controls in women exposed to dicyclomine during the first trimester (ie, 48/1024 [cases] vs 3200/49,258 [controls], RR = 1.04 [95% CI 0.82,1.30]).[21] However, dicyclomine failed to demonstrate independent or synergistic effectiveness in combination with doxylamine /pyridoxine for the treatment of NVP and was removed from the Bendectin preparation.

Teratogenicity studies of scopolamine in pregnancy are limited to 2 controlled observational studies: a prospective cohort of 309 first trimester exposures[21] and a record linkage study of 27 first trimester exposures.[11] Neither study associated scopolamine with an increased risk for malformations (ie, 14/309 [cases] vs 3234/49,973 [controls], RR = 1.05 [95% CI 0.70,1.59] and 1/27 exposed (malformation rate = 3.7%), respectively). No effectiveness trials for NVP have been published.

Dopamine Antagonists

A number of dopamine antagonists may be used to treat NVP: phenothiazines (eg, chlorpromazine, perphenazine, prochlorperazine, promethazine, and trifluoperazine), domperidone, droperidol, metoclopramide, and trimethobenzamide. Anecdotal case reports have associated first trimester phenothiazine use with major malformations. However, the bulk of evidence suggests that phenothiazines show no evidence of teratogenicity. Prospective cohort,[21-25] retrospective cohort,[26] case-control,[27, 28] and record-linkage studies[29] of patients (n = 2948) with exposure to various and multiple phenothiazines have failed to demonstrate an increased risk for major malformations (RR = 1.03 [95% CI 0.88,1.22]). However, it must be pointed out that the pooled studies exhibit heterogeneity, which appears to be explained by the study by Rumeau-Rouquette et al.[23] This is the only study that found a relationship between phenothiazine use and congenital anomalies; however, trimester of drug exposure and other potential confounders of the phenothiazine-malformation relationship were not accounted for. When this study is removed from the pooled data analysis, the remaining trials are homogeneous and find no association between phenothiazine use in pregnancy and major malformations $\chi^2 = 7.05$ with 6 df, pooled RR = 1.00 [95% CI 0.84,1.18]).

There have been 3 trials of various phenothiazines versus placebo for treatment of (usually severe) NVP.[30-32] Figure 1 shows that phenothiazines significantly decrease NVP. All 3 trials reported a significant reduction in vomiting, but the magnitude of improvement was very different among the studies. Therefore, what is at issue is the magnitude of effect, although the pooling of different phenothiazines may have affected the results, given that individual phenothiazines may act at distinct receptors or receptor subtypes.

Domperidone was not teratogenic in animals in doses greater than 100 times the recommended human dose,[33] but there are no published observational or trial data of its use in human pregnancy.

Only 1 study addresses the safety and effectiveness (for NVP) of first trimester use of droperidol. Eighty women with hyperemesis gravidarum were treated with droperidol and diphenhydramine in addition to an intravenous hydration protocol, and outcomes were compared with those of 73 women (with similarly severe NVP) exposed to a variety of other antiemetics.[34] There was no difference in malformations between groups (3 [droperidol/ diphenhydramine] and 2 [other medications]); however, the statistical power of the study was limited. The authors reported that women treated with the droperidol/diphenhydramine were less frequently readmitted and had shorter mean lengths of hospitalization. However, given the variety of agents administered to (the historical) controls and the use of treatment by protocol for the cases, droperidol cannot be considered effective or superior to other agents until randomized controlled trials are conducted.

Metoclopramide has not been extensively studied for treatment of NVP, even though in many countries it is commonly used in clinical practice.[35] Studies of the drugs' teratogenic potential are limited but reassuring. No malformations were reported among 4 first trimester exposures.[36, 37] The rate of malformations was not above baseline among 126 women enrolled in a prospective cohort study and exposed to metoclopramide in the first trimester.[38] In 2 retrospective record linkage studies of 501 women,[11, 39] there was no increase in major malformations above baseline and no pattern of defects was detected. No trials have been published to support the effectiveness of metoclopramide for NVP. If used, observational data suggest that side effects (including akathesia and other extrapyramidal symptoms) are common, although usually minor in severity.[40, 41]

Two cohort studies[21, 29] and 1 case-control trial[28] have been published on the safety of first trimester exposure to trimethobenzamide in human pregnancy. When combined, the pooled risk included unity (RR = 0.81 [95% CI 0.53,1.23]) and the trials were homogeneous (2 = 0.66 with 2 df). Hence, trimethobenzamide does not seem to pose a teratogenic risk to the fetus. In the single published trial for NVP,[42] trimethobenzamide alone or in combination with pyridoxine significantly improved symptoms of nausea and vomiting compared with placebo (pooled RR = 0.11 [95% CI 0.06,0.18]).

HT3 Antagonists

Ondansetron is the most widely used of this class of drugs. No developmental toxicity was seen in rats and rabbits at ondansetron doses of 70 times that given to humans.[43] No malformation was reported with first trimester exposure[44] or in the setting of a randomized controlled trial of 15 patients exposed during the first trimester.[45] In this same trial of intravenous ondansetron versus promethazine for treatment of severe NVP, ondansetron was not more beneficial than promethazine with respect to the following outcome measures: severity of nausea, daily weight gain, days requiring hospitalization, treatment failures, and voluntary use of the drug. The lack of statistical differences between groups did not seem to have resulted from low statistical power.

There are no controlled human studies on the safety of either granisetron or tropisetron in pregnancy. There are no randomized controlled trials on their effectiveness for NVP.

Corticosteroids

That corticosteroids (eg, dexamethasone, prednisolone) may be effective for NVP stemmed from the hypothesis that severe NVP may result from ACTH deficiency,[46] and from successful use of steroids for chemotherapy-induced emesis.[47]

In a recent meta-analysis, the pooled relative risk for major malformations in cohort[21, 48-52] and case-control[53] studies was not significantly increased (RR = 1.24 [95% CI 0.97,1.60] and 1.20 [95% CI 0.93,1.56], respectively). [53] However, a significant, but small, increase in oral clefts was found in pooled case-control studies examining the association between corticosteroid use and oral clefts[34, 54] (pooled RR = 3.19 [95% CI 2.05,4.95], 2 = 0.29

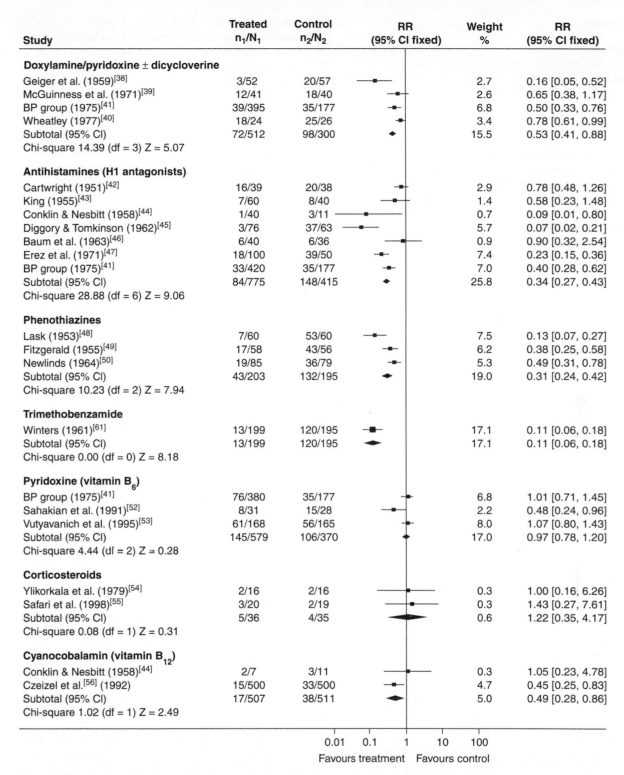

Study	Treated n_1/N_1	Control n_2/N_2	Weight %	RR (95% CI fixed)
Doxylamine/pyridoxine ± dicycloverine				
Geiger et al. (1959)[38]	3/52	20/57	2.7	0.16 [0.05, 0.52]
McGuinness et al. (1971)[39]	12/41	18/40	2.6	0.65 [0.38, 1.17]
BP group (1975)[41]	39/395	35/177	6.8	0.50 [0.33, 0.76]
Wheatley (1977)[40]	18/24	25/26	3.4	0.78 [0.61, 0.99]
Subtotal (95% CI)	72/512	98/300	15.5	0.53 [0.41, 0.88]
Chi-square 14.39 (df = 3) Z = 5.07				
Antihistamines (H1 antagonists)				
Cartwright (1951)[42]	16/39	20/38	2.9	0.78 [0.48, 1.26]
King (1955)[43]	7/60	8/40	1.4	0.58 [0.23, 1.48]
Conklin & Nesbitt (1958)[44]	1/40	3/11	0.7	0.09 [0.01, 0.80]
Diggory & Tomkinson (1962)[45]	3/76	37/63	5.7	0.07 [0.02, 0.21]
Baum et al. (1963)[46]	6/40	6/36	0.9	0.90 [0.32, 2.54]
Erez et al. (1971)[47]	18/100	39/50	7.4	0.23 [0.15, 0.36]
BP group (1975)[41]	33/420	35/177	7.0	0.40 [0.28, 0.62]
Subtotal (95% CI)	84/775	148/415	25.8	0.34 [0.27, 0.43]
Chi-square 28.88 (df = 6) Z = 9.06				
Phenothiazines				
Lask (1953)[48]	7/60	53/60	7.5	0.13 [0.07, 0.27]
Fitzgerald (1955)[49]	17/58	43/56	6.2	0.38 [0.25, 0.58]
Newlinds (1964)[50]	19/85	36/79	5.3	0.49 [0.31, 0.78]
Subtotal (95% CI)	43/203	132/195	19.0	0.31 [0.24, 0.42]
Chi-square 10.23 (df = 2) Z = 7.94				
Trimethobenzamide				
Winters (1961)[61]	13/199	120/195	17.1	0.11 [0.06, 0.18]
Subtotal (95% CI)	13/199	120/195	17.1	0.11 [0.06, 0.18]
Chi-square 0.00 (df = 0) Z = 8.18				
Pyridoxine (vitamin B_6)				
BP group (1975)[41]	76/380	35/177	6.8	1.01 [0.71, 1.45]
Sahakian et al. (1991)[52]	8/31	15/28	2.2	0.48 [0.24, 0.96]
Vutyavanich et al. (1995)[53]	61/168	56/165	8.0	1.07 [0.80, 1.43]
Subtotal (95% CI)	145/579	106/370	17.0	0.97 [0.78, 1.20]
Chi-square 4.44 (df = 2) Z = 0.28				
Corticosteroids				
Ylikorkala et al. (1979)[54]	2/16	2/16	0.3	1.00 [0.16, 6.26]
Safari et al. (1998)[55]	3/20	2/19	0.3	1.43 [0.27, 7.61]
Subtotal (95% CI)	5/36	4/35	0.6	1.22 [0.35, 4.17]
Chi-square 0.08 (df = 1) Z = 0.31				
Cyanocobalamin (vitamin B_{12})				
Conklin & Nesbitt (1958)[44]	2/7	3/11	0.3	1.05 [0.23, 4.78]
Czeizel et al.[56] (1992)	15/500	33/500	4.7	0.45 [0.25, 0.83]
Subtotal (95% CI)	17/507	38/511	5.0	0.49 [0.28, 0.86]
Chi-square 1.02 (df = 1) Z = 2.49				

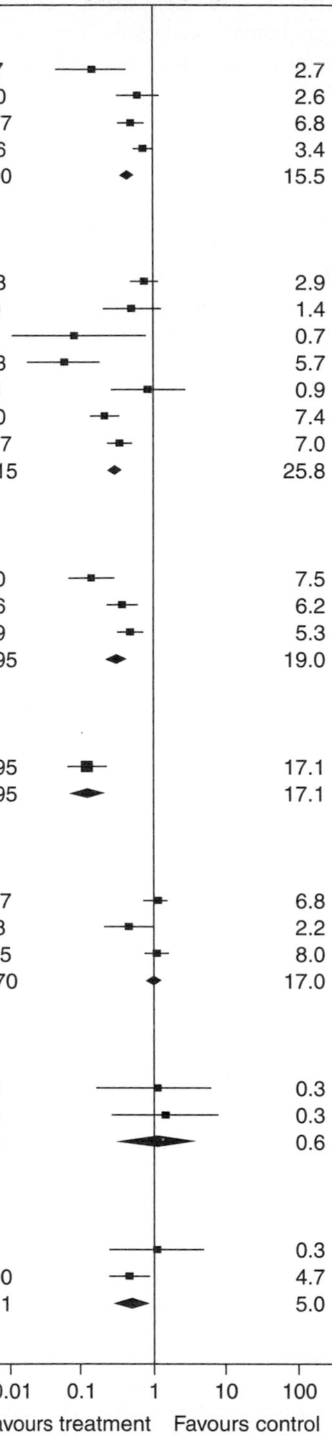

Figure 1. Effectiveness of various agents for nausea and vomiting in pregnancy. Reproduced with permission from Mazzotta and Magee.[19]

with 2 df). This raises the issue of whether there is a small teratogenic risk associated with first trimester exposure.

A number of reports have described successful use of corticosteroids for hyperemesis gravidarum.[47, 55-58] There are 3 randomized controlled trials on this topic. Figure 1 summarizes 2 trials in women with hyperemesis: Ylikorkala et al,[59] which compared intramuscular ACTH to placebo, and Safari et al,[60] which compared methylprednisolone to promethazine. The pooled results failed to reduce the number of subsequent readmissions to hospital compared with controls. More recently, oral prednisolone was compared with placebo in a double-blind, placebo-controlled trial of inpatients with hyperemesis.[61] This trial also failed to show a significant decrease in nausea or vomiting, although the steroid group had a greater sense of well-being, appetite, and weight gain.

Cannabinoids

Cannabinoids have been shown to relieve chemotherapy-induced nausea and vomiting; however, human studies on the use of cannabinoids in pregnancy, or for the treatment of NVP specifically, have not been conducted.

CONCLUSION

Despite evidence of fetal safety, most antiemetics are contraindicated in pregnancy. However, a risk-benefit analysis of the literature on safety and effectiveness of pharmacotherapy for nausea and vomiting of pregnancy (NVP) has failed to substantiate this practice.[19]

Evidence from controlled trials has shown that all the following are safe and effective for treatment of varying degrees of NVP: Bendectin/Diclectin (doxylamine, pyridoxine), antihistamine (H_1) blockers, and phenothiazines (as a group). The best approach is unknown because of the paucity of head-to-head comparisons for individual drugs. If success is not achieved with one of these agents, then it is reasonable to switch to another. Also, many of these agents may be used in combination (eg, antihistamines, pyridoxine, and metoclopramide, along with nonpharmacologic approaches).

When to treat a woman with NVP is probably as important an issue as what to use. Evidence suggests that quality of life may be impaired before severe physical symptoms appear. It is hoped that by highlighting the safe and effective therapies for NVP, consideration will be given to offering them to women with either mild to moderate physical symptoms or impaired psychosocial functioning.

We gratefully acknowledge the annual educational grant provided by Duchesnay, Incorporated, to the Motherisk Program, The Hospital for Sick Children, Toronto.

REFERENCES

1. Gadsby R, Barnie-Adshead AM, Jagger C. A prospective study of nausea and vomiting during pregnancy. Br J Gen Prac 1993;43: 245-8.
2. Vellacott ID, Cooke EJA, James CE. Nausea and vomiting in early pregnancy. Int J Gynaecol Obstet 1988;27:57-62.
3. Newman V, Fullerton JT, Anderson PO. Clinical advances in the management of severe nausea and vomiting during pregnancy. J Obstet Gynecol Neonatal Nurs 1993;22:483-90.
4. de laRonde S, Thirsk J, the SOGC Clinical Practice-Obstetrics Committee. Committee opinion: guidelines for the management of nausea and vomiting in pregnancy. J Soc Obstet Gynaecol Can 1996;18:255-7.
5. Jewell D, Young G. Treatments for nausea and vomiting in early pregnancy. In: Neilson JP, Crowther CA, Hodnett ED, Hofmeyr GJ, Keirse MJNC, editors. Pregnancy and childbirth module of The Cochrane Database of Systematic Reviews, (updated 04 March 1997). Available in The Cochrane Library (database on disk and CDROM). The Cochrane Collaboration; Issue 2. Oxford: Update Software; 1997. Updated quarterly.
6. Chandra K, Magee L, Einarson A, Koren G. Nausea and vomiting in pregnancy: results of a survey that identified interventions used by women to alleviate their symptoms. Submitted to J Psychosom Obstet Gynecol.
7. Koch K. Gastrointestinal factors in nausea and vomiting of pregnancy. Am J Obstet Gynecol 2002;186:S198-203.
8. Roscoe J. Accupressure and accustimulation bands for control of nausea: a brief review. Am J Obstet Gynecol 2002;186:S244-7.
9. Niebyl J. Overview of nausea and vomiting of pregnancy with an emphasis on vitamins and ginger. Am J Obstet Gynecol 2002;186:S253-5.
10. Schatz M, Petitti D. Anti-histamines and pregnancy. Ann Allergy Asthma Immunol 1997;78:157-9.
11. Briggs GG, Freeman RK, Yaffe SJ, editors. Drugs in pregnancy and lactation. 5th ed. Baltimore: Williams and Wilkins; 1998.
12. Seto A, Einarson T, Koren G. Pregnancy outcome following first trimester exposure to anti-histamines: meta-analysis. Am J Perinatology 1997;14;119-24.
13. Bendectin Peer Group. BioBasics International Peer Group Report, Merrell Dow Pharmaceuticals Inc, March 14, 1975. p. 559–637.
14. Cartwright EW. Dramamine in nausea and vomiting of pregnancy. West J Surg 1951;59:216-34.
15. Conklin FJ, Nesbitt REL. Buclizine hydrochloride for nausea and vomiting of pregnancy. Obstet Gynecol 1958;11:214-9.
16. King AG. The treatment of pregnancy nausea with a pill. Obstet Gynecol 1955;6:332-8.
17. Diggory PLC, Tomkinson JS. Nausea and vomiting in pregnancy. A trial of meclozine dihydrochloride with and without pyridoxine. Lancet 1962;2:370-2.
18. Erez S, Schifrin BS, Dirim O. Double-blind evaluation of hydroxyzine as an anti-emetic in pregnancy. J Reprod Med 1971;7:57-9.
19. Mazzotta P, Magee LA. A risk-benefit assessment of pharmacological and nonpharmacological treatment for nausea and vomiting of pregnancy. Drugs 2000;59:781-800.
20. McKeigne PM, Lamm SH, Linn S, Kutcher JS. Bendectin and birth defects. I. A meta-analysis of the epidemiologic studies. Teratology 1994;50:688-90.
21. Heinonen OP, Slone D, Shapiro S. Birth defects and drugs in pregnancy. Littleton, MA: Publishing Sciences Group; 1977.
22. Milkovich L, Van den Berg BJ. An evaluation of the teratogenicity of certain antinauseant drugs. Am J Obstet Gynecol 1976;125:244-8.
23. Rumeau-Rouquette C, Goujard J, Hud G. Possible teratogenic effect of phenothiazines in human beings. Teratology 1976; 15:57-64.
24. Kullander S, Kallen B. A prospective study of drugs and pregnancy. II. Anti-emetic drugs. Acta Obstet Gynecol Scand 1976; 55:105-11.
25. Moriarty AJ, Nance MR. Trifluoperazine and pregnancy. Can Med Assoc J 1963;88:375-6.
26. Nelson MM, Forfar JO. Associations between drugs administered during pregnancy and congenital abnormalities of the fetus. Br Med J 1971;1:523-7.
27. Greenberg G, Inman WHW, Weatherall JA, Adelstein AM, Haskey JC. Maternal drug histories and congenital abnormalities. Br Med J 1977;2:853-6.
28. Mitchell AA, Schwingl PJ, Rosenberg L, Louik C, Shapiro S. Birth defects in relation to Bendectin use in pregnancy. II. Pyloric stenosis. Am J Obstet Gynecol 1983;147:737-42.
29. Aselton P, Jick H, Milunsky A, Hunter JR, Stergachis A. Firsttrimester drug use and congenital disorders. Obstet Gynecol 1985;65:451-5.
30. Lask S. Treatment of nausea and vomiting of pregnancy with antihistamines. Br Med J 1953;1:652-3.
31. Fitzgerald JPB. The effect of promethazine in nausea and vomiting of pregnancy. N Z Med J 1955;54:215-8.
32. Newlinds JS. Nausea and vomiting in pregnancy: a trial of triethylperazine. Med J Aust 1964;51:234-6.
33. Shepard TH. Catalog of teratogenic agents. 7th ed. Baltimore: John Hopkins University Press; 1992.

34. Nageotte MP, Briggs GC, Towers CV, Asrat T. Droperidol and dipenhydramine in the management of hyperemesis gravidarum. Am J Obstet Gynecol 1996;174:1801-6.
35. Einarson A, Koren G, Bergman U. The treatment of nausea and vomiting in pregnancy. Eur J Obstet Gynecol Reprod Biol 1998;76:1-3.
36. Sidhu MS, Lean TH. The use of metodopramide (M axolon) in hyperemesis gravidarum. Proc Obstet Gynaecol Soc Singapore 1970;1:43-6.
37. Pinder RM, Brogden RN, Sawyer PR, Speight TM, Avery GS. Metoclopramide: a review of its pharmacological properties. Drugs 1976;12:81-131.
38. Berkovitch M, Elbirt D, Addis A, Schuler-Faccini L, Ornoy A. Fetal effects of metoclopramide therapy for nausea and vomiting of pregnancy. N Engl J Med 2000;343:445-6.
39. Sorenson HT, Nielsen GL, Christensen K, Tage-Jensen U, Ekbom A, Baron J, and the Euromap study group. Birth outcome following maternal use of metoclopramide. Br J Clin Pharmaco1 2000;49:264-8.
40. Buttino L Jr, Coleman SK, Bergauer NK, Gambon C, Stanziano GJ. Home subcutaneous metoclopramide therapy for hyperemesis gravidarum. J Perinatol 2000;20:359-62.
41. Poortinga E, Rosenthal D, Bagri S. Metoclopramide-induced akathisia during the second trimester of a 37-year-old woman's first pregnancy. Psychosomatics 2001;42:153-6.
42. Winters HS. Anti-emetics in nausea and vomiting of pregnancy. Obstet Gynecol 1961;18:753-6.
43. Tucker ML, Jaakson MR, Scales MDC. Ondansetron: pre-clinical safety evaluation. Eur J Cancer Clin Oncol 1989;25(Supp 1 1):S79-93.
44. Tincello DG, Johnstone MJ. Treatment of hyperemesis gravidarum with the 5-HT3 antagonist ondansetron (Zofran). Postgrad Med J 1996;72:688-9.
45. Sullivan CA, Johnson CA, Roach H, Martin RW, Stewart DK, Morrison JC. A pilot study of intravenous ondansetron for hyperemesis gravidarum. Am J Obstet Gynecol 1996;174:1565-8.
46. Wells CN. Treatment of hyperemesis gravidarum with cortisone. Am J Obstet Gynecol 1953;66:598-601.
47. Parry H, Martin K. Single dose iv dexamethasone: an effective anti-emetic in cancer chemotherapy. Cancer Chem Pharmacol 1991;28:231-2.
48. Mogadam M, Dobbins WO, Korelitz BI, Ahmed SW. Pregnancy in inflammatory bowel disease: effect of sulfasalazine and corticosteroid on fetal outcome. Gastroenterology 1981;80:72-6.
49. Proper AJ. Pregnancy and adrenocortical hormones. Br Med J 1962:967-72.
50. Warrdl DW, Taylor R. Outcome for the fetus of mothers receiving prednisolone during pregnancy. Lancet 1968;1:117-8.
51. Mintz G, Niz J, Gutierrez G, Garcia-Alonso A, Karchmer S. Prospective study of pregnancy in systemic lupus erythermatosus. Results of a multidisciplinary approach. J Rheumatol 1986;13:732-9.
52. Jacobson SJ, Pasmszak A, Koren G. Effects of prenatal exposure to prednisone: a prospective study. Ped Res 1997;41:348A.
53. Czeizel C, Rockenbauer M. Population-based case-control study of teratogenic potential of corticosteroids. Teratology 1997;56: 335-40.
54. Rodriguez-Pinilla E, Martinez-Firas ML. Corticosteroids during pregnancy and oral clefts: a case-control study. Teratology 1998; 58:2-5.
55. Taylor R. Successful management of hyperemesis gravidarum using steroid therapy. QJM 1996;89:103-7.
56. Nelson-Piercy C, de Swiet M. Corticosteroids for the treatment of hyperemesis gravidarum. Br J Obstet Gynaecol 1994; 101:1013-5.
57. Nelson-Piercy C, de Swiet M. Complications of the use of corticosteroids for the treatment of hyperemesis gravidarum. Br J Obstet Gynaecol 1995;102:507-9.
58. Magee LA, Redman CWG. An N-of-1 trial for treatment of hyperemesis gravidarum. Br J Obstet Gynaecol 1996;103:478-80.
59. Ylikorkala O, Kauppila A, Ollanketo ML. Intramuscular ACTH and placebo in the treatment of hyperemesis gravidarum. Acta Obstet Gynecol Scand 1979;58:453-5.
60. Safari HR, Fassett M J, Souter IC, Asulyman OM, Goodwin TM. The efficacy of methylprednisolone in the treatment of hyperemesis gravidarum: a randomized, double-blind, controlled study. Am J Obstet Gynecol 1998;179:921-4.
61. Nelson-Piercy C, Fayers P, de Swiet M. Randomised, doubleblind, placebo-controlled trial of corticosteroids for the treatment of hyperemesis gravidarum. Br J Obstet Gynaecol 2001; 108:9-15.

CHAPTER 44

FETAL GENITAL EFFECTS OF FIRST-TRIMESTER SEX HORMONE EXPOSURE: A META-ANALYSIS

Lalitha Raman-Wilms, Alice Lin-in Tseng, Suzanne Wighardt, Thomas R. Einarson, and Gideon Koren

Objective. To determine if first-trimester exposure to sex hormones, and oral contraceptives (OCs) specifically, is associated with an increased risk of external fetal genital malformations.

Data Sources. MEDLINE and Science Citation Index data bases were searched for the years 1966–1992 for relevant English-language articles on first-trimester sex-hormone exposure and fetal genital changes.

Methods of Study Selection. One hundred eighty-six articles were identified initially. Inclusion criteria were cohort or case-control studies, first-trimester sex-hormone exposure, and live infants or full-term stillborn infants with external genital malformations. Exclusion criteria were diethylstilbestrol exposure, spontaneous abortions, and teratogen exposure.

Data Extraction and Synthesis. The Methods section of each study was reviewed independently by two authors and two outside reviewers, using the above criteria. Fourteen studies, seven cohort and seven case-control, involving 65,567 women, met the criteria for meta-analysis. Extracted data were entered into 2 × 2 tables. The overall summary odds ratio (OR) was 1.09 (95% confidence interval [CI] 0.90–1.32); subanalysis of OC exposure identified an OR of 0.98 (95% CI 0.24–3.94).

Conclusion. There was no association between first-trimester exposure to sex hormones generally (or to OCs specifically) and external genital malformations. Thus, women exposed to sex hormones after conception may be assured there is no increased risk of fetal sexual malformation. (*Obstet Gynecol* 1995;85:141–9)

The first report of masculinization of female infants associated with maternal progestin treatment appeared in 1958.[1] Since then, a large number of sexual malformations have been reported[2–11] in infants exposed to various sex hormones during pregnancy. In 1971, Aarskog[12] claimed that progestins and medroxyprogester one given during early pregnancy could result in hypospadias, an observation that was supported by a few other studies.[13–16] However, others[17–19] have failed to show an association between hypospadias or other sexual malformations and fetal medroxyprogesterone or progestin exposure. Several subsequent attempts have been made to evaluate the relation between fetal sex hormone exposure and congenital malformations.[19–23] Most of the exposures in these studies were secondary to hormonal pregnancy tests, supportive hormonal therapy to maintain pregnancy, or inadvertent continuation of oral contraceptives (OCs) after conception.

No studies to date have specifically addressed the issue of fetal genital malformations secondary to sex-hormone exposure during the first trimester of pregnancy; as mentioned earlier, most information on this subject has been based on case reports.[1–11] Specific information is needed because of the number of women who inadvertently continue taking OCs after conception. In Europe and the United States, OCs are taken by 2–5% of women in early pregnancy.[20] In 1991, the MotheRisk Clinic in Toronto, Canada, received 175 calls (2.6% of all calls to the clinic) concerning the effects of OCs taken during pregnancy (data on file from MotheRisk Clinic, December 1992). Fear of fetal changes secondary to sex-hormone exposure may lead many women to consider terminating otherwise wanted pregnancies.

The purpose of the present meta-analysis was to determine if exposure to sex hormones in general, and to OCs specifically, during the first trimester of pregnancy is associated with an increased risk of external genital malformations in the fetus.

From the Faculty of Pharmacy and the Departments of Pediatrics and Pharmacology, University of Toronto, Toronto; and the MotheRisk Clinic, The Hospital for Sick Children, Canada.

METHODS

A computerized search was conducted to identify all relevant studies on the topic of fetal genital malformations as a result of sex-hormone exposure during pregnancy. Using MEDLINE, we searched for human studies published in the English language for the years 1966–1992 (August). The Science Citation Index was also searched. General MeSH headings used were adapted from the sex-hormone section of the Anatomic Therapeutic Chemical Classification[24]; the terms included: oral contraceptives, estrogens, and progestins. The MEDLINE term "sex hormones" was also used in the search. The list of genitourinary changes by Heinonen et al[25] was adapted to include only visible external genital malformations (Table 1). Additional genital malformations were obtained from lists of genitourinary malformations as classified in both the Birth Defects Encyclopedia[26] and the Birth Defects Compendium, Second Edition.[27] These terms were cross-referenced with the previously mentioned drug classes in our computer search. We also reviewed the April issues of *Pediatric Research* from 1980–1992 for relevant published and unpublished abstracts submitted to the Annual Meeting of the Society for Pediatric Research. Other sources were review articles, [21–23,28–56] textbooks,[26,27,57] and the references listed at the end of all searched articles.

The list of articles obtained was reviewed independently by four investigators. Because sexual changes were often not the main focus of the articles, they were not excluded based on the title alone. After reviewing at least the abstracts of the articles, clearly irrelevant papers were discarded. If the abstract or a preliminary review of the article suggested relevancy, the article was retrieved.

We used the following to select studies: 1) English-written cohort or case-control study design with exposed and nonexposed

Table 1
Visual Abnormalities of Sexual Differentiation*

Abnormal testes	Absent
	Aberrant
	Undescended (cryptorchidism)
Ambiguous genitalia	Pseudohermaphrodite
	Hermaphrodite
Hydrocele	
Hypoplasia penis (microphallus)	
Hypospadia	
Malformations of female genitalia	Imperforate hymen
	Absent vaginal opening
	Abnormal vagina
	Malformed vulva, absent external genitalia
	Enlarged clitoris
Malformations of male genitalia	Chordee
	Abnormal ventral foreskin
	Absent epididymis
	Hypoplastic prostate

* Adapted from Heinonen et al.[25]

groups, 2) fetal exposure to sex hormones during at least the first trimester of pregnancy and administration of sex hormones after the last menstrual period (LMP), 3) sex hormones, as defined previously in the MeSH headings, 4) the definition of external genital malformations as listed previously, 5) live infants and full-term stillbirths, and 6) sex hormone used as a single agent or in combination products, and any doses.

Exclusion criteria included: 1) diethylstilbestrol (DES) exposure, because problems from the use of this drug are well-known and it is no longer used in obstetric patients of childbearing age, 2) spontaneously aborted fetuses, because several inborn problems may be present in this group, 3) exposure to any known or suspected teratogens other than sex hormones, and 4) review articles or animal studies.

The Methods section of each study was reviewed independently by at least two of the authors, using the inclusion and exclusion criteria. After eliminating the names of authors and study locations to avoid bias, each of these sections was also given to two outside reviewers for independent review. The inclusion of the articles was agreed on by mutual consensus between reviewers, and reasons for exclusion were identified.

Data from each study were extracted independently by at least two of the authors, and a consensus was reached. If the results were so questionable that agreement could not be reached, we rejected the study. If studies had collected data for outcomes other than sexual malformations, only those consistent with the inclusion criteria were retrieved. Information abstracted included the following: cohort studies (the total number of infants exposed and not exposed to sex hormones in the first trimester and the number of infants who presented with genital malformations at birth in these groups), case-control studies (the total number of infants born with genital malformation), the total number of control infants, and the number of infants who had exposure and those with no exposure of sex hormones in the first trimester in utero. These data were entered into 2 × 2 tables. We also extracted the type of sex hormones used and the sex of the infants, if specified. For subgroup analysis, we also identified and analyzed cohort and case-control studies specifically involving OC exposure.

The *Q* statistic for homogeneity of effect was calculated to detect any systematic bias among the studies.[58] After the data were entered in 2 × 2 tables, risk ratios for cohort studies and odds ratios (ORs) for case-control studies were calculated. To determine the significance of individual studies, χ^2 and 95% confidence intervals (CI) were calculated. To get an estimate of the risk ratio for genital malformations in exposed versus unexposed infants, an overall summary OR was calculated using the method of Mantel and Haenszel.[59] Also, a 95% CI was calculated using the method described by Miettinen.[60] The equations and methods of these analyses have been described by Einarson et al.[61] Data from studies reporting OC use were extracted in a manner similar to that described previously. The OR and 95% CI were calculated, as well as a summary OR.

RESULTS

One hundred eighty-six articles published between 1962–1992 were identified; 73 of them appeared relevant on initial inspection. Twenty-three articles met our inclusion criteria; however, only 14 were included in our meta-analysis (Table 2).[13,15–19,62–69] Nine reports were excluded for various reasons, as described in Table 3.[14,70–77]

The 14 included papers were from various locations: North America (six), Israel (three), West Germany (one), Latin America (one), Sweden (one), Australia (one), and one multicenter study from eight countries. Seven were cohort studies, and the others were case-control studies. Data were collected prospectively in all of the cohort studies and retrospectively in all case-control studies. Five specifically addressed exposure to OCs in the first trimester. Other indications for sex hormone use included hormonal pregnancy tests and prevention of miscarriage. Table 2 lists the specific hormones investigated in each study. One study included hormonal use after the LMP. Eight studies were conducted in male infants alone and one specifically in females; sex was not specified in the other studies.

The case-control studies evaluated retrospectively any exposure to sex hormones in utero during the first trimester in infants who were born with particular genital changes. Information on babies with genital changes was obtained from birth registries. Mothers, and sometimes also physicians, were contacted to obtain information regarding sex hormone exposure during pregnancy. Patient charts were also reviewed for information.

The cohort studies compared outcomes for first-trimester sex-hormone exposed fetuses with respect to genital changes as defined in the inclusion criteria. In those studies, the researchers categorized fetuses as sex-hormone exposed or nonexposed, and prospectively followed the pregnancies to delivery. The infants were then examined for evidence of adverse outcome.

Table 4 presents 2 × 2 tables of all the cohort and case-control studies. Initial calculation of a Q statistic showed heterogeneity between the studies ($\chi^2 = 28.61$, $df = 13$, $P = .007$). One study[69] was identified as an outlier by the graphic method suggested by L'Abbe et al[78]; when this study was excluded from the overall analysis, the Q statistic showed homogeneity between the studies ($\chi^2 = 19.87$, $df = 12$, $P = .07$). However, inclusion of this study in the overall analysis did not significantly affect the overall OR or 95% CI (overall OR, excluding the Jacobson study.[69] : 1.01, 95% CI 0.83–1.23).

Table 2
Studies Meeting the Criteria for Meta-Analysis

REFERENCE NO.	AUTHORS	STUDY TYPE	GENITAL CHANGE(S) INVESTIGATED	SEX HORMONE(S) EXPOSURE
13	Monteleone et al, 1981	CC	Hypospadias	Sex hormones (not specified)
15	Kallen, 1988	CC	Hypospadias	OCs
16	Sweet et al, 1974	CC	Hypospadias	Estrogen, hydroxyprogesterone caproate
17	Polednak and Jenerich, 1983	CC	Hypospadias	Hormonal pregnancy tests, supportive hormone, OCs
18	Katz et al, 1985	CH	Hypospadias	Progestogens
			Hydrocele	
			Cryptorchidism	
			Mild epispadias	
			Enlarged clitoris	OCs
19	Harlap et al, 1985	CH	Hypospadias	
			Cryptorchidism	
			Hydrocele	
			Other male and female sexual changes	
62	Harlap et al, 1975	CH	Hydrocele	Estrogens, progesterones, abortifacients, miscellaneous
			Hypospadias	
			Cryptorchidism	
63	Mau, 1981	CH	Hypospadias	Progestin ± pregnancy test
64	Kallen et al, 1991	CC	Hypospadias	OCs
65	Yovich et al, 1988	CH	Hypospadias	OCs
			Cryptorchidism	Medroxyprogesterone
66	Beard et al, 1984	CC	Cryptorchidism	OCs
67	Harlap and Eldor, 1980	CH	Hypospadias	OCs
			Cryptorchidism	Pregnancy tests
			Hydrocele	
			Hermaphrodite	
			Other sex organ anomalies	
68	McBride et al, 1991	CC	Cryptorchidism (at 1 y)	Hormones to prevent miscarriage, other female hormones
69	Jacobson, 1962	CH	Clitoral enlargement	Norethindrone
			Labioscrotal fusion, phallic enlargement	

CC = case-control study; OCs = oral contraceptives; PH = cohort study.

Therefore, we decided to include it in our analysis because it was the study that showed the strongest positive correlation. Table 4 shows the results of significance tests for the studies analyzed. A significant association between sex hormones and genital malformations was identified in two case-control studies and in one cohort study. The summary OR was 1.09 (95% CI 0.90–1.32). The cohort and case-control studies were also analyzed separately (Table 5).

Five studies (two cohort and three case-control) investigated OC use in the first trimester. The summary OR for this subgroup was 0.98 (95% CI 0.24–3.94). During data collection, it was noticed that most genital malformations involved male infants, raising the question of a possible difference in incidence of genital malformations between males and females. Therefore, it was decided to examine these groups individually. Eight studies specifically addressed infant sex when investigating the epidemiology of genital malformations. Eight studies (two cohort and six case-control) dealt specifically with male infants; five examined the epidemiology of hypospadias, two assessed cryptorchidism, and one included nonspecific male genital changes. The summary OR for this subgroup was 1.11 (95% CI 0.04–29.21). Only one cohort study specifically addressed genital malformations in females and males separately. The individual risk ratio for the female subpopulation was 29.87 (95% CI 3.81–234.21).

DISCUSSION

Fetal malformations are nonprogressive structural defects that arise secondary to localized errors of morphogenesis during embryonic life. Etiologic causes are numerous and often difficult to determine conclusively. Spontaneous genetic malformations, such as those due to mutant genes or abnormal chromosome numbers, occur in about 1–3% of births.[79] Occasionally, fetal malformations are due to malignant environmental factors (ie, teratogens). In many instances, drugs can induce malformations of various forms and

Table 3
Studies Excluded From the Meta-Analysis

REFERENCE NO.	AUTHORS	REASON FOR REJECTION
14	Czeizel et al, 1979	Genetically predisposed hypospadiac male infants were included
70	Janerich et al, 1980	Included babies with various birth defects (not just genital) in control population
71	Torfs et al, 1981	Some mothers in each group received sex hormones Unable to detect from table if mothers of babies with genital changes received drug or not
72	Calzolari et al, 1986	Preterm live and still-births (from the 28th gestational week onward) were included
73	Depue, 1984	Unclear whether exposure occurred during the first trimester Unable to extract data
74	Cosgrove et al, 1977	DES included
75	Kallen and Winberg, 1982	Unable to extract data
76	Resseguie et al, 1985	Unable to extract data
77	Stoll et al, 1990	Women taking OCs before conception and in the first trimester were grouped together (ie, unable to identify first-trimester exposure)

DES = diethylstilbestrol; OCs = oral contraceptives.

Table 4
Results of Studies Comparing Genital Changes of Fetuses Exposed or Not Exposed to Sex Hormones in the First Trimester

REFERENCE NO.	EXPOSURE	CONGENITAL DEFECT YES	CONGENITAL DEFECT NO	χ^2	*P*
13	Yes	24	290	3.75	.006
	No	12	307		
15	Yes	5	43	0.75	.386
	No	6	109		
16	Yes	4	103	0.13	.718
	No	5	221		
17	Yes	21	78	0.69	.406
	No	27	72		
18	Yes	35	1573	0.01	.920
	No	26	1120		
19	Yes	24	826	0.45	.502
	No	917	26,874		
62	Yes	8	424	0.67	.413
	No	141	10,895		
63	Yes	8	551	1.32	.251
	No	25	3018		
64	Yes	16	830	0.61	.435
	No	11	835		
65	Yes	3	344	0.04	.841
	No	2	412		
66	Yes	14	53	5.13	.024
	No	99	173		
67	Yes	5	103	0.39	.532
	No	431	13,401		
68	Yes	2	242	0.86	.354
	No	10	478		
69	Yes	14	112	15.97	<.001
	No	1	184		
Total	Yes	183	5572		
	No	1713	58,099		

differing severity depending on fetal stage, intensity and duration of drug exposure, and sensitivity of fetal target tissues to the particular agent.

A recent meta-analysis by Bracken[22] failed to reveal a positive association between OC exposure and fetal malformations. However, most fetal malformations included in that meta-analysis were cardiac and limb defects; fetal genital malformations were not addressed specifically. Although genetic sex is determined at fertilization, morphologic sexual differentiation occurs later during embryonic life. This process is dependent on the presence of specific masculinizing or feminizing factors during certain periods of fetal development. It is theoretically possible that the presence of

Table 5
Summary Odds Ratios

STUDY TYPE	NO. OF STUDIES	SUBJECT EXPOSED	SUBJECT CONTROLS	ODDS RATIOS	95% CI
All studies	14	5755	59,812	1.09	0.90–1.32
Case-control[13,15–17,64,66,68]	7	1731	2,365	0.96	0.25–3.72
Cohort[18,19,62,63,65,67,69]	7	4030	57,447	1.20	0.16–8.90
Subanalyses					
OC exposure[15,17,19,64,67]	5	1931	42,660	0.98	0.24–3.94
Male infants only[13,15,16,63,64,66,68,69]	8	2259	5398	1.11	0.04–29.21
Female infants only[69]	1	59	99	29.87	3.81–234.21

CI = confidence interval; OC = oral contraceptive.

exogenous hormones during this formative phase could disturb the sexual differentiation process and result in fetal genital malformations.

Individual case reports on this subject are conflicting and inconclusive. To date, this issue has not been addressed specifically in any well-documented studies. Thus, there are still concerns regarding the potential association between inadvertent OC exposure and fetal genital malformations.

Our original interest was to determine the effects of OCs on the genital system of the developing fetus. However, we were limited by the relatively small number of epidemiologic studies involving OCs specifically. Most studies reporting sex-hormone exposure in early pregnancy included fetal exposure as a result of treatment of threatened or habitual abortion, hormonal pregnancy tests, inadvertent exposure to OCs because of unrecognized pregnancy, or treatment of premature onset of labor. Agents included progestins, estrogens, or combination agents. Therefore, we also included studies involving fetal estrogen and progestin exposure under the conditions listed earlier.

The sexual differentiation process begins at 6 weeks' gestation. By 12–14 weeks' gestation, differentiation of internal genital ducts and external genitalia along either male or female lines is complete.[80] Therefore, we considered exposure during the first trimester to be most important. One study[19] reported OC exposure after the LMP. In this case, discontinuation of OCs within approximately 2 weeks of the woman's LMP (ie, before her next ovulation and subsequent fertilization) could raise the possibility that fetal exposure to sex hormones did not occur. However, none of the studies reported any discontinuations within this time period.

Our meta-analysis showed no significant relationship (summary OR 1.09, 95% CI 0.90–1.32) between exposure to sex hormones during the first trimester and external genital malformations. The subanalysis of OCs showed no significant association between the exposure to OCs and sexual malformations (OR 0.98, 95% CI 0.24–3.94). This result is consistent with the meta-analysis performed by Bracken,[22] who found no increase in the risk of overall congenital malformations in the offspring of women exposed to OCs during pregnancy. However, two studies (one case-control[13] and one cohort[69]) showed a significant association, whereas one case-control study[66] showed a presumable protective effect.

The study by Monteleone et al[13] (OR 2.12, 95% CI 1.04–4.31) was conducted in six countries in Latin America. These infants had several associated major malformations involving limbs (27.7%), the central nervous system (15.4%), and gastrointestinal (23.1%) systems. The case infants were matched with nonmalformed children born at the same time and in the same hospital. However, possible disparities in other factors, such as maternal age, smoking, socioeconomic status, and use of other drugs were not reported. Therefore, infants who were more susceptible to genetic anomalies could have been inadvertently selected out in the case group, possibly explaining the high incidence of genital malformations observed. These results are thus suspect and require further studies to verify or disprove. In our opinion, decisions should generally not be based on a single study. The study by Jacobsen[69] (OR 23.0, 95% CI 2.98–177.3) has several inherent problems, discussed in detail subsequently under the subgroup of female genital changes.

The study by Beard et al[66] showed a protective effect of maternal sex-hormone exposure (OR 0.46, 95% CI 0.24–0.87). The authors used a central index to identify all male infants with cryptorchidism residing in Rochester between 1943–1973. Each case infant was matched with two control infants by the date of delivery and maternal age. Although exposure to progestins in both groups was similar, the control mothers had been exposed to more estrogens. Furthermore, it is not known whether the two groups were comparable with respect to socioeconomic status, alcohol use, and smoking during pregnancy. Information regarding the prevalence of other malformations in both groups was also not provided. All data were obtained solely from medical records dating back several decades. Because of these various factors, the reason for the apparent protective effect of hormone exposure during pregnancy is unclear.

The inherent development of the fetus is normally along female lines, requiring only the absence of male determinants. Therefore, the genital abnormality of female fetuses usually seen is masculinization after maternal exposure to elevated levels of androgens at the crucial stage of fetal development. On the other hand, male genital development consists of many more steps, which allows for potentially many more disorders of male sex differentiation. Thus, it is possible that the effects of female hormones on male and female embryos may be different. Therefore, we subanalyzed the incidence in male and female infants.

The subanalysis of male infants revealed no significant association between sex-hormone exposure and genital abnormalities (OR 1.11, 95% CI 0.04–29.21). However, one case-control study[13] showed significance (OR 2.12, 95% CI 1.04–4.31). The possible limitations of this study have already been discussed.

The only study in the female subanalysis[69] showed a highly significant relationship between maternal norethindrone therapy and sexual malformations of female fetuses (OR 29.87, 95% CI 3.81–234.21). However, this study had several inherent characteristics that raise questions about the validity of its conclusions. It was published approximately 30 years ago and was one of the first studies to develop from the case report format. High doses of norethindrone were administered to women for threatened abortion. Most patients received 10–40 mg/day, and doses as high as 120 mg/day were also given; this agent is still used today as an OC, but at a dose of only 0.35 mg/day. Furthermore, norethindrone had been shown previously to be associated with androgenic effects on the mothers and fetuses when administered for prolonged periods of time. The only data provided on the control mothers were the numbers exposed and not exposed to the drug. We extracted only data involving first-trimester hormonal exposure in case mothers, but were not able to be as selective with the control mothers since this information was not specified. Other confounding variables, such as socioeconomic status, alcohol, or tobacco use, were not addressed. Finally, this study involved a relatively small number of subjects.

Hence, there are many possible factors that could account for the high OR and significance value. However, the wide variation in the CI reflects the variability inherent within this study. Therefore, we recommend that these results be interpreted with caution. In fact, although the current package inserts for OCs do not specifically discuss genital changes in the fetus, they do state that studies with these agents do not suggest a teratogenic effect when taken inadvertently during early pregnancy.[81]

Certain factors should be kept in mind when evaluating our results. Seven of the 14 studies included in our meta-analysis were case-control in design. Certain factors inherent to this study design may affect the interpretation of their results, including recall of events during pregnancy, selection of samples based on voluntary reporting, and a change in the knowledge over time regarding factors considered to significantly affect the fetus.

Mothers of malformed children may understandably report exposure to sex hormones (or any drug) more often than mothers of healthy children.[82] The recall of the exact name of the hormone, the dosage, and the starting and stopping date of hormonal therapy are also difficult to establish retrospectively. Recall may be affected by the method of questioning; when asked open questions, women may not recall details as well as when questioned with respect to specific drug exposure. As a result, there could be a systematic bias toward reporting exposure.

The selection of samples in several retrospective studies was based on voluntary reporting. This method of data collection could affect the outcome of a study because milder cases of malformations may have not been reported. For example, some abnormalities (such as undescended testes) are so common that many physicians consider them to be "normal" variants. Also, reporting of factors regarding the mother may have evolved over time. For instance, factors presently considered to be relevant to fetal outcome, such as smoking and alcohol use during pregnancy, may not have been recognized previously. For example, Beard et al[66] collected data from as far back as 40 years, when smoking and alcohol patterns could have been different. In addition, the reporting of additional confounding factors, such as age, parity, socioeconomic conditions, and the use of other drugs, was not consistent among the studies. These factors may be of particular importance in our analyses, considering the various countries and cultural backgrounds in which the studies were conducted. Prior pregnancies may be important because the birth of one child with a birth defect may confer an increased risk of malformation in subsequent offspring.[83,84] In a similar fashion, the occurrence of a stillborn child may tempt the obstetrician to prescribe hormones in subsequent pregnancies.[48]

The timing of detection of genital malformations is also important. Some abnormalities decrease in prevalence with increasing age, whereas others increase. In general, approximately 50% of all congenital malformations are not ascertained until the child is 1 year old.[53] This factor is especially relevant in the studies assessing cryptorchidism. Because the testes normally descend between 7 months[1] gestation and the first several postnatal months, most cases of cryptorchidism resolve spontaneously by 1 year of age[80] Therefore, the detection of cryptorchidism at birth may not reflect the true incidence. In our analysis, only one study[68] included subjects with cryptorchidism present at 1 year of age. Although the other studies did not take this factor into account, cases of cryptorchidism were observed at the same time (ie, immediately after birth) in both the control and case groups; therefore, the overall OR should not be affected.

Although epidemiologic data regarding fetal malformations in both male and female infants are collected routinely, examination of the literature suggests that most epidemiologic studies involving fetal genital malformations are based on assessment of data involving primarily male infants. This may be due to many factors. There may be a greater awareness among pediatricians of potential genital malformations in male (eg, undescended testes) compared to female (eg, abnormal vulva, clitoris, or vagina) infants. In addition, the more internal nature of female genitalia makes detection of abnormalities more difficult, from both a physical and chronological standpoint; for instance, abnormalities such as vaginal inadequacy or imperforate hymen may not be detected until the first pelvic examination in adulthood. As mentioned previously, the steps involved in the development of male compared to female genitalia are more complex; therefore, it is possible that the male sexual differentiation process may be more susceptible to disruption by exposure to external sex hormones.

At present, the reasons for the uneven distribution between studies assessing males versus females are unclear. Developing male genitalia may in fact be more susceptible to the effects of exogenous sex hormones. On the other hand, this observation may be a reflection of better case ascertainment in male infants relative to female infants. This issue clearly indicates the need for more studies of infant girls exposed to sex hormones in utero.

REFERENCES

1. Wilkins L, Jones HW, Holman GH. Masculinzation of the female fetus associated with administration of oral and intramuscular progestins during gestation: Non-adrenal female pseudohermaphrodism. J Clin Endocrinol Metab 1958;18:559–85.
2. Bongiovanni AM, DiGeorge AM, Grumbach MM. Masculinization of the female infant associated with estrogen therapy alone during gestation. J Clin Epidemiol 1959;19:1004–11.
3. Fine E, Levin HM, McConnell EL. Masculinization of female infants associated with norethindrone acetate. Obstet Gynecol 1963;22: 210–3.
4. Grumbach MM, Ducharme JR, Moloshok RE. On the fetal masculinizing action of certain oral progestins. J Clin Endocrinol Metab 1959;19:1369–80.
5. Grumbach MM, Ducharme JR. The effect of androgens on fetal sexual development. Androgen-induced female pseudohermaphroditism. Fertil Steril 1960;11:157–80.
6. Hayles AB, Nolan RB. Masculinization of female fetus, possibly related to administration of progesterone during pregnancy: Report of two cases. Mayo Clin Proc 1958;33:200–3.
7. Hillman DA. Fetal masculinization with maternal progesterone therapy. Can Med Assoc J 1959;80:200–1.
8. Moncrieff A. Non-adrenal female pseudohermaphroditism associated with hormone administration in pregnancy. Lancet 1958;ii:267–8.
9. Mortimer PE. Female pseudohermaphroditism due to progestogens. Lancet 1960;ii:438–9.
10. Voorhess ML. Masculinization of the female fetus associated with norethindrone-mestranol therapy during pregnancy. J Pediatr 1967;71:128–31.
11. Wilkins L. Masculinization of female fetus due to use of orally given progestins. JAMA 1960;172:1028–32.
12. Aarskog D. Intersex conditions masquerading as simple hypospadias. Birth Defects 1971;7:122–30.
13. Monteleone RN, Castilla EE, Paz JE. Hypospadias: An epidemiological study in Latin America. Am J Med Genet 1981;10:5–19.
14. Czeizel A, Toth J, Erodi E. Aetiological studies of hypospadias in Hungary. Hum Hered 1979;29:166–71.
15. Kallen B. Case-control study of hypospadias based on registry information. Teratology 1988;38:45–50.
16. Sweet RA, Schrott HG, Kurland R, Culp OS. Study of the incidence of hypospadias in Rochester, Minnesota, 1940–1970, and a case-control comparison of possible etiologic factors. Mayo Clin Proc 1974;49:52–8.
17. Polednak AP, Janerich DT. Maternal characteristics and hypospadias: A case-control study. Teratology 1983;28:67–73.
18. Katz Z, Lancet M, Skornik J, Chemke J, Mogilner BM, Klinberg M. Teratogenicity of progestogens given during the first trimester of pregnancy. Obstet Gynecol 1985;65:775–80.

19. Harlap S, Shiono PH, Ramcharan S. Congenital abnormalities in the offspring of women who used oral and other contraceptives around the time of conception. Int J Fertil 1985;30:39–47.
20. Smithells RW. Oral contraceptives and birth defects. Dev Med Child Neurol 1981;23:369–72.
21. Ambani LM, Joshi NJ, Vaidya Ra, Devi PK. Are hormonal contraceptives teratogenic? Fertil Steril 1977;28:791–7.
22. Bracken MB. Oral contraception and congenital malformations in offspring: A review and meta-analysis of the prospective studies. Obstet Gynecol 1990;76:552–7.
23. Czeizel A. Are contraceptive pills teratogenic? Acta Morphol Hung 1980;28:177–88.
24. Anatomic Therapeutic Chemical (ATC) Classification Index. Section G03: Sex hormones and modulators of the genital system. World Health Organization Collaborating Centre for Drug Statistics Methodology. Oslo, Norway: World Health Organization, 1993.
25. Heinonen OP, Slone D, Shapiro S. Birth defects and drugs in pregnancy. Littleton, Massachusetts: Publishing Science Group Inc., 1977.
26. Buyse ML, ed. Birth defects encyclopedia. Dover, Massachusetts: The Center for Birth Defects Information Services, Inc., 1990.
27. Bergsma D, ed. Birth defects compendium. 2nd ed. New York: Alan R. Liss, Inc., 1979.
28. Aarskog D. Maternal progestins as a possible cause of hypospadias. N Engl J Med 1979;300:75–8.
29. Bongiovanni AM, McPadden AJ. Steroids during pregnancy and possible fetal consequences. Fertil Steril 1960;11:181–6.
30. Briggs MH, Briggs M. Sex hormone exposure during pregnancy and malformations. Adv Steroid Biochem Pharmacol 1979;7:51–89.
31. Chez RA. Proceedings of the symposium, "progesterone, progestins, and fetal development". Fertil Steril 1978;30:16–26.
32. American College of Obstetricians and Gynecologists Committee on Gynecologic Practice. Contraceptives and congenital anomalies. ACOG Committee opinion no. 62. Washington, DC: American College of Obstetricians and Gynecologists, 1988.
33. Dawson K. Side effects of oral contraceptives. Nurse Pract 1979;4:53–9.
34. Fraumeni JF. Chemicals in human teratogenesis and transplacental carcinogenesis. Pediatrics 1974;53:807–12.
35. Goldman AS, Bongiovanni AM. Induced genital anomalies. Ann N Y Acad Sci 1967;142:755–67.
36. Herbest AL. Diethylstilbestrol and other sex hormones during pregnancy. Obstet Gynecol 1981;58(Suppl):35–40S.
37. Huggins GR, Cullins VE. Fertility after contraception or abortion. Fertil Steril 1990;54:559–73.
38. Jirasek JE. Genital ducts and external genitalia: Development and anomalies. Birth Defects 1971;7:131–9.
39. Johnston GA. Health risks and effects of prenatal exposure to diethylstilbestrol. J Fam Pract 1983;16:51–4.
40. Jost A, Prepin J, Vigier B. Hormones in the morphogenesis of the genital system. Birth Defects 1977;13:85–97.
41. Kaplan SL, Grumbach MM. Pituitary and placental gonadotrophins and sex steroids in the human and sub-human primate fetus. Clin Endocrinol Metab 1978;7:487–11.
42. Kelsey FO. The importance of epidemiology in identifying drugs which may cause malformations–With particular reference to drugs containing sex hormones. Acta Morphol Hung 1980;28:189–95.
43. Mills JL, Bongiovanni AM. Effect of prenatal estrogen exposure on male genitalia. Pediatrics 1978;62:1160–5.
44. Neumann F, Elger W, Steinbeck H. Effects of oral contraceptives on the fetus. Lancet 1970;ii:1258–9.
45. Rumeau-Rouquette C, Goujard J, Kaminski M. Problems in conducting prospective surveys. Acta Morphol Hung 1980;28:167–75.
46. Schardein JL. Congenital abnormalities and hormones during pregnancy: A clinical review. Teratology 1980;22:251–70.
47. Shapiro S, Slone D. The effects of exogenous female hormones on the fetus. Epidemiol Rev 1979;1:110–23.
48. Simpson JL. Do contraceptive methods pose fetal risks? Res Front Fertil Regulation 1985;3:1–11.
49. Smithells RW. Oral contraceptives and birth defects. Dev Med Child Neurol 1981;23:369–72.
50. Stillman RJ. In utero exposure to diethylstilbestrol: Adverse effects on the reproductive tract and reproductive performance in male and female offspring. Am J Obstet Gynecol 1982;142:905–21.
51. Vande Wiele RL, Husami N, Dyrenfurth I. Progestogens in pregnancy. In: Diabetes and other endocrine disorders during pregnancy and in the newborn. New York: Alan R. Liss, Inc., 1976. 179–203.
52. Walker PA, Money J. Prenatal androgenization of females. A review. Horm Res 1972;3:119–128.
53. Anonymous. The effect of female sex hormones on fetal development and infant health. World Health Organ Tech Rep Ser No. 657, 1979.
54. Anonymous. The effect of female sex hormones on fetal development and infant health. World Health Organ Tech Rep Ser No. 657, 1981.
55. Wilson JG. Present status of drugs as teratogens in man. Teratology 1973;7:3–15.
56. Wilson JG, Brent RL. Are female sex hormones teratogenic? Am J Obstet Gynecol 1981;141:567–80.
57. Winter RM, Knowles SAS, Bieber RF, Baraitser M. The malformed fetus and stillbirth. A diagnostic approach. Toronto: John Wiley and Sons Ltd., 1988.
58. Der Simonian R, Charette LJ, McPeek B, Mosteller F. Reporting on methods in clinical trials. N Engl J Med 1982;306:1332–7.
59. Mantel N, Haenszel W. Statistical aspects of the analysis of data from retrospective studies of disease. J Natl Cancer Inst 1959;22:719–48.
60. Miettinen O. Estimability and estimation in case-referent studies. Am J Epidemiol 1976;103:226–35.
61. Einarson TR, Leeder JS, Koren G. A method for meta-analysis of epidemiological studies. Drug Intell Clin Pharm 1988;22:813–24.
62. Harlap S, Prywes R, Davies AM. Birth defects and estrogens and progesterones in pregnancy. Lancet 1975;i:682–3.
63. Mau G. Progestins during pregnancy and hypospadias. Teratology 1981;24:285–7.
64. Kallen B, Mastroiacovo P, Lancaster PA, et al. Oral contraceptives in the etiology of isolated hypospadias. Contraception 1991;44:173–82.
65. Yovich JL, Turner SR, Draper R. Medroxyprogesterone acetate therapy in early pregnancy has no apparent fetal effects. Teratology 1988;38:135–44.
66. Beard CM, Melton LJ, O'Fallon WM, Noller KL, Benson RC. Cryptorchism and maternal estrogen exposure. Am J Epidemiol 1984;120:707–16.
67. Harlap S, Eldor J. Births following oral contraceptive failures. Obstet Gynecol 1980;55:447–52.
68. McBride ML, Van den Steen N, Lamb CW, Gallagher RP. Maternal and gestational factors in cryptorchidism. Int J Epidemiol 1991; 20:964–70.
69. Jacobson BD. Hazards of norethindrone therapy during pregnancy. Am J Obstet Gynecol 1962;7:962–8.
70. Janerich DT, Piper JM, Glebatis DM. Oral contraceptives and birth defects. Am J Epidemiol 1980;112:73–9.
71. Torfs CP, Milkovich L, Van Den Berg BJ. The relationship between hormonal pregnancy tests and congenital anomalies: A prospective study. Am J Epidemiol 1981;113:563–74.
72. Calzolari E, Contiero MR, Roncarati E, Mattiuz PL, Volpato S. Aetiological factors in hypospadias. J Med Genet 1986;23:333–7.
73. Depue RH. Maternal and gestational factors affecting the risk of cryptorchidism and inguinal hernia. Int J Epidemiol 1984;13: 311–8.
74. Cosgrove MD, Benton B, Henderson BE. Male genitourinary abnormalities and maternal diethylstilbestrol. J Urol 1977;117:220–2.
75. Kallen B, Winberg I. An epidemiological study of hypospadias in Sweden. Acta Paediatr Scand Suppl 1982;293:1–21.
76. Resseguie LJ, Hick JF, Bruen JA, Noller KL, O'Fallon WM, Kurland LT. Congenital malformations among offspring exposed in utero to progestins, Olmsted County, Minnesota, 1936–1974. Fertil Steril 1985;43:514–9.
77. Stoll C, Alembik Y, Roth MP, Dott B. Genetic and environmental factors in hypospadias. J Med Genet 1990;27:559–63.

78. L'Abbe KA, Detsky As, O'Rourke K. Meta-analysis in clinical research. Ann Intern Med 1987;107:224–33.
79. Shepard TH. Human teratogenicity. Adv Pediatr 1986;33:225–68.
80. Fanaroff AA, Martin RJ, eds. Neonatal-perinatal medicine: Diseases of the fetus and infant. 4th ed. St. Louis: CV Mosby, 1987.
81. Brent RL. Editorial comment: Kudos to the Food and Drug Administration: Reversal of the package insert warning for birth defects for oral contraceptives. Teratology 1989;39:93–4.
82. Feldman Y, Koren G, Mattice K, Shear N, Pellegrini E, MacLeod SM. Determinants of recall and recall bias in studying drug and chemical exposure in pregnancy. Teratology 1989;40:37–45.
83. Taffel S. Congenital anomalies and birth injuries among live births: United States, 1973–74. Vital & Health Statistics—Series 21: Data from the National Vital Statistics System 1978;31:i–vi,1–58.
84. Simpson JL, Golbus MS, Martin AO, Sarto GE. Genetics in Obstetrics and gynecology. New York: Grune & Stratton, 1982.

Address reprint requests to:
Thomas R. Einarson, PhD
Faculty of Pharmacy
University of Toronto
19 Russell Street
Toronto, ON M5S 2S2
Canada

Received April 8, 1994.
Received in revised form August 8, 1994.
Accepted August 29, 1994.

Reprinted from Raman-Wilms L, Tseng AL, Wighardt S, Einarson TR, Koren G. Fetal genital effects of first-trimester sex hormone exposure: a meta-analysis. Obstet Gynecol 1995;85:141–9 with permission from Lippincott Williams & Wilkins.

CHAPTER 45

ASPIRIN CONSUMPTION DURING THE FIRST TRIMESTER OF PREGNANCY AND CONGENITAL ANOMALIES: A META-ANALYSIS

Eran Kozer, Shekoufeh Nikfar, Adriana Costei, Rada Boskovic, Irena Nulman, and Gideon Koren

Objective. The purpose of this study was to determine, on the basis of published reports, whether aspirin use during the first trimester of pregnancy is associated with an increased risk of congenital malformations.

Study Design: We reviewed the literature for published studies that reported exposure to aspirin during the first trimester of pregnancy and congenital malformations. Two reviewers independently determined whether a study should be included in the final analysis and extracted the data. We calculated the pooled odds ratio and 95% CI.

Results: Twenty-two studies met the inclusion criteria. In the eight studies that reported an overall risk, the risk of congenital malformations in offspring of women who were exposed to aspirin was not significantly higher than that in control subjects (odds ratio, 1.33; 95% CI, 0.94-1.89). However, a significantly increased risk of gastroschisis (odds ratio, 2.37; 95% CI, 1.44-3.88) was found.

Conclusion: We found no evidence of an overall increase in the risk of congenital malformations that could be associated with aspirin. Aspirin exposure during the first trimester may be associated with an increased risk of gastroschisis. (Am J Obstet Gynecol 2002;187:·1623-30.)

Keywords: Aspirin, pregnancy, congenital malformations, meta-analysis

Although new anti-inflammatory and analgesic drugs are available, aspirin (acetylsalicylic acid) is still widely used as an anti-inflammatory and analgesic drug. Exposure to aspirin during the first trimester occurs in 2% to 30% of all pregnancies.[1-4] During pregnancy, aspirin may be used as a nonprescription drug taken either for the relief of pain and fever or for specific indications (eg, collagen diseases,[5,6] recurrent fetal loss,[7] intrauterine growth retardation,[8] and the prevention of pregnancy-induced hypertension[9-11]).

Although animal studies[12-14] have shown that aspirin may increase the risk of congenital anomalies, data from human studies are conflicting. The results of several human studies suggested an increased risk of specific types of malformations (eg, congenital heart defects,[15] neural tube defects [NTDs],[16,17] hypospadias,[2] cleft palate,[17,18] gastroschisis,[19-23] central nervous system [CNS] defects,[17,24] and pyloric stenosis[17]). However, no increased risk of malformations was found in a large cohort study[3] and small randomized control studies.[25,26]

The objective of this study was to determine, on the basis of a systematic review of all published reports, whether the use of aspirin during the first trimester of pregnancy is associated with an overall increased risk of congenital malformations or an increased risk of specific anomalies.

METHODS

Data Sources

A search of the literature was done for studies that involved the effects of aspirin on the outcome of pregnancy. The following OVID (4.3.0) databases (and relevant segment dates) were searched electronically by a professional librarian in October 2000: MEDLINE (1966-2000), EMBASE (1980-2000), TOXLINE (1994-2000), and the EBM Reviews—Cochrane Database of Systematic Reviews (1991-2000). The MEDLINE search was repeated in April 2001. Reprotox (Reproductive Toxicology Center, Bethesda, Md; 2000), teratology texts,[27,28] and the bibliographies of all the included studies were searched manually.

The key words used to search for articles about the exposure to aspirin were *salicylic acid, pregnancy,* and *pregnancy complications*; the key words used to search for articles about the outcome were *neonatal diseases* and *abnormalities.* Key words were explored whenever possible.

The search was limited to sources that dealt with human pregnancy.

Study Selection

Controlled studies of human populations, both prospective and retrospective, were included for data analysis if they examined maternal exposure to aspirin during the first trimester of pregnancy and reported congenital malformations. Only full publications were considered.

Excluded were uncontrolled studies, case reports or case series of <6 patients, editorials, reviews, and animal studies. We also excluded studies that reported significant differences between exposed and control groups (eg, women who were exposed to aspirin and were treated with other drug therapies; the control group was not treated with other drug therapies). Studies that reported only premature closure of the ductus arteriosus as a primary outcome were excluded because this outcome is not associated with exposure to aspirin during the first trimester. Studies in languages other than English were excluded if they did not have an abstract in English.

From the Motherisk Program, Division of Clinical Pharmacology and Toxicology, Hospital for Sick Children, and the Department of Paediatrics, University of Toronto.

Supported by a grant from Pfizer, Inc, Groton, Conn, and Fetox International, Inc, Toronto, Ontario.

Table
Characteristics of the Studies Included in the Analysis

STUDY	YEAR	DESIGN	HOW ASPIRIN EXPOSURE WAS ESTABLISHED
Aselton et al[33]	1985	Cohort	Based on prescription given to the mothers
Correy et al[2]	1991	Cohort	Recorded by doctor in early antenatal period
Drongowski et al[21]	1991	Case control	Questionnaire distributed to mothers
Gierup and Lundkvist[22]	1979	Case control	Interview of mothers
Karkinen-Jääskeläinen and Saxén[29]	1974	Case control	Medical records and interview of mothers within the first weeks after delivery
Lynberg et al[16]	1994	Case control	Telephone interview of parents
Martinez-Frias et al[19]	1997	Case control	Interview of mothers within 3 days after birth
Nelson and Forfar[30]	1971	Case control	Interview of mothers before discharge from the maternity unit, review of medical records
Newman et al[34]	1977	Cohort	Review of medical records from a private clinic
Pattison et al[25]	2000	Randomized controlled	Patients assigned to aspirin 75 mg/d or placebo
Richards[17]	1972	Case control	Interview of mothers in the second month after delivery
Saxen[18]	1975	Case control	Medical records, interview of mothers within the first weeks after delivery
Shaw et al[31]	1998	Case control	Interview of mothers at 4.9 (average) months after birth
Siffel and Czeizel[35]	1995	Cohort	Interview at early pregnancy and at 12 weeks
Slone et al[3]	1976	Cohort	Interview during antenatal clinic visit
Tikkanen and Heinonen[32]	1990	Case control	Interview of mothers 3 mo (average) after delivery
Torfs et al[20]	1996	Case control	Interview of mothers
Turner and Collins[36]	1975	Cohort	Urine test for salicylates during pregnancy, interview of mothers immediately after birth
Werler et al[23]	1992	Case control	Interview of mothers within 6 mo after delivery
Werler et al[4]	1989	Case control	Interview of mothers
Winship et al[24]	1984	Case control	Mothers' medical records
Zierler and Rothman[15]	1985	Case control	Interview of mothers 14 mo (average) after birth, obstetric records

One reviewer screened all the abstracts, titles, and, if necessary, full reports and bibliographies that were found for inclusion in this review. On the basis of this preliminary screening, studies were chosen for detailed review by two reviewers who specialized in maternal-fetal toxicology and who applied the selection criteria and decided independently the studies that should be included in the final analysis. In cases of disagreement between the two reviewers, the decision was made on the basis of the assessment of a third reviewer. When multiple studies reported data for the same populations or subpopulations, only the study that reported the more comprehensive data was included.

Data Extraction

Using structured data collection forms, each of the reviewers extracted data independently and entered the data into 2 × 2 tables. Discrepancies were resolved by consensus.

Data Synthesis

We used the Cochrane Review Manager software (version 4.1, Update Software, Oxford) to calculate the pooled odds ratio (OR) and 95% CI, using the Mantel-Haenszel method, assuming a random-effect model.

RESULTS

On the basis of our search strategy, 1902 citations were identified; their titles and abstracts were reviewed. Of these citations, 180 studies were selected for detailed review. Twenty-two of these studies met the inclusion criteria: 15 case-control studies,[4,15-24,29-32] 6 cohort studies,[2,3,33-36] and 1 randomized control trial.[25] Characteristics of the included studies are presented in the Table.

Overall Rates of Malformation

Eight studies reported an overall rate of congenital malformations: 5 cohort studies,[3,33-36] 2 case-control studies,[17,30] and 1 randomized control study.[25] The risk of congenital malformations in the offspring of women who were exposed to aspirin was not significantly higher than that in the offspring of control subjects (OR, 1.33; 95% CI, 0.94-1.89; Fig 1). However, these studies were heterogeneous ($P = .016$).

When the pooled results of the case-control studies,[17,30] cohort studies,[3,33-36] and the randomized control[25] trial were analyzed separately, the results of the case-control studies showed a higher risk of malformations in exposed infants than in the nonexposed (OR, 1.64; 95% CI, 1.30-2.04), whereas analysis of the results of the cohort and randomized control studies indicated no such effect (OR, 1.03; 95% CI, 0.94-1.13; Fig 2). The studies were not heterogeneous for both subanalyses ($P = .38$ and $P = .63$, respectively).

Because the results of the study by Slone et al[3] had a huge impact on the combined results, we repeated the analysis of cohort and randomized control studies, excluding that study. The risk of congenital malformations among exposed offspring was not statistically significant (OR, 1.72; 95% CI, 0.69-4.3).

OUTCOMES REPORTED	DETECTION OF OUTCOME
Overall rate of malformations	Hospital charts review, clinical follow-up
Overall rate of malformations	Birth registry from Tasmania
Gastroschisis	Hospital charts review
Gastroschisis	Hospital charts review
CNS defects	Finnish Register of Congenital Malformations
NTDs	Metropolitan Atlanta Congenital Defect Program
Gastroschisis	Physician examination within 3 days after birth
Overall rate of malformations	Routine inspection within 10 days after birth, postmortem examination
Overall rate of malformations	Review of medical records from a private clinic
Overall rate of malformations	Prospective follow-up of newborn infants
Overall rate of malformations, CNS defects, cardiovascular defects, gastrointestinal defects, musculoskeletal defects, cleft lip/palate, pyloric stenosis	South Wales Survey of Congenital Defects
Cleft lip and/or palate	Finnish Register of Congenital Malformations
NTDs	California Birth Defect Monitoring Program
Overall rate of malformations	Mothers' report confirmed by physician
Overall rate of malformation, CNS malformation, cardiovascular malformations, musculoskeletal malformations, gastrointestinal malformations, hypospadias, respiratory malformations, eye or ear malformations	Pediatric examination after birth, follow-up in first year of life, autopsy reports
Cardiovascular malformations	Finnish Register of Congenital Malformations, Children's Cardiac Register
Gastroschisis	Hospital charts review by a pediatric geneticist
Overall rate of malformations	Physician examination after birth
Gastroschisis	Slone Epidemiology Unit Birth Defect Study
Congenital heart defect	Slone Epidemiology Unit Birth Defect Study
CNS defects	Birth defect registry and review of medical records
Congenital heart disease	New England Regional Infant Cardiac Registry

CNS Defects

Three case-control studies[17,24,29] and one cohort study[3] reported rates of CNS defects. The risk of congenital CNS defects was not significantly higher among offspring who were exposed to aspirin than among offspring who were not exposed (OR, 1.39; 95% CI, 0.89-2.16); however, the studies were heterogeneous (P = .054). Analysis of the results of case-control studies alone indicated a small, but significant risk of CNS defects (OR, 1.68; 95% CI, 1.23-2.30).

Three case-control studies[16,17,31] assessed the risk of NTDs in offspring of mothers who used aspirin during the first trimester. The estimated OR for NTDs in exposed infants was 2.2; however, the 95% CI was wide (0.93-5.17). The risk was not statistically significant, and the studies were heterogeneous (P = .002).

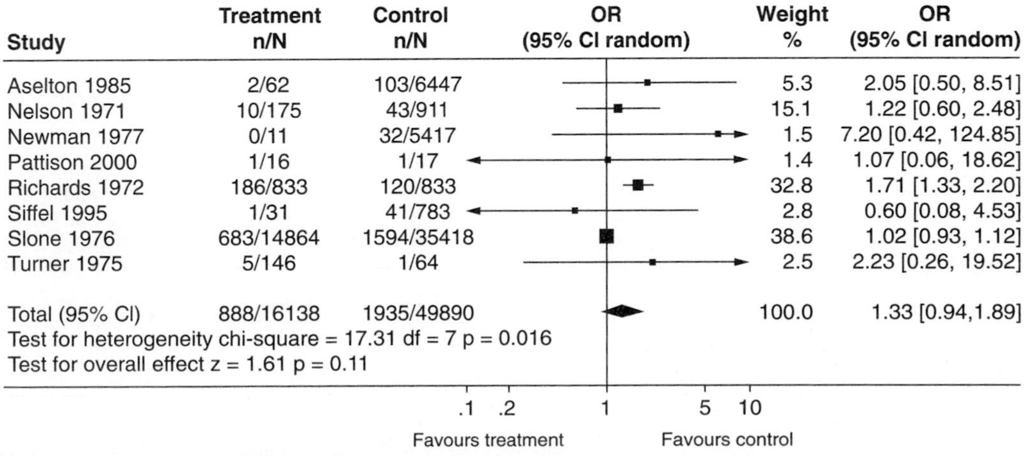
Study
Treatment n/N
Control n/N
OR (95% CI random)
Weight %
OR (95% CI random)
Aselton 1985 2/62 103/6447 5.3 2.05 [0.50, 8.51]
Nelson 1971 10/175 43/911 15.1 1.22 [0.60, 2.48]
Newman 1977 0/11 32/5417 1.5 7.20 [0.42, 124.85]
Pattison 2000 1/16 1/17 1.4 1.07 [0.06, 18.62]
Richards 1972 186/833 120/833 32.8 1.71 [1.33, 2.20]
Siffel 1995 1/31 41/783 2.8 0.60 [0.08, 4.53]
Slone 1976 683/14864 1594/35418 38.6 1.02 [0.93, 1.12]
Turner 1975 5/146 1/64 2.5 2.23 [0.26, 19.52]
Total (95% CI) 888/16138 1935/49890 100.0 1.33 [0.94,1.89]
Test for heterogeneity chi-square = 17.31 df = 7 p = 0.016
Test for overall effect z = 1.61 p = 0.11
.1
.2
1
5
10
Favours treatment
Favours control

Figure 1. OR for congenital malformations in offspring of mothers who were exposed to aspirin during the first trimester of pregnancy. Treatment refers to women who were exposed to aspirin in cohort studies or affected children in case control studies; Weight refers to the relative weight of each study in the combined results.

Study	Treatment n/N	Control n/N	Weight %	OR (95% CI random)
Aselton 1985	2/62	103/6447	0.4	2.05 [0.50, 8.51]
Newman 1977	0/11	32/5417	0.1	7.20 [0.42, 124.85]
Pattison 2000	1/16	1/17	0.1	1.07 [0.06, 18.62]
Siffel 1995	1/31	41/783	0.2	0.60 [0.08, 4.53]
Slone 1976	683/14864	1594/35418	99.0	1.02 [0.93, 1.12]
Turner 1975	5/146	1/64	0.2	2.23 [0.26, 19.52]
Total (95% CI)	692/15130	1772/48146	100.0	1.03 [0.94, 1.13]

Test for heterogeneity chi-square = 3.48 df = 5 p = 0.63

Test for overall effect z = 0.58 p = 0.6

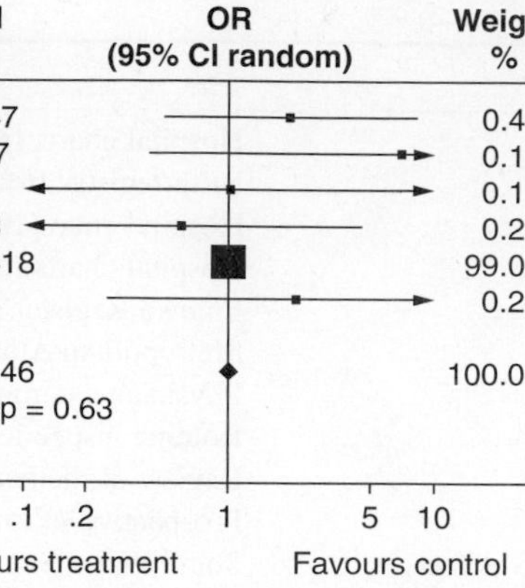

Figure 2. OR for congenital malformations in cohort and randomized controlled studies in offspring of mothers who were exposed to aspirin during the first trimester of pregnancy. Treatment refers to women who were exposed to aspirin in cohort studies or affected children in case control studies; Weight refers to the relative weight of each study in the combined results.

Subanalyses, excluding the study by Lynberg et al,[16] which compared offspring of mothers who had influenza with the offspring of healthy control subjects, was excluded from the analysis; the results showed a small, but statistically significant, risk of NTDs (OR, 1.46; 95% CI, 1.03-2.08).

Congenital Heart Defects

Six studies (4 case-control studies[4,15,17,32] and 2 cohort studies[3,36]) focused on aspirin and congenital heart defects. Data analysis showed no increased risk of congenital heart defects among exposed infants (OR, 1.01; 95% CI, 0.91-1.12; Fig 3). An increased risk of specific cardiac defects (conal septal defects) was suggested by Zierler and Rothman,[15] which could not be found in the study by Werler et al.[4] Because the definition of conal septal defects in these studies was different, the results could not be grouped together.

Gastroschisis

Five case-control studies[19-23] assessed the risk of gastroschisis in infants who were exposed to aspirin during the first trimester. The OR for gastroschisis was significant (OR, 2.37; 95% CI, 1.44-3.88; Fig 4).

Congenital Anomalies Reported in Only Two Studies

One cohort study[3] and one case-control study[17] reported rates of gastrointestinal malformations. The risk of malformations among exposed infants was not higher than that among unexposed infants (OR, 0.97; 95% CI, 0.62-1.51). However, the studies were heterogeneous ($P = .043$), possibly because of the different study designs.

When the data for the two case-control studies[17,18] that assessed the risk of cleft lip and palate among exposed infants were pooled, the OR was significant (OR, 2.87; 95% CI, 2.04-4.02).

One cohort study[3] and one case-control study[17] reported rates of musculoskeletal malformations. The risk for exposed infants was not higher than that for the control group (OR, 0.93; 95% CI, 0.77-1.13).

One cohort study[2] reported an increased risk of hypospadias in exposed infants. This association was not found in the other cohort study.[3] When the results of the studies were analyzed together, the risk of hypospadias among exposed infants was not statistically significant (OR, 1.82; 95% CI, 0.58-5.72).

Study	Treatment n/N	Control n/N	Weight %	OR (95% CI random)
Richards 1972	13/100	125/833	2.8	0.85 [0.46, 1.56]
Slone 1976	122/14864	282/35418	23.2	1.03 [0.83, 1.28]
Tikkanen 1990	41/408	75/755	6.6	1.01 [0.68, 1.51]
Turner 1975	4/146	1/64	0.2	1.77 [0.19, 16.20]
Werler 1989	364/1381	1856/6966	61.5	0.99 [0.86, 1.12]
Zierler 1985	36/298	67/738	5.7	1.38 [0.90, 2.11]
Total (95% CI)	580/17197	2406/44774	100.0	1.01 [0.91, 1.12]

Test for heterogeneity chi-square = 2.73 df = 5 p = 0.74

Test for overall effect z = 0.26 p = 0.8

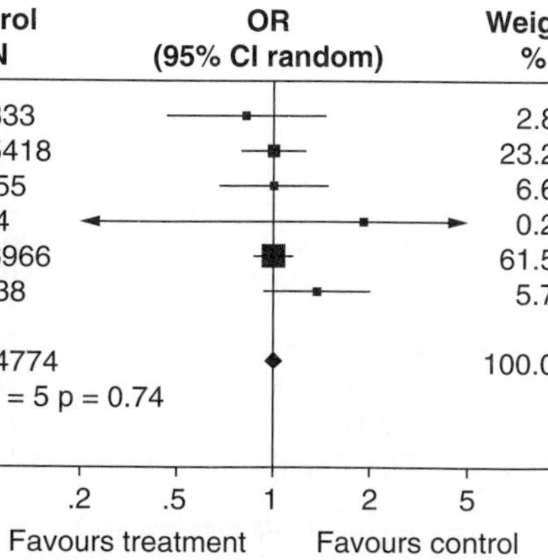

Figure 3. OR for cardiac malformations in offspring of mothers who were exposed to aspirin during the first trimester of pregnancy. Treatment refers to women who were exposed to aspirin in cohort studies or affected children in case control studies; Weight refers to the relative weight of each study in the combined results.

Study	Treatment n/N	Control n/N	Weight %	OR (95% CI random)
Drongowski 1991	10/16	8/32	13.4	5.00 [1.38, 18.17]
Glerup 1979	4/14	1/11	4.3	4.00 [0.38, 42.37]
Martinez-Friaz 1997	5/45	2/44	8.0	2.62 [0.48, 14.31]
Torts 1996	7/110	3/220	11.9	4.92 [1.25, 19.40]
Werler 1992	26/76	509/2142	62.4	1.67 [1.03, 2.71]
Total (95% CI)	52/261	523/2449	100.0	2.37 [1.44, 3.88]

Test for heterogeneity chi-square = 4.43 df = 4 p = 0.36
Test for overall effect z = 3.42 p = 0.0006

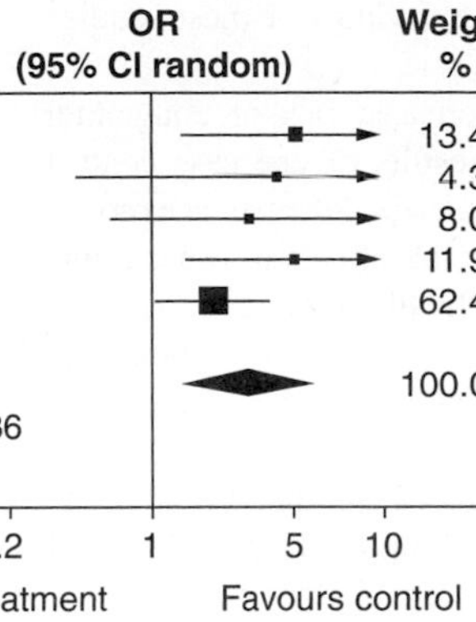

Figure 4. OR for gastroschisis in offspring of mothers who were exposed to aspirin during the first trimester of pregnancy. Treatment refers to women who were exposed to aspirin in cohort studies or affected children in case control studies; Weight refers to the relative weight of each study in the combined results.

Specific Congenital Anomalies Reported in Only a Single Study

A trend toward increased risk for pyloric stenosis (OR, 2.24; 95% CI, 1.00-5.03) was reported in only one case-control study.[17]

No increased risk of respiratory, eye, or ear malformations was reported in the study by Slone et al.[3] The incidence of these malformations was not reported in other studies.

No human study addressed the risk of diaphragmatic hernia in infants who were exposed to aspirin during the first trimester. However, a tally of the results of all identified cohort studies that reported on specific malformations revealed one case of diaphragmatic hernia in 532 exposed infants and none in the nonexposed group (n = 13,178).

COMMENT

When a drug that is commonly used by pregnant women has detrimental effects (even if they are small) on pregnancy outcome, that drug may have a significant impact on public health. Although such an effect of aspirin has been suggested,[17] a large cohort study[3] of >50,000 women, almost 15,000 of whom were exposed to aspirin during their first trimester, found no evidence of such an effect. When all the results of the studies that were selected for this meta-analysis were combined, we could not show an overall increased risk of congenital malformations. However, studies were heterogeneous and possibly reflected the different methods of the case control studies (which are more sensitive to detect rare events but may be more subject to bias) and the cohort and randomized control studies. The heterogeneity of the studies could result also from differences in the way malformations were detected and reported or the ages in which malformations were observed in different studies.

When the results of the two case-control studies[17,30] were pooled and analyzed separately from the others, a small but statistically significant risk of overall malformation was detected. Because one case-control study[17] used healthy infants as control subjects, recall bias, which may account for the higher reported rate of aspirin exposure among subjects, cannot be ruled out. However, other drugs such as antibiotics and sulfonamides that were used in that study were not associated with an increased risk of malformations, and the association of aspirin and congenital malformations remained significant after an adjustment for maternal disease.

Conclusions that are based on the findings of the cohort studies are also limited. For example, the definition of exposure to aspirin in the cohort study of Aselton et al[33] was based on the number of prescriptions that were filled. Because aspirin is used commonly as an over-the-counter medication, some of the control subjects could have been exposed to aspirin but may have been considered unexposed control subjects. On the other hand, in the study by Siffel and Czeizel,[35] exposure occurred only during the first 4 weeks of pregnancy and hence could not be expected to have an effect on malformations that developed later in the first trimester.

Randomized control studies were not subject to the limitations of the studies that were included in this meta-analysis. Indeed, large-scale randomized control studies[10,37-40] of aspirin use during pregnancy have been conducted to determine whether aspirin use prevents preeclampsia and intrauterine growth retardation, and improves pregnancy outcomes. However, because these women were enrolled in these studies during their second and third trimesters and because organogenesis takes place in the first trimester, these studies were not included in our meta-analysis.

In two[16,31] of the three case-control studies that assessed the risk of NTDs, mothers had a fever during the first trimester. In the study by Lynberg et al,[16] other drugs such as acetaminophen and antibiotics were also associated with increased risk of NTDs, which suggests that influenza and hyperthermia rather than aspirin itself could be risk factors for NTDs. Although the reason for aspirin use in the study by Shaw et al[31] was also fever, the cause of the fever could have been different. Because the reasons for aspirin use in the third case-control study were not reported,[17] it is possible that NTDs were associated with aspirin use because the use of aspirin is a marker for maternal hyperthermia. The small (and statistically insignificant) risk of NTDs reported in case-control studies should be viewed carefully in light of these limitations.

Although the exact number of NTDs in exposed infants was not reported, no increased risk of NTDs was reported in the cohort studies.[2,3]

When the results of all eligible studies were included, the risk of CNS defects was not significantly higher among exposed infants than among control infants. However, when the results of only case-control studies were included, we found a small, but statistically significant, risk of such defects. In one of these studies,[29] the exposed women took aspirin for fever. The limitations that are inherent in the differences in control populations and the definitions of aspirin exposure and in recall bias and the use of other drugs also apply to this analysis, so the findings of these studies should be interpreted with caution.

We found no evidence for an increased risk of congenital heart disease in exposed infants. The results of one case-control study suggested an increased risk of conal septal defects in exposed infants.[15] However, after adjustment for the effects of other drugs and maternal symptoms, the only statistically significant associations with aspirin exposure were aortic stenosis and hypoplastic left ventricle. Other drugs such as antibiotics and codeine were associated with an increased risk of specific malformations, which suggests that maternal disease could be a confounding factor in the observed associations. Indeed, maternal upper respiratory tract infection may be a risk factor for conal septal defect.[32]

Our analysis showed a small, but significant, risk of cleft palate and lip among exposed infants, based on the pooled results of two case-control studies.[17,18] These results, however, are subject to the limitations previously outlined. Moreover, in one of these studies,[18] the use of other drugs was associated also with an increased risk of cleft lip and palate, which suggests that other factors could have contributed to the observed association.

Because these results were based on the data from only two studies, the possibility of publication bias should be considered also. In such cases, one negative unpublished study would nullify the trend. The so-called file-drawer effect (the effect of not publishing negative studies) may make such a possibility viable.[41]

Gastroschisis is a rare congenital anomaly that occurs in 3 to 6 of every 100,000 births.[19,42] The increased risk of gastroschisis that was reported in all five case-control studies could not be detected, even in a very large cohort study (a sample of 147,000 in each group would have a power of 0.8 to show a 3-fold increase in risk, with an α level of .05).

However, these results should be interpreted with caution because of the limitations of the studies that are involved. In one study, mothers of infants with gastroschisis were of lower socioeconomic class and had used illegal drugs more often than the mothers of infants in the control group.[21] These factors may account for the findings instead of aspirin. In the study of Werler et al,[23] the diagnosis of gastroschisis was confirmed in only 58% of the cases, and other antipyretic drugs such as acetaminophen were associated with gastroschisis, which suggests that maternal disease could have contributed to the observed association. Two other studies used healthy infants as control subjects and their results were therefore more likely affected by recall bias.[19,20]

The analyzed studies did not indicate an increased risk of hypospadias or musculoskeletal or gastrointestinal defects. However, very few studies reported the incidence of these defects[2,3,17]: each of these effects was reported in only two studies, which makes a definitive conclusion difficult.

The fact that the overall congenital malformation rate was not higher among infants who were exposed to aspirin does not exclude the possibility of an increased risk of rare malformations, as suggested by some of the case-control studies. For example, the incidence of gastroschisis is 3 to 6 in 100,000 births; therefore, even if the risk among exposed infants tripled, it is unlikely it would be detected by a cohort study with 50,000 participants. However, because most studies in our analysis were observational, causality between aspirin use and congenital anomalies cannot be established, even when the analysis indicates an increased risk of malformations. It is possible that the clinical condition or the fever caused the malformations. A meta-analysis is limited by the data available in the literature. Because the dose of aspirin was not specified in most studies, we were unable to analyze the outcomes on the basis of doses.

We found no evidence of an overall increase in rates of major congenital malformations that were associated with aspirin. Exposure to aspirin may be associated with an increased risk of gastroschisis. An increased risk of other specific malformations (such as NTDs, CNS malformations, and cleft lip and palate) cannot be excluded and should be investigated further in studies of more rigorous design. These results would enable physicians to better inform women who have used aspirin during the first trimester of pregnancy. When considering aspirin as a treatment for high-risk pregnancies, one should consider the potential risks against the benefit.

We thank Editorial Services, the Hospital for Sick Children, Toronto, Ontario, Canada, for assistance in the preparation of this manuscript. E. K. was a fellow of the Research Training Centre, the Hospital for Sick Children; G. K. is a senior scientist of the Canadian Institute for Health Research and holder of the Research Leadership for Better Pharmacotherapy during Pregnancy and Lactation.

REFERENCES

1. Richards ID. Congenital malformations and environmental influences in pregnancy. Br J Prev Soc Med 1969;23:218-25.
2. Correy JF, Newman NM, Collins JA, Burrows EA, Burrows RF, Curran JT. Use of prescription drugs in the first trimester and congenital malformations. Aust N Z J Obstet Gynaecol 1991; 31:340-4.
3. Slone D, Siskind V, Heinonen OP, Monson RR, Kaufman DW, Shapiro S. Aspirin and congenital malformations. Lancet 1976;1:1373-5.
4. Werler MM, Mitchell AA, Shapiro S. The relation of aspirin use during the first trimester of pregnancy to congenital cardiac defects. N Engl J Med 1989;321:1639-42.
5. Landy HJ, Kessler C, Kelly WK, Weingold AB. Obstetric performance in patients with the lupus anticoagulant and/or anticardiolipin antibodies. Am J Perinatol 1992;9:146-51.
6. Passaleva A, Massai G, D'Elios MM, Livi C, Abbate R. Prevention of miscarriage in antiphospholipid syndrome. Autoimmunity 1992;14: 121-5.
7. Kwak JYH, Gilman-Sachs A, Beaman KD, Beer AE. Reproductive outcome in women with recurrent spontaneous abortions of alloimmune and autoimmune causes: preconception versus postconception treatment. Am J Obstet Gynecol 1992;166:1787-95.
8. Leitich H, Egarter C, Husslein P, Kaider A, Schemper M. A meta-analysis of low dose aspirin for the prevention of intrauterine growth retardation. Br J Obstet Gynaecol 1997;104:450-9.
9. Imperiale TF, Petrulis AS. A meta-analysis of low-dose aspirin for the prevention of pregnancy-induced hypertensive disease. JAMA 1991;266:260-4.
10. Collaborative Low-dose Aspirin Study in Pregnancy (CLASP) Collaborative Group. CLASP: a randomised trial of low-dose aspirin for the prevention and treatment of pre-eclampsia among 9364 pregnant women. Lancet 1994;343:619-29.
11. Beaufils M, Uzan S, Donsimoni R, Colau JC. Prevention of preeclampsia by early antiplatelet therapy. Lancet 1985;1:840-2.

12. DePass LR, Weaver EV. Comparison of teratogenic effects of aspirin and hydroxyurea in the Fischer 344 and Wistar strains. J Toxicol Environ Health 1982;10:297-305.
13. Klein KL, Scott WJ, Wilson JG. Aspirin-induced teratogenesis: a unique pattern of cell death and subsequent polydactyly in the rat. J Exp Zool 1981;216:107-12.
14. Robertson RT, Allen HL, Bokelman DL. Aspirin: teratogenic evaluation in the dog. Teratology 1979;20:313-20.
15. Zierler S, Rothman KJ. Congenital heart disease in relation to maternal use of Bendectin and other drugs in early pregnancy. N Engl J Med 1985;313:347-52.
16. Lynberg MC, Khoury MJ, Lu X, Cocian T. Maternal flu, fever, and the risk of neural tube defects: a population-based case-control study. Am J Epidemiol 1994;140:244-55.
17. Richards ID. A retrospective enquiry into possible teratogenic effects of drugs in pregnancy. Adv Exp Med Biol 1972;27:441-55.
18. Saxen I. Associations between oral clefts and drugs taken during pregnancy. Int J Epidemiol 1975;4:37-44.
19. Martinez-Frias ML, Rodriguez-Pinilla E, Prieto L. Prenatal exposure to salicylates and gastroschisis: a case-control study. Teratology 1997;56:241-43.
20. Torfs CP, Katz EA, Bateson TF, Lam PK, Curry CJ. Maternal medications and environmental exposures as risk factors for gastroschisis. Teratology 1996;54:84-92.
21. Drongowski RA, Smith RK Jr, Coran AG, Klein MD. Contribution of demographic and environmental factors to the etiology of gastroschisis: a hypothesis. Fetal Diagn Ther 1991;6:14-27.
22. Gierup J, Lundkvist K. Gastroschisis: a pilot study of its incidence and the possible influence of teratogenic factors. Z Kinderchir 1979;28:39-42.
23. Werler MM, Mitchell AA, Shapiro S. First trimester maternal medication use in relation to gastroschisis. Teratology 1992; 45:361-7.
24. Winship KA, Cahal DA, Weber JCP, Griffin JP. Maternal drug histories and central nervous system anomalies. Arch Dis Child 1984;59:1052-60.
25. Pattison NS, Chamley LW, Birdsall M, Zanderigo AM, Liddell HS, McDougall J. Does aspirin have a role in improving pregnancy outcome for women with the antiphospholipid syndrome? A randomized controlled trial. Am J Obstet Gynecol 2000;183:1008-12.
26. Laskin CA, Bombardier C, Hannah ME, et al. Prednisone and aspirin in women with autoantibodies and unexplained recurrent fetal loss. N Engl J Med 1997;337:148-53.
27. Briggs GG, Freeman RK, Yaffe SJ, editors. Drugs in pregnancy and lactation: a reference guide to fetal and neonatal risk. 5th ed. Baltimore (MD): Williams & Wilkins; 1998.
28. Shepard TH. Catalogue of teratogenic agents. 9th ed. Baltimore (MD): Johns Hopkins University Press; 1998.
29. Karkinen-Jääskeläinen M, Saxén L. Maternal influenza, drug consumption, and congenital defects of the central nervous system. Am J Obstet Gynecol 1974;118:815-8.
30. Nelson MM, Forfar JO. Associations between drugs administered during pregnancy and congenital abnormalities of the fetus. BMJ 1971;1:523-7.
31. Shaw GM, Todoroff K, Velie EM, Lammer EJ. Maternal illness, including fever and medication use as risk factors for neural tube defects. Teratology 1998;57:1-7.
32. Tikkanen J, Heinonen OP. Risk factors for cardiovascular malformations in Finland. Eur J Epidemiol 1990;6:348-56.
33. Aselton P, Jick H, Milunsky A, Hunter JR, Stergachis A. First-trimester drug use and congenital disorders. Obstet Gynecol 1985;65:451-5.
34. Newman NM, Correy JF, Dudgeon GI. A survey of congenital abnormalities and drugs in a private practice. Aust N Z J Obstet Gynaecol 1977;17:156-9.
35. Siffel C, Czeizel AE. Study of developmental abnormalities and deaths after human zygote exposure. Mutat Res 1995;334:293-300.
36. Turner G, Collins E. Fetal effects of regular salicylate ingestion in pregnancy. Lancet 1975;2:338-9.
37. Low-dose aspirin in prevention and treatment of intrauterine growth retardation and pregnancy-induced hypertension: Italian study of aspirin in pregnancy. Lancet 1993;341:396-400.
38. ECPPA (Estudo Colaborativo para Prevencao da Pre-eclampsia com Aspirina) Collaborative Group. ECPPA: randomised trial of low dose aspirin for the prevention of maternal and fetal complications in high risk pregnant women. Br J Obstet Gynaecol 1996;103:39-47.
39. Caritis S, Sibai B, Hauth J, et al. Low-dose aspirin to prevent preeclampsia in women at high risk: National Institute of Child Health and Human Development Network of Maternal-Fetal Medicine Units. N Engl J Med 1998;338:701-5.
40. Golding J. A randomised trial of low dose aspirin for primiparae in pregnancy: the Jamaica Low Dose Aspirin Study Group. Br J Obstet Gynaecol 1998;105:293-9.
41. Sutton AJ, Duval SJ, Tweedie RL, Abrams KR, Jones DR. Empirical assessment of effect of publication bias on meta-analyses. BMJ 2000;320:1574-7.
42. Calzolari E, Volpato S, Bianchi F, et al. Omphalocele and gastroschisis: a collaborative study of five Italian congenital malformation registries. Teratology 1993;47:47-55.

CHAPTER 46

FETAL SAFETY OF DRUGS USED IN THE TREATMENT OF ALLERGIC RHINITIS: A CRITICAL REVIEW

Cameron Gilbert,[1,2] *Paolo Mazzotta,*[1] *Ronen Loebstein,*[1] *and Gideon Koren*[1,2]

[1]*Motherisk Program, Division of Clinical Pharmacology and Toxicology, The Hospital for Sick Children, The University of Toronto, Toronto, Ontario, Canada* [2]*The Institute of Medical Science, The University of Toronto, Toronto, Ontario, Canada*

Abstract

Allergic rhinitis is the most common allergic disease. Pharmacological interventions are often not used in pregnancy because of alarming information in drug labels and patient information, even when evidence for safety exists.

Low-risk therapies could include immunotherapy, intranasal sodium cromoglycate (cromolyn sodium), beclometasone, budesonide and first-generation antihistamines. In a meta-analysis examining the safety of first-generation antihistamines in pregnancy, 200 000 first trimester exposures failed to show increased teratogenic risk. Loratadine is the most studied second-generation antihistamine (with a total patient cohort of 2147 women who were exposed) and does not appear to increase the risk of major congenital malformations; however, it has not been as well studied as the earlier antihistamines. Since desloratadine is the principal metabolite of loratadine, it can be assumed that a similar safety profile would fit for desloratadine as was described for loratadine although no direct human studies have been done.

Decongestants have not been conclusively proven to affect the fetal outcome and may be used for short-term relief when no other safer alternatives are available.

Intranasal corticosteroids have not been associated with an increase in congenital malformations in humans. Based on efficacy and the fact that there would be little systemic absorption, they can be considered a first-line treatment over oral antihistamines, decongestants and mast cell stabilisers; however, the number of controlled trials in pregnancy is limited. Intranasal corticosteroids are associated with minimal systemic effects in adults and are the most effective therapy for allergic rhinitis. Benefit-risk considerations must, therefore, be done but favour their first-line use during pregnancy.

Because fetal safety is paramount, recommendations should be based both on the safety of the drugs during pregnancy and the comparative efficacy of the agent in the treatment of the underlying condition. This review exemplifies the fact that there are many safe treatment options for the clinician when dealing with allergic rhinitis during pregnancy.

The symptoms of allergic rhinitis include itching, sneezing, rhinorrhoea and nasal congestion. It can be accompanied by symptoms in the eyes, ears and throat. Typically, there is a gradual decrease in the occurrence and severity of symptoms with age. Symptoms of allergic rhinitis develop before the age of 20 years in 80% of cases and, therefore, fetal safety data on pharmacological treatments are critical to a large number of women.[1] Allergic rhinitis is the most common allergic disease and has shown a prevalence of 42% in 6-year-old children.[1] Allergic diseases are estimated to affect 20–30% of women of childbearing age, making them the most common medical conditions to complicate pregnancy.[2,3]

In this review, we have updated our analysis published in *Drug Safety* in 1999, which examined the safety of different pharmacological interventions available to treat allergic rhinitis in pregnancy.[4] MEDLINE and EMBASE electronic databases were searched from 1966 to September 2004 to identify relevant observational studies. The keywords included the specific drug, generic and brand name, along with ‘rhinitis’ and ‘pregnancy’. We examined fetal outcome with respect to major and minor congenital malformations. We tried to highlight the gaps of knowledge and methodological issues that may have hindered the interpretation of existing data. We decided not to include homeopathy or other alternative treatments in this review.

PATHOPHYSIOLOGY OF ALLERGIC RHINITIS

General Mechanism of Allergic Rhinitis

The fluid in the nasal mucosa contains IgA and IgE. IgE antibodies fix to the mucosal and submucosal mast cells. With the introduction of an allergen into the nose, the mucosal and submucosal mast cells generate and release mediators, such as histamine, prostaglandin D_2 and leukotrienes, that are capable of producing tissue oedema, gland stimulation, sinusoidal congestion and sensory nerve activation, as well as late-phase reactions that lead to an influx of eosinophils. The intensity of the clinical response to inhaled allergens is correlated with the antigen dose and levels of specific IgE antibodies, as well as basophilic cell mediator releasability.[4] Once sensitised to allergens, exposures can trigger events that result in the symptoms of allergic rhinitis.[1]

Allergic Rhinitis and Pregnancy

Pregnancy has been demonstrated to affect certain mediators of the immediate hypersensitivity type reaction and their modulating factors. Plasma histamine levels in women with allergic conditions have been demonstrated to be significantly lower during the first trimester of pregnancy compared with postpartum levels.[5] Despite the theoretical protective effects of these changes on the course of allergic rhinitis, the actual clinical effects are unknown. More clinically relevant, pregnancy-related hormonal changes can lead to nasal mucosal congestion. This congestion is secondary to increased circulating blood volume and increased activity of the nasal mucosal cells, resulting in swelling and increased secretions.[6]

‘Vasomotor rhinitis of pregnancy’ is an entity that is characterised by nasal congestion limited to the gestational period, with more prominent symptoms during the second and third trimesters of pregnancy. It is important to note that, like asthma, pre-existing symptoms of chronic rhinitis may improve, worsen or remain unchanged during pregnancy. It has been reported that nasal symptoms in pregnant women who have allergic rhinitis tend to improve in 34%, worsen in

15% and remain unchanged in the remainder of the women.[7] Another common symptom related to rhinitis during pregnancy is ear fullness that is secondary to eustachian tube congestion.[4]

SAFETY DATA FOR PHARMACOLOGICAL INTERVENTIONS IN PREGNANCY

Rhinitis management may consist of allergen avoidance, pharmacological treatment or immunotherapy. The first trimester of pregnancy is the most critical time for fetal development. Most drugs are contraindicated during pregnancy by their manufacturers, based, for the most part, on the fact that there are little human data or fetal outcomes. It is only after sufficient human observational data that safety of drugs during pregnancy can be established. In the following sections, when discussing different pharmacological interventions, the rate of congenital malformations will be compared with the baseline rate of congenital malformations in the general population (1–5%, depending on the comparison group and methodology of the detection of malformations).[8] When congenital malformations have been reported, the defects are reviewed to determine whether there is a pattern that could suggest a drug effect.

Methodological Considerations

Many of the studies identified by us are quite small and have a low power to reveal a significant teratogenic effect of a drug. A number of the existing studies are too small to draw any conclusions; moreover, the quality of studies varies widely. For example, retrospective studies are likely to have poorer data collection and potential recall and re porting bias.

First-Generation Antihistamines

First-generation antihistamines are characterised by their longevity on the market and their potential for certain adverse effects. A summary of teratogenicity studies for first-generation antihistamines in humans and animals is given in table I and table II, respectively.

Several meta-analyses have been conducted by the Motherisk Program, which examined the safety of antihistamines used in the treatment of nausea and vomiting in pregnancy and other conditions and concluded that, as a class, they were safe to use during pregnancy.[28] Based on large numbers, no excess of any specific type of congenital malformations was detected.

Alkylamines. Alkylamines include chlorphenamine (chlorpheniramine), dexchlorpheniramine, brompheniramine and triprolidine.

The Collaborative Perinatal Project found 90 major/minor congenital malformations out of 1070 pregnancies with first trimester exposure to chlorphenamine.[8] A retrospective cohort study and a record linkage study (congenital malformation rate of 3.3%) both looked at exposure to chlorphenamine and failed to demonstrate an increased risk.[11]

Table I
Summary of Teratogenicity Studies for First-Generation Antihistamines in Humans

DRUG	EXPOSED[a]	CONTROL[b]	RELATIVE RISK (95% CI)	REFERENCE
Brompheniramine	10/65	3238/50 217	2.34 (1.31, 4.17)[c]	8
	5/172	100/6337	1.84 (0.76, 4.46)	9
	1/34	2/34	0.50 (0.05, 5.26)	10
Chlorphenamine (chlorpheniramine)	90/1070	3158/49 212	1.2 (0.98, 1.46)[c]	8
	4/257	101/6252	0.96 (0.36, 2.6)	9
	2/61	ND	ND	11
Dexchlorpheniramine	50/1080	ND	ND	
Triprolidine	6/384	74/6453	1.36 (0.6, 3.11)	12
	3/244	102/6265	0.76 (0.24, 2.36)	9
Diphenhydramine	20/599	6/599	1.56 (1.25, 1.94)	13
	49/595	3199/49 687	1.25 (0.95, 1.64)[c]	8
	1/361	79/6476	0.23 (0.03, 1.63)	12
	4/270	101/6239	0.92 (0.34, 2.47)	9
	80/1461	ND	ND	11
Tripelennamine	6/100	3242/50 182	0.81 (0.37, 1.76)[c]	8
Hydroxyzine	1/74	0/34	1.40 (0.06, 33.51)	14
	5/50	3243/50 232	1.57 (0.68, 3.62)[c]	8
	6/43	2/44	3.07 (0.66, 14.38)	15
	48/828	ND	ND	11
Clemastine	71/1617	ND	ND	11
	39/1230	549/16 967	0.98 (0.72, 1.33)	16
Azatadine	6/127	ND	ND	11
Cyproheptadine	12/285	ND	ND	11

a Number of major/minor fetal malformations in total number of pregnancies exposed to the drug.
b Number of major/minor fetal malformations in total number of pregnancies not exposed to the drug.
c Hospital-standardised relative risk.
ND = no data.

Table II
Results of Teratogenicity Studies for Antihistamines and Decongestants in Animals

DRUG	TERATOGENIC CORRELATION WITH DRUG	REFERENCE
First-generation antihistamines		
Brompheniramine	Negative	17
Chlorphenamine (chlorpheniramine)	Negative	17
Dexchlorpheniramine	Negative	11
Triprolidine	Negative	18
Diphenhydramine	Positive	19
	Negative	17
Tripelennamine	Negative	18
Hydroxyzine	Positive	20
	Negative	21
Clemastine	Negative	11
Azatadine	Negative	11
Cyproheptadine	Positive	22
	Negative	11
	Negative	23
Second-generation antihistamines		
Cetirizine	Negative	24
Astemizole	Positive	19
	Negative	17
Loratadine	Negative	25
Terfenadine	Negative	26
Oral decongestants		
Phenylephrine	Positive	17
Phenylpropanolamine	Negative	27
Ephedrine	Positive	11
Intranasal decongestants		
Phenylephrine	Positive	17

Dexchlorpheniramine is the dextrorotatory-isomer of chlorphenamine. In a retrospective record linkage study, 50 malformations out of 1080 exposed pregnancies were observed (congenital malformation rate of 4.6%) and no pattern of defects was detected.[11]

In recent guidelines published on the treatment of allergic rhinitis during pregnancy, chlorphenamine and dexchlorpheniramine are no longer recommended as first-line treatment.[29]

The Collaborative Perinatal Project identified 65 women exposed to brompheniramine in the first trimester of pregnancy. Ten congenital malformations occurred that represented an increased rate as compared with the general population (15% vs 5%).[8] This cohort is grossly underpowered to draw any conclusions. Also, there were no specific clusters of congenital malformations identified and the sample size was very small. The investigators also cautioned that their results did not demonstrate causation due to the lack of dose information and the variety of other exposures and underlying diseases in the women studied.[8] In contrast, yet another small cohort could not detect an increased risk for congenital malformations following first-trimester exposure.[9,10] Sixteen women took triprolidine in the first trimester as reported by the Collaborative Perinatal Project. However, the outcomes were not reported in this group.[8] Two other studies did not detect an increased risk for major congenital malformations when brompheniramine was taken in the first trimester.[9,12]

Ethanolamines. Ethanolamines include carbinoxamine, clemastine and diphendydramine. Studies on diphenhydramine provide contradicting results regarding development of congenital malformations. A retrospective study examining diphenhydramine in the first trimester of pregnancy found an increased incidence of cleft palate.[13] In addition, a record linkage study found an increase rate for congenital malformations when looking at 1000 women exposed during the first trimester (80 of 1461 women exposed), although no pattern of defects was found.[11] However, the first study was done retrospectively and, therefore, the participants might have been limited by their recall bias of drug use in their pregnancy and in addition confounding variables, such as other drug exposures, were not used as a matching criteria.[13] However, the Collaborative Perinatal Project and two retrospective cohort studies did not detect any increased risk for congenital malformations when women were exposed in the first trimester.[8,9,12] This combined cohort includes a total of 1226 exposed patients, which is an inadequate sample size to detect a specific malformation such as oral clefts (incidence of 1 in 1000). In addition, Nelson and Forfar,[30] in a retrospective cohort study looking at antihistamine use during the first trimester, could not find any association between major congenital malformations and the drugs. In this study, diphenhydramine was the second most commonly used drug.

In a record linkage study of clemastine, there was no increase in the rate of congenital malformations (71 of 1617 women exposed).[11] The data from the Swedish Medical Birth Registry include 1230 exposures to clemastine with a congenital malformation rate of 3.2%.[16] There are limited data on carbinox-amine use during pregnancy. The Collaborative Perinatal Project reported two exposures during the first-trimester; however, pregnancy outcomes were not reported.[8]

Ethylenediamine. The only ethylenediamine is tripelennamine and there are limited data of its exposure in pregnancy. The Collaborative Perinatal Project reported six major/minor congenital malformations of 100 first trimester exposures.[8]

Piperazines. The only drug in clinical use from piperazines is hydroxyzine. In a record linkage study, the rate of congenital malformations was 5.8%;[11] however, two early prospective cohort studies and one more recent one were all negative for an association between hydroxyzine exposure during pregnancy and birth defects, although these studies only included 167 exposures.[8,14,15]

Piperidines. There are limited data on piperidines use during pregnancy, although all reported data did not detect an increased rate of congenital malformations for women exposed to these drugs. A record linkage study looking at azatadine and cyproheptadine did not detect an association between these drugs and congenital malformations (6 of 127 exposed for azatadine and 12 of 285 exposed for cyproheptadine).[11] The Collaborative Perinatal Project also reported data on three women exposed to cyproheptadine, although no data on the pregnancy outcome was given.[8]

Second-Generation Antihistamines

Second-generation antihistamines are mainly lacking the central nervous adverse effects of their earlier counterparts and are, therefore, a first-choice treatment for allergic rhinitis; however, most of them lack large safety studies in pregnancy. A summary of teratogenicity studies for second-generation antihistamines in animals and humans is presented in table II and table III, respectively.

Astemizole. There is one published prospective cohort study on astemizole use during pregnancy. There was no association between first-trimester exposure to the drug and the occurrence of major congenital malformations.[31] However, it has been withdrawn in many countries because of cardiotoxicity.

Azelastine. There are no published studies of exposure during pregnancy.

Cetirizine. Cetirizine is an active metabolite of hydroxyzine. Given the negative teratogenicity findings for hydroxyzine (section 2.2.4), it is unlikely that cetirizine would be a serious concern for use in pregnancy. There is one published prospective cohort study of its use in pregnancy and the investigators did not find a statistically significant difference between exposed and control groups in the rates of major congenital malformations, although the study only included 33 exposed subjects.[15] The data from the Swedish Medical Birth Registry includes 917 exposures to cetirizine with no increased incidence of congenital malformations.[16]

Fexofenadine. Fexofenadine is a metabolite of terfenadine. There are no epidemiological studies in human pregnancy published; however, in animal studies it was found to be negative for teratogenicity at levels up to 47 times the therapeutic levels.[35] In rats with doses three times the human therapeutic levels, there was a decrease in the number of implantations and an increase in post-implantation loss. It was also found that there was a decrease in pup weight gain when mothers were administered fexofenadine.[35]

Loratadine. In a Swedish study, the incidence of hypospadias was twice that of the general population for children born to mothers who had taken loratadine (7 of 1796 women exposed to loratadine).[16,36] This has caused an international wave of concern as the drug is very widely used; however, despite its limited statistical power, it might well be a random effect. This rate was not confirmed in two other controlled studies that were both published in 2003, although both studies had small sample sizes. Neither study showed a significant difference in outcomes between the loratadine-exposed group and the controls. Moretti et al.[32] found a rate of 5 congenital malformations of 161 exposures in the exposed group versus 6 of 161 in control group. In the exposed group, there were no cases of hypospadias (there was one case of hypospadias in the nonexposed control group).[32] Diav-Citrin et al.[33] found the rate of major congenital malformations to be 2.3%, 4% and 3% for loratadine, the other anti histamine group and the non-teratogenic control group, respectively. Again, in this study there were no cases of hypospadias in the loratadine-exposed group.[33] The Centers for Disease Control and Prevention recently examined data from the NBDPS (National Birth Defects Prevention Study) and found no increased risk for second or third-degree hypospadias.[34,37]

Desloratadine. Desloratadine is the principal metabolite of loratadine. At 230-fold the area under the plasma concentration-time curve in humans at the recommended daily oral dose, animal studies were negative for teratogenicity.[38] However, as with loratadine the concerns regarding hypospadias have been aired, but not proven.[27]

Terfenadine. There have been four studies examining the safety of terfenadine in human pregnancy. In none of the four studies did the investigators find an increase in the rate of congenital malformations.[11,16,39,40] Specific data are available on three of the four studies. In the first study, a record linkage study, the rate of malformations was found to be 4.9% (51 of 1034 women exposed).[11] In the second study, a prospective controlled study, no congenital malformations were found, although a lower mean birth rate was seen among those exposed to terfenadine during the first trimester.[40] The data from the Swedish Medical Birth Registry include 917 exposures to terfenadine with a congenital malformation rate of 3.22%.[16] However, like astemizole, it has been withdrawn in many countries because of cardiotoxicity.

Other Antihistamines. Other second-generation antihistamines have not been well studied. There are no human or animal studies

Table III
Summary of Teratogenicity Studies for Second-Generation Antihistamines in Humans

DRUG	EXPOSED[a]	CONTROL[b]	RELATIVE RISK (95% CI)	REFERENCE
Cetirizine	2/33	2/38	1.15 (0.17, 7.73)	15
	36/917	552/17 280	1.22 (0.89, 1.69)	16
Astemizole	2/114	2/114	1 (0.14, 6.98)	31
Loratadine	61/1796	527/16 401	1.05 (0.83, 1.34)	16
	5/143	6/150	0.93 (0.48, 1.79)	32
	4/175	25/844	0.80 (0.32, 2.00)	33
	11/33	547/1957	1.29 (0.62, 2.68)[c]	34
Terfenadine	51/1031	ND		11
	37/1164	551/17 033	0.98 (0.72, 1.35)	16

a Number of major/minor fetal malformations in total number of pregnancies exposed to the drug.
b Number of major/minor fetal malformations in total number of pregnancies not exposed to the drug.
c Odds ratio as it was a case-control study.
ND = no data.

that could be located on acrivastine or mizolastine. One published animal study found no association between ebastine and congenital malformations at doses higher than those used in humans.[41]

Oral Decongestants

Oral decongestants are typically used alone or in conjunction with second-generation antihistamines. They include phenylephrine, phenylpropanolamine and pseudoephedrine. A summary of teratogenicity studies in humans and animals is given in table IV and table II, respectively.

Phenylephrine. There have been contradicting reports published regarding the safety of phenylephrine during pregnancy. The Collaborative Perinatal Project and a case-control study both found an association between the drug and the occurrence of congenital malformations.[42,46] However, a retrospective cohort study could not find any association between exposure to the drug and congenital malformations.[9] In two case-control studies that investigated the association between phenylephrine and cardiac defects, gastroschisis and vascular disruption defects, no association could be confirmed.[43,44]

Phenylpropanolamine. In two early studies, contradicting results were found on the association between phenylpropanolamine and congenital malformations. The Collaborative Perinatal Project found a positive occurrence between the drug and congenital malformations, although a retrospective cohort study did not.[8,9] Two other studies examined the risk of gastroschisis associated with phenylpropanolamine use in pregnancy. The results of the studies are contradicting;[44,45] however, a more recent study did not verify gastroschisis suspicions in 206 cases and 798 controls.[47] It must be considered that the viral illness causing the upper respiratory tract infection, and not the drug, may increase the risk for gastroschisis.

Pseudoephedrine. There have been numerous studies that examined the safety of pseudoephedrine during pregnancy and only one found a statistically significant association between the drug and congenital malformations. The Collaborative Perinatal Project,[8] two retrospective cohort studies,[9,12] one case-control study[45] and a record linkage study (malformation rate of 3.9%)[11] were not able to detect an association between the drug and any specific malformation. However, one case-control study found a statistically significant association between pseudoephedrine and gastroschisis and vascular disruption defects.[44] The relative risk for use in the first trimester was found to be 3.2.[44]

Ephedrine. In one published study, 373 women exposed to ephedrine in the first trimester had a congenital malformation rate of 4.6%.[8]

Intranasal/Ophthalmic Decongestants

The intranasal/ophthalmic decongestants are typically categorised based on their duration of action. For example, phenylephrine is a short-acting agent, naphazoline is an intermediate-acting agent and

Table IV
Summary of Teratogenicity Studies for Oral Decongestants in Humans

DRUG	EXPOSED[a]	CONTROL[b]	RELATIVE RISK (95% CI)	REFERENCE
Phenylephrine	102/1249	3146/49 033	1.23 (1.02, 1.49)[c]	8
	10/390	15/1254	1.70 (1.05, 2.78)	42
	6/301	99/6208	1.25 (0.55, 2.83)	9
	10/298	25/738	0.99 (0.58, 1.69)	43
	0/76	43/2142	0.32 (0.02, 5.13)	44[d]
	2/416	43/2142	0.27 (0.07, 1.05)	44[e]
Phenylpropanolamine	71/726	3177/49 556	1.40 (1.11, 1.75)[c]	8
	7/254	98/6255	1.76 (0.83, 3.75)	9
	4/76	74/2142	1.52 (0.57, 4.07)	44[d]
	19/416	74/2142	1.27 (0.84, 1.91)	44[e]
	5/110	1/220	2.57 (1.74, 3.8)	45
Pseudoephedrine	1/39	3247/50 243	0.35 (0.05, 2.42)[c]	8
	8/865	72/5972	0.77 (0.37, 1.59)	
	10/665	95/5844	0.93 (0.48, 1.77)	9
	9/76	79/2142	3.25 (1.68, 6.31)	44[d]
	26/416	79/2142	1.56 (1.1, 2.2)	44[e]
	9/110	9/220	1.54 (0.95, 2.52)	45
	37/940	ND		11
Ephedrine	17/373	3231/49 909	0.69 (0.43, 1.12)[c]	8

a Number of major/minor fetal malformations in total number of pregnancies exposed to the drug.
b Number of major/minor fetal malformations in total number of pregnancies not exposed to the drug.
c Hospital-standardised relative risk.
d Children born with gastroschisis.
e Children born with vascular disruption.
ND = no data.

oxymetazoline is a long-acting agent. A summary of the teratogenicity studies for these drugs in animals and humans can be found in table II and table V, respectively.

Short-Acting Decongestants. The only short-acting decongestant is phenylephrine and its safety data have already been reviewed in section 2.3.1. These agents have duration of action of up to 4 hours.

Intermediate-Acting Decongestants. Intermediate-acting decongestants include naphazoline and tetryzoline (tetrahydrozoline). These drugs have duration of action of 4–6 hours. There are limited documented data on the use of naphazoline and tetryzoline in pregnancy. The Collaborative Perinatal Project looked at 20 women exposed to naphazoline during pregnancy and one baby was born with a malformation. Three women were exposed to tetryzoline during pregnancy, but the outcomes of these pregnancies were not recorded.[8] A case-control study that looked at the association of these drugs with gastroschisis could not confirm any association.[44]

Long-Acting Decongestants. Long-acting decongestants have duration of action of up to 12 hours. This class includes oxymetazoline and xylometazoline. In two published studies, one retrospective and one case-control, neither drug was found to be significantly associated with congenital malformations.[9,44] The Collaborative Perinatal Project reported two exposures to oxymetazoline and eight exposures to xylometazoline; however, there were no data on the outcomes of the pregnancies.[8] Both drugs are widely used by pregnant women.

Ophthalmic Antihistamines

Ophthalmic antihistamines include antazoline, levocabastine and pheniramine. There have been no epidemiological studies in human pregnancy done on any of these drugs except for pheniramine. The Collaborative Perinatal Project monitored 831 women who were exposed to pheniramine during the first trimester of pregnancy and did not detect an increase in congenital malformations.[11]

Inhaled/Intranasal Corticosteroids

The most common corticosteroids used to treat allergic rhinitis are beclometasone, budesonide, dexamethasone, flunisolide, fluticasone propionate, mometasone and triamcinolone.

There are very few population studies on the safety of inhaled or intranasal corticosteroids during pregnancy. In a prospective study looking at the safety of beclometasone in 40 women during the first trimester, the incidence of congenital malformations was not significantly different from the baseline rate (1 of 43 live births).[48] In an earlier study examining the safety of beclometasone in first-trimester exposure, there were no congenital defects found that were attributed to the drug.[49] A record linkage study looking at beclometasone exposure during the first trimester could not detect an increased rate for congenital malformations (16 of 395 women exposed).[29]

In 2014 pregnancies exposed to inhaled budesonide, 76 infants in the exposed group had a congenital malformation. The investigators compared this rate of 3.8% to the rate of congenital malformations in the general population (3.5% used in this study) and concluded that it is unlikely that there is any no increased risk.[50] Analysis of the data from the manufacturer's postmarketing surveillance did not find clustering of defects.[11] This large sample size and low congenital malformation rate makes it unlikely that the malformations were caused by the drug.

In a randomised, double-blind, placebo-controlled study that looked at the efficacy of fluticasone propionate nasal spray in pregnancy, no effects on the outcomes of the pregnancies were found.[51] The budesonide studies[50] were conducted in pregnant women with asthma where systematic exposure to the inhaled drug was much longer than that encountered in allergic rhinitis.

Table V
Summary of Teratogenicity Studies for Ophthalmic Antihistamines and Intranasal/Ophthalmic Decongestants in Humans

DRUG	EXPOSED[a]	CONTROL[b]	RELATIVE RISK (95% CI)	REFERENCE
Pheniramine	68/831	3180/49 451	1.24 (0.98, 1.56)[c]	8
Phenylephrine	0/76	8/2142	1.61 (0.11, 23.96)	44[d]
	1/416	8/2142	0.68 (0.11, 4.34)	44[d]
Naphazoline	1/20	3247/50 262	0.61 (0.09, 4.13)[c]	8
	0/76	2/2142	4.83 (0.38, 61.24)	44[d]
	0/416	2/2142	1.02 (0.08, 12.87)	44[e]
Tetryzoline (tetrahydrozoline hydrochloride)	0/76	2/2142	4.83 (0.38, 61.24)	44[d]
	0/416	2/2142	1.02 (0.08, 12.87)	44[e]
Oxymetazoline	2/155	103/6354	0.80 (0.2, 3.2)	9
	0/76	18/2142	0.76 (0.05)	44[d]
	4/416	18/2142	1.12 (0.46, 2.73)	44[e]
Xylometazoline	5/207	100/6302	1.52 (0.63, 3.7)	9
	0/76	6/2142	2.07 (0.14, 30.14)	44[d]
	1/416	6/2142	0.88 (0.14, 5.4)	44[e]

a Number of major/minor fetal malformations in total number of pregnancies exposed to the drug.
b Number of major/minor fetal malformations in total number of pregnancies not exposed to the drug.
c Hospital-standardised relative risk.
d Children born with gastroschisis.
e Children born with vascular disruption.

Mast Cell Stabilisers

Sodium Cromoglycate (Cromolyn Sodium). Intranasal sodium cromoglycate (cromolyn sodium) is a mast cell stabiliser used for the prophylaxis of allergic rhinitis. In two studies, one intervention study and one record linkage study, no association between the drug and congenital malformations were found. In the first study, 296 women were treated with sodium cromoglycate in the first trimester (4 babies were born with malformations to 296 women exposed).[52] In the second study, 7 babies were born with malformations to 191 women exposed to sodium cromoglycate.[11] In a third study, there were reassuring data on 151 first-trimester exposures to intranasal and/or inhaled sodium cromoglycate in pregnancy.[53]

Nedocromil. Nedocromil has similar pharmacological action to sodium cromoglycate. In animal studies at doses 800 times the human maintenance dose, nedocromil was not found to be teratogenic.[54]

Lodoxamide. There are no reported controlled teratogenicity studies in human pregnancy.

Immunotherapy

Allergen immunotherapy is primarily used in patients with chronic symptoms of allergies or hay fever. It differs from pharmacotherapy in that immunotherapy is preventative rather than used to treat symptoms. There have been a number of case reports of women who have used immunotherapy during pregnancy for the treatment of allergic rhinitis, hay fever and dust and pollen asthma without any adverse outcomes reported.[55-59] The Collaborative Perinatal Project did not detect an increase in the rate of major congenital malformations with the use of desensitisation vaccines during pregnancy. However, a statistically significant increase was reported with the use of specific desensitisation vaccines (i.e. house dust extract, poison oak extract and poison ivy extract).[8] Two retrospective cohort studies did not find any association between the use of major congenital malformations.[60,61] One earlier study found an association between spontaneous abortions and pregnant women exposed to desensitising vaccines and one investigator published a case report of a woman who had an injection of grass pollen vaccine and had a spontaneous abortion.[62,63] The WHO published standards with regards to the use of immunotherapy treatment in pregnancy and it was not contraindicated; however, the WHO did advise to refrain from increasing the dose during pregnancy to prevent an anaphylactic accident.[29] A summary of teratogenicity studies for immunotherapy can be found in table VI.

Table VI
Summary of Teratogenicity Studies for Immunotherapy in Humans

EXPOSED[a]	CONTROL[b]	RELATIVE RISK (95% CI)	REFERENCE
6/64	3242/50 218	1.32 (0.61, 2.83)[c]	8[d]
3/14	3242/50 218	4.25 (1.52, 11.87)[c]	8[e]
3/115	3/119	1.03 (0.21, 5.02)	60
0/105	1/60	1.72[f]	61

a Number of major/minor fetal malformations in total number of pregnancies exposed to the drug.
b Number of major/minor fetal malformations in total number of pregnancies not exposed to the drug.
c Hospital-standardised relative risk.
d Allergy desensitisation vaccine.
e Specific desensitisation vaccine.
f Mantel-Haenszel χ^2 value, $p = 0.37$.

CONCLUSIONS

Pharmacological interventions in pregnancy always require a benefit-risk examination of the drug and the underlying condition. Guidelines for the treatment of allergic rhinitis have been published by the ARIA-WHO (Allergic Rhinitis and its Impact on Asthma – in collaboration with WHO).[29] This review exemplifies the fact that there are more than a few treatments available for use during pregnancy with no increased risk for congenital malformations. These treatments are summarised in table VII.

Low-risk therapies could include immunotherapy, intranasal sodium cromoglycate, beclometasone, budesonide and first-generation antihistamines. In a meta-analysis that examined the safety of first-generation antihistamines in pregnancy, 200 000 first-trimester exposures failed to show increased teratogenic risk.[28] Loratadine is the most studied second-generation antihistamine and does not appear to increase the risk of major congenital malformations; however, it has not been as well studied as the earlier antihistamines.

Decongestants have not been conclusively proven to affect the fetal outcome and may be used for short-term relief when no other safer alternatives are available.

Intranasal corticosteroids have not been associated with an increase in congenital malformations in humans. Based on efficacy,[64,65] they can be considered a first-line treatment over oral antihistamines, decongestants and mast cell stabilisers; however, the number of controlled trials in pregnancy is limited. Intranasal corticosteroids are associated with minimal systemic effects in

Table VII
Summary of Medications for the Management of Allergic Rhinitis in Pregnancy

EVIDENCE OF SAFETY	RECOMMENDATIONS
First-line safety	Avoidance of allergens Immunotherapy[a] Intranasal sodium cromoglycate (cromolyn sodium) Intranasal beclometasone, budesonide First-generation antihistamines chlorphenamine (chlorpheniramine) tripelennamine hydroxyzine
Second-line safety	Decongestants[b] phenylephrine oxymetazoline Second-generation antihistamines loratadine astemizole cetirizine
Of unproven safety in the first trimester of pregnancy	Fexofenadine

a Only if patient has initiated therapy prior to pregnancy.
b For acute relief only.

adults and are the most effective therapy for allergic rhinitis. Benefit-risk considerations must, therefore, be done but favour their first-line use during pregnancy.

Untreated rhinitis during pregnancy may exacerbate existing asthma and, therefore, adversely affect the pregnancy outcome, hence it is important to consider treatment.[66] Untreated rhinitis may also be a problem for the pregnancy by interfering with maternal eating, sleeping and emotional well being. Moreover, it may cause snoring during pregnancy, which has been associated with pregnancy-induced hypertension and intrauterine growth retardation.[67] Although women often choose not to be treated because of unfounded fears of teratogenicity, the option of intervention with drugs should not be discounted given the growing body of evidence on safety. Physicians should follow evidence-based, rather than emotionally based, medicine.

ACKNOWLEDGEMENTS

Dr G. Koren holds the Ivey Chair in Molecular Toxicology at the University of Western Ontario. Mr C. Gilbert is supported by the Government of Ontario/Edward Dunlop Foundation Scholarship in Science and Technology. No sources of funding were used to assist in the preparation of this review. Dr P. Mazzotta and Dr R. Loebstein have no conflicts of interest that are directly relevant to the content of this review.

REFERENCES

1. Skoner DP. Allergic rhinitis: definition, epidemiology, pathophysiology, detection, and diagnosis. J Allergy Clin Immunol 2001; 108 (1 Suppl.): S2-8.
2. Mabry RL. Intranasal steroid injection during pregnancy. South Med J 1980; 73 (9): 1176-9.
3. Mabry RL. Rhinitis of pregnancy. South Med J 1986; 79 (8): 965–71.
4. Mazzotta P, Loebstein R, Koren G. Treating allergic rhinitis in pregnancy: safety considerations. Drug Saf 1999; 20 (4): 361-75.
5. Beeley L. Adverse effects of drugs in later pregnancy. Clin Obstet Gynaecol 1981; 8 (2): 275-90.
6. Sorri M, Hartikainen-Sorri AL, Karja J. Rhinitis during pregnancy. Rhinology 1980; 18 (2): 83-6.
7. Schatz M, Zeiger RS. Diagnosis and management of rhinitis during pregnancy. Allergy Proc 1988; 9 (5): 545-54.
8. Heinonen OP, Slone D, Shapiro S. Birth defects and drugs in pregnancy. Littleton (MA): Publishing Sciences Group, 1977.
9. Aselton P, Jick H, Milunsky A, et al. First-trimester drug use and congenital disorders. Obstet Gynecol 1985; 65 (4): 451-5.
10. Seto A, Einarson T, Koren G. Evaluation of brompheniramine safety in pregnancy. Reprod Toxicol 1993; 7 (4): 393-5.
11. Briggs GG, Freeman RK, Yaffe S. Drugs in pregnancy and lactation. 5th ed. Baltimore (MD): Williams and Wilkins, 1998.
12. Jick H, Holmes LB, Hunter JR, et al. First-trimester drug use and congenital disorders. JAMA 1981; 246 (4): 343-6.
13. Saxen I. Cleft palate and maternal diphenhydramine intake [letter]. Lancet 1974; I (7854): 407-8.
14. Erez S, Schifrin BS, Dirim O. Double-blind evaluation of hydroxyzine as an antiemetic in pregnancy. J Reprod Med 1971;7 (1): 35-7.
15. Einarson A, Bailey B, Jung G, et al. Prospective controlled study of hydroxyzine and cetirizine in pregnancy. Ann Allergy Asthma Immunol 1997; 78 (2): 183-6.
16. Kallen B. Use of antihistamine drugs in early pregnancy and delivery outcome. J Matern Fetal Neonatal Med 2002; 11 (3): 146-52.
17. Schardein JL. Chemically induced birth defects. New York: Marcel Dekker Inc, 1993.
18. Physicians' Desk Reference. Montvale (NJ): Medical Economics Company, 1989.
19. Sciallia AR, Lione A. Pregnancy effects of specific medications used to treat asthma and immunological diseases. In: Schatz M, Zeiger RS, Claman HN, editors. Asthma and immunological diseases in pregnancy and early infancy. New York: Marcel Dekker Inc., 1998.
20. King CT, Howell J. Teratogenic effect of buclizine and hydroxizine in the rat and chlorcyclizine in the mouse. Am J Obstet Gynecol 1966; 95 (1): 109-11.
21. Steffek AJ, King CT, Wilk AL. Abortive effects and comparative metabolism of chlorcyclizine in various mammalian species. Teratology 1968; 1 (4): 399-406.
22. Shepard TH. Catalog of teratogenic agents. Baltimore (MD): The John Hopkins University Press, 1998.
23. Pfeifer Y, Sadowsky E, Sulman FG. Prevention of serotonin abortion in pregnant rats by five serotonin antagonists. Obstet Gynecol 1969; 33 (5): 709-14.
24. Kamijima M, Sakai KK, et al. Reproductive and developmental toxicity studies of cetirizine in rats and rabbits. Clin Rep 1994; 28: 1877-903.
25. Claritin [product information]. Memphis (TN): Schering-Plough Healthcare Products Inc., 2002.
26. Gibson JP, Huffmann KW, Newberne JW. Preclinical safety studies with terfenadine. Arzneimittel Forschung 1982; 32 (9a): 1179-84.
27. Loratadine, desloratadine and pregnancy: don't use, risk of hypospadias. Prescrire Int 2003; 12 (67): 183.
28. Seto A, Einarson T, Koren G. Pregnancy outcome following first trimester exposure to antihistamines: meta-analysis. Am J Perinatol 1997; 14 (3): 119-24.
29. Bousquet J, Van Cauwenberge P, Khaltaev N. Allergic rhinitis and its impact on asthma. J Allergy Clin Immunol 2001; 108 (5 Suppl.): S147-334.
30. Nelson MM, Forfar JO. Associations between drugs administered during pregnancy and congenital abnormalities of the fetus. BMJ 1971; 1 (5748): 523-7.
31. Pastuszak A, Schick B, D'Alimonte D, et al. The safety of astemizole in pregnancy. J Allergy Clin Immunol 1996; 98 (4): 748-50.
32. Moretti ME, Caprara D, Coutinho CJ, et al. Fetal safety of loratadine use in the first trimester of pregnancy: a multicenter study. J Allergy Clin Immunol 2003; 111 (3): 479-83.
33. Diav-Citrin O, Shechtman S, Aharonovich A, et al. Pregnancy outcome after gestational exposure to loratadine or antihistamines: a prospective controlled cohort study. J Allergy Clin Immunol 2003; 111 (6): 1239-43.
34. Centers for Disease Control and Prevention (CDC). Evaluation of an association between loratadine and hypospadias: United States, 1997–2001. MMWR Morb Mortal Wkly Rep 2004; 53 (10): 219-21.
35. Allegra [product information]. Kansas City (MO): Aventis Corporation, 2003.
36. Kallen B, Olausson PO. Monitoring of maternal drug use and infant congenital malformations: does loratadine cause hypospadias? Int J Risk Saf Med 2001; 14: 115-9.
37. Yoon PW, Rasmussen SA, Lynberg MC, et al. The National Birth Defects Prevention Study. Public Health Rep 2001; 116 Suppl. 1: 32–40.
38. Clarinex [product information]. Kenilworth (NJ): Schering Corporation, 2002.

39. Schick B, Hom M, Librizzi R, et al. Terfenadine (Seldane) exposure in early pregnancy [abstract]. Teratology 1994; 49 (5): 417.
40. Loebstein R, Lalkin A, Addis A, et al. Pregnancy outcome after gestational exposure to terfenadine: a multicenter, prospective controlled study. J Allergy Clin Immunol 1999; 104 (5): 953-6.
41. Aoki Y, Terada Y. Reproductive and developmental toxicity studies of ebastine (2): teratogenicity study in rats. Yakuri to Chiryo 1994; 22: 1193-1215.
42. Rothman KJ, Fyler DC, Goldblatt A, et al. Exogenous hormones and other drug exposures of children with congenital heart disease. Am J Epidemiol 1979; 109 (4): 433-9.
43. Zierler S, Rothman KJ. Congenital heart disease in relation to maternal use of Bendectin and other drugs in early pregnancy. N Engl J Med 1985; 313 (6): 347-52.
44. Werler MM, Mitchell AA, Shapiro S. First trimester maternal medication use in relation to gastroschisis. Teratology 1992; 45 (4): 361-7.
45. Torfs CP, Katz EA, Bateson TF, et al. Maternal medications and environmental exposures as risk factors for gastroschisis. Teratology 1996; 54 (2): 84-92.
46. Mitchell AA, Schwingl PJ, Rosenberg L, et al. Birth defects in relation to bendectin use in pregnancy: II. Pyloric stenosis. Am J Obstet Gynecol 1983; 147 (7): 737-42.
47. Werler MM, Sheehan JE, Mitchell AA. Maternal medication use and risks of gastroschisis and small intestinal atresia. Am J Epidemiol 2002; 155 (1): 26-31.
48. Greenberger PA, Patterson R. Beclomethasone diproprionate for severe asthma during pregnancy. Ann Intern Med 1983; 98 (4): 478-80.
49. Brown HM, Storey G. Beclomethasone dipropionate aerosol in long term treatment of perennial and seasonal asthma in children and adults: a report of five and a half years experience in 600 asthmatic patients. Br J Clin Pharmacol 1977; 4: 259S-67S.
50. Kallen B, Rydhstroem H, Aberg A. Congenital malformations after the use of inhaled budesonide in early pregnancy. Obstet Gynecol 1999; 93 (3): 392–5.
51. Ellegard EK, Hellgren M, Karlsson NG. Fluticasone propionate aqueous nasal spray in pregnancy rhinitis. Clin Otolaryngol 2001; 26 (5): 394-400.
52. Wilson J. Disodium cromoglicate use during pregnancy. Acta Ther 1982; 8 (2 Suppl.): 45-51.
53. Schatz M, Zeiger RS, Harden K, et al. The safety of asthma and allergy medications during pregnancy. J Allergy Clin Immunol 1997; 100 (3): 301-6.
54. Compendium of Pharmaceuticals and Specialties. Ottawa (ON): Canadian Pharmacists Association, 2004.
55. Chester SW. Pregnancy and the treatment of hay fever, allergic rhinitis and pollen asthma. Ann Allergy 1950; 8 (6): 772-3.
56. Jensen K. Pregnancy and allergic diseases. Acta Allergol 1953; 6 (1): 44–53.
57. Maietta AL. The management of the allergic patient during pregnancy. Ann Allergy 1955; 13 (5): 516-22.
58. Schaefer G, Silverman F. Pregnancy complicated by asthma. Am J Obstet Gynecol 1961; 82: 182-91.
59. Negrini AC, Molinelli G. On desensitizing therapy during pregnancy [in Italian]. Folia Allergol (Roma) 1970; 17 (2): 181-5.
60. Metzger WJ, Turner E, Patterson R. The safety of immunotherapy during pregnancy. J Allergy Clin Immunol 1978; 61 (4): 268-72.
61. Shaikh WA. A retrospective study on the safety of immunotherapy in pregnancy. Clin Exp Allergy 1993; 23: 857-60.
62. Derbes VJ, Soderman WA. Reciprocal influence of bronchial asthma and pregnancy. Am J Med 1946; 1: 367-75.
63. Francis N. Abortion after grass pollen injection. J Allergy 1941; 12: 559-63.
64. Weiner JM, Abramson MJ, Puy RM. Intranasal corticosteroids versus oral H1 receptor antagonists in allergic rhinitis: systematic review of randomised controlled trials. BMJ 1998; 317 (7173): 1624-29.
65. Yanez A, Rodrigo GJ. Intranasal corticosteroids versus topical H1 receptor antagonists for the treatment of allergic rhinitis: a systematic review with meta-analysis. Ann Allergy Asthma Immunol 2002; 89 (5): 479-84.
66. Schatz M, Zeiger RS. Asthma and allergy in pregnancy. Clin Perinatol 1997; 24 (2): 407-2.
67. Franklin KA, Holmgren PA, Jonsson F, et al. Snoring, pregnancy-induced hypertension, and growth retardation of the fetus. Chest 2000; 117 (1): 137-141.

USE OF PROTON PUMP INHIBITORS DURING PREGNANCY AND RATES OF MAJOR MALFORMATIONS: A META-ANALYSIS

Shekoufeh Nikfar, Mohammad Abdollahi,† Myla E. Moretti,* Laura A. Magee,* and Gideon Koren**

Proton pump inhibitors are used to treat gastroesophageal reflux, a symptom common in pregnancy. The aim of this study was to systematically analyze the available data on the risk for malformations following use of these agents in the first trimester of pregnancy. Medline, EMBASE, published abstracts, and reference lists were searched for articles reporting on proton pump inhibitor use in pregnancy. Summary relative risks and 95% confidence intervals (95% CI) were calculated using the Mantel-Haenszel method. Five cohort studies met the inclusion criteria for this meta-analysis. With almost 600 exposed pregnancies, the overall relative risk was 1.18 with a 95%CI of 0.72–1.94. In conclusion, proton pump inhibitors do not present a major teratogenic risk when used in recommend doses. These data are reassuring for the countless patients who have used these agents in the early part of their pregnancies.

Keywords: pregnancy; drug-induced malformations; omeprazole; antiulcer agents; proton pump inhibitors.

Gastroesophageal reflux disease (GERD) in pregnancy presents a special challenge for the clinician, predominantly because of the potential side effects of pharmacologic interventions on the fetus. The symptoms and complications of peptic ulcer disease can be quite significant during pregnancy. It is commonly recommended that dyspepsia or pyrosis during pregnancy should be treated first with dietary and lifestyle changes, together with antacids or sucralfate. Therapy with H_2-receptor antagonists or proton pump inhibitors (PPIs), such as omeprazole, can be considered in patients with refractory symptoms, although not approved for this use (1, 2).

Omeprazole is a benzimidazole that suppresses gastric acid secretion by binding to the proton pump of the parietal cells. Omeprazole has been effective in the short-term treatment of duodenal, gastric, and esophageal ulcers and may offer a useful alternative to conventional therapy. In combination with antimicrobials, as dual- and triple-drug regimens, omeprazole therapy can achieve high cure rates in the treatment of *Helicobacter pylori*-associated peptic ulcer disease. The duration of therapy ranges from two to four weeks for duodenal ulcers and from four to eight weeks for gastric ulcers or duodenal ulcer patients who smoke. Omeprazole is generally well tolerated and is significantly more effective than H_2-blockers.

During the last few years there has been a steep increase in the use of omeprazole for common gastrointestinal disorders. With sales of over six billion worldwide (3), it is a best selling pharmaceutical, and because more than half of all pregnancies are unplanned, an increasing number of women of reproductive age may be inadvertently exposed to omeprazole in pregnancy. Since the drug was demonstrated to cross both animal and human placentas (4, 5), its fetal safety needs to be clarified. Omeprazole is presently classified as a "C" in the FDA pregnancy category, indicating that animal reproduction studies have not shown unequivocally its fetal safety and that not enough human data are available.

From the *The Motherisk Program, Hospital for Sick Children, Toronto, Canada; and †Faculty of Pharmacy, University of Toronto, Canada.

Supported by a grant from CIHR and AstraZeneca Ltd, Sweden; Gideon Koren is a Senior Scientist of CIHR and holder of the Research Leadership in Better Pharmacotherapy During Pregnancy and Lactation.

According to the manufacturer (6), omeprazole did not produce impairment of rat fertility at parenteral doses of up to 138 mg/kg/day, which is 345 times the recommended human dose. Teratology studies in rats at this dose and in rabbits at half this dose did not produce an increase in congenital anomalies. In both species, other embryotoxicities occurred at these doses. A similar finding in rats was reported by other investigators (7). The objective of the present study was to review systematically all the studies performed in human pregnancy where women used PPIs, and omeprazole specifically, during the first trimester in order to examine rates of congenital malformations and provide a more definitive estimate of fetal safety.

MATERIALS AND METHODS

We searched Medline and EMBASE databases for studies that reported the use of omeprazole and other PPIs, including lansoprazole and pantoprazole, in pregnancy. The dates from year of drug release to August 2001 were searched using the MeSH terms and key words: pregnancy, pregnancy outcome, abnormalities—drug induced, birth defect, teratogen, congenital abnormalities, proton pump inhibitors, omeprazole, lansoprazole, and pantoprazole. The reference list from retrieved articles was reviewed for additional applicable studies. Citations from abstracts or meeting proceedings, which were published, were also reviewed.

Two reviewers independently reviewed the retrieved articles and performed data extraction into 2 × 2 tables. Studies were excluded if they did not report on the rates of major malformations, did not include a comparison group of pregnant women not exposed to PPIs, or did not report on first trimester exposure to the drugs. In cases where only a single group was available for comparison (ie, there was no control group), the summary relative risk could not be computed. However, using the method proposed by Einarson (8), a summary incidence rate for major malformations was calculated.

All included studies were pooled and weighted. The data were analyzed using Cochrane's Review Manager version 4.1. Relative risks (RR) and 95% confidence intervals (95%CI) were calculated using the Mantel-Haenszel method. A chi-square test was used to test for heterogeneity.

Table 1
Characteristics of Included Studies

		SUBJECTS	
STUDY	STUDY TYPE	PPI EXPOSED	NOT EXPOSED
Källén 1998 (11)	Prospective cohort	275	255
Lalkin et al., 1998 (12)	Prospective cohort	78	98
Moretti (personal commun.)	Prospective cohort	63	75
Nielsen et al., 1999 (10)	Retrospective cohort	38	13,327
Ruigómez et al., 1999 (9)	Retrospective cohort	139	1,575
Källén, 2001 (13)	Prospective cohort	863	not reported

Results

Five studies met the inclusion criteria and were included in the meta-analysis (Table 1). Among the included studies, all were cohort studies ascertaining pregnancy outcome with either registry linkage (9–11) or by direct interview with the mother (12, M. Moretti, personal communication). A total of 593 infants were exposed to PPIs, most often omeprazole. The summary relative risk for all major malformations among any PPI exposure was 1.18 with a 95% CI of 0.72–1.94, a nonsignificant relative risk ($P = 0.7$) (Figure 1). For the four studies where data for omeprazole only could be extracted (9, 11, 12, M. Moretti, personal communication), the summary relative risk was 1.05 with a 95% CI of 0.59–1.85, also indicating a nonsignificant relative risk for malformations (Figure 2). The chi-square tests for heterogeneity ($P = 0.94$ and 0.89, respectively) indicate that the studies were not significantly heterogeneous and could be combined.

The data originally published by Källén in 1998 (11) were subsequently published in 2001 (14) with a significantly larger number of omeprazole-exposed pregnancies but no control group (Table 1). This report was included in the calculation of a summary incidence rate for malformations among the four cohorts included in the omeprazole analysis (9, 12, 13). Overall, a rate of 2.8% (95%CI 1.8–3.8) for malformations was observed.

Descriptive data on the PPI-exposed women is available only from the two studies based at The Motherisk Program (12, M. Moretti, personal communication). In the study by Lalkin et al. (12), the indication for omeprazole was listed as reflux esophagitis and heartburn in 27% of cases, peptic ulcer in 26% of cases, and gastritis in 19% of cases. Moretti (personal communication) reported, among the omeprazole cases, that the median dose was 20 mg/day with a range of 10–80 mg/day. The mean duration of therapy was 15.3 weeks, ranging between 3 days and 42 weeks (the entire pregnancy).

DISCUSSION

Omeprazole is currently very widely used for peptic disease all over the world. Our meta-analysis suggests that PPI, and specifically omeprazole, exposure during the first trimester of pregnancy does not pose an important teratogenic risk. The relative risk was close to unity and the confidence interval is tight, with a maximum of less than twofold increased risk.

The upper confidence interval in this study does not quite reach twofold risk. If there were an equal number of cases and controls, one would need over 700 cases to show a doubling of teratogenic risk. Here, with such a large number of controls, the sample has well over 80% power to detect a twofold difference, if one existed. The fact that none of the five available human cohort studies found a significant association between exposure during the first trimester and risk of major malformation is reassuring and is further supported by the homogeneity of the studies. In addition, the meta-analytic summary incidence rate for major malformations (2.8%; 95%CI 1.8–3.8), was well within the range expected among the general population. These results are consistent with the animal data as well as with the available human case reports (14–16). Further evidence of human safety in late pregnancy is demonstrated by the use of omeprazole as a premedication for cesarean section, where no short-term adverse effects were seen in the offspring (5, 17, 18).

Although more and larger cohorts examining the effects of this drug in human pregnancy are required to determine if a small teratogenic risk exists, analysis of over 1100 exposed infants has given no indication for concern. We conclude that PPIs, particularly omeprazole, are reasonable therapeutic options for treatment of peptic ulcer disease in pregnancy, particularly when antacids and H_2-blockers have been found to be ineffective.

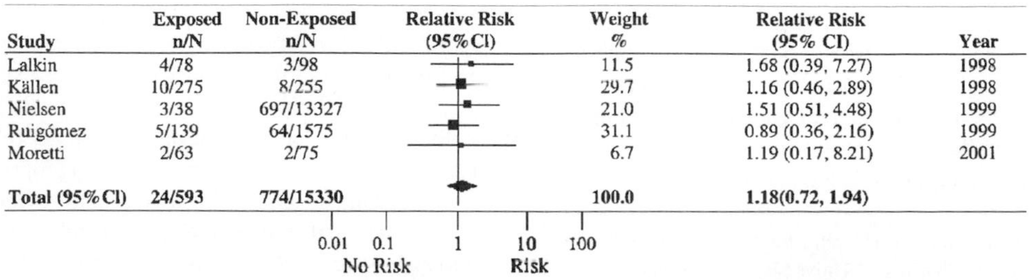
Study
Exposed n/N
Non-Exposed n/N
Relative Risk (95% CI)
Weight %
Relative Risk (95% CI)
Year
Lalkin 4/78 3/98 11.5 1.68 (0.39, 7.27) 1998
Källen 10/275 8/255 29.7 1.16 (0.46, 2.89) 1998
Nielsen 3/38 697/13327 21.0 1.51 (0.51, 4.48) 1999
Ruigómez 5/139 64/1575 31.1 0.89 (0.36, 2.16) 1999
Moretti 2/63 2/75 6.7 1.19 (0.17, 8.21) 2001
Total (95% CI) 24/593 774/15330 100.0 1.18(0.72, 1.94)
0.01 0.1 1 10 100
No Risk
Risk

Figure 1. Individual and summary relative risks for studies including all proton-pump inhibitor exposures.

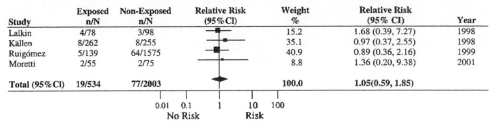

Study	Exposed n/N	Non-Exposed n/N	Relative Risk (95% CI)	Weight %	Relative Risk (95% CI)	Year
Lalkin	4/78	3/98		15.2	1.68 (0.39, 7.27)	1998
Källen	8/262	8/255		35.1	0.97 (0.37, 2.55)	1998
Ruigómez	5/139	64/1575		40.9	0.89 (0.36, 2.16)	1999
Moretti	2/55	2/75		8.8	1.36 (0.20, 9.38)	2001
Total (95% CI)	**19/534**	**77/2003**		**100.0**	**1.05(0.59, 1.85)**	

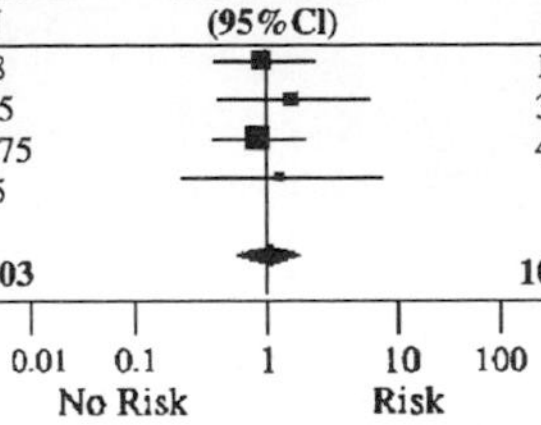

Figure 2. Individual and summary relative risks for omeprazole data only.

REFERENCES

1. Cappell MS, Garcia A: Gastric and duodenal ulcers during pregnancy. Gastroenterol Clin North Am 27:169–195, 1998.
2. Charan M, Katz PO: Gastroesophageal reflux disease in pregnancy. Curr Treat Options Gastroenterol 4:73–81, 2001.
3. AstraZeneca: Annual report. AstraZeneca, 2000.
4. Ching MS, Morgan DJ, Mihaly GW, Hardy KJ, Smallwood RA: Placental transfer of omeprazole in maternal and fetal sheep. Dev Pharmacol Ther 9:323–331, 1986.
5. Moore J, Flynn RJ, Sampaio M, Wilson CM, Gillon KR: Effect of single-dose omeprazole on intragastric acidity and volume during obstetric anaesthesia. Anaesthesia 44:559–562, 1989.
6. Merck: Product information: Prilosec Omeprazole. West Point, Pennsylvania, Merck & Company, 2000.
7. Shimazu H, Matsuoka T, Ishikawa Y, Imanishi M, Fujii T: Reproductive and developmental toxicity study of omeprazole sodium in rats. Pharmacometrics 49:573–592, 1995.
8. Einarson TR: Pharmacoeconomic applications of metaanalysis for single groups using antifungal onychomycosis lacquers as an example. Clin Ther 19:559–569, 1997.
9. Ruigómez A, Garcia Rodriguez LA, Cattaruzzi C, Troncon MG, Agostinis L, Wallander MA, Johansson S: Use of cimetidine, omeprazole, and ranitidine in pregnant women and pregnancy outcomes. Am J Epidemiol 150:476–481, 1999.
10. Nielsen GL, Sorensen HT, Thulstrup AM, Tage-Jensen U, Olesen C, Ekbom A: The safety of proton pump inhibitors in pregnancy. Aliment Pharmacol Ther 13:1085–1089, 1999.
11. Källén B: Delivery outcome after the use of acid-suppressing drugs in early pregnancy with special reference to omeprazole. Br J Obstet Gynaecol 105:877–881, 1998.
12. Lalkin A, Loebstein R, Addis A, Ramezani-Namin F, Mastroiacovo P, Mazzone T, Vial T, Bonati M, Koren G: The safety of omeprazole during pregnancy: a multicenter prospective controlled study. Am J Obstet Gynecol 179:727–730, 1998.
13. Källén BA: Use of omeprazole during pregnancy—no hazard demonstrated in 955 infants exposed during pregnancy. Eur J Obstet Gynecol Reprod Biol 96:63–68, 2001.
14. Harper MA, McVeigh JE, Thompson W, Ardill JE, Buchanan KD: Successful pregnancy in association with Zollinger-Ellison syndrome. Am J Obstet Gynecol 173:863–864, 1995.
15. Tsirigotis M, Yazdani N, Craft I: Potential effects of omeprazole in pregnancy. Hum Reprod 10:2177–2178, 1995.
16. Brunner G, Meyer H, Athmann C: Omeprazole for peptic ulcer disease in pregnancy. Digestion 59:651–654, 1998.
17. Rocke DA, Rout CC, Gouws E: Intravenous administration of the proton pump inhibitor omeprazole reduces the risk of acid aspiration at emergency cesarean section. Anesth Analg 78:1093–1098, 1994.
18. Stuart JC, Kan AF, Rowbottom SJ, Yau G, Gin T: Acid aspiration prophylaxis for emergency Caesarean section. Anaesthesia 51:415–421, 1996.

CHAPTER 48

THE SAFETY OF NITROFURANTOIN DURING THE FIRST TRIMESTER OF PREGNANCY: META-ANALYSIS

S Ben David,[1] T Einarson,[2] Y Ben David,[1] I Nulman,[1] A Pastuszak,[1] and G Koren[1]
[1]Motherisk, Division of Clinical Pharmacology/Toxicology, Department of Pediatrics and Research Institute, The Hospital for Sick Children, 555 University Ave, Toronto M5G 1X8, Canada;
[2]Department of Pediatrics, Pharmacology, Pharmacy and Medicine, The University of Toronto, Toronto, Canada
(Received 20 May 1994; accepted 7 February 1995)

Summary – Asymptomatic bacteriuria is common during pregnancy and may adversely affect both the mother and her fetus. Nitrofurantoin (NF) has been long recognized as an effective agent in both nonpregnant and pregnant women suffering from urinary tract infections. This meta-analysis was conducted in order to evaluate the safety of NF ingested during early pregnancy. Of twenty-two studies, only four met the inclusion criteria and their analysis could not demonstrate any significant correlation between NF ingestion and fetal malformation. The pooled odds ratio was 1.29 with 95% confidence interval 0.25–6.57. Although the number and quality of the studies included are limited, we thought it important to present the existing data. More extensive controlled studies are urgently needed in order to increase the significance of our study.

nitrofurantoin/safety/pregnancy/meta-analysis

INTRODUCTION

In 1958 Kass was the first to address the incidence of asymptomatic bacteriuria in pregnancy. His findings were corroborated by others showing that 6 to 7% of all pregnant women have clinically significant bacteriuria during their first prenatal visit (Kass, 1962). Urinary tract infection (UTI) during pregnancy, whether symptomatic or asymptomatic, is of great importance both to the pregnant mother and to the fetus. As high as 30% of patients with UTI during pregnancy progress to pyelonephritis (Kincaid-Smith and Bullen, 1965; Le Blanc and McGanity, 1964). This is more common among untreated patients and may be related to the urinary stasis occurring as a result of the compression effect of the growing uterus, changes in the hormonal milieu, as well as the increase in the levels of glucose, amino acids and degraded hormones which facilitate urine bacterial growth (Beydoun, 1985; Chng and Hall, 1982; Dafnis and Sabatini, 1992). Pyelonephritis during pregnancy is most likely to occur during the third trimester and is associated with increased risk of prematurity, low birth weight and perinatal death, as well as other maternal complications such as preeclampsia, anemia and chorioamnionitis (Brumfitt, 1975; Stuart *et al*, 1965; Naeye, 1986; Romero *et al*, 1989). The observation that treatment of symptomatic and asymptomatic UTI during pregnancy has been associated with 50% reduction of the risk of pyelonephritis (Tencer, 1982) and the fact that 20–43% of the patients who develop UTI have previously had UTI in the past, suggests that screening of women during early pregnancy or even prior to conception followed by preemptive treatment of the positive patients is recommended. Furthermore, some authors suggest that women with history of UTI should be on prophylactic antibiotics prior to conception or as soon as pregnancy has been diagnosed. An effective antibiotic should have minimal side effects and no teratogenicity.

Nitrofurantoin (NF) is an effective agent with high specificity for the urinary tract. The low levels attained in maternal serum and fetal compartment are an advantage when used during pregnancy (Pfau and Sacks, 1992; Chng and Hall, 1982; Lucas and Cunningham, 1993; MacDonald *et al*, 1983). Its toxicity rates to the mother have been very low, but its safety for the fetus during early pregnancy has not been determined yet by any randomized clinical trial. In the absence of a large prospective randomized study that would address this issue, we undertook to review all published reports that examined the safety of NF in pregnancy and to perform meta-analysis of all eligible studies. The objective of our study is to determine whether a relationship exists between maternal ingestion of NF during pregnancy and subsequent increases in rates of major fetal malformations.

PATIENTS AND METHODS

We retrieved all studies published in the medical literature that have examined the relationship between first trimester ingestion of NF and the presence of major or minor fetal malformations. Nitrofurantoin ingestion was defined as first trimester administration of any dose of the drug and for any period of time. In order to be included in this analysis, a study could be either a cohort or a case control. In addition to a treatment group, the study had to include a control group that did not receive NF and that was assessed in a similar manner. The following papers were excluded from meta-analysis: case reports, editorials, animal studies and studies in which data could not be extracted specifically for NF. Studies which did not present sufficient data on the treated and controlled groups were also excluded. Data accepted for analysis were pooled and the pooled odds ratio was calculated using the Mantel and Hanszel procedure (Mantel and Hanszel, 1959). The Medline database was searched using the key words: nitrofurantoin, fetal abnormality, fetal anomaly, malformations, teratogenicity and pregnancy. In addition, standard textbooks were checked for references that might not have been included in the Medline search. The inclusion criteria are delineated in table I. We reviewed all "method" sections with the names of the authors, journals, publishers and sites of the studies, without knowing the results. The data were reviewed independently by two investigators. In

Table I
Criteria for Inclusion of Studies in this Meta-Analysis

PARAMETER	CRITERION
Presentation	Any language
Subjects	Human studies
	First trimester maternal nitrofurantoin exposure
	Nonexposed control group
Outcome	Major or minor fetal malformation

Table II
Studies Meeting the Criteria for Inclusion in the Meta Analysis

STUDY	STUDY TYPE	DATA COLLECTION	MALFORMATION DESCRIBED
Heiley *et al* (1983)	C[c]	R	Any malformation
Heinonen and Sloan (1977)	C	R	Any malformation
Nesbitt and Young (1957)	C	P[p]	Any fetal effect
Pellegrini and Koren (1994)	C	R[r]	Any malformation

[c] Cohort; [p] prospective; [r] retrospective.

addition we searched the Motherisk data base for women seen prospectively in our clinic during the first trimester, for whom the pregnancy outcome was verified. Each case was matched by age (± 2 years) to several women exposed to non-teratogens who were seen prospectively during the first trimester of pregnancy.

RESULTS

The first study mentioning nitrofurantoin (NF) as an antibiotic treatment during pregnancy was published by Everett *et al* (1956). Since then 22 studies have been published in the literature in different languages. Eighteen studies did not meet the inclusion criteria for different reasons. The most common reason for excluding a study was the absence of a control group or a well-defined study group (Aubry *et al*, 1978; Everett *et al*, 1956; House *et al*, 1969; Jacobs, 1975; LeBlanc and Mcganity, 1965; Mintz *et al*, 1986; Nelson and Forfar, 1971; Neumann, 1981; Sandahl, 1985; Schreiber, 1971). Other reasons for exclusion were: 1) NF was given during second and third trimester and not during first trimester (Cameron and Krantz, 1969; Le Blanc and McGanity, 1964; Perry *et al*, 1967); 2) no definite information about anomalies incidence (House *et al*, 1969; Piper and Mitchel, 1991; Gordon, 1972); and 3) case reports and studies where NF is not the main topic (Cavallari *et al*, 1978; Connaughton and Daw, 1970; Olshan and Faustman, 1989). In most of these studies the patients were exposed to NF during the second or third trimester of pregnancy and not during the first trimester. Furthermore all rejected studies did not include a matched control group, thus not eligible for our analysis. Three studies were eligible to be included in this meta-analysis and the Motherisk cohort formed the fourth study (table II). In the first study (Nesbitt and Young, 1957), 71 pregnant women were treated with NF. Thirty of them were treated during the first and second trimesters for seven days on average. The control group was composed of 40 patients who were treated during the third trimester. This study did not find any fetal anomalies among both the study and control groups. Heinonen (1977) investigated the teratogenicity of different drugs in a well designed prospective cohort study of 50,000 mothers. Among 3,248 malformed children, he found six to be exposed to NF during the first four months of their fetal life. Among the 50,282 normal children 83 were exposed to NF during the same period of time. The calculated crude relative risk was 1.17. Heiley *et al* (1983) reported a retrospective analysis evaluating the safety of NF to human fetuses. Fetal and neonatal death, malformations, prematurity, low birth weight, low Agpar scores and jaundice were investigated. The control group was considered to be the American statistics for 1973–4 and 1977–8. Twenty-nine patients were exposed to NF during the first trimester of pregnancy, most of them for at least ten days. No fetal anomalies were found among the study group as compared to 8.11 cases per 1,000 live births in the control group. In Motherisk during the past few years we had nine pregnant women exposed to NF during the first trimester of pregnancy prospectively ascertained by the program (Pellegrini and Koren, 1994). In one of them an imperforated anus was diagnosed. All other babies were born with no abnormality. As a control group we had 72 consecutive pregnant women who were exposed to nonteratogens during the first trimester of pregnancy. Two out of the 72 patients delivered malformed babies, one with a cardiac anomaly and the second with a bilateral club foot. Tables II and III present the four studies included in the meta-analysis. The odds ratios (OR) are calculated along with the 95% confidence interval for each study. In the first study (Nesbitt and Young, 1957) the number of malformed fetuses in both the study and control groups was 0. In order to calculate the OR we added the number 1/2 to each cell frequency before obtaining the ratio. Of all possible numbers which might be added or substracted from the cell frequencies, 1/2 is the number which reduces the bias of the estimate to a minimum (Sheehe, 1966). The number of patients used in each study was vastly different. In order to avoid any possible bias for one study over the other three, we calculated the OR of three of the four studies while omitting one study each time. The calculated OR showed no significant difference between the study and control groups (OR = 1.2, 2.00, 1.25, 1.08, correspondingly). Figure 1 presents on a logarithmic scale the OR with the 95% confidence intervals of the four studies. Values greater than one indicate an increased teratogenic risk of NF. It is evident from this figure that overall there was no significant difference between the study and control groups with respect to rates of fetal malformations.

DISCUSSION

Despite impressive progress in the understanding of the pathogenesis and treatment of UTI during pregnancy, the extent to which this infection affects maternal and perinatal health remains controversial. Of major concern are the possible deleterious effects on the fetus (Naeye, 1986). For this reason it is well accepted to treat symptomatic UTI during pregnancy and some authors suggest that every

Table III
Results of Studies Comparing the Outcome of Fetuses Exposed or Not Exposed Exposed to Nitrofurantoin

STUDY	EXPOSURE	CONGENITAL DEFECTS ODDS YES	NO	TOTAL	RATIO	95% CI_{CI-}
Heiley *et al* (1983)	Yes	0	29	29	1.98	0.11–35.1
	No	811	99,189	10,000		
	Total	811	99,218	10,029		
Heinonen and Sloan (1977)	Yes	6	83	89	1.17	0.49–2.51
	No	3,242	50,199	56,683		
	Total	3,248	50,282	56,772		
Nesbitt and Young (1957)	Yes	0	30	30	1.36	0.037–70
	No	0	41	41		
	Total	0	71	71		
Pellegrini and Koren (1994)	Yes	1	8	9	4.37	0.36–53.8
	No	2	70	72		
	Total	3	78	81		

CI– 95% confidence interval.

bacteriuria during pregnancy, whether symptomatic or asymptomatic should be treated. Furthermore prophylaxis treatment to high risk groups was considered by others. Therefore treatment should be simple to use with minimal side effects and toxicity for both the mother and the fetus. It is crucial that the agent used not induce major malformations, so it can be safely used during embriogenesis.

Nitrofurantoin is an antibiotic agent with a wide range of antimicrobial activity against both Gram negative and positive organisms. Its bacteriostatic effect can be achieved at a concentration of 32 μg/ml especially in an acidic urine. It crosses the placenta very rapidly but in small quantity and readily disappears from the fetal circulation (Perry and LeBlanc, 1967). Nitrofurantoin is highly effective against *E Coli, Klebsiella* and *Aerobacter* infection but less effective against *Proteus* and *Pseudomonas.* The compliance with this oral antibiotic, given one to two times daily, is good. Meta-analysis gives an overall odds ratio that describes the relationship between a drug and an outcome (Einarson *et al,* 1988). The advantage of this method is in aggregation of results from individual studies in a systematic, thorough and quantitative manner, which is less prone to bias than the classical review of available studies. As a primary endpoint for our meta-analysis we have chosen the rates of major malformations, as any increase in teratogenic potential in humans would preclude the drug from use during gestation.

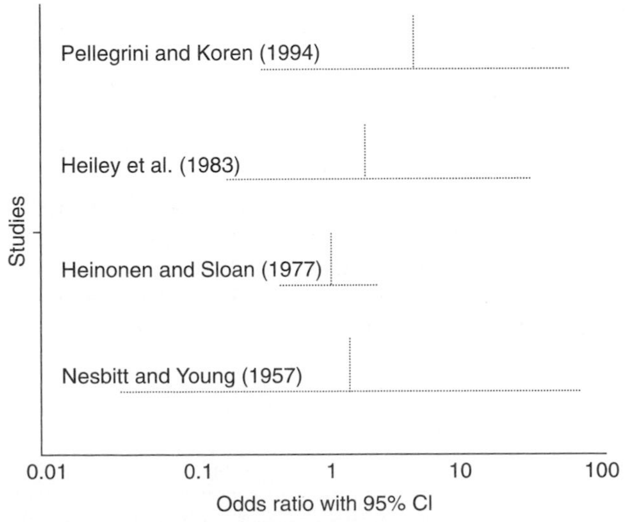

Figure 1. Odds ratio along with 95% confidence interval for each study.

In general, available studies ranged over four decades. However, the overall risk for major malformations has not changed during this period. The fact that only four studies could be included in this analysis while scores had to be excluded, attests to the poor quality of most of the research in this area. It also reflects the grim reality that women are easily orphaned from the benefits of effective therapies even when their health and their babies' health necessitate such drugs. The scarce number of studies limit the statistical power of our study to detect an OR smaller than 2 or 3. The total relative risk of exposure to NF was 1.7. This means that for a power of 80% at least 2,045 patients are required in each study group in order to reach valid statistical conclusions and for a relative risk of 2.0 (which was the maximum calculated, omitting the Heinonen study) 1,000 patients need to be included in each study group. Neither the results from any of the individual studies nor the combined results from all the studies together showed a significant correlation between exposure to NF and fetal malformations. Although the data are not optimal for meta-analysis, we thought it important to evaluate the existing data and combine the different studies in the absence of any prospective study. In conclusion we believe that prospective controlled studies with optimal scientific rigor are urgently needed in order to verify the safety of nitrofurantoin.

ACKNOWLEDGMENTS

Supported in part by Procter and Gamble Pharm, Toronto. The author G Koren is a Career Scientist of the Ontario Ministry of Health.

REFERENCES

Aubry RH, Shah A, Cuenca VG. Managing bacteriuria in the high risk obstetric patient. *Female Patient* 1978;3:66–9.

Beydoun SN. Morphologic changes in the renal tract in pregnancy. *Clin Obstet Gynecol* 1985;28:249–56.

Brumfitt W. The effects of bacteriuria in pregnancy on maternal and fetal health. *Kidney Int* 1975;8:S113–9.

Cameron WJ, Krantz KE. Urinary tract infection in pregnancy. *Obstet Gynecol Digest* 1969;11:36–44.

Cavallari V, Granese D, Batolo D, Montanari G. Contributo allo studio delle malformazione sirenoidi. *Folia Hered Pathol* 1978;27(2):25–37.

Chng PK, Hall MH. Antenatal prediction of urinary tract infection in pregnancy. *Br J Obstet Gynaecol* 1982;89:8–11.

Connaughton J, Daw E. Three cases of Cyclopia. *Br J Clin Pract* 1970;24:37–9.

Dafnis E, Sabatini S. The effect of pregnancy on renal function, physiology and pathophysiology. *Am J Med Sci* 1992;303:184–205.

Einarson TR, Leeder JS, Koren GA. Method for meta-analysis of epidemiological studies. *Drug Intell Clin Pharm* 1988;22:813–24.

Everett SD, Edward CP, Jose GV. Treatment of urinary tract infections in obstetrics and gynecology patients with nitrofurantoin. *Am J Obstet Gynecol* 1956;71:399–401.

Gordon SF. Asymptomatic bacteriuria of pregnancy. *Clin Med* 1972;79:22–4.

Heiley FJ, Fort H, Williams JC, Hammer B. Foetal safety of nitrofurantoin macrocrystals therapy during pregnancy: a retrospective analysis. *J Int Med Res* 1983;11:364–9.

Heinonen OP, Slone D. Antimicrobial and antiparasitic agents. *In:* Kaufman DW, eds. *Birth effects and drugs in pregnancy*. Littleton, Mass: Publishing Sciences Group, 1977;296–313.

House TE, Williams BL, Meares GM, Hester LL. Pregnancy complicated by urinary tract infections. *Obstet Gynecol* 1969;34:670–4.

Jacobs D. Maternal drug ingestion and congenital malformations. *S Afr Med J* 1975;49:2073–80.

Kass EH. Pyelonephritis and bacteriuria: a major problem in preventive medicine. *Ann Intern Med* 1962;56:46–51.

Kincaid-Smith P, Bullen M. Bacteriuria in pregnancy. *Lancet* 1965;1:395–9.

Le Blanc AL, McGanity WJ. The impact of bacteriuria in pregnancy-a survey of 1300 pregnant patients. *Biol Med* 1964a;22:336–47.

Le Blanc AL, McGanity WJ. Bacteriuria in pregnancy. Preliminary report. *Tex State J Med* 1964b;60:137–45.

LeBlanc A, McGanity WJ. A survey of bacteriuria in pregnancy. *In:* Kass EH, ed. *Progress in pyelonephritis.* Philadelphia: Davis A Company, 1965;58–63.

Lucas MJ, Cunningham FG. Urinary infection in pregnancy. *Clin Obstet Gynecol* 1993;36:855–68.

MacDonald P, Alexander D, Catz C, Edelman R. Summary of a workshop on maternal genitourinary infections and the outcome of pregnancy. *J Infect Dis* 1983;147:596–605.

Mantel N, Hanszel W. Statistical aspects of the analysis of data from retrospective studies of disease. *JNCI* 1959;22:719–48.

Mintz G, Niz J, Gutierrez G, Garcia-Alonso A, Karchmer S. Prospective study of pregnancy in systematic lupus erythematosus. Results of a multidisciplinary approach. *J Rheumatol* 1986;13:732–9.

Naeye RL. Causes of the excessive rates of perinatal mortality and prematurity in pregnancies complicated by maternal urinary tract infections. *N Engl J Med* 1979;300:819–23.

Naeye RL. Urinary tract infections and the outcome of pregnancy. *Adv Nephrol* 1986;15:95–102.

Nelson MM, Forfar JO. Associations between drugs administered during pregnancy and congenital abnormalities of the fetus. *Br Med J* 1971;1:523–7.

Nesbitt REL, Young JE. Urinary tract infections during pregnancy and the puerperium. *Obstet Gynecol* 1957;10:89–94.

Neumann HJ. Klinish-aetiologische und tierexperinentell-teratolgische untersuchungen aetiologie von missbildugen unter besonderer beruecksichtigung der lippen-kiefer-gaumensegel spalte. *Stomatol DDR* 1981;31:82–95.

Olshan AF, Faustman EM. Nitrosatable drug exposure during pregnancy and adverse pregnancy outcome. *Int J Epidemiol* 1989;18: 891–9.

Pellegrini EM, Koren G. *In:* Koren G, eds. *Maternal fetal toxicology. Motherisk I. A new model for counseling in reproductive toxicology.* New York: Marcel Dekker Inc, 1994;707–27.

Perry JE, LeBlanc AL. Transfer of nitofurantoin across the human placenta. *Tex Rep Biol Med* 1967;25:265–8.

Perry JE, Toney JD, Le Blanc AL. Effect of nitrofurantoin on the human fetus. *Tex Rep Biol Med* 1967;25:270–2.

Pfau A, Sacks TG. Effective prophylaxis for recurrent urinary infections during pregnancy. *Clin Infect Dis* 1992;14:810–4.

Piper JM, Mitchel EF. Prenatal exposure to prescribed drugs in Tennessee Medicaid, 1983–1988. *Paediatr Perinat Epidemiol* 1991;5: 402–9.

Pitkin RM. Morphological changes in pregnancy. *In:* Buchsbaum HJ, Schmidt JD, eds. *Gynecologic and Obstetric in Urology*. Philadelphia: Saunders, 1978;375–81.

Romero R, Oyarzun E, Mazor M, Sirtori M, Hobbins JC, Bracken M. Meta-analysis of the relationship between asymptomatic bacteriuria and preterm delivery/low birth weight. *Obstet Gynecol* 1989;73:576–82.

Sandahl B. A prospective study of drug use, smoking and contraceptives during early pregnancy. *Acta Obstet Gynecol Scand* 1985;64: 381–6.

Schreiber W. Medikamente in der Schwagerschaft. *Med Klin* 1971;66:686–8.

Sheehe PR. Combination of log relative risk in retrospective studies of disease. *Am J Public Health* 1966;56:1745–50.

Stuart KL, Cummins GTM, Chin WA. Bacteriuria, prematurity and the hypertensive disorders of pregnancy. *Br Med J* 1965;1:554–6.

Tencer J. Asymptomatic bacteriuria: a long-term study. *Scand J Urol Nephrol* 1982;22:31–4.

Reprinted from Ben David S, Einarson T, Ben David Y, Nulman I, Pastuszak A, Koren G. The safety of nitrofurantoin during the first trimester of pregnancy: meta-analysis. Fundam Clin Pharmacol.1995; 9: 503–7 with permission from Blackwell Publishing.

CHAPTER 49

SAFETY OF METRONIDAZOLE IN PREGNANCY: A META-ANALYSIS

Pascale Burtin, Anna Taddio, Omer Ariburnu, Thomas R. Einarson, and Gideon Koren

Objective. Our purpose was to determine from published experience in humans whether metronidazole exposure during the first trimester of pregnancy is associated with an increased teratogenic risk.
Study Design. All published articles reporting on metronidazole use during pregnancy were screened by two independent reviewers to select those including pregnant patients exposed during the first trimester and comparing the outcomes of their pregnancies with that of patients either not exposed to metronidazole or exposed only during the third trimester. The outcome under consideration was the occurrence of birth defects in live-born infants. The overall odds ratios of first-trimester exposure versus no first-trimester exposure was calculated by combining the selected studies in a meta-analysis according to the procedure of Mantel and Haenszel.
Results. From 32 identified studies, 7 met the inclusion criteria for meta-analysis. Six were prospective and included 253 women exposed to the drug in the first trimester of pregnancy; one was retrospective and reported on 1083 exposed women. The overall weighted odds ratio of exposure versus no exposure during the first trimester calculated by meta-analysis of the 7 studies was 0.93 (95% confidence interval 0.73 to 1.18). The odds ratio calculated from the 6 prospective studies was 1.02 (95% confidence interval 0.48 to 2.18).
Conclusion. Metronidazole does not appear to be associated with an increased teratogenic risk. (AM J OBSTET GYNECOL 1995;172:525-9.)

Keywords: Metronidazole, teratogenicity, meta-analysis

Metronidazole is the drug of choice for the treatment of trichomoniasis,[1] a common infection affecting millions of women during the reproductive age. Despite its having been in clinical use for more than three decades, the question of its safe use during pregnancy has not been fully addressed. Metronidazole passes freely through the placental barrier.[2] It has been shown to be nonteratogenic in mice, rats and guinea pigs; however, it is mutagenic for bacteria and carcinogenic in mice after long-term use.[3] Carcinogenicity has never been reported in humans, [4] and to date the only published reports of adverse pregnancy outcome are three cases of midline facial defects that occurred after exposure of the mothers to metronidazole between 5 and 7 weeks of gestation).[5,6] Two reviews based on qualitative assessment of the literature concluded that there is a lack of evidence for teratogenicity of metronidazole. [7,8] However, physicians and patients alike hesitate to use metronidazole, especially at the time of embryogenesis during the first trimester of pregnancy, thus often prolonging the infection and the discomfort associated with it.

Moreover, because half of the pregnancies in North America are unplanned and in view of the common use of metronidazole by sexually active women, thousands of women every year are being exposed to it during the first trimester of pregnancy. Lack of decisive, authoritative knowledge on the safety of the drug during embryogenesis is causing high levels of anxiety to women and their families and possibly leading to termination of otherwise wanted pregnancies. The objective of the current study was to determine from published experience in humans whether a relationship exists between maternal consumption of metronidazole during the first trimester of pregnancy and increased rates of birth defects in the offspring.

From the Motherisk Program, Division of Clinical Pharmacology and Toxicology, Department of Pediatrics and Research Institute, The Hospital For Sick Children, and the Departments of Pediatrics and Pharmacology and the School of Pharmacy, University of Toronto. Dr. Koren is a Career Scientist of the Ontario Ministry of Health. *Dr. Burtin was supported by a grant from the Association Française pour la Recherche Thérapeutique, Paris, France.*

METHODS

We retrieved all medical literature published on metronidazole use during pregnancy since its release in 1959. This retrieval was initiated by a MEDLine review with the key words *metronidazole, pregnancy,* and *teratogenicity* and by consultation of three teratology textbooks (Schardein,[9] Briggs et al.,[10] and Shepard[11]). Because many articles related to metronidazole were published before 1966 (the Medline starting year), we completed the search by systematically investigating all references from all extracted articles.

This procedure allowed us to identify 32 articles reporting original data. Full lists are available on request. All dealt with metronidazole use for *Trichomonas vaginalis* and reported experience with oral treatment courses of 7 to 10 days, either alone (15 studies) or in association with intravaginal administration (17 studies). Fourteen articles specifically addressed the topic of metronidazole use during pregnancy, and 18 articles reported cases of metronidazole use during pregnancy in the context of a broader study.

A preliminary review of these articles revealed that the vast majority reported follow-up data of cohorts of pregnant patients treated with metronidazole but did not compare the outcomes of their pregnancies with those of controls unexposed to the medication. However, several studies that did not have an unexposed group included patients exposed to metronidazole during the third trimester of pregnancy, at a stage when dysmorphologic development cannot occur. These patients had the same disease, trichomoniasis, as those treated during the first trimester; they were recruited among the same population and at the same period of time. For all these reasons we decided that they could constitute acceptable comparison groups for those exposed to the drug during the first trimester.

Two independent reviewers, who had nonmedical backgrounds and thus no a priori opinion on the outcome of this analysis, evaluated the studies for appropriate inclusion in the meta-analysis according to the following criteria: (1) inclusion of at least 10 patients exposed to metronidazole during the first trimester of pregnancy; (2) inclusion of either a group of pregnant women not exposed to metronidazole or a group of women exposed only during the third trimester of pregnancy; this group should have had at least 10 patients; (3) report of the number of malformations observed in live-born infants in each of these groups.

If the nature of the observed malformations was described, the reviewers characterized them as minor or major according to the list described by Heinonen et al.[12] Reported spontaneous abortions and stillbirths were examined, but they were not considered as "birth defects." Data were extracted in the form of 2 × 2 tables; they contained for each study the absolute numbers of pregnancies reported as having resulted or not resulted in live-born offspring with birth defects.

Meta-analysis included only studies meeting all three criteria, with consideration of the number of major malformations rather than the total number of malformations whenever both types of data were available.

Statistical Methods

The outcomes of the studies were combined according to the procedure of Mantel and Haenszel,[13,14] which provides summary odds ratios and their confidence intervals. Homogeneity among studies was tested with the Breslow and Day test.[15] Significance of the results of individual studies was evaluated by χ^2 with Yates' correction whenever relevant. A two-tailed probability level of ≤ 0.05 was considered statistically significant for all tests.

RESULTS

From the 32 screened studies, 7 met the three inclusion criteria for meta-analysis[16-22] All were cohort studies; 6 were prospective and reported series ranging between 13 and 79 pregnant women exposed to metronidazole during the first trimester[16-21]; 1 was a historic cohort based on computerized Medicaid records that reported the data of > 1000 exposed women.[22] In the four studies in which description of the observed birth defects was available, [16, 17, 19, 21] the respective rates of major birth defects in the control group were 2.3%, 3.8%, 1.4%, and 1.8%. In the study of Heinonen et al., [20] birth defects were defined as any major or minor malformation observed in children born after four lunar months of gestation, whether live or dead; the rate of such birth defects in the control group was 6.4%. In the study of Rosa et al., [22] the concept of birth defect was not defined and the rate in the control group was 6.3%.

The 25 remaining reports were excluded for the following reasons: (1) Eight studies included none or < 10 patients exposed to metronidazole during the first trimester of pregnancy; (2) 11 studies did not state at what stage of pregnancy the patients received metronidazole; 6 studies either did not report the outcome of pregnancies or reported the outcome globally without detailing the time of exposure during pregnancy.

Table I presents the basic data and analyses of the seven studies that contribute to the meta-analysis. For each study the number of children with first-trimester exposure to metronidazole are

Table I
Results of Individual Studies Included in Meta-Analysis

SERIES	EXPOSURE	BIRTH DEFECTS YES	BIRTH DEFECTS NO	TOTAL	ODDS RATIO	χ^2	SIGNIFICANCE
Scott-Gray [16]	T1	0	79	79	0	1.57	$p = 0.21$
	T3	4	100	104			
	Total	4	179	183			
Robinson and Merchandani [17]	T1	0	14	14	0	0.158	$p = 0.69$
	T3	4	172	176			
	Total	4	186	190			
Rodin and Hass [18]	T1	0	13	13	–	–	–
	T3	0	19	19			
	Total	0	32	32			
Peterson et al. [19]	T1	0	54	54	0.45	0.025	$p = 0.87$
	T3	1	73	74			
	Total	1	127	128			
Heinonen et al. [20]	T1	4	27	31	2.15	1.20	$p = 0.27$
	NE	3,244	47,007	50,251			
	Total	3,248	47,034	50,282			
Morgan [21]	T1	1	61	62	0.91	0.21	$p = 0.65$
	NE	5	278	283			
	Total	6	339	345			
Rosa et al. [22]	T1	63	1,020	1,083	0.92	0.42	$p = 0.52$
	NE	6,501	96,755	103,256			
	Total	6,564	97,775	104,339			

T1, Exposed during first trimester; *T3*, exposed during third trimester; *NE*, nonexposed.

shown, separated into those reported to have birth defects and those without reported birth defects. Only 3 of the 7 studies reported any children with birth defects and first-trimester exposure to metronidazole. The number of children with either third-trimester exposure to metronidazole or no exposure to metronidazole are also shown, separated into those reported to have birth defects and those without reported birth defects. The study by Rodin and Hass[18] was the only study to have no children with birth defects in the comparison group. For each study the odds ratio, the χ^2, and the p value are shown. Odds ratios for the 7 studies ranged from 0 to 2.15. None of the odds ratios were statistically significantly different from 1 (i.e., 95% confidence limits included 1.0), and none of them detected a significantly increased risk of birth defects among the children exposed to metronidazole during the first trimester. The major birth defects reported in these studies are listed in Table II. None of them detected a significantly increased risk of birth defects in women exposed during the first trimester of pregnancy, either because the odds ratio was close to 1 or because the numbers of patients were insufficient for conclusion.

The overall weighted odds ratio of exposure versus no exposure during the first trimester calculated by meta-analysis of the 7 studies was 0.93 (95% confidence interval 0.73 to 1.18), indicating no increased teratogenic risk after first-trimester exposure to metronidazole (Fig. 1). There was no statistically significant heterogeneity among the 7 studies (χ^2 with 6 degrees of freedom = 4.30, $p = 0.636$). However, because the historic cohort study differed from the other studies in method and sample size, meta-analysis was repeated after exclusion of this study. The overall weighted odds ratio calculated from the 6 prospective studies was 1.02 (95% confidence interval 0.48 to 2.18), thus leading to the same conclusion.

When the total number of reported birth defects was taken into account for all 7 studies rather than the number of major malformations, the overall odds ratio was 0.96 (95% confidence interval 0.75 to 1.22).

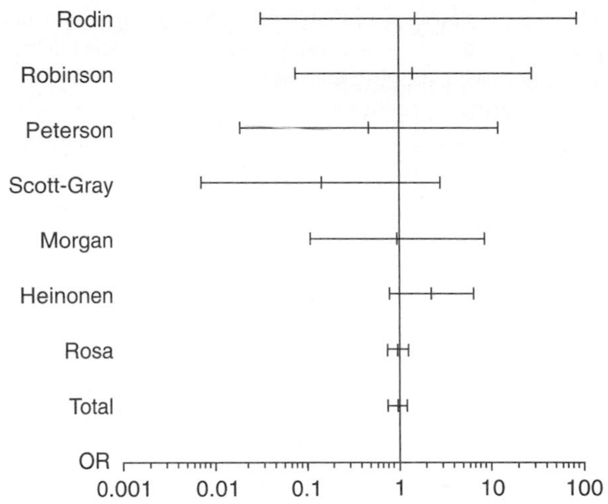

***Figure 1.** Metronidazole exposure during first trimester of pregnancy and birth defects. Odds ratios of exposed versus unexposed women calculated from individual studies and from their combination in a meta-analysis (Total).*

COMMENT

During the last decade, meta-analysis has emerged as a powerful method for combining the data of similar studies. The strength of this method is in its ability to increase the sample size and thus the statistical power. Because major malformations occur rarely, most studies including even 200 cases and a similar number of controls lack statistical power to show a relative risk of 2 to be significant. When we look at specific malformations, which occur much more rarely, very large cohorts are needed.

In the current analysis we have taken an operational choice of including studies that did not have an unexposed group but did have an identified group of pregnant women exposed to metronidazole only during the third trimester of pregnancy. The primary end point of interest was the rate of major malformations, and third-trimester exposure to metronidazole cannot cause a normal child to become malformed; hence this group can safely be designated as controls.

The published data used for this meta-analysis do not offer sufficient information for analysis of other reproductive end points, such as rates of stillbirth or spontaneous abortions. Detailed report of these events was available in four studies regarding stillbirths and in three studies regarding spontaneous abortions. In one of them

Table II
List of Major Malformations Reported in Live-Born Infants in 4 of 7 Studies Included in Meta-Analysis

SERIES	FIRST TRIMESTER EXPOSURE	CONTROLS
Scott-Gray [16]	–	1 Anencephaly 1 Microcephaly plus cephalomeningocele 1 Multiple defects (hemimelia, common truncus,absence of ductus arteriosus) 1 Hydrocephalus
Robinson and Mirchandani [17]	–	1 Hydrocephalus 1 Harelip and cleft palate 1 Congenital dislocation of hip 1 Clubfoot
Peterson et al. [19]	–	1 Hydrocephalus
Morgan [21]	1 Anencephaly plus myelomeningocele	2 Anencephaly 1 Idiopathic hydrops fetalis 1 Renal anomaly 1 Congenital short femur

(Scott-Gray [16]) a case of spontaneous abortion after first-trimester exposure to the drug also was associated with a cardiac defect and another case was a stillbirth caused by anencephaly, for which the time of exposure to metronidazole was not stated. If these two events are considered as birth defects linked with first-trimester exposure to metronidazole ("worst case scenario"), the overall odds ratio of the 6 prospective studies is 1.21 (95% confidence interval 0.57 to 2.54), which still represents no significantly increased risk. In many instances metronidazole is used as a single dose; it is safe to assume that the lack of teratogenicity in studies with a course of 7 to 10 days can be generalized for single-dose exposures.

An important criticism against meta-analysis is that of combining well-designed studies with poorly designed ones. In analyzing the available studies we had some questions about the data of the large retrospective study. [22] It assumed that the 47% of women who enrolled through Medicaid only after the first trimester had not previously had metronidazole during that pregnancy. The calculation of the relative risk of exposed versus nonexposed mothers is based on that assumption. However, because of the large size of the cohort and the low rate of exposure to metronidazole (1.9%), the rate of malformations in the nonexposed group was likely to be almost identical to the rate of malformations in the entire cohort, so that this approximation should not have affected the result. However, we repeated the meta-analysis after exclusion of this study and still came to a similar relative risk. This points out the argument made by many analysts that the quality of a study does not appear to affect the overall direction of the results. In a recent meta-analysis of antihistamine use in pregnancy (Seto A, Einarson TR, Leeder JS, Koren G. Unpublished observations), we added a quality score to the analysis and still arrived at identical results.

Another major limitation of meta-analysis is publication bias (i.e., the fact that studies concluding in one way may be less easily published than studies concluding another way). However, in the case of metronidazole it would be extremely unlikely that studies concluding a significantly increased teratogenic risk would not have been published. Furthermore, none of the 25 studies not included in our meta-analysis reported high rates of major birth defects among offspring born to mothers exposed to metronidazole. The three cases of midline facial defects [5, 6] constituted the only reported cluster of malformations; however, this association was not confirmed by any other report and can probably be attributed to chance.

In summary, our study indicates that, on the basis of an analysis of 30 years' experience, metronidazole does not appear to be associated with an increased teratogenic risk. Pregnant women in need of this drug should be encouraged to use it, and those exposed during pregnancy should be reassured, so that unnecessary terminations of pregnancy, on the basis of misinformation, can be prevented.

REFERENCES

1. Lossick JG, Kent HL. Trichomoniasis: trends in diagnosis and management. Am J Obstet Gynecol 1991 ; 165:1217-22.
2. Heisterberg L. Placental transfer of metronidazole in the first trimester of pregnancy. J Perinat Med 1984;12:43-5.
3. Roe JFC. A critical appraisal of the toxicology of metronidazole. In: Phillips I, Collier J, eds. Metronidazole, proceedings, Geneva, Switzerland, April 1979. New York: Academic Press, 1979:215-22.
4. Beard CM, Noller KL, O'Fallon M, Kurland LT, Dockerty MB. Lack of evidence for cancer due to use of metronidazole. N Engl J Med 1979;301:519-22.
5. Cantu JM, Garcia-Cruz D. Midline facial defect as a teratogenic effect of metronidazole. Birth Defects 1982;18: 85-8.
6. Greenberg F. Possible metronidazole teratogenicity and clefting. Am J Med Genet 1985;22:825.
7. Berget A, Weber T. Metronidazole and pregnancy. Ugeskri Laeger 1972;134:2085-9.
8. Royer ME. Innocuité du métronidazole prescrit pendant la grossesse. Med Maladie Infect 1983;13:727-9.
9. Schardein JL. Chemically induced birth defects. New York: Marcel Dekker, 1985:411-4.
10. Briggs CG, Freeman RK, Yaffe SJ. Drugs in pregnancy and lactation. 3rd ed. Baltimore: Williams & Wilkins, 1990:430-3.
11. Shepard TH. Catalog of teratogenic agents. 7th ed. Baltimore: Johns Hopkins University Press, 1992:1446.
12. Heinonen OP, Slone D, Shapiro S. Birth defects and drugs in pregnancy. Littleton, Massachusetts: PSG Publishing, 1977:447-55.
13. Einarson TR, Leeder JS, Koren G. A method for metaanalysis of epidemiological studies. Drug Intell Clin Pharm 1988;22:813-24.
14. Mantel N, Haenszel W. Statistical aspects of the analysis of data from retrospective studies of disease. J Natl Cancer Inst 1959;22:719-48.
15. Breslow NE, Day NE. Statistical methods in cancer research. Volume 1: the analysis of case-control studies. Lyon, France: International Agency for Research in Cancer, 1980; IARC Scientific Publications no 32.
16. Scott-Gray M. Metronidazole in obstetric practice. Obstet Gynecol 1964;71:82-5.
17. Robinson SC, Mirchandani G. Trichomonas vaginalis. V. Further observations on metronidazole (including infant follow-up). Am J Obstet Gynecol 1965;93:502-5.
18. Rodin P, Hass G. Metronidazole in pregnancy. Br J Vener Dis 1966;42:210-2.
19. Peterson W, Stauch J, Ryder C. Metronidazole in pregnancy. Am J Obstet Gynecol 1966;94:343-9.
20. Heinonen OP, Slone D, Shapiro S. Birth defects and drugs in pregnancy. Littleton, Massachusetts: PSG Publishing, 1977:296-302.
21. Morgan IFK. Metronidazole treatment in pregnancy. In: Phillips I, Collier J, eds. Metronidazole, proceedings, Geneva, Switzerland, 1979. London: The Royal Society of Medicine, 1979:245-7.
22. Rosa FW, Baum C, Shaw M. Pregnancy outcomes after first-trimester vaginitis drug therapy. Obstet Gynecol 1987;69:751–5.

Reprinted from Burtin P, Taddio A, Ariburnu O, Einarson TR, Koren G. Safety of metronidazole in pregnancy: a meta-analysis. Am J Obstet Gynecol 1995;172:525-9 with permission from Elsevier.

CHAPTER 50

RISKS AND BENEFITS OF β-RECEPTOR BLOCKERS FOR PREGNANCY HYPERTENSION: OVERVIEW OF THE RANDOMIZED TRIALS

Laura A. Magee,[a] Einat Elran.[a] Shelley B. Bull,[b] Alexander Logan,[b] and Gideon Koren[a]

[a]*Motherisk Program, Division of Clinical Pharmacology/Toxicology, The Hospital for Sick Children, Toronto, Ont., Canada*

[b]*Samuel Lunenfeld Research Institute, Mount Sinai Hospital, Toronto, Ont., Canada*

Received 16 December 1998; accepted 23 February 1999

Abstract

Objective. Examine the benefits/risks of β-blockers for pregnancy hypertension. *Study design*: Meta-analysis of relevant trials identified by comprehensive literature review (1966–97).

Results. Included were 30 trials for pregnancy hypertension, and four others for perinatal outcomes only. For mild chronic hypertension treated throughout pregnancy (n = 2 trials), oral β-blockers (compared with no therapy) were associated with an inconsistent increase in small for gestational age (SGA) infants (OR 2.46 [1.02, 5.92]). For mild-moderate 'late-onset' pregnancy hypertension (i.e. either chronic treated only late in pregnancy, or pregnancy-induced) (n = 8 trials), oral β-blockers (compared with no therapy) were associated with a decrease in severe hypertension (OR 0.27 [0.16, 0.45]), borderline decrease in development of proteinuria (OR 0.69 [0.48, 1.02]), decrease in RDS (OR 0.33 [0.13, 0.85]), but a borderline increase in SGA infants (OR 1.47 [0.96, 2.26]). β-blockers were equivalent to other agents (n=15 trials). For severe 'late-onset' pregnancy hypertension (n=5 trials), i.v. labetalol produced less maternal hypotension (OR 0.13 [0.03, 0.71]) and fewer cesareans (OR 0.23 [0.13, 0.63]) than i.v. hydralazine/diazoxide.

Conclusions. It is not clear that the benefits outweigh the risks when β-blockers are used to treat mild to moderate chronic or pregnancy-induced hypertension, given the unknown overall effect on perinatal outcomes. For severe 'late-onset' pregnancy hypertension, i.v. labetalol is safer than i.v. hydralazine or diazoxide.

Keywords: Adrenergic β-antagonists; Pregnancy complications; Severe hypertension; Randomized controlled trial

INTRODUCTION

β-Blockers are effective antihypertensive agents that have become accepted first-line therapy for all types of pregnancy hypertension [1]. Early in their use during pregnancy, case series described perinatal morbidity such as intrauterine growth restriction (IUGR), respiratory depression, as well as neonatal bradycardia, hypoglycemia and hypothermia [2]. Consistent with these reports were the pharmacology of β-blockers and the knowledge that catecholamine levels are greatest in the first days of life and play an important role in neonatal adaptation [3]. However, given the retrospective nature of the data, it was not clear that the observed morbidity was due to β-blockers rather than the underlying maternal disease for which the β-blockers had been prescribed.

Randomized controlled trials (RCTs) should provide the best evidence for establishing a causal link between β-blocker treatment and maternal and perinatal outcomes. *Qualitative* reviews of relevant RCTs have been published [4], but this approach is recognized to be potentially biased because it examines the statistical significance of results of individual studies, without considering their statistical power. Using a quantitative approach, the Cochrane Group has published its assessment of the use of antihypertensive drugs in pregnancy in a series of monographs [5–8] and concluded: (i) oral β-blockers for preeclampsia reduce the incidence of severe hypertension but may also increase the incidence of IUGR [5]; (ii) oral β-blockers are no more effective than methyldopa [6]; and (iii) intravenous (i.v.) labetalol for severe preeclampsia results in less maternal hypotension than diazoxide [8]. However, some trials were misclassified; for example, reviews of treatment of preeclampsia [5,6] included two trials which enrolled only patients with chronic hypertension. Secondly, in their analysis, differences in participants, interventions, and outcome definitions, and their impact on treatment effect were not examined. When between-trial heterogeneity in these characteristics is not taken into account, misleading conclusions can be reached [9] and clinicians may have difficulties in extrapolating the results to their clinical practice [10].

This overview was undertaken to relate measurable characteristics of participants, interventions, and outcome definitions to demonstrated effects of β-blockers for pregnancy hypertension. This would both clarify the current state of knowledge regarding management of pregnancy hypertension, and identify priorities for future research.

METHODS

Identification and Selection of Trials

The following were searched for published RCTs: (i) Medline (1966–Dec. 1997; key words: adrenergic beta-antagonists, maternal mortality, pregnancy, pregnancy complications, perinatology, neonatology, infant newborn diseases, infant, infant mortality); (ii) Excerpta Medica (1989–92) to identify *Clinical and Experimental Hypertension* (now *Hypertension in Pregnancy*) which was hand-searched for 1992–97; (iii) Science Citation Index (1990–94 which was available locally on computerized disk); (iv) bibliographies of retrieved papers; and (v) a standard toxicology text[2]. Titles, abstracts and/or photocopies of the methods of retrieved papers were screened and data abstracted independently by two reviewers who corroborated their findings (i.e. double-checked their data and resolved disagreement through discussion). The most up-to-date data were abstracted from duplicate publications. Inclusion criteria were English/French language, human pregnancy, RCT, β-blocker (including labetalol, a drug with α- and β-blocking activity) versus non-β-blocker/no therapy, and assessment of the effectiveness of maternal antihypertensive therapy and/or perinatal risk. Studies with clearly inadequate methods of randomization (e.g. randomization by alternate allocation) were included only in a sensitivity analysis. β-Blockers were considered as a class, given the fact that their effects are receptor mediated. Trials of β-blockers for indications other than pregnancy hypertension were included only in the evaluation of perinatal mortality and morbidity. Trials of single drug administration were accepted if β-blockers could be expected to be in the maternal–fetal bloodstream at delivery and affect neonatal health. Short-term treatment trials were excluded from analysis of end-points which they could not theoretically impact (i.e. prematurity, small for gestational age (SGA) infants, admission to hospital prior to delivery, and development of proteinuria (see below)). Abstracts without companion publications were included only in a sensitivity analysis, as a potential source of trials that did not demonstrate a treatment effect. Abstracted data were entered into 2 × 2 tables using StatXact software [11] for IBM-compatible computers. Entry was double-checked.

Outcome definitions that were not standardized were documented at data abstraction and considered as potential sources of between-study variation (e.g. SGA was defined as <3, <5 or <10 centiles, or <250 in Usher's curve). *Maternal* outcomes were severe hypertension, additional antihypertensive therapy, admission to hospital prior to delivery, development of preeclampsia or proteinuria (as a surrogate for preeclampsia), cesarean section, placental abruption, and the need for patients to discontinue their randomized drug due to maternal side effects. *Perinatal* outcomes were perinatal mortality, prematurity (not examined when there was routine induction of labor or in i.v. β-blocker trials which delivered patients shortly after starting treatment), SGA infants, admission to special care nursery (SCN) (for trials that did not practice routine admission), and neonatal bradycardia, hypotension, hypoglycemia, hypothermia, low Apgar scores, and respiratory distress syndrome (RDS) (outcomes classified as apnea, 'asphyxia' or respiratory depression were excluded).

Meta-Analysis

By convention [12], the summary statistic for each RCT '*i*' was the odds ratio (ψ_i). Pooling of trial results in the form of a summary odds ratio (denoted OR) and 95% confidence interval (CI) was based on the fixed effects model using the Mantel Haenszel method [13] with the Robins–Breslow–Greenland (RBG) confidence interval [14]. Exact methods were used when the data were sparse, that is when no events were observed among β-blocker or control groups. Trials in which no outcomes were observed in either arm were not informative for analysis. A multiplicative model was chosen, as it is stable over a wide range of reported event rates. This model assumed that between-trial variation in outcome was due to chance alone; therefore, this variation was disregarded when weights for individual trials were estimated. The null hypothesis (of no between-trial variation) was not rejected (and the pooling of outcomes was considered valid) if the asymptotic *p* value for the Breslow–Day test for homogeneity of all ψ_i values was less than 0.05; when exact methods were used for the odds ratio, the Zelen test of homogeneity was employed. An OR of 1 reflected the absence of a β-blocker effect. An OR <1 reflected fewer events among β-blocker groups, and an OR >1 reflected excess events among β-blocker groups. Results were considered to be significant when the 95% CI for the odds ratio did not include 1.

For ease of interpretation, significant results were also expressed in terms of the absolute risk reduction, called the 'number need to treat' (NNT) (Appendix A) [12], which referred to the number of patients one would need to treat with β-blockers to cause one (adverse or favorable) event; the median p_2 (event rate among controls) of included trials was used in the calculation because the distribution of p_2 for various outcomes was not normally distributed. The lower and upper limits of the 95% CI for NNT were calculated by using the respective lower and upper limits of the 95% CI of the OR.

Reporting bias for each outcome was estimated as the proportion of trials that reported an outcome, of all that could have reported that outcome. For example, admission to hospital prior to delivery was not a potential outcome among trials of hospitalized patients who were treated with i.v. β-blockers.

Ideally, publication bias should have been based on all included trials. However, variation in reporting of outcomes made this impossible. For each outcome, both (i) calculation of the fail-safe N (N_{fs}) [15] (Appendix A) which estimates the number of trials that would have to be uncovered to negate a statistically significant finding and (ii) plots of $\ln(\psi_i)$ versus sample size were performed. Publication bias was taken to be demonstrated either by (i) an N_{fs} less than the number of trials included in the analysis that did report that outcome or (ii) a relative paucity of studies with OR ≥ 1 (i.e. $\ln(\psi_i)>0$) corresponding to those in the left upper quadrant of a $\ln(\psi_i)$ versus sample size plot. Given that investigators tend not to report (and journals tend not to publish) studies which did not show beneficial therapeutic effects, it was assumed that publication bias would be reflected by failure to publish (especially small) trials that did not demonstrate a beneficial therapeutic effect of β-blockers on maternal or perinatal outcomes [16]. Otherwise, results were considered to be robust to reporting and publication biases.

Grouping of Trials and Subgroup Analyses

Trials were grouped according to the nature of the hypertensive process: (1) those that enrolled and treated with oral β-blockers only pregnant women with mild-to-moderate chronic hypertension; (2) those that enrolled and treated with oral β-blockers women with mild-to-moderate hypertension presenting later in pregnancy (be it chronic or pregnancy-induced); and (3) those that enrolled patients with severe (usually pregnancy-induced) hypertension requiring parenteral therapy. There were several reasons for analysis of the data in this way. Firstly, the rationale for separating chronic hypertension from PIH is based on different underlying pathophysiology and potential duration of treatment (i.e. throughout pregnancy in many cases versus after 20 weeks' gestation, respectively). Secondly, although a clear distinction between the two types of hypertension would have been ideal, many hypertension trials failed to distinguish between chronic hypertension needing treatment only later in pregnancy, and pregnancy-induced hypertension (proteinuric or non-proteinuric), as the distinction may become clear only months after delivery. Trials with these participants were designated 'late-onset' pregnancy hypertension trials. Thirdly, parenteral therapy for patients with acute, severe (usually proteinuric) hypertension (i.e. category (iii) above) should be considered separately given that the urgency of treatment dictates a different route of drug administration and duration of therapy. Groups (i) and (ii) were also subdivided according to whether β-blockers were compared with placebo/no therapy or other antihypertensive therapy; the former addresses the question of whether therapy is beneficial overall, whereas the latter defines whether β-blockers are preferable to other agents. It follows from the aforementioned arguments that pooling of results of all trials for each outcome was not performed.

The following were considered as explanatory variables, for each grouping of trials: *characteristics of participants* (severity of hypertension), *intervention* (route of administration, type of β-blocker (i.e. selective/non-selective, and agent used), therapy of controls, goal and duration of treatment, and fall in mean arterial pressure (MAP)), and *outcome definitions*. Hypertension was defined as mild (dBP of 90–99 or MAP of ≤107 mmHg), moderate (dBP 100–109 or MAP 108–129) or severe (dBP ≥ 110 or MAP ≥ 130) according to mean severity at enrollment. It was expected that 'fall in MAP' would be related to fall in maternal blood pressure, but 'fall in MAP' was examined specifically because of the historical obstetric concern that lowering blood pressure will lower placental perfusion and cause intrauterine growth restriction. Such subgroup analyses were planned in light of the potentially low statistical power of tests to detect heterogeneity.

The relationship between $\ln(\psi_i)$ and continuous explanatory variables was assessed by weighted least-squares regression using weights from the fixed effects model analysis. Pearson R^2 >20% (with $P \le 0.10$) was (arbitrarily) taken to suggest a relationship between $\ln(\psi_i)$ and a trial characteristic. The relationship between $\ln(\psi_i)$ and categorical variables was assessed by arranging the 95% CI of $\ln(\psi_i)$ for each trial according to the categories of the explanatory variable (e.g. route of drug administration); the CI values were then compared visually. Secondly, the event rate in each β-blocker group (p_1, y-axis) was plotted against that in the control group (p_2, x-axis) using different plotting symbols to denote the categories of interest [17]; no β-blocker effect was reflected by a symmetrical distribution of data points relative to the line of unity, whereas excess points *below* the line reflected excess events among controls and excess points above the line reflected excess events among β-blocker treated cases. These analyses were planned because of the anticipated low statistical power of trials of pregnancy hypertension.

RESULTS

Characteristics of Trials

Of the 3096 papers screened, 32 trials in 40 publications [18–58] met the inclusion criteria; two trials [39,48] each with two β-blocker treatment arms were included as four data sets to bring the total number of trials to 34. Most trials (20/32) were retrieved from Medline. Articles were excluded for the following reasons: not pregnancy (n = 2083), animal data or in vitro (n = 129); not English or French (n = 194); not RCT (n = 519); outcomes assessed neither maternal nor perinatal benefit/risk (n = 91); no β-blocker exposure among cases (n = 6); β-blocker treatment of control groups (n = 5); duplicate publications (n = 27); abstracts with no companion articles (n = 4) [59–62]; and other (n = 6). The latter were for inadequate methods of randomization [63,64], results not presented by randomized group [65,66], and trials in which most patients would have cleared β-blockers before delivery [67,68].

Thirty trials [18–54] studied β-blockers for treatment of pregnancy hypertension. Four additional trials examined either the effect of β-blockers on the hypertensive response to endotracheal intubation [55,56], attenuation of side effects of ritodrine tocolysis [57], or management of dysfunctional labor [58]; these studies were included only in the evaluation of perinatal outcomes. No trial of β-blockers for other medical problems (e.g. maternal thyrotoxicosis) was located. Eleven trials [21,35,36,47–49,54–58] had not been included in previous overviews [5–8].

Table 1 shows selected characteristics of included trials, arranged according to management of the following: (i) chronic hypertension treated with oral β-blockers throughout pregnancy, (ii) 'late-onset' hypertension amenable to oral antihypertensive therapy; and (iii) severe 'late-onset' hypertension requiring parenteral therapy. There were only two trials that enrolled patients with mild chronic hypertension (Butters et al. [23], Sibai et al. [37]) and treated for over 25 weeks with a goal of decreasing dBP to <90 mmHg. Other trials enrolled patients with 'late-onset' pregnancy hypertension (presenting late in the second trimester or third trimester) and randomized them to oral β-blockers or either placebo/no therapy (n = 8 trials) or other antihypertensive therapy (usually methyldopa) (n = 15 trials). With the exception of Ref. [46], all trials enrolled women with mild-to-moderate hypertension. The goal was a dBP<86–90 mmHg in all but one trial [35] in which most patients received i.v. antihypertensive therapy to get dBP<100 mmHg. Mean treatment duration was 8.7 weeks (reported by 15/23 trials). The mean fall in MAP (reported by 15/23 trials) was 4.8 mmHg greater among β-blocker treated groups than among controls. Acute, severe 'late-onset' hypertension was treated with either i.v. labetalol vs. hydralazine (n = 4 trials) or diazoxide (n = 1 trial). The treatment goal was a diastolic BP<100 mmHg in preparation for imminent delivery (i.e. mean treatment duration of 2.3 h (5/5 trials)). The mean fall in MAP was 6.3 mm lower among labetalol-treated groups than among the comparison group. Labetalol was the most common β-blocker prescribed orally (9/25 trials overall) and i.v. (5/5). Drugs were used in standard therapeutic doses.

The median sample size of included trials was only 22 patients per group (range, 3–97) (Table 1). There was usually no description of randomization method (70%), allocation blinding (61%), or outcome assessment blinding (67%) (Table 1). Only the tendency to report allocation blinding improved over time (not presented). No effect was seen of methodological quality (assessed by allocation blinding) on outcome (not presented).

Outcome definitions varied considerably, but for only neonatal bradycardia (discussed below) did outcome definition have an impact on treatment effect. Severe hypertension was defined as a dBP>100 mmHg [21,22,35,47], dBP>110 mmHg [24,25,27,28,32–34], a sudden rise in BP requiring urgent delivery [26,40,42], or failure to meet treatment goals before imminent delivery [49–53]. The need for additional antihypertensive therapy was defined as the addition of ancillary therapy to randomized treatment or withdrawal due to severe hypertension [23,43].

Table 1
Characteristics of Randomized Trials of β-Blockers in Pregnancy[a]

TRIAL	NO. OF WOMEN	TYPE OF HTN[b]	SEVERITY OF HTN	DRUG ROUTE	TREATMENT CASES	TREATMENT CONT.	DURATION (WEEKS)	OUTCOME BLINDING	FALL MAP[c] (mmHg)
Chronic hypertension									
Butters et al. [23]	29	Chronic	Mild	Oral	aten	Placebo	23.15	Double	4.66
Sibai et al. [37]	176	Chronic	Mild	Oral	lab	None	27.60	None	–
'Late-onset' pregnancy hypertension									
Oral β-bl vs. placebo/no therapy:									
Cruickshank et al. [18–20]	114	Mixed	Mild	Oral	lab	None	4.23	None	–
Bott-Kanner et al. [21]	60	Mixed	Mild	Oral	pind	Placebo	9.45	Double	4.06
Plouin et al. [22]	154	PIH	Mild	Oral	oxpren	Placebo	10.15	Double	1.33
Pickles et al. [24,25]	144	PIH	Mild	Oral	lab	Placebo	3.54	Double	5.87
Sibai et al. [26]	186	PIH	Mild	Oral	lab	None	2.95	None	7.99
Hogstedt et al. [27,28]	161	Mixed	Mild	Oral	metop	None	7.57	None	6.00
Wichman et al. [29–31]	52	Mixed	Mild	Oral	metop	Placebo	5.00	Double	–
Rubin et al. [32–34]	120	PIH	Mild	Oral	aten	Placebo	5.20	Double	–
Oral β-bl vs. other drugs									
Hjertberg et al. [35]	20	PIH	mod	Oral	lab	Hydral	–	None	–
Oumachigui et al. [36]	30	PIH	mod	Oral	metop	MD	–	None	3.37
Plouin et al. [38]	176	Mixed	Mild	Oral	lab	MD	11.81	None	1.00
Lardoux (lab) et al. [39]	42	Mixed	Mild	Oral	lab	MD	–	None	–
Lardoux (aceb) et al. [39]	42	Mixed	Mild	Oral	aceb	MD	–	None	–
Rosenfeld et al. [40]	44	Mixed	Mild	Oral	pind + hydral	Hydral	–	None	1.50
Ellenboggen et al. [41]	32	PIH	mod	Oral	pind	MD	5.43	None	15.77
Gallery et al. [42]	183	Mixed	Mild	Oral	oxpren	MD	8.58	None	–
Livingstone et al. [43]	28	Mixed	Mild	Oral	propran	MD	–	None	5.10
Fidler et al. [44]	98	Mixed	mod	Oral	oxpren	MD	7.55	None	1.01
Lamming et al. [45]	26	PIH	Mild	Oral	lab	MD	2.95	None	10.80
Redman [46]	72	Mixed	severe	Oral	lab	MD	4.39	None	−1.66
Jannet et al. [47]	100	Mixed	mod	Oral	metop	nicard	9.0	None	–
Paran et al. (prop) [48]	32	Mixed	mod	Oral	prop + hydral	Hydral	–	None	2.50
Paran et al. (pind) [48]	34	Mixed	mod	Oral	pind + hydral	Hydral	–	None	0.60
'Late-onset' pregnancy hypertension, i.v. therapy									
Bhorat et al. [49]	34	PIH	severe	i.v.	lab	Hydral	0.04	None	0.83
Mabie et al. [50,51]	21	Mixed	severe	i.v.	lab	Hydral	0.01	None	−7.80
Ashe et al. [52]	20	Mixed	severe	i.v.	lab	Hydral	0.02	None	−12.00
Michael [53]	90	Mixed	severe	i.v.	lab	diazox	0.16	None	–
Garden et al. [54]	6	Mixed	severe	i.v.	lab	Hydral	0.24	None	–
β-bl for other indications									
Ramanathan et al. [55]	25	PIH [d]	mod	i.v.	lab	None	0.0006	none	–
Tunstall [56]	10	n/a [d]	n/a [d]	i.v.	propran	Placebo	0.0001	Double	–
Ross et al. [57]	17	n/a [d]	n/a [d]	Oral	metop	Placebo	–	Double	–
Sanchez-Ramos et al. [58]	96	n/a[d]	n/a [d]	i.v.	prop	Placebo	0.024	Double	–

[a] Ordered according to therapeutic approach. aceb (acebutolol), aten (atenolol), βbl (β-blocker), β_1-sel. (β_1-selective), diazox (diazoxide), Cont. (controls), HTN (hypertension), hydral (hydralazine), ISA (intrinsic sympathomimetic activity), lab (labetalol), metop (metoprolol), MD (methyldopa), mod (moderate), nicard (nicardipine), oxpren (oxprenolol), PIH (pregnancy-induced hypertension), pind (pindolol), propran (propranolol).

[b] Defined as 'chronic' (antedating pregnancy or diagnosed before 20 weeks), PIH (pregnancy-induced, whether proteinuric or not), 'mixed' (when participants had 'late-onset pregnancy hypertension that could have been either chronic or PIH).

[c] Fall MAP (Fall in MAP in {β-blocker}–{Control} groups).

[d] These trials studied the effect of β-blockers on the hypertensive reaction to endotracheal intubation (Ramanathan et al. [55], Tunstall [56]), the side effects of ritodrine (Ross et al. [57]), or dysfunctional labor (Sanchez-Ramos et al. [58]).

Admission to hospital prior to delivery was for dBP>100 mmHg [29–31], dBP>110 mm [22,38,44], or was not stated [32,34]. Proteinuria was defined as 'greater than trace' [44,46], >1 + or 0.25 g/l [18–20,22,27,28], >2 + or 0.5 g/l [21,38,41], or was not defined at all [24,25,45,47]; preeclampsia per se was defined as hypertension, proteinuria, and hyperuricemia [37,29–31]. Perinatal mortality was defined as death of a fetus weighing >500 g or a newborn up to 4 weeks after birth. Prematurity was defined as GA at delivery <37 weeks in all but one trial [32,34] which used a cut-off of <36 weeks. SGA was defined as BW<10th percentile for GA [18–20,22–26,32–35,46,47], <5th percentile for GA [38], <250 in Usher's curve [40], or not defined at all [27,28,37]. Neonatal bradycardia was defined as neonatal HR <120 bpm [24,25,32–35,53], or not defined at all [27,28,38,43,47,54,55]. Neonatal hypotension was defined as a sBP<30–40 mmHg [35,50,51] or not at all [53,55]. Neonatal hypothermia was defined as a temperature <36°C [40] or not at all [47]. Neonatal hypoglycemia was defined as <1.4 mM [24,25,32–34], ≤1.7 mM [27,28,35,40], <2.0 mM [50,51], <2.2 mM [39], or not at all [37,43,47,52,53,55].

OR and 95% CI

There was no association between β-blocker type (e.g. β_1-selectivity) and outcome (not presented).

Mild Chronic Hypertension. Only patients with mild chronic hypertension were enrolled. Table 2 shows that no significant therapeutic effects of β-blockers were demonstrated on maternal outcomes; no data were provided for the incidence of severe hypertension, admission to hospital prior to delivery, or the need to change drugs due to maternal side effects, despite a mean treatment duration of over 25 weeks.

The only demonstrated effect of β-blockers on perinatal outcomes was an increased incidence of SGA infants; however, the two trials included differed significantly in their effects. Butters et al. [23], in a small trial of long-term atenolol versus placebo, revealed a dramatic increase in SGA infants among atenolol-treated patients (OR of 54.6, 95% CI [2.8, 1111.1]). There were two withdrawals from the placebo group because of uncontrolled hypertension, and the remaining controls had relatively normal mean birthweight (3530 g, SD not reported). However, even if both withdrawals from the control arm had been delivered of SGA infants, the odds ratio for SGA infants would still have been significantly increased (i.e. OR of 10.0, 95% CI [2.0, 50.0]). In contrast, the other trial of long-term labetalol versus no therapy [37] failed to reveal (or even suggest) an adverse effect of labetalol on fetal growth (i.e. 6/85 [labetalol] vs. 7/89 [no therapy]).

Mild-to-Moderate 'Late-Onset' Pregnancy Hypertension. All participants in β-blockers versus placebo/no therapy trials had mild 'late-onset' hypertension severity. Table 3 shows that when compared with placebo/no therapy, β-blockers decreased the incidence of severe hypertension (NNT of 10, 95% CI [8,14]) and additional antihypertensive therapy (NNT of 9, 95% CI [8,13]). These results were unlikely to be due to publication bias given that more trials than included in this subgroup analysis (i.e. 6.9 vs. 6 [severe hypertension] (respectively) and 7.1 vs. 6 [additional therapy] (respectively)) would have to be uncovered to negate the findings. Treatment was also associated with less frequent admission to hospital prior to delivery; however, there was more variation between trials that could be expected by chance alone and all were published prior to the advent of obstetric day units. β-Blockers were associated with a borderline decrease in the development of proteinuria; however, significant between-trial variation in outcome was detected and remained unexplained by variation in participants, interventions or outcome definitions.

β-Blockers did not affect perinatal mortality; this analysis included data from the non-hypertension trial by Ross et al. [57]. β-Blockers were associated with a borderline increase in SGA infants and a significant decrease in the incidence of RDS (NNT of 21, 95% CI [16, 99]; N_{fs} of 4.7, compared with 4 included), despite having no effect on the incidence of prematurity. Although β-blockers were not associated with a significant increase in neonatal bradycardia,

Table 2
Randomized Trials of Oral β-blockers for Mild Chronic Hypertension[a]

OUTCOME	NO. OF TRIALS (n = 2)	β-BLOCKER EVENT RATE	CONTROL EVENT RATE	POOLED OR [95% CI]	P^b
Maternal					
Additional therapy	2	5/102	12/107	0.41 [0.14, 1.20]	0.33
Developed proteinuria	1	14/86	14/90	1.06 [0.47, 2.37]	n/a
Cesarean section	1	30/86	29/90	1.12 [0.60, 2.13]	n/a
Placental abruption	1	2/86	2/90	1.05 [0.14, 7.61]	n/a
Perinatal					
Perinatal mortality	2	2/112	1/112	1.99 [0.18, 22.30]	0.39
Prematurity	1	10/85	8/89	1.35 [0.51, 3.60]	n/a
SGA infants	2	16/100	7/104	**2.46 [1.02, 5.92]**	**0.0008**
Neonatal hypoglycemia	1	2/85	1/90	2.14 [0.19, 24.10]	n/a
Low Apgar scores	1	4/85	4/89	1.05 [0.25, 4.35]	n/a

[a] Bold type refers to statistical significance (P<0.05). Additional therapy, additional antihypertensive therapy; df, degrees of freedom; n/ a, not applicable; SGA, small for gestational age.

[b] P value for Breslow–Day test of homogeneity, with df = {(no. of trials)–1}.

Table 3
Randomized Trials of Oral β-Blockers Versus Placebo/No Therapy for Mild 'Late-Onset' Pregnancy Hypertension[a]

OUTCOME	NO. OF TRIALS (n = 8)	β-BLOCKER EVENT RATE	CONTROL EVENT RATE	POOLED OR [95% CI]	P^b
Maternal					
Severe hypertension	6	23/412	71/413	**0.27 [0.16, 0.45]**	0.62
Additional therapy	6	32/412	81/413	**0.32 [0.21, 0.50]**	0.73
Admitted prior to delivery	3	80/150	98/141	**0.52 [0.33, 0.83]**	**0.0006**
Developed proteinuria	7	70/366	93/369	0.69 [0.48, 1.02]	0.19
Cesarean section	6	94/347	106/363	0.89 [0.64, 1.24]	0.09
Placental abruption	2	3/170	0/170	0.00 [0.00, 2.40]	n/a
Changed drugs due to maternal side effects	6	9/371	4/382	2.28 [0.69, 7.54]	0.59
Perinatal					
Perinatal mortality[c]	9	8/503	9/519	0.87 [0.33, 2.28]	0.38
Prematurity	5	52/335	66/349	0.79 [0.53, 1.18]	0.21
SGA infants	6	56/414	41/423	1.47 [0.96, 2.26]	0.35
Admission to SCN	4	74/275	69/253	0.95 [0.66, 1.37]	0.34
Neonatal bradycardia	3	23/193	12/188	1.88 [0.89, 3.95]	**0.01**
Neonatal hypoglycemia	3	14/207	18/209	0.74 [0.35, 1.53]	0.30
Low Apgar scores	3	4/180	7/178	0.56 [0.16, 1.93]	0.30
RDS	4	6/283	22/284	**0.33 [0.13, 0.85]**	0.93

[a] Bold type refers to statistical significance (P<0.05). Additional therapy, additional antihypertensive therapy; df, degrees of freedom; n/ a, not applicable; RDS, respiratory distress syndrome; SCN, special care nursery; SGA, small for gestational age.

[b] P value for Breslow–Day test of homogeneity, with df = {(no. of trials)–1} unless no events were recorded among one group, in which case Zelen statistic for homogeneity is reported.

[c] Includes data from non-pregnancy hypertension trial [57].

trial results were heterogeneous; Fig. 1 shows that outcomes from Rubin and co-workers [32–34] were discordant with the others; this trial specified continuous monitoring of neonatal heart rate, and no intervention was required for the bradycardia diagnosed. No data were reported on the incidence of neonatal hypotension or hypothermia.

Participants in β-blockers versus other antihypertensive therapy trials had 'late-onset' hypertension of mild-moderate severity, with one exception [46]. Table 4 shows that β-blockers had no impact on maternal or perinatal outcomes when compared with other agents (usually methyldopa). The inconsistencies in outcomes between trials were difficult to explain. Of note, neither β-blocker type, nor type of comparator drug, explained the variation in effectiveness of blood pressure control. Definitions of proteinuria were also not informative. Finally, none of the trials that reported maternal side effects was double-blinded.

Severe 'Late-Onset' Pregnancy Hypertension. Table 5 shows that i.v. labetalol was no more effective than hydralazine or diazoxide in decreasing severe hypertension or additional antihypertensive therapy. However, labetalol was also associated with less maternal hypotension (NNT of 6, 95% CI [6, 21]) and fewer cesarean sections (NNT of 3.3, 95% CI [2.1, 9.5]), regardless of whether the comparator drug was hydralazine or diazoxide. The N_{fs} was 5.8 trials, compared with the 5 included. The results were not explained by hydralazine dosing schedule (i.e. bolus injection or infusion), and insufficient information was available on the indications for operative delivery. Perinatal mortality did not differ

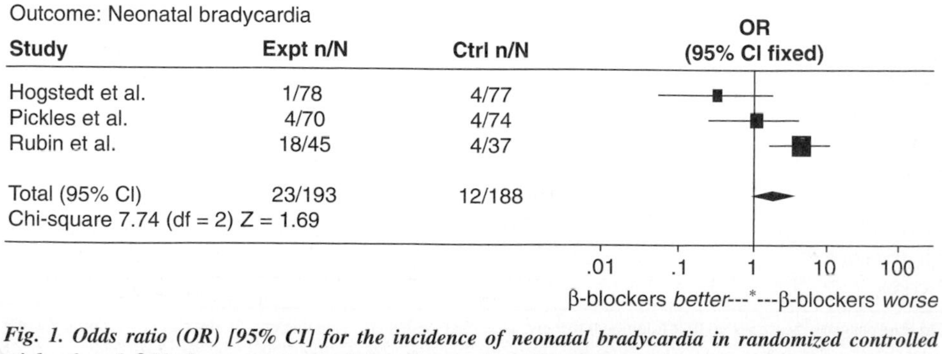

Fig. 1. Odds ratio (OR) [95% CI] for the incidence of neonatal bradycardia in randomized controlled trials of oral β-blockers versus placebo/no therapy for mild 'late-onset' pregnancy hypertension. The results of Rubin et al. [32–34] differ from those of Hogstedt et al. [27,28] and Pickles et al. [24,25].

Table 4
Randomized Trials of Oral β-Blockers Versus Other Antihypertensives for Primarily Mild to Moderate 'Late-Onset' Pregnancy Hypertension[a]

OUTCOME	NO. OF TRIALS (n = 15)	β-BLOCKER EVENT RATE	CONTROL EVENT RATE	POOLED OR [95% CI]	P^b
Maternal					
Severe hypertension	4	32/178	30/169	1.36 [0.76, 2.44]	**0.04**
Additional therapy	11	114/418	102/397	1.10 [0.79, 1.55]	**0.0006**
Admitted prior to delivery	2	83/139	82/133	0.93 [0.56, 1.54]	0.30
Developed proteinuria	6	28/226	30/222	0.98 [0.57, 1.71]	**0.02**
Cesarean section	10	144/371	125/344	1.12 [0.83, 1.52]	0.79
Changed drugs due to maternal side effects	7	7/244	2/234	2.49 [0.46, 13.34]	**0.04**
Perinatal					
Perinatal mortality	15	9/555	19/531	0.45 [0.22, 1.12]	0.65
Prematurity	5	44/164	32/146	1.32 [0.78, 2.22]	0.97
SGA infants	6	55/288	57/258	0.84 [0.55, 1.29]	0.34
Admission to SCN	3	32/183	29/171	0.89 [0.52, 1.52]	0.50
Neonatal bradycardia	3	0/90	0/82	Not informative	n/a
Neonatal hypotension	1	0/9	0/11	Not informative	n/a
Neonatal hypothermia	1	3/23	5/21	0.46 [0.09, 2.20]	n/a
Neonatal hypoglycemia	5	9/88	12/86	1.18 [0.49, 2.81]	0.23
Low Apgar scores	4	13/172	9/162	1.34 [0.55, 3.25]	0.55
RDS	2	**16/47**	9/45	2.01 [0.77, 5.22]	0.77

[a] Bold type refers to statistical significance ($P<0.05$). Additional therapy, additional antihypertensive therapy; df, degrees of freedom; n/ a, not applicable; RDS, respiratory distress syndrome; SCN, special care nursery; SGA, small for gestational age.

[b] P value for Breslow–Day test of homogeneity, with df = {(no. of trials) –1} unless no events were recorded among one group, in which case Zelen statistic for homogeneity is reported.

Table 5
Randomized Trials of i.v. Labetalol Versus Hydralazine/Diazoxide for Severe 'Mixed' Pregnancy Hypertension[a]

OUTCOME	NO. OF TRIALS (n = 7)	β-BLOCKER EVENT RATE	CONTROL EVENT RATE	POOLED OR [95% CI]	P^b
Maternal					
Severe hypertension	4	13/113	8/91	1.57 [0.59, 4.21]	**0.05**
Additional therapy	3	1/73	1/71	1.00 [0.05, 18.57]	n/ a
Maternal hypotension	4	1/101	14/81	**0.13 [0.03, 0.71]**	0.98
Cesarean section	5	63/175	76/167	**0.28 [0.13, 0.63]**	0.08
Placental abruption	1	0/13	1/6	Invalid	n/ a
Changed drugs due to maternal side effects	1	0/18	0/16	Invalid	n/ a
Perinatal					
Perinatal mortality[c]	7	4/111	8/98	0.37 [0.09, 1.46]	0.20
Admission to SCN[c]	2	1/64	1/57	0.96 [0.06, 15.78]	n/ a
Neonatal bradycardia[c]	4	0/45	0/30	Invalid	n/ a
Neonatal hypotension[c]	3	0/75	1/63	Invalid	n/ a
Neonatal hypothermia	1	0/14	0/11	Invalid	n/ a
Neonatal hypoglycemia[c]	5	2/99	1/74	1.21 [0.11, 13.07]	0.24
Low Apgar scores[c]	5	4/85	4/71	0.69 [0.19, 2.49]	**0.018**
RDS	3	8/63	6/56	1.03 [0.33, 3.23]	0.18

[a] Bold type refers to statistical significance ($P < 0.05$). Additional therapy, additional antihypertensive therapy; df, degrees of freedom; n/ a, not applicable; RDS, respiratory distress syndrome; SCN, special care nursery; SGA, small for gestational age.

[b] P value for Breslow–Day test of homogeneity with df {(no. of trials)–1}, not applicable when only one trial included in analysis.

[c] Includes data from non-pregnancy hypertension trials: Ramanathan et al. [55], Sanchoz-Ramos et al. [58], and/or Tunstall [56].

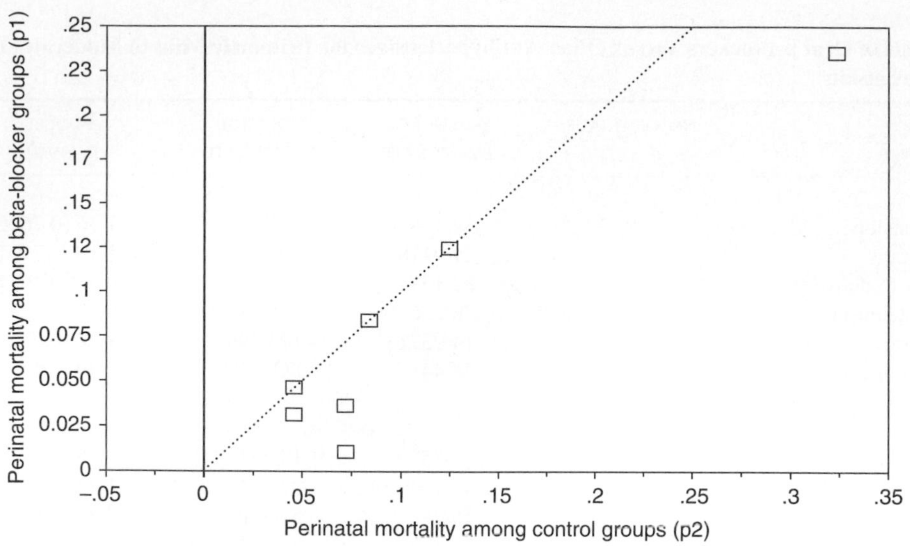

Fig. 2. Bivariate plot of perinatal mortality rates for i.v. labetalol (p_1, y-axis) versus hydralazine/diazoxide (p_2, x-axis) groups. An excess of data points below the dotted line of unity reflects more perinatal mortality among control groups.

significantly between groups, although Fig. 2 shows that the bivariate plot of event rates favors labetalol. Finally, the lack of homogeneity for low Apgar scores was attributable to Tunstall's trial which was small (n = 10 patients) and did not relate the significance of the low Apgar scores to other neonatal outcomes (e.g. admission to SCN).

Meta-Regression

Overall, β-blocker-induced falls in MAP were associated with less severe hypertension (R^2 = 0.49, P = 0.03) and a borderline increase in SGA infants (R^2 = 0.41, P = 0.06); no effect was seen on proteinuria (R^2 = 0.19, P = 0.25). No effect of duration of therapy was seen on SGA infants (R^2 = 0.23, P = 0.23).

Impact of Including Trials with Clearly Inadequate Methods of Randomization

Most trials described unclear methods of randomization. Therefore, the two reports excluded because of alternate allocation [63,64] were included in a sensitivity analyses. Both trials fell into the group of trials that administered oral β-blocker versus other antihypertensive therapy for 'late-onset' pregnancy hypertension. Marlettini et al. [63] reported on two trials for treatment of mild PIH: atenolol versus verapamil slow release (SR) (n = 50) and pindolol versus verapamil SR (n = 44). El-Qarmalawi et al. [64] randomized patients with mild PIH to pindolol or verapamil SR (n = 104). Analysis of outcomes was unchanged with two exceptions. β-Blockers were shown to be less effective antihypertensives than calcium channel blockers (OR of 0.40, 95% CI [0.20, 0.79]); the effects of Marlettini et al. were consistent with those of Jannet et al., the only β-blocker versus calcium channel blocker trial in the main analysis. Abstracts without companion publications provided little useful data, but when their data were included in analysis of severe hypertension, perinatal mortality, and SGA infants, results were not changed (not presented).

DISCUSSION

This meta-analysis updates previous quantitative overviews [5–8] with the inclusion of 11 new trials and relates measurable characteristics of participants, interventions, and outcome definitions to demonstrated effects of β-blockers when used primarily for treatment of pregnancy hypertension.

The data from this meta-analysis may aid practicing clinicians in several clinical situations: (1) chronic hypertension considered for treatment throughout pregnancy; (2) mild-moderate 'late-onset' pregnancy hypertension (i.e. either chronic hypertension requiring treatment only later in pregnancy, or mild-to-moderate pregnancy-induced hypertension) amenable to orally administered treatment later in pregnancy; and (3) severe 'late-onset' pregnancy hypertension requiring parenteral antihypertensive therapy and imminent delivery.

Mild Chronic Hypertension

There are only two trials that provided data on β-blocker therapy for chronic hypertension, in women who are planning pregnancy or are in early pregnancy. No beneficial effects were seen on maternal outcomes examined, although neither trial reported the relevant outcomes of uncontrolled hypertension or admission to hospital prior to delivery. There was uncertainty as to the perinatal risks of therapy given the discordant and inexplicable findings of a β-blocker-associated increase in SGA infants. Therefore, it is unclear that the benefits of β-blocker therapy outweigh the potential risks. Consideration should be given to use of antihypertensive treatment only when blood pressure reaches a level (i.e. close to 170/110 mmHg) [69]) which is clearly dangerous to the mother over the short term. If therapy is instituted, then pending future data, labetalol may be a better β-blocker to use than atenolol, although methyldopa is still considered by professional organizations to be the drug of first choice [1]. No data were provided on teratogenicity (i.e. induction of structural or functional defects) after first trimester exposure, making it necessary for practitioners to seek observational data on this matter [2].

Mild-to-Moderate 'Late-Onset' Pregnancy Hypertension

Eight trials of oral β-blockers versus placebo/no therapy for mild 'late-onset' pregnancy hypertension revealed, not surprisingly, that β-blockers significantly improved maternal outcomes, but had an uncertain impact on perinatal outcomes.

β-Blockers significantly improved control of maternal blood pressure, and the incidence of severe hypertension. Although β-blocker treatment decreased admission to hospital prior to delivery, the clinical significance of this is uncertain given that the trials were conducted prior to the onset of obstetrical day units. Although β-blockers were associated with a borderline decrease in the incidence of proteinuria (a surrogate endpoint for preeclampsia), it was not clear that this represented a decrease in proteinuric preeclampsia. Statistical power was low, but there was no relationship between either the incidence of proteinuria and lowering of blood pressure, or β-blocker treatment and preeclampsia-related perinatal mortality and prematurity.

β-Blocker therapy significantly decreased RDS without a concomitant decrease in prematurity. The mechanism by which this occurred is a matter of conjecture, and could be related to either a direct effect of β-blockers on type II pneumocytes, the borderline increase in SGA infants, or reporting bias. Secondly, β-blockers were associated with a borderline increase in the incidence of SGA infants, which is a risk factor for perinatal morbidity and survival with handicap. Finally, although trials differed in their effect estimates for neonatal bradycardia, what was actually defined was a pharmacological (rather than a clinically significant) effect of β-blockers on neonatal heart rate.

Therefore, it is unclear that the benefits of β-blocker therapy outweigh the risks for mild-to-moderate 'late-onset' pregnancy hypertension. Consideration should be given to treat only severe hypertension until the relative benefits and risks to mother and fetus are better defined.

Given the uncertainty about whether β-blocker therapy is better than no therapy, it follows that it is premature to discuss comparisons with other antihypertensive agents. However, the 15 relevant published trials revealed that oral β-blockers were equivalent to methyldopa, so there is a choice of available agents (Table 1). Although β-blockers were less effective antihypertensives than calcium channel blockers (i.e. either nicardipine or verapamil SR), this finding requires cautious interpretation given the inadequate methods of randomization in the two trials included only in a sensitivity analysis (Marlettini et al. [63], El-Qarmalawi [64]).

Severe 'Late-Onset' Pregnancy Hypertension

In the five relevant trials of β-blockers (all labetalol) versus either hydralazine or diazoxide, labetalol was associated with less maternal hypotension, fewer cesarean sections, and no excess of perinatal mortality. This review provides more justification for the use of labetalol (rather than hydralazine) when parenteral therapy is used to control severe hypertension and no contraindications to β-blockers exist. No trial compared labetalol (or another β-blocker) with nifedipine, which is now commonly used for acute, severe hypertension.

The limitations of this meta-analysis relate to process, as well as the data on which the meta-analysis was based. Study selection may have been improved by contacting experts about unpublished trials and authors for missing information; nevertheless, significant results appeared large enough to be true regardless of publication and/or reporting biases. Although the OR (which is less immediately understandable than the relative risk (RR)) was used as the summary statistic, the NNT was also calculated for significant results. It was not possible to consider an overall measure of perinatal morbidity as a primary outcome, given variation in and incompleteness of reporting; therefore, the meta-analysis had limited statistical power to rule out important β-blocker effects on most perinatal morbidities.

Finally, even meta-analyses that meet high standards may be misleading when compared with large, definitive trials [70]; therefore, the results presented here should be regarded primarily as uncertainty- and caution-generating for clinicians, and hypothesis-generating for researchers.

ACKNOWLEDGEMENTS

L.A.M. was supported by a Duncan Gordon International Fellowship of the Hospital for Sick Children's Foundation, and a Detweiler Travelling Fellowship from the Royal College of Physicians and Surgeons of Canada. S.B.B. is a National Health Research Scholar of the National Health Research Development Program (Health Canada). G.K. was a Career Scientist of the Ontario Ministry of Health. Research supported by grants from Physicians' Services Incorporated Foundation, for correspondence/requests for reprints. As always, to P.v.D. for his valuable feedback and undying support.

Equations

(1) Number needed to treat (NNT) to cause or prevent one event [12]

$$\mathrm{NNT} = \frac{1-[p_2 \times (1-\mathrm{OR})]}{p_2 \times (1-\mathrm{OR}) \times (1-p_2)}$$

where p_2 is the median event rate among control groups.
(2) Fail-safe N (N_{fs}) [15]

$$N_{\mathrm{fs}} = \frac{N_{\mathrm{o}}(d_{\mathrm{o}} - d_{\mathrm{c}})}{d_{\mathrm{o}} - d_{\mathrm{fs}}},$$

where N_{o}, number of studies included in the overview; d_{o}, ln(OR), (i.e. obtained from the n_{o} trials in the overview); d_c ln(OR) of all studies (published and unpublished; taken to be small (i.e. 0.2) according to Cohen's classification [71]; d_{fs} ln(OR) of unpublished studies (taken to be zero).

REFERENCES

[1] National High Blood Pressure Education Program Working Group. Report on high blood pressure in pregnancy. Am J Obstet Gynecol 1990;163:1691–712, (Review).

[2] Briggs GG, Freeman RK, Yaffe SH, editors, Drugs in pregnancy and lactation, 4th ed, Baltimore: Williams & Wilkins, 1994.

[3] Sulyok E. Endocrine factors in the neonatal adaptation. Acta Physiol Hung 1989;74(3-4):329–39.

[4] Sibai BM. Treatment of hypertension in pregnant women. New Engl J Med 1996;335(4):267–268.

[5] Collins R, Duley L. Beta-blockers in the treatment of pre-eclampsia. In: Enkin MW, Keirse MJNC, Renfrew MJ, Neilson JP, editors. Pregnancy and childbirth module. 'Cochrane Database of systematic Reviews': Review No. 03998, 20 April 1993. Published through 'Cochrane Updates on Disk'. Oxford: Update Software, 1993, Disk Issue 2.

[6] Collins R, Duley L. Beta-blockers vs. methyldopa in the treatment of pre-eclampsia. In: Enkin MW, Keirse MJNC, Renfrew MJ, Neilson JP, editors. Pregnancy and childbirth module. 'Cochrane Database of Systematic Reviews': Review No. 03999, 20 April 1993. Published through 'Cochrane Updates on Disk'. Oxford: Update Software, 1993, Disk Issue 2.

[7] Collins R, Duley L. Labetalol vs hydralazine in severe pregnancy-induced hypertension. In: Enkin MW, Keirse MJNC, Renfrew MJ, Neilson JP, editors. Pregnancy and childbirth module. 'Cochrane Database of Systematic Review': Review No. 04392, 7 May 1992. Published through 'Cochrane Updates on Disk'. Oxford: Update Software, 1993, Disk Issue 2.

[8] Collins R, Duley L. Intravenous labetalol vs. i.v. diazoxide in severe preeclampsia. In: Enkin MW, Keirse MJNC, Renfrew MJ, Neilson JP, editors. Pregnancy and childbirth module. 'Cochrane Database of Systematic Reviews': Review No. 04400, 20 April 1993,. Published through 'Cochrane Updates on Disk'. Oxford: Update Software, 1994, Disk Issue 1.

[9] Sharp SH, Thompson SG, Altman DG. The relation between treatment benefit and underlying risk in meta-analysis. Br Med J 1996;313:735–8.

[10] Thompson SG. Why sources of heterogeneity in meta-analysis should be investigated. Br Med J 1994;309:1351–5.

[11] StatXact 3 for Windows; statistical software for exact nonparametric inference. CYTEL Software Corporation, Cambridge, USA, 1995.

[12] Sackett DL, Deeks JJ, Altman DG. Down with odds ratios! Evidence-Based Med 1996;1(6):164–6.

[13] Fleiss JL. The statistical basis of meta-analysis. Stat Methods Med Res 1993;2:121–45.

[14] Robins J, Breslow N, Greenland S. Estimators of the Mantel–Haenszel variance consistent in both sparse data and large strata limiting models. Biometrics 1986;42:311–23.

[15] Orwon RG. A fail-safe N for effect size in meta-analysis. J Educ Stat 1983;8(2):157–9.

[16] Begg CB. A measure to aid in the interpretation of published clinical trials. Stat Med 1985;4:1–9.

[17] Demets DL. Methods for combining randomized clinical trials: Strengths and limitations. Stat Med 1987;6:341–8.

[18] Cruikshank DJ, Campbell D, Robertson AA, MacGillivary I. Intrauterine growth retardation and maternal labetalol treatment in a random allocation controlled study. J Obstet Gynaecol 1992;12:223–7.

[19] Cruikshank DJ, Robertson AA, Campbell DM, MacGillivary I. Maternal obstetric outcome measured in a randomised controlled study of labetalol in the treatment of hypertension in pregnancy. Clin Exp Hypertens Pregnancy 1991;B10(3):333–44.

[20] Cruickshank DJ, Robertson AA, Campbell DM, MacGillivray I. Does labetalol influence the development of proteinuria in pregnancy hypertension? A randomised controlled study. Eur J Obstet Gynecol Reprod Biol 1992;45:47–51.

[21] Bott-Kanner G, Hirsch M, Friedman S et al. Antihypertensive therapy in the management of hypertension in pregnancy-A clinical double-blind study of pindolol. Clin Exp Hypertens Pregnancy 1992;B11 (2/3):207–20.

[22] Plouin PF, Breart G, Llado J et al. A randomized comparison of early with conservative use of antihypertensive drugs in the management of pregnancy-induced hypertension. Br J Obstet Gynaecol 1990;97: 134–41.

[23] Butters L, Kennedy S, Rubin PC. Atenolol in essential hypertension during pregnancy. Br Med J 1990;301:587–9.

[24] Pickles CJ, Symonds EM, Broughton Pipkin F. The fetal outcome in a randomized double-blind controlled trial of labetalol versus placebo in pregnancy-induced hypertension. Br J Obstet Gynaecol 1989; 96:38–43.

[25] Pickles CJ, Broughton Pipkin F, Symonds EM. A randomised placebo controlled trial of labetalol in the treatment of mild to moderate pregnancy induced hypertension. Br J Obstet Gynaecol 1992;99:964–8.

[26] Sibai BM, Gonzalez AR, Mabie WC, Moretti M. A comparison of labetalol plus hospitalization versus hospitalization alone in the management of preeclampsia remote from term. Obstet Gynecol 1987;70:323–7.

[27] Hogstedt S, Lindeberg S, Axelsson O et al. A prospective controlled trial of metoprolol-hydralazine treatment in the hypertension during pregnancy. Acta Obstet Gynecol Scand 1985;64:505–10.

[28] Hogstedt S, Lindberg B, Lindeberg S, Ludviksson K. Effect of metoprolol on fetal heart rate patterns during pregnancy and delivery. Clin Exp Hypertens Pregnancy 1984;B3:152.

[29] Wichman K, Ryden G, Karlberg BE. A placebo controlled trial of metoprolol in the treatment of hypertension in pregnancy. Scand J Clin Lab Invest 1984;169:90–5.

[30] Wichman K, Karlberg BE, Ryden G. Metoprolol in the treatment of mild to moderate hypertension in pregnancy effects on the mother. Clin Exp Hypertens Pregnancy 1985;B4(2and3):141–56.

[31] Wichman K, Ezitis J, Finnstrom O, Ryden G. Metoprolol in the treatment of hypertension in pregnancy: effects on the newborn baby. Clin Exp Hypertens Pregnancy 1984;B3:153.

[32] Rubin PC, Butters L, Clark D et al. Obstetric aspects of the use in pregnancy-associated hypertension of the β-adrenoreceptor antagonist atenolol. Am J Obstet Gynecol 1984;150:389–92.

[33] Rubin PC, Butters L, Clark DM, Reynolds B, Sumner DJ, Steedman D, Low RA, Reid JL. Placebo-controlled trial of atenolol in treatment of pregnancy-associated hypertension. Lancet 1983;1:431–4.

[34] Rubin PC, Butters L, Reynolds B, Low RAL. Atenolol in the management of pregnancy associated hypertension: Obstetric and paediatric aspects. Clin Exp Hypertens Pregnancy 1984;B3:154.

[35] Hjertberg R, Faxelius G, Lagercrantz H. Neonatal adaptation in hypertensive pregnancy: a study of labetalol vs hydralazine treatment. J Perinat Med 1993;21:69–75.

[36] Oumachigui A, Verghese M, Balachander J. A comparative evaluation of metoprolol and methyldopa in the management of pregnancy-induced hypertension. Indian Heart J 1992;44(1):39–41.

[37] Sibai BM, Mabie WC, Shamsa F, Villar MA, Anderson GD. A comparison of no medication versus methyldopa or labetalol in chronic hypertension during pregnancy. Am J Obstet Gynecol 1990; 162:960–7.

[38] The Labetalol Methyldopa Study Group, Plouin PF, Breart G, Maillard F, Papiernik E, Relier JP. Comparison of antihypertensive efficacy and perinatal safety of labetalol and methyldopa in the treatment of hypertension in pregnancy: a randomized controlled trial. Br J Obstet Gynaecol 1988;95:868–76.

[39] Lardoux H, Blazquez G, Leperlier E, Gerard J. Essai ouvert, comparatif, avec tirage au sort pour le traitement de l'HTA gravidique moderee: methyldopa, acebutolol, labetalol. Arch Mal Coeur 1988;81(Suppl HTA):137–40.

[40] Rosenfeld J, Bott-Kanner G, Boner G et al. Treatment of hypertension during pregnancy with hydralazine monotherapy or with combined therapy with hydralazine and pindolol. Eur J Obstet Gynecol Reprod Biol 1986;22:197–204.
[41] Ellenbogen A, Jaschevatzky O, Davidson A, Anderman S, Grunstein S. Management of pregnancy-induced hypertension with pindolol-comparative study with methyldopa. Int J Gynaecol Obstet 1986;24:3–7.
[42] Gallery EDM, Ross MR, Gyory AZ. Antihypertensive treatment in pregnancy: analysis of different responses to oxprenolol and methyldopa. Br Med J 1985;291:563–6.
[43] Livingstone I, Craswell PW, Bevan EB. Propranolol in pregnancy; three year prospective study. Clin Exp Hypertens Pregnancy 1983;B2(2):341–50.
[44] Fidler J, Smith V, Fayers P, DeSwiet M. Randomised controlled comparative study of methyldopa and oxprenolol in treatment of hypertension in pregnancy. Br Med J 1983;286:1927–30.
[45] Lamming GD, Broughton Pipkin F, Symonds EM. Comparison of the alpha and beta blocking drug, labetalol, and methyldopa in the treatment of moderate and severe pregnancy-induced hypertension. Clin Exp Hypertens Pregnancy 1980;A2(5):865–95.
[46] Redman CWG. A controlled trial of the treatment of hypertension in pregnancy: labetalol compared with methyldopa. In: International Congress Series, Vol. vol. 591, Amsterdam: Excerpta Medica, 1978, pp. 101–10.
[47] Jannet D, Carbonne B, Sebban E, Milliez J. Nicardipine versus metoprolol in the treatment of hypertension during pregnancy: a randomized comparative trial. Obstet Gynecol 1994;84:354–9.
[48] Paran E, Holzberg G, Zmora E, Insler V. β-adrenergic blocking agents in the treatment of pregnancy-induced hypertension. Int J Clin Pharmacol Ther 1995;33(2):119–23.
[49] Bhorat IE, Naidoo DP, Rout CC, Moodley J. Malignant ventricular arrhythmias in eclampsia: a comparison of labetalol with dihydralazine. Am J Obstet Gynecol 1993;168:1292–6.
[50] Mabie WC, Gonzalez AR, Sibai BM, Amon E. A comparative trial of labetalol and hydralazine in the acute management of severe hypertension complicating pregnancy. Obstet Gynecol 1987;70:328–33.
[51] Mabie WC, Gonzalez-Ruiz A, Amon E, Sibai BM. A comparative trial of labetalol and hydralazine for acute management of severe hypertension complicating pregnancy. Clin Exp Hypertens Pregnancy 1987;B6:91.
[52] Ashe RG, Moodley J, Richards AM, Philpott RH. Comparison of labetalol and dihydralazine in hypertensive emergencies of pregnancy. SAMJ 1987;71:354–6.
[53] Michael CA. Intravenous labetalol and intravenous diazoxide in severe hypertension complicating pregnancy. Aust NZ J Obstet Gynaecol 1986;26:26–9.
[54] Garden A, Davey DA, Dommisse J. Intravenous labetalol and intravenous dihydralazine in severe hypertension in pregnancy. Clin Exp Hypertens Pregnancy 1982;B1(2and3):371–83.
[55] Ramanathan J, Sibai BM, Mabie WC, Chauhan D, Ruiz AG. The use of labetalol for attenuation of the hypertensive response to endotracheal intubation in preeclampsia. Am J Obstet Gynecol 1988;159: 650–4.
[56] Tunstall ME. The effect of propranolol on the onset of breathing at birth. Br J Anaesth 1969;41(9):792.
[57] Ross MG, Nicolls E, Stubblefield PG, Kitzmiller JL. Intravenous terbutaline and simultaneous β1-blockade for advanced premature labor. Am J Obstet Gynecol 1983;147:897.
[58] Sanchez-Ramos L, Quillen MJ, Kaunitz AM. Randomized trial of oxytocin alone and with propranolol in the management of dysfunctional labor. Obstet Gynecol 1996;88:517–20.
[59] Li CY, Lao TT, Yu KM, Wong SP, Leung CF. The effect of labetalol on mild pre-eclampsia. In: Proceedings of 7th World Congress of Hypertension in Pregnancy, Perugia, Italy, 1990, p. 191.
[60] Hjertberg P, Belfrage P, Faxelius G, Lagercrantz H. Neonatal outcome in infants <1500 g; a randomized study of labetalol- vs. dihydralazine-treated hypertensive pregnant women. In: Proceedings of 7th World Congress of Hypertension in Pregnancy, Perugia, Italy, 1990, p. 191.
[61] Thorley KJ. Randomised trial of atenolol and methyldopa in pregnancy related hypertension. Clin Exp Hypertens Pregnancy 1984;B3:168.
[62] Walker JJ, Bonduelle M, Calder AA. The effect of maternal labetalol on the neonate. Clin Exp Hypertens 1984;B3:150.
[63] Marlettini MG, Crippa S, Morselli-Labate AM, Contrarini A, Orlandi C. Randomized comparison of calcium antagonists and beta-blockers in the treatment of pregnancy-induced hypertension. Curr Ther Res 1990;48(4):684–94.
[64] El-Qarmalawi AM, Morsy AH, Al-Fadly A, Obeid A, Hashem M. Labetalol vs. methyldopa in the treatment of pregnancy-induced hypertension. Int J Gynecol Obstet 1995;49:125–30.
[65] Hjertberg R, Faxelius G, Belfrage P. Comparison of outcome of labetalol or hydralazine therapy during hypertension in pregnancy in very low birth weight infants. Acta Obstet Gynecol Scand 1993;72:611–5.
[66] Walker JJ, Crooks A, Erwin L, Calder AA. Labetalol in pregnancy-induced hypertension: fetal and maternal effects. In: Riley A, Symonds EM, editors, The investigation of labetalol in the management of hypertension in pregnancy. Proceedings of a symposium at the Royal College of Physicians in London, International Congress Series, Vol. vol. 591, Amsterdam: Excerpta Medica, 1982, pp. 148–60.
[67] Walker JJ, Greer I, Calder AA. Treatment of acute pregnancy-related hypertension; labetalol and hydralazine compared. Postgrad Med J 1983;59(Suppl 3):168–70.
[68] Harper A, Murnaghan GA. Maternal and fetal haemodynamics in hypertensive pregnancies during maternal treatment with intravenous hydralazine or labetalol. Br J Obstet Gynaecol 1991;98:453–9.
[69] Kyle PM, Redman CWG. Comparative risk-benefit assessment of drugs used in the management of hypertension in pregnancy. Drug Safety 1992;7(3):233–4.
[70] Borzak S, Ridker PM. Discordance between meta-analyses and large-scale randomized, controlled trials. Ann Intern Med 1995;123: 873–7.
[71] van den Anker JN, de Groot R, Broerse HM et al. Assessment of glomerular filtration rate in preterm infants by serum creatinine: comparison with inulin clearance. Pediatrics 1995;96(6):1156–8.

CHAPTER 51

THE SAFETY OF ORAL HYPOGLYCEMIC AGENTS IN THE FIRST TRIMESTER OF PREGNANCY: A META-ANALYSIS

Sheryl J. Gutzin,[1] Eran Kozer,[2] Laura A. Magee,[3] Denice S. Feig,[1] and Gideon Koren[2]

[1]Department of Medicine, Mount Sinai Hospital and University of Toronto; [2]Motherisk Program and Department of Pediatrics. The Hospital for Sick Children and University of Toronto, Toronto, Ontario; [3]Department of Medicine, University of British Columbia and Division of Specialized Women's Health, Children's and Women's Health Centre of British Columbia, Vancouver, British Columbia

SJ Gutzin, E Kozer, LA Magee, DS Feig, G Koren. The safety of oral hypoglycemic agents in the first trimester of pregnancy: A meta-analysis. Can J Clin Pharmacol 2003;10(4):179–183.

Objective. To examine the relationship between first-trimester exposure to oral hypoglycemic agents (OHAs), congenital anomalies and neonatal mortality, accounting for the potential confounding effect of maternal glycemic control.

Method. A meta-analysis was conducted by searching the literature for studies reporting on women with type II diabetes mellitus, first-trimester exposure to OHAs and either major malformations and/or neonatal mortality. Glycemic control monitoring was noted. Studies were reviewed by two reviewers and disagreement was resolved by consensus. Odds ratios and risk differences were calculated to determine the risk of major malformations and neonatal mortality between those exposed and those not exposed to OHAs.

Results. Ten studies met the inclusion criteria. There was no significant difference in the rates of major malformations between those exposed and those not exposed to OHAs; the odds ratio was 1.05 (95% CI 0.65 to 1.70) and the risk difference was 0.00 (95% CI –0.03 to 0.03). For studies reporting glycemic control, the odds ratio for major malformations between those exposed and those not exposed to OHAs was 1.06 (95% CI 0.62 to 1.81). For neonatal death, the odds ratio was 1.16 (95% CI 0.67 to 2.00) and the risk difference was –0.03 (95% CI –0.17 to 0.12). The studies did not provide sufficient detail to determine which OHA(s) were associated with adverse neonatal outcomes.

Conclusions. First-trimester exposure to OHAs did not significantly increase rates of major malformations or neonatal death. However, the studies were heterogeneous and care must be taken in interpreting the results. Further studies are needed to address the safety of OHAs in the first trimester with concomitant good glycemic control.

Keywords: Diabetes; Oral hypoglycemic agents; Pregnancy

Oral hypoglycemic agents (OHAs) have been avoided in pregnancy due to concerns about fetal teratogenicity following first-trimester exposure. Specific OHAs have been suggested to cause anomalies in human case reports and animal studies (1-3). These primarily include cardiovascular (transposition of great vessels, ventricular septal defect, atrial septal defect, patent ductus arteriosus), central nervous system (anencephaly, spina bifida, hydrocephaly) and renal (agenesis, cystic kidneys) defects (4,5). The reported increased risk of major malformations in women with diabetes is up to fourfold of a baseline risk of 1% to 3% in those without diabetes (1). Glycemic control, however, has also been implicated as an etiological factor for congenital malformations in women with diabetes. Poor glycemic control is known to be associated with an increased number of malformations in individuals with insulin-dependent diabetes in a dose-dependent fashion (6-9). Near normalization of glycemic control is associated with elimination of this increased risk (7,10).

The prevalence of all types of diabetes (type I, type II and gestational) in women of childbearing age is 4%. Women with type II diabetes account for 8% of these pregnancies and may be exposed to OHAs during the first trimester of pregnancy (11). Fifty per cent of pregnancies are unplanned and, therefore, some women with type II diabetes may inadvertently be taking these medications in the first trimester. Metformin is being used to increase fertility among women with polycystic ovarian syndrome. Spontaneous pregnancies may occur during treatment with metformin (12). Furthermore, in some countries, insulin is not widely available for women with type II diabetes. Discontinuing OHAs with resultant worsened glycemic control may be more teratogenic than continuing these medications.

To date, the teratogenic potential of OHAs has not been addressed by a systematic review. This meta-analysis is aimed at examining the relationship between first-trimester exposure to OHAs, and congenital anomalies and/or neonatal mortality, accounting for the potential confounding effect of maternal glycemic control.

METHODS

A search of the literature was conducted using Medline (1966–2000), Embase (1980–2000), the Cochrane database of systematic reviews, teratology texts (1-3), and bibliographies of retrieved papers and books. The keywords pregnancy, diabetes; diabetes mellitus; diabetes mellitus, non-insulin dependent; and polycystic ovary syndrome were used to search for studies on the disease. The keyword oral hypoglycemic agents (including sulfonylureas and bigunides) was used to search for studies on exposure. As well, the keywords abnormalities; drug-induced, pregnancy complications; neonatal diseases and abnormalities; infant mortality; and hypoglycemia were used to search for studies on the outcome. The keywords were exploded where possible. The search was limited to human pregnancy and English language. Studies were included if they enrolled women with type I or type II diabetes mellitus, or gestational diabetes, reported on first-trimester exposure to any type of OHAs and reported on the incidence of either major malformations and/or neonatal death. Whether studies reported on glycemic control monitoring was noted. Other potential confounding variables abstracted were maternal age, weight, race, comorbidities (eg, hypertension), and complications of labour and delivery. Uncontrolled studies, case reports or case series with less than six women, editorials, reviews and animal studies were excluded. All abstracts, titles and, if necessary, full reports and bibliographies were reviewed by one reviewer, and a random subset of 5% were also reviewed by a second reviewer. Based on this screening, studies were chosen for detailed review. Using structured data collection forms, data were extracted independently by each reviewer and disagreements resolved by consensus. Studies with the most comprehensive data were included if patient information was presented in duplicate reports.

Glycemic control was rated as 'adequate' for the study group if one or more of the following criteria were met for the group mean: Hemoglobine A1c (HbA1c) less than 8% (7), fasting blood glucose less than 6.7 mmol/L(10), random blood glucose less than 11.1 mmol/L, and/or two-hour postprandial blood glucose less than 11.1 mmol/L. If studies reported glycemic measurements above these cutoffs, glycemic control was considered to be 'inadequate.'

The quality of cohort and case-controlled studies was rated according to a priori criteria(13). Data were entered into 2 × 2 tables. Peto odds ratios (95% C1) and risk differences were calculated using the Cochrane Review Manager software (Revman 4.1, Cochrane, Denmark). Risk differences were reported because of the rarity of major malformations and neonatal deaths, leading to a number of empty cells in the 2 × 2 odds ratio tables.

RESULTS

The literature search yielded 4376 citations on initial screening. Twenty-two reports were chosen for detailed review. Ten studies were considered to be eligible (14-23). Studies were excluded if they had less than six subjects, no patients with first-trimester OHAs exposure (24-28), an unclear number of patients exposed to OHAs (29), data duplicated in other published studies (30-33) or no control group (34). There was initial disagreement regarding whether three of the 22 studies chosen for detailed review merited inclusion (14,17,34). This was resolved by consensus.

The 10 studies reported on 471 women exposed to OHAs and 1344 women not exposed to OHAs. There were three prospective cohort studies (17,20,22), three retrospective cohorts (14,19,23), three case series (15,16,18) and one case–control study (21). Eight studies were conducted at a single centre (15-22) and two were multicentre studies (14,23). Cases and controls were recruited from obstetric and endocrine clinics, except for one study from South Africa in which it was not stated (17). Two studies had financial support from pharmaceutical companies (17,20), three were funded by national, university or diabetic association sources (14,18,22), and funding was not stated for five studies (15,16,19,21,23). In terms of the quality of studies, six were 'poor' (14-19), two were 'fair' (20,23), and two were 'good' (21,22).

Most women in the studies had type II diabetes [14,16,17,20–23]. Women with type I diabetes (23), gestational diabetes (first diagnosed with diabetes in pregnancy) (14,16,18) and impaired glucose tolerance (23) were also present in some studies. The type of diabetes was not defined clearly in two studies (15,19). Three studies did not provide any demographic information for the women enrolled (16,19,20), and two studies did not differentiate between those exposed and not exposed to OHAs for the information (age, weight or race) that was provided (17,23). In one study, there was a greater number of black women (42 out of 60) in the control group than in the exposed group and greater number of Indian women (24 out of 37) in the exposed group (14) than in the control group; however, it was not clear which of these groups had adverse outcomes. This study also did not provide the mean age or weight. The only other study reporting details on race had 11 Mexican-American women, six white women and three 'other' women out of 20 in the OHAs exposed group compared with 20 Mexican-American women, 13 white women and seven 'other' women out of 40 in the nonexposed group (21). Four studies provided information on age (range 31 years to 34 years); however, there was no significant difference between OHAs exposed and nonexposed women (15,18,21,22). Mean parity was also not significantly different between groups in the two studies that reported this information (2.2 exposed, 1.9 control (21); 2.5 exposed, 2.3 control (22)). One study provided information about alcohol, smoking or drug use (five of 147 OHAs exposed, 7.7 of 185 control), and medications (14 of 147 OHAs exposed, 13.7 of 185 control) (22). However, details about what medications were used was not provided. Information on comorbidities was not provided by any studies.

With regard to glycemic control, three studies had 'inadequate' glycemic control (14,21,22); however, there was no significant difference between OHAs-exposed and nonexposed groups, and there was no within-study differences. For instance, in one study, the monitoring method involved hyperglycemic symptoms, glycosuria and fasting blood glucose, where "good" control was defined as being symptom free, having minimal glycosuria and a fasting glucose that was normal or reduced from previous levels. The exposed and control groups had good control in 32% and 34% of patients, respectively (14). In one study monitoring HbA1c, the level was reported to be between 8.8±2.7% for exposed versus 8.3±2.4% for the control group (21), while in another study HbA1c was 8.2±0.2% for both groups (22). Although glycemic control was stated to have been monitored in four other studies by postprandial, random or fasting glucose, or HbA1c (17,18,20,23), the quality of the glycemic control could not be assessed because of incomplete or absent information.

The OHAs used varied in the studies and included chlorpropamide (eight), tolbutamide (six), glyburide (one), glipizide (two), acetohexamide (one), glibenclamide (three), metformin (five) and phenformin (three). Studies with multiple agents (sulfonylureas and biguanides) did not provide details about which specific drug(s) were associated with adverse neonatal outcome (14,15,17,19-23). Information about birth weight, gestational age at delivery, minor neonatal malformations, neonatal hypoglycemia, hypocalcemia, hyperglycemia and other neonatal outcomes were rarely and inconsistently reported across studies and were not statistically analyzed (18,20). Information on maternal disease, such as pre-eclampsia and labour and delivery complications, was not available in many studies (15,16,18-23). In one study it was noted that the caesarean section rate was similar between groups(14), while another study commented on similar labour and delivery complications between groups (17).

Major malformations reported included cardiovascular (interatrial septum aneurysm [23], interventricular defect [23], atrial septal defect [19,21], patent ductus arteriosus [16,19], congenital heart block [19], Fallot's tetralogy [17,19], transposition of great vessels [19], ventricular septal defect [19,21], aortic coarctation [21], central nervous system (spina bifida [19], cerebral diplegia [19], microcephalic [14,19], anencephaly [19,21], encephalocele [19], hydrocephalus [23]), skeletal (sacral dysgenesis [19–21,23], cleft palate [19], vertebral anomalies

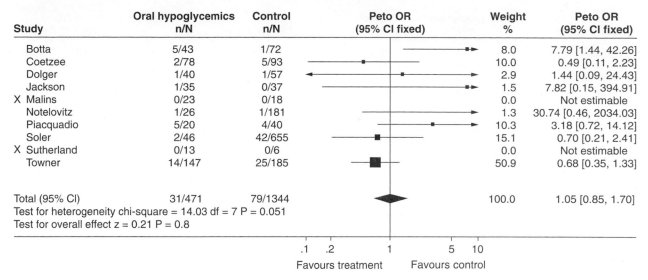

Study	Oral hypoglycemics n/N	Control n/N	Weight %	Peto OR (95% CI fixed)
Botta	5/43	1/72	8.0	7.79 [1.44, 42.26]
Coetzee	2/78	5/93	10.0	0.49 [0.11, 2.23]
Dolger	1/40	1/57	2.9	1.44 [0.09, 24.43]
Jackson	1/35	0/37	1.5	7.82 [0.15, 394.91]
X Malins	0/23	0/18	0.0	Not estimable
Notelovitz	1/26	1/181	1.3	30.74 [0.46, 2034.03]
Piacquadio	5/20	4/40	10.3	3.18 [0.72, 14.12]
Soler	2/46	42/655	15.1	0.70 [0.21, 2.41]
X Sutherland	0/13	0/6	0.0	Not estimable
Towner	14/147	25/185	50.9	0.68 [0.35, 1.33]
Total (95% CI)	31/471	79/1344	100.0	1.05 [0.85, 1.70]

Test for heterogeneity chi-square = 14.03 df = 7 P = 0.051
Test for overall effect z = 0.21 P = 0.8

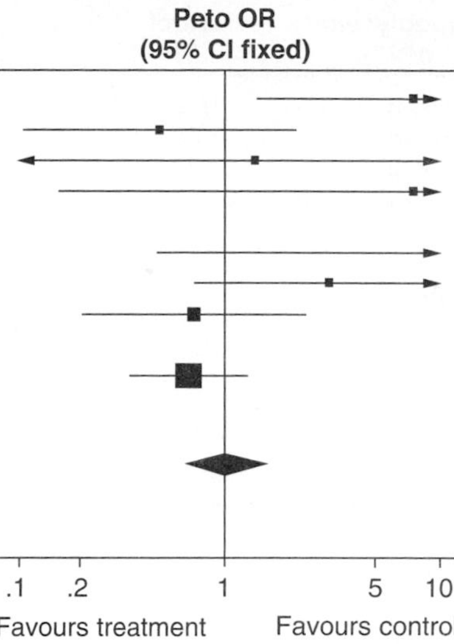

Figure 1. Odds ratio (OR) for major malformations in women exposed to oral hypoglycemic agents in the first trimester and women not exposed to oral hypoglycemic agents in the first trimester

[21]), gastrointestinal (Hirschprung's disease [19], imperforate anus (19), stricture lower ileum [19], deficient diaphragm [20,21], choanal atresia [17]) and genitourinary (renal agenesis [19], polycystic kidneys [19], hypoplastic kidney [19]) malformations.

There was no significant difference in the rate of major malformations between those exposed to OHAs and those not exposed (n = 10 studies, odds ratio 1.05, 95% CI 0.65 to 1.70) (Figure 1). The test for heterogeneity was significant (P = 0.05). The overall risk difference for major malformation between the exposed and control groups was 0.00 (95% CI –0.03 to 0.03, P = 0.35). The rates of neonatal death did not differ significantly between groups (n = 6 studies, odds ratio 1.16, 95% CI 0.67 to 2.00) Figure 2) (14-16, 18,20,21). However, the results were statistically and graphically heterogeneous (P = 0.0006). The overall risk difference for neonatal death was –0.03 (95% CI –0.17 to 0.12) and the studies were heterogeneous (P = 0.0002).

We were unable to explain the heterogeneity in the results among the studies by accounting for glycemic control. The odds ratio between studies with glycemic control rating was not significantly different for major malformations (1.06, 95% CI 0.62 to 1.81; exposed 27 of 336, nonexposed 35 of 433) (14,18,20-23). The odds ratio for major malformations of the three studies with 'poor' glycemic control was also not significantly different, 0.93 (95% CI 0.51 to 1.70; exposed 20 of 202, nonexposed 29 of 262) (14,21,22). For neonatal death, the odds ratio for the four studies reporting glycemic control was 2.19 (95% CI 1.17 to 4.09; 32 of 146 exposed, 20 of 176 nonexposed) (14,18,20,21). The heterogeneity in the results was also not explained by the study quality. Figure 3 shows that in the analysis of major malformations including only studies with 'good-fair' quality, the results were similar to the group in total; odds ratio 1.02 (95% CI 0.60 to 1.75; 26 of 288 exposed, 35 of 390 nonexposed) and risk difference 0.00 (95% CI –0.04 to 0.05; 26 of 288 exposed, 35 of 390 nonexposed) (20-23).

DISCUSSION

There was no significant difference in rate of major malformations or neonatal death among women with first-trimester exposure to OHAs when compared to nonexposed women. This finding was present even in the few studies that factored in glycemic control (albeit poor) for major malformations (14,18,20–23). However, P for

Study	Treatment n/N	Control n/N	Weight %	Peto OR (95% CI fixed)
Coetzee	12/78	4/93	28.1	3.67 [1.31, 10.27]
Dolger	0/40	7/57	12.4	0.18 [0.30, 0.77]
Jackson	16/35	10/37	32.7	2.22 [0.85, 5.78]
Malins	1/23	6/18	11.4	0.14 [0.03, 0.69]
Piacquadio	3/20	0/40	10.9	1.61 [0.31, 8.46]
Sutherland	1/13	2/6	4.5	0.16 [0.01, 2.13]
Total (95% CI)	33/209	33/251	100.0	1.16 [0.67, 2.00]

Test for heterogeneity chi-square = 21.85 df = 7 P = 0.0006
Test for overall effect z = 0.52 P = 0.6

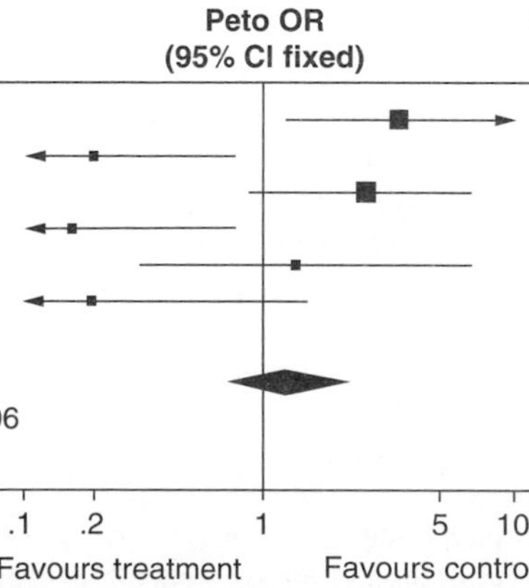

Figure 2. Odds ratio (OR) for neonatal death in women exposed to oral hypoglycemic agents in the first trimester and women not exposed to oral hypoglycemic agents in the first trimester

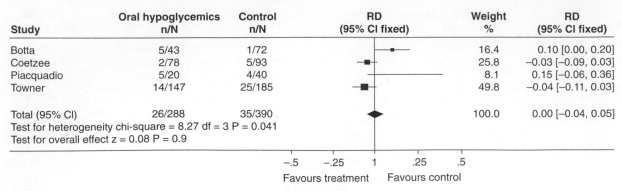

Study	Oral hypoglycemics n/N	Control n/N	Weight %	RD (95% CI fixed)
Botta	5/43	1/72	16.4	0.10 [0.00, 0.20]
Coetzee	2/78	5/93	25.8	−0.03 [−0.09, 0.03]
Piacquadio	5/20	4/40	8.1	0.15 [−0.06, 0.36]
Towner	14/147	25/185	49.8	−0.04 [−0.11, 0.03]
Total (95% CI)	26/288	35/390	100.0	0.00 [−0.04, 0.05]

Test for heterogeneity chi-square = 8.27 df = 3 P = 0.041
Test for overall effect z = 0.08 P = 0.9

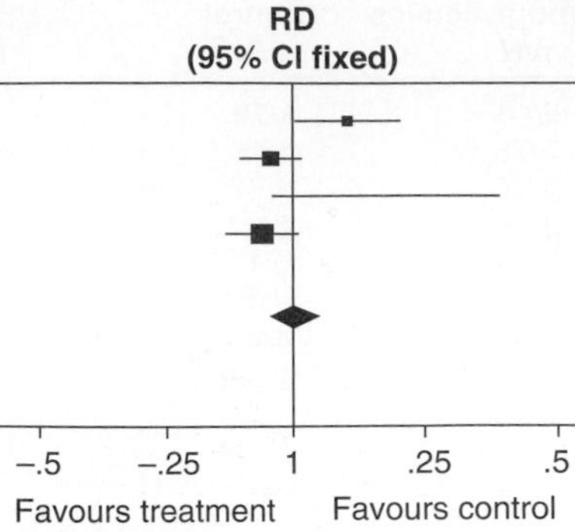

Figure 3. Risk difference (RD) for major malformations in 'good-fair' quality studies of women exposed to oral hypoglycemic agents in the first trimester and women not exposed to oral hypoglycemic agents in the first trimester

heterogeneity was significant for odds ratio for overall major malformations and neonatal death, and for the risk difference for neonatal death. This suggests that care must be taken in interpreting the results because the combined studies were heterogeneous. There were no within-study or between-study differences identified for glycemic control to explain the heterogeneity. There was no significant differences between 'poor' to 'good-fair' quality studies. The heterogeneity may reflect different agents, patient populations and patient selection. In addition, the existing studies did not report on many characteristics that may cause heterogeneity, including smoking, alcohol intake and body weight, among others.

Neonatal death was significantly increased in studies with reported glycemic control (which was poor) (2,19). However, one of the four studies in this analysis had a high perinatal mortality rate attributable to poor glycemic control in the early phase of the study and later changed to a stricter regimen, making interpretation difficult (20). Another study had a high rate of neonatal death in the OHAs and insulin groups, suggesting perhaps a different standard of care at the time (14).

Individual studies have conflicting results regarding the safety of OHAs in pregnancy. Some report higher rates of major malformations in women exposed to OHAs (14,16,21,23). However, many studies have not found this to be the case (15,17–20,22,25,28,34,35). These studies are heterogeneous, using different agents and doses, and direct comparison has been difficult. Many studies did not take into consideration glycemic control and even in those that did, the quality of the control is not readily evident. These factors influence how the results of these studies may be interpreted, as hyperglycemia has been associated with major malformations.

A recent randomized, controlled study by Langer et al (35) has shown that glyburide use for gestational diabetes in the second and third trimester does not increase maternal or fetal complications compared with insulin. There was no difference in the incidence of macrosomia or neonatal hypoglycemia. Similarly, there was no significant difference in glycemic control between glyburide versus insulin (35). Although this study did not include first-trimester exposure OHAs and, therefore, does not discuss congenital malformations, it brings forward the notion of alternative methods of treatment with the focus on appropriate glycemic control.

There are a number of weaknesses in our systematic review. Most of the studies available were of poor quality, included multiple agents, and did not comment on type of drug or dosage used for any given malformation. Only studies that were published in English were included in the present review, therefore, evidence published in other languages might have been missed. There are inherent weaknesses in meta-analyses of observational design, such as the incorporation of potential biases and flaws of individual studies, and reporting bias (36). Observational studies may lack information about important confounding variables (particularly, glycemic control in this study). Because more weight was assigned to one study in the present systematic review (22), potential biases inherent in it may have magnified the results. Even with preferential weighting towards studies with higher exposure/event rates, the effect of biases is potentially more serious in examining phenomena of low exposure rates (eg, malformations).

An ideal trial to study the safety of OHAs in the first trimester of pregnancy would be randomized, controlled and double blinded. A group of patients with type II diabetes should be treated with an OHA to achieve optimal glycemic control. Rates of adverse effects should be compared with a matched control group not exposed to OHAs, but with the same glycemic control achievable with insulin. This is not currently feasible from a safety or ethical point of view because of the potential teratogenic effects of OHAs. Hence, to date, the best available information is from observational studies of patients who have been inadvertently exposed to OHAs and those treated with OHAs intentionally in a nonrandomized fashion.

Because of the weaknesses of the available data discussed above, this systemic review cannot be relied upon for clinical decision-making. If our findings are confirmed, they would have widespread implications. More women than ever with type II diabetes mellitus are of childbearing age and may become pregnant on OHAs (11,37). This study suggests that the risk of major malformations and/or neonatal death may not be as great as that previously reported, and it would appear that the use of OHAs in later pregnancy may be safe (35). The use of OHAs in early pregnancy may warrant further evaluation, especially in environments where resources are insufficient to provide diabetic antenatal care with insulin and when OHA-exposed pregnancy is diagnosed after the first trimester. Until further information is available, women exposed to OHAs in early pregnancy should undergo detailed fetal structural scanning and receive close antepartum care.

ACKNOWLEDGEMENTS

EK was supported by a Fellowship from the Research Training Centre, The Hospital for Sick Children, Toronto, Ontario. GK is a senior scientist of the Canadian Institutes for Health Research.

REFERENCES

1. Schardein JL. Chemically Induced Birth Defects, 2nd edn. New York: Marcel Dekker Inc, 1993.
2. Briggs GG, Freeman RK, Yaffe SJ. Drugs in Pregnancy and Lactation, 5th edn. Baltimore: Williams & Wilkins, 1998.
3. Shepard TH. Catalog of Teratogenic Agents, 9th edn. Baltimore: The John Hopkins University Press, 1998.
4. Becerra JE, Khoury MJ, Cordero JF, Erickson JD. Diabetes mellitus during pregnancy and the risks for specific birth defects: A population-based case-control study. Pediatrics 1990;85:1-9.
5. Simpson JL, Elias S, Martin AO, Palmer MS, Ogata ES, Radvany RA. Diabetes in pregnancy, Northwestern University series (1977–1981). Am J Obstet Gynecol 1983;146:263-8.
6. Miller E, Hare JW, Cloherty JP, et al. Elevated maternal hemoglobin A1c in early pregnancy and major congenital anomalies in infants of diabetic mothers. N Engl J Med 1981;304:1331-4.
7. Mills JL, Knopp RH, Simpson JL, et al. Lack of relation of increased malformation rates in infants of diabetic mothers to glycemic control during organogenesis. N Engl J Med 1988;318:671-6.
8. Greene MF, Hare JW, Cloherty JP, Benacerraf BR, Soeldner JS. First-trimester hemoglobin A1c and risk of major malformation and spontaneous abortion in diabetic pregnancy. Teratology 1989;39:225-31.
9. Kitzmiller JL, Gavin LA, Gin GD, Jovanovic-Peterson L, Main EK, Zigrang WD. Preconception care of diabetes: Glycemic control prevents congenital anomalies. JAMA 1991;265:731-6.
10. Rosenn B, Miodovnik M, Combs A, Khoury J, Siddiqui TA. Glycemic thresholds for spontaneous abortion and congenital malformations in insulin-dependent diabetes mellitus. Obstet Gynecol 1994;84:515-20.
11. Engelau MH, Herman WH, Smith PJ, German RR, Aubert RE. The epidemiology of diabetes and pregnancy in the U.S., 1988. Diabetes *Care* 1995;18:1029-33.
12. Velazquez EM, Mendoza S, Hamer T, Sosa F, Gluek CJ. Metformin therapy in polycystic ovary syndrome reduces hyperinsulinemia, insulin resistance, hyperandrogenemia, and systolic blood pressure, while facilitating normal menses and pregnancy. Metabolism 1994; 43:647-54.
13. Harris RP, Helfand M, Woolf SH, et al, for the Methods Work Group, Third U.S. Preventative Services Task Force. Current Methods of the U.S. Preventative Services Task Force. A Review of the Process. Am J Prev Med 2001;20:21-35.
14. Jackson WP, Campbell GD, Notelovitz M, Blumsohn D. Tolbutamide and chlorpropamide during pregnancy in human diabetics. Diabetes 1962;11(Suppl):98-101.
15. Malins JM, Cooke AM, Pyke DA, Fitzgerald MG. Sulfonylurea drugs in pregnancy. Br Med J 1964;2:187.
16. Dolger H, Bookman JJ, Nechemias C. Tolbutamide in pregnancy and diabetes. J Mt Sinai Hosp 1969;36:471-4.
17. Notelovitz M. Sulfonylurea therapy in the treatment of the pregnant diabetic. S Afr Med J 1971;45:226-9.
18. Sutherland HW, Bewsher PD, Cormack JD, et al. Effect of moderate dosage of chlorpropamide in pregnancy on fetal outcome. Arch Dis Child 1974;49:283-91.
19. Soler NG, Walsh CH, Malins JM. Congenital malformations in infants of diabetic mothers. QJM 1976;45:303-13.
20. Coetzee EJ, Jackson WP. Oral hypoglycaemics in the first trimester and fetal outcome. S Afr Med J 1984;65:635-7.
21. Piacquadio K, Hollingsworth DR, Murphy H. Effects of in-utero exposure to oral hypoglycemic drugs. Lancet 1991;338:866-9.
22. Towner D, Kjos SL, Leung B, et al. Congenital malformations in pregnancies complicated by NIDDM. Diabetes Care 1995;18:1446-51.
23. Botta RM. Congenital malformations in infants of 517 pregestational diabetic mothers. Ann Ist Super Sanita 1997;33:307-11.
24. Sutherland HW, Stower JM, Cormack JD, Bewsher PD. Evaluation of chlorpropamide in chemical diabetes diagnosed during pregnancy. Br Med J 1973;3:9-13.
25. Douglas CP, Richards R. Use of chlorpropamide in the treatment of diabetes in pregnancy. Diabetes 1967;16:60-91.
26. Temesio P, Belitzky R, Gallego L, Martell M, Pose SV. Congenital malformations in diabetic offspring. Acta Diabet Lat 1977;14:192-8.
27. Moss JM, Conner EJ. Pregnancy complicated by diabetes. Report of 102 pregnancies including eleven treated with oral hypoglycemic drugs. Med Ann DC 1965;34:253-60.
28. Dolger H, Bookman JJ, Nechemias, C. The diagnostic and therapeutic value of tolbutamide in pregnant diabetics. Diabetes 1962;11(Suppl): 97-8.
29. Day RE, Insley J. Maternal diabetes mellitus and congenital malformation. Arch Dis Child 1976;51:935-8.
30. Coetzee EJ, Jackson WP. Metformin in management of pregnant insulin-dependent diabetics. Diabetologia 1979;16:241-5.
31. Coetzee EJ, Jackson WP. Diabetes newly diagnosed during pregnancy: A 4-year study at Groote Schuur Hospital. S Afr Med J 1979; 56:467-75.
32. Coetzee EJ, Jackson WP. Pregnancy in established non-insulin-dependent diabetics. A five-and-a-half-year study at Groote Schuur Hospital. S Afr Med J 1980;58:795-802.
33. Coetzee EJ, Jackson WP. The management of non-insulin-dependent diabetes during pregnancy. Diabetes Res Clin Pract 1986;1:281-7.
34. Hellmuth E, Damm P, Molsted-Pedersen, L. Congenital malformations in offspring of diabetic women treated with oral hypoglycaemic agents during embryogenesis. Diabet Med 1994;11:471-4.
35. Langer O, Conway DL, Berkus MD, Xenakis EM, Gonzales O. A comparison of glyburide and insulin in women with gestational diabetes mellitus. N Engl J Med 2000;343:1134-8.
36. Borzak S, Ridker PM. Discordance between meta-analyses and large-scale randomized, controlled trials. Examples from the management of acute myocardial infarction. Ann Intern Med 1995;123:873-7.
37. Harris MI, Hadden WC, Knowler WC, Bennett PH. Prevalence of diabetes and impaired glucose tolerance and plasma glucose levels in U.S. population aged 20–74 yr. Diabetes 1987;36:523-34.

Reprinted from Gutzin SJ, Kozer E, Magee LA, Feig DS, Koren G. The safety of oral hypoglycemic agents in the first trimester of pregnancy: a meta-analysis. Can J Clin Pharmacol 2003;10:179-83 with permission.

CHAPTER 52

PREGNANCY OUTCOME AFTER FIRST-TRIMESTER EXPOSURE TO METFORMIN: A META-ANALYSIS

Cameron Gilbert,[a] Maria Valois,[b] and Gideon Koren[a]

[a] Motherisk Program, Division of Clinical Pharmacology and Toxicology, The Hospital for Sick Children, The University of Toronto; and [b] The Scarborough Hospital, Toronto, Ontario, Canada

Abstract

Objective. To conduct a systematic review and meta-analysis of pregnancy outcome after metformin use for polycystic ovary syndrome (PCOS), because the efficacy of metformin has been demonstrated in the treatment of infertility caused by PCOS, whereas the fetal safety of metformin has received very little attention, and the few studies addressing this issue are limited by small sample sizes.
Design. Meta-analytic review.
Setting. All pertinent studies in MEDLINE and EMBASE from 1966 to September 2004.
Patient(s). Women with PCOS or diabetes.
Intervention(s). Exposure to metformin in the first trimester of pregnancy.
Main Outcome Measure(s). Major malformations.
Result(s). Eight studies were included in the meta-analysis, with an odds ratio of 0.50 (95% confidence interval, 0.15, 1.60). After adjustment for publication bias, metformin treatment in the first trimester was associated with a statistically significant 57% protective effect. After pooling the studies, the malformation rate in the disease-matched control group was approximately 7.2%, statistically significantly higher than the rate found in the metformin group (1.7%).
Conclusion(s). On the basis of the limited data available today, there is no evidence of an increased risk for major malformations when metformin is taken during the first trimester of pregnancy. Large studies are needed to corroborate these preliminary results. (Fertil Steril® 2006;86:658–63. ©2006 by American Society for Reproductive Medicine.)

Keywords: Metformin, pregnancy, pregnancy outcome, congenital malformations, biguanide, PCOS, polycystic ovary syndrome, diabetes, fertility, Stein and Leventhal syndrome

Metformin currently is approved by the US Food and Drug Administration for use in the treatment of type 2 diabetes (1). Its off-label use in the treatment of infertility caused by polycystic ovary syndrome (PCOS) has been growing over the past decade. This poses a problem because the fetal safety of metformin has not been established.

Polycystic ovary syndrome is defined by the presence of at least 2 out of the following 3 criteria: chronic oligoovulation or anovulation, hyperandrogenism, and polycystic ovaries on imaging. Approximately 5%–7% of women of reproductive age have PCOS (2), and it is the most common cause of anovulatory infertility (3). The causes of PCOS are unknown (3); however, insulin resistance with resultant hyperinsulinemia is prominent in this condition. The clinical presentation of subfertility and oligomenorrhea that is accompanied by hirsutism can be explained by two mechanisms: first, the increase in insulin stimulates an increase in androgen production in the ovary. Second, insulin also induces a decrease in the hepatic production of sex hormone-binding globulin, leading to an increase in free androgen level. This leads to the typical clinical manifestation (4).

Biguanides and thiazolidinediones decrease the amount of glucose produced by the liver and sensitize peripheral tissues to insulin. Hence, there is a mechanistic rationale to use these drugs to treat the hyperinsulinemia associated with PCOS. Thiazolidinediones, specifically troglitazone, have been shown to cause fatal liver failure in human beings and are still US Food and Drug Administration pregnancy class C, because in animal studies, fetal death and growth retardation have been documented (5). Sales of troglitazone are currently not authorized in the United States or Canada. There are two drugs in the biguanide class: metformin and phenformin. Phenformin was found to be teratogenic in animal models, whereas metformin was not (6).

Metformin has been used increasingly in the treatment of infertility secondary to PCOS (7, 8). Oligomenorrhea, a frequent feature of PCOS, may lead to a delay in the diagnosis of pregnancy. Therefore, despite the fact that most fertility experts discontinue metformin as soon as a diagnosis of pregnancy is confirmed, it is not unusual for women with PCOS to be exposed to metformin during part or the entire period of embryogenesis (9). There also have been studies examining metformin efficacy in reducing first-trimester pregnancy loss (10) and in reducing the incidence of gestational diabetes in women with PCOS (11).

These are not new indications; these are off-label use with no regulatory approval. Oral hypoglycemic drugs have been contraindicated in pregnancy because of their ability to cause fetal hyperinsulinemia and neonatal hypoglycemia. The teratogenic potential of oral hypoglycemic agents has been a subject of debate in literature (1–5). The objective of the present study was to determine whether metformin treatment during pregnancy is associated with an increased risk of major malformations.

MATERIALS AND METHODS

A systematic review was conducted with all pertinent studies that were found in MEDLINE and EMBASE that examined metformin and pregnancy outcome from 1966 to September 2004. The search strategy included the terms *teratogens, fetal development, pregnancy,*

Table 1
Inclusion and Exclusion Criteria

Inclusion criteria
At least first-trimester exposure to metformin.
Studies could be a prospective, retrospective, or a case–control study; however, there had to be a control group.
Data on rates of major malformations.
Studies written in any language.

Exclusion criteria
Review or letter to the editor.
Animal studies.
Studies with no control group or with an inappropriate control group.
Women with exposures to other known teratogens or other maternal disorders that might affect pregnancy outcome.

Gilbert. First-trimester exposure to metformin. Fertil Steril 2006.

abnormalities, metformin, biguanide, polycystic ovary syndrome, and *PCOS.* Articles were excluded from the analysis if they did not have either adequate disease-matched control groups or data on the outcome of the pregnancy with respect to major malformations and exposure to the drug in at least the first trimester. The control groups consisted of disease-matched women who were not treated with metformin. The inclusion–exclusion criteria are presented in Table 1. Meta-analysis was conducted using Review Manager 4.2 software (Review Manager [RevMan] [computer program]. Version 4.2 for Windows. Oxford, England: The Cochrane Collaboration, 2002).

Initially, rates of malformations were compared in all controlled studies, and subsequently, the data were analyzed separately according to the disease (diabetes or PCOS). Finally, because of the relatively small numbers, we also pooled all study and control subjects into a 2 × 2 table and compared malformation rates. The primary outcome measure was the pooled odds ratio (OR) for major malformations.

A funnel plot of the data was drawn with the effect size plotted against the sample size for each study. Subsequently, the Begg and Mazumdar (12) test for publication bias was used.

RESULTS

Tables 2 and 3 list, respectively, the included studies (9–11, 13–17) and the excluded studies. For all excluded studies, the rationale for exclusion is given, and for all included studies, the type of study is specified.

Eight studies met the inclusion criteria, and an additional five uncontrolled studies were included in the calculation of overall malformation rate. First-trimester exposure to metformin was not associated with an increased rate of major malformations. The OR for major malformations (including all studies with disease-matched controls) was 0.50 (95% confidence interval [CI]: 0.15, 1.60; Fig. 1). Subanalysis was conducted to separate studies into those with diabetic subjects and those with PCOS subjects (Figs. 2 and 3, respectively). With 28 subjects in the treatment group, the OR for the diabetic group was 0.85 (95% CI: 0.14, 5.11). With 139 subjects in the treatment group for PCOS, the OR was 0.33 (95% CI: 0.07, 1.56).

A funnel plot of the data shows an overall effect estimate of 0.50. Using the Begg and Mazumdar (12) test for publication bias, there was a significant publication bias ($\tau = 0.8$, $P = .05$), with smaller studies showing more apparent teratogenic effect of metformin. Adjustment of the funnel plot to account for this bias and calculation of an ideal pooled OR were conducted by using the *Trim and Fill* method proposed by Duval and Tweedie (18). Pseudovalues were added to the funnel plot that represent unpublished studies that are equal in size to the two small studies (Piacquadio et al. [14] and Hellmuth et al. [15]) but have opposite results. An updated funnel plot showed an adjusted pooled OR of 0.43.

Some studies had to be excluded because they had an insufficient control group even though they had subjects exposed to metformin in the critical time period. We therefore also calculated an overall malformation rate that can be compared with that of the general population (1%–5%) (19). The overall malformation rate of exposed pregnancies (including studies without

Table 2
Metformin Studies Included in the Meta-Analysis

REFERENCE NO.	AUTHOR	STUDY TYPE	DATA COLLECTION	MALFORMATION DESCRIBED
13	Coetzee and Jackson	C	R	None
14	Piacquadio et al.	C	R	None
15	Hellmuth et al.	C	R	None
11	Glueck et al.	C (self as control)	P	None
16	Vandermolen et al.	C (RCT with placebo)	P	None
10	Jakubowicz et al.	C	R	Achondrodysplasia
17	Sahin et al.	C (RCT)	P	None
9	Gargaun et al.	C	R	Club foot, one kidney, and no bone in left thumb

Note: C = cohort; P = prospective; R = retrospective.
Gilbert. First-trimester exposure to metformin. Fertil Steril 2006.

Table 3
Metformin Studies Excluded from the Meta-Analysis

AUTHOR GROUP	REASON FOR EXCLUSION
Balen	Review
Barbieri	Review
Ben-Haroush et al.	Review
Ben-Haroush et al.	Review
Cardone	Review
Cedars	Review
Clemens et al.	Review
Coetzee et al.	No given time of recruitment
Coetzee et al.	Not in first trimester
Collins et al.	Review
Costello and Eden	Review
De Leo et al.	No outcomes
De Leo et al.	No outcomes
Delvigne and Rozenberg	Review
Devendra et al.	Review
Dhont	Review
Diamanti-Kandarakis et al.	No outcomes
ESHRE Capri Workshop Group	Review
Fleming et al.	No outcomes
Genazzani et al.	No outcomes
George et al.	No outcomes
Glueck et al.	No control, no outomes
Glueck et al.	No control group
Glueck et al.	No control
Haas et al.	Review
Hague et al.	Letter
Harborne et al.	Review
Heard et al.	No pregnancy outcomes, no control
Holt	Review
Homburg	Review
Ibanez et al.	No outcomes
Kjotrod et al.	IVF
Kocak et al.	No outcomes
Ledger and Skull	Review
Lord et al.	Review
Malkawi et al.	No outcomes
Malkawi and Qublan	No outcomes
Massin et al.	Review
McCarthy et al.	Review
Merlob et al.	Review
Morin-Papunen et al.	No outcomes
Nestler et al.	No outcomes
Ng et al.	No outcomes
Norman et al.	Review
Papoushek	Review
Riddle	Review
Saleh and Khalil	Review
Sarlis et al.	Case report
Seale et al.	Case report
Seli and Duleba	Review
Simmons et al.	Review
Stadtmauer et al.	No outcomes
Stadtmauer et al.	No outcomes
Stadtmauer et al.	Review
Sturrock et al.	No outcomes
Tasdemir et al.	No outcomes
Teelucksingh et al.	Case report
Tran et al.	Review
Velazquez et al.	No metformin during pregnancy
Velazquez et al.	No control, no outcomes
Yarali et al.	No outcome data
Glueck et al.	No control group
Glueck et al.	No control group
Glueck et al.	No control group
Glueck et al.	No control group

Gilbert. First-trimester exposure to metformin. Fertil Steril 2006.

relevant controls) was 1.01% (5 malformations in 496 first-trimester exposures), as compared with 7.5% in the disease-matched control group ($P < .01$).

DISCUSSION

On the basis of eight small studies available now, metformin does not appear to be unsafe for use during pregnancy with respect to major malformations. As with any drug use in pregnancy, it is challenging to establish the safety of metformin use in the first trimester considering the background incidence of malformations in the general population and the confounder of the underlying diseases (PCOS and diabetes) that have been linked to increased rates of malformations. During pregnancy, extra care must be taken to ensure the safety of the unborn child. Meta-analytical summaries of existing studies therefore are of importance to monitor fetal safety.

Although it yields a reassuring trend, this study exemplifies the need for more research on metformin during pregnancy. It was our initial goal to examine all possible adverse pregnancy outcomes including spontaneous abortion, stillbirth, major malformations, minor anomalies, intrauterine growth retardation, or preterm labor. Because of the paucity of data, however, we were limited to focusing only on major malformations. Most studies reported on clinical markers (i.e., success in conceiving), and when women became pregnant, they were excluded from many studies and hence there were no reports of their pregnancy outcome.

It must be noted that some of the older studies included were not well controlled for potential confounders. These confounders may be relevant in studying diabetic patients taking metformin. For example, in the study performed by Coetzee and Jackson (13), patients had suboptimal metabolic control of their diabetes at the time of exposure to oral hypoglycemic agents (OHGA). Yet there were no major malformations reported in patients taking metformin, and those investigators concluded that biguanides can be safely used in the first trimester of pregnancy (13). Piacquadio et al. (14) reported that Hemoglobin A1c (HbA_{1c}) levels did not differ between exposed and disease-matched control mothers, at 8.8% vs. 8.3% at their first visit (between 7 and 28 weeks of gestation) and at 7.3% vs. 7.3% in their last visit before delivery. Even though these values are

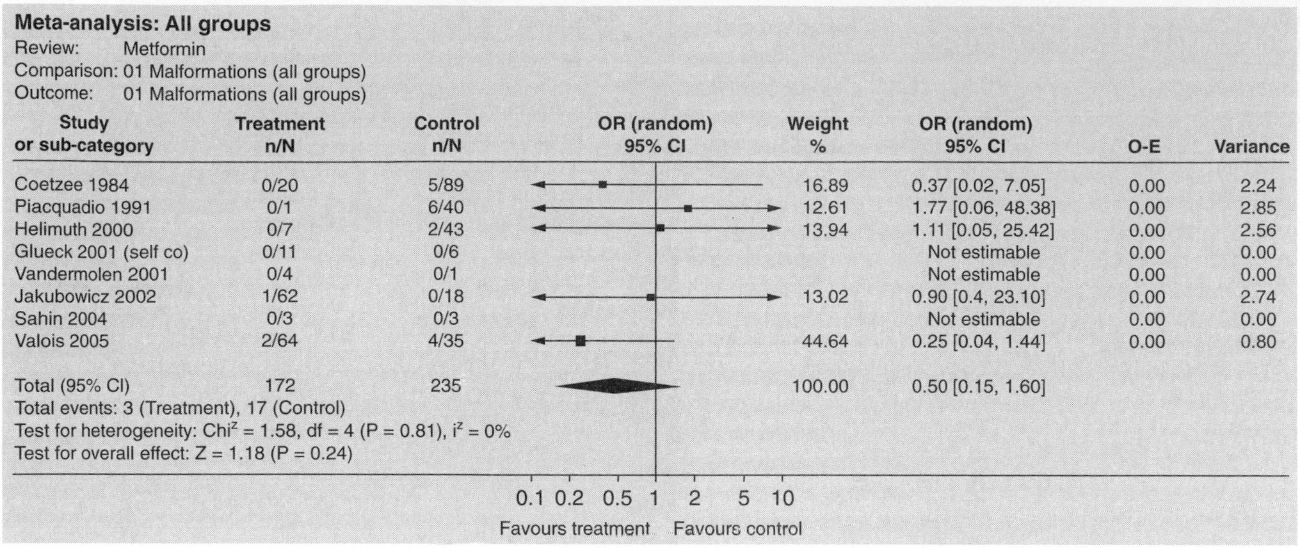

Gilbert. First-trimester to metformin. Fertil Steril 2006.

Figure 1. Meta-analysis of all studies.

properly matched, they are still above recommended levels, which introduces the confounder of poorly controlled underlying disease in their conclusion of increased teratogenic risk with OHGA.

The metformin cohort of Hellmuth et al. (15) included only seven (of 50) exposed women who were taking metformin during the first trimester of pregnancy. Levels of HbA_{1c} were available in 29 patients in the study, although one cannot identify them. In that study, women in the metformin group were significantly more obese. However, there were no malformations among the seven women who were exposed to metformin during the first trimester of pregnancy. The control groups consisted of women with polycystic ovaries untreated with metformin.

The mean malformation rate in the untreated group was approximately 7.2%. This is in the expected range for diabetic women, approximately two to three times the baseline rate in the general population (14). The rate found in the metformin group was 1.7%, which is well within the baseline rate for malformations in the general population. It could be argued that the low malformation rate in the metformin group may represent underreporting. But it is conceivable that underreporting also would occur in the disease matched control group.

Although the present data are reassuring, there is still limited documentation of pregnancy outcome with metformin exposure. Because of the limited published data, this study examined only major malformations. Until other outcomes such as spontaneous abortions, stillbirth, minor anomalies, intrauterine growth retardation, and preterm labor are properly addressed, the use of metformin in pregnancy cannot be assumed to be safe.

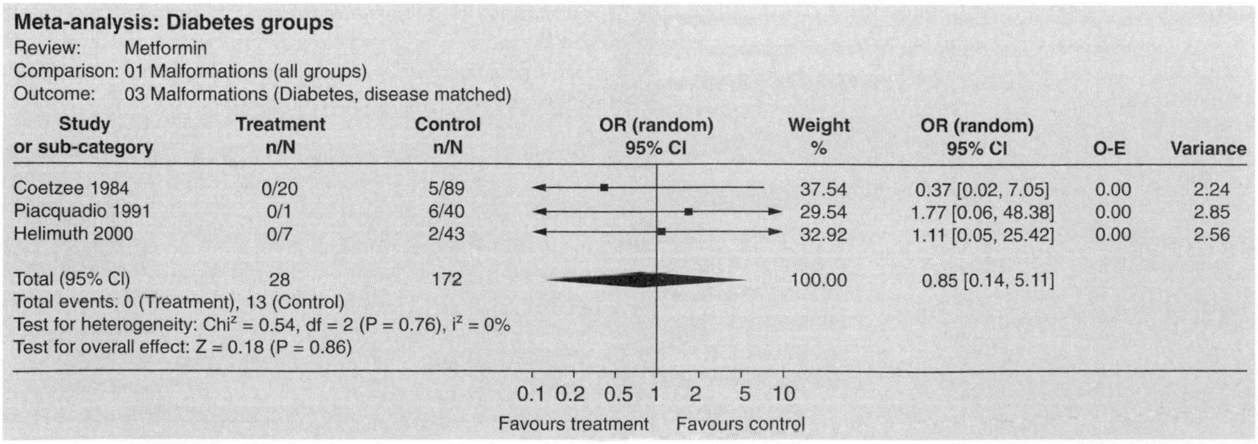

Gilbert. First-trimester to metformin. Fertil Steril 2006.

Figure 2. Meta-analysis of diabetes studies.

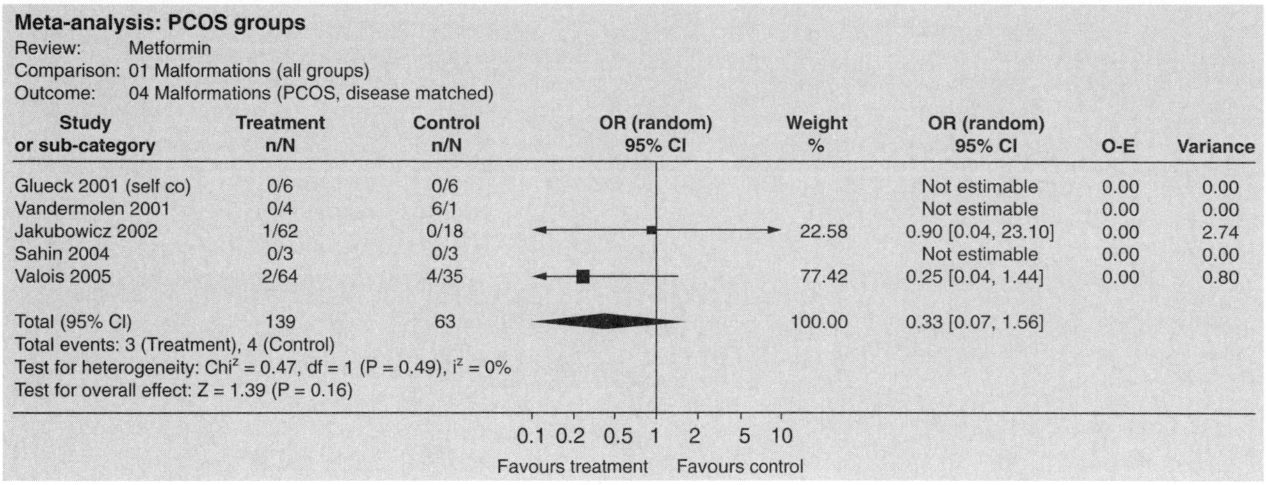

Gilbert. First-trimester to metformin. Fertil Steril 2006.

Figure 3. Meta-analysis of PCOS studies.

REFERENCES

1. Botta RM. Congenital malformations in infants of 517 pregestational diabetic mothers. Ann 1st Super Sanita 1997;33(3):307–11.
2. Hellmuth E, Damm P, Molsted-Pedersen L. Congenital malformations in offspring of diabetic women treated with oral hypoglycaemic agents during embryogenesis. Diabet Med 1994;11(5):471–4.
3. Hellmuth E, Damm P, Molsted-Pedersen L. Oral hypoglycaemic agents in 118 diabetic pregnancies. Diabet Med 2000;17(7):507–11.
4. Piacquadio K, Hollingsworth DR, Murphy H. Effects of in-utero exposure to oral hypoglycaemic drugs. Lancet 1991;338(8771):866–9.
5. Towner D, Kjos SL, Leung B, Montoro MM, Xiang A, Mestman JH, et al. Congenital malformations in pregnancies complicated by NIDDM. Diabetes Care 1995;18(11):1446–51.
6. Denno KM, Sadler TW. Effects of the biguanide class of oral hypoglycemic agents on mouse embryogenesis. Teratology 1994;49:260–6.
7. Ben Haroush A, Yogev Y, Fisch B. Insulin resistance and metformin in polycystic ovary syndrome. Eur J Obstet Gynecol Reprod Biol 2004; 115:125–33.
8. McCarthy EA, Walker SP, McLachlan K, Boyle J, Permezel M. Metformin in obstetric and gynecologic practice: a review. Obstet Gynecol Surv 2004;59:118–27.
9. Gargaun S, Ryan E, Greenblatt E, Fettes I, Shapiro H, Padjen A, et al. Pregnancy outcome in women with polycystic o to metformin. Can J Clin Pharmacol 2003;10:149.
10. Jakubowicz DJ, Iuorno MJ, Jakubowicz S, Roberts KA, Nestler JE. Effects of metformin on early pregnancy loss in the polycystic ovary syndrome. J Clin Endocrinol Metab 2002;87:524–9.
11. Glueck CJ, Wang P, Kobayashi S, Phillips H, Sieve-Smith L. Metformin therapy throughout pregnancy reduces the development of gestational diabetes in women with polycystic ovary syndrome. Fertil Steril 2002;77:520–5.
12. Begg CB, Mazumdar M. Operating characteristics of a rank correlation test for publication bias. Biometrics 1994;50:1088–101.
13. Coetzee EJ, Jackson WP. Oral hypoglycaemics in the first trimester and fetal outcome. S Afr Med J 1984;65:635–7.
14. Piacquadio K, Hollingsworth DR, Murphy H. Effects of in utero exposure to oral hypoglycaemic drugs. Lancet 1991;338:866–9.
15. Hellmuth E, Damm P, Molsted-Pedersen L. Oral hypoglycaemic agents in 118 diabetic pregnancies. Diabet Med 2000;17:507–11.
16. Vandermolen DT, Ratts VS, Evans WS, Stovall DW, Kauma SW, Nestler JE. Metformin increases the ovulatory rate and pregnancy rate from clomiphene citrate in patients with polycystic ovary syndrome who are resistant to clomiphene citrate alone. Fertil Steril 2001;75:310–5.
17. Sahin Y, Yirmibes U, Kelestimur F, Aygen E. The effects of metformin on insulin resistance, clomiphene-induced ovulation and pregnancy rates in women with polycystic ovary syndrome. Eur J Obstet Gynecol *Reprod Biol* 2004;113:214–20.
18. Duval S, Tweedie R. Trim and fill: a simple funnel-plot-based method of testing and adjusting for publication bias in meta-analysis. Biometrics 2000;56:455–63.
19. Koren G. Maternal-fetal toxicology: a clinician's guide. New York, NY: Marcel Dekker, 2001.

CHAPTER 53

PREGNANCY OUTCOME FOLLOWING FIRST TRIMESTER EXPOSURE TO ANTIHISTAMINES: META-ANALYSIS

Arnold Seto, Tom Einarson, and Gideon Koren

Motherisk Program, Division of Clinical Pharmacology and Toxicology, Department of Pediatrics and Research Institute, The Hospital for Sick Children, Toronto, Faculties of Medicine and Pharmacy, University of Toronto

Abstract

To determine the relative risk for major malformations associated with antihistamine (H_1 blockers) exposure in the first trimester of pregnancy, a literature search of all studies examining the association between antihistamines and major malformations for the period 1960 to 1991 was conducted, followed by meta-analysis. Odds ratio was calculated using the Mantel–Haenszel method. Twenty-four controlled studies met the inclusion criteria with more than 200,000 participating women. The summary odds ratio of major malformations associated with antihistamines taken during the first trimester was 0.76 (95% CI: 0.60–0.94). This analysis indicates that H_1 blockers used mainly for morning sickness during the first trimester do not increase the teratogenic risk in humans and may, in fact, be associated with a protective effect. More study is needed to verify the possibility that by preventing vomiting, antihistamines may ensure better metabolic conditions to the fetus and thus may reduce some birth defects. Alternatively, it is possible that pregnancies characterized by vomiting are associated with better outcome due to other reasons, such as hormonal status or placental function. Women suffering from morning sickness which is not controlled by nonpharmacological methods can safely use antihistamines.

Keywords: Pregnancy; antihistamine, H_1 blockers; malformations; birth defects

During early pregnancy, women receive more prescriptions of antihistamines than for any other agent except vitamins.[1] Antihistamines are used during early pregnancy mainly to treat morning sickness. The critical stage of organogenesis may be adversely affected by drugs and environmental agents, leading in some cases to birth defects.

Although antihistamines have been widely prescribed to large numbers of pregnant women, their safety has not been unequivocally established and some studies reported increased teratogenic risk. The removal of Bendectin® (doxylamine-pyridoxine) from the American market by its manufacturer in 1983 due to the litiginous atmosphere surrounding it, highlights public sensitivity to potential teratogenic risk. Following the removal of Bendectin, which was the most commonly used agent for morning sickness by American women, the rates of hospitalization due to hyperemesis gravidarum doubled, underscoring the serious consequences of wrongly perceiving a drug as a human teratogen when it is needed by large numbers of women.[2]

The objective of the present study was to review all controlled studies of antihistamine use in early pregnancy using meta-analysis to quantify the relative risk of major malformations associated with their use.

METHODS

A literature search was conducted to collect studies reporting antihistamine use during the first trimester of pregnancy. Using a bibliographic retrieval service with the Medline database, literature published between 1960–1991 was extracted based on the following key words: Pregnancy, antihistamine, antinauseant, antiemetic, cough/cold, morning sickness, hyperemesis gravidarum, nausea, vomiting, hypersensitivity, allergy, adverse fetal outcome, malformation, congenital abnormalities, birth defect, and teratogen.

Antihistamines (H_1 blockers) were defined as any compound with H_1 receptor antagonist action as its principal intended effect (Table 1). Any compound indicated for the treatment of allergies, nausea, vomiting, cough/cold, and respiratory disorders was reviewed, as was any compound listed under the ATC (anatomic therapeutic classification subclass of R06A, pp. 51–52, 1989).

Articles found in this review were obtained and photocopied. The Methods section of each article was cut out and identifying markers of the study such as authors' names and institutions were removed to prevent selection bias. The articles were cut and pasted onto a data collection sheet and presented to two reviewers for selection into analysis according to criteria outlined in Table 2. Statistical analysis included calculation of pooled odds ratio by the method of Mantel–Haenszel. Homogeneity was calculated using Mantel–Haenszel Chi-square.[3]

RESULTS

The Medline database search yielded 109 articles dealing with antihistamines in pregnancy. The 24 accepted papers are listed in Table 3.[4–27] Eighty-five papers[28–112] were rejected according to our exclusion criteria (animal studies, case reports, review articles, editorial comments, obstetric aspects, duplicate articles, or irrelevant).

The 24 studies meeting our inclusion criteria had over 200,000 women enrolled. The summary odds ratio for major malformations in offspring of women exposed to antihistamines during the first trimester was 0.76 (95% CI: 0.6–0.94). Chi-square test for homogeneity yielded a c^2 = 512 (df=23, p<0.01). Outliers were examined using residuals and three studies were identified: Eskenazi et al.,[12] Gibson et al.,[19] and Jick et al.[20] All three papers dealt exclusively with Bendectin in pregnancy. Exclusion of these studies did not change the overall odds ratio or confidence intervals significantly.

Table 1
ATC List of Antihistamines

R06		SYSTEMIC ANTIHISTAMINES	
R06A			
R06AA	**Aminoalkyl Ethers**	**R06AD**	**Phenothiazine**
Derivatives			
R06AA01	diphenhydramine	R06AD01	alimemazine
R06AA02	clemastine	R06AD02	promethazine
R06AA04	diphenhydramine, combinations	R06AD03	thiethylperazine
R06AA05	clemastine, combinations	R06AD04	methdilazine
R06AA06	bromaxine, combinations	R06AD05	promethazine, combinations
R06AA07	diphenylpyraline combination	R06AD06	alimemazine, combinations
R06AB	**Substituted Alkylamines**	**R06AE**	**Piperazine Derivatives**
R06AB01	brompheniramine	R06AE01	cyclizine
R06AB02	dexchlorpheniramine	R06AE04	meclozine
R06AB03	clorpheniramine	R06AE05	cyclizine, combinations
R06AB51	brompheniramine, combinations	R06AE55	meclozine, combinations
R06AB52	chlorpheniramine, combinations	**R06AK**	combination of antihistamines
R06AB53	dexbrompheniramine, combination	**R06AX**	various systemic antihistamines
R06AB54	pheniramine, combination	R06AX01	cyproheptadine
R06AC	**Substituted Ethylene Diamines**	R06AX02	antazoline
R06AC01	tripelennamine	R06AX03	azatadine
R06AC02	mepyramine, combinations	R06AX04	astemizole
		R06AX05	terfenadine
		R06AX06	loratadine
		R06AX07	dimethethiazide mesylate
		R06AX08	triprolidine, combinations
		R06AX09	azamdine, combinations

DISCUSSION

Approximately 60% of all women experience nausea and vomiting during the first trimester of their pregnancy, and about half of them are treated with antihistamines for that end. Our analysis indicates that there is no positive association between the use of antihistamines in the first trimester of pregnancy and the rates of major malformations. An overall odds ratio of 0.76 with 95% confidence intervals of 0.6 to 0.94 indicates an apparent 24% protective effect. The ability to prove lack of teratogenic effect of antihistamines is of utmost importance, because many women and their physicians are reluctant to treat effectively morning sickness due to the perception of teratogenic risk.[113] Our analysis included over 200,000 investigated women in 24 different studies, and therefore it has an unprecedent power to reject the suggestion of teratogenic potential of this class of drugs.

Table 2
Inclusion and Exclusion Criteria

INCLUSION CRITERIA	EXCLUSION CRITERIA
1) Human subjects	1) animal data
2) Maternal exposure to antihistamines in pregnancy	2) stillbirths as outcome measure
3) Nonexposed control group	3) abortions as outcome measure
4) Outcome—malformation	4) case reports
5) Presentation of exposed and nonexposed rates of outcome	5) reviews

The suggestion that antihistamines may have a protective effect against some major malformations has not been examined in the past. Severe nausea and vomiting can be often debilitating and rarely even life-threatening. It is biologically conceivable that suboptimal maternal nutrition, combined with dehydration and electrolyte imbalances resulting from hyperemesis gravidarum, may create suboptimal conditions for embryonic growth. Animal studies have demonstrated maternal nutritional deficiencies during gestation to result in an increased risk of malformations in the offspring.[114] In humans, hyperemesis gravidarum has been associated with increased risk of central nervous system malformations, and eye ear malformations.[115] Hence, it is possible that by preventing the untoward results of nausea and vomiting, antihistamines may have protective fetal effects. This possibility will have to be further addressed by future research.

An alternative explanation is that pregnancies characterized by vomiting are biologically different from those not exhibiting vomiting, leading the former to a better prognosis. The idea that vomiting signals better pregnancy outcome has been forwarded in the past,[116] however, these studies did not outline the antiemetic drugs used by the participating women.

In summary, pregnant women suffering from morning sickness and its consequences, which does not respond to nonpharmaological methods, can safely use antihistamines.

Table 3
Characteristics of the 24 Studies Included in the Meta-Analysis

	SIGNIFICANCE OF INDIVIDUAL 2 × 2 TABLES OUTCOME				
EXPOSURE	MALFORMATION		NO MALFORMATIONS		TOTAL
yes	A		B		n1
no	C		D		n0
Total	m1		m0		N
STUDY REF	**A**	**B**	**C**	**D**	**N**
14	35	1939	39	1935	3948
6	15	145	151	766	1077
7	1435	3207	9263	18339	32244
22	19	561	24	57	661
8	2	39	3	74	118
9	35	71	230	461	797
10	203	1749	131	4222	6305
4	251	6319	5274	38438	50282
11	14	847	91	5557	6509
15	32	679	162	4323	5196
12	44	78	659	1634	2415
13	31	589	1208	21149	22977
16	31	344	93	1222	1690
17	24	46	366	1208	1644
18	52	121	240	607	1020
19	2	1362	4	3886	5254
20	78	1607	245	5526	7456
21	24	2231	56	4526	6837
23	12	9	184	398	603
24	76	88	760	748	1672
25	6	1186	70	6671	7933
26	28	1685	31	1682	3426
27	11	2207	21	2197	4436
5	1	33	2	32	68

REFERENCES

1. Bonati M, Tognoni G. Drug use in pregnancy: A preliminary report of the International Co-operative Drug Utilization Study. Pharmaceutisch Weekblad Scientific edition 1990;12:75–8.
2. Skalnick A. Key witness against morning sickness drug faces scientific fraud charges. JAMA 1990;263:1468–73.
3. Einarson T, Leeder J, Koren G. A method for meta-analysis of epidemiological studies. Drug Intell Clin Pharm 1988;22:813–24.
4. Heinonen OP, Slone D, Shapiro S. *Birth Defects and Drugs in Pregnancy*. Littleton MA: PSG Publishing; 1977.
5. Seto A, Einarson T, Koren G. Evaluation of brompheniramine safety in pregnancy. Reprod Toxicol 1993;7:393–5.
6. Nelson M. Forfar J. Associations between drugs administered during pregnancy and congenital abnormalities of the fetus. Brit Med J 1971;1:523–7.
7. Ayd FJ. Haloperidol: Fifteen years of clinical experience. Dis Nerv Syst 1972;33:459–69.
8. Nora J, Nora A, Sommerville R, Hill R, McNamara D. Maternal exposure to potential teratogens. JAMA 1967.
9. Mellin G, Katzenstein M. Meclozine and fetal abnormalities. Brit Med J 1963;26:222–3.
10. Miklovich L, Van den Berg B. An evaluation of the teratogenicity of certain antinauseant drugs. Amer J Obstet Gynecol 1976; 125:244–8.
11. Aselton P, Jick H. Additional followup of congenital limb disorders in relation to Bendectin use. JAMA 1983;250:33–4.
12. Eskenazi B. Bracken M. Bendectin (Debendox) as a risk factor for pyloric stenosis. Am J Obstet Gynecol 1982;144:919–24.
13. Fleming DM, Knox JDE, Crombie DL. Debendox in early pregnancy and fetal malformation. Br Med J 1981;283:99–101.
14. Michaelis J, Michaelis H, Gluck E, Koller S. Prospective study of suspected associations between certain drugs administered during early pregnancy and congenital malformations. Teratology 1983;27:57–64.
15. Morelock S, Hingson R, Kayne H, et al. Bendectin and fetal development: A study at Boston City Hospital. Am J Obstet Gynecol 1982;142:209–13.

16. Rothman KJ, Fyler DC, Goldblatt A, Kreidberg MB. Exogenous hormones and other drug exposures of children with congenital heart disease. Am J Epidermiol 1979;109:433–9.
17. Zierler S, Rothman KJ. Congenital heart disease in relation to maternal use of Bendectin and other drugs in early pregnancy. N Engl J Med 1985;313:347–52.
18. Aselton PJ, Jick H. Additional followup of congenital limb disorders in relation to Bendectin use. JAMA 1983;250:33–4.
19. Gibson GT, Colley DP, McMichael AJ, Hartshorne JM. Congenital anomalies in relation to the use of doxylamine/dicyclomine and other antenatal factors. Med J Aust 1981;1:410–14.
20. Jick H, Holmes LB, Hunter JR, Madsen S, Stergachis A. First trimester drug use and congenital disorders. JAMA 1981; 246:343–6.
21. General Practitioner Clinical Trials. Drugs in pregnancy survey. Practitioner 1963;191:775–80.
22. Golding J, Vivian S, Baldwin JA. Maternal anti-nauseants and clefts of lip and palate. Hum Toxicol 1983;2:63–73.
23. Greenberg G, Inman WHW, Weatherall JAC, Adalstein AM, Haskey JC. Material drug histories and congenital abnormalities. Br Med J 1977;2:853–6.
24. Newman NM, Correy JF, Dudgeon GI. A survey of congenital abnormalities and drugs in a private practice. Aust NZ J Gynaecol 1977;17:156–9.
25. Smithells RW, Sheppard S. Teratogenicity testing in humans: A method of demonstrating safety of Bendectin. Teratology 1978;17:31–6.
26. Bunde CA, Bowles DM. A technique for controlled survey of case records. Curr Ther Res 1963;5:245–8.
27. Kullander S, Kallen B. A prospective study of drugs and pregnancy. II. Anti-emetic drugs. Acta Obstet Gynecol Scand 1976;55:105–11.
28. Auerbach C, Barrow M. Urogenital abnormalities produced in rat fetuses with chlorcyclizine. Teratology 1972;5:23–31.
29. Barrow M, Rowland C. Prolonged gestation in the rat and its usefulness in experimental teratology. Teratology 1969;2:261–74.
30. Brandes J. First-trimester nausea and vomiting as related to outcome of pregnancy. Obstet Gynecol 1967;30:427–31.
31. Brown N, Fabro S. The value of animal teratogenicity testing for predicting human risk. Clin Obstet Gynecol 1983;26:467–77.
32. Busse W. Chronic rhinitis. A systematic approach to diagnosis and treatment. Postgrad Med 1983;73:325–9, 333–5.
33. Bierme S, Bierme R. Antihistamines in hydrops foetalis. Lancet 1967;1:574.
34. Carroll J, Moir R. Use of promethazine hydrochloride in obstetrics. JAMA 1958;168:2218–24.
35. Carter M, Wilson F. Ancoloxin and fetal abnormalities. B Med J 1962;2:1609.
36. Charles A, Blumenthal L. Promethazine hydrochloride therapy in severely Rh-sensitized pregnancies. Obstet Gynecol 1982;60: 627–30.
37. Choid N, Klaponski F. On neural-tube defects: An epidemiological elicitation of etiological factors. Neurology 1970;20:399–400.
38. Corby D, Schulman I. The effects of antenatal drug administration on aggregation of platelets of newborn infants. Ped Pharmacol Ther 1971;79:307–313.
39. Cordero J, Oakley GJ. Drug exposure during pregnancy: Some epidemiologic considerations. Clin Obstet Gynecol 1983;26: 418–28.
40. Crawford L, Cohen R. Therapy for allergic rhinitis. Comprehen Ther 1985;11:60–9.
41. David A, Goodspeed A. Ancoloxin and fetal abnormalities. Brit Med J 1963;1:121.
42. David M, Doyle E. First trimester pregnancy. Am J Nurs 1976;76:1945–8.
43. Diggory P, Tomkinson J. Meclozine and fetal abnormalities. Lancet 1962;2:1222–3.
44. Dipalma J. Drugs for nausea and vomiting of pregnancy. Am Fam Phy 1983;28:272–4.
45. Donnai D, Harris R. Unusual fetal malformations after antiemetics in early pregnancy. Br Med J 1978;1:691–2.
46. Failor H, Huffman M. Dystonic reactions to phenothiazine drugs. 1965;26:714–7.
47. Forfar J, Nelson M. Epidemiology of drugs taken by pregnant women: Drugs that may affect the fetus adversely. Clin Pharmacol Ther 1973;14:632–41.
48. Gibbs D. Diseases of the alimentary system: Nausea and vomiting. Brit Med J 1976;2:1489–92.
49. Gibson J, Staples R, Larson E, Kuhn W, Holtkamp D, Newberne J. Teratology and reproduction studies with an antinauseant. Toxicol Appl Pharmacol 1968;13:439–47.
50. Goldberg J, Golbus M. The value of case reports in human teratology. Am J Obstet Gynecol 1986;154:479–82.
51. Greenberger P, Patterson R. Safety of therapy for allergic symptoms during pregnancy. Ann Inter Med 1978;89:234–7.
52. Guillozet N. Drug risks in pregnancy revisited. J Fam Pract 1977;4:1043–52.
53. Gusdon JJ. The treatment of erythroblastosis with promethazine hydrochloride. J Reprod Med 1981;26:454–8.
54. Hill R. Drugs ingested by pregnant women. Clin Pharmacol Ther 1973;14:654–9.
55. Holt G, Mabry R. ENT medications in pregnancy. Otolaryng-Head and Neck Surg 1983;91:338–41.
56. Huff P. Safety and drug therapy for nausea and vomiting of pregnancy. J Fam Pract 1980;11:969–70.
57. Iuliucci J, Gautieri R. Morphine-induced fetal malformations. II. Influence of histamine and diphenydramine. J Pharm Sci 1971;60:420–5.
58. Jaffe P, Liberman M, McFadyen I, Valman H. Incidence of congenital limb-reduction deformities. Lancet 1975;1:526–7.
59. Kasperlik-Zaluska A, Migdalska B, Hartwig W, et al. Two pregnancies in a woman with Cushing's syndrome treated with cyproheptadine. Brit J Obstet Gynecol 1980;87:1171–3.
60. Khir A, How J, Bewsher P. Successful pregnancy after cyproheptadine treatment for Cushing's disease. Eur J Obstet Gynecol Reprod Biol 1982;13:343–7.
61. King C. Teratogenic effects of meclizine hydrochloride on the rat. Science 1963;141:353–4.
62. King C, Weaver S, Derr J. Benzhydrylpiperazine antihistamines, hydramnios, and congenital malformations in the rat. Am J Obstet Gynecol 1965;93:563–5.
63. King C, Howell J. Teratogenic effect of buclizine and hydroxyzine in the rat and chlorcyclizine in the mouse. Am J Obstet Gynecol 1966;95:109–11.
64. Klingberg M, Papier C, Hart J. Birth defects monitoring. Am J Indust Med 1983;4:309–28.
65. Kucera J. Congenital anomalies. Teratology 1971;4:492.
66. Leathem A. Safety and efficacy of antiemetics used to treat nausea and vomiting in pregnancy. Clin Pharm 1986;5:660–8.
67. Lewis J, Weingold A. The use of gastrointestinal drugs during pregnancy and lactation. Am J Gastroenterol 1985;80:912–23.
68. Levin S. Problems and pitfalls in conducting epidemiological research in the area of reproductive toxicology. Am J Indust Med 1983;4:349–64.
69. McBride W. Cyclizine and congenital abnormalities. Brit Med J 1963;27:1157–8.
70. McColl J. Dimenhydrinate in pregnancy. Can Med Assoc J 1963;88:861.
71. Milton-Thompson G. Anti-nauseant drugs. Practitioner 1979; 223:516–9.
72. Montminy M, Teres D. Shock after phenothiazine administration in a pregnancy patient with a pehochromocytoma. J Reprod Med 1983;28:159–61.
73. Muller L, Korte A, Madle S. Mutagenicity testing of doxylamine succinate, an antinauseant drug. Toxicol Lett 1989;49:79–86.
74. Niebyl J. Therapeutic drugs in pregnancy. Caution is the watchword. Postgrad Med 1984;75:165–6.

75. Niebyl J. Therapeutic drugs in pregnancy. Postgrad Med 1984;75: 169–72.
76. Okafor B. Tracheostomy in the management of pediatric airway problems. ENTJ 1983;62:28–33.
77. Patterson S. Our bundle or responsibility. Presidential address. Am J Obstet Gynecol 1984;149:245–50.
78. Polednak AP. Uses of available record systems in epidemiologic studies of reproductive toxicology. Am J Indust Med 1983;4:329–48.
79. Posner H, Graves A, King C, Wilk A. Experimental alteration of the metabolism of chlorcyclizine and the incidence of cleft palate in rats. 1967;155:494–505.
80. Posner H, Darr A, Barrow M. Anomalies of the internal organs and diminished calcification of vertebrae in fetuses after benzhydrylpiperazine treatment of pregnant rats. Toxicol Appl Pharmacol 1970;17:76–82.
81. Posner H, Darr A. Fetal edema from benzhydrylpiperazines as a possible cause of oral-facial malformations in rats. Toxicol Appl Pharmacol 1970;17:67–75.
82. Ratten G. The use of drugs in pregnancy and labor. Austr Fam Phys 1978;7:1118–9.
83. Riffel H, Nochimson D, Paul R, Hon E. Effects of meperidine and promethazine during labor. Obstet Gynecol 1973;42:738–45.
84. Shepard T. *Catalog of Teratogenic Agents*. Baltimore, MD: The Johns Hopkins University Press; 1986
85. Rodriguez-Gonzalez M, Lima Perez M, Sanabria Negrin J. The effect of cyproheptadine chlorhydrate on rat embryonic development. Teratogenesis Carcinog Mutagen 1983;3:439–46.
86. Sadusk JJ, Palmisano P. Evaluation of the teratogenic effect of meclizine in man. JAMA 1965;194:987–9.
87. Saxen I. Epidemiology of cleft lip and palate. An attempt to rule out chance correlations. Br J Prevent Soc Med 1975;29:103–10.
88. Schardein J, Hentz D, Petrer J, Kurtz S. Teratogenesis studies with diphenhydramine HCI. Toxicol Appl Pharmacol 1971;18:971–6.
89. Schenkel B, Vorherr H. Non-prescription drugs during pregnancy: Potential teratogenic and toxic effects upon embryo and fetus. J Reprod Med 1974;12:27–45.
90. Schmid B, Hauser R, Donatsch P. Effects of cyproheptadine on the rat yolk sac membrane and embryonic development in vitro. Xenobiotica 1985;15:695–9.
91. Shapiro S, Kaufman D, Rosenberg L, et al. Meclizine in pregnancy in relation to congenital malformations. Br Med J 1978,1:483.
92. Stahlmann R, Neubert D. Which drugs are allowed, which should one avoid, which are contraindicated? Gynakologe 1987;20:129–36.
93. Steffek A, King C, Derr J. The comparative pathogenesis of experimentally induced cleft palate. J Oral Ther Pharmacol 1966;3:9–16.
94. Villumsen A. Congenital malformations. Teratology 1971;4:503.
95. Von Almen W, Miller JJ. “T’s and Blues” in pregnancy. J Reprod Med 1986;31:236–9.
96. Walters W, Humphrey M. Common medical disorders in pregnancy and their treatment.
97. Walters W. The management of nausea and vomiting during pregnancy. Med J Aust 1987;147:290–1.
98. Watson G. Meclozine and fetal abnormalities. Brit Med J 1962;1:1446.
99. Wheatley D. Treatment of pregnancy sickness. Brit J Obstet Gynaecol 1977;84:444–7.
100. Whyatt P. Astemizole in pregnancy. Austr Fam Phys 1986;15: 382–4.
101. Wilk A, Steffek A, King C. Norchlorcyclizine analogs: Relationship of teratogenic activity to in vitro cartilage binding. J Pharmacol Exp Ther 1970;171:118–26.
102. Wilk A, King C, Pratt RJ. Enhancement of chlorcyclizine teratogenicity in the rat by coadministration of calcium chelating agents. Teratology 1978;18:193–8.
103. Wilk A, King C, Pratt R. Chlorcyclizine induction of cleft palate in the rat: Degradation of palatal glycosaminoglycans. Teratology 1978;18:199–209.
104. Barcellona P. Investigations on the possible teratogenic effects of trazodone in rats and rabbits. Bollett Chim Farmac 1970;109: 323–32.
105. Brandstater S, Grillmaier J. Various presuppositions for epidemiologic studies on the relation between hyperemesis, use of antiemetics in pregnancy and fetal defects. Geburtshilfe Und Frauenheilkunde 1972;32:227–9.
106. De Rom R. Meclizine and congenital malformations. Geburtschilfe Und Frauenheilkunde 1966;26:565–7.
107. Guskova T, Golovanova V. Effect of embryogenesis of a new antiallergic agent bikarfen (Rus). Farmakologiia I Toksikologiia 1981;44:721–3.
108. Karchmer S, Ontiveros E, L’opes Garcia R. Placental function and pharmacologic damage to the fetus (Spa). Maternidade e Infancia 1971;30:169–82.
109. Kitschke H, Kuemmerle H. Pharmacotherapy in pregnancy. Part 4. Antidiabetics, antiemetics, neuroleptics and hormones. Munchener Medizinische Wochenschrift 1980;122:44–5.
110. Litta R, Rainone R, Zingariello L. A case of incomplete amelia. Pediatria 1983;91:287–93.
111. Peszynski-Drews C. Modern views on the pathogenetic mechanisms of experimental labiopalatal clefts. Pediatria Polska 1974;49:85–92.
112. Koren G. *Maternal-Fetal Toxicology*, 2nd ed. New York and Basel: Marcel Dekker, Inc.; 1994
113. Rosenzweig S, Blaustein FM. Cleft palate in A/J mice resulting from restraint and deprivation of food and water. Teratology 1971;3: 47–51.
114. Warkany J, Petering H. Congenital malformations of the brain caused by short zinc deficiencies in rats. Am J Ment Defic 1973;77: 645–53.
115. Depue RH, Bernstein L, Ross RK, Judd HL, Henderson BE. Hyperemesis gravidarum in relation to estradiol levels, pregnancy outcome, and other maternal factors: A seroepidemiologic study. Amer J Obstet Gynecol 1987;156:1137–41.
116. Brandes JM. First trimester nausea and vomiting as related to outcome of pregnancy. Obstet Gynecol 1967;30:427–31.

Reprinted from Seto A, Einarson T, Koren G. Pregnancy outcome following first trimester exposure to antihistamines: meta-analysis. Am J Perinatol. 1997; 14:119–24 with permission.

CHAPTER 54

EVALUATION OF BROMPHENIRAMINE SAFETY IN PREGNANCY

Arnold Seto, Tom Einarson, and Gideon Koren

EVALUATION OF BROMPHENIRAMINE SAFETY IN PREGNANCY

At the Motherisk Program in Toronto, gestational exposures of most frequent concern have been antibiotics, followed by analgesics and antihistamines (1). Until now, there has been no clear overall statement regarding fetal toxicity following antihistamine exposure because of conflicting reports. Within the reports on H_1 antagonists, there is very little information concerning the reproductive and developmental toxicity of brompheniramine. The published data collected in the Boston Collaborative Perinatal (1958–1965) Project (2) reported a statistically significant association between the use of brompheniramine during pregnancy and an increase in the incidence of birth defects. Of the 50,000 mother–child pairs examined in that study, 11 of the 65 brompheniramine-exposed pregnancies (17%) had detectable malformations at birth, with syndactyly observed in three of the brompheniramine-exposed pregnancies. That incidence of malformations yielded a relative risk of 2.34 ($P < 0.05$) for brompheniramine. The relative risk values for the other antihistamines investigated in that study ranged from 0.81 to 1.25, all nonsignificant. Although the risk for brompheniramine malformations was statistically significant, the authors cautioned that it may have been a chance finding and that larger numbers were needed to provide a definitive conclusion.

Nonetheless, based on that report, women have been generally advised not to take brompheniramine during pregnancy. However, because about one half of the pregnancies in North America are unplanned, the problem becomes quite different. Women who perceive a risk for malformation may elect to terminate an otherwise wanted pregnancy. Because antihistamines are widely used in a variety of cold and allergy remedies (1), a very large number of unborn babies are exposed in utero to these agents. In another report, Aselton and Jick (3) studied the prevalence of certain major congenital disorders among liveborn infants of 6,509 mothers. Brompheniramine had a relative risk of 1.8 (95% CI, 0.8 to 4.4), which was not statistically significant. These authors hypothesized that the observed lower rate in their study when compared to the Boston report (2) was due to their exclusion of some minor malformations that were included in the previous cohort.

Because of these conflicting reports and since only a few studies have addressed the question of the teratogenic potential of brompheniramine, we performed a prospective study to determine the teratogenic potential of gestational exposure to brompheniramine, followed by meta-analysis of all available cohorts.

Prospective Controlled Study

We conducted a prospective cohort study comparing the outcome of brompheniramine-exposed pregnancies to dimenhydrinate-exposed pregnancies. Dimenhydrinate was chosen as a control drug because it is the agent of choice for treating nausea and vomiting in pregnancy and has not been found to be associated with increased risk for birthd efects (2). Being an H_1 antihistamine, it interacts with the same receptors as brompheniramine.

Data for the cohort study were extracted from the database of the Motherisk program at the Hospital for Sick Children in Toronto. Pregnant women who contacted Motherisk prospectively regarding first trimester exposure to brompheniramine and dimenhydrinate between September 1986 and August 1991 were included in this study. Patients were matched for age of the mother (within 2 years), cigarette smoking, and alcohol exposure to women exposed during the first trimester to dimenhydrinate.

The Motherisk database identified 65 women who had ingested brompheniramine during the first trimester of pregnancy. However, only 34 could be contacted for follow-up. Mean age of mothers at birth was 31 ± 3.8 years (range 21 to 37); they had on average 2.5 ± 1.4 pregnancies (range 1 to 6) with 1.1 ± 1.0 previous children (range 0 to 4).

There was one major malformation, pulmonary valve stenosis, among the 34 brompheniramine-exposed infants. In the control group, there were two major malformations reported, namely, pyloric stenosis and cerebral palsy. The odds ratio for major malformation was 0.5 with a 95% confidence interval of –0.37 to 1.03.

Meta-Analysis

A computerized Medline search (1960–1991) was conducted to identify all papers examining the use of brompheniramine in pregnancy using the key words pregnancy, antihistamine, antinauseant, antiemetic, cough-cold product, adverse fetal outcome, malformation, congenital abnormalities, teratogen, morning sickness, hyperemesis gravidarum, nausea, vomiting, hypersensitivity, and allergy. Included in this meta-analysis were studies that compared maternal brompheniramine exposure during the first trimester of pregnancy in humans with a nonexposed control group. Outcome rates for major malformations must have been presented. An overall odds ratio was calculated using the Mantel-Haenszel equation (4). A 95% confidence interval was calculated using Miettinen's method (5,8).

The literature review identified three other studies that addressed the issue of brompheniramine exposure in pregnancy and congenital malformations (2,3,6). However, two of those articles were excluded from analysis. The study by Heinonen and coworkers (2) could not be initially included because it did not separate major from minor malformations. The study by Jick and coworkers (6) was duplicated in the later study by Aselton and coworkers (3). The paper by Aselton and coworkers (3) reported 5 malformations in 172 brompheniramine exposures and 105 in the 6209 controls. The odds ratio was 1.74 (95% CI, 0.70 to 4.32). Thus, only two studies relating brompheniramine in pregnancy to major malformations were initially extracted and analyzed. When the two studies were combined, the summary odds ratio was 1.4 (95% CI, 0.61 to 3.23). Chi-square homogeneity was not significant ($\chi^2 = 1.85$, df = 2, $P > 0.05$).

The study of Heinonen and coworkers (2), which indicated a significant association between brompheniramine exposure and congenital malformations, was not included in the above meta-analysis because those authors did not separate major and minor malformations. Such an approach may be misleading and lacks a sound theoretical basis. However, three cases of syndactyly classified as major malformation were reported by the Heinonen study. This fact was obtained from REPROTOX®, an on-line reproductive toxicology database. If this information were included in the meta-analysis, the summary odds ratio for malformations would still remain nonsignificant (OR = 0.96, 95% CI, 0.49 to 1.89). Not knowing whether any other major malformations were identified in the Heinonen study, we attempted to determine how many major malformations would be required in that study in order for the summary odds ratio to be significant. We calculated that 10 of the 11 (90.1%) reported malformations must be classified as major in order for the summary odds ratio to reach statistical significance (lower 95% confidence limit = 1.09). That percentage would be extremely unlikely because the same authors reported that the proportion of major malformations as a percentage of all malformations in the class of antihistamines was only 65% (2). In other words, if only 2 out of the 11 observed malformations were minor, then the summary odds ratio would be nonsignificant. Hence, even the inclusion of the data from Heinonen's study would not result in a significant association between brompheniramine exposure in pregnancy and risk for major malformations.

Due to the small sample size (34 pairs), the power of the present cohort study (15%) was not adequate to rule out some increased risk of brompheniramine. However, the power of the combined studies calculated according to the method of Munoz and Rosner (9) was 92.2%. As a result, we believe it is likely that there is no clinically important increased teratogenic risk from brompheniramine exposure during the first trimester.

It does not appear to us justified to label brompheniramine as an H_1-blocker more toxic to the fetus than other compounds of the same class of drugs. It is of interest that, although used quite widely, no attempts have been made during the past two decades to ascertain the validity of the single report by Heinonen on brompheniramine (2). Not only was the drug "contraindicated" for use in pregnancy (7), but despite Heinoinen and coworkers' cautioning against premature conclusions, their study has led to high levels of anxiety among pregnant women who had used brompheniramine before they realized they had conceived. Continuous, prospective followup of brompheniramine exposures by additional Teratogen Information Services will be important to verify the present results.

REFERENCES

1. Koren G. Maternal–fetal toxicology, a clinicians' guide. New York: Marcel Dekker; 1990.
2. Heinonen O, Sloane D, Shapiro S. Birth defects and drugs in pregnancy. Littleton, Massachusetts: PSG Publishing; 1977.
3. Aselton P, Jick H, Milkunsky A, Hunter JR, Stergachis A. First-trimester drugs use and congenital disorders. Obstet Gynecol. 1985;65:451–5.
4. Mantel MH, Haenszel W. Statistical aspects of the analysis of data from retrospective studies of disease. JNCI. 1959;22:718–48.
5. Glass GV. Integrating findings: the meta-analysis of research. Rev Res Educ. 1978;316:351–79.
6. Jick H, Hunter JR, Madsen S, Stergachis A. First-trimester drug use and congenital disorders. JAMA. 1981;246:343–6.
7. Briggs GG, Freeman RK, Yaffe SJ. Drugs in pregnancy and lactation. Baltimore: Williams and Wilkins; 1986.
8. Meittinen O. Estimability and estimation in case–referent studies. Am J Epidemiol. 1976;103:226–35.
9. Munoz A, Rosner B. Power and sample size for a collection of 2 × 2 tables. Biometrics. 1984;40:995–1004.

Reprinted from Seto A, Einarson T, Koren G. Evaluation of brompheniramine safety in pregnancy. Reprod Toxicol 1993;7:393–5 with permission from Elsevier.

CHAPTER 55

BIRTH DEFECTS AFTER MATERNAL EXPOSURE TO CORTICOSTEROIDS: PROSPECTIVE COHORT STUDY AND META-ANALYSIS OF EPIDEMIOLOGICAL STUDIES

Laura Park-Wyllie,[1] Paolo Mazzotta,[2] Anne Pastuszak,[3] Myla E. Moretti,[2] Lizanne Beique,[1] Laura Hunnisett,[2] Mark H. Friesen,[1] Sheila Jacobson,[2] S. Kasapinovic,[2] Debra Chang,[2] Orna Diav-Citrin,[2] David Chitayat,[4] Irena Nulman,[2] Thomas R. Einarson,[1] and Gideon Koren[2]

[1]Faculty of Pharmacy, University of Toronto, Toronto, Canada [2]Motherisk Program, Division of Clinical Pharmacology and Toxicology, Research Institute, Hospital for Sick Children, CIBC World Market Children's Miracle Chair in Child Health Research and University of Toronto, Toronto, Canada M5G 1X8 [3]Fetal Diagnosis and Treatment Centre, University of Toronto, Toronto, Canada [4]Department of Genetics, Toronto General Hospital, Toronto, Canada

Abstract

Background. Corticosteroids are first-line drugs for the treatment of a variety of conditions in women of childbearing age. Information regarding human pregnancy outcome with corticosteroids is limited.
Methods. We collected prospectively and followed up 184 women exposed to prednisone in pregnancy and 188 pregnant women who were counseled by Motherisk for nonteratogenic exposure. The primary outcome was the rate of major birth defects. A meta-analysis of all epidemiological studies was conducted. The Mantel-Haenszel summary odds ratio was calculated for the pooled studies with 95% confidence intervals. A cumulative summary odds ratio was also calculated by combining studies in chronological order. Chi-squared for homogeneity was determined to establish the comparability of the studies.
Results. In our prospective study, there was no statistical difference in the rate of major anomalies between the corticosteroid-exposed and control groups. In the meta-analysis, the Mantel-Haenszel summary odds ratio for major malformations with all cohort studies was 1.45 [95% CI 0.80, 2.60] and 3.03 [95% CI 1.08, 8.54] when Heinonen et al. ('77) was removed. This suggests a marginally increased risk of major malformations after first-trimester exposure to corticosteroids. In addition, summary odds ratio for case-control studies examining oral clefts was significant (3.35 [95% CI 1.97, 5.69]).
Conclusions. Although prednisone does not represent a major teratogenic risk in humans at therapeutic doses, it does increase by an order of 3.4-fold the risk of oral cleft, which is consistent with the existing animal studies.

Teratology 62:385–392, 2000.

INTRODUCTION

Prednisone, a glucocorticoid used in the treatment of asthma, transplantation, collagen vascular, and other disorders, has been shown to cross the human placenta (Pasqualini et al., '70; Beitins et al., '72; Levitz et al., '78; Renisch et al. '78; Crowley et al., '95). Large doses administered to pregnant mice, rats and rabbits during organogenesis have caused cleft palate in the exposed offspring (Fainstat, '54; Pinsky and DiGeorge, '65; Walker et al., '71). The same teratogenic effect on the developing palates is observed in mice given the naturally occurring glucocorticoid, cortisone (Baxter and Fraser, '50).

Direct extrapolation from animals to humans is tenuous. In several case reports, women were treated during the first trimester with prednisone for a plethora of diseases, including Hodgkin's disease (Schilsky et al., '81), leukemia (Sinykin and Kaplan, '62; Dara et al., '81), renal transplantation (Nolan et al., '74; Coulam et al., '82; diMalatesta et al., '93), systemic lupus erythematosus (SLE) (Tozman et al., '80; Jones et al., '86), antiphospholipid antibodies (Tabbutt et al., '94), asthma (Fitzsimmons et al., '86), rheumatoid arthritis (Wright et al., '82), regional enteritis (Kraus, '75), glomerulonephritis (Coté et al., '74) and idiopathic thrombocytopenic purpura (Al-Mofada et al., '94). Although a variety of birth defects in their offspring were reported, there was no consistent pattern of embryopathy. The increased incidence of low birth weight and stillbirths may be attributable to the underlying maternal condition for which the steroids were administered.

The most rigorous epidemiologic data come from those observational and interventional studies in which women with unexplained recurrent fetal loss (Lockshin et al., '89; Cowchock et al., '92; Out et al., '92; Silveira et al., '92; Carp et al., '93; Silver et al., '93) or autoimmune thrombocytopenia (Karpatkin et al., '81) were either randomized or allocated to receive prednisone throughout pregnancy. In these publications, there was no evidence to suggest that incidence of oral cleft was elevated above the baseline risk. In light of the paucity of controlled trials or prospective studies, we investigated in a prospective observation study the relative fetal safety of maternal prednisone therapy. In addition, we conducted a meta-analysis to determine the risk, if any, of steroid use on the fetus with respect to major malformations and, more specifically, oral clefts (cleft lip with or without cleft palate, or cleft palate alone).

SUBJECTS AND METHODS

Prospective Study

This was a prospective observational cohort study in which the exposed patients were women who voluntarily telephoned the Motherisk Program, Toronto, Canada, for information about the fetal safety/risk from use of prednisone by the mother during pregnancy. Women were included in the exposed cohort if they had taken systemic prednisone for any indication in the first trimester and if their exposure details and medical history had been collected during the first trimester at the time they called for a consultation with one of our teratology information counselors and documented on the clinic's standardized intake forms.

As the unexposed group, we chose a cohort of pregnant women who voluntarily contacted the Motherisk Program for safety/risk information about either topical retinoic acid for uncomplicated acne, or oral astemizole for seasonal allergies, neither of which has been associated with an increased risk of major malformations (Pastuszak et al., '96; Shapiro et al., '97). This comparison group was intended to represent the baseline population of pregnant women.

We collected the following information prospectively, from every caller: dose, indication, and dates of initiation and discontinuation of the medication of concern, as well as obstetric, medical, and genetic history and drug exposure of the mother. Approximately 1 year after the expected date of delivery, as calculated by the date of the last menstrual period, all patients were telephoned by a Motherisk team member who collected details about the outcome of pregnancy, birth weight, and presence or absence of birth defects, and perinatal and neonatal complications. Follow-up details were corroborated subsequently by written documentation from the child's physician.

The primary outcome of interest was the rate of major birth defects after the use of corticosteroids, which was compared between the two groups. If etiologies other than corticosteroids were considered to have caused the specific malformation (i.e., genetic syndromes or maternal infections), these cases were excluded from calculation of malformation rates that could be attributed to corticosteroid use. The reports of all anomalies were reviewed and classified as major or minor malformations according to Heinonen et al. ('77) and Holmes ('99), with major malformations including abnormalities that are life-threatening, that require surgical intervention, or that have serious cosmetic ramifications.

All data were entered into a spreadsheet for statistical analysis using Statview™ SE + Graphics (Abacus Concepts, Berkeley, CA, 1987) for Macintosh computers. For the two group comparisons of continuous data, a single factor factorial, a *t*-test was used and the Fisher's least significant difference post-hoc test for multiple comparisons was used to identify mean differences between groups. Categorical data were compared using chi-square analysis or Fisher exact test, when appropriate.

Meta-Analysis

The databases Medline (1966–December 1999), EMBASE (1988–October 1999), and Current Contents (Jan–Dec 1999) were searched using the following criteria. The search items congenital anomalies, drug induced, teratogen, and birth defect were combined using the Boolean operator odds ratio (OR). The search item glucocorticosteroid was combined with the previous search using the Boolean operator AND. A preliminary review of the titles (and abstracts when available) was made to determine whether the article was relevant to our topic. Abstracts of meetings published in the journals *Teratology* and *Pediatric Research* for 1995–1998 were also reviewed to cover new studies potentially not published yet as full papers. Bibliographies were reviewed for retrieved articles to identify any additional relevant articles. The reviewers were blinded by eliminating all reference to the authors, journal, and study location. This was done to reduce the potential bias in the selection of articles, data extraction, and quality assessment.

Controlled studies that examined first-trimester human systemic exposure for any corticosteroids, any doses, all indications, any duration, and all languages were included. Both case-control and cohort studies were acceptable for analysis; however, studies consisting of fewer than 10 corticosteroid-treated patients were excluded. Again, major malformations were defined, using the criteria described by Heinonen et al. ('77) and Holmes ('99). Trials examining topical or inhaled steroids were excluded. A third author was used as an arbitrator in the case of discrepancies between raters. Inclusion of studies was agreed on by mutual consensus between reviewers and the reasons for exclusion were identified. The same procedure was followed during the data extraction and quality assessment scoring. Accepted studies had to report on the rates of major malformations in the corticosteroid and control groups. Data from the accepted studies were extracted in the form of 2 × 2 tables. The following four values were extracted from each study: number of neonates exposed to corticosteroids exhibiting major malformations, number of neonates exposed to corticosteroids without major malformations, number of neonates not exposed to corticosteroids with malformations, and number of neonates not exposed to corticosteroids without malformations. In the case of a woman with multiple pregnancies, each pregnancy was considered an independent event. Stillbirths and abortions were excluded from data extraction unless the study specifically mentioned assessment of malformations. The following demographic data of all the accepted studies were recorded where available: disease of the mother, number of neonates, types and doses of corticosteroid used, and type of birth defect.

Abstracted data were entered into 2 × 2 tables using the Cochrane Review Manager version 4.0.3. software for IBM compatible computers. For each of the studies, a Mantel-Haenszel summary and cumulative OR (with a 95% confidence interval [CI]) was calculated. The null hypothesis (of no variation in outcome between n studies) was not rejected (and the pooling of outcomes was considered valid) if the chi-square test of homogeneity was less than the upper 95th percentile of the chi-square distribution with {n-1} degrees of freedom (df). An OR of 1 reflected no effect of exposure on fetal outcome, whereas an OR > 1 reflected an increased risk of malformations among corticosteroid-exposed groups.

A sensitivity analysis was performed to determine the association between corticosteroids exposure and oral cleft. In addition, we calculated an incidence rate of major malformations from the included studies in addition to the studies that were rejected only because they had no control groups but that otherwise met the inclusion criteria. Assessment of the quality of the studies was performed using a quality assessment score for epidemiological studies published by our group (Seto, '93). Inter-rater agreement was measured for inclusion of articles, data extraction and quality assessment of articles. The correlation between the quality of scores for our studies and the OR was tested in order to determine whether the quality of the studies was biasing our results. The mean, raw mean, and meta-analytic mean were calculated for the incidence rate of major malformations.

RESULTS

Prospective Study

During 1985–1995, 184 women met inclusion criteria and completed the postnatal follow-up. In the Motherisk cohort, corticosteroids were used for Crohn's disease (by 34 women, 18%), asthma

(30, 16%), ulcerative colitis (28, 15%), rheumatoid arthritis (18, 10%), Bell's palsy (7, 4%), transplant (8, 4%), lupus (20, 11%), sarcoidosis (4, 2%), and other indications (35, 19%). Although duration, dose and route of prednisone exposure varied, 138 (75%) women were exposed in the first trimester of pregnancy (Table 1). Compared with the unexposed, women exposed to corticosteroids were more likely to be primigravida and identify themselves as smokers. The rates of previous terminations of pregnancy and reported patterns of alcohol consumption between the two groups were not different statistically (Table 2). In the exposed group, 184 women delivered 157 infants (3 sets of twins); the controls included 188 women who delivered 171 live-born infants.

The rate of live-born infants was similar in the exposed and control groups (157/187 vs 171/188, $P = 0.06$). However, the number of elective pregnancy terminations was higher in the exposed group (16/187 vs 2/188, $P = 0.002$) (Table 3). There was one stillbirth among the controls and a fetal death (≥26 weeks) in each of the study and control groups. The proportion of male to female infants was similar between the two groups. When compared with controls, babies born to exposed mothers were smaller (mean 3,112 g vs 3,428 g, $P = 0.0001$), born earlier (mean 38 weeks vs 39.5 weeks, $P = 0.0001$) and more likely to be premature (27/158 vs 9/172, $P = 0.0001$). Despite these differences, the majority of infants in both groups were AGA (139/157 and 158/168, respectively, $P = 0.2$) and there was no preponderance of SGA or LGA babies (Table 3). There was no statistical difference in the rate of vaginal or cesarean section deliveries between the groups. When pregnancies resulting in multiple births were temporarily excluded from analysis of gestational age at birth and weight, mean differences remained different statistically.

There was no statistical difference in the rate of major anomalies between the groups (exposed: 4/111, controls: 3/172; $P = 0.3$) (Table 4). The major defects reviewed by the dysmorphologist and presented in Table 5 show no consistent phenotype, when examined by group of exposure. Only malformations that could possibly be attributable to the corticosteroids were included in the statistical comparison. A malformation with a genetic etiology and another due to maternal infection were excluded from the calculation of malformation rates (Table 5).

Table 1
Characteristics of Prednisone Exposure (*n = 184*) in the Prospective Study

CHARACTERISTIC	MEAN OR PROPORTION
Therapy duration (wk)	21 ± 16 (161)*
Daily dose (mg)	27 ± 29 (173)*
Route	
p.o.	165/167 (99%)
i.v.	1/167 (0.5%)
p.o + i.v	1/167 (0.5%)
Exposure	
≤13 wk	38/184 (21%)
≤26 wk	16/184 (9%)
13–26 wk	11/184 (6%)
throughout	84/184 (45%)
>13 wk	22/184 (12%)
>26 wk	13/184 (7%)
Polytherapy	122/182 (67%)
Prednisone + amniosalicylic acid	38/124 (31%)
Prednisone + azathioprine	13/124 (10%)
Prednisone + other	73/124 (59%)

* Number in parentheses represents total number of cases in which value was known.

Table 2
Baseline Characteristics of Mothers in the Prospective Study and Groups*

CHARACTERISTIC	CORTICOSTEROIDS (*n* = 184)	CONTROLS (*n* = 188)	*P*
Maternal age (yr)	30 ± 5 (186)	31 ± 5 (186)	0.0003
Gravidity 1	75 (41%)	86 (46%)	0.6
Gravidity 2	112 (61%)	102 (54%)	
Parity 0	83 (45%)	51 (27%)	0.0003
Parity 1	104 (56%)	137 (73%)	
Prior miscarriages 0	153 (83%)	151 (80%)	0.99
Prior miscarriages 1	34 (18%)	37 (20%)	
Previous abortions 0	173 (94%)	175 (93%)	0.99
Previous abortions 1	14 (8%)	13 (7%)	
No smoking	154 (83%)	175 (93%)	0.01
No alcohol use	152 (82%)	141 (75%)	0.3

* Information was missing for some patients regarding various characteristics.

Meta-Analysis

There were 455 articles identified from the search of the literature. The main reasons for excluding studies were case reports, reviews, case series, absence of a control arm, inadequate reporting of fetal outcome, and inability to verify first-trimester exposure. Eight studies were excluded from the analysis because they lacked a control group; however, these studies reported sufficient information to calculate an incidence rate, but not OR (Wells, '53; Kenny et al., '66; Yackel et al., '66; Walsh and Clark, '67; Morris, '69; Hack et al., '72; Schatz, et al., '75; Mercado et al., '95). Three studies were excluded because the number of treated patients was less than 10. Ten studies met our inclusion criteria and were entered into the meta-analysis (Table 6).

Of the 10 accepted studies, six were cohort studies and four were case-control studies. The time frame of study publications was 1962–1999. The studies included women with varying underlying diseases including rheumatoid arthritis, systemic lupus erythematosus, ankylosing spondylitis, asthma, inflammatory bowel disease, and arthropathy. Study sample sizes ranged from 22 to more than 50,000 neonates. The specific corticosteroids and dosage regimens used by the mothers were not detailed in 3 of the 10 studies (Heinonen et al., '77; Robert et al., '94; Carmichael and Shaw, '99). Four studies examined the effects of fetal exposure to corticosteroids and other medications (Mogadam et al., '81; Rodriguez-Pinilla and Martinez-Frias, '98; Carmichael and Shaw, '99; Park-Wyllie et al., '00), while the remaining six studies followed women who were presumably only on corticosteroids. Of the four case-control studies, one focused solely on the presence of oral clefts as pregnancy outcome for women exposed to corticosteroids in the first-trimester (Rodriguez-Pinilla and Martinez-Frias, '98). When performing the Mantel-Haenszel summary OR of cohort studies examining major malformations, statistical significance was

Table 3
Pregnancy Outcome Characteristics in the Prospective Study*

OUTCOME	CORTICOSTEROIDS (n = 187)[a]	CONTROLS (n = 188)	P
Live-born infants	157 (85%)	171 (91%)	0.06
Miscarriage <26 wk	13 (7%)	13 (7%)	NS
Medical abortion	16 (9%)	2 (1%)	0.002
Fetal death/stillbirth ≥26 wk	1 (0.5%)	2 (1%)	NS
Male:female	86:68	81:84	0.7
Gestational age (wk)	38 ± 3 (157)	39.5 ± 2 (172[b])	0.0001
Premature (<37 wk)	27/158 (17%)	9/172 (5%)	0.0001
Birth weight (g)	3112 ± 684 (157)	3428 ± 578 (172[b])	0.0001
AGA:SGA:LGA	139:11:7	158:4:6	0.3
Vaginal delivery	112/155 (72%)	131/172 (76%)	0.9

AGA, appropriate for gestational age; SGA, small for gestational age (<3rd percentile); LGA, large for gestational age (>97th percentile).

[a] With three sets of twins in this cohort, the number of outcomes is greater than the number of pregnancies (n = 184).

[b] Gestational age of stillborn included in this mean value

* Information may be missing on some end points in a few cases.

not achieved (cumulative OR = 1.45 [95% CI 0.81–2.60]), and the trials were homogeneous (Fig. 1). However, of the six studies included, Heinonen et al. ('77) did not separate major and minor malformations in the exposed group. Since one of our primary outcomes was major malformation rates in corticosteroid-exposed pregnancies compared with nonteratogen controls, the analysis was repeated without Heinonen's study, yielding marginally significant results: the Mantel-Haenszel summary OR was 3.03 [95% CI 1.08, 8.54] (Fig. 1).

Specific malformations reported by the cohort studies are listed in Table 7. The pooled sample of malformations in fetuses exposed to corticosteroids revealed that cleft palate was the most commonly reported anomaly with three cases being identified, compared with none among the controls. There were 4 case control studies examining the risk of oral clefts. All four had a significantly increased OR, with an overall OR of 3.35 [95%CI 1.97, 5.69] (Fig. 2). The specific phenotype of clefts was as follows; isolated cleft palate (4 cases), isolated cleft lip (6 cases), cleft lip and palate (5 cases) and cleft lip without palate specified (10 cases).

For both cohort and case-control studies, the Spearman's ρ did not show a significant correlation between the quality of the studies and their OR (r = –0.32). An incidence rate of 3.5% was calculated using the meta-analytic means and the means of 15 studies, including those without control groups, that could not be included in the formal meta-analysis. The raw average showed a very similar incidence rate of 3.9%.

Table 4
Classification of Birth Defect Status Between Groups in the Prospective Study*

	CORTICOSTEROIDS (n = 111)	CONTROLS (n = 172)	P
No anomalies	107 (96.4%)	169 (98%)	
Major anomalies[a]	4 (3.6%)	3 (2%)	0.3

[a] Only anomalies that could possibly be attributable to corticosteroids are included (see Table 5).

* Rates are calculated only for fetuses exposed in utero to corticosteroids during the first trimester of pregnancy

DISCUSSION

Although the list of epidemiologically proven human teratogens is small, labeling a medication as the cause of a major birth defect has serious clinical implications. In situations in which known teratogens are drugs of choice (e.g., carbamazepine, coumadin, isotretinoin, lithium, methotrexate, phenytoin, valproic acid), evidence-based risk assessment is important for the woman, in order to make an informed decision upon the future of the pregnancy.

Prospective Study

While prednisone has never been proved to be a human teratogen, there are clinicians who extrapolate animal studies to suggest that the drug can cause cleft lip or palate and subsequently counsel their patients to avoid therapy during pregnancy. This may have been a factor in some of the 16 exposed women, who chose to terminate their pregnancies after prednisone exposure.

Prednisone is used for a variety of indications by women of reproductive age, making it very likely that risk assessment will be sought by many who intend to conceive while on prednisone therapy. The positive predictive value of animal testing for teratogenicity in humans is not high (Jelovsek, et al., '89). Interspecies pharmacodynamic differences may account for the difference in susceptibility between humans and animals. Glucocorticoids may mediate their teratogenic effect in animals through a receptor that does not exist in the human embryonic palate (Pratt, '85).

In light of the limited number of published pregnancy outcomes after prednisone use for recurrent fetal loss, our study reports rates of major malformations for women exposed to prednisone and is the first and largest prospective study to specifically compare the

Table 5
Description of All Recorded Major Anomalies in Infants in the Prospective Study

ABNORMALITY	GROUP	PREDNISONE EXPOSURE
Polydactyly (family history)[a]	Exposed	5 mg/day throughout + 50 mg/day azathioprine
Hirschsprung's disease	Exposed	80 mg/day from 2–2 3/7 wk
Double outlet right ventricle, valvar and subvalvar pulmonary stenosis, hypothyroidism, hypospadias	Exposed	30 mg/day from 0–4.5 wk
Multiple birth defects, congenital toxoplasmosis[a]	Exposed	Unknown dose from 12–12.5 wk + cotrimoxazole
Undescended testicle (full term; required intervention)	Exposed	25 mg/day throughout + 80 mg/day ASA + 50 mg progesterone in 1st trimester
Cleft palate, hypospadias	Exposed	15 mg/day throughout + 200 mg/day carbamazepine, 40 mg/day nifedipine, 100 mg/day atenolol
Aortic valve stenosis	Control	None
Pyloric stenosis	Control	None
Dysplastic kidney (in the stillborn child)	Control	None

[a] Two cases were excluded from the analysis because etiology of malformation was known (genetic history and maternal infection).

Table 6
Summary of Patient, Drug, and Size of Study for Studies Included in the Meta-Analysis

STUDY/YEAR	STUDY TYPE	PATHOLOGY OF MOTHER	NO. OF CASES	CORTICOSTEROID(S)	DOSE (PREDNISOLONE EQUIVALENT)
Popert '62	Cohort	Rheumatoid arthritis, SLE, ankylosing spondylitis, psoriatic arthropathy	22	Prednisolone, cortisone, corticotropin	2.5–27.5 mg/day
Warrell and Taylor '68	Cohort	Asthma, eczema, ulcerative colitis, SLE, urticaria, sarcoidosis	69	Prednisolone	2.5–40 mg/day
Heinonen et al., '77	Cohort	N/A	50,282	Corticosteroid and/ or corticotropin	N/A
Mogadam et al., '81	Cohort	Inflammatory bowel disease	521	Corticosteroid or corticosteroid + sulfasalazine	N/A
Mintz et al., '86	Cohort	SLE	204	Prednisone	10 mg/day
Robert et al., '94	Case control	N/A	1,448	Corticosteroids	N/A
Czeizel and Rockenbauer '97	Case control	Asthma, hay fever, rheumatoid arthritis, Addison's disease, subfertility	56,557	Dexamethasone, prednisone, cortisone, betamethasone, methylpred-nisolone, triamcinolone	5–100 mg/day
Rodriguez-Pinilla and Martinez-Frias, '98	Case control	N/A	12,304	Prednisolone, hydrocortisone, prednisone, triamcinolone	10–30 mg/day
Carmichael and Shaw, '99	Case control	Crohn's disease, asthma, lupus	1,396	Prednisone, cortisone, dexamethazone, triamcinolone	N/A
Park-Wyllie et al., '00 (present study)	Cohort	Crohn's disease, ulcerative colitis, rheumatoid arthritis, SLE, and other	372	Prednisone	5–80 mg/day

SLE, systemic lupus erythematosus; N/A, not available.

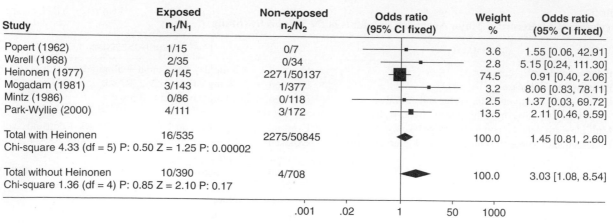

Study	Exposed n_1/N_1	Non-exposed n_2/N_2	Odds ratio (95% CI fixed)	Weight %	Odds ratio (95% CI fixed)
Popert (1962)	1/15	0/7		3.6	1.55 [0.06, 42.91]
Warell (1968)	2/35	0/34		2.8	5.15 [0.24, 111.30]
Heinonen (1977)	6/145	2271/50137		74.5	0.91 [0.40, 2.06]
Mogadam (1981)	3/143	1/377		3.2	8.06 [0.83, 78.11]
Mintz (1986)	0/86	0/118		2.5	1.37 [0.03, 69.72]
Park-Wyllie (2000)	4/111	3/172		13.5	2.11 [0.46, 9.59]
Total with Heinonen	16/535	2275/50845		100.0	1.45 [0.81, 2.60]
Chi-square 4.33 (df = 5) P: 0.50 Z = 1.25 P: 0.00002					
Total without Heinonen	10/390	4/708		100.0	3.03 [1.08, 8.54]
Chi-square 1.36 (df = 4) P: 0.85 Z = 2.10 P: 0.17					

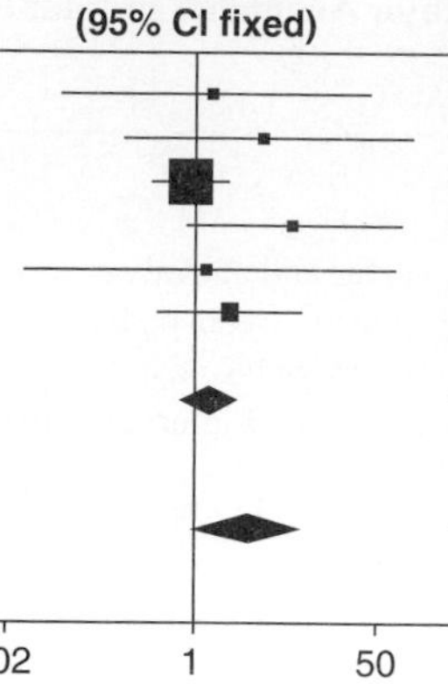

Fig. 1. Individual and cumulative Mantel-Haenszel summary odds ratio for corticosteroid-exposed cohort studies for major malformations with and without the Heinonen et al. ('77) analysis.

rate of major defects between exposed women and a nonexposed cohort. The observed rates of anomalies (3.6% and 2%, respectively) are within the expected baseline rate. Although this study is limited by its sample size and by the lack of information on the 16 elective terminations, it is reassuring that among the major defects that could possibly be attributed to corticosteroids, there was no apparent pattern that would suggest causality.

Meta-Analysis

To our knowledge, no systematic analysis examining the relationship between first-trimester exposure of corticosteroids and rates of major malformations has been published. Lack of well-designed trials that specifically address major malformations compound the controversy surrounding corticosteroid-induced malformations. The animal studies and case studies suggesting an association with cleft palate prompted us to review critically the existing evidence. Most available studies examining corticosteroid association with major malformations were small, and quite a few are old.

Meta-analysis has emerged as a powerful method for systematic review and aggregation of studies with similar methodologies and endpoints, especially when the outcome of interest is rare and the effect size is relatively small. The strengths and weaknesses of meta-analysis for reproductive risk have been reviewed by us (Einarson, '88). It is possible that synthesizing studies of different qualities decrease the validity of the overall estimate. Very rarely are all the studies clear with respect to definitions of major malformations, and confounders. Because negative studies (those finding no increase in malformation rates) are more likely not to be published, it is possible that the true odds ratio would be lower if all negative studies were identified.

The cumulative OR for cohort and case-control studies included in the meta-analysis showed a nonsignificant increased risk of major malformations associated with corticosteroid exposure, with the very large study by Heinonen et al. ('77) and a significant risk without this study (Fig. 1). A subanalysis of the cohort studies that specified the malformations revealed three cases of cleft palate among 390 corticosteroid exposures compared with no cases of cleft palate among 708 unexposed fetuses. Some of the studies could not be used because they did not contain any details as to the nature of the major malformations. Of the four case-control studies identified, one focused on the association between corticosteroid use in the first-trimester and the incidence of oral clefts. Separately and when combined, the four studies produced a significant summary OR for oral clefts, and the trials were homogeneous.

Although our meta-analysis did could only detect an increased risk of major malformations without the largest trial, it did show a greater than threefold increase in the risk of oral clefts specifically, when the fetus was exposed to corticosteroids during the first trimester. Moreover, there is evidence of excess of cleft palate cases among cohort studies, which is consistent with the existing animal experience (Schardein, '93), where cleft palate is the primary malformation induced. Taken together, these data make epidemiological sense, as oral clefts comprise only a small part of all major malformations. More studies will be needed to determine which cleft phenotype is associated with corticosteroids and whether it is cleft lip with or without palate or cleft palate alone, or both. There

Table 7
List of Malformations Reported in Exposed and Unexposed Infants from the Cohort Studies Included in the Meta-Analysis

CORTICOSTEROID-TREATED GROUP	CONTROL GROUP
Cleft palate[a]	Aortic valve stenosis
Cleft palate[a] + microglossia	Pyloric stenosis
Cleft palate[a] + hypospadias	Dysplastic kidneys
Congenital deafness	Spina bifida
Anencephaly (2 cases)	Other malformations (undefined)
Left ventricular atresia (died within 1 month)	
Hirschsprung's disease	
Double outlet right ventricle + valvar and subvalvar pulmonary stenosis + hypospadias	
Undescended testicles	
Other malformations undefined (6 cases)	

[a] All cleft palates were isolated (without cleft lip).

Study	Exposed n_1/N_1	Non-exposed n_2/N_2	Odds ratio (95% CI fixed)	Weight %	Odds ratio (95% CI fixed)
Robert (1994)	7/35	125/1413		41.9	2.58 [1.10, 6.02]
Czeizel (1997)	4/37	1219/36913		18.9	3.55 [1.26, 10.03]
Rodriguez (1998)	5/14	1179/12290		14.9	5.24 [1.75, 15.65]
Carmichael (1999)	9/662	3/734		24.3	3.36 [0.91, 12.46]
Total (95% CI)	25/748	2526/51350		100.0	3.35 [1.97, 5.69]

Chi-square 1.02 (df = 3) P: 0.80 Z = 4.46 P: 0.3

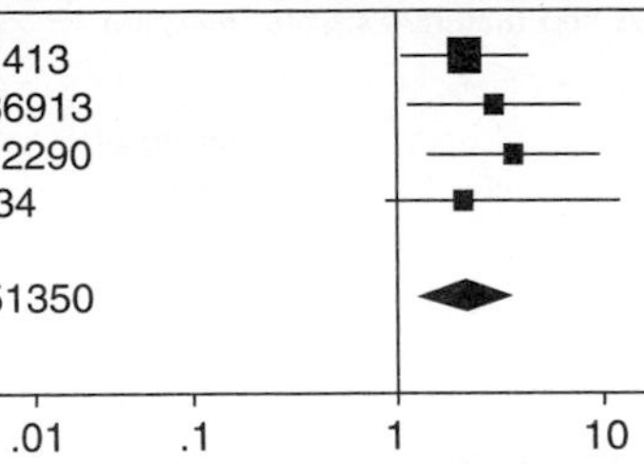

Fig. 2. Individual and cumulative Mantel-Haenszel summary odds ratio for corticosteroid-exposed case-control studies focusing on oral clefts.

appears to be no pattern from the findings presented here. The apparent increased risk of oral clefts caused by corticosteroids has to be balanced against potentially serious implications for the mother and indirectly to the fetus if steroid therapy is discontinued or not initiated. Since oral clefts occur at about 1:1,000 births, this increased risk will have a minimal effect on the overall malformation rate of 3% in newborn infants. Our study may permit clinicians to make a more informed decision on the use of corticosteroid therapy in pregnancy, which shows a small but significantly increased risk of oral clefts after first-trimester exposure.

LITERATURE CITED

al-Mofada SM, Osman MEE, Kides E, al-Momen AK, al-Herbish AS, al-Mobaireek K. 1994. Risk of thrombocytopenia in the infants of mothers with idiopathic thrombocytopenia. Am J Perinatol 11:423–426.

Baxter H, Fraser FC. 1950. Production of congenital defects in offspring of female mice treated with cortisone. McGill Med J 19:245–249.

Beitins IZ, Bayard F, Ances IG, Kowarski A, Migeon CJ. 1972. The transplacental passage of prednisone and prednisolone in pregnancy near term. J Pediatr 81:936–945.

Carmichael SL, Shaw GM. 1999. Maternal corticosteroid use and risk of selected congenital anomalies. Am J Med Genet 86:242–244.

Carp HJ, Menashe Y, Frenkel Y, et al. 1993. Lupus anticoagulant. Significance in habitual first-trimester abortion. J Reprod Med 38: 549–552.

Coté CJ, Meuwissen HJ, Pickering R. 1974. Effects on the neonate of prednisone and azathioprine administered to the mother during pregnancy. J Pediatr 85:324–328.

Coulam CB, Zincke H, Sterioff S. 1982. Pregnancy after renal transplantation: estrogen secretion. Transplantation 33:556.

Cowchock FS, Reece EA, Balaban D, Branch DW, Plouffe L. 1992. Repeated fetal losses associated with antiphospholipid antibodies. Am J Obstet Gynecol 166:1318–1323.

Cox D, Hinkley DV. 1974. Theoretical statistics. London: Chapman Hall.

Crowley P. 1995. Antenatal corticosteroid therapy: a meta-analysis of the randomized trials, 1972 to 1994. Am J Obstet Gynecol 173: 322–335.

Czeizel AE, Rockenbauer M. 1997. Population-based case-control study of teratogenic potential of corticosteroids. Teratology 56:335–340.

Dara P, Slater LM, Armentrout SA. 1981. Successful pregnancy during chemotherapy for acute leukemia. Cancer 47:845.

Doig RK, Cox OM. 1956. Cleft palate following cortisone therapy in early pregnancy. Lancet 2:730.

Fainstat T. 1954. Cortisone induced congenital cleft palate in rabbits. Endocrinology 55:502–508.

Framarino di Malatesta ML, Poli L, Pierucci F, Paolucci A, Prestagostini R, Di Nicuolo A, Berloco P, Alfani D, Piccioni MG, Veneziano M, Cortesini L, Marzetti L. 1993. Pregnancy and kidney transplantation: clinical problems and experience. Transplant Proc 25:2188–2189.

Fraser FC, Fainstat TD. 1951. The production of congenital defects in the offspring of pregnant mice treated with cortisone: a progress report. Pediatrics 8:527–533.

Gleicher N. 1986. Pregnancy and autoimmunity. Acta Haematol 76: 68–77.

Hack M, Brish M, Serr D, Insler V, Salomy M, Lunenfeld B. 1972. Outcome of pregnancy after induced ovulation follow-up of pregnancies and children born after clomiphene therapy. JAMA 220: 1329–1333.

Harper PS. 1993. Practical genetic counselling. 4th Ed. Oxford: Butterworth-Heinemann.

Harris JWS, Ross IP 1956. Cortisone therapy in early pregnancy: relation to cleft palate. Lancet 1:1045–1047.

Heinonen OP, Slone D, Shapiro S, editors. 1977. Birth defects and drugs in pregnancy. Littleton, MA: Publishing Sciences Group.

Holmes LB. 1999. Need for inclusion and exclusion criteria for the structural abnormalities recorded in children born from exposed pregnancies. Teratology 59:1–2.

Jelovsek FR, Mattison DR, Chen JJ. 1989. Prediction of risk for human developmental toxicity: how important are animal studies for hazard identification? Obstet Gynecol 74:624–636.

Jones MM, Lidsky MD, Brewer EJ, Yow MD, Williamson WD. 1986. Congenital cytomegalovirus infection and maternal systemic lupus erythematosus. Arthritis Rheum 29:1402–1404.

Kaplan C, Daffos F, Forestier F, Tertian G, Catherine N, Pons JC, Tchernia G. 1980. Fetal platelet counts in thrombocytopenic pregnancy. Lancet 336:979–982.

Karpatkin M, Porges RF, Karpatkin S. 1981. Platelet counts in infants of women with autoimmune thrombocytopenia. N Engl J Med 305: 936–939.

Kenny FM, Preeyasombat C, Spaulding JS, Migeon CJ. 1966. Cortisol production rate. Pediatrics 37:960–966.

Kraus AM. 1975. Congenital cataract and maternal steroid ingestion. J Pediatr Ophthalmol 12:107–108.

Levitz M, Jansen V, Dancis J. 1978. The transfer and metabolism of corticosteroids in the perfused human placenta. Am J Obstet Gynecol 132:363–366.

Lockshin MD, Druzin ML, Qamar T. 1989. Prednisone does not prevent recurrent fetal death in women with antiphospholipid antibody. Am J Obstet Gynecol 160:439–443.

Mercado AB, Wilson RC, Cheng KC, Wei JQ, New MI. 1995. Prenatal treatment and diagnosis of congenital adrenal hyperplasia owing to steroid 21-hydroxylase deficiency. J Clin Endocrinol Metab 80: 2014–2020.

Mintz G, Niz J, Gutierrez G, Garcia-Alonso A, Karchmer S. 1986. Prospective study of pregnancy in systemic lupus erythematosus. Results of a multidisciplinary approach. J Rheumatol 13:732–739.

Mogadam M, Dobbins WO, Korelitz BI, Ahmed SW. 1981. Pregnancy in inflammatory bowel disease: effect of sulfasalazine and corticosteroid on fetal outcome. Gastroenterology 80:72–76.

Morris WI. 1969. Pregnancy in rheumatoid arthritis and systemic lupus erythematosus. Aust NZ Obstet Gynecol 9:136–144.

Nolan GH, Sweet RL, Laros RK, Roure CA. 1974. Renal cadaver transplantation followed by successful pregnancies. Obstet Gynecol 43:732.

Out HJ, Bruinse HW, Christiaens G, van Vliet M, de Groot PG, Nieuwenhuis HK, Derksen RH. 1992. A prospective, controlled multicenter study on the obstetric risks of pregnant women with antiphospholipid antibodies. Am J Obstet Gynecol 167:26–32.

Pasqualini JR, Nguyen BL, Uhrich F, Wiqvist N, Diczfalusy E. 1970. Cortisol and cortisone metabolism in the human placental unit at midgestation. J Steroid Biochem 1:209–219.

Pastuszak A, D'Alimonte D, Koren G. 1996. Astemizole use and pregnancy outcome. J Allergy Clin Immunology 98:124–126.

Pinsky L, DiGeorge AM. 1965. Cleft palate in the mouse: a teratogenic index of glucocorticoid potency. Science 147:402–403.

Popert AJ. 1962. Pregnancy and adrenocortical hormones. BMJ 967–972.

Pratt RM 1985. Receptor-dependent mechanisms of glucocorticoid and dioxin-induced cleft palate. Environ Health Perspect 61:35–40.

Rai RS, Regan L, Clifford K, Pickering W, Dave M, Mackie I, McNally T, Cohen H. 1995. Antiphospholipid antibodies and β2-glycoprotein-I in 500 women with recurrent miscarriage: results of a comprehensive screening approach. Hum Reprod 10:2001–2005.

Renisch JM, Simon JN, Karow WG, Gandelman R. 1978. Prenatal exposure to prednisone in humans and animals retards intrauterine growth. Science 202:436–438.

Robert E, Vollset SE, Botto L, Lancaster PAL, Merlob P, Mastroiacovo P, Cocchi G, Ashizawa M, Sakamoto S, Orioli I. 1994. Malformation surveillance and maternal drug exposure: the MADRE project. Int J Risk Safety Med 6:75–118.

Rodriguez-Pinilla E, Martinez-Frias ML. 1998. Corticosteroids during pregnancy and oral clefts: a case-control study. Teratology 58:2–5.

Rubins JM, Woll JE. 1981. Immune thrombocytopenic purpura. NY State Med J 81:1743–1747.

Schardein JL 1993. Chemically induced birth defects. 2nd Ed. New York: Marcel Dekker. p 307–310.

Schatz M, Patterson R, Zeitz S, Rourke J, Melam H. 1975. Corticosteroid therapy for the pregnant asthmatic patient. JAMA 233: 804–807.

Schilsky RL, Sherins RJ, Hubbard SM, Wesley MN, Young RC, De Vita VT. 1981. Long-term follow-up of ovarian function in women treated with MOPP chemotherapy for Hodgkin's disease. Am J Med 71:552.

Seto AH. 1993. Meta-analysis of adverse neonatal effects due to maternal exposure to antihistamines. Thesis. Faculty of Pharmacy, University of Toronto.

Shapiro L, Pastuszak A, Curto G, Koren G. 1997. Safety of first trimester exposure to topical tretanoic: a prospective cohort study. Lancet 350:1143–1144.

Silveira LH, Jara LJ, Saway S, Martinez-Osuna P, Seleznick MJ, Angel J, O'Brien W, Espinoza LR. 1992. Prevention of anticardiolipin antibody-related pregnancy losses with prednisone and aspirin. Am J Med 93:403–411.

Silver RK, MacGregor SN, Sholl JS, Hobart JM, Neerhof MG, Ragin A. 1993. Comparative trial of prednisone plus aspirin vs. aspirin alone in the treatment of anticardiolipin antibody-positive obstetric patients. Am J Obstet Gynecol 169:1411–1417.

Sinykin MB, Kaplan H. 1962. Leukemia in pregnancy. Obstet Gynecol 83:220–234.

Tozman ECS, Urowitz MB, Gladman DD. 1980. Systemic lupus erythematosus and pregnancy. J Rheumatol 7:624–632.

Walker B. 1971. Induction of cleft palate in rats with anti-inflammatory drugs. Teratology 4:39–42.

Walsh DS, Clark FR. 1967. Pregnancy in patients on long-term corticosteroid therapy. Scott Med J 12:302–306.

Warrell DW, Taylor R. 1968. Outcome for the foetus of mothers receiving prednisolone during pregnancy. Lancet 1:117–118.

Wells CN. 1953. Treatment of hyperemesis gravidarum with cortisone. Am J Obstet Gynecol 598–601.

Wright CG, Rouse RC, Weinberg AG, Hubbard DG. 1982. Vaterite otoconia in two cases of otoconial membrane dysplasia. Ann Otol 91:193–199.

Yackel DB, Kempers RD, McConahey WM. 1966. Adrenocorticosteroid therapy in pregnancy. Am J Obstet Gynecol 96: 985–989.

Reprinted from Park-Wyllie L, Mazzotta P, Pastuszak A, Moretti ME, Beique L, Hunnisett L, Friesen MH, Jacobson S, Kasapinovic S, Chang D, Diav-Citrin O, Chitayat D, Nulman I, Einarson TR, Koren G. Birth defects after maternal exposure to corticosteroids: prospective cohort study and meta-analysis of epidemiological studies. Teratology 2000;62:385–92 with permission.

CHAPTER 56

PREGNANCY OUTCOME AFTER CYCLOSPORINE THERAPY DURING PREGNANCY: A META-ANALYSIS[1]

Benjamin Bar Oz,[2] Richard Hackman,[2] Tom Einarson,[2,3] and Gideon Koren[2]
The Motherisk Program, Division of Clinical Pharmacology/Toxicology, The Hospital for Sick Children, Toronto, Department of Pediatrics, Pharmacology, Medicine and Genetics, and the School of Pharmacy, The University of Toronto, Toronto, Canada

Background. Cyclosporine (CsA) therapy must often be continued during pregnancy to maintain maternal health in such conditions as organ transplantation and autoimmune disease. This meta-analysis was performed to determine whether CsA exposure during pregnancy is associated with an increased risk of congenital malformations, preterm delivery, or low birthweight.
Methods. Various health science databases were searched to identify relevant articles. Articles selected for inclusion in the study were required to be free of any apparent selection bias and report outcomes in at least 10 newborns exposed to CsA in utero, specifically commenting on the presence or absence of congenital malformations. Article selection and data extraction were performed by two independent reviewers, with adjudication in cases of disagreement. To assess risks of CsA exposure, a summary odds ratio was calculated. Prevalence of malformations was calculated as a rate for all cyclosporine-exposed live births and for the subgroups identified. Ninety-five percent confidence intervals were constructed for both the odds ratio and prevalence rates.
Results. Fifteen studies (6 with control groups of transplant without use of cyclosporine; total patients: 410) met the inclusion criteria for major malformations, 10 for preterm delivery (4 with control groups; total patients: 379) and 5 for low birth weight (1 with control groups; total number of patients: 314). The calculated odds ratio of 3.83 for malformations did not achieve statistical significance (CI 0.75–19.6). The overall prevalence of major malformations in the study population (4.1%) also did not vary substantially from that reported in the general population. OR for prematurity [1.52 (CI 1.00–2.32)] did not reach statistical significance although the overall prevalence rate was 56.3%. The OR for low birth weight [1.5 (CI 0.95–2.44 based on 1 study)].
Conclusions. CsA does not appear to be a major human teratogen. It may be associated with increased rates of prematurity. More research is needed to evaluate whether cyclosporine increases teratogenic risk.

INTRODUCTION

Cyclosporine (Sandimmune, Neoral, Novartis, Basel, Switzerland) is a selective immunosuppressive agent that attenuates T cell-mediated responses (*1*, *2*) by preventing formation of interleukin-2 (IL-2) (*3–5*). As a result, cyclosporine is a unique agent for preventing graft rejection in organ transplant recipients (*1*, *6*). Since its introduction for this indication in the early 1980s, cyclosporine has profoundly advanced survival (*6*) in transplant recipient, and is now a standard component of most immunosuppressant regimens used to prevent graft rejection in transplant recipients (*7*).

Transplantation can return normal gonadotrophic function in organ recipients, enabling patients to conceive or father children (*8*). Transplant recipients include women of childbearing age (*5*) and children who may survive to their reproductive years (*9*). The first pregnancy after kidney transplantation occurred in 1958 (*8*), and, since then, pregnancies have also been reported in patients with kidney-pancreas, liver, heart, heart-lung, and bone marrow grafts (*10*). By 1997, an estimated 5000 pregnancies had occurred in transplant patients (*11*). Approximately 1 in 50 female kidney transplant recipients of child-bearing age will become pregnant (*8*). Of liver transplant patients, about 30% are female, and of these, 75% are in their reproductive years (*5*). Approximately 10% of cardiac graft recipients are women in their childbearing years (*12*). The use of cyclosporine in transplantation has contributed greatly to the survival of these individuals.

In addition to its success in the transplant population, cyclosporine can also be effective in the treatment of autoimmune diseases such as systemic lupus erythematosus, and rheumatoid arthritis (*4*, *13*), and psoriatic arthritis (*13*) when these diseases are refractory to conventional therapies. These conditions also occur frequently in women in their reproductive years (*4*, *13*, *14*), and can remain active or worsen during pregnancy (*13*, *14*) or flare shortly after childbirth (*4*), thus making continued treatment necessary.

Organ transplantation and autoimmune diseases represent conditions where ongoing immunosuppression is required to maintain patient health. Because these groups include women with reproductive potential, consideration of the effects of this drug on the fetus is required if the drug is continued during pregnancy. Although pregnancy may be regarded by some as a period of immunological tolerance, because the fetus is likened to an allograft, there is no evidence to demonstrate that transplant rejection occurs with less frequency or allows reduction or cessation of immunosuppressant treatment, such that therapy must be maintained (*9*). Although patients with autoimmune diseases may elect to forego immunosuppression or, in the case of rheumatoid arthritis, actually experience disease remission during pregnancy (*14*), the effects of cyclosporine exposure on the fetus are still of concern if the drug was administered before the patient was aware of her pregnancy.

Although there are conflicting reports regarding the extent of placental transfer of cyclosporine (*13*), a range of 37–64% of maternal levels has been suggested (*9*), indicating that clinically significant amounts of drug do reach the fetus. Other immunosuppressants have been associated with teratogenic effects (*15*). In particular, several other antirheumatic drugs, such as cyclophosphamide, 6-mercaptopurine, and methotrexate, are usually avoided during pregnancy (*13*).

[1] Motherisk is Supported by Novartis Ltd., Barcelona. GK is a Senior Scientist of the Canadian Institutes for Health Research.

[2] The Motherisk Program, Division of Clinical Pharmacology/Toxicology, The Hospital for Sick Children, Toronto, Department of Pediatrics, Pharmacology, Medicine and Genetics.
[3] The School of Pharmacy.

Cyclosporine is classified as having a "C" category risk by the FDA; that is, although risk to the fetus has not been ruled out in human and/or animal studies, benefits of use may exceed risk (*4*). Unfortunately, no systematic overview of the use of cyclosporine in pregnancy has been conducted to date; and, in fact, there are few controlled studies of immunosuppressive drugs in pregnancy (*13*). In particular, no such studies exist to address the prevalence of congenital malformations, prematurity and being small for gestational age, which are leading causes of neonatal morbidity and mortality and can have medical, surgical, or cosmetic implications for the surviving child (*16*). A meta-analysis that pools the best available evidence can help quantify the reproductive risks after in utero exposure to cyclosporine. Knowledge of relative risk of outcomes will aid the patient in making informed decisions regarding the decision to become pregnant and/or continue cyclosporine during pregnancy. Reported in the literature are two maternal deaths that resulted from discontinuation of immunosuppressive agents in transplant recipients (*7*) as well as an anecdotal observation of serious consequences of interruption of therapy in other maternal chronic illnesses (*14*).

The primary objective of this study was to determine if cyclosporine exposure in utero is associated with increased risk of congenital malformations, premature delivery or small for gestational age births.

METHODS

Eligible Articles

Eligible articles were identified by searching the Medline, EMBASE, International Pharmaceutical Abstracts, Toxline, Cochrane, and Current Contents databases using variations of the keywords *cyclosporine*, *pregnancy*, *teratogen*, and *malformation*. Articles of all languages were included in the search. An attempt was made to retrieve all citations through the database search from local hospitals and university libraries.

Human studies included for analysis in this systematic review were required to 1) describe at least 10 live births that were exposed to cyclosporine during the first trimester of pregnancy; 2) report on malformations (presence, absence, and/or descriptions), and/or rates of prematurity (<37 weeks of gestation) and/or small for gestational age; and 3) represent a comprehensive sample which appeared to be free of selection bias (e.g., case series and cohort studies were eligible). All case reports, editorials, letters, and review articles were excluded. In selecting eligible articles, retrieved articles were screened by two independent reviewers according to the inclusion criteria; where the reviewers disagreed, the article was referred to a third judge to break the tie. All accepted studies were used for calculation of prevalence rate. For calculation of odds ratios we included studies that described a control group of mother-child pairs with transplantation, but without the use of cyclosporine.

Data extracted from eligible articles included the site of the published study (to enable detection of duplicate publications or data overlap), the indication for cyclosporine, the trimester of exposure, and, for each regimen cited in the study, the number of patients, pregnancies, live births, and malformations noted. In extracting data, eligible articles were screened by two independent reviewers, with disagreements being settled through discussion or adjudicated by a judge.

Calculations and Statistical Analysis

To determine if CSA exposure is associated with an increased prevalence of malformations, prematurity, or smaller for gestational age birth, eligible studies that describe a control group of pregnancies without CSA exposure were identified. The number of malformations in both the CSA-exposed and unexposed live births was used to construct 2×2 tables. A χ_2 test was performed to test for homogeneity, and a Mantel-Haenszel summary odds ratio was calculated to assess the risk of malformations with CSA exposure. Subsequently, a power analysis was performed to determine the number of studies and patients required to demonstrate statistical significance. This was done by adding hypothetical studies of average size and prevalence rates to the data present until statistical significance was achieved (i.e., the lower limit of the 95% confidence interval became or exceeded the value of 1).

Data from all eligible studies were then used to calculate overall prevalence rates for malformations. The overall prevalence rate was calculated by dividing the total number of pathological observations (e.g., malformations) by the total number of live births in CSA-exposed pregnancies. All prevalence rates were reported as percentage of malformations per CSA-exposed live birth, with 95% confidence intervals constructed for each rate.

RESULTS

Literature Search

More than 300 citations were located from the databases searched, of which 212 articles were retrieved. From these articles, 134 were excluded (51 case reports, 31 reviews, 52 irrelevant articles). Of the remaining 79 articles, 62 were rejected because they did not meet inclusion criteria, or were duplicate publications. Although 19 articles met the inclusion criteria, data could not be extracted from 4, leaving 15 articles that could be used to calculate prevalence rates (*17–31*); these are described in Tables 1–3. Some of these articles described a control group, and were used to calculate the summary odds ratio. All studies were used to calculate the prevalence of each end point.

Risk Ratio

The summary odds ratio for congenital malformations was 3.83, with a 95% confidence interval of 0.75–19.6 (NS). This was based on 6 studies reporting on 410 patients. Power analysis revealed that only 631 additional live births would be required to yield a statistically significant odds ratio of 3.83. The χ_2 test for homogeneity was 0.42 ($P = 0.93$), indicating that the studies used to compose the summary odds ratio were not significantly different, and their results could be pooled. (Table 4). The prevalence rate of malformations (4.1% or 14 of 339 babies) (95% CI 2.6–7%) was not substantially different from the figure typically described in population-based studies.

The odds ratio for preterm delivery (1.50) (CI 1.00–2.32) was not significant based on 4 studies with 379 patients. The pooled studies were found to be heterogeneous. Power analysis revealed that 447 more patients would be needed for this OR to be significant. The prevalence of prematurity based on 10 studies was 56.3% (CI 37.8–74.7%). The risk for low birth weight (OR of 1.53) (CI0.95–2.44) was not significant based on one study with 314 patients, with 43% of the cyclosporine-exposed infants suffering from low birth weight in the prevalence study.

Table 1
Articles Used in the Analysis of Congenital Malformations

AUTHOR	SITE	DATES OF STUDY	COMPARISON GROUP AVAILABLE?	TYPE OF TRANSPLANT RECEIVED
Aichberger	Austria	1974 –1991	No	Kidney
Armenti	USA	1991 –1993	Yes	Kidney
Barrou	International	Pre-1994	No	Pancreas, kidney
Bererhi	France	1968 –1981 and 1985–1995	Yes	Kidney
Crawford	USA	Pre-1993	No	Kidney, liver
Framarino di Malatesta	Italy	Pre-1993	No	Kidney
Haugen	Norway	1974 –1991	Yes	Kidney
Muirhead	Canada	1977–1988	Yes	Kidney
Nojima	Japan	1973 –1995	Yes	Kidney
Randomski	USA	Pre-1995	No	Kidney, heart, liver
Sabagh	Saudi Arabia	1984 –1994	No	Kidney
Scantlebury	USA	1977 –1988	No	Liver
Talaat	Sweden	1977 –1992	Yes	Kidney-pancreas, liver
Ville	France	1985 –1992	No	Liver
Wu	Germany	1988 –1996	No	Liver

DISCUSSION

The overall prevalence rate for malformations among cyclosporine-exposed live births in this analysis was somewhat more than the range of 2–3% reported for the general population (*16*), and is consistent with a recent international summary (n = 629 pregnancies in transplant recipients) prepared by the manufacturer that describes a 3% prevalence rate for congenital malformations (*10*). Our overall prevalence rates calculated likely represent the extreme possible values, where the "pooled" prevalence represents the case in which each exposure has equal weight and the "averaged" prevalence reflects the case where each study has equal weight, regardless of sample size. The OR of 3.8 may reflect a beta error and indicates that more human experience needs to be gathered before the potential teratogenic risk of cyclosporine can be accurately calculated. Only two additional studies with a similar effect size would be needed for this OR to become statistically significant.

Because the control groups consisted of transplanted women treated with other medications, this should correct for maternal disease factors and yield a closer estimate of the risk/safety of cyclosporine itself. Our analysis reveals high rates of preterm delivery among children of transplanted mothers, and a trend toward higher prevalence of intrauterine growth retardation.

It is essential to acknowledge the limitations inherent in this systematic review. The quality of the results generated was limited by the nature of data available, the study design and confounding factors specific to the transplant population. For obvious ethical reasons, there are no randomized controlled human trials that study teratogenicity. The available data included by us regarding teratogenic outcomes in pregnant women are derived from case-control and cohort studies, none of which are without limitations (*15*). In these studies, no direct causal relationship can be established between malformation observed and drug under investigation. Because our study employed only published data, which is subject to publication and selection biases, our results may not reflect the true incidence of malformations. Our analysis was limited to studies which described comprehensive, complete samples of patients, and appeared to include all-comers. We excluded case reports, letters and small case series (n<10) to avoid anecdotal reporting and duplication, as well as to obtain a more accurate prevalence rate.

Table 2
Articles Used in Analysis of Premature Delivery

AUTHOR	SITE	DATES OF STUDY	COMPARISON GROUP AVAILABLE?	TYPE OF TRANSPLANT RECEIVED
Aichberger	Austria	1974–1991	No	Kidney
Barrou	International	Pre-1994	No	Pancreas, kidney
Haugen	Norway	1974–1991	Yes	Kidney
Muirhead	Canada	1977–1988	Yes	Kidney
Nojima	Japan	1973–1995	Yes	Kidney
Radomski	USA	1991–1995	Yes[a]	Kidney, liver, heart
Sabagh	Saudi Arabia	1984–1994	No	Kidney
Scantlebury	USA	1977–1988	No	Liver
Ville	France	1985–1993	No	Liver
Wu	Germany	1988–1996	No	Liver

[a] For kidney transplant patients only.

Table 3
Articles Used in Analysis of Low Birth Weight

AUTHOR	SITE	DATES OF STUDY	COMPARISON GROUP AVAILABLE?	TYPE OF TRANSPLANT RECEIVED
Aichberger	Germany	1974–1991	No	Kidney
Nojima	Japan	1973–1995	Yes	Kidney
Radomski	USA	1991–1995	No	Kidney, liver, heart
Ville	France	1985–1993	No	Liver
Wu	Germany	1988–1996	No	Liver

However, this strict inclusion criteria resulted in a small sample size study of only several hundred live births in patients receiving cyclosporine.

Another limitation of the published data is the absence of referenced or standard classifications of major or minor malformations. Reports of malformations varied among studies based on how the researchers defined a malformation. No all studies reported malformation rates, although some did so in a manner that made it difficult or impossible to attribute the malformations to either the cyclosporine-exposed or the control group. In some cases, an estimate of the live births of cyclosporine-treated mothers was necessary; however, because this occurred only twice with small numbers, our conservative estimation is unlikely to affect the results significantly. This limitation is partially remedied by the fact that for calculation of odds rations, the control group had been collected in a similar manner, with similar methodology of collection of malformations.

Our systematic review did not include unpublished data (i.e., dissertations, registries from the manufacturer, or individual transplant/autoimmune centers) because of the concern that inclusion of such data would result in duplicate reports of cases (*32*). Excluding unpublished data may have overestimated our prevalence rate if positive findings were more likely to be published than negative findings. However, given the importance of any information regarding teratogenicity, we assumed that both negative and positive results would be equally published.

There are many other factors unique to organ transplant recipients that may have also influenced the prevalence of congenital malformations observed. First, pregnancies in transplant patients are considered high risk. Poor graft function, hypertension, and elevated serum creatinine prepregnancy have been associated with poorer pregnancy outcomes, such as prematurity and low birth weight (*33*, *34*). In turn, premature and low birth weight babies seem to present more frequently with malformations than the general population (*33*). In calculating odds ratio for prematurity and low birth weight, the control groups were also based on transplanted women. However, the studies did not allow control for variabilities in maternal morbidity.

A higher incidence of rejection episodes during pregnancy has also been noted in patients whose immunosuppressive therapy included cyclosporine compared with those receiving other regimens (*33*). This may be due to lower cyclosporine levels during pregnancy (*15*). Subtherapeutic levels may result from alterations in cyclosporine metabolism and distribution (*15*), or reduced medication compliance secondary to the patient's fear of effects of immunosuppresants on the developing fetus. As discussed above, graft dysfunction may predispose to prematurity or low birth weight that may then result in increased malformations. Cyclosporine levels were not evaluated in our study, but it is possible that the observed results are due to changes in pharmacokinetics of cyclosporine during pregnancy rather than direct toxic effects of the drug upon the fetus.

Many renal transplant patients also have diabetes. Renal transplant patients were by far the largest group represented in our study (84.8% of live births). Poorly controlled diabetes has been associated with an increased incidence of congenital malformations (3–22%) (*35–37*). Drug-treated diabetes is more common among transplant patients treated with cyclosporine (*33*), our results may reflect the consequences of that disease state, as opposed to fetal effects of cyclosporine.

Transplant patients often require a combination of immunosuppressive medications. In our study, few patients received cyclosporine alone for immunosuppression. More commonly, cyclosporine was combined with prednisone and/or azathioprine; therefore the potential for teratogenicity secondary to these concomitant medications must also be considered. Both prednisone and azathioprine have shown teratogenic potential in animal studies and cross the human placenta readily (*15*). Each may therefore have the potential to cause malformations in humans. For example, prednisone has been associated with a clinically significant increase in cleft palate (*38*). Although the odds ratio in our analysis compared cyclosporine exposure outcomes to noncyclosporine exposure outcomes, it may reflect the effect of the combined exposure to cyclosporine and other concurrent immunosuppressants.

A large proportion of renal transplant patients are also hypertensive and require therapy for this condition (*33*). Certain

Table 4
Results Summary

PARAMETER OF INTEREST	ODDS RATIO (95% CI)	PREVALENCE RATE (95% CI)
Malformation	3.83 (0.75–19.6) (6 studies)	4.1% (2.6–7.0) (15 studies)
Preterm birth	1.52 (1.00–2.32) (4 studies)	56.3% (37.8–74.7) (10 studies)
Low birth weight	1.60 (0.95–2.44) (1 study)	43.0% (22.8–63.3) (5 studies)

antihypertensives, such as ACE inhibitors (*36*), are associated with malformations in newborns, although other antihypertensives, including selected calcium channel blockers (felodipine, nifedipine, diltiazem) and diuretics, have shown teratogenic potential in animal studies. A higher incidence of hypertension has been observed in cyclosporine exposed patients compared to noncyclosporine users (*15, 33*). Hypertension is also a commonly recognized side effect of cyclosporine. Our studies report patients treated for hypertension, but do not consistently report the antihypertensive(s) used. Thus, our results may be reflecting the teratogenicity of concurrent antihypertensive medications.

In general, any number of medications that this patient population may have taken chronically or acutely during pregnancy may have affected the results seen. Our study was not able to control for all medications used and therefore teratogenicity secondary to concomitant medications is a possibility. Last, different types of organ transplant may confer different fetal risks. However, at this stage the sample size is too small to sub analyze the data by different types of organ transplant.

Our results with respect to malformation rates are not quantitatively different from those generated by the National Transplantation Pregnancy Registry data, in showing that, overall, cyclosporine use is not associated with a substantially higher overall prevalence of major malformations (*39*). However, the meta-analysis allows estimations of odds ratios, and it is quite possible that will a larger sample size, the OR of 3.24 may become statistically significant. The significant trend for low birth weight with cyclosporine, after controlling for transplant itself, should be corroborated carefully by larger numbers.

In summary, the results of our analysis suggest a trend towards increased risk of congenital malformations among infants born to transplant recipients who received cyclosporine throughout their pregnancy. The small sample size may have contributed to the inability to achieve statistical significance. Further study is warranted to adequately quantify or approximate the fetal risks of in utero exposure to cyclosporine. Clinicians caring for transplanted patients should be encouraged to publish results of such registries to allow the larger sample size needed to draw more concrete conclusions. Such studies should report on concomitant medications, concurrent disease states, severity of maternal illness, and other confounders as identified.

REFERENCES

1. Burckart GJ, Venkataramanan R, Ptachcinski RJ. Overview of transplantation. In: DiPiro JT, Talbert RL, Yee GC et al, eds. Pharmacotherapy: A Pathophysiologic Approach, 3rd ed. Stamford, CT: Appleton and Lange, 1997; 129.
2. Salomon DR. The use of immunosuppressive drugs in kidney transplantation. Pharmacother 1991; 11: 153S.
3. Khaliq Y. Neoral® cyclosporine: its role after Sandimmune®. Pharm Prac (insert) June 1997.
4. Ramsey-Goldman R, Schilling E. Immunosuppressive drug use during pregnancy. Rheum Dis Clin North Am 1997; 23: 133.
5. Fleschler RG, Sala DJ. Pregnancy after renal transplantation. JOGNN 1995; 24: 413.
6. Weber M, Deng S, Olthoff K et al. Organ transplantation in the twenty-first century. Urol Clin North Am 1998; 25: 51.
7. Sims CJ. Organ transplantation and immunosuppressive drugs in pregnancy. Clin Obstet Gynecol 1991; 34: 100.
8. Penn I, Makowski EL, Harris P. Parenthood following renal transplantation. Kidney Int 1980; 18: 221.
9. Laifer SA, Guido RS. Reproductive function and outcome of pregnancy after liver transplantation in women. Mayo Clin Proc. 1995; 70: 388.
10. Lamarque V, Leleu MF, Monka C, et al. Analysis of 629 pregnancy outcomes in transplant recipients treated with Sandimmun. Trans Proc 1997; 29: 2480.
11. Esplin MS, Branch DW. Immunosuppressive drugs and pregnancy. Obstet Gynecol Clin North Am 1997; 24: 601.
12. Shen AY-J, Mansukhani PW. Is pregnancy contraindicated after cardiac transplantation? Int J Cardiol 1997; 60: 151.
13. Bermas BL, Hill JA. Effects of immunosuppressive drugs during pregnancy. Arth Rheum 1995; 38: 1722.
14. Dombroski RA. Autoimmune disease in pregnancy. Med Clin North Am 1989; 73: 605.
15. Huynh LA, Min DI. Outcomes of pregnancy and the management of immunosuppressive agents to minimize fetal risks in organ transplant patients. Ann Pharmacother 1994; 28: 1355.
16. Bianchi DW. Genetic issues presenting it the nursery. In: Cloherty JP, Stark AR, eds. Manual of neonatal care, 4th ed. Philadelphia: Lippincott-Raven Publications, 1998; 81.
17. Aichberger C, Lechner W, Ofner D, et al. Zum problem der schwanger-schaft nach nierentransplantation. Wien Klin Wochenschr 1993; 195: 723.
18. Armenti VT, Ahlswede KM, Ahlswede BA, et al. National Transplantation Prengancy Registry—outcomes of 154 pregnancies in cyclosporine-treated female kidney transplant recipients. Transplantation 1994; 57: 502.
19. Barrou BM, Gruessner AC, Sutherland DER, et al. Prengancy after pancreas transplantation in the cyclosporine era. Transplantation 1998; 65: 524.
20. Bererhi L, Bedrossian J, Metivier F, et al. Pregnancy in kidney transplantation: past and present experience. Transplant Proc 1997; 29: 2478.
21. Crawford JS, Johnson K, Jones KL. Pregnancy outcome after transplantation in women maintained on cyclosporine immunosuppression (abstract). Reprod Toxicol 1993; 7: 156.
22. Framarino di Malatesta ML, Poli L, Pierucci. A, et al. Prengancy and kidney transplantation: clinical problems and experience. Transplant Proc 1993; 25: 2188.
23. Haugen G, Fauchald P, Sodal G, et al. Pregnancy outcomes in renal allograft recipients in Norway. Acta Obstet Gynecol Scand 1994; 73: 541.
24. Muirhead N, Sabharwal AR, Rieder MJ, et al. The outcome of pregnancy following renal transplantation—the experience of a single center. Transplantation 1992; 54: 429.
25. Nojima M, Ihara H, Ichikawa Y, et al. Influence of pregnancy on graft function after renal transplantation. Transplant Proc 1996; 28: 1582.
26. Sabagh TO, Eltorkey MM, EI Awad MA et al. Outcome of pregnancy in renal transplant recipients taking cyclosporin A. J Obs Gyn 1995; 15: 226–9.
27. Scantlebury V, Gordon R, Tzakis A, et al. Childbearing after liver transplantation. Transplantation 1990; 49: 317–321.
28. Talaat KM, Tyden G, Bjorkman U et al. Thirty successful pregnancies in organ transplant recipients: a single-center experience. Transplant Proc 1994; 26: 1773.
29. Ville Y, Fernandez H, Samuel D et al. Prengancy in liver transplant recipients: course and outcome in 19 cases. Am J Obs Gyn 1993; 168: 896–902.

30. Wu A, Nashan B, Messner U et al. Outcome of 22 successful pregnancies after liver transplantation. Clin Transplant 1998; 12: 454–64.
31. Radomski JS, Ahlswede BA, Jarrell BE, et al. Outcome of 500 pregnancies in 335 female kidney, liver, and heart transplant recipients. Transplant Proc 1995; 27: 1089.
32. Einarson TR, Leeder JS, Koren G. A method for meta-analysis of epidemiological studies. Drug Intell Clin Pharm 1998; 22: 813.
33. Armenti VT, Moritz MJ, Davison JM. Medical management of the pregnant transplant recipient. Adv Renal Replace Ther 1998; 5 (1): 14.
34. Salmela K, Kyllonen L, Eklund B, et al. Thirty years of renal transplant in Helsinki. In: Tersaki Y, Cecka B, eds. Clinical Transplantation. Helsinki, Finland: 1994; 219.
35. Marden PM, Smith DW, McDonald MJ. Congenital anomalies in the newborn infant, including minor variations. J Ped 1964; 64 (3): 357.
36. McCombs J. Therapeutic considerations in pregnancy and lactation. In: DiPiro JT, Talbert RL, Yee GC, et al, eds. Pharmacotherapy: a pathophysiologic approach, 3rd ed.. Stamford, CT: Appleton and Lange, 1997; 1565.
37. Reece EA, Eriksson UJ. The pathogenesis of diabetes-associated congenital malformations. Obstet Gynecol Clin North Am 1996; 23 (1): 29.
38. Park-Wyllie L, Mazzotta P, Pastuszak A, et al. Birth defects after maternal exposure to corticosteroids: prospective cohort study and meta-analysis of epidemiological studies. Teratology 2000; 62: 385.
39. Armenti VT, Radomski JS, Moritz MJ, Branch KR, McGrory CH, Coscia LA. Report from the National Transplantation Pregnancy Registry (NTPR): outcomes of pregnancy after transplantation. Clin Transplant 1997; 3: 101.

Received 7 September 1999.
Revision Requested 21 November 1999.
Accepted 25 April 2000.

CHAPTER 57

SYSTEMATIC REVIEW OF RANDOMIZED CONTROLLED TRIALS AND COHORT STUDIES ON PREGNANCY OUTCOME FOLLOWING ANTIRETROVIRAL TREATMENT IN PREGNANCY

Alejandro A. Nava-Ocampo,[1] Haleh Talaie,[1,2] and Gideon Koren[1]

[1]The Motherisk Program, Division of Clinical Pharmacology & Toxicology, The Hospital for Sick Children, Toronto ON, Canada, and [2]Shahid Beheshti University of Medical Sciences, Poison Center of Loghman General Hospital, Tehran, Iran

Abstract

Objective. To evaluate the clinical literature on the effects of antiretroviral therapy (ART) on pregnancy outcome.

Methods. A search in PubMed, MEDLINE, and the Cochrane Controlled Trials Register (from inception to 2005) was conducted for randomized controlled trials (RCTs) and cohort studies assessing maternal and fetal safety of antiretroviral therapy (ART) in HIV-infected pregnant women. The rates of cesarean sections, premature deliveries, very premature deliveries, low birth weight, very low birth weight, fetal death, and of major malformations were abstracted as study outcomes. Odds ratios were calculated for each outcome. Meta-analysis was conducted for studies with similar methodologies by using the random effects model and exact stratified analysis.

Results. Five published RCTs and 13 cohort studies met the inclusion criteria. In RCTs, women were exposed to ART mainly during the prenatal or intrapartum periods. Similar rates of preterm deliveries between treated and placebo groups were reported and no risk of fetal deaths was associated to ART exposure during pregnancy. In the cohort studies, reduced rates of premature deliveries, babies born with low birth weight, and fetal deaths were observed among HIV-infected treated women in comparison to untreated patients.

Conclusions. This systematic review suggests that ART administered in pregnancy does not increase the rate of adverse fetal outcomes whereas it may result in better fetal outcomes.

Keywords: Antiretroviral agents, cohort studies, embryonic and fetal development, randomized clinical trials.

INTRODUCTION

According to the World Health Organization, by the end of 2005, the global estimate of human immunodeficiency virus (HIV) infection resulted in 25 million deaths and 40 million persons living infected.[1] About half of all HIV transmission occurs among people aged 15–24 years, and 5000–6000 young people become infected every day.[2] Accounting for nearly half of all infections worldwide, there are approximately 18 million women living with HIV in 2006.[3] Since most women and men continue to be sexually active even after receiving a diagnosis of HIV infection, pregnancies among infected women are not uncommon.[4]

While it is globally recommended to treat pregnant women with HIV to ensure maternal health and prevent vertical transmission, the information on the safety of antiretroviral therapy (ART) during pregnancy is mostly based on single-arm studies or pregnancy registries based on medical voluntary reports. Relevant information regarding the safety use of ART in pregnancy has also been found in controlled cohort studies on ART in pregnancy. However, the contribution of randomized controlled trials (RCTs) of drug efficacy, where safety is also included in the evaluations, appear limited to a few number of studies in pregnant women. Therefore, available information on the potential teratogen risk at therapeutic doses of ART administered during pregnancy requires more clarification in order to critically analyze the published studies.

Correspondence: Dr. Gideon Koren, The Motherisk Program, The Hospital for Sick Children, 555 University Ave., Toronto, Ontario M5G 1X8, Canada. Fax: 1 416 813 7562. *E-mail address:* gkoren@sickkids.ca

This study aimed to systematically review the published RCTs and cohort studies on HIV-pregnant women exposed to ART in order to estimate the odds ratio for teratogenicity and other adverse maternal and fetal outcomes of women exposed to the ART during pregnancy in comparison to a group of HIV-pregnant women either receiving placebo or untreated.

METHODS

Data Sources

From their inception to December 31, 2005, a search was conducted in the following databases: PubMed, EMBASE, Cochrane Central Register of Control Trials, and Ovid MEDLINE. In the references listed in the retrieved articles, we also searched potentially relevant studies for this systematic review. Language was not used as a limit in any search.

Study Selection and Data Abstraction

As a first approach, we searched for published RCTs and prospective or retrospective controlled cohort studies reporting on fetal and pregnancy outcomes of HIV-infected pregnant women when compared against placebo (for RCTs) or against either no antiretroviral drugs or placebo (for cohort studies). Our search strategy identified 256 citations (Figure 1). Thereafter, two of the investigators screened independently the titles and abstracts of each citation in order to identify, as our inclusion criteria, the studies reporting any

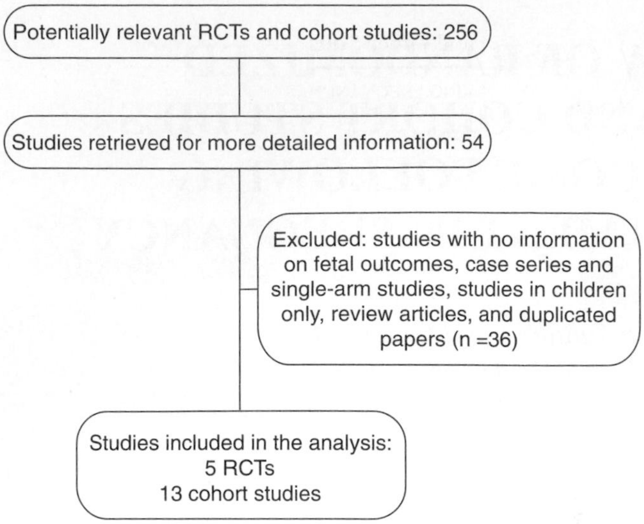

Figure 1. Study flow.

of the following outcomes: rates of premature deliveries, very premature deliveries, low birth weight, very low birth weight, fetal death, or major malformations. The rate of cesarean sections was also documented in this systematic review but was not considered as part of our inclusion criteria. When the abstract did not allow the investigators to achieve any conclusion on the selection process, the manuscript was retrieved and checked.

This process yielded 51 full-text publications identified by one or both screeners for full review plus 3 additional publications that were identified by means of review papers and expert opinion (total = 54 papers). The studies were retrieved and reviewed by two of the authors to verify that they were RCTs or cohort studies of ART administered to HIV-infected pregnant women. Disagreements between reviewers in the selection process were resolved by consensus. At this step, 7 RCTs and 13 cohort studies met the inclusion criteria and were revised to verify whether they contained the study outcomes mentioned above. Of the seven RCTs, three manuscripts reported different aspects of the Pediatric AIDS Clinical Trial Group Protocol 0.76; only the first published report was selected. Therefore, 5 RCTs and 13 cohort studies were included in the data abstraction (Figure 1).[5–22] During the different steps of the review and selection processes, the authors' names and addresses were removed from the abstracts and manuscripts.

Quantitative Data Synthesis

Odds ratios (OR) were calculated for each outcome between treated and placebo groups (for RCTs) or between treated and no ART groups (for cohort studies); where possible, the OR for pooled data was also calculated. Only one article was published in a language other than English (in Spanish), but we did not find any problem with data abstraction. A meta-analysis was conducted for studies with similar methodologies by using the random effects model and exact stratified analysis by means of StatsDirect v.2.2.5 (Cheshire, United Kingdom). Homogeneity test (Wolf Q index) and test for bias from regression of normalized effect versus precision were also computed.

RESULTS

Of the five RCTs included in this systematic review, zidovudine (ZDV) was evaluated in four and nevirapine in the other one. Women were exposed to ART mainly during the prenanatal or intrapartum periods. The cohort studies included different ART drugs: ZDV, didanosine (ddI), nevirapine, stavudine, lamivudine, nelfinavir, saquinavir, indinavir, and ritonavir. Some cohort studies included the highly active antiretroviral therapy (HAART), a combination of a nucleoside reverse transcriptase inhibitor, a non-nucleoside reverse transcriptase inhibitor, and a protease inhibitor. However, the study groups were generally reported as "no ART" and "ART" groups.

In the 13 cohort studies, time and duration of drug exposure varied widely. In one of the studies, the exposure occurred throughout pregnancy, in another during the second and third trimester, in one during the first trimester, in yet another one during the third trimester only, and in seven studies the time at which exposure occurred was not specify (Table 1). One of the cohort studies was comparing placentae from control women and women with HIV either treated or untreated, and the gestational age at which drug exposure occurred was not specified. The other study was a mortality register and exposure to ART occurred at different times from the first to the third trimester.

Three RCTs specified the rates of cesarean sections and showed similar rates in the treated and placebo arms (Table 2). In the cohort studies, however, more cesarean sections were performed among women receiving ART, with a pooled OR of 2.26 (95% CI 1.98 to 2.58).

Preterm deliveries (≤37 weeks of gestational age) were reported in three RCTs (Table 3), and the risk was similar between the treated and placebo arms [pooled OR 0.99 (95% CI 0.77 to 1.27)]. Very preterm deliveries (≤32 weeks of gestational age) were reported in only one study comparing nevirapine to placebo; similar rates between groups were observed. The pooled data of eight cohort studies reporting premature deliveries demonstrated a protective effect of ART administration during pregnancy on prematurity (Table 3). In contrast, meta-analysis of the cohort studies found similar rates of preterm deliveries between the treated and untreated groups (Figure 2) probably affected by the higher risk of preterm deliveries observed in the two studies where ART included protease inhibitors as well as for the methodological problems found by repeatedly using the control group in three of the studies included in the meta-analysis for pairing them with the different treatments. Very preterm deliveries (≤32 weeks of gestational age) were reported in three cohort studies and showed a protective effect by ART (Table 3).

Similar rates of low birth weight (≤2500 g) in the treated and placebo groups were found in the RCTs (Table 4 and Figure 3). Although the studies resulted homogenous (Wolf Q index: 4.4), bias indicator was significant in the meta-analysis [intercept (approximate 95% CI): -2.4 (-3.5 to -1.4)]. In addition, an RCT showed similar rates of babies born with very low birth weight between ART and control groups. The cohort and other studies found that ART administered during pregnancy was associated with decreased rates of babies born with low birth weight (Table 4 and Figure 4). However, the studies showed similar rates of babies born with very low birth weight (≤1500 g) (Table 4).

In reporting malformation rates, no increased risk of major malformations associated with ART exposure during pregnancy was identified by RCTs or by cohort studies (Table 5). According

Table 1
Length of Drug Administration in HIV-Infected Pregnant Women in Cohort and Other Studies

	PERIOD OF EXPOSURE DURING PREGNANCY			
	FIRST TRIMESTER	SECOND TRIMESTER	THIRD TRIMESTER	NOT SPECIFIED/UNCLEAR
RCTs				
Connor et al., 1994*			+	
Shaffer et al., 1999†			+	
Wiktor et al., 1999†			+	
Dabis et al., 1999†			+	
Dorenbaum et al., 2002†			+	
Cohort studies				
Dickover et al., 1996		+	+	
Mandelbrot et al., 1998				+
Simonds et al., 1998				+
Italian Register, 1999	+	+	+	
ECS: Swiss cohort, 2000				+
Jungmann et al., 2001†				+
Cooper et al., 2002				+
Tuomala et al., 2002				+
Arnold et al., 2003				+
Mayaux et al., 2003			+	
ECS, 2003				+
Other studies				
Lindegren ML et al., 2000				+
Villegas Castrejon et al., 1999	+	+	+	

* Other aspects of this RCT were published later.
† ART was administered in the prenatal or during intrapartum periods only.

to the RCTs, the overall rate of major malformations was 2% in the control group and 2.3% in the ART exposed group. Similar overall rates of major malformations were reported in the cohort studies: 2% and 1.7%, respectively. However, one of the studies showed that the simultaneous exposure to ART and folate antagonists (co-trimoxazole and pyrimethamine) during pregnancy was associated with an increased risk of malformations.

The three RCTs that reported the rate of fetal deaths found no increased risk associated with ART exposure during pregnancy (Table 6). The studies were homogeneous (Wolf Q index: 4.5) and

Table 2
Rates of Cesarean Sections Among HIV-Infected Pregnant Women Exposed to Antiretroviral Therapy

		NO EXPOSED TO ART		EXPOSED TO ART		
	TREATMENT	WITHOUT EVENT	WITH EVENT	WITHOUT EVENT	WITH EVENT	OR (95% CI)
RCTs						
Connor et al., 1994	Placebo vs. ZDV	151	51	142	59	1.23 (0.77 to 1.96)
Shaffer et al., 1999	Placebo vs. ZDV	171	24	156	32	1.46 (0.79 to 2.71)
Wiktor et al., 1999	Placebo vs. ZDV	133	2	132	2	1.01 (0.07 to 14.1)
Pooled data		*455*	*77*	*430*	*93*	*1.28 (0.91 to 1.8)*
Cohort and other studies						
Mandelbrot et al., 1998	No ART vs ZDV	1,594	283	625	247	2.23 (1.82 to 2.71)
Villegas et al., 1999	No ART vs:	6	1			
	ZDV			4	3	4.5 (0.23 to 274.8)
	ZDV + ddI			4	3	4.5 (0.23 to 274.8)*
Cooper et al., 2002	No-ART vs ART	324	72	878	268	1.37 (1.02 to 1.86)
Mayaux et al., 2003	No-ART vs ART	79	13	1,390	685	2.99 (1.64 to 5.91)
Pooled data		2003	369	2,901	1,206	2.26 (1.98 to 2.58)

No ART: none antiretroviral therapy; ddI: didanosine; ZDV: zidovudine

Table 3
Rates of Premature Deliveries in HIV-Infected Pregnant Women Exposed to ART in Cohort Studies

		NO EXPOSED TO ART		EXPOSED TO ART		
	TREATMENT	WITHOUT EVENT	WITH EVENT	WITHOUT EVENT	WITH EVENT	OR (95% CI)
RCTs						
a) ≤37 weeks						
Connor et al., 1994	Placebo vs ZDV	196	13	190	16	1.27 (0.56 to 2.95)
Dabis et al., 1999	Placebo vs ZDV	152	22	156	12	0.53 (0.23 to 1.17)
Dorenbaum et al., 2002	Placebo vs Nevirapine	510	119	517	125	1.04 (0.78 to 1.38)
Pooled data		*858*	*154*	*863*	*153*	*0.99 (0.77 to 1.27)*
b) ≤32 weeks						
Dorenbaum et al., 2002	Placebo vs Nevirapine	619	9	632	10	1.09 (0.39 to 3.1)
Cohort studies						
≤37 weeks						
Mandelbrot et al., 1998	No ART vs ZDV	1,674	206	799	62	0.63 (0.46 to 0.85)
Simonds et al., 1998	No ART vs ZDV	659	186	155	32	0.73 (0.47 to 1.12)
Italian Register, 1999	No ART vs ZDV	136	34	32	6	0.75 (0.24 to 2.02)
ECS: Swiss cohort, 2000	No ART vs:	2,375	444			
	Mono ART			462	93	1.08 (0.83 to 1.38)
	ART-PI			147	41	1.49 (1.01 to 2.16)
	ART + PI			72	29	2.15 (1.33 to 3.4)
Cooper et al., 2002	No ART vs ART	311	85	954	192	0.74 (0.55 to 0.99)
Tuomala et al., 2002	No ART vs: Mono-ART	915	228	1,336	254	0.76 (0.62 to 0.93)
	Any ART combination			453	80	0.71 (0.53 to 0.94)
	Any Mono-ART			1,789	334	0.75 (0.62 to 0.91)
	ART-PI			341	55	0.65 (0.46 to 0.90)
	ART + PI			112	25	0.90 (0.54 to 1.43)
ECS, 2003	No ART vs: Mono-ART	1,221	221	390	75	1.06 (0.79 to 1.42)
	ART-PI			182	49	1.49 (1.03 to 2.12)
	ART + PI			137	51	2.06 (1.41 to 2.95)
Mayaux et al., 2003	No ART vs ART	83	9	2,072	3	0.01 (0.002 to 0.06)
Pooled data		*7,374*	*1,413*	*9,433*	*1,381*	*0.76 (0.70 to 0.83)*
≤32 weeks						
Cooper et al., 2002	No ART vs ART	313	83	947	199	0.79 (0.59 to 1.07)
Tuomala et al., 2002	No ART vs:	1107	36			
	Mono-ART			1542	48	0.96 (0.60 to 1.53)
	Any ART combination			517	16	0.95 (0.49 to 1.78)
	Any Mono-ART			2,059	64	0.96 (0.62 to 1.49)
	ART-PI			396	10	0.78 (0.34 to 1.62)
	ART + PI			131	6	1.41 (0.48 to 3.46)
Mayaux et al., 2003	No ART vs ART	83	9	1,930	145	0.64 (0.32 to 1.49)
Pooled data		*1,503*	*128*	*7,552*	*448*	*0.70 (0.57 to 0.86)*

Mono-ART: antiretroviral therapy with one drug only; No ART: none antiretroviral therapy; ddI: didanosine; PI: protease inhibitors; ZDV: zidovudine

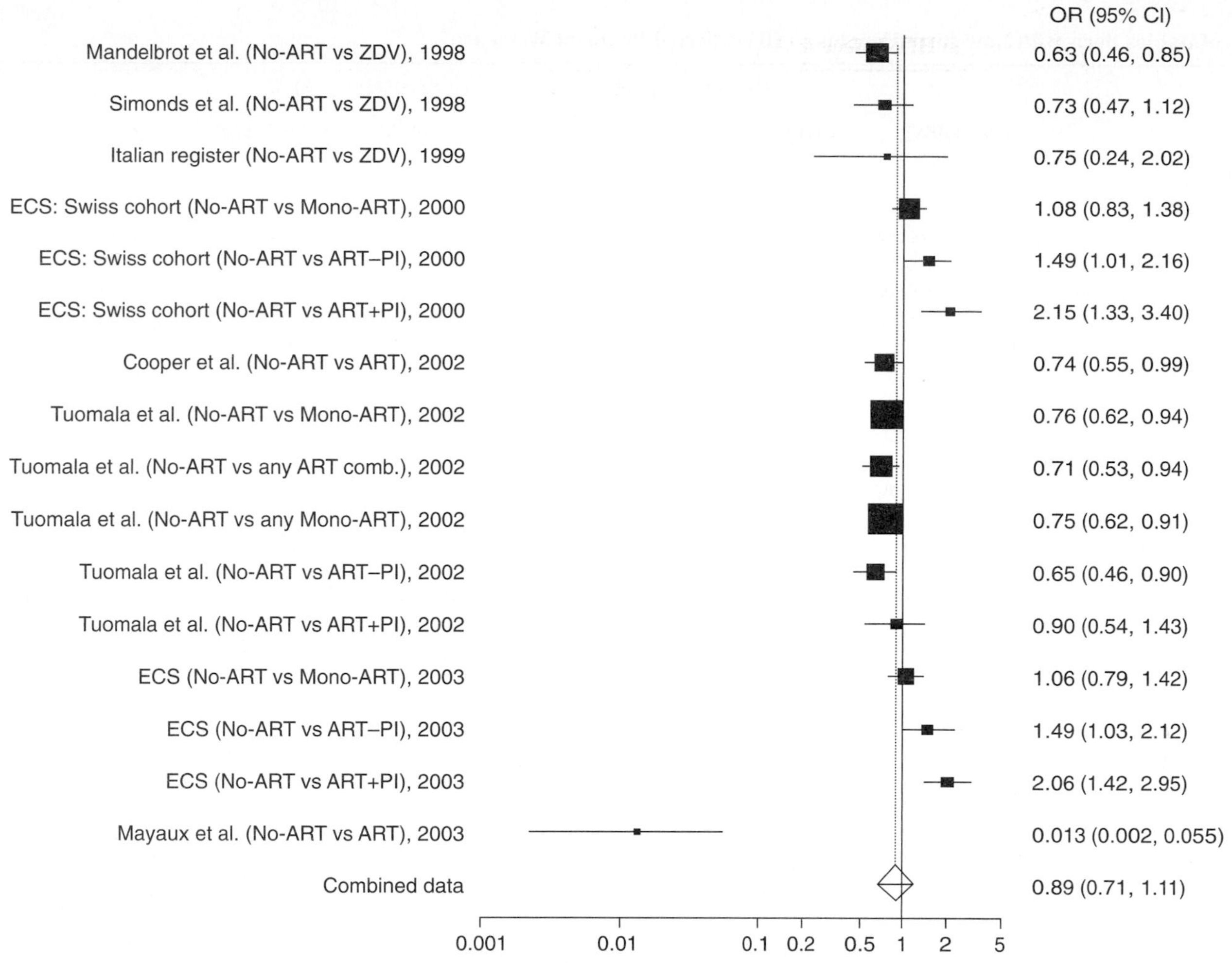

***Figure 2.** Meta-analysis of the rates of deliveries ≤37 weeks of gestational age, as reported in cohort studies. Abbreviations: Any ART comb: any combination of drugs used for ART; ECS: European Collaborative Study; Mono-ART: antiretroviral therapy with one drug only; No-ART: none antiretroviral therapy; PI: protease inhibitors; ZDV: zidovudine.*

the intercept was not biased (1.3 [-8.5 to 11]). The cohort studies showed a protective effect for fetal deaths when ART was used in pregnancy (Table 6), reducing the rate of fetal deaths from 2% among control HIV-infected pregnant women to 0.7% among women treated with ART during pregnancy.

The cohort studies included in the meta-analysis of the rates of deliveries at ≤37 weeks, malformations and fetal deaths showed positive heterogeneity. In contrast, the cohort studies included in the meta-analysis of the rates of deliveries ≤32 weeks and of babies born with birth weight ≤2500 g or ≤1200 g showed negative heterogeneity, meaning a homogenous pattern of the results among the studies. Of meta-analyzed data, no evaluation resulted with positive bias indicator as judged by the intercept of regression between normalized effects and precision.

DISCUSSION

This study aimed at addressing a critical question on the safety for the mother and the developing fetus of ART administered to HIV-pregnant women. Exposure to ART at different gestational ages, especially during the first trimester of pregnancy, may potentially increase the risk of congenital malformations. Such data are critical in counseling women with HIV infection in the context of continuing the pregnancy. However, we have identified only a limited number of placebo-controlled RCTs testing the effectiveness of ART in preventing vertical HIV transmission to also obtain information on safety of ART during pregnancy. Furthermore, the RCTs were monotherapy studies with ZDV or nevirapine. This reality is understandable in the light of the absolute rejection of giving placebo to women with HIV after the original ZDV study has shown the drug to be superior to placebo.[5,23] By restricting this review to only randomized placebo-controlled studies, we could leave behind some relevant information that can be learned from, for example, cohort studies. Yet, cohort studies cannot control for numerous confounders pertinent to pregnancy outcome. It is conceivable that pregnant women with HIV infection who were not offered ART may differ in other potentially relevant characteristics, such as socioeconomic status and rates of poverty, other diagnostic tests, medications, prenatal care, and so on, to those who received treatment.

We found a large variability in the methods of the cohort studies, including gestational age at which exposure to ART occurred as well as the drugs administered as part of the ART. Such limitations

Table 4
Rate of Babies Born with Low Birth Weights to HIV-Infected Pregnant Women

		NO EXPOSED TO ART		EXPOSED TO ART		
	TREATMENT	WITHOUT EVENT	WITH EVENT	WITHOUT EVENT	WITH EVENT	OR (95% CI)
RCTs						
a) ≤2500 g						
Connor et al., 1994	Placebo vs ZDV	176	33	181	25	0.74 (0.40 to 1.34)
Shaffer et al., 1999	Placebo vs ZDV	177	18	177	11	0.61 (0.25 to 1.41)
Wiktor et al., 1999	Placebo vs ZDV	117	18	118	11	0.61 (0.25 to 1.43)
Dabis et al., 1999	Placebo vs ZDV	159	31	166	28	0.87 (0.48 to 1.57)
Dorenbaum et al., 2002	Placebo vs Nevirapine	567	75	567	86	1.15 (0.81 to 1.62)
Pooled data		*1,196*	*175*	*1,209*	*161*	*0.91 (0.72 to 1.15)*
b) ≤1500 g						
Connor et al., 1994	Placebo vs ZDV	205	4	203	3	0.76 (0.11 to 4.54)
Cohort and other studies						
≤2500 g						
Simonds et al., 1998	No ART vs ZDV	608	237	146	41	0.72 (0.48 to 1.06)
Italian Register, 1999	No ART vs ZDV	144	33	30	7	1.02 (0.35 to 2.64)
Villegas et al., 1999	No ART vs:	7	0			
	ZDV			6	1	Undefined
	ZDV + ddI			5	2	Undefined
Cooper et al., 2002	No ART vs ART	313	83	947	199	0.79 (0.59 to 1.07)
Tuomala et al., 2002	No ART vs:	930	213			
	Mono-ART			1,332	258	0.85 (0.69 to 1.04)
	Any ART combination			465	68	0.64 (0.47 to 0.86)
	Any Mono-ART			2,123	326	0.67 (0.55 to 0.81)
	ART-PI			355	41	0.50 (0.34 to 0.73)
	ART + PI			110	27	1.07 (0.66 to 1.69)
ECS, 2003	No ART vs. ART	1,176	289	714	160	0.91 (0.73 to 1.14)
Pooled data		*3,178*	*855*	*6,233*	*1,130*	*0.67 (0.61 to 0.74)*
≤1500 g						
Tuomala et al., 2002	No ART vs:	1118	25			
	Mono-ART			1556	34	0.98 (0.56 to 1.72)
	Any ART combination			530	3	0.25 (0.05 to 0.84)
	Any Mono-ART			2073	50	1.08 (0.65 to 1.83)
	ART-PI			387	9	1.04 (0.42 to 2.33)
	ART + PI			130	7	2.41 (0.86 to 5.87)
Pooled data		*1118*	*25*	*4676*	*103*	*0.99 (0.63 to 1.60)*

ART-PI: ART without protease inhibitors; ART + PI: ART plus a protease inhibitor; ddI: didanosine; Mono-ART: antiretroviral therapy with one drug only; No ART: none antiretroviral therapy; ZDV: zidovudine

should have contributed in the positive heterogeneity of several subanalyses. The quality of the studies and the details provided in the cohort studies should improve for helping us to learn from them. Importantly, we found that in most of the RCTs, drug therapy was administered only at the end of pregnancy and, therefore, the effect of this intervention on most pregnancy outcomes is expected to be negligible, as clearly demonstrated in our analysis.

In most developing countries, the access to ART may be very difficult. However, the administration of ZDV during the third trimester or a single dose of nevirapine before delivery may result in an important reduction in mother-to-child transmission. In addition, the knowledge that these ART regiments do not produce a higher risk of malformations or preterm deliveries could add to justifying their use in pregnant women in countries with limited

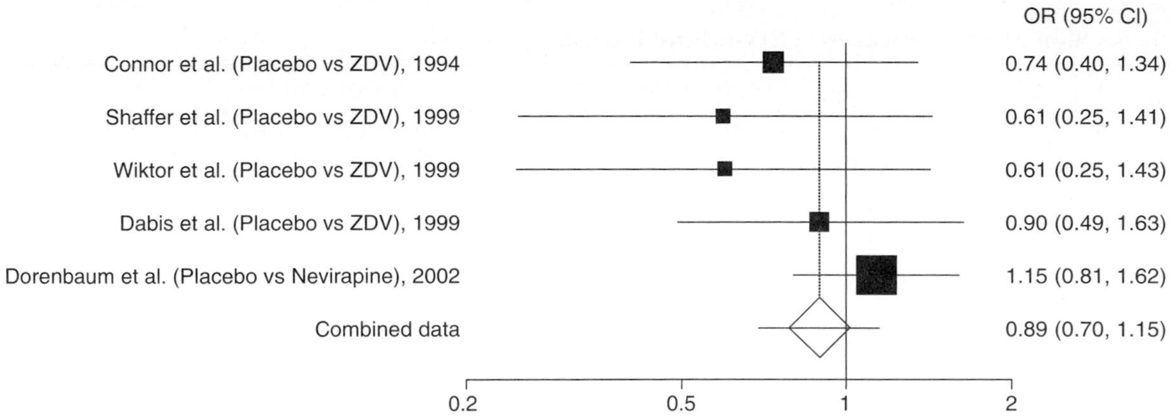

Figure 3. Meta-analysis of the rates of babies with birth weigh ≤2500 g, as reported in RCTs. For abbreviations, see Figure 2.

resources. Caution, however, should be practiced since children born to HIV-infected women receiving ZDV during pregnancy may be at risk for mitochondrial dysfunction.[24]

We found that the rates of cesarean sections as well as fetal deaths were similar in the treated and placebo groups of RCTs. In contrast, a higher rate of cesarean sections was observed in the treated arms of the cohort studies. Although cesarean section rates may vary with the time of the study, that is, recent studies may have higher rates because of an increased awareness of the benefits of cesarean sections, randomization and blindness of RCTs should have contributed to balance the rate of cesarean sections between treated and control groups. Their current recommendation is in favor of cesarean section in HIV-infected women, and it is therefore conceivable that treated women were offered cesarean sections two- to threefolds more often than those who did not receive ART in the cohort studies.[25]

In the systematic review based on cohort studies of ART in HIV-infected pregnant women, we found that the therapy does not only lack of deleterious effects in the mother and her baby but may exert protective effects against premature deliveries, babies born with low birth weight, and fetal deaths. However, an increased risk of malformations was found in a study with ART and folate antagonists during pregnancy. Because the latter drugs may increase the risk of birth defects, the findings reported in the study of Jungmann et al. were more likely due to the effects of folate antagonists and not to the ART.[15,26–28] We were unable to locate RCTs comparing highly active ART (HAART) versus placebo in HIV-infected pregnant women.

Benign and self-limited hyperlactatemia may occur in up to half of children exposed to nucleoside analogues, and may probably increase the risk of future hemangiomas.[29,30]

Our results support two previous extensive studies evaluating the rates of maternal toxicity and obstetric outcomes by type and duration of ART during pregnancy in HIV-infected women, adverse events were found to be uncommon.[31,32] In addition, the new recommendations of the International AIDS Society-USA panel only

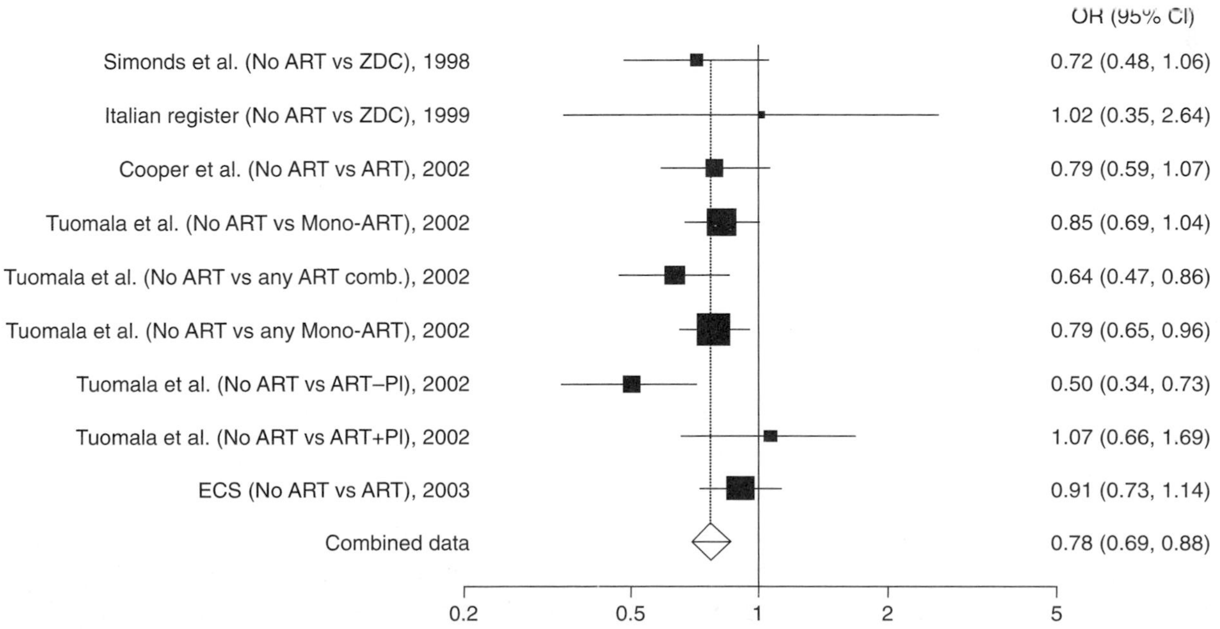

Figure 4. Meta-analysis of the rates of babies born with birth weigh ≤2500 g, as reported in cohort studies. For abbreviations, see Figure 2.

Table 5
Rate of Babies Born with Malformations to HIV-Infected Pregnant Women

	TREATMENT	NO EXPOSED TO ART		EXPOSED TO ART		OR (95% CI)
		WITHOUT EVENT	WITH EVENT	WITHOUT EVENT	WITH EVENT	
RCTs						
Connor et al., 1994	Placebo vs ZDV	204	5	201	5	1.01 (0.23 to 4.48)
Shaffer et al., 1999	Placebo vs ZDV	192	3	183	5	1.75 (0.33 to 11.4)
Wiktor et al., 1999	Placebo vs ZDV	131	6	134	2	0.33 (0.03 to 1.87)
Dabis et al., 1999	Placebo vs ZDV	199	1	195	5	5.1 (0.56 to 242.5)
Pooled data		*726*	*15*	*713*	*17*	*1.5 (0.54 to 2.5)*
Cohort studies						
Jungmann et al., 2001	No ART/FA vs:	142	6			
	ART + FA			10	3	6.93 (0.98 to 38.97)
	ART or FA			34	0	Undefined
Arnold et al., 2003*	No ART vs ART	16	4	22	1	0.19 (0.003 to 2.15)
ECS, 2003	No ART vs ART	1,484	24	893	13	0.90 (0.42 to 1.85)
Pooled data		*1,642*	*34*	*959*	*17*	*0.86 (0.45 to 1.59)*

ZDV: zidovudine

Table 6
Rates of Fetal Death Among HIV-Infected Pregnant Women Exposed to ART

	TREATMENT	NO EXPOSED TO ART		EXPOSED TO ART		OR (95% CI)
		WITHOUT EVENT	WITH EVENT	WITHOUT EVENT	WITH EVENT	
RCTs						
Connor et al., 1994	Placebo vs ZDV	206	3	201	5	1.71 (0.33 to 11.13)
Shaffer et al., 1999	Placebo vs ZDV	195	0	187	1	Undefined
Wiktor et al., 1999	Placebo vs ZDV	127	10	128	8	0.79 (0.26 to 2.32)
Dabis et al., 1999	Placebo vs ZDV	204	7	202	1	0.14 (0.003 to 1.14)
Pooled data		*732*	*20*	*718*	*15*	*0.76 (0.36 to 1.59)*
Cohort studies						
Italian Register, 1999	No ART vs ZDV	176	1	37	0	Undefined
Lindegren et al., 2000	No ART vs:	890	37			
	ZDV			4,476	36	0.19 (0.12 to 0.32)
	ZDV + Lamivudine			676	3	0.11 (0.02 to 0.34)
	Other ART			2,652	20	0.18 (0.10 to 0.32)
Tuomala et al., 2002	No ART vs:	1,136	7			
	Mono-ART			1,579	11	1.13 (0.40 to 3.45)
	Any ART combination			532	1	0.31 (0.006 to 2.39)
	Any Mono-ART			2,111	12	0.92 (0.33 to 2.77)
	ART-PI			395	1	0.41 (0.009 to 3.22)
	ART + PI			137	0	Undefined
Mayaux et al., 2003	No ART vs ART	90	2	2,062	13	0.28 (0.006 to 2.63)
Pooled data		*2,292*	*47*	*14,657*	*97*	*0.32 (0.22 to 0.47)*

Mono-ART: antiretroviral therapy with one drug only; No ART: none antiretroviral therapy; ZDV: zidovudine address concerns about exposure to tenofovir and fetal bone formation and contraindicate efavirenz in the first trimester of pregnancy based on case reports linking exposure to therapeutic doses of efavirenz and neural tube defects.[33] However, in a pregnancy registry maintained by a collaboration of manufacturers of antiretroviral drugs (The Antiretroviral Pregnancy Registry), of 244 first-trimester exposures to efavirenz, only 6 cases accounting for a prevalence of 2.5% (95% CI 0.9% to 5.3%) of congenital defects were reported.[34] Although negative criticisms may be addressed for both type of evidence on efavirenz (case reports and spontaneous-report registries), these contrasting examples further emphasize the need to discuss how to obtain the best evidence about drug safety in pregnancy in future studies, especially where there is a clear dilemma between treating HIV-infected pregnant women with the most effective available drugs and the risk of teratogenicity.

In summary, this systematic review suggests that ART administered late in pregnancy does not increase the rate of adverse fetal adverse outcomes, that is, premature deliveries, low birth weight, and fetal death. However, information obtained from RCTs was based on monotherapy with zidovudine or nevirapine administered late in pregnancy whereas in developed countries, HIV-infected pregnant women should be receiving HAART as the standard of care and therefore our findings may not be applied to counsel women exposed to such therapy. In addition, although included cohort studies did not contain critical details about drug exposure, our study found that ART not only lacked of fetal deleterious effects but was associated with lesser rates of premature and very premature deliveries, low birth weight, and fetal death. However, the risk of malformation may increase with the coadministration of ART and folate antagonists and therefore this subgroup of treatment should be considered in separate of the rest when counseling women exposed to these drugs.

In addition, we believe that the inclusion of a "no-ART" arm in cohort studies should be questioned and that at least ZDV or nevirapine should be administered to HIV-infected pregnant women. However, there is an urgent need to discuss the future of research in drug safety among pregnant women to be capable for obtaining the best evidence-based information. However, under the alarming perspective of worldwide spread of HIV infection, neither RCTs nor cohort studies have provided satisfactory information and therefore our findings would require to be updated once more carefully designed studies may become available and the quality of publications in this field have improved. Until more information becomes available, prenatal counseling should preferably be supported by available recommendations for use of ART in pregnant HIV-1-infected women.[32,35,36] However, efforts to update such guidelines with new evidence about safety of new ART in pregnancy should be made before counseling HIV-infected pregnant women.

ACKNOWLEDGEMENTS

The study was sponsored by the Canadian Institutes for Health Research (CIHR); GK is a Senior Scientist of the CIHR and holds the Ivey Chair in Molecular Toxicology at the University of Western Ontario; HT was supported in Canada at The Motherisk Program, Hospital for Sick Children, Toronto, by a special grant from the Iran Health Ministry through Dr Yadegarinia. The study was not supported in any form by any pharmaceutical company.

REFERENCES

1. UNAIDS/WHO. AIDS Epidemic Update: December 2005 report. URL: *www.unaids.org/epi/2005/doc/report.asp* Accessed: December 12, 2006.
2. Ross D, Dick B, Ferguson J. Preventing HIV/AIDS in young people: a systematic review of the evidence from developing countries. Geneva: UNAIDS Inter-agency Task Team on Young People, WHO Technical Report Series. 2006.
3. UNAIDS/WHO. The Global Coalition on Women and AIDS. URL: http://womenandaids.unaids.org. Accessed: December 12, 2006.
4. Cohan D. Perinatal HIV: special consideration. *Top HIV Med.* 2003;11:200–213.
5. Connor EM, Sperling RS, Gelber R, et al. Reduction of maternal-infant transmission of human immunodeficiency virus type 1 with zidovudine treatment. Pediatric AIDS Clinical Trials Group Protocol 076 Study Group. *N Engl J Med.* 1994;331:1173–1180.
6. Shaffer N, Chuachoowong R, Mock PA, et al. Short-course zidovudine for prenatal HIV-1 transmission in Bangkok, Thailand: a randomized controlled trial. *Lancet.* 1999;353:773–780.
7. Wiktor SZ, Ekpini E, Karon JM, et al. Short-course oral zidovudine for prevention of mother-to-child transmission of HIV-1 in Abidjan, Côte d'Ivoire: a randomized trial. *Lancet.* 1999;353:781–785.
8. Dabis F, Msellati P, Meda N, et al. 6-month efficacy, tolerance, and acceptability of a short regimen of oral zidovudine to reduce vertical transmission of HIV in breastfed children in Côte d'Ivoire and Burkina Faso: a double-blind placebo-controlled multicentre trial. *Lancet.* 1999;353:786–792.
9. Dorenbaum A, Cunningham CK, Gelber RD, et al. Two-dose intrapartum/newborn nevirapine and standard antiretroviral therapy to reduce perinatal HIV transmission: a randomized trial. *JAMA.* 2002;288:189–198.
10. Dickover RE, Garratty EM, Herman SA, et al. Identification of levels of maternal HIV-1 RNA associated with risk of perinatal transmission: effect of maternal zidovudine treatment on viral load. *JAMA.* 1996;275:599–605.
11. Mandelbrot L, Le Chenadec J, Berrebi A, et al. Perinatal HIV-1 transmission: interaction between zidovudine prophylaxis and mode of delivery in the French Perinatal Cohort. *JAMA.* 1998;280:55–60.
12. Simonds RJ, Steketee R, Nesheim S, et al. Impact of zidovudine use on risk and risk factors for perinatal transmission of HIV. Perinatal AIDS Collaborative Transmission Studies. *AIDS.* 1998;12: 301–308.
13. The Italian register for HIV Infection in Children. Rapid disease progression in HIV-1 perinatally infected children born to mothers receiving zidovudine monotherapy during pregnancy. *AIDS.* 1999;13:927–933.
14. European Collaborative Study. Exposure to antiretroviral therapy in utero or early life: the health of uninfected children born to HIV-infected women. *J Acquir Immune Defic Syndr.* 2003;32:380–387.
15. Jungmann EM, Mercey D, DeRuiter A, et al. Is first trimester exposure to the combination of antiretroviral therapy and folate antagonists a risk factor for congenital abnormalities? *Sex Transm Infect.* 2001;77:441–443.

16. Cooper ER, Charurat M, Mofenson L, et al. Combination antiretroviral strategies for the treatment of pregnant HIV-1-infected women and prevention of perinatal HIV-1 transmission. *J Acquir Immune Defic Syndr.* 2002;29:484–494.
17. Tuomala RE, Shapiro DE, Mofenson LM, et al. Antiretroviral therapy during pregnancy and the risk of an adverse outcome. *N Engl J Med.* 2002;346:1863–1870.
18. Arnold S, Degani N, King S. Lack of adverse events associated with pre- and postnatal antiretroviral therapy exposure: a retrospective review of 43 children followed up at 4-7 years of age. *AIDS Patient Care STDs.* 2003;17:53–55.
19. Mayaux MJ, Teglas JP, Blanche S; French Pediatric HIV Infection Study Group. Characteristics of HIV-infected women who do not receive preventive antiretroviral therapy in the French Perinatal Cohort. *J Acquir Immune Defic Syndr.* 2003;34:338–343.
20. European Collaborative Study; Swiss Mother and Child HIV Cohort Study. Combination antiretroviral therapy and duration of pregnancy. *AIDS.* 2000;14:2913–2920.
21. Lindegren ML, Rhodes P, Gordon L; Perinatal Safety Review Working Group, and State and Local Health Department HIV/AIDS Surveillance Programs. Drug safety during pregnancy and in infants. Lack of mortality related to mitochondrial dysfunction among perinatally HIV-exposed children in pediatric HIV surveillance. *Ann N Y Acad Sci.* 2000;918:222–235.
22. Villegas Castrejon H, Mayon Gonzalez J, Paredes Vivas Y, et al. Response of fetal macrophages in the placenta of pregnant HIV-positive patients with and without antiretroviral treatment (in Spanish). *Ginecol Obstet Mex.* 1999;67:196–206.
23. Lurie P, Wolfe SM. Unethical trials of interventions to reduce perinatal transmission of the human immunodeficiency virus in developing countries. *N Engl J Med.* 1997;337:853–856.
24. Poirier MC, Divi RL, Al-Harthi L, et al. Long-term mitochondrial toxicity in HIV-uninfected infants born to HIV-infected mothers. *JAIDS.* 2003;33:175–183.
25. ACOG Committee Opinion. Number 219, August 1999. Washington, DC: The American College of Obstetricians and Gynecologists.
26. Hernandez-Diaz S, Werler MM, Walker AM, et al. Folic acid antagonists during pregnancy and the risk of birth defects. *N Engl J Med.* 2000;343:1608–1614.
27. Hernandez-Diaz S, Werler MM, Walker AM, et al. Neural tube defects in relation to use of folic acid antagonists during pregnancy. *Am J Epidemiol.* 2001;153:961–968.
28. Czeizel AE, Rockenbauer M, Sorensen HT, Olsen J. The teratogenic risk of trimethoprim-sulfonamides: a population based case-control study. *Reprod Toxicol.* 2001;15:637–646.
29. Noguera A, Fortuny C, Muñoz-Almagro C, et al. Hyperlactatemia in human immunodeficiency virus-uninfected infants who are exposed to antiretrovirals. *Pediatrics.* 2004;114:e598–e603.
30. De Santis M, Cavaliere AF, Caruso A, et al. Hemangiomas and other congenital malformations in infants exposed to antiretroviral therapy in utero. *JAMA.* 2004;291:305.
31. Watts DH, Balasubramanian R, Maupin RT Jr, et al. Maternal toxicity and pregnancy complications in human immunodeficiency virus-infected women receiving antiretroviral therapy: PACTG 316. *Am J Obstet Gynecol.* 2004;190:506–516.
32. Tuomala RE, Watts DH, Li D, et al. Improved obstetrics outcomes and few maternal toxicities associated with antiretroviral therapy, including highly active antiretroviral therapy during pregnancy. *J Acquir Immune Defic Syndr.* 2005;38:449–473.
33. Hammer SM, Saag MS, Schechter M, et al. Treatment for adult HIV infection: 2006 recommendations of the International AIDS Society-USA panel. *JAMA.* 2006;296:827–843.
34. Antiretroviral Pregnancy Registry Steering Committee. The antiretroviral pregnancy registry interim report for 1 January 1989 through 31 January 2006. Registry Coordinating Center: Wilmington, NC, 2003. URL: *http://www.apregistry.com* Accessed: December 12, 2006.
35. Perinatal HIV Guidelines Working Group. Public Health Service Task Force recommendations for use of antiretroviral drugs in pregnant HIV-1-infected women for maternal health and interventions to reduce perinatal HIV-1 transmission in the United States. Rockville, MD: Public Health Service Task Force; 2005.
36. Talaie H, Nava-Ocampo AA, Koren G. Motherisk update: antiretroviral treatment of maternal HIV infection. *Can Fam Physician.* 2004;50:865–868.

CHAPTER 58

NEURODEVELOPMENT OF CHILDREN EXPOSED IN UTERO TO TREATMENT OF MATERNAL MALIGNANCY

I Nulman,[1,2,3,4] D Laslo,[1] S Fried,[4] E Uleryk,[3] M Lishner,[1] and G Koren[1,2,3,4]

[1]*Motherisk Program Division of Clinical Pharmacology/Toxicology;* [2]*Department of Pediatrics;* [3]*The Hospital for Sick Children and* [4]*University of Toronto, Toronto, Canada*

Summary. Cancer is the second most common cause of death during the reproductive years, complicating approximately 1/1000 pregnancies. The occurrence of cancer during gestation is likely to increase as a result of a woman's tendency to delay childbearing. Improved diagnostic techniques for malignancies increases detection of cancer during pregnancy. Malignant conditions during gestation are believed to be associated with an increase in poor perinatal and fetal outcomes that are often due to maternal treatment. Physicians should weigh the benefits of treatment against the risks of fetal exposure. To date, most reports have focused on morphologic observations made very close to the time of delivery with little data collected on children's long-term neurodevelopment following in utero exposure to malignancy and treatment. Because the brain differentiates throughout pregnancy and in early postnatal life, damage may occur even after first trimester exposure. The possible delayed effects of treatment on a child's neurological, intellectual and behavioural functioning have never been systematically evaluated. The goal of this report was to summarize all related issues into one review to facilitate both practitioners' and patients' access to known data on fetal risks and safety.

Keywords: malignancy; child development; antineoplastic medications; radiation; glucocorticoids; bromocriptine

METHODS

The data presented in this paper are based on a Medline search of the literature from 1966 to May 2001 and a Cancerlit search from 1983 to May 2001. Both searches were performed on Ovid Medline. The search strategy combined the following four concepts using available MeSH terms:

Concept 1 (exp pregnancy or exp pregnancy complication); and
Concept 2 (exp developmental disabilites or exp 'behaviour and behaviour mechanisms' or exp cognition disorders); and
Concept 3 (exp antibiotics, anthracycline or exp antibiotics, antineoplastic, exp antineoplastic agents, or antineoplastic agents, combined or exp antineoplastic agents, hormonal or exp antineoplastic and immunosuppressive agents or exp radioisotopes or exp anesthetics or prednisone or bromocriptine or glucocorticoids or exp estrogens); and
Concept 4 (exp neoplasms).

The search was not limited to specific languages, age groups or human studies. The studies were reviewed for details on fetal brain development evidenced postnatally by different physical, neurological and neurodevelopmental tests.

MATERNAL CANCER

Whether an association of maternal cancer with pregnancy has an undesirable effect on neurodevelopment in later childhood remains largely unknown. Metastasis to the placenta and/or fetus is very rare (Gililland and Weinstein, 1983; Potter, 1970). Melanoma is the most frequent of the few malignancies that do metastasize to the placenta and fetus (Gililland et al, 1983). Live born children exposed to such malignancies tend to die within a 1 day to 10 month period. Comprehensive reports about physical and mental health of the surviving children are not available.

The cancer patient has an increased tendency to experience febrile illnesses due to infections and/or as a result of the tumour itself. The relationship between hyperthermia, fetal brain development, and the incidence of impairment in human children has not been fully addressed. However, many human studies do support the hypothesis that maternal fever in early pregnancy is associated with an increased risk of NTDs and microphthalmia (Chambers et al, 1998; Miller et al, 1978; Layde et al, 1980; Clarren et al, 1979).

Malignancies may also be associated with maternal malnutrition and adverse neonatal outcome (Metcoff et al, 1981; Brown et al, 1981). Although animal studies have shown that severe maternal undernutrition can result in stillbirths and increased perinatal mortality, retrospective analyses of human data obtained during historical periods of starvation have shown little or no adverse fetal effects (Pritchard et al, 1985). Several studies have suggested that severe ketoacidosis due to dehydration or severe weight loss may pose an additional risk to the developing fetus (Naeye et al, 1981). On the other hand, analysis of males at age 19 born to mothers starved during pregnancy failed to document any differences in IQ score between these boys and the general male population (Stein et al, 1972).

SURGERY

Surgical interventions may be required for the evaluation and treatment of malignancies diagnosed in pregnancy. Each year about 0.5% to 2% of pregnant women in North America undergo surgery for reasons unrelated to their pregnancy and approximately 7000 to 30 000 of these women are in the first trimester of pregnancy (Sylvester et al, 1994), a critical time for the development of the central nervous system (CNS) (Webster et al, 1988). This is also the time period when the woman may not be aware of her pregnancy. Some women are occupationally exposed to anaesthetics throughout gestation. Little is known about neurodevelopmental outcomes due to exposure in either surgical or occupational conditions. During surgery the fetus is exposed to a potential risk from the effects of anaesthetic agents in addition to complications that may arise during or as a result of maternal surgery. Surgery in pregnancy is often associated with hypotension, hypoxia, coagulation, metabolic disturbances, and decreased utero-placental perfusion secondary to prolonged maintenance in the supine position. Each of these conditions can threaten fetal well being (Doll et al, 1988).

There are studies that establish the safety of the most commonly used anaesthetic agents during pregnancy, including nitrous oxide, enflurane, barbiturates, and narcotics (Schardein, 1985). Friedman (1988) reviewed possible teratogenic effects of general anaesthetics, local anaesthetics, and occupational exposure to anaesthetic gases. He concluded that data available on these agents do not suggest a major teratogenic risk in humans.

Kallen and Mazze (1990), in a case control study, assessed the pregnancy outcome of 2252 infants born to women who had surgery in the first trimester. Six neonates (expected number = 2.5) had a definite diagnosis of neural tube defect (NTD). Five of these 6 mothers were operated on in the fourth and fifth weeks of gestation, the window of exposure in which NTDs may take place. Sylvester (1994), in a large population-based case-controlled study, evaluated whether exposure to maternal general anaesthesia is associated with an increase in fetal CNS abnormalities. Twelve of 694 mothers with infants who had CNS defects reported having first trimester surgery with anaesthesia. Thirty-four of the 2984 controls were exposed to general anaesthesia at the same time of gestation (OR = 1.7, 95% CI-0.8,3.3). The strongest association was observed between exposure to anaesthesia and hydrocephalus, as well as eye defects. Although available studies have indicated that the CNS is the most sensitive organ to surgical and anaesthetic damage, none of the studies have addressed later childhood neurodevelopment or cognition. Functional CNS abnormalities may exist even when structural abnormalities are not observed.

MEDICATIONS

Cytotoxic Drugs

The common denominator of anti-cancer drugs is the ability to affect cell division adversely. Therefore, the same qualities that make those compounds desirable for cancer therapy, may also render them detrimental to the developing embryo. The dose of medication and time of exposure are critical during embryogenesis when susceptibility to teratogenic agents is high (Webster et al, 1988). A number of studies focused on congenital malformations at the time of delivery, and concluded that when chemotherapy is administered to women before conception or after the first trimester, in the majority of cases normal births are experienced (Harada, 1978; Gililland and Weinstein, 1983; Doll et al, 1988; Cantini and Yanes, 1984). These conclusions may not apply to the CNS, which develops throughout gestation and postnatally. Xenobiotics, including some heavy metals, ethanol and cocaine, are known to adversely affect CNS development during the second and third trimester (Koren et al, 1994; Harada, 1978).

Cognitive and behavioural functioning of children exposed in utero to chemotherapy at different periods of gestation remain largely undefined. Available data are based on small series and case reports. These reports suggest that gross and mental development of children exposed in utero to chemotherapy appears to be normal, but most authors did not conduct formal motor, cognitive and behavioural tests. As a result, they may have missed the opportunity to detect more subtle neurodevelopmental abnormalities. In case reports of women who were treated with a variety of chemotherapeutic agents and the developmental outcome was reported, the infants presented normal growth and developmental milestones at 3–21 months following delivery (Odom et al, 1990). However, Reynoso (1987) and Cantini (1984) reported 2 children with mental and or growth retardation born to mothers treated in pregnancy for acute leukaemia.

Presented below are the data concerning late effects of chemotherapy on children's neurodevelopment (Table 1). Blatt et al (1980) assessed retrospectively pregnancy outcome in patients who received aggressive moderate to high-dose combination chemotherapy for various oncologic diseases. Two patients conceived during treatment, which was continued for the first 2 months of gestation, and two other women started chemotherapy in the second and third trimester respectively. At the time of evaluation, the offspring ranged in age from several days to 12 years. Development was evaluated using the Denver Developmental Screening Test, and school performance was ascertained by history. Growth and development as well as school performance appeared to be normal in these children.

The peak incidence of Hodgkin's disease occurs during the reproductive years. Therefore, it is not surprising that there have been more reports on long-term follow-up for Hodgkin's disease than for other malignancies. Baisogolov and Shishkin (1985) reported on the pregnancy outcome of 78 retrospectively collected patients with Hodgkin's disease who delivered 89 children. The data were collected from the parents by local paediatricians. Twenty-one women conceived while undergoing chemotherapy. The psychomotor development of the case children was not different from that of the controls (children of healthy mothers). Seventeen out of 19 school-aged children were considered as 'good' or 'excellent' students. Twelve of these children were good in mathematics, 6 were in advanced programs to study foreign languages, 4 studied music, and 10 were good in sports. Another 7 children were gifted in other areas. A study conducted in Poland reported on the outcome of 20 pregnancies in 16 women with Hodgkin's disease (Balcewicz-Sablinska et al, 1990). In three pregnancies, cytostatic treatment was given after the first trimester. The course and labour of the observed pregnancies were normal. All babies were born healthy and were followed for a period of 6 years. The development of these children was reported to be normal, although formal psychological assessments were not performed.

The pregnancy outcome of women with haematologic malignancies, screened between 1970 and 1986, was presented by Aviles et al (1991). Forty-three children were born to 43 mothers who were treated with chemotherapy for non-Hodgkin's lymphoma, Hodgkin's disease, acute leukaemia, or chronic granulocytic leukaemia. Nineteen women received chemotherapy during the first trimester. The children's ages ranged from 3 to 19 years in 1989 at the time of testing. They were evaluated by physical and neurological examination in a 'blinded' manner. Evaluation of the children's school performance was obtained from their teachers. The Wechsler and Bender-Gestalt tests were administered to the children according to their ages, and the results were compared with those of 25 children of similar age and socioeconomic class. The children in the study group were not different from their controls in any of the measured tests.

Leukaemia occurs in approximately one out of 100 000 pregnancies (Caligiuri and Mayer, 1989). Aviles and Niz (1988) examined 17 offspring of patients with acute leukaemia treated during pregnancy. Chemotherapy was given during the pregnancy in each case, including 11 cases during the first trimester. The treatment of acute leukaemia was not modified due to the pregnancy and these

Table 1
In Utero Exposure to Chemotherapeutic Agents

INDICATION	AUTHORS	TIME OF EXPOSURE IN PREGNANCY	STUDY DESIGN	SAMPLE SIZE $n = 111$	AGE ASSESSED	MEDICATIONS	TESTS	RESULTS
Different forms of malignancies	Blatt et al, 1980	Preconceptionally or 1st trimester	Retrospective	4	1 month to 12 years old	Combined chemotherapy	Denver Developmental Screening Test. School reports	Normal development and school performance
Hodkin's disease	Baisogolov and Shishkin, 1985	–	Retrospective	19	1 to 14 years old	Combined chemotherapy	Parent and school reports	Normal development
Hodgkin's disease	Balcewicz-Sablinska et al, 1990	1st trimester	Retrospective	3	Up to age 6	MOPP	No formal testing	Normal development
Hodgkin's disease	Aviles et al, 1991	1st and 2nd trimesters	Retrospective, controlled	15	3 to 17 years	MOPP, ABVD	Wechsler and Bender-Gestalt cognitive tests. School report	Not different from controls
Haematological malignacies	Aviles et al, 1991	1st trimester, 2nd and 3rd trimester	Retrospective, controlled	43	3 to 19 years	Combination chemotherapy	Wechsler and Bender-Gestalt cognitive tests. School report	Not different from controls
Acute leukaemia	Aviles et al, 1988	1st trimester or sometime during pregnancy	Retrospective, controlled	17	4 to 22 years	Combination chemotherapy	Wechsler and Bender-Gestalt cognitive tests. School reports	Not different from controls
Rheumatic disease	Kozlowsky et al, 1990	1st trimester	Retrospective	5	3.7 to 16.7 years	Low-dose methotrexate	Parent reports	Normal development
Occupational exposure	Medkova 1991	Preconceptionally and/or during pregnancy	Retrospective, controlled	5	–	Low dose cytostatics	No formal testing	Normal development

patients received at least 80% of the planned dose. Neurological, intellectual and visual-motor-perceptual assessments were performed on the offspring (who ranged in ages between 4 to 22 years), their siblings, and unrelated controls. All children were given the Wechsler or the Bender–Gestalt test according to their age. No differences were detected between the groups on any of the tests. Kozlowski et al (1990) reviewed retrospectively the outcome of first-trimester exposure to low-dose methotrexate in eight patients with rheumatic disease. The duration of treatment ranged from 2 to 20 weeks of gestation. The women were given 7.5 to 10 mg methotrexate weekly. Five full-term live babies were born with a mean follow-up age of 11.5 years (range 3.7–16.7 years). All children reached normal growth and neurodevelopment. None of the children had learning disabilities. One child with speech impairment improved after speech therapy. Unfortunately, the methods of mental assessments were not reported.

The outcome of occupational chemotherapy exposure during pregnancy was addressed by Medkova (1991). The author reported on the pregnancy outcome and neurodevelopment of health personnel's children exposed to small doses of cytostatic medications. Sixty-one children were born to the healthcare workers on the oncology unit. In this group, exposure to antineoplastic agents was proven in five mothers and five fathers. Attention was paid to the children's physical development and possible incidence of dyslexia or dysgraphia. No abnormalities in these areas were found. Formal cognitive tests and statistical comparisons were not reported.

In summary, the data presented regarding late effects of chemotherapy on children's neurodevelopment are incomplete and are hampered by a lack of population-based, well designed studies. It is important to note that the paucity of neurobehavioural and cognitive studies in older children is due to limited late follow-up. The majority of available reports have focused on immediate maternal and fetal pregnancy outcomes, not considering later neu rodevelopment as a primary end point, thus using a crosssectional rather than longitudinal approach. The studies which did address long-term neurodevelopmental aspects typically used retrospective design in order to recruit a sufficient number of cases. Notwithstanding the limitations, these studies are very important as they represent the only existing source of information on the neurodevelopmental outcome of in utero exposure to cytotoxic therapy. The general impression, based on these reports, is that chemotherapy does not have a major impact on later child neurodevelopment. Methodologically, retrospective studies tend to show more adverse outcome than prospective studies, due to reporting bias (e.g.: parents of children with adverse outcome are more likely to report than those with normal outcome). Hence, negative retrospective studies are reassuring. With the increased use of cancer medications in nonmalignant conditions (e.g.: transplant, collagen diseases), it may be possible to recruit larger numbers of children for prospective, longitudinal studies and delineate abnormal outcomes induced by the malignancy itself.

Glucocorticoids

Glucocorticoids are part of the treatment protocol for many malignancies. They are also used as immunosupressive treatment in organ transplantation and for fetal lung maturation when preterm delivery is suspected. Most comprehensive studies on the neurodevelopmental effects of glucocorticoids were done in late pregnancy. Animal studies indicate that corticosteroids are associated with cognitive and behavioural abnormalities when administered during pregnancy. This has raised concerns about their use in humans (Trautman et al, 1995; Meaney et al, 1982; Angelucci et al, 1985). Table 2 presents the longterm effects of glucocorticoids used in gestation.

A prospective pilot study that investigated the long-term neurodevelopmental effects of prenatal exposure to dexamethasone (DEX) was conducted by Trautman et al (1995). The authors followed 26 children (ranging in age from 6 months to 5.5 years) whose mothers took DEX during pregnancy from weeks 1 to 21. The mothers took DEX for 2–29 weeks for the treatment of fetal risk for congenital adrenal hyperplasia (CAH). The offspring were compared with 14 children who were also at risk for CAH, but had not been exposed to DEX. The authors attempted to separate the effects of maternal disease by controlling for the same medical condition without treatment. The results indicated that DEX-exposed children were less likely to be cognitively delayed on a comprehension-conceptualization measure of development and that DEX-exposed 2- to 3-year-old children ($n = 14$) displayed more internalizing behaviour than unexposed children of the same age ($n = 4$). DEX-exposed children also exhibited a tendency to show higher avoidance behaviour and to be more shy and emotional and less sociable than unexposed children. No other significant differences were reported.

Pregnancy outcome and long-term follow-up with DEX used as an immunosuppressive agent taken throughout pregnancy for the treatment of lupus erythematosus (21 children) and heart transplant patients (29 children) were reported (Tincani et al, 1992; Wagoner et al, 1993). The authors indicated that the offspring were doing well at follow-up, but no formal cognitive or behavioural tests were conducted.

The literature on exposure to DEX in late pregnancy suggests that there are no significant cognitive differences between exposed and non-exposed children (MacArthur et al, 1982; Veszelovsky et al., 1981; Collaborative Group on Antenatal Steroid Therapy, 1984). The Collaborative Group on Antenatal Steroid Therapy (1984) was a prospective, randomized, placebo controlled, double-blinded study on the use of antenatal DEX for the prevention of respiratory distress syndrome in infants. The authors evaluated 200 children at 9, 18, and 36 months of age. The Bayley Scales and McCarthy Scales of Children's Abilities were used to assess cognitive and motor development. The results indicated that there were no significant differences in head circumference, cognitive, developmental or neurologic functioning between the placebo and the steroid treatment groups. The authors concluded that there were no detectable effects within the first 3 years of life in children who were exposed antenatally to DEX.

MacArthur et al (1982) conducted a double-blind, controlled study investigating the cognitive and psychosocial development of children whose mothers were treated antenatally with betamethasone during preterm labour. A total of 250 children, 139 in the betamethasone group and 111 in the control group, were studied through to age 7. The authors used well-established measures of cognitive, academic, and psychosocial development. Their results suggested that there were no significant differences in the cognitive or psychosocial development between the two groups.

The NIH Consensus Conference in 1994 (Anonymous, 1995) summarized data on the effects of corticosteroids for fetal maturation and perinatal outcomes. The results from available studies did not indicate any evidence of adverse long-term outcomes associated with the use of single doses of glucocorticoids for lung maturation in the areas of motor, cognitive, language, memory, concentration,

Table 2
Children Exposed in Utero to Glucocorticoids

INDICATION	AUTHOR	TIME OF EXPOSURE IN PREGNANCY	STUDY DESIGN	SAMPLE SIZE $n = 540$	AGE ASSESSED	SUBSTANCE	DURATION OF SUBSTANCE USE	TESTS	RESULTS
Lung maturation **in Hungarian	Veszelovszky et al, 1981	3rd trimester	Retrospective, controlled	125	12–36 months	Dexamethasone		Neurological and psychological	No difference from the control group
Fetal lung maturation	MacArthur et al, 1981 and 1982	3rd trimester	Prospective, controlled	139	Age 4 and 6	Betamethasone		Stanford-Binet Intelligence Scale, Frostig Visual Perception Test, Vineland Social Maturity Scale, Illinois Test of Psycholinguistic Abilities, Peabody Vocabulary Test, Raven's Matrices, Bender-Gestalt Test	No difference from the control group
Fetal lung maturation	Collaborative Group on Antenatal Steroid Therapy (1984)	3rd trimester	Prospective, randomized, placebo controlled, double-blind	200	36 months	Dexamethasone		Bayley Scales, McCarthy Scales	No difference from the control group
Fetal lung maturation	NIH Consensus Conference, 1995	3rd trimester	Analysis of available data		up to age 12	Corticosteroids			No increased risk of long-term neuro-developmental impairment
Maternal SLE	Tincani et al, 1992	Throughout pregnancy	Prospective	21	1–85 months	Fluocortolone plus aspirin and azathioprine (if needed)		No formal tests	No long-term consequences
Maternal heart transplants	Wagoner et al, 1993	During pregnancy	Prospective	29	3 months to 6.5 years	Corticosteroids plus other immuno-suppresives		No formal tests	All children reported to be in good health
Fetal congenital adrenal hyperplasia	Trautman et al, 1995	Started from week 1 to 21 weeks of gestation	Porspective, controlled pilot study	26	6 months to 5.5 years	Dexamethasone	2–29 weeks	Denver Developmental Questionnaire, Minnesota Child Development Inventory, Child Behaviour Checklist, Temperament Questionnaire, EAS Temperament Survey	More shy, emotional, less sociable, and a trend for greater avoidance than control group. No differences in cognitive abilities.

or scholastic achievement skills. There is however evidence that repeated doses, similar to what is encountered in cancer chemotherapy are associated with microcephaly and low birth weight.

The results of a prospective control study by French et al (1999) point to a reduction in head circumference when repeated courses of corticosteroids were given in late pregnancy. Although smaller head circumference may be associated with impaired cognitive outcome, the investigator did not report cognitive impairment.

In conclusion, although the literature on the impact of corticosteroids administration in pregnancy on fetal development is reassuring, more information is required on long-term effects of these substances on the CNS development.

Bromocriptine

Bromocriptine is an alkaloid that functions as a dopamine receptor agonist suppressing prolactine production and is the treatment of choice for pituitary tumours during pregnancy. Pregnancy outcome and children's functioning in long-term follow-up (up to age 9 years) in hundreds of children exposed in utero to bromocriptine were reported (Turkalj et al, 1982; Konopka et al, 1983; Nader, 1990) with no significant findings. However, no reports of formal tests of cognitive and behavioural functioning are available.

RADIATION

Radiation is widely used in the diagnosis and treatment of malignancies. Based on live birth rate statistics in the US, about 33 000 women each year are exposed to diagnostic abdominal radiation in early pregnancy (US Department of Health and Human Services, 1976). The developing embryo and fetus are extremely sensitive to ionizing radiation (Brent, 1980). Fetal structures exhibit various susceptibilities to ionizing radiation and the human brain seems to be the most sensitive organ. The CNS maintains its sensitivity to radiation throughout gestation and into the neonatal period, when morphological changes can still be observed. Ionizing radiation is a CNS teratogen and is a recognized cause of mental retardation. It has been suggested to be a more serious fetal risk than maternal cancer following in utero exposure (Hoel, 1987). The lowest dose of radiation that produces significant behavioural changes postnatally at any gestational day is 0.2 Gy (Schull et al, 1990).

Although radiation is one of the most studied environmental hazards in animal species, there are very few human studies available. Brent (1980) hypothesized that a radiation dose as low as 50 rad (0.5 Gy) in humans may be harmful to the fetus, especially to its CNS. Dekaban (1968), in a retrospective analysis, reported that 22 infants who were exposed to radiation in the third to twentieth week of gestation for treatment purposes, were microcephalic and/or mentally retarded. Woo et al (1992) reported results of 16 women treated for nodular sclerosing Hodgkin's disease. Seven women were treated during the first trimester, 10 in the second, and 8 in the third. Sixteen women received 35–40 Gy for supradiaphragmatic nodes. The uterus was shielded by a 4 to 5 hold-value layer of lead. The estimated dose to the mid-fetus ranged from 1.4 to 5.5 cGY for 6 MV photons and 10 to 13.6 cGY for cobalt 60. All 16 patients subsequently delivered full-term normal infants, who, at the time of assessment, were found to be physically and mentally normal. Formal cognitive tests were not reported.

The experience at Hiroshima and Nagasaki is the most commonly sited source of knowledge considering long-term effects of radiation on the human embryo and fetus. These population based studies addressed relationships between dose of radiation and gestational age. Analysis of the data of survivors of the atomic bombings in Japan using refined estimates of the absorbed fetal dose demonstrated that the highest risk of brain damage occurred at 8–15 weeks of gestational age (Otake and Schull, 1984). These data were consistent with a linear dose-response model, which did not indicate the existence of a threshold level.

In contrast, the data collected for in utero exposures after the fifteenth week of gestation were not linearly related to dose, suggesting that a nonlinear model with a threshold dose for radiation effects best fits the data for this period of gestation. Radiation exposure before the eighth week of gestation and after the twenty-fifth week was not associated with an increased risk of mental retardation. Yoshimaru et al (1991) assessed school performance of prenatally exposed survivors of the atomic bombings using the DS86 dosimetry system and found that damage to the fetus exposed at 16–25 weeks after fertilization appeared similar to that seen in the 8–15 week group. Other studies of this population also suggest that radiation exposure in utero may affect intelligence test scores, with the greatest sensitivity during the eighth to fifteenth week of gestation (Mettler et al, 1985). One estimate of the doseresponse relationship was a 20-point loss of IQ for each additional 1 Gy of exposure. The relationship between dose and intelligence test scores is not yet well-established, and the findings have to be refined to a demonstrable level of statistical significance or clinical relevance (Mettler et al, 1985). Jensh and Brent (1987) demonstrated a downward shift in the Gaussian distribution of IQ with an estimated probability coefficient indicating a loss of 30 IQ points per 1 Gy fetal dose at 8–15 weeks after conception. A similar, but smaller shift to lower intelligence was detectable following exposure at 6–25 weeks of gestation, but not at other periods of pregnancy. Several reports did not find mental retardation in 19 children exposed to 0.015 and 0.1 Gy and among 1458 children exposed to low diagnostic doses of radiation (Meyer and Tonascia, 1981). However, behavioural tests were not performed and these results should be interpreted with caution because of methodological limitations of the study design. Conversely, in a case control study, Granoth (1979) assessed the association of diagnostic X-ray examinations with the occurrence of CNS defects and found a significant increase in anencephaly, hydrocephaly, and microcephaly when the study group is compared with matched control infants. The cognitive and behavioural effects of low-dose prenatal diagnostic radiation has not been elucidated. As well, it is unknown whether there are behavioural sequelae due to exposure to radiation in the area of the electromagnetic spectrum. To date it is believed that fetal exposure to less than 0.05 Gy does not increase the teratogenic risk (Jensh and Brent, 1986).

In summary, ionizing radiation fulfills all of Wilson's criteria for a teratogen (Vorhees, 1986). Being neurotropic, radiation is capable of producing behavioural teratogenic effects that are demonstrable at doses below those causing obvious structural malformations (Vorhees, 1986).

In addition to the classic triad produced by a teratogenic substance, ionizing radiation was observed to cause obvious behavioural alternations in animals. As suggested by Jensh and Brent (1986) the inseparable radiation teratogenic effect on behaviour must be added to the triad thus creating a 'tetrad'.

CONCLUSION

Malignancy poses a difficult challenge to both patients and physicians, creating a conflict between optimal maternal therapy and fetal well-being. However, most malignant conditions are not absolute contraindications for pregnancy. Unfortunately, neurodevelopmental and behavioural effects, both important parts of the teratogenic spectrum regarding drug or treatment safety, have been only sparsely addressed. Mental health effects, which act as strong predictors of a child's quality of life, merit closer attention, as does the cognitive and behavioural effects of these drugs. At the present time little is known on the long term mental health effects in young children exposed in utero to treatment for maternal cancer. However, existing studies on cancer chemotherapy beyond the first trimester have failed to show neurotoxicity. In contrast, repeated doses of corticosteroids and radiation are definitely teratogenic. Further research is required to assess the behavioural teratology of cancer and its management.

REFERENCES

Angelucci L, Patacchioli FR, Scaccianoce S, Di Sciull A, Maccari S and Cardillo A (1985) A model for later-life effects of perinatal drug exposure: Maternal hormone mediation. *Neurobehav Toxicol Teratol* 7: 511–517.

Anonymous (1995) Effect of corticosteroids for fetal maturation on perinatal outcomes. NIH Consensus Development Panel on the Effect of Corticosteroids for Fetal Maturation on Perinatal Outcomes. *JAMA* **273:** 413–418.

Aviles A and Niz J (1988) Long-term follow-up of children born to mothers with acute leukemia during pregnancy. *Med Pediatr Oncol* **16:** 3–6.

Aviles A, Zepeda G and Cruz J (1991) Hodgkin's disease during pregnancy. Study of late effects in the newborn. *Bol Med Hosp Infant Mex* **48:** 622–626.

Baisogolov GD and Shishkin IP (1985) Course of pregnancy and condition of infants born to patients treated for lymphogranulomatosis [Russian]. *Med Radiol (Mosk)* **30:** 35–37.

Balcewicz-Sablinska K, Ciesluk S, Kopec I, Slomkowski M and Maj S (1990) Analysis of pregnancy, labor, child development and disease course in women with Hodgkin's disease. *Acta Haematol Pol* **21:** 72–80.

Blatt J, Mulvihill JJ, Ziegler JL, Yong RC and Poplack DG (1980) Pregnancy outcome following cancer chemotherapy *Am J Med* **69:** 828–832.

Brent RL (1980) Radiation teratogenesis. *Teratology* **21:** 281–298.

Brown JE, Jacobson HN, Askue LH and Peick MG (1981) Influence of pregnancy weight gain on the size of infants born to underweight women. *Obstet Gynecol* **57:** 13–17.

Caligiuri MA and Mayer RJ (1989) Pregnancy and Leukemia. *Semin Oncol* **16:** 388–396.

Cantini E and Yanes B (1984) Acute myelogenous leukemia in pregnancy. *South Med J* **77:** 1050–1052.

Chambers CD, Johnson KA, Dick LM, Felix RJ and Jones KL (1998) Maternal fever and birth outcome: a prospective study. *Teratology* **58:** 251–257.

Clarren SK, Smith DW, Harvey MA and Ward KH (1979) Hyperthermia: a prospective evaluation of a possible teratogenic agent in man. *J Pediatr* **95:** 81–83.

Collaborative Group on Antenatal Steroid Therapy (1984) Effects of antenatal dexamethasone administration in the infant: long-term follow-up. *J Pediatr* **104:** 259–267.

Dekaban AS (1968) Abnormalities in children exposed to x-radiation during various stages of gestation: tentative timetable of radiation injury to the human fetus. *J Nucl Med* **9:** 412–477.

Doll DC, Ringenberg QS and Yarbo JW (1988) Management of cancer during pregnancy. *Arch Intern Med* **148:** 2058–2064.

French NP, Hagan R, Evans SF, Godfrey MRN and Newnham J (1999) Repeated antenatal corticosteroids: Size at birth and subsequent development. *Am J Obstet Gynecol* **180:** 114–121.

Friedman JM (1988) Teratogen update: anesthetic agents. *Teratology* **37:** 69–77.

Gililland J and Weinstein L (1983) The effects of cancer chemotherapeutic agents on the developing fetus. *Obstet Gynecol Surv* **38:** 6–13.

Granoth G (1979) Defects of the central nervous system in Finland. IV Associations with diagnostic X-ray examinations. *Am J Obstet Gynecol* **133:** 191–194.

Harada M (1978) Congenital Minamata disease: intrauterine methylmercury poisoning. *Teratology* **18:** 285–288.

Hoel DG (1987) Radiation risk estimation models. *Environ Health Perspect* **75:** 105–107.

Jensh RP and Brent RL (1986) Effects of 0.6-Gy prenatal X irradiation on postnatal neurophysiologic development in the Wistar rat. *Proc Soc Exp Biol Med* **181:** 611–619.

Jensh RP and Brent RL (1987) The effect of low level prenatal X-irradiation on postnatal development in the Wistar rat. *Proc Soc Exp Biol Med* **184:** 256–263.

Kallen B and Mazze RI (1990) Neural tube defects and first trimester operations. *Teratology* **41:** 717–720.

Konopka P, Raymond JP, Merceron RE and Seneze J (1983) Continuous administration of bromocriptine in the prevention of neurological complications in pregnant women with prolactinomas. *Am J Obstet Gynecol* **146:** 935–938.

Koren G and Nulman I (1994) Teratogenic Drugs and Chemicals in Humans. In: *Maternal Fetal Toxicology: Clinician's Guide*, 2nd edn, Koren G (ed.) pp 33–48. Marcel Dekker: New York.

Kozlowski RD, Steinbrunner JV and MacKenzie AH (1990) Outcome of first-trimester exposure to low-dose methotrexate in eight patients with rheumatic disease. *Am J Med* **88:** 589–592.

Layde PM, Edmonds LD and Erickson JD (1980) Maternal fever and neural tube defects. *Teratology* **21:** 105–108.

MacArthur BA, Howie RN, Dezoete JA and Elkins J (1982) School progress and cognitive development of 6-year old children whose mothers were treated antenatally with betamethasone. *Pediatrics* **70:** 99–105.

Meaney MJ, Stewart J and Beatty WW (1982) The influence of glucocorticoids during the neonatal period on the development of play-fighting in Norway rat pups. *Horm Behav* **16:** 475–491.

Medkova J (1991) Analysis of the health condition of the children born to the personnel exposed to cytostatics at an oncology unit. *Acta Univ Palacki Olomuc Fac Med* **130:** 323–332.

Metcoff J, Costiloe JP, Crosby W, Bentle L, Seshachalam D, Sandstead HH, Bodwell CE, Weaver F and McClain P (1981)

Maternal nutrition and fetal outcome. *Am J Clin Nutr* **34:** 708–721 (Suppl 4).

Mettler FA and Moseley RD (1985) *Medical Effects of Ionizing Radiation* pp 206–209. Grune & Stratton: New York.

Meyer MB and Tonascia J (1981) Long term effects of prenatal x-ray of human females. *Am J Epidemiol* **114:** 317–326.

Miller P, Smith DW and Shepard TH (1978) Maternal hyperthermia as a possible cause for anencephaly. *Lancet* **1:** 519–521.

Nader S (1990) Pituitary disorders and pregnancy. *Semin Perinatol* **14:** 24–33.

Naeye RL and Chez RA (1981) Effects of maternal acetonuria and low pregnancy weight gain on children's psychomotor development. *Am J Obstet Gynecol* **139:** 189–193.

Odom LD, Plouffe L and Butler WJ (1990) 5-Fluorouracil exposure during the period of conception: Report on two cases. *Am J Obstet Gynecol* **163:** 76–77.

Otake M and Schull WJ (1984) In utero exposure to A-bomb radiation and mental retardation: a reassessment. *Br J Radiol* **57:** 409–414.

Potter JF and Schoeneman M (1970) Metastasis of maternal cancer to the placenta and fetus. *Cancer* **25:** 380–388.

Pritchard JA, MacDonald PC and Gant NF (1985) *Williams Obstetrics*, 17th edn. Appleton-Century-Crofts: Norwalk, CT.

Reynoso EE, Sheperd FA, Messner HA, Farquharson HA, Garvey MB and Baker MA (1987) Acute leukemia during pregnancy: the Toronto Leukemia.

Study group experience with long-term follow-up of children exposed in utero to chemotherapeutic agents. *J Clin Oncol* **5:** 1098–1106.

Schardein JL (1985) Cancer chemotherapeutic agents. In: *Chemically Induced Birth Defects*, Schardein JL (ed.) pp 467. Marcel Dekker: NY and Basel.

Schull WJ, Norton S and Jensh RP (1990) Ionizing radiation and the developing brain. *Neurotoxicol Teratol* **12:** 249–260

Stein Z, Susser M, Saenger G and Marolla F (1972) Nutrition and mental performance. *Science* **178:** 708–713.

Sylvester GC, Khoury MJ, Lu X and Erickson D (1994) First-trimester anesthesia exposure and the risk of central nervous system defects: A population-based case-control study. *Am J Public Health* **84:** 1757–1760.

Tincani A, Faden D, Tarantini M, Lojacono A, Tanzi P, Gastaldi A, Di Mario C, Spatola L, Cattaneo R and Balestrieri G (1992) SLE and pregnancy: a prospective study. *Clin Exp Rheumatol* **10:** 439–446.

Trautman PD, Meyer-Bahlburg HF, Postelnek J and New MI (1995) Effects of early prenatal dexamethasone on the cognitive and behavioral development of young children: results of a pilot study. *Psychoneuroendocrinology* **20:** 439–449.

Turkalj I, Braun P and Krupp P (1982) Surveillance of bromocriptine in pregnancy. *JAMA* **247:** 1589–1591.

US Department of Health and Human Services: Vital Statistics of the Unites Stat, 1976. Bol. Natality. Hyattsville, MD, National Center for Health Statistics, 1980.

Veszelovszky I, Farkasinszky T, Nogy J, Bodis L and Szilard J (1981) Psychological and neurosomatic follow-up studies of children of mother treated with dexamethasone. *Orv Hetil* **122:** 629–631.

Vorhees CV (1986) Principles of behavioural teratology. In: *Handbook of Behavioural Teratology*, Riley EP and Vorhees CV (eds) pp 23–48. Plenum Press: New York.

Wagoner LE, Taylor DO, Olsen SL, Price GD, Rasmussen LG, Larsen CB, Scott JR and Renlund DG (1994) Immunosuppressive therapy, management, and outcome of heart transplant recipients during pregnancy. *J Heart Lung Transplant* **12:** 993–1000.

Webster WS, Lipson AH and Sulik KK (1988) Interference with gastrulation during the third week of pregnancy as a cause of some facial abnormalities and CNS defects. *Am J Med Genet* **31:** 505–512.

Woo SY, Fuller LM, Cundiff JH, Bondy ML, Hagemeister FB, McLanghlin P, Velasquez WS, Swan F, Rodriguez MA and Cabanillas F (1992) Radiotherapy during pregnancy for clinical stages IA-IIA Hodgkin's disease. *Int J Radiat Oncol Biol Phys* **23:** 407–412.

Yoshimaru H, Otake M, Fujikoshi Y and Schull WJ (1991) Effect on school performance of prenatal exposure to Hiroshima atomic bomb. *Nippon Eiseigaku Zasshi* **46:** 747–754.

Reprinted from Nulman I, Laslo D, Fried S, Uleryk E, Lishner M, Koren G. Neurodevelopment of children exposed in utero to treatment of maternal malignancy. Br J Cancer 2001; 85: 1611–8 with permission.

CHAPTER 59

BENZODIAZEPINE USE IN PREGNANCY AND MAJOR MALFORMATIONS OR ORAL CLEFT: META-ANALYSIS OF COHORT AND CASE-CONTROL STUDIES

Lisa R. Dolovich, Antonio Addis, J M Régis Vaillancourt, J D Barry Power, Gideon Koren, and Thomas R. Einarson

Faculty of Pharmacy, University of Toronto, Toronto, Ontario, Canada M5S 2S2
Lisa Dolovich, PharmD candidate
J M Régis Vaillancourt, PharmD candidate
J D Barry Power, PharmD candidate
MotheRisk Program, Division of Clinical Pharmacology and Toxicology, Hospital for Sick Children, University of Toronto, Toronto, Ontario, Canada M5G 1X8
Antonio Addis, research fellow
Gideon Koren, director of MotheRisk and clinical pharmacology
Faculty of Pharmacy, Hospital for Sick Children, University of Toronto, Toronto, Ontario, Canada M5S 2S2
T R Einarson, professor of social and administrative pharmacy

Abstract

Objective. To determine if exposure to benzodiazepines during the first trimester of pregnancy increases risk of major malformations or cleft lip or palate.
Design. Meta-analysis.
Setting. Studies from 1966 to present.
Subjects. Studies were located with Medline, Embase, Reprotox, and from references of textbooks, reviews, and included articles. Included studies were original, concurrently controlled studies in any language.
Interventions. Data extraction and quality assessment were done independently and in duplicate.
Main outcome measures. Maternal exposure to benzodiazepines in at least the first trimester; incidence of major malformations or oral cleft alone, measured as odds ratios and 95% confidence intervals with a random effects model.
Results. Of over 1400 studies reviewed, 74 were retrieved and 23 included. In the analysis of cohort studies fetal exposure to benzodiazepine was not associated with major malformations (odds ratio 0.90; 95% confidence interval 0.61 to 1.35) or oral cleft (1.19; 0.34 to 4.15). Analysis of case-control studies showed an association between exposure to benzodiazepines and development of major malformations (3.01; 1.32 to 6.84) or oral cleft alone (1.79; 1.13 to 2.82).
Conclusions. Pooled data from cohort studies showed no association between fetal exposure to benzodiazepines and the risk of major malformations or oral cleft. On the basis of pooled data from case-control studies, however, there was a significant increased risk for major malformations or oral cleft alone. Until more research is reported, level 2 ultrasonography should be used to rule out visible forms of cleft lip.

INTRODUCTION

Benzodiazepines are commonly used for anxiety, insomnia, and epilepsy. Their use is substantial, even by pregnant women. Bergman et al found that 2% of pregnant women in the United States who were receiving Medicaid benefits filled one or more prescriptions for benzodiazepines during pregnancy.[1] As about half of pregnancies in the United States are unplanned,[2] many women may inadvertently expose the fetus to benzodiazepines during the first trimester. Therefore, women require valid information regarding the risks of benzodiazepine use during pregnancy to avoid exposure to teratogens but also to ensure that they are not denied medication during pregnancy because of unfounded fear of unknown consequences.

Antepartum exposures to benzodiazepines have been associated with teratogenic effects (for instance, facial cleft, skeletal anomalies) in some animal studies[3 4] but not others.[5 6] Early case-control studies in humans found that maternal benzodiazepine exposure increased the risk of fetal cleft lip and cleft palate.[7 8] Subsequent reports implicated benzodiazepines as the cause of major malformations[9–11] and a benzodiazepine syndrome similar to fetal alcohol syndrome.[9 12 13] Numerous studies, however, have refuted these findings.[1 14–16] These contradictory results have led to considerable controversy surrounding the use of benzodiazepines in pregnancy. We carried out a meta-analysis to examine whether exposure to benzodiazepines during at least the first trimester is associated with increased risk of major malformations or oral cleft.

METHODS

Data Sources

We systematically searched Medline (1966 to December 1997 via Ovid), Embase (1980 to December 1997), Reprotox (a database of reviews on reproductive toxicity topics), references in textbooks on drugs in pregnancy, references of included studies, and review articles. "Benzodiazepine(s)" (exploded as a subject heading or the various preparations put in as textwords) was combined with the following words as subject headings or textwords: fetal diseases, infant, fetal organ maturity, cleft lip, cleft palate, major malformations, and prenatal exposure.

The Toronto based MotheRisk Program, a consultation service for drug, chemical, and radiation exposure during pregnancy, helped to locate unpublished papers and provided one unpublished study and one abstract. The original authors provided unpublished data.

Study Selection

Searches were reviewed or completed independently and in duplicate. Cohort or case-control studies in any language considered pertinent were retrieved and included if they examined the relation between human maternal exposure to benzodiazepines in at least the first trimester and major malformations or oral cleft alone and included an unexposed concurrent control group. Major malformations were those described by Heinonen et al, which, among others, include cleft palate and cleft lip.[17] Hereafter "oral cleft" is used for cleft lip or cleft palate, or both. Studies examining only certain subtypes of malformations or studies in patients with epilepsy were included but considered separately from the main analysis. Only studies where exposure occurred during the first trimester were considered as the fetus is most susceptible to teratogens during the period between the 1st and 8th weeks of organogenesis, the lip forms between weeks 4 and 8, and the oral palate forms between weeks 5 and 12. Studies were excluded if they were case series or reports, editorials, reviews, animal studies or used only stillbirths or abortions or the data could not be extracted.

All published studies deemed suitable were retrieved. Unpublished studies were treated methodologically in the same way as published studies. The methods sections with study identifiers removed were reviewed independently and in duplicate to determine inclusion. Consensus or a third party whose decision was final resolved disagreements.

Data Extraction

Once the study was included data were extracted and quality assessed independently and in duplicate. Discrepancies were resolved through consensus. Study quality was assessed by using predetermined criteria. These aspects of study quality are provided in the results section as descriptive information.

Data Analysis

Studies of different design—namely, cohort and case-control studies—were analysed separately because of differing threats to their internal validity.[18 19] Data were analysed by calculating the odds ratio and 95% confidence interval with a random effects model.[20] We also calculated χ^2 tests for heterogeneity.[21] Further sensitivity analyses were performed for case-control studies to assess the impact of recall bias through the use of normal babies compared with malformed babies as controls.

In a further examination of homogeneity of effects we plotted the data with the rates of malformations in the control groups on the X axis and in the exposed subjects on the Y axis as suggested by L'Abbé et al.[22] We first visually inspected the plot for evidence of obvious outliers. We then regressed the malformation rate in the exposed group on that of the controls. The slope of that regression line was compared with the null hypothesis (that is, a slope of 1) by using standard techniques as a test for effects. We also examined residuals to determine if any observations were outliers (that is, > 1.96 SE) from a statistical point of view. Publication bias was examined through visual inspection of a funnel plot whereby odds ratios were plotted against study sample size.

RESULTS

Over 1400 studies were considered. Most were not retrieved because two independent reviewers considered that they did not relate to the question under review. Of the studies considered, 74 studies were retrieved and 51 of these were excluded. Studies were excluded because they had no concurrent control group (18), they did not examine major malformations (9), they were carried out on animals (1), benzodiazepines were not studied (1), exposure was not during the first trimester (1), studies were review articles or commentaries (5), data presented were duplicated in an included trial (6), results for benzodiazepines were not reported separately from other agents (5), only a range of results were reported (1), only partial data were provided (2), benzodiazepine exposure was not linked to malformations (1), and the study was not available in North America (1). A complete list of excluded studies is available from the authors. Thirteen studies that examined major malformations,[11 13 14 23–32] 11 studies that examined oral cleft alone,[1 7 10 13 27 30 31 33–36] and three studies that examined other specific malformations[37–39] were included (some providing information for more than one evaluation). One study unpublished at the time of consideration has since been published.[26]

Of the 23 included studies, 20 (87%) predefined exposure[1 10 11 13 14 23 25-28 30-39] and 22 (96%) predefined the outcome.[1 7 10 11 13 14 23 25–32 34–40] Exposure was ascertained mainly through interview with the mother (61% of studies)[7 10 14 25–30 33 34 36 38] and outcome was confirmed mainly by using physician examination or records (44% of studies)[11 13 14 25 28 30 32 34 39 40] or malformation registries (30% of studies).[7 10 29 31 35–37] Equal diagnostic examination between exposed and unexposed groups occurred in all but three studies.[14 25 35] Hartz et al gathered and confirmed information about malformed babies from different sources but did not do so for control babies.[14] Czeizel et al sent surveys to up to three controls if initial controls did not respond.[35] Laegreid et al used blood samples to confirm benzodiazepine exposure and had blood sample results for 78% of cases but only 66% of controls.[25]

Various benzodiazepines were used or prescribed, although 48% of the studies (11/23) examined the use of chlordiazepoxide or diazepam only.[10 11 14 23 28 30 32–34 37 40] Only two studies provided any information regarding the duration of maternal exposure.[25 26] The indications for use were infrequently provided.[11 25 26 41] Sixty one percent (14/23) of studies reported concurrent use of at least some prescription medications.[1 10 11 13 25 26 28–32 37–39]

Associations with Major Malformations

Data pooled from seven cohort studies did not show an association between fetal exposure to benzodiazepines during pregnancy and major malformations (odds ratio 0.90; 95% confidence interval 0.61 to 1.35; homogeneity $\chi^2 = 1.74$; $P = 0.62$; table 1, figure 1).[11 14 23–27] Two cohort studies carried out in patients with epilepsy were located. Results of both were not significant.[30 31]

Combination of four case-control studies showed that major malformations were associated with the use of benzodiazepines during pregnancy (3.01; 1.32 to 6.84; $\chi^2 = 9.87$; $P = 0.008$).[13 28 29 32]

Table 1
Association of Major Malformations in Fetuses with Prenatal Benzodiazepine Exposure

	EXPOSED		NOT EXPOSED		
FIRST AUTHOR (YEAR)	NO MALFORMED	TOTAL	NO MALFORMED	TOTAL	ODDS RATIO (95% CI)
Cohort studies					
Non-epileptic patients:					
Milkovich (1974)[11]	5	86	10	229	1.35 (0.45 to 4.07)
Crombie (1975)[23]	3	200	382	19 143	0.75 (0.24 to 2.35)
Hartz (1975)[14]	11	257	2179	46 233	0.90 (0.49 to 1.66)
Kullander (1976)[24]	2	89	198	5 664	0.63 (0.16 to 2.60)
Laegreid (1992)[25]	1	17	1	29	1.75 (0.10 to 29.92)
Pastuszak (1996)[26]	1	106	3	115	0.36 (0.04 to 3.47)
Ornoy (1997)[27]	9	335	10	363	0.97 (0.39 to 2.43)
Combined effect					0.90 (0.61 to 1.35)*
Epileptic patients:					
Nakane (1980)[30]	16	117	42	490	1.69 (0.91 to 3.13)
Robert (1986)[31]	0	4	8	144	1.78 (0.09 to 35.94)
Case-control studies					
Greenberg (1977)[29]	36	60	800	1 612	1.52 (0.9 to 2.58)
Bracken (1981)[28]	39	72	1331	4 266	2.61 (1.63 to 4.16)
Noya (1981)[32]	1	24	0	24	3.13 (0.12 to 80.68)
Laegreid (1990)[13]	8	10	10	68	23.20 (4.29 to 125.55)
Combined effect					3.01 (1.32 to 6.84)†

* $\chi^2 = 1.74$; $P = 0.62$.
† $\chi^2 = 9.87$; $P = 0.008$.

All included case-control studies that evaluated major malformations used normal babies as controls so subgroup analyses based on types of controls could not be done. Regression analyses for both cohort and case-control studies showed no obvious heterogeneity.

Associations with Oral Cleft

Data pooled from three cohort studies showed no relation between fetal exposure to benzodiazepines during pregnancy and oral cleft (1.19; 0.34 to 4.15; $\chi^2 = 0.01$; $P = 0.997$; table 2, figure 2).[1 27 33] The analysis of six case-control studies produced a significant odds ratio for oral cleft of 1.79 (1.13 to 2.82; $\chi^2 = 11.39$; $P = 0.01$).[7 10 13 34–36] Subgroup analysis of the case-control studies with normal babies as controls showed no significant association with oral cleft (1.63; 0.89 to 2.96; $\chi^2 = 3.81$; $P = 0.15$).[7 13 35] Similarly, no significant association was found in analyses of case-control studies with malformed babies as controls (2.03; 0.88 to 4.71; $\chi^2 = 6.90$; $P = 0.10$).[10 34 36] Regression analyses for both cohort and case-control studies showed no obvious heterogeneity.

In general, for the analyses of major malformation and oral cleft the risks for case-control studies were grouped at a different end of the distribution than the risks for cohort studies, showing that the relative risks within each study design are of the same magnitude but the absolute differences in risk are of a different order of magnitude between studies (case-control about 10 times greater than cohort). This finding suggests a possible systematic difference between study designs. Funnel plot analyses produced funnel shaped plots, indicating that there was no obvious publication bias.

Two case-control studies examined the association of benzodiazepine use with fetal cardiac malformations. One showed no association between exposure and outcome; the other did.[37 38] One study examined benzodiazepine use with malformations of the central nervous system and did not find any association between exposure and outcome.[39]

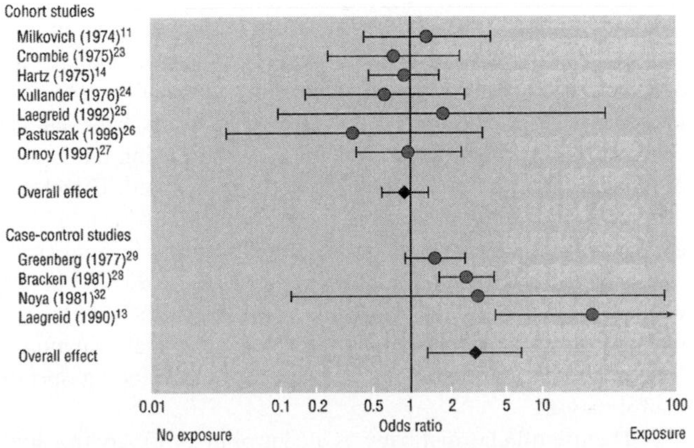

Figure 1. Association of major malformations with prenatal exposure to benzodiazepines.

DISCUSSION

Data taken from cohort studies showed no significant association between benzodiazepines taken during the first trimester and either

Table 2
Results of Studies Examining Association of Specific Malformations with Prenatal Exposure to Benzodiazepines

AUTHOR (YEAR)	EXPOSED NO MALFORMED	EXPOSED TOTAL	NOT EXPOSED NO MALFORMED	NOT EXPOSED TOTAL	ODDS RATIO (95% CI)
Cohort studies (oral cleft)					
Non-epileptic patients:					
Shiono (1984)[33]	1	854	31	32 395	1.22 (0.17 to 8.98)
Bergman (1992)[1]	0	1354	62	102 985	1.21 (0.17 to 8.71)
Ornoy (1997)[27]	0	335	0	363	1.08 (0.07 to 17.39)
Combined effect					1.19 (0.34 to 4.15)*
Epileptic patients:					
Nakane (1980)[30]	3	117	12	490	1.05 (0.29 to 3.78)
Robert (1986)[31]	0	4	1	144	10.63 (0.38 to 298.57)
Case-control studies					
Oral cleft:					
Safra (1975)[10]	7	16	42	262	4.07 (1.44 to 11.54)
Saxen (1975)[7]	27	40	511	1 044	2.17 (1.11 to 4.24)
Rosenberg (1983)[34]	13	67	590	3 011	0.99 (0.54 to 1.82)
Rodriguez (1986)[36]	8	61	442	7 990	2.58 (1.22 to 5.45)
Czeizel (1987-88)[35]	48	91	1153	2 311	1.12 (0.74 to 1.71)
Laegreid (1990)[13]	2	10	4	68	4.00 (0.63 to 25.43)
Combined effect					1.79 (1.13 to 2.82)†
Cardiac malformations:					
Tikkanen (1992)[37]	2	10	404	1 152	0.46 (0.10 to 2.19)
Correa-Villasenor (1994)[38]	57	92	3318	6 855	1.74 (1.14 to 2.65)
Malformations of central nervous system:					
Winship (1984)[39]	14	750	14	750	1.00 (0.47 to 2.11)

* $\chi^2 = 0.01$; $P = 0.997$.
† $\chi^2 = 11.39$; $P = 0.01$.

major malformations or malformations of the oral cleft alone. However, data from case-control studies showed a small but significant increased risk for these events. This finding may reflect the substantially higher sensitivity of case-control studies to examine the risk of specific malformations or it may be chance.

The tests of heterogeneity also showed that the cohort studies were not heterogeneous for both major malformation and oral cleft, whereas the case-control studies for oral cleft were heterogeneous, which decreases the reliability of these marginally significant results.

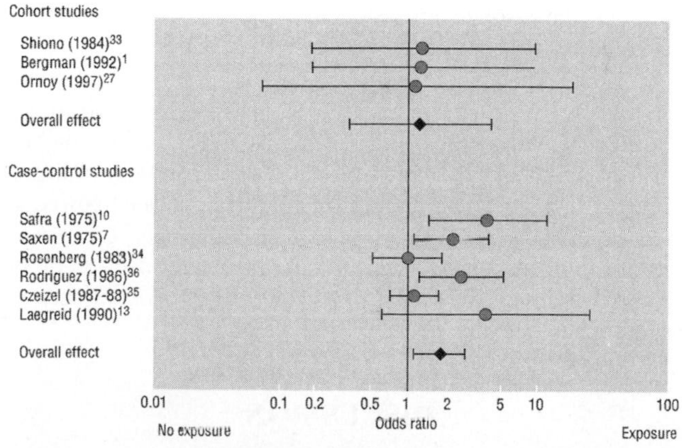

Figure 2. Association of oral cleft with prenatal exposure to benzodiazepines.

A case series of eight children exposed to benzodiazepines in utero suggested the existence of a benzodiazepine syndrome.[9] This syndrome was described as dysmorphic features, growth aberrations, and abnormalities of the central nervous system.[9 12 13] Our results, however, do not confirm the presence of this syndrome. Even before this report alternative causes for these findings, such as Zellweger syndrome or other genetic abnormalities, have been suggested.[42]

Possible Confounding and Bias

Concomitant exposure to other medications can result in an overestimation of the risk of benzodiazepines. Fourteen studies, eight of which were case-control, allowed exposure to other potentially teratogenic medications.[1 10 11 13 25 26 28–32 37–39] This large number confounds the results. In most studies no information on duration or indication for use of benzodiazepines was provided. Therefore it was difficult to determine if any of the populations included have an increased or decreased risk of major malformations. Studies that evaluated the risk of fetal malformations in women with epilepsy were separated from the main analysis as fetuses born to such women already have an increased risk of major malformations.[43] Information is lacking regarding the risk of developing specific malformations.

The use of a normal baby as a control in a case-control study can produce recall bias, as mothers of malformed babies may be more likely to recall exposures than mothers of normal babies. The subgroup analysis that compared benzodiazepine use in mothers of healthy babies as controls compared with mothers of malformed babies as controls produced similar effect sizes, suggesting that recall bias did not have a large effect on study outcome.

The present meta-analysis has several limitations. The number of reports was relatively small and may have limited the power of our analysis. Also, although the overall sample was large, most cases for analyses of both oral cleft and major malformations were derived from only three studies.[1 14 23] With regard to assessment of malformations, the studies used wide ranging definitions for identification of malformations to be considered. When we examined the association of benzodiazepines with cleft lip and cleft palate we had to combine these two malformations as "oral cleft" because many studies combined these malformations as one entity and it was not possible to stratify the data.[1 10 13 36]

KEY MESSAGES

- Pooled data from cohort studies showed no apparent association between fetal exposure to benzodiazepines and the risk for major malformations or oral cleft
- Data from case-control studies showed that risk for major malformations or oral cleft alone was increased
- Until more studies are done, it is prudent to perform level 2 ultrasonography to rule out visible forms of cleft lip

This study differs from previous reviews. Altshuler et al reported an association between benzodiazepines and oral cleft, but the review included studies that did not have any control groups or studies that did not have concurrent control groups.[44] That method of analysis may have seriously increased the strength of association found and the heterogeneity found when studies were combined and thereby produced different results. McElhatton provided a narrative review that succinctly summarised the opposing information, but because the studies presented were not combined systematically or quantitatively the conclusions remain controversial and inconclusive.[45]

CONCLUSIONS

Because women commonly use benzodiazepines and half of all pregnancies are unplanned, counselling of women on the safety of such exposure is clinically important. Pooled data from cohort studies showed no apparent association between benzodiazepine use and the risk for major malformations or oral cleft alone. There was, however, a small but significantly increased risk for oral cleft according to data from the available case-control studies. More case-control studies examining these events are needed especially because the available studies are not homogeneous. Even when the "worst case scenario" is assumed, benzodiazepines do not seem to be major human teratogens, but because some cases of cleft lip can be visualised by fetal ultrasound level 2 ultrasonography should be used to rule out this malformation.

This project was completed as part of a requirement for a doctor of pharmacy course on critical appraisal, PHM 605, at the University of Toronto.

Contributors: LRD coordinated the study, including discussion of core ideas, design of study, information retrieval, study selection, data extraction, statistical analysis, data analysis and interpretation, and writing the paper; AA participated in discussion of core ideas, design of study, sugy selection, data extraction, data nalaysi and interpretation, and editing the paper; JMRV and JDBP participated in discussion of core ideas, designing the study, information retrieval, study selection, data extraction, and writing the paper; GK and TRE helped initiate the project, participated in research design, analysis and interpretation and in editing the paper. LD will act as guarantor for the study.

Funding: No additional funding.

Conflict of interest: None.

REFERENCES

1. Bergman U, Rosa FW, Baum C, Wiholm BE, Faich GA. Effects of exposure to benzodiazepine during fetal life. *Lancet* 1992;340:694-6.
2. Skrabanek P. Smoking and statistical overkill. *Lancet* 1992;340: 1208-9.
3. Miller RP, Becker BA. Teratogenicity of oral diazepam and diphenylhydantoin in mice. *Toxicol Appl Pharmacol* 1975;32:53-61.
4. Walker BE, Patterson A. Induction of cleft palate in mice by tranquillizers and barbiturates. *Teratology* 1974;10:159-63.
5. Beall JR. Study of the teratogenic potential of oral diazepam and SCH 12041. *Can Med Assoc J* 1972;106:1061.
6. Chesley S, Lumpkin M, Schatzki A, Galpern WR, Greenblatt DJ, Shader RI, et al. Prenatal exposure to benzodiazepine. I. Prenatal exposure to lorazepam in mice alters open-field activity and GABA receptor function. *Neuropharmacology* 1991;30:53-8.
7. Saxen I, Saxen L. Association between maternal intake of diazepam and oral clefts. *Lancet* 1975;ii:498.
8. Saxen I, Lahti A. Cleft lip and palate in Finland: incidence, secular, seasonal, and geographical variations. *Teratology* 1974;9:217-24.
9. Laegreid L, Olegard R, Walstrom J, Conradi N. Teratogenic effects of benzodiazepine use during pregnancy. *J Pediatr* 1989;114:126-31.
10. Safra MJ, Oakley GP. Association between cleft lip with or without cleft palate and prenatal exposure to diazepam. *Lancet* 1975;ii: 478-80.
11. Milkovich L, van den Berg BJ. Effects of prenatal meprobamate and chlordiazepoxide hydrochloride on human embryonic and fetal development. *N Engl J Med* 1974;291:1268-71.
12. Laegreid L, Olegard R, Wahlstrom J, Conradi N. Abnormalities in children exposed to benzodiazepines in utero. *Lancet* 1987;i:108-9.
13. Laegreid L, Olegard R, Conradi N, Hagberg G, Wahlstrom J, Abrahamsson L. Congenital malformations and maternal consumption of benzodiazepines: a case-control study. *Dev Med Child Neurol* 1990;32:432-41.
14. Hartz SC, Heinonen OP, Shapiro S, Siskind V, Slone D. Antenatal exposure to meprobamate and chlordiazepoxide in relation to malformations, mental development, and childhood mortality. *N Engl J Med* 1975;292:726-8.
15. St Clair SM, Schirmer RG. First trimester exposure to alprazolam. *Obstet Gynecol* 1992;80:843-6.
16. Jick H, Holmes LB, Hunter JR, Madsen S, Stergachis A. First trimester drug use and congenital disorders. *JAMA* 1981;246:343-6.

17. Heinonen OP, Sloane D, Shapiro S. *Birth defects and drugs in pregnancy: maternal drug exposure and congenital malformations.* Littleton, Massachusetts: Publishing Sciences Group, 1977.
18. Horwitz RI, Feinstein AR. Methodologic standards and contradictory results in case-control research. *Am J Med* 1979;66:556-64.
19. Levine M, Walter S, Lee H, Haines T, Holbrook A, Moyer V. Users' guides to the medical literature. IV. How to use an article about harm. *JAMA* 1994;271:1615-9.
20. DerSimonian R, Laird N. Meta-analysis in clinical trials. *Cont Clin Trials* 1986;7:177-88.
21. Fleiss JL. The statistical basis of meta-analysis. *Stat Methods Med Res* 1993;2:121-45.
22. L'Abbe KA, Detsky AS, O'Rourke K. Meta-analysis in clinical research. *Ann Intern Med* 1987;107:224-33.
23. Crombie DL, Pinsent RJ, Fleming DM, Rumeau-Rouquette C, Goujard J, Huel G. Fetal effects of tranquilizers in pregnancy. *N Engl J Med* 1975;293:198-9.
24. Kullander S, Kallen B. A prospective study of drugs and pregnancy. I. Psychopharmaca. *Acta Obstet Gynecol Scand* 1976;55:25-33.
25. Laegreid L, Hagberg G, Lundberg A. Neurodevelopment in late infancy after prenatal exposure to benzodiazepines—a prospective study. *Neuropediatrics* 1992;23:60-7.
26. Pastuszak A, Milich V, Chan S, Chu J, Koren G. Prospective assessment of pregnancy outcome following first trimester exposure to benzodiazepines. *Can J Clin Pharmacol* 1996;3:167-71.
27. Ornoy A, Moerman L, Lukashova I, Arnon J. The outcome of children exposed in-utero to benzodiazepines. *Teratology* 1997;55:102A.
28. Bracken MB, Holford TR. Exposure to prescribed drugs in pregnancy and association with congenital malformations. *Obstet Gynecol* 1981;58:336-44.
29. Greenberg G, Inman WH, Weatherall JA, Adelstein AM, Haskey JC. Maternal drug histories and congenital abnormalities. *BMJ* 1977;ii:853-6.
30. Nakane Y, Okuma T, Takahashi R, Sato Y, Wada T, Sato T, et al. Multi-institutional study on the teratogenicity and fetal toxicity of antiepileptic drugs: a report of a collaborative study group in Japan. *Epilepsia* 1980;21:663-80.
31. Robert E, Lofkvist E, Mauguiere F, Robert JM. Evaluation of drug therapy and teratogenic risk in a Rhone-Alpes district population of pregnant epileptic women. *Eur Neurol* 1986;25:436-43.
32. Noya CA. Epidemiological study on congenital malformations. *Rev Cubana Hig Epidemiol* 1981;19:200-10.
33. Shiono PH, Mills JL. Oral clefts and diazepam use during pregnancy. *N Engl J Med* 1984;311:919-20.
34. Rosenberg L, Mitchell AA, Parsells JL, Pashayan H, Louik C, Shapiro S. Lack of relation of oral clefts to diazepam use during pregnancy. *N Engl J Med* 1983;309:1282-5.
35. Czeizel A. Lack of evidence of teratogenicity of benzodiazepine drugs in Hungary. *Reprod Toxicol* 1987-88;1:183-8.
36. Rodriguez PE, Salvador PJ, Garcia AF, Martinez FM. Relationship between benzodiazepine ingestion during pregnancy and oral clefts in the newborn: a case-control study. *Med Clin* 1986;87:741-3.
37. Tikkanen J, Heinonen OP. Congenital heart disease in the offspring and maternal habits and home exposures during pregnancy. *Teratology* 1992;46:447-54.
38. Correa-Villasenor A, Ferencz C, Neill CA, Wilson PD, Boughman JA. Ebstein's malformation of the tricuspid valve: genetic and environmental factors. *Teratology* 1994;50:137-47.
39. Winship KA, Cahal DA, Weber JP, Griffin JP. Maternal drug histories and central nervous system anomalies. *Arch Dis Child* 1984;59:1052-60.
40. Gregroire G, Derderian F, LeLorier J. Selecting the language of the publications included in a meta-analysis: is there a tower of Babel bias? *Pharmacoepidemiol Drug Safety* 1994;3:S18.
41. Viggedal G, Hagberg BS, Laegreid L, Aronsson M. Mental development in late infancy after prenatal exposure to benzodiazepines—a prospective study. *J Child Psychol Psychiatry* 1993;34:295-305.
42. Winter RM. In utero exposure to benzodiazepines. *Lancet* 1987;i:627.
43. Samrem EB, van Duijn CM, Hiilesmaa VK, Klepel H, Bardy AH, Mannagetta GB, et al. Maternal use of antiepileptic drugs and the risk of major congenital malformations: a joint European prospective study of human teratogenesis associated with maternal epilepsy. *Epilepsia* 1997;38:981-90.
44. Altshuler LL, Cohen L, Szuba M, Burt VK, Gitlin M, Mintz J. Pharmacologic management of psychiatric illness during pregnancy: dilemmas and guidelines. *Am J Psychiatry* 1996;153:592-606.
45. McElhatton PR. The effects of benzodiazepine use during pregnancy and lactation. *Reprod Toxicol* 1994;8:461-75.

(Accepted 11 June 1998)

CHAPTER 60

SAFETY OF FLUOXETINE DURING THE FIRST TRIMESTER OF PREGNANCY: A META-ANALYTICAL REVIEW OF EPIDEMIOLOGICAL STUDIES

Antonio Addis and Gideon Koren

From Regional Drug Information Centre (CRIF), Laboratory for Mother and Child Health, Istituto di Ricerche Farmacologiche 'Mario Negri', Milano, Italy; and Motherisk Program, Division of Clinical Pharmacology and Toxicology, The Hospital for Sick Children, Toronto, Canada

Abstract

Background. This study was designed to examine whether there is an increased risk for major malformations following the use of fluoxetine during the first trimester of pregnancy.

Methods. Published and unpublished reports were identified through computerized and manual searches of bibliographical databases, reference lists from primary articles, and letters to editors, agencies, foundations and content experts. Meta-analysis was undertaken of prospective controlled and uncontrolled studies on the use of fluoxetine during first trimester of pregnancy.

Results. The pooled relative risk and 95% confidence interval for major malformations does not suggest an association between the use of fluoxetine during the first trimester and an increased risk of major malformations. Combination of controlled and uncontrolled studies shows a weighted risk of 2·6% (95% CI 1–4·2%). The summary odds ratio from the two controlled studies (OR = 1·33, 95% CI 0·49–3·58) was not significant. Homogeneity testing shows that the effect sizes are similar throughout all studies. Power analysis indicates that 26 controlled studies of similar size, would be required, to reverse this finding.

Conclusions. The use of fluoxetine during the first trimester of pregnancy is not associated with measurable teratogenic effects in human.

INTRODUCTION

An estimated 8 to 20% women develop clinical symptoms of depression at some time during their lives, for which drug therapy is often required (Weissman *et al.* 1991; Kessler *et al.* 1993). Fluoxetine (Prozac®) was approved in the United States for the treatment of major depression in 1987 and has become the world's largest-selling antidepressant. Due to this trend and because 50% of pregnancies are unplanned (Skrabanek, 1992), numerous women will be involuntarily exposed to fluoxetine during the first trimester of their pregnancy. The lack of data on the potential foetal safety of fluoxetine has created anxiety among women, their families and physicians. In 1993 Pastuszak and colleagues published a study comparing 128 pregnant women treated with fluoxetine with 128 women exposed to non-teratogenic drugs (e.g. acetaminophen, penicillins, dental X-rays) and with 74 treated with tricyclic antidepressants, showing that neither fluoxetine nor tricyclic antidepressants taken during the first trimester were associated with an increased risk of congenital malformations (Pastuszak *et al.* 1993). Recently, Chambers and colleagues reported on their cohort of women (228 cases; 254 non-teratogenic exposed controls) taking fluoxetine during pregnancy (Chambers *et al.* 1996). Despite the fact that this study did not show an increase of risk for major malformations, a variety of international agencies have decided to caution women against the use of this drug during pregnancy.

The objective of our review was to summarize the results of all original studies investigating the risk for major malformations after fluoxetine use during the first trimester of pregnancy using a meta-analytical approach, in order to allow risk estimation based on all available data to date.

METHOD

Literature Search

A computerized literature search was performed using MEDLINE and EMBASE (up to August 1996) bibliographic databases. A search strategy using a combination of 'pregnancy' or 'abnormalities drug induced' and 'fluoxetine' keywords (Medical Subject Headings) was undertaken. REPROTOX® and Current Content® databases were also searched up to November 1996. All abstracts retrieved were reviewed to identify articles related to fluoxetine exposure during the first trimester and major malformations. In addition, an extensive manual search was conducted by reviewing references for all retrieved articles and selected review articles (Cooper, 1988; Rand, 1991; De Cuypere *et al.* 1992; Schwartz & Brotman, 1992; Altshuler & Szuba, 1994; Schorr & Richardson, 1995; Altshuler *et al.* 1996; Miller, 1996) to ensure that all potentially eligible articles were identified for analysis. The criteria for inclusion of studies in this analysis were: human exposure to any dosage of fluoxetine during the first trimester of pregnancy, and prospective report of outcome of pregnancy. The term 'prospective' means that all cases in a given study had to be collected before any outcome was known. Major malformations were defined as 'abnormalities resulting from abnormal formation of tissue leading to a compromise of function or requiring surgical correction'. Since studies that report retrospective exposure are considered biased in term of ascertainment of the relative risk, we have excluded them from our analysis.

Statistical Methods

Cohort studies with or without control groups were pooled to calculate the meta-analytical weighted average of foetal risk for major malformations. Data were combined using a random effects model, modified for use with single groups (Der Simonian & Laird, 1986). The results are point estimated with 95% confidence interval that incorporates both within and between study variance. χ^2 and P values for homogeneity of the studies were calculated using standard statistical methods.

For cohort studies with control groups we calculated a Mantel–Haenszel summary odds ratio and an overall 95% confidence interval, which indicates a reasonable estimate of the risk ratio for major malformations in treated versus untreated subjects (Einarson *et al.* 1988). Power analysis was performed by calculating the number of studies with the same power of those identified that would be needed to bring the relative risk to significance.

RESULTS

Thirty-one references for papers that reported the use of fluoxetine during pregnancy (published between 1988 and 1996) were identified. Of these papers 27 (87%) were excluded because of the following reasons: not original studies (Cooper, 1988; Matthews *et al.* 1991; Rand, 1991; De Cuypere *et al.* 1992; Schwartz & Brotman, 1992; Anonymous, 1993; Altshuler & Szuba, 1994; Edwards, 1994; Kacew, 1994; Mortola, 1994; Nightingale, 1994; Lee & Donaldson, 1995; Schorr & Richardson, 1995; Altshuler *et al.* 1996; Miller, 1996) i.e. reviews, guidelines or notes; case reports (Sichel *et al.* 1993; Spencer, 1993; Livingston *et al.* 1994; Franko & Hilsinger, 1995; Vendittelli *et al.* 1995); retrospective cohorts (Edwards *et al.* 1994; Rosa, 1994) i.e. prescription data monitoring or retrospective design; letters or abstracts followed by full articles (Schick-Boschetto & Zuber, 1992; Chambers *et al.* 1993; Goldstein & Marvel, 1993; Nulman & Koren, 1996); exposure during the third trimester only (Goldstein, 1995). Four original studies were conducted with a prospective design and two of these had control groups (matched in one of them). The analysis, therefore included 367 women (average per study: 91.7; range 11–162) exposed to fluoxetine during the first trimester. The meta-analytical weighted average of foetal risk for major malformations from all the prospective studies is shown in Table 1. The mean value of 2.6% represents the ratio of the number of infants with major malformations to the number who were live-born and is well within the expected rate of major malformations in the general population. The test of homogeneity, ($\chi^2 = 0{\cdot}81$, df = 3; $P = 0{\cdot}85$), showed that all studies detected an effect size of similar magnitude and direction.

Two studies used the same kind of controls defined as 'non-teratogenic'. In both studies those women were exposed during pregnancy to drugs and procedures not considered teratogenic (e.g. acetaminophen, dental radiography). Both of the two controlled studies recruited patients through two different Teratology Information Services. These just recently became a new source of data for prospective observational research. Pregnant women taking prescription drugs (e.g. fluoxetine) voluntarily call the centre for risk-assessment counselling. Since the exposure data are recorded prospectively the probability of recall bias is reduced and followup of exposed pregnancies can extend well beyond parturition. Control groups were selected from those women who contacted the same Teratology Information Services but who had non-teratogenic exposure.

Maternal characteristics (age, obstetric history, ethanol and cigarette use and previous pregnancy outcomes (spontaneous and elective abortions abortion, etc.) were compared to test differences between fluoxetine cases and controls.

The Mantel–Haenszel summary odds ratio extracted from the two prospective controlled studies is shown in Fig. 1. Here too, the test of homogeneity ($\chi^2 = 0.04$, df = 1; $P = 0.85$) revealed no heterogeneity between the two studies, although the analysis, based only on two reports, is limited.

Major malformations are considered rare events with an incidence range of 1–3% of all pregnancies (Stevenson, 1993). Thus, with 367 women included in this analysis between 4 to 11 major malformations would be expected; 10 cases of major malformations were observed. A review of these malformations has revealed no homogeneic pattern with relatively common malformations prevailing as expected (Table 2).

Power analysis shows that it would take 26 controlled studies with similar size, to make the measurable effect size statistically significant.

DISCUSSION

Although fluoxetine is one of the most widely prescribed drugs of the last decade, dat on its safety during pregnancy are not readily available. Despite the documented necessity of antidepressant therapy for many women during pregnancy and the efforts spent on the study of the efficacy of fluoxetine, pregnant women exposed to this drug remain a population 'orphan' of safety data. In this context, an objective summary of the present data on the foetal safety of fluoxetine during pregnancy may avoid unnecessary discontinuation of therapy, or unjustified termination of pregnancy, due to high perception of teratogenic risk (Koren *et al.* 1989).

Table 1
Prospective Studies Measuring Major Malformations After Exposure to Fluoxetine During the First Trimester of Pregnancy

STUDY	NO. MAJOR MALFORMATIONS/NO. EXPOSED	(%)	TYPE OF STUDY
Pastuszak *et al.* (1993)	2/98	2	Cohort study, with controls
Brunel *et al.* (1994)	0/11	0	Cohort study, no controls
McElhatton *et al.* (1996)	2/96	2·1	Cohort study, no controls
Chambers *et al.* (1996)	6/162	3·7	Cohort study, with controls
Meta-analytical weighted average	2·6% (95% CI 1–4·2%)		

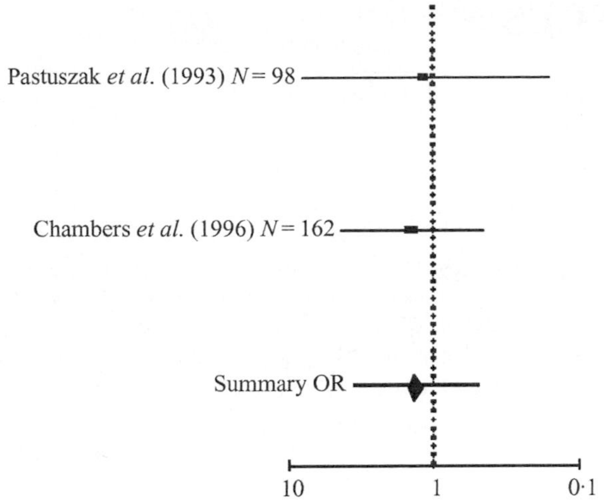

Fig. 1. Mantel–Haenszel summary odds ratio extracted from the two prospective controlled studies.

Since retrospective studies that report drug exposure may introduce major ascertainment bias of the relative risk, we have excluded them from our present analysis. However, the two retrospective reports identified by us, also failed to show an increased risk of malformations. (Edwards *et al.* 1994; Rosa, 1994).

Meta-analysis is a well established strategy useful to clarify the status of therapeutic modalities and objectively combine and quantify a potential risk from a number of epidemiological studies (Einarson *et al.* 1988).

The rate of major malformations, calculated from meta-analytical weighted average in live births exposed to fluoxetine during the first trimester was within the expected normal range (1 to 3%). Sub-analysis of the two controlled studies confirmed that the cases of malformations were comparable to the control groups. The non-homogenous pattern of malformation reflects the distribution of major malformation in the general population.

A limitation of this analysis is the small number of studies that exist. However, the fact that it would take 26 more studies of the same size to make the measurable effect size statistically significant, and the homogeneity of the effect size in the existing studies strongly suggests that fluoxetine is not a major human teratogen, and probably does not increase the baseline teratogenic risk in a clinically important manner.

In the study by Chambers *et al.* (1996) the rate of minor malformations, prematurity, decreased body weight, and neonatal complications were high among infants exposed to the drug throughout gestation, but not during the first trimester. The lack of a control group of pregnant women with depression not treated with fluoxetine (e.g. with tricyclic antidepressants) did not allow for the determination of whether the above differences, shown by Chalmers and colleagues were caused by continuous use of fluoxetine or were due to the severity of disease. That is, women who need the drug throughout gestation are substantially different in their characteristics from those who can discontinue therapy after pregnancy has been diagnosed. In an attempt to separate the effects of fluoxetine from those of maternal depression and other confounders, Pastuszak *et al.* (1993) used as controls, women who were exposed to tricyclic antidepressants (TCA) during the first trimester of pregnancy. No differences between fluoxetine exposure and TCA exposure were identified, with respect to the rate of major malformations.

This meta-analysis did not address the safety of fluoxetine in terms of developmental toxicity. However, we have recently shown that the neurodevelopment of children exposed *in utero* to fluoxetine is similar to that of controls in a large number of domains including IQ, language and behaviour (Nulman *et al.* 1997). Similar results were obtained when children exposed only during the first trimester were compared with those exposed throughout gestation. These data, in conjunction with the present meta-analysis indicate that there is no evidence that the use of fluoxetine during the first trimester of pregnancy increases the baseline risk for major malformations.

An abstract of the preliminary analysis of this study was submitted at the International Conference of the Organization of Teratology Information Services, June 1997, Palm Beach, Florida, USA; and at the Symposium of the International Society of Pharmacoepidemiology, August 1997, at Walt Disney, Florida, USA.

Table 2
Congenital Malformations in Live Born Infants Who were Prenatally Exposed to Fluoxetine

	STUDY/NO. OF WOMEN EXPOSED				
MALFORMATIONS	PASTUSZAK 1993 (*N* = 98)	MCELHATTON 1996 (*N* = 96)	BRUNEL 1994 (*N* = 11)	CHAMBERS 1996 (*N* = 162)	TOTAL (*N* = 367) *N* (%)
Cardiac defects					
Ventricular septal	1	1	–	2*	4 (1)
Atrial septal	–	–	–	1	1 (0·3)
Genitourinary					
Hypospadias	–	1	–	1	2(0·6)
Gastrointestinal					
Jejunal obstruction	1	–	–	–	1 (0·3)
Miscellaneous					
Nasal dermoid sinus	–	–	–	1	1 (0·3)
Coccygeal dermal sinus	–	–	–	1	1 (0·3)

* One ventricular septal defect with bilateral cryptorchidism.

REFERENCES

Altshuler, L. L. & Szuba, M. P. (1994). Course of psychiatric disorders in pregnancy: Dilemmas in pharmacologic management. *Neurologic Clinics* **12,** 613–35.

Altshuler, L. L., Cohen, L., Szuba, M. P., Burt, V. K., Gitlin, M. & Mintz, J. (1996). Pharmacologic management of psychiatric illness during pregnancy: dilemmas and guidelines. *American Journal Psychiatry* **153,** 492–606.

Anonymous (1993). Depression in women: ACOG technical bulletin number 182 – July 1993. *International Journal of Gynaecology and Obstetrics* **43,** 203–211.

Brunel, P., Vial, T., Roche, I., Bertolotti, E. & Evreux, J. C. (1994). First-trimester exposure to antidepressant drugs. Result of a follow-up. *Therapie* **49,** 117–122.

Chambers, C. D., Johnson, K. A. & Jones, K. L. (1993). Pregnancy outcome in women exposed to fluoxetine. *Teratology* **47,** 386.

Chambers, C. D., Johnson, K. A., Dick, L. M., Felix, R. J. & Jones, K. L. (1996). Birth outcomes in pregnant women taking fluoxetine. *New England Journal of Medicine* **335,** 1010–1015.

Cooper, G. L. (1988). The safety of fluoxetine: an update. *British Journal of Psychiatry* **3,** 77–86.

De Cuypere, G., Rombaut, P. & Van Moffaert, M. (1992). Congenital malformations caused by psychotropic drugs in pregnancy. *Acta Neuropsychiatrica* **4,** 77–85.

Der Simonian, R. & Laird, N. (1986). Meta-analysis in clinical trials. *Controlled Clinical Trials* **7,** 177–188.

Edwards, J. G. (1994). Selective serotonin reuptake inhibitors in the treatment of depression. *Prescribers' Journal* **34,** 197–204.

Edwards, J. G., Inman, W. H., Wilton, L. & Pearce, G. L. (1994). Prescription-event monitoring of 10,401 patients treated with fluvoxamine. *British Journal of Psychiatry* **164,** 387–395.

Einarson, T. R., Leeder, S. T. & Koren, G. (1988). A method for meta-analysis of epidemiological studies. *Drug Intelligent Clinical Pharmacology* **22,** 813–824.

Franko, D. & Hilsinger, E. (1995). Depression and bulimia in a pregnant woman. *Harvard Review of Psychiatry* **2,** 282–287.

Goldstein, D. J. (1995). Effect of third trimester fluoxetine exposure on the newborn. *Journal of Clinical Psychopharmacology* **15,** 417–420.

Goldstein, D. J. & Marvel, D. E. (1993). Psychotropic medication during pregnancy: risk to the fetus. *Journal of American Medical Association* **270,** 2177.

Kacew, S. (1994). Fetal consequences and risks attributed to the use of prescribed and over-the-counter (OTC) preparations during pregnancy. *International Journal of Clinical Pharmacology and Therapeutics* **32,** 335–343.

Kessler, R. C., McGonagle, K. A., Swartz, M., Blazer, D. G. & Nelson, C. B. (1993). Sex and depression in the National Comorbidity Survey. I : Lifetime prevalence, chronicity and recurrence. *Journal of Affective Disorders* **29,** 85–96.

Koren, G., Bologa, M., Long, D., Feldman, Y. & Shear, N. (1989). Perception of teratogenic risk by pregnant women exposed to drugs and chemicals during the first trimester. *American Journal of Obstetric and Gynecology* **160,** 1190–1194.

Lee, A. & Donaldson, S. (1995). Drug use in pregnancy: psychiatric and neurological disorders – Part 1. *Pharmaceutical Journal* **254,** 87–90.

Livingston, J. C., Johnstone, W. M. & Hadi, H. A. (1994). Electroconvulsive therapy in a twin pregnancy: a case report. *American Journal of Perinatology* **11,** 116–118.

McElhatton, P. R., Garbis, H. M., Elefant, E., Vial, T., Bellemin, B., Mastroiacovo, P., Arnon, J., Rodriguez-Pinilla, E., Schaefer, C., Pexieder, T., Merlob, P. & Dal Verme, S. (1996). The outcome of pregnancy in 689 women exposed to therapeutic doses of antidepressants. A collaborative study of the European Network of Teratology Information Services (ENTIS). *Reproductive Toxicology* **10,** 285–294.

Matthews, D. A., Manu, P. & Lane, T. J. (1991). Evaluation and management of patients with chronic fatigue. *American Journal Medical Science* **302,** 269–277.

Miller, L. J. (1996). Psychopharmacology during pregnancy. *Primary Care Update for Obstetric Gynecology* **3,** 79–86.

Mortola, J. F. (1994). A risk-benefit appraisal of drugs used in the management of premenstrual syndrome. *Drug Safety* **10,** 160–169.

Nightingale, S. L. (1994). Fluoxetine labeling revised to identify phenytoin interaction and to recommend against use in nursing mothers. *Journal of American Medical Association* **271,** 1067.

Nulman, I. & Koren, G. (1996). The safety of fluoxetine during pregnancy and lactation. *Teratology* **53,** 304–308.

Nulman, I., Rovet, J., Stewart, D. E., Wolpin, J., Gaudner, A., Theis, J. G. W., Kullin, N. & Koren, G. (1997). Neurodevelopment of children exposed in utero to antidepressant drugs. *New England Journal of Medicine* **336,** 258–262.

Pastuszak, A., Schick-Boschetto, B., Zuber, C., Feldkamp, M., Pinelli, M., Sihn, S., Donnenfeld, A., McCormack, M., Leen-Mitchell, M., Woodland, C., Gardner, A., Horn, M. & Koren, G. (1993). Pregnancy outcome following first-trimester exposure to fluoxetine. *Journal of American Medical Association* **269,** 2246–2248.

Rand, E. H. (1991). Choosing an antidepressant to treat depression. *American Family Physician* **43,** 847–854.

Rosa, F. (1994). Medicaid antidepressant pregnancy exposure outcomes. *Reproductive Toxicology* **8,** 444–445.

Schick-Boschetto, B. & Zuber, C. (1992). Fluoxetine exposure in early human pregnancy. *Teratology* **45,** 460.

Schorr, S. J. & Richardson, D. (1995). Psychiatric emergencies. *Obstetric Gynecological Clinics of North American* **22,** 369–383.

Schwartz, J. T. & Brotman, A. W. (1992). A clinical guide to antipsychotic drugs. *Drugs* **44,** 981–992.

Sichel, D. A., Cohen, L. S., Dimmock, J. A. & Rosenbaum, J. F. (1993). Postpartum obsessive compulsive disorder: a case series. *Journal of Clinical Psychiatry* **54,** 156–159.

Skrabanek, P. (1992). Smoking and statistical overkill. *Lancet* **340,** 1208–1209.

Spencer, M. J. (1993). Fluoxetine hydrochloride (Prozac) toxicity in a neonate. *Pediatrics* **92,** 721–722.

Stevenson, R. E. (1993). Causes of human anomalies: an overview and historical perspective. In *Human Malformations and Related Anomalies* (ed. R. E. Stevenson), pp. 3–20. Oxford University Press : New York.

Vendittelli, F., Alain, J., Nouvaille, Y., Brosset, A. & Tabaste, J. L. (1995). A case of lipomeningocele reported with fluoxetine (and alprazolam, vitamins B1 and B6, heptaminol) prescribed during pregnancy. *European Journal of Obstetrics, Gynecology and Reproductive Biology* **38,** 85–86.

Weissman, M. M., Bruce, M. L., Leaf, P. I., Florio, L. P. & Holzer, C. III (1991). Affective disorders. In *Psychiatric Disorders in America* (ed. N. Robins and D. Reiger), pp. 53–80. Free Press: New York.

Reprinted from Addis A, Koren G. Safety of fluoxetine during the first trimester of pregnancy: a meta-analytical review of epidemiological studies. Psychol Med 2000;30:89–94 with permission.

CHAPTER 61

ANTIDEPRESSANT USE DURING PREGNANCY AND THE RATES OF SPONTANEOUS ABORTIONS: A META-ANALYSIS

Michiel EH Hemels, Adrienne Einarson, Gideon Koren, Krista L. Lanctôt, and Thomas R. Einarson

Background. Due to the high prevalence of depression in women of childbearing age and coupled with the fact that approximately 50% of the pregnancies are unplanned, there is a high chance that these women have been exposed to antidepressants in early pregnancy.

Objective. To determine baseline rates of spontaneous abortions (SAs) and whether antidepressants increase those rates.

Methods. Rates of SAs in women taking antidepressants compared with non-depressed women were combined into a relative risk using a random effects model. MEDLINE, EMBASE, Healthstar, Toxline, Psychlit, Cochrane database, and Reprotox were searched for studies published in any language from 1966 to 2003. Key words used to identify articles included pregnancy outcome, abortion, miscarriage, spontaneous, antidepressant, depression, and the generic names of each antidepressant and class. Bibliographies, review articles, and reference lists from studies were also used to identify potential articles expected to provide evidence of safety of antidepressants in pregnancy.

Results. Of 15 potential articles, 6 cohort studies of 3567 women (1534 exposed, 2033 nonexposed) provided extractable data. All matched on important confounders. Tests found no heterogeneity (χ^2 3.13; p = 0.98), and all quality scores were adequate (>50%). The baseline SA rate (95% CI) was 8.7% (7.5% to 9.9%; n = 2033). For antidepressants, the rate was 12.4% (10.8% to 14.1%; n = 1534), significantly increased by 3.9% (1.9% to 6.0%); RR was 1.45 (1.19 to 1.77; n = 3567). No differences were found among antidepressant classes.

Conclusions. Maternal exposure to antidepressants may be associated with increased risk for SA; however, depression itself cannot be ruled out.

Keywords: antidepressants, depression, spontaneous abortion.
Ann Pharmacother 2005;39:803-9.
Published Online, 22 Mar 2005, *www.theannals.com*, DOI 10.1345/aph.1E547

A substantial number of women of childbearing age suffer from depression. Prevalence estimates, evaluated by clinical assessment on the basis of structured criteria, vary between 4% and 17.6%.[1,2] Recently, 3472 pregnant women were screened prospectively for depressive symptoms using the Centre for Epidemiologic Studies Depression Scale. In that study, 20% of the women scored above the cutoff for depressive symptoms.[3] The incidence of prenatal depression appears to be increased in the first trimester, suggesting that this trimester may be the time of maximum vulnerability to depression.[4]

Untreated maternal depression and depressive symptoms have been associated with risks for negative pregnancy outcomes. These outcomes included major fetal growth retardation, preterm birth, lower birth weight, smaller head circumference, and lower Apgar scores.[5-10] These outcomes, in turn, have been associated with mortality, increased risk of severe neurologic morbidity, and mental retardation.[11-13] Although there are several possible mechanisms by which depression during pregnancy could affect neonatal outcome, no causal connections have been established.[5] However, increased serum cortisol and catecholamine levels, which are typically observed in depressed patients, may affect placental function by altering uterine blood flow and inducing uterine irritability.[14,15] A dysfunction in mood could lead to disturbances of the hypothalamic–pituitary–adrenal axis, resulting in deficiencies of glucose metabolism, which may also directly affect fetal development.[16,17]

Predisposing factors for depression during pregnancy include personal or family history of affective illness. However, for about one-third of the women who become depressed during pregnancy, it was their first episode. Other risk factors include marital dysfunction or dissatisfaction, young age, inadequate psychosocial supports, recent adverse life events, lower socioeconomic status or minimal education, unwanted pregnancy, and a larger number of children.[18,19]

In 1993, Pastuszak et al.[20] reported that women taking antidepressants incurred higher rates of spontaneous abortions (SAs), although the results were not statistically significant. Subsequently, several studies investigated this topic as a secondary pregnancy outcome and found similar results. However, no conclusive statements have been made, primarily because the increase in rates was not statistically significant, which may be due to small sample sizes in these studies.[21-23]

In a review of the literature, Garciá-Enguídanos et al.[24] estimated that the incidence of SAs was about 12–15% in the general population. Furthermore, after including early pregnancy losses, the general incidence was about 17–22%. The authors pointed out that there were many suggested risk factors. However, 2 etiologic factors that were acknowledged by all researchers were uterine congenital malformations and parental balanced chromosomal rearrangements such as trisomy.

A thorough literature search failed to identify definitively the baseline risk for SAs in healthy pregnant women. In the studies examining antidepressant use during pregnancy, the exposed group was in the range of 12–15%. However, the comparison group rates were much lower (7–9%).[21-23] One reason for the lack of data for SAs may be a lack of control of possible contributing and confounding variables. Possible major confounding variables are caffeine intake, smoking, age, alcohol use, socioeconomic status, stress, and previous SA.[24-27]

A need exists to ascertain whether antidepressants are associated with an increased risk for SAs when used in early pregnancy. The objective of our study was to combine data from all prospective

Author information provided at the end of the text.
This research represents a part of the thesis written by Dr. Hemels for the Degree of Master of Science from the Graduate Department of Pharmacology, University of Toronto.

studies to date that examined the rates of SAs in pregnant women exposed to antidepressants in a meta-analysis.

METHODS

A comprehensive literature search was undertaken to identify all published papers reporting on SAs in women aged 18–45 years taking antidepressants for depression (comorbidities ≤25%/no comedications). Additionally, only patients with continuous exposure to antidepressant monotherapy (any dose) during the first 20 weeks of gestation were included. SA was defined as the unwanted loss of a fetus within the first 20 weeks of gestation. Antidepressants were defined as all drugs in category N06A of the Anatomic Therapeutic Chemical classification of the World Health Organization.[28] Included were the selective serotonin-reuptake inhibitors (SSRIs; citalopram, fluoxetine, fluvoxamine, paroxetine, sertraline), dual action agents (DAAs; nefazodone, trazodone, venlafaxine), tricyclics (TCAs; amitriptyline, amoxapine, clomipramine, desipramine, doxepin, imipramine, maprotiline, nortriptyline, protriptyline, trimipramine), and monoamine oxidase inhibitors (moclobemide, phenelzine, tranylcypromine). Acceptable comparison groups were non-depressed pregnant women not exposed to antidepressants or drugs associated with teratogenicity or which possess abortifacient properties.

Cohort studies were included, with observational (including interviews, survey) research design as well as database analyses. Excluded were studies reporting on patients with manic or mixed depression, bipolar disorders (I and II), cyclothymic disorders, or who concomitantly showed psychotic features. We also excluded studies reporting maternal exposure to other risk factors, data reported in abstracts, reports from proceedings or symposia, and nonoriginal research.

MEDLINE, EMBASE, Healthstar, Toxline, Psychlit, Cochrane database, and Reprotox were searched for studies published in any language from 1966 to 2003. Key words used to identify articles included pregnancy outcome, abortion, miscarriage, spontaneous, antidepressant, depression, and the generic names of each antidepressant and class. Bibliographies, review articles, and reference lists from studies were also used to identify potential articles expected to provide evidence of safety of antidepressants in pregnancy.

Studies were selected in a stepwise approach. In a comprehensive initial search, information in titles and abstracts was compared against the preset criteria. Next, included articles were retrieved and thoroughly examined. Possible reasons for rejection were non-original research, ineligible outcome measure, no data of interest, noncomparative study, data not extractable, and/or other/miscellaneous. Results were compared with those of a second reviewer. Discrepancies were settled through consensus discussion, with unresolved disputes adjudicated by a third reviewer whose judgment was considered final.

After final selection of articles for inclusion in the meta-analysis, the same 2 reviewers independently extracted data from the accepted studies onto a collection sheet. Discrepancies in data extraction were resolved in the same manner as for article identification.

After entering the data from each study into 2 × 2 tables, individual risk ratios and 95% confidence intervals were calculated. Before pooling results, we examined for heterogeneity of effects by calculating χ^2. Results were then pooled using the random-effects model developed by Cochran.[29] As subgroup analyses, SA rates were determined for individual classes of antidepressants.

Because outputs like risk ratios may be difficult to interpret, the number needed to treat to harm (NNTH) was also calculated. The NNTH estimates the number of patients who would need to be exposed to an antidepressant to produce one additional SA. The confidence interval was calculated using the limits of the confidence interval on the risk ratio.[30]

The presence of publication bias was evaluated with the funnel plot–based trim-and-fill method.[31-35] This algorithm is based on the qualitative approach using the funnel plot. The asymmetric outlying part of the funnel is trimmed off after the number of studies that are in the asymmetric part are counted. The symmetric remainder is then used to estimate the true center of the funnel. Then, the trimmed studies and their (presumed) missing counterparts are replaced symmetrically around the meta-analytic average. The final estimate of the true mean, and also its variance, are then based on the filled funnel plot and compared with its original value to assess the impact.[34]

Because the funnel plot requires judgment and has no associated statistical test, we also applied the Begg and Mazumdar[36] test, which complements the funnel graph, examining the agreement between effect estimates and their variances by calculating Kendall's τ. In this way, it exploits the fact that publication bias will tend to induce a correlation between these 2 factors; thus, a significant τ would indicate the presence of publication bias.

The quality of individual studies may affect the overall interpretation of meta-analysis results. Based on critical appraisal systems, a scoring sheet was developed to assess study quality.[37-39] The checklist contains 29 questions in total and requires the reviewer to answer yes or no to each item, scoring 1 point for each yes and 0 points for each no. Thus, the highest score is 29. Questions that are not applicable to a specific article are eliminated, the total score being calculated based on the total answerable questions. The questions in the checklist are separated into 7 categories, each representing a section within the article. Categories include research design, subjects, exposure, analysis, confounders and bias, methods, and results.

We decided that descriptors would assist in judging the quality. The scores were therefore divided into quartiles as follows: <25% = very poor, 25–49% = poor, 50–75% = acceptable, and >75% = good quality. Descriptive statistics, such as the mean and range, were used to quantitatively determine the studies. A copy of the checklist appears in Appendix I. To avoid potential bias, all identifying information (eg, authors, institutions, journal, country) was removed from the articles by an independent third party. Two independent, blinded raters performed scoring. Scores were compared between raters, with differences settled through consensus. In the case of disagreement, a third judge was enlisted as final adjudicator.

To determine the validity of the quality scoring, the interrater reliability between the 2 reviewers was measured using κ, with statistical significance set at 0.05.[40,41] It was decided a priori that a κ value of 0.8 would be deemed satisfactory to establish reliability. Furthermore, to ensure the quality of the meta-analysis, a cut-off point in quality score <50% was used to exclude studies from the meta-analysis.

RESULTS

The initial search yielded 156 potential articles; however, after the titles and abstracts were evaluated, only 15 remained. Of those 15, 9 were rejected[42-50]; 5 presented no data for the control group or a control group was not present, [42-46] 3 did not report data of interest,[47-49] and data could not be extracted from one study.[50] That left 6 articles that met the inclusion criteria and provided usable data[20-23,51,52] with 11 different data sets (ie, some reported on >1 group, different drugs or classes of drugs). Table 1 describes the accepted studies and their characteristics.

Table 1
Description of Included Studies and Their Characteristics

REFERENCE	QUALITY SCORE (%)	INDICATION, DRUG	NONEXPOSED SUBJECTS	PRIMARY OUTCOME	MATCHING VARIABLES	EXPOSURE HISTORY	EXPOSURE DEFINITION	OUTCOME VERIFICATION
Einarson et al. (2003)[21] Canada	66	depressed trazodone/ nefazodone, dose NS	NT	MM	disease, age, smoking alcohol, time of call	medical indication for drug use, dose, frequency/ timing of administration, maternal demographics, obstetrical history	occurring during oranogenesis (4–14th wk)	telephone interview and examination of medical record
Einarson et al. (2001)[22] Canada	69	depressed venlafaxine 75 mg/day (37.5–300)	SSRI, depressed, NT	MM	age, smoking status, alcohol use	medical indication for drug use, dose, frequency/ timing of administration, maternal demographics, obstetrical history	occurring during organogenesis	telephone interview and examination of medical record
Kulin et al. (1998)[23] Canada	72	depressed SSRIs: sertraline 50 mg/day, paroxetine 30 mg/day, fluvoxamine 50 mg/day	NT	MM	NS	medical indication for drug use; SSRI dose schedule and length of therapy; other therapy; smoking and alcohol; medical, obstetric, and genetic history; exposure to environmental toxins	occurring during first trimester	telephone interview and examination of medical record
Chambers et al. (1996)[51] US	83	depressed (77%) fluoxetine 28 ± 15 mg/day	NT	major and minor struc-tural anoma-lies or perinatal compla-cations	age	dosage, dates, and indications for all medications, caffeine, vitamins, occupational exposures, infectious/ chronic disease, prenatal testing, use of recreational drugs, tobacco, alcohol	occurring during first trimester	telephone interview and examination of medical record
Pastuszak et al. (1993)[20] Canada	79	depressed fluoxetine 25.8 mg/day (range 10–80)	TCA NT	birth defects	age	obstetric, medical, genetic, and drug exposure history	occurring during first trimester	telephone interview and examination of medical record
McElhatton et al. (1996)[52] Europe	66	depressed TCA, dose NS	non-TCA NT	pregnancy outcomes[a]	NS	medical and obstetric history	throughout pregnancy	questionnaire and telephone interview

MM = major malformations; NS = not stated; NT= non-teratogenic; SSRI = selective serotonin-reuptake inhibitor; TCA = tricyclic antidepressant.

[a] Including spontaneous and therapeutic abortions, fetal death, malformations, and neonatal disorders.

The overall test for heterogeneity of effects was nonsignificant ($\chi^2 = 3.13$; $p = 0.978$), suggesting that results could reasonably be combined. As well, tests for individual classes of antidepressants were not significant (SSRIs $\chi^2 = 1.16$, $p = 0.948$; TCAs $\chi^2 = 0.79$, $p = 0.672$; DAAs $\chi^2 = 0.01$, $p = 0.971$).

The funnel plots (not shown) for the 11 sets of data showed that there existed a lack of small negative studies. The Begg–Mazumdar test confirmed this observation that publication bias was present ($t = 0.491$; $p = 0.04$). The meta-analytic risk ratio was 1.45 (95% CI 1.19 to 1.77, n = 3567; Table 2); however, after adjustment, it changed only slightly to 1.36 (95% CI 1.15 to 1.61). Thus, although publication bias appeared to be present, the results of the meta-analysis were not affected. Overall, the quality of the included articles was rated as acceptable (Table 1). Kappa between the 2 raters was 0.86 ($Z = 11.32$; $p < 0.001$), which was considered acceptable.

Table 3 summarizes all of the rates of interest. The baseline rate of SAs, as estimated by the group not exposed to antidepressants, was 8.7%. The risk for SAs in depressed pregnant women who were exposed to antidepressants during the pregnancy was 12.4%. Exposure to antidepressants was associated with an average increase of 3.9% (95% CI 1.9% to 6.0%), with a corresponding risk ratio of 1.45. This means that, for antidepressants in general, the NNTH was 26. Nonsignificant differences were found between antidepressant classes in risk ratios.

DISCUSSION

To our knowledge, as of March 7, 2005, this is the first meta-analysis to examine the risk for SA in pregnant women (3567) exposed to antidepressants. Although this meta-analysis indicates that maternal exposure to antidepressants may be associated with a significantly increased risk for SA, depression per se may also be associated with abortive properties.

Despite a great volume of literature on the subject, we were able to include only a relatively small number of cohort studies. Six studies with a total of 11 treatment arms reporting rates on SA were included in the analysis. Women were exposed to drugs from 3 therapeutic classes (SSRIs, TCAs, DAAs). Because there was sufficient power to detect a difference, one may assume that there is no important clinical difference between SAs compared with those women in the non-exposed groups.

Some of the studies included in the meta-analysis matched the patients for age, smoking status, alcohol use, and time of the call. None of the studies, however, investigated the patient's reproductive history. Regan et al.[26] prospectively followed 630 women to estimate the overall incidence of SA prior to 20 weeks of gestation. Initially, the overall risk was 12% (50/407 pregnancies). After stratification with respect to the patients' reproductive history, this rate was 4% (3/73) for women who had a history of consistently successful pregnancies and 24% (24/98) among women with unsuccessful histories, whereas the incidence of loss of pregnancy among women whose last pregnancy had aborted was 19% (40/214). Therefore, it may be possible that the results of our studies are biased; however, in which direction remains unknown. The strength of our study was the use of comparative groups that were enrolled in the same fashion, thus eliminating some of this bias.

An interesting finding was that all meta-analytic risk rates in the antidepressant exposure group were approximately the same (12.4–12.8%). This may indicate that it is the disease that is associated with the increased risk for abortion and not the treatment. If the treatment were the cause, one would expect there to be differences in the classes (SSRIs, TCAs, DAAs), as they differ in their mechanisms of action.

Table 2
Meta-Analysis Results by Study Arms

	EXPOSED GROUP			NONEXPOSED GROUP				
REFERENCE	SA	NO SA	RATE	SA	NO SA	RATE	RR	95% CI
DAAs								
Einarson et al. (2003)[21]	20	127	0.14	12	135	0.08	1.67	0.85 to 3.28
Einarson et al. (2001)[22]	18	132	0.12	11	139	0.07	1.64	0.80 to 3.35
SSRIs								
Einarson et al. (2001)[22]	16	134	0.11	11	139	0.07	1.45	0.70 to 3.03
Kulin et al. (1998)[23]	30	237	0.11	21	246	0.08	1.43	0.84 to 2.43
Chambers et al. (1996)[51]	23	146	0.14	22	232	0.09	1.57	0.91 to 2.73
Pastuszak et al. (1993)[20]	10	64	0.14	5	69	0.07	2.00	0.72 to 5.57
	19	109	0.15	10	118	0.08	1.90	0.92 to 3.93
McElhatton et al. (1996)[52]	12	80	0.13	28	235	0.11	1.23	0.65 to 2.31
TCAs								
Pastuszak et al. (1993)[20]	9	65	0.12	5	69	0.07	1.80	0.63 to 5.12
McElhatton et al. (1996)[52]	12	97	0.11	28	235	0.11	1.03	0.55 to 1.96
	23	151	0.13	28	235	0.11	1.24	0.74 to 2.08
Meta-analysis (all drug classes)	192	1342	0.124	181	1852	0.087	1.45	1.19 to 1.77

DAAs = dual-action agents; SA = spontaneous abortion; SSRIs = selective serotonin-reuptake inhibitors; TCAs = tricyclic antidepressants.

Table 3
Meta-Analytic Results by Drug Classes

			DRUG GROUP			COMPARISON GROUP			META-ANALYTIC RR			
CLASS	STUDIES	N	RATE (n)	95% CI	χ^2 HETEROGENEITY	RATE (n)	95% CI	χ^2 HETEROGENEITY	RATE (n)	95% CI	χ^2 HETEROGENEITY	NNTH (95% CI)
Overall	11	3567	12.4% (1534)	10.8 to 14.1	2.29 (p = 0.994)	8.7% (2033)	7.5 to 9.9	5.31 (p = 0.99)	1.45% (3567)	1.19 to 1.77	3.13 (p = 0.978)	26 (17 to 53)
SSRIs	6	2016	12.4% (880)	10.2 to 14.5	1.76 (p = 0.881)	8.4% (1136)	6.8 to 10.0	2.15 (p = 0.828)	1.52% (2016)	1.17 to 1.98	1.16 (p = 0.948)	23 (14 to 67)
TCAs	3	957	12.3% (357)	8.9 to 15.7	0.31 (p = 0.855)	10.0% (600)	7.6 to 12.4	1.47 (p = 0.481)	1.23% (957)	0.84 to 1.78	0.79 (p = 0.672)	43 (NS)
DAAs	2	594	12.8% (297)	9.0 to 16.5	0.17 (p = 0.679)	7.7% (297)	4.7 to 10.8	0.07 (p = 0.789)	1.65% (594)	1.02 to 2.69	0.001 (p = 0.971)	20 (10 to 500)

DAAs = dual-action agents; NNTH = number needed to treat to harm; SSRIs = selective serotonin-reuptake inhibitors; TCAs = tricyclic antidepressants.

A limitation was that institution bias may be present, as two-thirds of the studies were produced by the Motherisk Program at the Hospital for Sick Children in Toronto. Therefore, it could be possible that, methodologically, these 4 studies have more in common with each other compared with the other 2.

As previously discussed, SA rates in the population range between 12% and 15%. According to this study, the meta-analytic rate (12.4%) falls within this range of published rates. A few non-controlled prospective studies have been published reporting similar rates in women exposed to antidepressants during their pregnancy. One evaluated outcomes of pregnancies with confirmed first-trimester fluoxetine exposure in the Eli Lilly pregnancy registry.[43] In that study, SAs were reported in 110 of the 796 (13.8%) pregnancies, which is slightly higher than our SSRI rate of 12.4%.

There are other limitations: most importantly, the time of exposure among the studies varied. This is especially true with women identified through teratogen information services, where women initiate a call to the service requesting information regarding a drug used during pregnancy. If a woman taking an antidepressant becomes pregnant and suffers an SA early on, she would not call the service and therefore would not be included in the study, thus lowering the rates. Currently, the Motherisk Program enrolls all women in both groups within one week of the time of her call; however, this was only done in the trazodone/nefazodone study. In that study, the differences were greater between the exposed and comparison groups than in the other investigations. Despite this, even in the other studies that did not match for time of call, the comparison group was recruited in the same way as the exposed group, and there were still more SAs in the exposed group.

As this is an observational study, the current analysis was subjected to all limitations associated with such studies. For example, in one study, the authors stated that some of the women might have reported an SA when, in fact, they had electively terminated the pregnancy.[20] Other bias could enter through the time of enrollment, as many abortions occur early in the first trimester. Therefore, our reported rates for both groups may have been underestimated.

We were unable to locate any studies of women who were depressed and not receiving any pharmacotherapy, which may solve the question whether the drug or depression is associated with this increase in SA. The ideal study would be to enroll 4 groups of women including depressed, taking antidepressants; depressed, not taking antidepressants; not depressed, taking antidepressants; and not depressed, not taking antidepressants. However, this type of study would be difficult to carry out at a teratogen information service because women usually do not call these services unless they are taking a drug and want information on the safety of that medication in pregnancy.

CONCLUSIONS

Maternal exposure to antidepressants may be associated with a significantly increased risk for SAs. However, the underlying depression could also be a contributing factor. Women and their healthcare providers should use this information cautiously in deciding whether to treat depression pharmacologically during pregnancy. Further research is needed to reach definitive conclusions. Depressed pregnant women should be treated with antidepressants if appropriate to ensure optimal mental health for both mothers and babies.

Michiel EH Hemels Drs MSc, at time of writing, MSc Student, Department of Pharmacology, Faculty of Medicine, University of Toronto, Toronto, Ontario, Canada; Motherisk Program, Hospital For Sick Children, Toronto

Adrienne Einarson RN, Assistant Director, Motherisk Program, Hospital For Sick Children

Gideon Koren MD, Professor, Department of Pharmacology, Faculty of Medicine, University of Toronto, Hospital For Sick Children

Krista L Lanctôt PhD, Assistant Professor, Department of Pharmacology, University of Toronto

Thomas R Einarson PhD, Associate Professor, Leslie Dan Faculty of Pharmacy, University of Toronto

REFERENCES

1. O'Hara MW. Social support, life events, and depression during pregnancy and the puerperium. Arch Gen Psychiatry 1986;43:569-73.
2. Kitamura T, Shima S, Sugawara M, Ioda MA. Psychological and social correlates of the onset of affective disorders among pregnant women. Psychosom Med 1993;23:967-75.
3. Marcus SM, Flynn H, Blow FC, Barry KL. Depressive symptoms among pregnant women screened in obstetric settings. J Women Health 2003;12:373-80.
4. Jarrahi-Zadeh A, Kane FJJ, Van de Castle RL, Lachenbruch PA, Ewing JA. Emotional and cognitive changes in pregnancy and early puerperium. Br J Psychiatry 1969;115:797-805.
5. Goldenberg RL, Gotlieb SJ. Social and psychological factors and pregnancy outcome. In: Complications of pregnancy: medical, surgical, gynaecologic, psychosocial and perinatal. Philadelphia: Williams and Wilkins, 1991:80-95.
6. Zax M, Sameroff AJ, Babigian HM. Birth outcomes in the offspring of mentally disordered women. Am J Orthopsychiatry 1977;47:218-9.
7. Zuckerman B, Amaro H, Bauchner H, Cabral H. Depressive symptoms during pregnancy: relationship to poor health behaviors. Am J Obstet Gynecol 1989;160:1107-11.
8. Orr ST, Miller CA. Maternal depressive symptoms and the risk of poor pregnancy outcome. Review of the literature and preliminary findings. Epidemiol Rev 1995;17:165-71.
9. Steer RA, Scholl TO, Hediger ML, Fischer RL. Self-reported depression and negative pregnancy outcomes. J Clin Epidemiol 1992;45:1093-9.
10. Zuckerman B, Bauchner H, Parker S. Maternal depressive symptoms during pregnancy, and newborn irritability. J Dev Behav Pediatr 1990;11:190-4.
11. Thorngren-Jerneck K, Herbst A. Low 5-minute Apgar score: a population-based register study of 1 million term births. Obstet Gynecol 2001;98:1-7.
12. McGrath M, Sullivan M. Birth weight, neonatal morbidities, and school age outcomes in full-term and preterm infants. Issues Comprehens Pediatr Nurs 2002;25:231-54.
13. Allen MC. Preterm outcomes research: a critical component of neonatal intensive care. Ment Retard Dev D R 2003;8:221-33.

14. Glover V. Maternal stress or anxiety in pregnancy and emotional development of the child. Br J Psychiatry 1997;171:105-6.
15. Teixeira JM, Fisk NM, Glover V. Association between maternal anxiety in pregnancy and increased uterine artery resistance index: cohort based study. BMJ 1999;318:153-7.
16. Uno H, Lohmiller L, Thieme C. Brain damage induced by prenatal exposure to dexamethasone in fetal rhesus macaques. 1. Hippocampus. Brain Res Develop Brain Res 1990;53:157-67.
17. Uno H, Eisele S, Sakai A. Neurotoxicity of glucocorticoids in the primate brain. Horm Behav 1994;28:336-48.
18. Gotlib IH, Whiffen VE, Mount JH. Prevalence rates and demographic characteristics associated with depression in pregnancy and the postpartum. J Consult Clin Psychol 1989;57:269-74.
19. Klein MH, Essex MJ. Pregnant or depressed? The effect of overlap between symptoms of depression and somatic complaints of pregnancy on rates of major depression in the second trimester. Depression 1994;2:1994-5.
20. Pastuszak A, Schick-Boschetto B, Zuber C, Feldkamp M, Pinelli M, Sihn S, et al. Pregnancy outcome following first-trimester exposure to fluoxetine (Prozac). JAMA 1993;269:2246-8.
21. Einarson A, Bonari L, Voyer-Lavigne S, Addis A, Matsui D, Johnston Y, et al. A multicentre prospective controlled study to determine the safety of trazodone/nefazodone use during pregnancy. Can J Psychiatry 2003; 48:106-10.
22. Einarson A, Fatoye B, Sarkar M, Lavigne SV, Brochu J, Chambers C, et al. Pregnancy outcome following gestational exposure to venlafaxine: a multicenter prospective controlled study. Am J Psychiatry 2001;158:1728-30.
23. Kulin NA, Pastuszak A, Sage SR, Schick-Boschetto B, Spivey G, Feldkamp M, et al. Pregnancy outcome following maternal use of the new selective serotonin reuptake inhibitors: a prospective controlled multicenter study. JAMA 1998;279:609-10.
24. Garciá-Enguídanos A, Valero J, Luna S, Domínguez-Rojas V. Risk factors in miscarriage: a review. Eur J Obstet Gyn R B 2002;102:111-9.
25. Kesmodel U, Wisborg K, Olson FS, Henriksen TB, Secher NJ. Moderate alcohol intake in pregnancy and the risk of spontaneous abortion. Alcohol Alcoholism 2002;37:87-92.
26. Regan L, Braude PR, Trembath PL. Influence of past reproductive performance on risk of spontaneous abortion. BMJ 1989;26:541–5.
27. Cnattingius S, Signorello L, Anneren G, Clausson B, Ekborn A, Ljunger E, et al. Caffeine intake and the risk of first-trimester spontaneous abortions. N Engl J Med 2000;343:1839-45.
28. Anatomic Therapeutic Chemical classification of drugs. Oslo: World Health Organization Collaborating Center for Drug Utilization, 2004.
29. Cochran WG. The combination of estimates from different experiments. Biometrics 1954;10:101-29.
30. Bjerre LM, LeLorier J. Expressing the magnitude of adverse effects in case control studies: "The number of patients needed to be treated for one additional patient to be harmed." BMJ 2000;320:503-6.
31. Egger M, Smith GD, Schneider M, Mindcer C. Bias in meta-analysis detected by a simple, graphical test. BMJ 1997;315:629-34.
32. Sterne JAC, Egger M, Davey G. Investigating and dealing with publication and other biases in meta-analysis. BMJ 2001;323:101-8.
33. Sterne JAC, Egger M. Funnel plots for detecting bias in meta-analysis: guidelines on choice of axis. J Clin Epidemiol 2001;54: 1046-55.
34. Duval S, Tweedie R. Trim and fill: a simple funnel-plot–based method of testing and adjusting for publication bias in meta-analysis. Biometrics 2000;56:455-63.
35. Sutton AJ, Song F, Gilbody SM, Abrams KR. Modelling publication bias in meta-analysis: a review. Stat Methods Med Res 2000;9: 421-45.
36. Begg CB, Mazumdar M. Operating characteristics of a rank correlation test for publication bias. Biometrics 1994;50:1088-101.
37. Elwood JM. Critical appraisal of a cohort study. In: Causal relationships in medicine. 1st ed. Oxford: Oxford University Press, 1988:184-210.
38. Lichtenstein MJ, Mulrow CD, Elwood PC. Guidelines for reading case–control studies. J Chronic Dis 1987;40:893-903.
39. Feinstein AR. Observer variability. In: Clinical epidemiology. The architecture of clinical research. Philadelphia: WB Saunders, 1985:632-48.
40. Fleiss J. Measuring nominal scale agreement among many raters. Psychol Bull 1971;76:378-82.
41. Fleiss J, Nee J, Landis J. The large sample variance of kappa in the case of different sets of raters. Psychol Bull 1979;86:974-77.
42. Nulman I, Rovet J, Stewart DE, Wolpin J, Gardner HA, Theis JGW, et al. Neurodevelopment of children exposed in utero to antidepressant drugs. N Engl J Med 1997;336:258-62.
43. Goldstein DJ, Corbin LA, Sundell KL. Effects of first-trimester fluoxetine exposure on the newborn. Obstet Gynecol 1997;89:713-8.
44. Goldstein DJ, Sundell KL, Corbin LA. Birth outcomes in pregnant women taking fluoxetine. N Engl J Med 1997;336:872-3.
45. Shakir S. Data. Southampton, UK: Drug Safety Research Unit, 1999.
46. Brunel P, Vial T, Roche I, Bertolotti E, Evreux JC. Follow-up of 151 pregnant women exposed to antidepressant treatment (MAOI excluded) during organogenesis. Therapie 1994;49:117-22.
47. Ericson A, Kallén B, Wiholm B. Delivery outcome after the use of antidepressants in early pregnancy. Eur J Clin Pharmacol 1999;55: 503-8.
48. Emslie G, Judge R. Tricyclic antidepressants and selective serotonin reuptake inhibitors: use during pregnancy, in children/adolescents and in the elderly. Acta Psychiatr Scand Suppl 2000;403:26-34.
49. Goldstein DJ. Effects of third trimester fluoxetine exposure on the newborn. J Clin Psychopharmacol 1995;15:417-420.
50. Webster J, Chandler J, Battistutta D. Pregnancy outcomes and health care use: effects of abuse. Am J Obstet Gynecol 1996;174:760-7.
51. Chambers CD, Johnson KA, Dick LM, Felix RJ, Jones KL. Birth outcomes in pregnant women taking fluoxetine. N Engl J Med 1996;335: 1010-5.
52. McElhatton PR, Garbis HM, Elefant E, Vial T, Bellemin B, Mastroiacovo P, et al. The outcome of pregnancy in 689 women exposed to therapeutic doses of antidepressants. A collaborative study of the European Network of Teratology Information Services (ENTIS). Reprod Toxicol 1996;10:285-94.

EXTRACTO

INTRODUCCIÓN: Debido a la alta prevalencia de depresión en mujeres en edad fértil y con pareja, y al hecho de que el 50% de los embarazos no son planificados, existe una alta probabilidad de que estas mujeres hayan sido expuestas al uso de antidepresivos durante las primeras fases del embarazo.
OBJETIVO: Determinar las tasas basales de aborto espontáneo (AE) y si los antidepresivos aumentan estos niveles.
MÉTODOS: Los niveles de AE en las mujeres que tomaban antidepresivos comparados con los de las mujeres sin depresión se combinaron en un riesgo relativo utilizando los modelos de efectos aleatorios. Para la identificación de los estudios de cohortes se utilizaron las bases de datos MEDLINE, EMBASE, Healthstar, Toxline, Psychlit, Cochrane database, and Reprotox publicados durante el período 1966–2003.
RESULTADOS: De los 15 artículos potenciales, 6 estudios de cohortes de 3567 mujeres (1534 expuestas, 2033 no expuestas) proporcionaron datos para el análisis. Todos ellos fueron apareados por variables de confusión importantes. Las pruebas no encontraron heterogeneidad (χ^2 3.13; $p = 0.98$); todas las puntuaciones de calidad fueron adecuadas (>50%). La tasa basal de AE (CI 95%) fue del 8.7% (7.5%–9.9%; $n = 2033$); para las mujeres en tratamiento con antidepresivos, el nivel fue de 12.4% (10.8%–14.1%; $n = 1534$), con un incremento significativo del 3.9% (1.9%–6.0%); RR 1.45 (1.19–1.77; $n = 3567$). No se encontraron diferencias entre los distintos tipos de antidepresivos.
CONCLUSIONES: La exposición materna a los antidepresivos podría estar asociada a un incremento del riesgo de AE, aunque la depresión por si misma no puede ser descartada.

Corinne Zara Yahni

Appendix I. Checklist for Quality Scoring

Author and title of article: ______________________________
Reviewer: ______________________________

QUESTIONS	YES	NO	NA
Research Design			
Was research design model stated? (eg, cohort study)			
Was research question stated explicitly?			
Was exposure mentioned by name/definition?			
Was exposure well described?			
Was the outcome described by diagnostic procedure/definition?			
Was study population described?			
Subjects			
Was source of cohort identified?			
Was study group defined?			
Was outcome defined/described?			
Was follow-up appropriate for study purpose?			
Exposure			
Was duration of exposure described?			
Was quantity/dosage of exposure stated?			
Was the appropriate time of exposure measured?			
Was exposure verified?			
Analysis			
Was method of data collection mentioned? (eg, interview, questionnaire, record review)			
If an interviewer or record review was used, was there information on whether these observers were blinded?			
Was there a correct time relationship?			
Was conclusion drawn from data?			
Confounders and Bias			
Was information on the presence of possible confounding variables stated?			
Were possible sources of bias investigated?			
Were methods for dealing with confounders used and mentioned?			
Was the influence of bias on the results described?			
Methods			
Were analytic methods described? (statistical methods)			
Did controls undergo the same diagnostic procedures as the cases?			
Results			
Was nonresponse rate stated?			
Was main result described?			
Was there a dose–response relationship?			
Were appropriate results given? (eg, OR, RR)			
Was confidence interval stated?			

NA = not applicable.

RÉSUMÉ

INFORMATION DE BASE: La prévalence élevée de la dépression chez les femmes en âge de procréer, jumelée à la non planification des naissances dans approximativement 50% des cas, résulte en un risque élevé que ces femmes soient exposées aux antidépresseurs en début de grossesse.
OBJECTIF: Déterminer les taux de base d'avortement spontané et évaluer si la prise d'antidépresseurs pendant la grossesse augmente ces taux.
MÉTHODOLOGIE: Les taux d'avortement spontané chez des femmes prenant des antidépresseurs comparativement à ceux observés chez des femmes non atteintes de dépression ont été combinés pour produire un risque relatif en utilisant un modèle d'effets aléatoires. Les bases de données MEDLINE, EMBASE, Healthstar, Toxline, Psychlit, Cochrane database, et Reprotox ont été questionnées pour retrouver les études de cohortes publiées entre 1966–2003.
RÉSULTATS: Un total de 15 études de cohortes a été identifié. De celles-ci, 6 études regroupant en tout 3567 femmes (1534 exposées, 2033 non exposées) ont fourni des données extractibles. Toutes ces études pouvaient être couplées pour les variables confondantes importantes. Seulement les données pour les femmes exposées de façon continue à un agent antidépresseur unique durant les 20 premières semaines de la grossesse ont été retenues. L'avortement spontané était défini comme une perte fœtale non désirée au cours des 20 premières semaines de gestation. Les tests statistiques n'ont pas détecté d'hétérogénéité (χ^2 3.13; p = 0.98); tous les scores de qualité étaient adéquats (>50%). Le taux de bases d'avortements spontanés (IC 95%) était de 8.7% (7.5% à 9.9%, n = 2033) alors qu'il était de 12.4% (10.8% à 14.1%; n = 1534) chez les femmes exposées aux antidépresseurs. L'augmentation du risque de 3.9% (1.9% à 6.0%) était significative. Le risque relatif observé était de 1.45 (1.19 à 1.77; n = 3567). Aucune différence n'a été observée entre les différentes classes d'antidépresseurs.
CONCLUSIONS: L'exposition maternelle aux antidépresseurs peut être associée à une augmentation du risque d'avortement spontané. Cependant, l'effet négatif de la dépression elle-même sur le risque d'avortement spontané ne peut être exclu.

Marie-Claude Vanier

CHAPTER 62

NEWER ANTIDEPRESSANTS IN PREGNANCY AND RATES OF MAJOR MALFORMATIONS: A META-ANALYSIS OF PROSPECTIVE COMPARATIVE STUDIES†

Thomas R. Einarson[1,‡] *and Adrienne Einarson*[2]

[1]*Faculty of Pharmacy, Department of Clinical Pharmacology, Faculty of Medicine, University of Toronto, Ont., Canada*

[2]*The Motherisk Program, Division of Clinical Pharmacology, The Hospital for Sick Children, Ont., Canada*

Summary

Background. A substantial number of women of childbearing age suffer from depression. Despite this, relatively little is known about the safety of antidepressant use during pregnancy.

Purpose. We conducted a meta-analysis of prospective comparative cohort studies to quantify the relationship between maternal exposure to the newer antidepressants and major malformations.

Methods. We searched Medline, Embase and Reprotox from 1996 to the present for studies comparing outcomes in first trimester exposures to citalopram, escitalopram, fluoxetine, fluvoxamine, paroxetine, sertraline, reboxetine, venlafaxine, nefazodone, trazodone, mirtazapine and bupropion to those of non-exposed mothers. Data were combined using a random effects model; heterogeneity was tested with χ^2, and publication bias with a funnel plot and the Begg–Mazumdar statistic.

Results. Twenty-two studies were identified, 15 were rejected (4 reviews, 4 without comparison groups, 2 third trimester exposures, 2 retrospective database studies, 2 case reports and 1 duplicate); 7 studies (n = 1774) met inclusion criteria. Effects were not heterogeneous ($\chi^2 = 2.04$, $p = 0.92$); funnel plot and test ($\tau = -0.24$, $p = 0.45$) indicated no publication bias. The summary relative risk was 1.01 (95% CI: 0.57–1.80).

Conclusions. As a group, the newer antidepressants are not associated with an increased risk of major malformations above the baseline of 1–3% in the population.

Keywords: teratogenicity; congenital malformations; antidepressants; SSRIs; SNRIs; pregnancy; clinical toxicology

INTRODUCTION

A substantial number of women of childbearing age suffer from depression. Recently, a prevalence study was published in which 3472 pregnant women were screened for depressive symptoms using the Centre for Epidemiologic Studies Depression scale. The authors found that 20% of the women surveyed scored above the cutoff score for depressive symptoms.[1] This statistic coupled with the fact that at least 50% of pregnancies are unplanned means that a relatively large number of women will use an antidepressant in pregnancy, especially in the early stages.

The Committee on Research on Psychiatric treatments of The American Psychiatric Association identified treatment of major depression during pregnancy as a priority area in clinical management. Based on this recommendation, a position paper was published on the risk-benefit decision making for treatment of depression during pregnancy. The authors concluded that there was no evidence to implicate antidepressants as causing harm to an unborn baby and that a pregnant woman should be treated as long as the benefits and possible risks are well explained to her.[2]

Few studies exist in the literature on pregnancy outcome following exposure to the newer antidepressants in pregnancy, especially studies with comparison groups.

Those that have been published are comprised of sample sizes of 150 cases or less, which allows us at most, to be able to detect only a fourfold increase in risk for major malformations above the baseline of 1–3%. There is considerable criticism in the literature that there is insufficient information in these studies to be able give an accurate risk assessment to a pregnant woman and her physician, leading women to discontinue a needed antidepressant when she becomes pregnant.

Information is limited, because these types of studies are difficult and time consuming, with few groups undertaking this particular form of research. Therefore, if all these small studies could be combined, there would be more information to enable women and their health care providers to make an evidence-based decision on whether or not to take these antidepressants during pregnancy. The objective of our study was to combine all of the studies to date that examined the rates of major malformations in infants whose mothers took one of the newer antidepressants during pregnancy.

METHODS

We performed a meta-analysis of the literature. We accepted only prospective cohort studies that compared outcomes from exposed women with those from non-exposed women. The drugs of interest

† No conflict of interest was declared.

‡ Thomas Einarson is an Associate Professor in The Faculty of Pharmacy at The University of Toronto and Adrienne Einarson is The Assistant Director of The Motherisk Program at The Hospital for Sick Children in Toronto.

included the currently available[4] SSRIs (citalopram, escitalopram, fluoxetine, fluvoxamine, paroxetine and sertraline), SNRIs (venlafaxine), dual action drugs (nefazodone, trazodone and mirtazapine) or selective noradrenaline re-uptake inhibitors (reboxetine and bupropion). Excluded were the tricyclics and related drugs (e.g. maprotiline, amoxepine and lofepramine) and the MAOIs (phenelzine, tranylcypromine, isocarboxazid and moclobemide). We also excluded botanicals and related compounds such as St. John's Wort and tryptophan.

Individuals who were included were pregnant women exposed to any of the drugs of interest during the first trimester of pregnancy. Those exposed to known teratogens or fetotoxic substances were excluded. Outcomes were considered only for live births. The outcome of interest was major structural or functional malformations, including those requiring surgery to correct.

We searched Medline, Embase and Reprotox databases from 1966 to the present using keywords teratogenicity, malformation, congenital deformity, antidepressant and all of the generic names of the drugs of interest. There was no language restriction. Two reviewers independently searched and consensus agreement was used to settle discrepancies. Data were extracted in a similar fashion.

Data were combined into a summary risk ratio using a random effects model, with heterogeneity of effects tested using χ^2 Publication bias was examined visually using a funnel plot and statistically using the method of Beggand Mazumdar.[4]

Quality of articles was assessed using a 29-item checklist based on work by Feinstein,[5] Lichtenstein *et al.*[6] and Elwood[7] Reviewers assigned a score of 1 if the item I present in the paper and 0 if it absent. Nonapplicable items were not considered in the scoring. The quality score was expressed as a percentage of items present in the article. Inter-rater reliability was assessed by calculating kappa. The criterion for acceptable reliability was a significant kappa ($p < 0.05$) that was >0.8. Scores above 50% were considered acceptable.

RESULTS

Fifteen studies were rejected: 4 were reviews,[8–11] 4 lacked comparison groups,[12–15] 2 dealt only with third trimester exposures,[16,17] 2 retrospective database studies,[18,19] 2 were case reports[20,21] and 1 was a duplicate that appeared in abstract form.[22] The two database studies had further problems in that one did not examine pregnancy outcomes and the other did not have a comparison group.

Seven studies with 1774 patients met the inclusion criteria.[23–29] Table 1 presents those studies and their characteristics. The heterogeneity statistic was nonsignificant ($\chi^2 = 2.04$, $p = 0.92$), suggesting that results could reasonably be combined. The funnel plot (not shown) did not provide evidence of obvious publication bias. The Begg–Mazumdar test confirmed this observation with small and non-significant results ($\tau = -0.24$, $p = 0.45$).

Table 2 lists the malformations noted in the accepted studies, categorised according to group. The summary risk ratio was 1.01 (95% CI: 0.57–1.80), indicating no elevated risk. The average rate in both the exposed group and comparison group was 2.0%, which falls in the middle of the baseline risk rate of 1 to 3%. We had greater than 90% power to detect a relative risk of 2.5, with an assumed baseline risk of 2% and alpha error of 5%, and more than 80% power to detect a threefold difference if the baseline risk is as low as 1%.

We further conducted analyses for individual drugs. Results are presented in Table 3. We could not obtain results for fluvoxamine, paroxetine or sertraline because they were not presented separately by Kulin *et al.*[26] The only risk ratio that was above 2 was that of venlafaxine. However, the malformation rate in the exposed group was 1.6%, which was well within the range of 1 to 3% found in non-exposed babies.

DISCUSSION

To our knowledge, this is the first study to examine all the prospective comparative studies of the newer antidepressants in pregnancy that have entered the market since fluoxetine was introduced in the 1980s. We did this by performing a meta-analysis that showed there was no increase risk in the baseline rate of 1 to 3% for major malformations. The available sample size of 1774 women was adequate to rule out these drugs as major teratogens. However, we were unable to examine specific defects that occur less frequently than 1/240 exposures, according to the rule of threes.[30]

The malformations that were detected did not consistently present any one malformation or cluster of malformations. The observed anomalies (e.g. ventricular septal defect, hypospadias and cleft palate) were among the most commonly reported problems. If these drugs were teratogenic, then a single deformity or syndrome would be expected. However, those reported vary widely and affect a number of different unrelated body systems, including (among others) the heart, liver, brain, intestine and genital tract (Table 2).

It must be noted, however, that we only examined rates of malformations, not other outcomes such as the possible long-term neurobehavioral effects of these drugs or other more subtle effects. As well, we did not examine other important variables, such as birth weight, head circumference, pre maturity or other problems of the newborn or the mother.

The study does have its limitations. Most of the studies (5/7, 71%) that we used were produced by the Motherisk Program in Toronto and another came from a comparable service in San Diego. The women who contact these services tend to be highly educated, well informed and motivated to contact a counselling service. Thus, these women may not be typical of the entire population of women of childbearing age. Some would also see as a major limitation that one or both of the authors were involved with 3/7 studies included in the meta-analysis and with each other (husband and wife). We understand that normally this may create a bias because the appraisers may not wish to exclude any of their own studies. However, in this case because we were including studies that would qualify for the highest level of evidence, we chose only prospective cohorts with a comparative group. We then discovered that there were only seven of these types of studies in the literature and five of them came from Motherisk. We would like to state categorically that anyone could have performed this analysis and produced the same results.

The drugs that we studied belong to a variety of chemical families that differ in their mechanisms of action. What they have in common is that they all are used to treat depression (among other disorders). However, they exert their effects through different pathways and influence different neural receptors.

On the other hand, no single molecule stood out from the others in terms of toxicity. Malformation rates ranged from 0 for bupropion[29] to 4.1% in Kulin's study, which examined sertraline, paroxetine and fluvoxamine.[26] Fluoxetine, the oldest and most

Table 1
Statistical Summary of Individual Studies and Overall Results

FIRST AUTHOR	YEAR	QUALITY SCORE (%)	COUNTRY	DRUGS EXAMINED	AVERAGE DAILY DOSE OR RANGE (MCD) (mg)	EXPOSED GROUP		COMPARISON GROUP		RELATIVE RISK	95% CONFIDENCE LIMITS	
						m/n	RATE (%)	m/n	RATE (%)		LOWER	UPPER
Pastuszak *et al.*[23]	1993	79	Canada, U.S.A.	Fluoxetine	25.8	2/98	2.0	2/110	1.8	1.12	0.16	7.82
Chambers *et al.*[24]	1996	83	U.S.A.	Fluoxetine	26.8	6/174	3.4	6/226	2.7	1.30	0.43	3.96
Goldstein *et al.*[25]	1997	62	Worldwide	Fluoxetine	10–80	1/28	3.6	0/6	0	—	—	—
				Fluvoxamine	10–60 (50)							
Kulin *et al.*[26]	1998	72	Canada	Paroxetine	10–60 (30)	9/222	4.1	9/235	3.8	1.06	0.43	2.62
			U.S.A., Brazil	Sertraline	25–250 (50)							
Einarson *et al.*[27]	2001	69	Canada, Italy, U.S.A.	Venlafaxine	37.5–300 (75)	2/125	1.6	1/137	0.7	2.19	0.20	23.88
Einarson *et al.*[28]	2003	66	Canada, Italy	Nefazodone	NS	2/121	1.7	4/131	3.1	0.54	0.10	2.90
			U.S.A.	Trazodon								
Chan *et al.*[29]	2004	69	Canada, U.S.A.	Bupropion	NS	0/72	0	2/89	2.2	0.25	0.01	5.06
Overall						22/830	2.0	24/934	2.0	1.01	0.57	1.80

MCD, most common dose; m/n, number of malformations/number in sample; NS, not stated.

Table 2
Major Malformations Reported in Women Exposed to Antidepressants

FIRST AUTHOR	EXPOSED GROUP	COMPARISON GROUP
Pastuszak *et al.*[23]	Jejunal obstruction	Pulmonary atresia
	Ventricular septal defect	Ventricular septal defect
Chambers *et al.*[24]	Ventricular septal defect (2)	Ventricular septal defect
	Atrial septal defect	Hypospadias (2)
	Nasal dermoid sinus	Bilateral inguinal hernia
	Coccygeal dermoid sinus	Cleft palate
	Hypospadias	
Goldstein *et al.*[25]	Hepatoblastoma	Nil
Kulin *et al.*[26]	Double urinary collecting system (2)	
	Cardiac malformations (2)	Cardiac malformations (4)
	Absent corpus callosum	Inguinal hernia (2)
	Bilateral club foot	Undescended testicle
	Ear malformation	Ectopic kidney
	Ovarian cyst	Vesicourethral reflux
	Pyloric stenosis	
Einarson *et al.*[27]	Hypospadias	Congenital heart defect
	Neural tube defect and club foot	
Einarson *et al.*[28]	Hirschsprung disease	Urethral stenosis
	Neural tube defect	Hypospadias
		Pyloric stenosis
		Ventricular septal defect
Chan *et al.*[29]	Nil	

studied drug had a relative risk of 1.19 (95%CI: 0.47–3.00) when the three studies were combined, while both nefazodone/trazodone [28] and bupropion[29] had relative risks below unity. Venlafaxine had the highest relative risk of 2.19, but the rate in the comparison group was 0.7%, which is below the usual range.[27] Therefore, this low denominator inflated the relative risk for venlafaxine, which had a malformation rate of 1.6%, third lowest among all of the drugs and well within the normal expected range.

This is important information to add to the literature on the safety of the use of the newer antidepressants during pregnancy.

Table 3
Risk Ratios for Individual Drugs

DRUG	RR	95%CI	STUDIES	PATIENTS
Bupropion	0.25	0.01–5.06	1	99
Fluoxetine	1.19	0.47–3.00	3	300
Nefazodone/ trazodone	0.54	0.10–2.90	1	147
Venlafaxine	2.19	0.20–23.88	1	125

Depression is a serious and often debilitating illness and women should not be expected to discontinue their antidepressant for lack of information, simply because they are pregnant. Abrupt discontinuation of a needed antidepressant during pregnancy has been associated with a number of negative consequences, including suicidal ideation and hospitalisation.[31] In addition, women should not necessarily be switched to another antidepressant that may not be appropriate for them, simply because there is more information on pregnancy outcomes.

Pregnancy is a time of relative mental instability for all women, and for women with depression it can be more difficult if their depression is untreated, for both mother and baby.[32] Women and their health care providers will now have more evidence-based information to make an informed decision on whether or not to continue taking one of the newer classes of antidepressant during pregnancy.

SUMMARY

This meta-analysis of all published prospective comparative studies found no association between first trimester exposure to the newer antidepressants and an increase in the rates of major malformations. Women with depression who are pregnant or planning pregnancy and their physicians, can use this evidence-based information to enable them to weigh the risks and benefits of treatment with antidepressants.

REFERENCES

1. Marcus SM, Flynn HA, Blow FC, Barry KL. Depressive symptoms among pregnant women screened in obstetric settings. *J Womens Health* 2003; **12:** 373–380.
2. Altshuler LL, Cohen L, Szuba MP, *et al.* Pharmacological management of psychiatric illness during pregnancy: dilemmas and guidelines. *Am J Psychiatry* 1997; **154:** 718–719.
3. BritishNational Formulary (47th edn). British Medical Association and Royal Pharmaceutical Society of Great Britain: London, March 2004.
4. Begg CB, Mazumdar M. Operating characteristics of a rank correlation test for publication bias. *Biometrics* 1994; **50:** 1088–1101.
5. Feinstein AR. Observer variability. In *Clinical Epidemiology: The Architecture of Clinical Research.* W.B. Saunders Company: Philadelphia, 1985; 632–648.
6. Lichtenstein MJ, Mulrow CD, Elwood PC. Guidelines for reading case-control studies. *J Chronic Dis* 1987; **40:** 893–903.
7. Elwood JM. Critical appraisal of a cohort study. *In Causal Relationships in Medicine* (1st edn). Oxford University Press: Oxford, 1988; 184–210.
8. Cohen LS, Rosenbaum JF. Psychotropic drug use during pregnancy: weighing the risks. *J Clin Psychiatry* 1998; **59:** 18–28.
9. Kulin NA, Pastuszak A, Koren G. Are the new SSRIs safe for pregnant women? *Can Fam Physician* 1998; **44:** 2081–2083.
10. Nonacs R, Cohen LS. Assessment and treatment of depression during pregnancy: an update. *Psychiatr Clin N Am* 2003; **26:** 547–562.
11. Stewart DE. Antidepressant drugs during pregnancy and lactation. *Int Clin Psychopharmacol* 2000; **15:** S19–S24.
12. Brunel P, Vial T, Roche I, Bertolotti E, Evreaux JC. Firsttrimester exposure to antidepressant drugs: result of a follow-up. *Therapie* 1994; **49:** 117–122.
13. Hendrick V, Smith LM, Suri R, Hwang S, Haynes D, Altshuler L. Birth outcomes after exposure to antidepressant medication. *Am J Obstet Gynecol* 2003; **188:** 812–815.
14. McElhatton PR, Garbis HM, Elefant E, *et al.* The outcome of pregnancy in 689 women exposed to therapeutic doses of antidepressants: a collaborative study of the European Network of Teratology Information Services (ENTIS). *Reprod Toxicol* 1996; **10:** 285–294.
15. Reiff-Eldridge R, Heffner CR, Ephross SA, Tennis PS, White AD, Andrews EB. Monitoring pregnancy outcomes after prenatal drug exposure through prospective pregnancy registries: a pharmaceutical company commitment. *Am J Obstet Gynecol* 2000; **82:** 59–63.
16. Goldstein DJ. Effects of third trimester fluoxetine exposure on the newborn. *J Clin Psychopharmacol* 1995; **15:** 417–420.
17. Costei AM, Kozer E, Ho T, Ito S, Koren G. Perinatal outcome following third trimester exposure to paroxetine. *Arch Pediatr Adolesc Med* 2002; **156:** 1129–1132.
18. Malm H, Martikainen J, Klaukka T, Neuvonen PJ. Prescription drugs during pregnancy and lactation—a Finnish register-based study. *Eur J Clin Pharmacol* 2003; **59:** 127–133.
19. Rosa F. Medicaid antidepressant pregnancy exposure outcomes. *Reprod Toxicol* 1994; **8:** 444–445.
20. Rybakowski JK. Moclobemide in pregnancy. *Pharmacopsychiatry* 2001; **34:** 82–83.
21. Simhandl C, Zoghlami A. Mirtazapine use during emergency. *Neuropsychiatrie* 1999; **13:** 145–147.
22. Chambers CD, Johnson KA, Jones KL. Pregnancy outcome in women exposed to fluoxetine. *Teratology* 1993; **47:** 386.
23. Pastuszak A, Schick-Boschetto B, Zuber C, et al. Pregnancy outcome following first-trimester exposure to fluoxetine (Prozac). *JAMA* 1993; **269:** 2246–2248.
24. Chambers CD, Johnson KA, Dick LM, Felix R, Jones KL. Birth outcomes in pregnant women taking fluoxetine. *N Engl J Med* 1996; **335:** 1010–1015.
25. Goldstein DJ, Corbin LA, Sundell KL. Effects of first-trimester fluoxetine exposure on the newborn. *Obstet Gynecol* 1997; **89:** 713–718.
26. Kulin NA, Pastuszak A, Sage SR, *et al.* Pregnancy outcome following maternal use of the new selective serotonin reuptake inhibitors: a prospective controlled multicenter study. *JAMA* 1998; **279:** 609–610.
27. Einarson A, Fatoye B, Sarkar M, *et al.* Pregnancy outcome following gestational exposure to venlafaxine: a multicenter prospective controlled study. *Am J Psychiatry* 2001; **158:** 1728–1730.
28. Einarson A, Bonari L, Voyer-Lavigne S, *et al.* A multicentre prospective controlled study to determine the safety of trazodone and nefazodone use during pregnancy. *Can J Psychiatry* 2003; **48:** 106–110.
29. Chan B, Koren G, Fayez I, *et al.* Pregnancy outcome of women exposed to bupropion during pregnancy: a prospective comparative study. (in press) *Am J Obstetrics and Gynecology* 2004.
30. Dieck GS, Glasser DB, Sachs RM. A view from industry. In *Pharmacoepidemiology* (2nd edn), Strom BL (ed.). John Wiley and Sons: Chichester, 1994; 75.
31. Einarson A, Selby P, Koren G. Abrupt discontinuation of psychotropic drugs during pregnancy: fear of teratogenic risk and impact of counselling. *J Psychiatry Neurosci* 2001; **26:** 44–48.
32. Bennett HA, Einarson A, Taddio A, Koren G, Einarson TR. Prevalence of depression during pregnancy: systematic review. *Obstet Gynecol* 2004; **103:** 698–709.

CHAPTER 63

MAJOR MALFORMATIONS WITH VALPROIC ACID

Gideon Koren, Alejandro A. Nava-Ocampo, Myla E. Moretti, Reuven Sussman, and Irena Nulman

Abstract

Question. Increasing numbers of pregnant patients are treated with valproic acid, not just for epilepsy, but also for psychiatric conditions. Are there teratogenic risks other than the risk of spina bifida?
Answer. It has now become evident that valproic acid might cause more than just neural tube defects (NTDs). In a systematic review of all cohort studies intended to answer this question, higher rates of major malformations (and not just NTDs) were found in most studies. The calculated relative risk was 2.59 when compared with other antiepileptic drugs and was 3.77 when compared with risk in the general population. There is compelling evidence that the risk is dose dependent. The risks appear to begin increasing at doses of 600 mg/d and to become more prominent at doses above 1000 mg/d.

Résumé

Question. Un nombre grandissant de patientes enceintes suivent un traitement à l'acide valproïque, non seulement pour l'épilepsie, mais aussi pour des problèmes psychiatriques. Y a-t-il des risques tératogènes autres que celui du spina bifida?
Réponse. Il est maintenant devenu évident que l'acide valproïque peut causer plus que des défauts du tube médullaire. Dans une synthèse critique de toutes les études de cohortes conçues pour répondre à cette question, des taux plus élevés de malformations majeures (ne se limitant pas au tube médullaire) ont été observés dans la plupart des études. Le risque relatif calculé se situait à 2,59 en comparaison de celui observé avec d'autres médicaments contre l'épilepsie et à 3,77 par rapport au risque dans la population en général. Des données scientifiques convaincantes indiquent que le risque dépend de la dose. Le risque semble commencer à augmenter avec des doses de 600 mg/j et à devenir plus prépondérant à des doses de plus de 1 000 mg/j.

Soon after valproic acid was introduced to clinical use for epilepsy, cases emerged suggesting an increased risk of neural tube defects (NTDs), particularly of spina bifida, among offspring exposed to the drug in early gestation.[1,2] The experimental animal work by Nau and colleagues was very important in establishing that valproic acid caused development of NTDs.[3] The overall risk for NTDs has been estimated at 2%. While this looks like a low rate, it virtually doubles the overall risk for major malformations in the general population from its usual 1% to 3%. Because NTDs can be detected in utero in most cases by detailed ultrasonography and by measuring levels of alpha-fetoproteins in maternal serum or amniotic fluid, women treated with valproic acid in early gestation should be informed of these diagnostic options.

Over the last 15 years, an increasing number of anecdotal reports and case series have suggested that valproic acid causes malformations other than NTDs, including limb and cardiac anomalies. Until recently, a lack of controlled or large-scale studies precluded corroboration of these impressions. To complicate the situation, increasing numbers of women are now receiving valproic acid as part of treatment for a variety of psychiatric conditions.[4]

Over the last few years, larger cohort studies of pregnancy outcome among women exposed to valproic acid in pregnancy have been published, now allowing us to evaluate the overall rates of teratogenic risk of valproic acid.

We searched the MEDLINE, EMBASE, and Cochrane databases from 1978, when reports on valproic acid use in pregnancy began to emerge, to December 31, 2005. We selected controlled cohort studies that reported the use of valproic acid during the first trimester of pregnancy and that had a comparison group of women treated with other antiepileptic drugs, untreated epileptic women, or healthy women representing the general population of pregnant women. To be included in our analysis, the studies had to describe rates of major malformations among the study and comparison groups. Several studies had comparison groups, but the papers did not allow extraction of these numbers. Individual and summary relative risks were calculated with the Mantel-Haenszel random effect test using Cochrane's Review Manager (version 4.2). We calculated the relative risk for major malformations among babies exposed to valproic acid alone or in combination with other anticonvulsant drugs during embryogenesis as compared with babies exposed to other anticonvulsants, or babies of unexposed healthy control subjects.

MALFORMATION RATES

Based on more than 1700 exposed babies reported in 11 cohort studies, exposure to monotherapy with valproic acid was associated with a relative risk of 2.59 for major malformation (95% confidence interval [CI] 2.11 to 3.17) when compared with monotherapy using other anticonvulsant drugs (Figure 1A).[5-15] Based on more than 1300 exposed babies, the relative risk was 3.16 (95% CI 2.17 to 4.60) when compared with untreated epileptic patients (Figure 1B).[7,8,10,13,14,16-18] Although less frequently reported, when compared with the general population of healthy control subjects the relative risk of major congenital malformations among patients receiving monotherapy with valproic acid was 3.77 (95% CI 2.18 to 6.52)(Figure 1C).[5,6,9] This means that women exposed to valproic acid monotherapy during embryogenesis have more than 2.5 times the risk of having babies with malformations and that this trend is highly significant ($P < .001$).

When valproic acid was administered as part of anticonvulsant *polytherapy,* the number of exposed babies was lower than those exposed to valproic acid monotherapy, yet the relative risk also increased significantly over that of other anticonvulsant drugs (1.84 [95% CI 1.34 to 2.52]), untreated epilepsy (3.24 [95% CI 2.06 to 5.08]), and healthy control subjects (3.35 [95% CI 1.87 to 6.01]) (Figure 2).[5,6,8-14,18] Valproic acid polytherapy regimens varied greatly, and combinations with all commercially available treatments were reported.

A)

STUDY	TREATMENT SAMPLE/TOTAL	CONTROL SAMPLE/TOTAL	WEIGHT %	RR N (95% CI)
Tanganelli and Regesta,[5] 1992	0/6	3/72	0.50	1.49 (0.09, 26.01)
Samren et al,[6] 1997	6/21	20/159	6.53	2.27 (1.03, 5.01)
Canger et al,[7] 1999	6/44	12/269	4.76	3.06 (1.21, 7.72)
Kaneko et al,[8] 1999	9/81	30/419	8.20	1.55 (0.77, 3.14)
Samren et al,[9] 1999	9/158	21/741	7.04	2.01 (0.94, 4.31)
Mawer et al,[10] 2002	1/14	1/29	0.56	2.07 (0.14, 30.74)
Meischenguiser et al,[11] 2004	3/21	3/62	1.76	2.95 (0.64, 13.52)
Wide et al,[12] 2004	26/268	42/988	18.48	2.28 (1.43, 3.65)
Artama et al,[13] 2005	28/263	24/968	14.66	4.29 (2.53, 7.28)
Morrow et al,[14] 2006	44/715	47/1753	25.30	2.30 (1.54, 3.43)
Wyszynski et al,[15] 2005	16/149	31/1048	12.21	3.63 (2.04, 6.47)
TOTAL (95% CI)	**148/1740**	**234/6508**	**100.00**	**2.59 (2.11, 3.17)**

B)

STUDY	TREATMENT SAMPLE/TOTAL	CONTROL SAMPLE/TOTAL	WEIGHT %	RR N (95% CI)
Canger et al,[7] 1999	6/44	0/25	1.76	7.51 (0.44, 128.00)
Kaneko et al,[8] 1999	9/81	3/98	8.52	3.63 (1.02, 12.96)
Mawer et al,[10] 2002	1/14	0/1	1.75	0.40 (0.02, 6.85)
Kaaja et al,[16] 2003	4/61	2/239	4.98	7.84 (1.47, 41.79)
Adab et al,[17] 2004	7/63	4/101	9.75	2.81 (0.86, 9.20)
Artama et al,[13] 2005	28/263	26/939	45.60	3.84 (2.30, 6.44)
Morrow et al,[14] 2006	44/715	8/227	24.05	1.75 (0.83, 3.65)
Vajda and Eadie,[18] 2005	19/110	1/40	3.59	6.91 (0.96, 49.94)
TOTAL (95% CI)	**118/1351**	**44/1670**	**100.00**	**3.16 (2.17, 4.60)**

C)

STUDY	TREATMENT SAMPLE/TOTAL	CONTROL SAMPLE/TOTAL	WEIGHT %	RR N (95% CI)
Tanganelli and Regesta,[5] 1992	0/6	4/128	3.77	2.05 (0.12, 34.39)
Samren et al,[6] 1997	6/21	12/158	39.88	3.76 (1.58, 8.96)
Samren et al,[9] 1999	9/158	29/2000	56.35	3.93 (1.89, 8.15)
TOTAL (95% CI)	**15/185**	**45/2286**	**100.00**	**3.77 (2.18, 6.52)**

RR—relative risk (random).

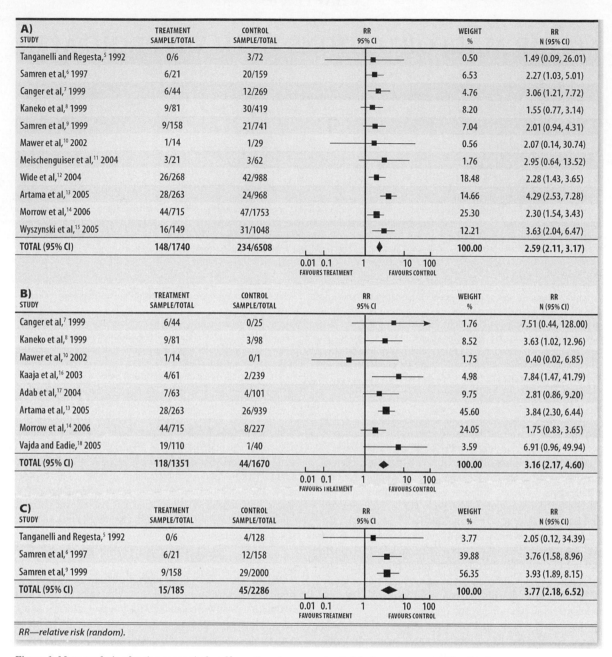

Figure 1. Meta-analysis of major congenital malformations in women treated during pregnancy with valproic acid monotherapy: Rates are compared with those of A) women treated with other anticonvulsant monotherapies, B) untreated epileptic women, and C) healthy control subjects.

DOSE DEPENDENCE

Several studies [6-10,13,14,18-21] performed subanalyses evaluating dose effects. Most suggested that the risk for major congenital malformations was dose dependent, with risks increasing statistically at 600 mg/d.[9,14] The largest attributable risks, however, were seen when doses exceeded 1000 mg/d.

NEUROBEHAVIOURAL RISK

Several studies have compared child development and cognitive deficits among children exposed in utero to valproic acid with those among children exposed to other anticonvulsant drugs.[17,22-25] Although variation in study designs, outcomes, and cognitive tests precluded synthesis of these data into meta-analyses, all researchers reported developmental delays and cognitive deficits associated with valproic acid use in pregnancy. The most prominent effect was on verbal intelligence quotient (IQ). Two of the studies, however, noted that mothers taking valproic acid had had lower levels of education,[23,24] which could predict lower levels of cognitive functioning among their children. Another study [17] found that frequent tonic-clonic seizures in pregnancy were significantly associated with a lower verbal IQ (P =.007). More neurodevelopment studies are needed to control for confounders affecting child development, such as maternal IQ and socioeconomic class.

CONCLUSION

A 3-fold increase in major congenital malformations above the general population is associated with use of valproic acid in early

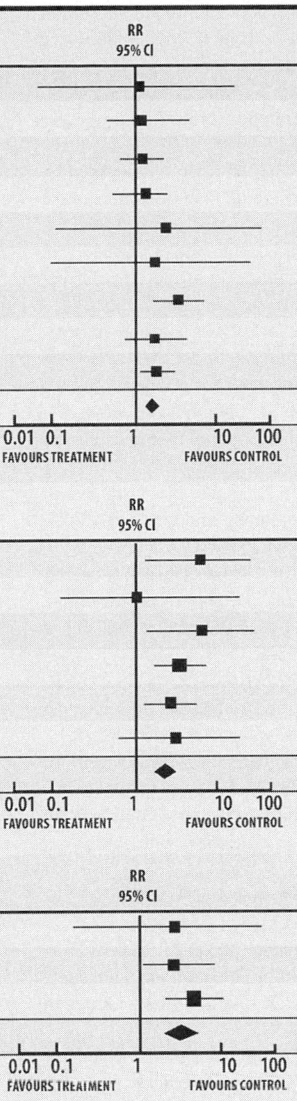

A) STUDY	TREATMENT SAMPLE/TOTAL	CONTROL SAMPLE/TOTAL	WEIGHT %	RR N (95% CI)
Tanganelli and Regesta,[5] 1992	0/4	3/40	1.27	1.17 (0.07, 19.53)
Samren et al,[6] 1997	5/26	7/42	9.30	1.15 (0.41, 3.26)
Kaneko et al,[8] 1999	11/86	30/299	23.89	1.27 (0.67, 2.44)
Samren et al,[9] 1999	8/136	14/322	14.04	1.35 (0.58, 3.15)
Mawer et al,[10] 2002	1/5	0/5	1.12	3.00 (0.15, 59.89)
Meischenguiser et al,[11] 2004	0/2	2/29	1.28	2.00 (0.12, 32.72)
Wide et al,[12] 2004	12/42	7/100	13.57	4.08 (1.73, 9.64)
Artama et al,[13] 2005	9/98	4/82	7.71	1.88 (0.60, 5.89)
Morrow et al,[14] 2006	27/304	16/414	27.82	2.30 (1.26, 4.19)
TOTAL (95% CI)	**73/703**	**83/1333**	**100.00**	**1.84 (1.34, 2.52)**

B) STUDY	TREATMENT SAMPLE/TOTAL	CONTROL SAMPLE/TOTAL	WEIGHT %	RR N (95% CI)
Kaneko et al,[8] 1999	11/86	3/98	13.11	4.18 (1.21, 14.49)
Mawer et al,[10] 2002	1/5	0/1	2.64	1.00 (0.06, 15.99)
Kaaja et al,[16] 2003	4/65	2/239	7.22	7.35 (1.38, 39.26)
Artama et al,[13] 2005	9/98	26/939	38.15	3.32 (1.60, 6.87)
Morrow et al,[14] 2006	27/304	8/227	34.18	2.52 (1.17, 5.44)
Vajda and Eadie,[18] 2005	6/55	1/40	4.70	4.36 (0.55, 34.84)
TOTAL (95% CI)	**58/613**	**40/1544**	**100.00**	**3.24 (2.06, 5.08)**

C) STUDY	TREATMENT SAMPLE/TOTAL	CONTROL SAMPLE/TOTAL	WEIGHT %	RR N (95% CI)
Tanganelli and Regesta,[5] 1992	0/4	4/128	4.40	2.87 (0.18, 46.29)
Samren et al,[6] 1997	5/26	12/158	37.15	2.53 (0.97, 6.59)
Samren et al,[9] 1999	8/136	29/2000	58.45	4.06 (1.89, 8.70)
TOTAL (95% CI)	**13/166**	**45/2286**	**100.00**	**3.35 (1.87, 6.01)**

RR—relative risk (random).

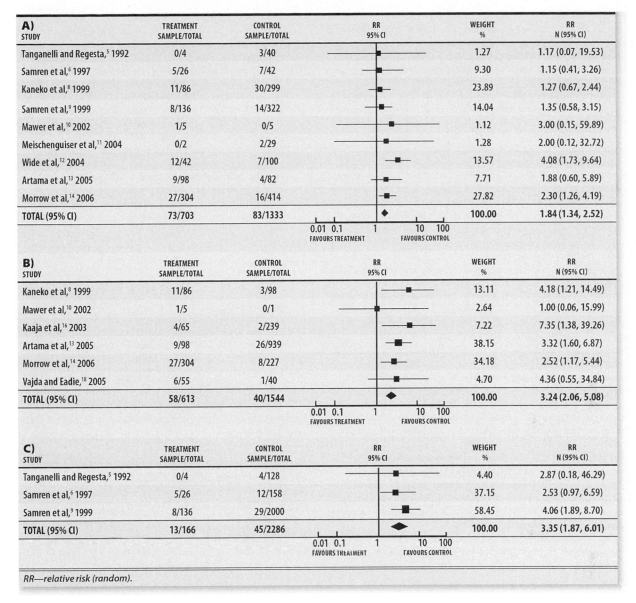

Figure 2. Meta-analysis of major congenital malformations among women treated during pregnancy with valproic acid polytherapy: Rates are compared with those of A) women treated with other polytherapies, B) untreated epileptic women, and C) healthy control subjects.

pregnancy. Consequently, practitioners should inform women of increased risk of malformation and of potentially higher risk of cognitive deficits when valproic acid is used in early pregnancy, especially at high doses. A combination of high-resolution ultrasonography, measuring maternal serum levels of alpha-fetoprotein, and (if necessary) fetal echocardiography between weeks 16 and 18 of pregnancy sometimes helps to evaluate major malformations.

REFERENCES

1. Robert E, Guibaud P. Maternal valproic acid and congenital neural tube defects. *Lancet* 1982;2:937.
2. Lammer EJ, Sever LE, Oakley GP Jr. Teratogen update: valproic acid. *Teratology* 1987;35:465–73.
3. Nau H, Zierer R, Spielmann H, Neubert D, Gansau C. A new model for embryotoxicity testing: teratogenicity and pharmacokinetics of valproic acid following constant-rate administration in the mouse using human therapeutic drug and metabolite concentrations. *Life Sci* 1981;29:2803–14.
4. Koren G, Kennedy D. Safe use of valproic acid during pregnancy [Motherisk Update]. *Can Fam Physician* 1999;45:1451–3.
5. Tanganelli P, Regesta G. Epilepsy, pregnancy, and major birth anomalies: an Italian prospective, controlled study. *Neurology* 1992;42(4 Suppl 5):89–93.
6. Samren EB, van Duijn CM, Koch S, Hiilesmaa VK, Klepel H, Bardy AH, et al. Maternal use of antiepileptic drugs and the risk of major congenital malformations: a joint European prospective study of human teratogenesis associated with maternal epilepsy. *Epilepsia* 1997;38:981–90.

7. Canger R, Battino D, Canevini MP, Fumarola C, Guidolin L, Vignoli A, et al. Malformations in offspring of women with epilepsy: a prospective study. *Epilepsia* 1999;40:1231–6.
8. Kaneko S, Battino D, Andermann E, Wada K, Kan R, Takeda A, et al. Congenital malformations due to antiepileptic drugs. *Epilepsy Res* 1999;33:145–58.
9. Samren EB, van Duijn CM, Christiaens GC, Hofman A, Lindhout D. Antiepileptic drug regimens and major congenital abnormalities in the offspring. *Ann Neurol* 1999;46:739–46.
10. Mawer G, Clayton-Smith J, Coyle H, Kini U. Outcome of pregnancy in women attending an outpatient epilepsy clinic: adverse features associated with higher doses of sodium valproate. *Seizure* 2002;11: 512–8.
11. Meischenguiser R, D'Giano CH, Ferraro SM. Oxcarbazepine in pregnancy: clinical experience in Argentina. *Epilepsy Behav* 2004;5: 163–7.
12. Wide K, Winbladh B, Kallen B. Major malformations in infants exposed to antiepileptic drugs in utero, with emphasis on carbamazepine and valproic acid: a nationwide, population-based register study. *Acta Paediatr* 2004;93:174–6.
13. Artama M, Auvinen A, Raudaskoski T, Isojarvi I, Isojarvi J. Antiepileptic drug use of women with epilepsy and congenital malformations in offspring. *Neurology* 2005;64:1874–8.
14. Morrow J, Russell A, Guthrie E, Parsons L, Robertson I, Waddell R, et al. Malformation risks of antiepileptic drugs in pregnancy: a prospective study from the UK Epilepsy and Pregnancy Register. *J Neurol Neurosurg Psychiatry* 2006;77:193–8.
15. Wyszynski DF, Nambisan M, Surve T, Alsdorf RM, Smith CR, Holmes LB. Increased rate of major malformations in offspring exposed to valproate during pregnancy. *Neurology* 2005;64:961–5.
16. Kaaja E, Kaaja R, Hiilesmaa V. Major malformations in offspring of women with epilepsy. *Neurology* 2003;60:575–9.
17. Adab N, Kini U, Vinten J, Ayres J, Baker G, Clayton-Smith J, et al. The longer term outcome of children born to mothers with epilepsy. *J Neurol Neurosurg Psychiatry* 2004;75:1575–83.
18. Vajda FJ, Eadie MJ. Maternal valproate dosage and foetal malformations. *Acta Neurol Scand* 2005;112:137–43.
19. Vajda FJ, O'brien TJ, Hitchcock A, Graham J, Cook M, Lander C, et al. Critical relationship between sodium valproate dose and human teratogenicity: results of the Australian register of anti-epileptic drugs in pregnancy. *J Clin Neurosci* 2004;11:854–8.
20. Omtzigt JG, Los FJ, Grobbee DE, Pijpers L, Jahoda MG, Brandenburg H, et al. The risk of spina bifida aperta after first-trimester exposure to valproate in a prenatal cohort. *Neurology* 1992;42(4 Suppl 5):119–25.
21. Lindhout D, Meinardi H, Meijer JW, Nau H. Antiepileptic drugs and teratogenesis in two consecutive cohorts: changes in prescription policy paralleled by changes in pattern of malformations. *Neurology* 1992;42 (4 Suppl 5):94–110.
22. Vinten J, Adab N, Kini U, Gorry J, Gregg J, Baker GA. Neuropsychological effects of exposure to anticonvulsant medication in utero. *Neurology* 2005;64:949–54.
23. Eriksson K, Viinikainen K, Monkkonen A, Aikia M, Nieminen P, Heinonen S, et al. Children exposed to valproate in utero—population based evaluation of risks and confounding factors for long-term neurocognitive development. *Epilepsy Res* 2005;65:189–200.
24. Gaily E, Kantola-Sorsa E, Hiilesmaa V, Isoaho M, Matila R, Kotila M, et al. Normal intelligence in children with prenatal exposure to carbamazepine. *Neurology* 2004;62:28–32.
25. Adab N, Jacoby A, Smith D, Chadwick D. Additional educational needs in children born to mothers with epilepsy. *J Neurol Neurosurg Psychiatry* 2001;70:15–21.

MOTHERISK

Motherisk questions are prepared by the Motherisk Team at the Hospital for Sick Children in Toronto, Ont. Dr Koren is Director; Dr Nava-Ocampo, Ms Moretti, and Dr Nulman are members; and Mr Sussman is a student in the Motherisk Program. Dr Koren holds the Ivey Chair in Molecular Toxicology at the University of Western Ontario in London and is supported by the Research Leadership for Better Pharmacotherapy during Pregnancy and Lactation and, in part, by a grant from the Canadian Institutes of Health Research.

Do you have questions about the effects of drugs, chemicals, radiation, or infections in women who are pregnant or breastfeeding? We invite you to submit them to the Motherisk Program by fax at 416 813-7562; they will be addressed in future Motherisk Updates.

Published Motherisk Updates are available on the College of Family Physicians of Canada website (www.cfpc.ca) and also on the Motherisk website (www.motherisk.org).

Reprinted from Koren G, Nava-Ocampo AA, Moretti ME, Sussman R, Nulman I. Major malformations with valproic acid. Can Fam Physician 2006;52: 441–2, 444, 447 with permission.

INDEX

Page numbers followed by *f* or *t* indicate figures or tables, respectively.

N